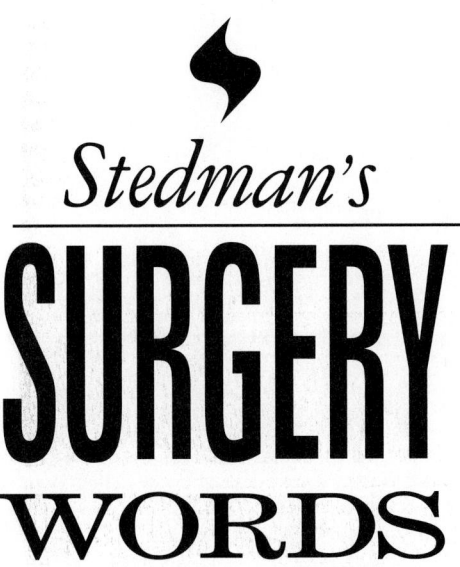

Stedman's
SURGERY
WORDS

INCLUDES
ANATOMY, ANESTHESIA,
& PAIN MANAGEMENT

THIRD EDITION

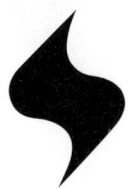

Stedman's

SURGERY
WORDS

INCLUDES
ANATOMY, ANESTHESIA,
& PAIN MANAGEMENT

THIRD EDITION

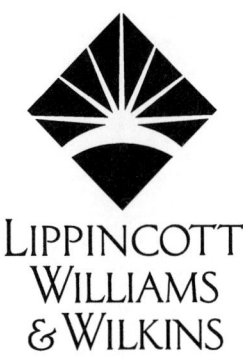

LIPPINCOTT
WILLIAMS
& WILKINS

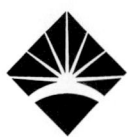

Publisher: Julie K. Stegman
Senior Product Manager: Eric Branger
Associate Managing Editor: Steve Lichtenstein
Production Coordinator: Jason Delaney
Typesetter: Josephine Bergin
Printer & Binder: Malloy Litho, Inc.

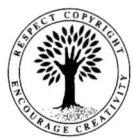

Printed in the United States of America

Third Edition, 2006

Library of Congress Cataloging-in-Publication Data

Stedman's surgery words : includes anatomy, anesthesia & pain management.— 3rd ed.
    p. ; cm.— (Stedman's word books)
Includes bibliographical references.
ISBN 0-7817-6179-4
1. Surgery--Terminology.. [. Surgery--Terminology--English. WO 15 S8124 2006]] I.
Lippincott Williams & Wilkins. II. Series.
RD16.S74 2006
617'.001'4—dc22

2005012513

05 06 07
1 2 3 4 5 6 7 8 9 10

Contents

Acknowledgements

An important part of our editorial process is the involvement of medical transcriptionists — as advisors, reviewers, and/or editors.

We extend special thanks to Jeanne Bock, CSR, MT; and Nicole Peck, CMT, for editing the manuscript, helping resolve many difficult questions, and contributing material for the appendix sections. We are grateful to our MT Editorial Advisory Board members, including Marty Cantu, CMT; Helen Littrell; Robin Koza; and Wendy Ryan, RHIT, who were instrumental in the development of this reference. They recommended sources and shared their valuable judgment, insight, and perspective.

We also extend thanks to Jeanne Bock for working on the appendix. Additional thanks to Helen Littrell for performing the final prepublication review. Other important contributors to this edition include Susan Bartolucci, CMT; Shemah Fletcher; and Beverly S. Oberline, CMT.

And, as always, Lisa Fahnestock played an integral role in the process by reviewing the content files for format, updating the database, and providing a final quality check. Special thanks also to Josephine Bergin for her assistance with the typesetting.

As with all our Stedman's word references, this resource incorporates the suggestions and expertise of our many contacts in the medical transcriptionist community. Thanks to all of our advisory board participants, reviewers, and editors; AAMT meeting attendees; and others who have written us with requests and comments — keep talking, and we'll keep listening.

Editor's Preface

One of the most wonderful (and frustrating) truths about medical transcription is that it is an ever-changing environment because it involves a living language. Oh, yes, sometimes we find that aspect of the profession frustrating as it relates to style — just when we got used to q.d. (no longer using QD) we are told the correct handling is to change to daily — but the ever-changing aspect is also wonderful because there are new challenges every day. We do not work in an environment where the widget is built the same way day in and day out. Instead, every report tells a different story, using terminology preferred by the dictator and reflective of the specifics of their specialty and regional location.

The wording used to describe a medical procedure performed in Washington State may look very different when dictated by a medical professional in Washington, DC. Likewise, that medical procedure, though dictated at the exact same medical facility, may sound very different when dictated by a physician educated and trained in California compared with a physician who has previously worked in Maine. And that certainly makes for an eventful and interesting work day for the medical transcriptionist!

Those in our profession are referred to as medical language specialists, and most of us have chosen the profession of medical transcription because of our passion for words. We find it so very interesting when we notice the differences discussed above and we are known to experience extreme pleasure upon hearing a new term and documenting the same in a reliable source! These differences extend into how we research new terminology as well. Although our desks still are dominated by the presence of word books, dictionaries, and medical journals and newsletters, the internet also augments our research. As few as 5-10 years ago, books and journals were our only source for new terminology. Today we use Google to search manufacturers' and pharmaceutical websites for new products and drugs, as well as PubMed to review journal articles for verification of general medical terminology and procedures. Working as remote transcriptionists from the facilities we transcribe for, we need to use the

AMA's website to look up the spelling of doctors' names across the country. Does a day go by that we aren't pulling a book off our bookshelf or pulling up a website to verify something in a report?

While we all enjoy surfing the internet and discovering new nuggets of medical information, time is always of great importance, which is why we are so excited about the publication of Stedman's Surgery Words, Third Edition. This edition is an impressive compilation of new and existing surgical, anatomical, pain management, and anesthesia terms that would be heard in all medical specialties. We believe this book will minimize the need for a user to search in other resources, either hard copy or electronic, for verification of terminology. For a complete listing of equipment, you will find Stedman's Equipment Words, Fourth Edition, an invaluable tool and companion book to Stedman's Surgery Words, Third Edition.

The appendix section of this book has been enhanced with many new anatomical illustrations that will assist the user in confirming the accuracy of what is heard in the dictated report by confirming the anatomical location of the terminology. We have added images from many medical specialties, to include plastic surgery, dermatology, cardiology, pulmonology, pediatrics, and orthopedics. Also included are new sample reports to provide a comprehensive (though not all-inclusive) sampling of operative reports encountered in today's medical field.

This new edition of Stedman's Surgery Words, Third Edition, like all Stedman's word books, is made possible through the efforts of many people. We would like to thank the many medical transcriptionists who have contributed new terminology, the Editorial Advisory Board, Steve Lichtenstein, and Lisa Fahnestock for their dedication to and hard work on this project.

Jeanne Bock, CSR, MT
Nicole G. Peck, CMT

Publisher's Preface

Stedman's Surgery Words, Third Edition, offers an authoritative assurance of quality and exactness to the wordsmiths of the healthcare professions — medical transcriptionists, medical editors and copyeditors, health information management personnel, court reporters, and the many other users and producers of medical documentation.

We have received many requests for updates to *Stedman's Surgery Words*. As a result, we have published this new edition that includes surgical, anatomical, anesthesia, and pain management terminology. In this new edition, we have opted to omit equipment terminology. You will find *Stedman's Equipment Words, Third Edition* to be an excellent companion source for verifying equipment terminology.

In *Stedman's Surgery Words, Third Edition*, users will find thousands of words as they relate to the specialties of surgery, gross anatomy, anesthesia, and pain management. Users will also find terms for protocols, diagnostic and therapeutic procedures, new techniques, lab tests, clinical research terms, as well as abbreviations with their expansions. The appendix sections provide anatomical illustrations with useful captions and labels, sample reports, common terms by procedure, a pain glossary, pain management techniques, an explanation of dermatomes, American Academy of Pain Management (AAPM)-accredited pain programs, and drugs by indication.

This compilation of more than 90,000 entries, fully cross-indexed for quick access, was built from a base vocabulary of approximately 66,000 medical words, phrases, abbreviations, and acronyms. The extensive A-Z list was developed from the database of *Stedman's Medical Dictionary, 27th Edition*, and supplemented by terminology found in current medical literature (see References on page xx).

We at Lippincott Williams & Wilkins strive to provide you with the most up-to-date and accurate word references available. Your use of this word book will prompt new editions, which we will publish as often as updates and revisions justify. We welcome your suggestions for improvements, changes, corrections, and additions — whatever will make this Stedman's product more useful to you. Please complete the postpaid card at the back of this book, and send your recommendations care of "Stedman's" at Lippincott Williams & Wilkins.

Explanatory Notes

Medical transcription is an art as well as a science. Both approaches are needed to correctly interpret the dictation of a physician, whose language is a product of education, training, and experience. This variety in medical language means that there are several acceptable ways to express certain terms, including jargon. Stedman's Surgery Words, Third Edition, provides variant spellings and phrasings for many terms. These elements, in addition to complete cross-indexing, make *Stedman's Surgery Words, Third Edition*, a valuable resource for determining the validity of terms as they are encountered.

Alphabetical Organization

Alphabetization of main entries is letter by letter as spelled, ignoring punctuation, spaces, prefixed numbers, or other characters. For example:

chlormerodrin accumulation test
2-chloroprocaine
Cho anterior cruciate ligament reconstruction

Terms beginning or ending with Greek letters show the Greek letters spelled out and listed alphabetically. For example:

beta, β
b. adrenoreceptor
b. hemolytic streptococci infection

In subentry alphabetization, the abbreviated singular form or the spelled-out plural form of the noun main entry word is ignored.

Format and Style

All main entries are in boldface to expedite locating a sought-after term, to enhance distinction between main entries and subentries, and to relieve the textual density of the pages.

Irregular plurals and variant spellings are shown on the same line as the singular or preferred form of the word. For example:

acetabulum, pl. acetabula
discectomy, diskectomy

Hyphenation

As a rule of style, multiple eponyms (e.g., Mears-Rubash approach) are hyphenated. Also, hyphens have been added between a manufacturer and one or more eponyms (e.g., Vital-Metzenbaum dissecting scissors). Please note that in many cases, hyphenation is a question of style, not of accuracy, and thus is a matter of choice.

Possessives

Possessive forms have been dropped in this reference for the sake of consistency and conformance with the guidelines of the American Association for Medical Transcription (AAMT) and other groups. Please note, however, that in many cases, retaining the possessive, like hyphenating, is a question of style, not of accuracy, and thus is a matter of choice. To form the possessive of a word, simply add the apostrophe or apostrophe "s" to the end of the word.

Cross-indexing

The word list is in an index-like main entry-subentry format that contains two combined alphabetical listings:

(1) A noun main entry-subentry organization, which is typical of the A-Z section of medical dictionaries like *Stedman's*:

malignancy
  hepatic m.
  hereditary m.
  metastatic m.

reconstruction
  mandibular r.
  nasal r.
  microsurgical r.

(2) An *adjective* main entry-subentry organization, which lists words and phrases as you hear them. The main entries are the adjectives or modifiers in a multiword term. The subentries are the nouns around which the terms are constructed and to which the adjectives or modifiers pertain:

mucinous
  m. adenocarcinoma
  m. ascites
  m. cystic neoplasm (MCN)

regional
  r. anesthetic technique
  r. block
  r. flap

This format provides the user with more than one way to locate and identify a multiword term. For example:

end
  e. expiratory

expiratory
  end e.

algorithm
  registration a.

registration
  r. algorithm

It also allows the user to see together all terms that contain a particular descriptor, as well as all types, kinds, or variations of a noun entity. For example:

hand
   h. massage
   h. ventilation
   h. ratio

knee
   k. anatomy
   k. arthroplasty
   k. dislocation

Wherever possible, abbreviations are separately defined and cross-referenced. For example:

ICU
   intensive care unit

intensive
   i. care unit (ICU)

unit
   intensive care u. (ICU)

References

In addition to the manufacturers' literature we gather at various medical meetings, scientific reports from hospitals, and the lists of our MT Editorial Advisory Board members (from their daily transcription work), we used the following sources for new terms in *Stedman's Surgery Words, Third Edition.*

Books

Abram SE, Haddox JD. The Pain Clinic Manual, 2nd Edition. Philadelphia: Lippincott Williams & Wilkins, 2000.

Baker RJ, Fischer JE, eds. Mastery of Surgery, 4th Edition. Philadelphia: Lippincott Williams & Wilkins, 2001.

Ballantyne GH, Marescaux J, Giulianotti PC, eds. Primer of Robotic & Telerobotic Surgery. Philadelphia: Lippincott Williams & Wilkins, 2004.

Ballantyne J. The Massachusetts General Handbook of Pain Management, 2nd Edition. Philadelphia: Lippincott Williams & Wilkins, 2002.

Barash PG, Cullen BF, Stoelting RK. Clinical Anesthesia, 4th Edition. Philadelphia: Lippincott Williams & Wilkins, 2000.

Chung KW. Gross Anatomy, 5th Edition. Philadelphia: Lippincott Williams & Wilkins, 2005.

Corman ML. Colon and Rectal Surgery, 5th Edition. Philadelphia: Lippincott Williams & Wilkins, 2005.

Drake E. Sloane's Medical Word Book, 4th Edition. Philadelphia: Saunders, 2001.

General Surgery/GI Words and Phrases. Modesto, CA: Health Professions Institute, 2001.

Greenfield LJ, Mulholland MW, Oldham KT, Zelenock GB, Lilemoe KD. Surgery: Scientific Principles and Practice, 3rd Edition. Philadelphia: Lippincott Williams & Wilkins, 2001.

Hiatt JL, Gartner LP. Textbook of Head and Neck Anatomy, 3rd Edition. Philadelphia: Lippincott Williams & Wilkins, 2000.

Hollinshead WH. Anatomy for Surgeons, The Head and Neck, 3rd Edition. Philadelphia: Lippincott Williams & Wilkins, 1982.

Inabnet WB, DeMaria EJ, Ikramuddin S, eds. Laparoscopic Bariatric Surgery. Philadelphia: Lippincott Williams & Wilkins, 2005.

Jaffe RA, Samuels SI, eds. Anesthesiologist's Manual of Surgical Procedures, 3rd Edition. Philadelphia: Lippincott Williams & Wilkins, 2004.

Kalimi R, Faber LP, eds. Clinical Scenarios in Thoracic Surgery. Philadelphia: Lippincott Williams & Wilkins, 2004.

Lance LL. Quick Look Drug Book 2002. Baltimore: Lippincott Williams & Wilkins, 2002.

Lawrence PF. Essentials of General Surgery, 3rd Edition. Philadelphia: Lippincott Williams & Wilkins, 1999.

Loeser JD, Butler SH, Chapman CR, Turk DC. Bonica's Management of Pain, 3rd Edition. Philadelphia: Lippincott Williams & Wilkins, 2000.

McCaffery M, Pasero C. Pain Clinic Manual, 2nd Edition. Philadelphia: Saunders, 1999.

Olson T. A.D.A.M. Student Atlas of Anatomy. Philadelphia: Lippincott Williams & Wilkins, 1996.

Pain Management Made Incredibly Easy! Philadelphia: Lippincott Williams & Wilkins, 2003.

Schwartz SI, Shires GT, Spencer FC, Galloway AC. Principles of Surgery, 7th Edition. Columbus: McGraw-Hill, 1998.

Slinger PD, ed. Progress in Thoracic Anesthesia. Philadelphia: Lippincott Williams & Wilkins, 2004.

Stedman's Medical Dictionary, 27th Edition. Baltimore: Lippincott Williams & Wilkins, 2000.

Stedman's Surgery Words. Baltimore: Lippincott Williams & Wilkins, 1998.

Taylor J. Comprehensive Sports Injury Management: From Examination of Injury to Return to Sport. Austin: Pro-Ed, 2003.

Tessier C. The AAMT Book of Style. Modesto, CA: AAMT, 1995.

Tessier C. The Surgical Word Book, 2nd Edition. Philadelphia: Saunders, 1991.

Upchurch Jr, GR, Henke PK, eds. Clinical Scenarios in Vascular Surgery. Philadelphia: Lippincott Williams & Wilkins, 2005.

Valentine JR, Wind GG. Anatomic Exposures in Vascular Surgery, 2nd Edition. Philadelphia: Lippincott Williams & Wilkins, 2003.

Vera Pyle's Current Medical Terminology, 9th Edition. Modesto, CA: Health Professions Institute, 2003.

Whyte-Ferguson L, Gerwin R, eds. Clinical Mastery in the Treatment of Myofascial Pain. Philadelphia: Lippincott Williams & Wilkins, 2005.

CD

Lippincott's Interactive Anesthesia Library v3.0. Philadelphia: Lippincott Williams & Wilkins, 2001.

Image Sources

Abraham SE and Haddox JD. The Pain Clinic Manual, 2nd Edition. Philadelphia: Lippincott Williams & Wilkins, 2000.

Agur, AMR, Lee, MJ. Grant's Atlas of Anatomy, 10th Edition. Baltimore: Lippincott Williams & Wilkins, 1999.

Caldwell S, Pikesville, MD. From Stedman's Medical Dictionary, 27th Edition. Baltimore: Lippincott Williams & Wilkins, 2000.

Cousins MJ, Bridenbaug PO eds. Neural Blockade in Clinical Anesthesia and Management of Pain. Philadelphia: Lippincott-Raven Publishers; 1997.

Georgiade NG, Riefkohl R, Levine LS, Georgiade, GS. Plastic, Maxillofacial and Reconstructive Surgery, 3rd Edition. Baltimore: Williams & Wilkins, 1996.

LifeART Emergency 4, CD-ROM. Baltimore, Lippincott Williams & Wilkins.

LifeART Equipment 4, CD-ROM. Baltimore, Lippincott Williams & Wilkins.

LifeART Nursing 1-2, CD-ROM. Baltimore, Lippincott Williams & Wilkins.

LifeART Pediatrics 1, CD-ROM. Baltimore, Lippincott Williams & Wilkins.

LifeART Super Anatomy Collections 3-8, CD-ROM. Baltimore, Lippincott Williams & Wilkins.

MediClip Clinical Cardiopulmonary, CD-ROM. Baltimore, Lippincott Williams & Wilkins.

MediClip Human Anatomy 1-3, CD-ROM. Baltimore: Lippincott, Williams & Wilkins.

Mikki Senkarik, San Antonio, TX. From Pillitteri A, PhD, RN, PNP. Maternal & Child Health Nursing: Care of the Childbearing & Childrearing Family, 3rd Edition. Philadelphia: Lippincott Williams & Wilkins, 1998.

Mikki Senkarik, San Antonio, TX. From Stedman's Medical Dictionary, 27th Edition. Baltimore: Lippincott Williams & Wilkins, 2000.

Neil O. Hardy. Westport, CT and Susan Caldwell. Pikesville, MD. From Stedman's Medical Dictionary, 27th edition. Baltimore: Lippincott Williams & Wilkins, 2000.Smeltzer SC & Bare BG. Brunner & Suddarth's Textbook of Medical Surgical-Nursing, 8th Edition. Philadelphia: JB Lippincott Company, 1996.

Ward L, Salt Lake City, UT. From Fuller J, RN, PhD & Schaller-Ayers J, RN, MNSc, PhD. A Nursing Approach, 2nd Edition. Philadelphia: J.B. Lippincott Company, 1994.Willis MC. Medical Terminology: The Language of Health Care. Baltimore: Williams Wilkins, 1996.

Journals

Anesthesia & Analgesia. Baltimore: Lippincott Williams & Wilkins, 2005.

Anesthesiology. Baltimore: Lippincott Williams & Wilkins, 2001.

Annals of Surgery. Baltimore: Lippincott Williams & Wilkins, 1999-2005.

Clinical Journal of Pain. Baltimore: Lippincott Williams & Wilkins, 1999-2005.

Colon and Rectal Surgery. Baltimore: Lippincott Williams & Wilkins, 2004-2005.

Computer Aided Surgery. New York: John Wiley & Sons, Inc., 1997-2000.

Journal of the American College of Surgeons. New York: Elsevier Science, 1997-2005.

Laparoscopic Update. Baltimore: Lippincott Williams & Wilkins, 1998-2001.

Latest Word. Philadelphia: Saunders, 1999-2001.

Surgical Laparoscopy Endoscopy & Percutaneous Techniques. Baltimore: Lippincott Williams & Wilkins, 1999-2001.

Topics in Pain Management. Baltimore: Lippincott Williams & Wilkins, 2001.

Websites

http://www.aapainmanage.org./search/FacilSearch.php

http://carecure.rutgers.edu/spinewire/Articles/SpinalLevels.html

http://my.webmd.com/index

http://surgery.medscape.com/Home/Topics/surgery/surgery.html

http://www.aapainmange.org

http://www.anesthesiology.org

http://www.asahq.org

http://www.aspmn.org

http://www.centerwatch.com

http://www.facs.org

http://www.gasnet.com

http://www.hpisum.com

http://www.laparoscopy.com

http://www.lapsurgery.com

http://www.mtdaily.com

http://www.mtdesk.com

http://www.mtmonthly.com

http://www.nccn.org/patients/patient_gls/_english/_pain/3_treatment.asp

http://www.nci.nih.gov/cancertopics/treatment/types-of-treatment

http://www.pain.com

http://www.sciwire.com

http://www.sls.org

http://www.theasgs.org

http://www.ussurg.com

http://www.webmd.com

α (*var. of* alpha)

A
  ampere
  apex

AA
  anterior apical
  atrial activity
    AA segment

AAA
  abdominal aortic aneurysm

AAC
  acute acalculous cholecystitis

AACLR
  arthroscopic anterior cruciate ligament
  reconstruction

AANA
  American Association of Nurse
  Anesthetists

Aaron sign

AAST
  American Association for the Surgery of
  Trauma

AB
  anterior basal
    AB segment

ab
  ab externo filtering operation
  ab externo incision
  ab interno incision

ABA
  allergic bronchopulmonary aspergillosis
  American Board of Anesthesiology

Abbe
  A. flap
  A. operation
  A. vaginal construction

Abbe-Estlander
  A.-E. flap
  A.-E. operation

Abbe-McIndoe
  A.-M. procedure
  A.-M. vaginal reconstruction

Abbe-McIndoe-Williams procedure
Abbe-Wharton-McIndoe procedure
Abbott
  A. esophagogastroscopy
  A. esophagogastrostomy
  A. knee approach
  A. method

Abbott-Carpenter posterior approach
Abbott-Gill
  A.-G. epiphysial plate exposure
  A.-G. osteotomy

Abbott-Lucas shoulder operation

abbreviated
  A. Injury Scale (AIS)
  A. Injury Score (AIS)

ABC
  airway, breathing, circulation

abdomen
  accordion a.
  acute surgical a.
  apertures of a.
  boatlike a.
  boat-shaped a.
  carinate a.
  concave a.
  diffusely tender a.
  distended a.
  doughy a.
  exquisitely tender a.
  fascia of a.
  flabby a.
  flat a.
  hostile a.
  hyperdistended a.
  hyperresonant a.
  navicular a.
  nondistended a.
  pendulous a.
  postlymphangiography a.
  postsurgical a.
  protuberant a.
  prune-belly a.
  resonant a.
  scaphoid a.
  soft a.
  splinting of a.
  stiff a.
  surgical a.
  tympanitic a.

abdominal
  a. abscess
  a. adhesiolysis
  a. adipose tissue
  a. agitation
  a. air collection
  a. angina
  a. angiography
  a. aorta
  a. aortic aneurysm (AAA)
  a. aortic artery
  a. aortic plexus
  a. aponeurosis
  a. approach
  a. apron
  a. brace position
  a. canal
  a. carcinoma

abdominal (*continued*)
  a. cardiac reflex
  a. cavity
  a. circulation
  a. colectomy
  a. colic
  a. compartment syndrome
  a. complication
  a. content
  a. cramp
  a. cutaneous nerve entrapment syndrome
  a. distention
  a. domain
  a. drainage
  a. evisceration
  a. examination
  a. exploration
  a. external oblique muscle
  a. fasciocutaneous flap
  a. fat
  a. fat pad
  a. film
  a. fissure
  a. fluid collection
  a. fluid wave
  a. girth
  a. guarding
  a. gunshot wound
  a. gutter
  a. hemorrhage
  a. hydatid disease
  a. hysterectomy
  a. hysteropexy
  a. hysterotomy
  a. imaging
  a. impalement
  a. incisional hernia
  a. incision dehiscence
  a. internal oblique muscle
  a. iron deposition
  a. irradiation
  a. kidney
  a. lavage
  a. lipectomy
  a. lymph node biopsy
  a. malignancy
  a. midline incisional hernioplasty
  a. migraine
  a. muscle deficiency syndrome
  a. myomectomy
  a. nephrectomy
  a. ostium
  a. panniculus
  a. paracentesis
  a. peritoneum
  a. pool
  a. pregnancy
  a. pressure

  a. pressure technique
  a. procedure
  a. proctocolectomy
  a. pull-through
  a. pulse
  a. rectopexy
  a. reflux
  a. region
  a. respiration
  a. respiratory motion
  a. rigidity
  a. ring
  a. sac
  a. sacrocolpopexy
  a. sacropexy
  a. salpingo-oophorectomy
  a. salpingotomy
  a. section
  a. sonography
  a. space
  a. splenectomy
  a. stoma
  a. stool
  a. structure
  a. tap
  a. tenderness
  A. Trauma Index (ATI)
  a. tumor
  a. vascular accident
  a. view
  a. viscus
  a. volume
  a. wall closure
  a. wall fistula
  a. wall hernia
  a. wall incision
  a. wall lifting
  a. wall mass
  a. wall mobility
  a. wall rhabdomyosarcoma
  a. wall venous pattern
  a. wound closure
  a. x-ray (AXR)
  a. zone
abdominalis
abdominal-perineal resection
abdominal-sacral colpoperineopexy
abdominis
abdominocentesis
abdominocystic
abdominogenital
abdominohysterectomy
abdominohysterotomy
abdominoinguinal incision
abdominojugular reflux
abdominopelvic
  a. abscess
  a. cavity
  a. irradiation

a. mass
a. splanchnic nerve
a. viscus
abdominoperineal
a. excision
a. proctectomy
a. resection (APR)
abdominoplasty
abdominosacral resection
abdominoscopy
abdominoscrotal
abdominothoracic
a. arch
a. incision
abdominovaginal hysterectomy
abdominovesical
abducens nerve
abducent
abduction
a. deformity
a. external rotation test
a. osteotomy
a. traction technique
abduction-external
a.-e. rotation
a.-e. rotation fracture
abductor
a. digiti minimi opponensplasty
a. digiti quinti opponensplasty
a. hallucis muscle
a. longus muscle
a. magnus muscle
a. osteotomy
a. pollicis brevis muscle
a. pollicis longus muscle
a. pollicis longus tendon
abductorplasty
flexor pollicis longus a.
Smith flexor pollicis longus a.
abductory wedge osteotomy
Abell-Kendall method
Abell method
Aberdeen knot
Abernethy
A. fascia
A. operation
A. sarcoma
aberrancy
acceleration-dependent a.
aberrant
a. bile duct
a. bronchial origin

a. ductule
a. ganglion
a. goiter
a. obturator artery
a. obturator vein
a. pancreas
a. regeneration
a. third nerve degeneration
a. tissue
a. umbilical stomach
a. vessel
aberration
angle of a.
chromatic lens a.
color a.
coma a.
curvature a.
dioptric a.
distantial a.
distortion a.
intraventricular a.
lateral a.
lens a.
longitudinal a.
meridional a.
monochromatic a.
newtonian a.
oblique a.
optical a.
regeneration a.
sexual a.
spherical lens a.
ventricular a.
ability
tumor-targeting a.
ablate
ablation
accessory conduction a.
adrenal a.
androgen a.
atrioventricular junctional a.
carbon dioxide laser plaque a.
catheter a.
celiac alcohol a.
cold forceps a.
cold snare a.
Concept a.
contact laser a.
continuous wave laser a.
coronary rotational a.
cryogenic a.
cryosurgical a.

NOTES

3

ablation *(continued)*
    direct current shock a.
    electrical catheter a.
    endometrial a.
    endoscopic mucosal a.
    ethanol a.
    excimer laser a.
    fast-pathway radiofrequency a.
    His bundle a.
    homogeneous a.
    Kent bundle a.
    laparoscopic uterine nerve a.
    laser uterosacral nerve a.
    liver wire TC a.
    marrow a.
    mucosal a.
    Nd:YAG laser a.
    needle a.
    neoadjuvant total androgen a.
    nerve rootlet a.
    organ a.
    ovarian a.
    panretinal a.
    parathyroid tumor a.
    percutaneous ethanol a.
    percutaneous radical cryosurgical a.
    percutaneous radiofrequency
      catheter a.
    percutaneous tumor a.
    peripheral panretinal a.
    photothermal laser a.
    pituitary a.
    pulsed laser a.
    radiofrequency catheter a. (RFCA)
    radiofrequency thermal a. (RFTA)
    radioiodine a.
    rectoscopic endometrial a.
    renal cyst a.
    rollerball endometrial a.
    rotational a.
    slow-pathway a.
    stereotactic surgical a.
    surgical estrogen a.
    temperature-controlled radiofrequency
      tissue a.
    a. therapy
    thermal a.
    thyroid nodule a.
    tissue a.
    toric a.
    transcatheter a.
    transurethral needle a. (TUNA)
    tumor a.
    valve a.
    visual laser a.
ablative
    a. cardiac surgery
    a. laser angioplasty
    a. laser therapy

    a. procedure
    a. technique
ABMT
    autologous bone marrow transplant
    autologous bone marrow transplantation
ABMTR
    Autologous Bone and Marrow Transplant
      Registry
abnormal
    a. bleeding
    a. clotting
    a. cytology
    a. fetal urogenital tract
    a. mammogram
    a. parathyroid gland
    a. preoperative localization signal
abnormality, pl. **abnormalities**
    anatomic a.
    bleeding a.
    caliceal a.
    clotting a.
    cytologic a.
    dislocation contour a.
    diverticulation a.
    DNA ploidy a.
    electrical activation a.
    electrolyte a.
    extremity a.
    genetic a.
    ictal a.
    limb reduction a.
    mammographic a.
    migration a.
    mucosal a.
    nondermatomal sensory a. (NDSA)
    nonpalpable mammographic a.
    oral cavity a.
    persistent breast a.
    pulmonary vascular a.
    regional wall motion a.
    renal a.
    reproductive tract a.
    rostrocaudal extent signal a.
    skeletal a.
    soft tissue a.
    structural a.
    suspicious a.
    tissue texture a.
    urinary tract a.
    vascular a.
    ventilation/perfusion a.
    ventricular depolarization a.
abnormally
    a. feeding blood vessel
    a. hyperplastic gland
ABO barrier
aborad
aboral direction

abortion
    menstrual extraction a.
abortive infection
above-elbow (AE)
    a.-e. amputation (AEA)
above-knee (AK)
    a.-k. amputation (AKA)
    a.-k. amputation conversion
ABPC
    argon beam plasma coagulation
ABPI
    ankle-brachial pressure index
ABPM
    American Board of Pain Medicine
abraded wound
Abraham iridotomy
Abraham-Pankovich tendo calcaneus repair
Abrami disease
abrasion
    a. arthroplasty
    bobby-pin a.
    a. chondroplasty
    corneal a.
    perioperative corneal a.
    traumatic corneal a.
abrasive
    a. brush biopsy
    a. point
Abrikosov tumor
abrupt hemodynamic collapse
ABS
    American Board of Surgery
abscess
    abdominal a.
    abdominopelvic a.
    actinomycotic brain a.
    acute a.
    amebic hepatic a.
    anal a.
    anastomotic a.
    anorectal a.
    aponeurotic a.
    appendiceal a.
    arthrifluent a.
    axillary a.
    Bezold a.
    bicameral a.
    blind a.
    bone a.
    bowel a.
    brain a.

    breast a.
    Brodie metaphysial a.
    buccal space a.
    button a.
    caseous a.
    cerebral a.
    chronic subareolar a.
    cold a.
    collar-button a.
    colonic a.
    corneal a.
    crypt a.
    cuff a.
    deep interloop a.
    diffuse a.
    Douglas a.
    draining a.
    dry a.
    echinococcal liver a.
    encapsulated brain a.
    enteroperitoneal a.
    epidural a.
    extradural a.
    fecal a.
    fluctuant a.
    a. formation
    frontal a.
    gallbladder wall a.
    gas a.
    gas-forming liver a.
    gravitation a.
    growth plate a.
    hepatic a.
    Highmore a.
    horseshoe a.
    hot a.
    hypostatic a.
    infraorbital space a.
    intermesenteric a.
    intersphincteric a.
    intraabdominal a.
    intradural a.
    intrahepatic a.
    intramural a.
    intramuscular a.
    intraosseous a.
    intraperitoneal a.
    ischiorectal a.
    kidney a.
    lacunar a.
    liver a.
    local a.

NOTES

abscess *(continued)*
    localized a.
    lumbar epidural a.
    mesentery a.
    metaphysial a.
    metastatic a.
    midpalmar a.
    migrating a.
    miliary a.
    missile track a.
    necrotic a.
    pancreatic a.
    paranephric a.
    parapharyngeal space a.
    pelvic a.
    perforating a.
    perianal fistula a.
    periappendiceal a.
    periesophageal a.
    perihepatic a.
    perineal a.
    perinephric a.
    perirectal a.
    peritoneal cavity a.
    periumbilical a.
    periureteral a.
    periurethral a.
    phlegmonous a.
    pilonidal a.
    point of a.
    postoperative a.
    premasseteric space a.
    prevertebral space a.
    pterygomandibular space a.
    pyogenic hepatic a.
    residual a.
    retrocecal a.
    retroperitoneal-iliopsoas a.
    retrorectal a.
    a. ring
    ring a.
    satellite a.
    soft tissue a.
    space of Retzius a.
    spinal epidural a. (SEA)
    stercoral a.
    sterile a.
    stitch a.
    subdiaphragmatic a.
    subdural a.
    subgaleal a.
    subhepatic a.
    sublingual space a.
    submandibular space a.
    submasseteric space a.
    submental space a.
    subperiosteal a.
    subphrenic a.
    supralevator perirectal a.

    tuberculous a.
    tuboovarian a.
    wandering a.
    wound a.
abscise
abscission
    corneal a.
absence
    microscopic a.
absent
    a. bowel sounds
    a. bow tie sign
    a. gag reflex
    a. peristalsis
    a. respiration
Absidia **infection**
absolute
    a. construction
    a. curative resection
    a. humidity
    a. noncurative resection
absorbable surgical suture
absorbent
    a. point
    a. vessel
absorptiometry
absorption
    external a.
    nutrient a.
    reservoir mucosal a.
    systemic a.
absorptive cell
abut
abutment
    implant a.
    screw-type a.
    subperiosteal implant a.
AC
    acromioclavicular
ACAD
    atherosclerotic carotid artery disease
acalculous cholecystitis
acantha
acanthion
acanthocytosis
acanthoid
acantholysis
ACAS
    Asymptomatic Carotid Atherosclerosis
    Study
accelerans
accelerated
    a. arteriolar gas embolization
    a. respiration
    a. transplant rejection
acceleration
    angular a.
    fetal growth a.
    fetal heart rate a.

growth a.
a. injury
tibial a.
a. time
acceleration/deceleration injury
acceleration-dependent aberrancy
accelerator
a. fiber
linear a. (LINAC)
a. nerve
accentuation
paramagnetic enhancement a.
access
cavity a.
a. cavity
central venous a.
cutdown a.
a. emergency
exit a.
extrahepatic a.
a. flap
minimally invasive surgical a.
percutaneous a.
peritoneal a.
a. preparation
root canal a.
side-entry a.
surgical a.
transcervical tubal a.
transcutaneous a.
transjugular liver a.
vascular a.
venous a.
ventricular a.
accessible lesion
accessory
a. adrenal
a. breast
a. cephalic vein
a. conduction ablation
a. duct stenting
a. muscle activity
a. nerve
a. nerve root
a. nerve trunk
a. nipple
a. obturator artery
a. palatine canal
a. pancreas
a. pancreatic duct
a. papillotomy
a. parotid gland

a. plantar ligament
a. process
a. root canal
a. spleen
a. suprarenal gland
a. thyroid gland
a. tubercle
a. venous sinus of Verga
a. volar ligament
accident
abdominal vascular a.
cerebrovascular a.
intraoperative vascular a.
vascular a.
accidental
a. hemorrhage
a. hypothermia
a. pulp exposure
accommodation
a. curve
a. disorder
a. reflex
accordion
a. abdomen
a. graft
a. sign
Accreditation Council for Graduate Medical Education (ACGME)
accretion line
accumulation
collagen a.
third space fluid a.
accuracy
diagnostic a.
subvoxel a.
ACE
angiotensin-converting enzyme
antegrade continence enema
ACE inhibitor
Ace-Colles frame technique
acellular
a. mass
a. pannus tissue
acentric relation
acestoma
acetabula (*pl. of* acetabulum)
acetabular
a. artery
a. augmentation graft
a. branch
a. cavity
a. cup arthroplasty

NOTES

acetabular *(continued)*
    a. cup extractor
    a. extensile approach
    a. lip
    a. notch
    a. protrusio deformity
    a. reinforcement ring
    a. retractor
    a. rim fracture
acetabuloplasty
    Pemberton a.
    shelf a.
acetabulum, pl. **acetabula**
    notch of a.
acetohydroxamic acid irrigation
acetowhite
    a. lesion
    a. test
acetylcholine (Ach)
    a. receptor
ACGME
    Accreditation Council for Graduate
    Medical Education
Ach
    acetylcholine
achalasia
    a. balloon dilation
    a. cardiae
    esophageal a.
Achilles
    A. bursa
    A. tendon
    A. tendon rupture
Achillis
    bursa A.
    tendo A.
achondrogenesis
achondroplasia
    homozygous a.
achondroplastic
achondroplasty
achromic patch
acid
    amino a.
    a. anhydride method
    a. aspiration
    a. etch bonding technique
    gastric chloric a.
    a. gland
    a. guanidine thiocyanate-phenol-
      chloroform method
    a. hemolysis
    mefenamic a.
    phenylethylbarbituric a.
    a. reflux
    retinoic a.
    stomach a.
acid-base
    a.-b. balance

    a.-b. disturbance
    a.-b. equilibrium
    a.-b. status
    a.-b. value
acid-etched restoration
acidic fibroblast growth factor
acidification treatment
acidosis
    concomitant a.
    hepatocellular a.
    lactic a.
    local a.
    metabolic a.
    renal tubular a.
acinar tissue
acinous
    a. cell carcinoma
    a. gland
acinus, pl. **acini**
    lobular a.
Ackerman-Proffitt classification of malocclusion
ACL
    anterior cruciate ligament
    ACL reconstruction
    ACL repair
ACLR
    anterior cruciate ligament reconstruction
acneform
    a. lesion
    a. rash
acorn treatment
Acosta classification
acoupedic method
acoustic
    a. canal
    a. foramen
    a. method
    a. nerve
    a. neuroma
    A. Neuroma Registry
    a. pharyngometry
    a. pressure
    a. quantification
    a. reflection measurement
    a. reflectometry
    a. rhinometry
    a. shadowing
    a. stimulation study
    a. stimulation test
AC-PC
    anterior commissure-posterior
    commissure
    AC-PC line
acquired
    a. centric relation
    a. cornification disorder
    a. deformity
    a. diverticulum

a. eccentric jaw relation
a. hernia
acquisition
image a.
multiple gated a. (MUGA)
acral lentiginous melanoma (ALM)
Acrel ganglion
acridine orange method
acrobrachycephaly
acrocephalia
acrocephalic
acrocephalopolysyndactyly
acrocephalosyndactyly (type I-IV)
acrocephalous
acrocephaly
acrocyanosis
acrodysplasia
acrofacial syndrome
acromegaly
acromial
a. arterial network
a. artery
a. articular facies
a. articular surface
a. branch
a. bursa
a. extremity
a. process
acromioclavicular (AC)
a. articulation
a. disc
a. injury classification
a. joint dislocation
a. joint repair
a. ligament
a. pin fixation
a. space
acromiocoracoid
acromiohumeral
acromion
acromionectomy
Armstrong a.
acromioplasty
anterior a.
McLaughlin a.
McShane-Leinberry-Fenlin a.
Neer a.
acromioscapular
acromiothoracic
a. approach
a. artery
acroosteolysis

ACS
American College of Surgeons
ACT
activated clotting time
actinomycetoma
actinomycoma
actinomycotic brain abscess
actinomyoma
action
anesthesia a.
a. of anesthetic
ball valve a.
a. line
nonstereospecific a.
peripheral antinociceptive a.
stereospecific a.
ActiPatch therapy
Actiq
activated
a. clotting time (ACT)
a. coagulation time
a. protein C resistance
activating solution
activation
baroreflex a.
cortical a.
egg a.
hemostatic a.
hypothalamic a.
a. map-guided surgical resection
a. moment
neuronal nicotinic receptor a.
neutrophil a.
presynaptic and postsynaptic
nicotinic a.
very late a.
activation-sequence mapping
activator
a. modification
recombinant tissue-type
plasminogen a. (RTPA, rtPA)
active
a. appliance therapy
a. assistive motion therapy
a. chronic inflammation
a. core cooling
a. hemorrhage
a. reciprocation
a. source of bleeding
a. specific immunotherapy (ASI)
a. systemic bacterial infection
actively bleeding varix

NOTES

activity
>accessory muscle a.
antithrombotic a.
atrial a. (AA)
channel a.
duodenal migrating a.
efferent nerve a.
inspiratory intercostal a.
jejunal fasting motor a.
mitotic a.
motor a.
opioid antinociceptive a.
a. pattern analysis
postprandial motor a.
pulseless electrical a. (PEA)
sympathetic nerve a. (SNA)

actuation
>direct mechanical ventricular a.

acuminatum, pl. **acuminata**
>condyloma a.

acuology
acupressure
>Korean hand a.

acupuncture
>a. anesthesia
auricular a.

acusection
acustimulation antiemetic prophylaxis
acute
>a. abscess
a. acalculous cholecystitis (AAC)
a. allergic extrinsic alveolitis
a. allograft rejection
a. aortic dissection
a. blood transfusion
a. calculous cholecystitis
a. cardiac event
a. cellular rejection
a. and chronic inflammation
a. colonic pseudoobstruction
a. compression triad
a. coronary syndrome
a. digestive bleeding
a. disconnection syndrome
a. fracture
a. gastric mucosal lesion
a. graft-versus-host disease
a. hemorrhagic inflammation
a. hemorrhagic ulceration
a. hepatic coma
a. hepatic rupture
a. inflammatory exudate
a. inflammatory membrane
a. intermittent porphyria
a. intestinal obstruction
a. ischemic stroke
a. isovolemic hemodilution
a. limb ischemia (ALI)

>A. Low Back Pain Screening Questionnaire (ALBPSQ)
a. lung rejection
a. mesenteric venous thrombosis
a. normovolemic hemodilution (ANH)
a. pancreatitis (AP)
a. physiologic assessment and chronic health evaluation
a. physiology and chronic health evaluation (APACHE)
a. physiology prognostic scoring index
a. presentation
a. pyogenic membrane
a. radiation pneumonitis
a. recurrent rhabdomyolysis
a. rejection of liver transplant
a. respiratory distress syndrome (ARDS)
a. respiratory failure
a. severe isovolemic anemia
a. subdural hematoma
a. suppurative thyroiditis
a. surgical abdomen
a. symptom
a. toxicity
a. traumatic lesion
a. tubular necrosis (ATN)
a. tumor lysis syndrome (ATLS)
a. vascular rejection
a. wound

acyltransferase
>lecithin-cholesterol a. (LCAT)

acystia
adactylous
adactyly
adamantine membrane
adamantinoblastoma
adamantinocarcinoma
adamantinoma
adamantinum
Adams
>A. hip operation
A. position
A. procedure

Adam's apple
adaptable
adaptation
>arterial a.
a. disease
a. syndrome of Selye

adaptational approach
adaptive
>a. correction
a. relaxation

adaxial
addiction
>a. acknowledgment scale

a. potential scale
A. Severity Index
Addison
  A. maneuver
  A. point
additional canal
additive interaction
additivity
adduction
  a. deformity
  a. osteotomy
  a. traction technique
adduction-internal rotation deformity
adductor
  a. canal
  a. hiatus
  a. longus muscle rupture
  a. magnus tendon
  a. tenotomy
adductovarus deformity
adenectomy
adenoacanthoma
adenoameloblastoma
adenocanthoma
adenocarcinoma
  alveolar a.
  ampullary a.
  anaplastic a.
  anular a.
  appendiceal a.
  bile duct a.
  bronchial a.
  bronchiolar a.
  bronchioloalveolar a.
  bronchogenic a.
  cervical a.
  colonic a.
  colorectal a.
  cystic a.
  duct cell a.
  duodenal a.
  endometrial a.
  esophageal a.
  gastric a.
  infiltrating duct a.
  invasive a.
  kidney a.
  medullary a.
  mesonephric a.
  metastatic a.
  mucinous a.
  ovarian clear cell a.

pancreatic a.
peritoneal a.
primary a.
prostatic a.
renal a.
sebaceous a.
secretory a.
serous a.
signet-ring a.
spontaneous a.
stomach a.
sweat gland a.
undifferentiated a.
uterine a.
vaginal a.
vulvar adenoid cystic a.
adenochondroma
adenocystic carcinoma
adenocystoma
adenodiastasis
adenoepithelioma
adenofibroma
adenofibromyoma
adenohypophysial
adenohypophysis
adenoid
  a. cystic carcinoma
  a. pad
  a. squamous cell carcinoma
  a. tumor
adenoidal pad
adenoidal-pharyngeal-conjunctival (A-P-C)
  a.-p.-c. virus
adenoidectomy
  lateral a.
  tonsillectomy and a.
adenoleiomyofibroma
adenolipoma
adenolymphocele
adenolymphoma
adenolysis
adenoma
  adnexal a.
  adrenal a.
  bile duct a.
  a. of breast
  bronchial a.
  colonic a.
  colorectal a.
  double a.'s
  ductal a.

NOTES

adenoma (*continued*)
    duodenal a.
    ectopic parathyroid a.
    fibroid a.
    hepatic a.
    kidney a.
    malignant a.
    monoclonal a.
    papillary a.
    parathyroid a.
    pituitary a.
    prostatic a.
    renal a.
    a. sebaceum
    sessile a.
    single a.
    sporadic pituitary a.
    sweat gland a.
    thyroid a.
    tracheal a.
    tubulovillous a.
    upper a.
    well-localized a.
adenoma-hyperplastic polyp ratio
adenoma-nonadenoma ratio
adenomatosis
    endocrine a.
adenomatous
    a. hyperplasia
    a. polyp
    a. polyposis coli (APC)
adenomectomy
adenomyosarcoma
adenopathy
    axillary a.
    cervical a.
    metastatic a.
    retroperitoneal a.
adenosarcoma
adenose
adenosine-regulating agent
adenosine triphosphate (ATP)
adenosis
    sclerosing a.
adenosquamous carcinoma
adenotomy
adenotonsillectomy
adenoviral
    a. infection
    a. transfer
adenovirus infection
adequate hydration
adherence obstruction
adherent
    a. leukoma
    a. zone
adhesed
adhesiectomy

adhesiolysis
    abdominal a.
adhesion
    anomalous mesenteric a.
    attic a.
    banjo-string a.
    a. barrier
    cell-cell a.
    cell-extracellular matrix a.
    dense a.
    fibrinous a.
    fibrous a.
    filmy a.
    a. formation
    hard a.
    intraabdominal a.
    intraperitoneal a.
    laparoscopic lysis of a.'s
    a. lysis
    lysis of a.'s
    membranous a.
    peritoneal a.
    piano-wire a.
    primary a.
    secondary a.
    serologic a.
    tenacious a.
adhesiotomy
adhesive
    a. arachnoiditis
    a. band
    a. bandage
    a. bonding
    a. capsulitis
    a. disease
    a. ileus
    a. inflammation
    a. otitis media
    a. peritonitis
    a. resin-bonded bridge
    a. resin-bonded cast restoration
    a. small bowel obstruction
    a. syndrome
adipectomy
adipocele
adipodermal graft
adipolysis
adipose
    a. body
    a. capsule
    a. connective tissue
    a. fold
    a. graft
    a. infiltration
    a. tissue extract
aditus
adjunct
    surgical a.
    a. therapy

adjunctive
 a. balloon angioplasty
 a. chemotherapy
 a. screw fixation
 a. sedation
 a. suppressive medical therapy

adjustable
 a. gastric banding
 a. ring gastroplasty
 a. suture strabismus surgery

adjuvant
 anesthesia a.
 a. chemoradiation therapy
 a. chemotherapy
 a. diagnostic modality
 a. drug therapy
 a. irradiation
 a. nephrectomy
 a. radiotherapy
 a. regimen

Adkins
 A. spinal fusion
 A. technique spinal arthrodesis

Adler operation

admaxillary gland

admedial

administered
 spinally a.

administration
 altering route of a.
 buccal drug a.
 concomitant a.
 drug a.
 epidural a.
 interpleural a.
 intraocular a.
 intraoperative clonidine a.
 intraperitoneal drug a.
 intraspinal a.
 intrathecal a.
 intravenous a.
 oral a.
 oxygen a.
 parenteral a.
 postischemic a.
 preischemic a.
 route of a.
 sequential a.
 transdermal a.
 transnasal a.
 vasodilator a.

admixture
 a. lesion
 venous a.

adnexa
 ocular a.

adnexal
 a. adenoma
 a. carcinoma
 a. infection
 a. mass
 a. metastasis

adnexectomy

adnexopexy

adrenal
 a. ablation
 accessory a.
 a. adenoma
 a. androgen
 a. body
 a. branch
 a. capsule
 a. carcinoma
 a. cortex
 a. cystic mass
 a. feminization syndrome
 a. gland
 a. gland biopsy
 a. hemorrhage
 a. incidentaloma
 Marchand a.
 a. medulla graft
 a. medulla transplantation
 a. metastasis
 a. pathology
 a. pheochromocytoma
 a. primary aldosteronism
 a. vein

adrenalectomy
 bilateral total a.
 complete a.
 endoscopic a.
 ipsilateral a.
 laparoscopic a.
 laparoscopic anterior a.
 open a.
 transperitoneal laparoscopic a.

adrenergic

adrenic

adrenocortical
 a. carcinoma
 a. extract

adrenoprival

NOTES

adrenoreceptor
    alpha a.
    beta a.
Adson
    A. anterior transperitoneal approach
    A. maneuver
    A. test
Adson-Coffey scalenotomy
adsorption theory of narcosis
adsternal
adterminal
adult
    a. cardiovascular surgery
    a. familial hyaline membrane
      disease
    a. intussusception
    a. patient
    a. polycystic liver disease
    a. population
    a. recipient
    a. respiratory distress syndrome
      (ARDS)
    a. scoliosis surgery
    a. wandering spleen
adulthood astrocytoma
adult-to-adult living related donor living
   transplant
advance
    a. directive
    a. to regular diet
advanced
    a. cardiac mapping
    a. disease
    a. hyperspectral analysis
    a. local invasion
    a. retroperitoneal rhabdomyosarcoma
    a. therapeutic endoscopy
    a. trauma life support (ATLS)
    a. tumor perforation
advancement
    a. flap
    a. flap graft
    Johnson pronator a.
    LeFort III facial a.
    mandibular osteotomy a.
    mucosal a.
    a. procedure
    a. of rectal flap
    transanal pouch a.
    V-Y a.
advancer
    rotator cuff a.
adventitia
adverse
    a. effect
    a. event
AE
    above-elbow
    aryepiglottic

AEA
    above-elbow amputation
Aeby
    A. muscle
    A. plane
aerobe
    Gram-negative a.
aerobic
    a. flora
    a. Gram-negative organism
    a. infection
    a. metabolism
    a. respiration
aerobilia
aerocele
aerocystoscopy
aerodigestive tract
aerodynamic size
aerosol
    inhalation a.
    respirable a.
    a. therapy
aerosolized
    a. medication
    a. pollutant exposure
AESOP
    automated endoscopic system for optimal
      positioning
AESOP-assisted laparoscopic surgery
aesthetic (*var. of* esthetic)
aesthetics (*var. of* esthetics)
A-exotropia
AFBG
    aortofemoral bypass graft
affect
    congruent a.
afferens
afferent
    a. blockade
    a. clot
    a. glomerular arteriole
    a. jejunostomy
    a. limb
    a. loop syndrome
    a. lymphatic vessel
    PGA a.
    PJA a.
    a. projection
    a. spinal
    a. vagal
    a. vasodilation
affrication
AFH
    anterior facial height
afterload
    decreased a.
    a. reduction
afterloading technique
afterpain, after-pain

aganglionic rectum
aganglionosis
    total colonic a.
agar diffusion method
age
    a., distant metastases, extent of local size (AMES)
    fertilization a.
Agee force-couple splint reduction
agenesis
    tracheal a.
agenetic fracture
agent
    adenosine-regulating a.
    alpha-adrenergic a.
    alpha-sympatholytic a.
    anesthetic induction a.
    antiadhesion a.
    antibacterial a.
    antifibrinolytic a.
    antifungal a.
    antimotility a.
    antineoplastic a.
    beta-sympathomimetic a.
    cavity lining a.
    chemoprevention a.
    chemopreventive a.
    endogenous algogenic a.
    hemostatic a.
    inhalation a.
    neuroleptic a.
    neuromuscular blocking a.
    oral antimotility a.
    prothrombogenic a.
    sympatholytic a.
    sympathomimetic a.
    thrombolytic a.
    topical antibacterial a.
    topical hemostatic a.
    vasodilator a.
    ventilation a.
    volatile anesthetic a.
age-related macular degeneration
agglutinant
agglutinate
agglutination technique
aggregate gland
aggregation
    platelet a.
aggressive
    a. lesion

    a. renal angiomyolipoma
    a. surgical approach
aging degenerative change
agitation
    abdominal a.
    emergence a.
Agliette supracondylar osteotomy
aglossia-adactylia syndrome
aglossostomia
agminate gland
agnathia
agnathous
Agnew
    A. canthoplasty
    A. operation
Agnew-Verhoeff incision
agonadal
agonal
    a. clot
    a. respiration
agonist
    alpha-1-adrenergic a.
    alpha-2-adrenergic a.
    alpha-adrenergic receptor a.
    alpha-2-adrenoreceptor a.
    beta-adrenergic a.
    beta-receptor a.
    muscarinic a.
    opioid a.
Agrikola operation
AH
    atypical hyperplasia
ahaustral
Ahern knot
AHI
    Arthritis Helplessness Index
air
    bowel loop a.
    a. collection
    colonic a.
    a. critical care transport
    a. cyst
    a. embolism
    a. embolus
    a. enema
    a. entrainment
    a. entry
    a. exchange
    expired a.
    extrapleural a.
    free a.
    a. injection

NOTES

air *(continued)*
> inspired a.
> a. insufflation
> intramural colonic a.
> intramyocardial a.
> intraperitoneal a.
> minimal a.
> oxygen in a.
> a. plethysmography
> a. sac
> a. sinus
> a. space
> a. space disease
> a. test
> a. vesicle

air-bone-tissue boundary
airborne infection
airbrasive technique
air-contrast barium enema
air-filled loop
air-fluid
> a.-f. exchange
> a.-f. line

air-gap technique
airplane position
airway
> anatomic a.
> anatomical a.
> a., breathing, circulation (ABC)
> a. caliber
> a. compromise
> a. elastance
> esophageal obturator a.
> a. gas monitoring
> intubating laryngeal mask a.
> large mask a.
> laryngeal mask a. (LMA)
> a. management
> nasal a.
> nasopharyngeal a.
> a. obstruction
> a. occlusion technique
> oral pharyngeal a.
> oropharyngeal a.
> a. pattern
> pediatric a.
> pharyngeal a.
> a. pressure (AP)
> a. pressure release ventilation (APRV)
> a. protection
> a. reactivity
> a. responsiveness
> a. score
> a. shunting
> a. smooth muscle (ASM)
> a. suction
> surgical a.

AIS
> Abbreviated Injury Scale
> Abbreviated Injury Score

Aitken epiphysial fracture classification
AJCC
> American Joint Committee on Cancer
> AJCC TNM tumor classification

Ajmalin liver injury
AJPBD
> anomalous junction of pancreatobiliary duct

AK
> above-knee

AKA
> above-knee amputation

Akerlund deformity
Akin
> A. bunionectomy
> A. procedure
> A. proximal phalangeal osteotomy

Akiyama procedure
ala, pl. **alae**
> sacral a.

alanine
> a. aminotransferase (ALT)

alanine amino transaminase (ALT)
Alanson amputation
alar
> a. base reduction
> a. cartilage
> a. fascia
> a. fold
> a. groove
> a. incision
> a. lamina
> a. ligament
> a. reconstruction
> a. spine
> a. wedge excision

alarm
alba
Albarran
> A. gland
> A. y Dominguez tubule

Albee spinal fusion
Albert-Lembert gastroplasty
Albert suture technique
Albinus muscle
ALBPSQ
> Acute Low Back Pain Screening Questionnaire

Albrecht bone
Albright-Chase arthroplasty
Albright synovectomy
albugineotomy
albumin
> radiolabeled serum a.

Alcock canal

alcohol
    a. dependence scale
    a. fixation
    a. used disorders identification test
alcohol-fixed gastric biopsy
alcoholic
    a. coma
    a. liver
Alcon aspiration
Alden loop gastric bypass
Alder-Reilly anomaly
aldosterone-producing carcinoma
aldosteronism
    adrenal primary a.
Aldrete score
Aldridge sling procedure
Aldridge-Studdefort urethral suspension
alertness/sedation score
Alexander
    A. incision
    A. operation
    A. technique
Alexander-Adams
    A.-A. hysteropexy
    A.-A. uterine suspension
algesimeter
Al-Ghorab
    A.-G. modification
    A.-G. procedure
alginate
algiomotor
algodystrophy
algology
algorithm
    nonrigid registration a.
    registration a.
algoscopy
ALI
    acute limb ischemia
alien hand sign
aligner
    incision a.
alignment
    extramedullary a.
    normal anatomic a.
alimentarium
alimentary
    a. apparatus
    a. canal
    a. limb
    a. tract
    a. tract duplication

alimentation
    central venous a.
    enteral a.
    forced a.
    intravenous a.
    peripheral intravenous a.
    rectal a.
    total parenteral a.
alinasal
aliquorrhea
    spontaneous a.
aliquot
alkaline
    a. phosphatase-antiphosphatase
    a. reflux
Alken approach
alkylation resistance
Allain method
allantoic
    a. circulation
    a. sac
allele
Allen
    A. correction
    A. maneuver
    A. operation
    A. reduction
    A. test
allergen exposure
allergic
    a. bronchopulmonary aspergillosis
    (ABA)
    a. fungal sinusitis
    a. inflammation
    a. manifestation
    a. shock
allergy
    latex a.
Allgöwer stitch
alligator skin
all-inside repair
Allis
    A. maneuver
    A. sign
Allis-Abramson breast biopsy
Allison
    A. gastroesophageal reflux repair
    A. GE reflux correction
    A. hiatal hernia repair
    A. procedure
    A. suture technique

NOTES

Allman acromioclavicular injury classification
allocation
> dynamic storage a.
> fresh tissue a.
> static storage a.
> storage a.
> a. of treatment

allodynia
> compression-evoked a.

allogenic, allogeneic
> a. blood
> a. blood component
> a. blood transfusion
> a. bone
> a. bone graft
> a. bone marrow
> a. fetal graft
> a. transplantation

allogenous bone graft
allograft
> a. corneal rejection
> cryopreserved heart-valve a.
> a. extraction
> femoral cortical ring a.
> functioning a.
> hepatic a.
> intestinal a.
> liver a.
> organ a.
> osteoarticular a.
> osteochondral a.
> pancreaticoduodenal a.
> renal a.
> strut a.
> a. transplantation

allografting
> nerve a.
> peripheral nerve a.

allokeratoplasty
allongement
allopathic keratoplasty
alloplastic chin augmentation
alloplasty
all-or-nothing phenomenon
allotransplantation
> inlet a.
> liver a.

alloy restoration
Allport operation
ALM
> acral lentiginous melanoma

ALND
> axillary lymph node dissection

alone
> pancreas transplant a. (PTA)
> pancreatic transplantation a. (PTA)

Alonso-Lej classification

alopecia
> pressure a.
> traction a.

alpha, α
alpha-adrenergic
> a.-a. agent
> a.-a. antagonist
> a.-a. receptor
> a.-a. receptor agonist

alpha-1-adrenergic
> a.-1-a. agonist
> a.-1-a. antagonist

alpha-2-adrenergic
> a.-2-a. agonist
> a.-2-a. receptor
> a.-2-a. receptor antagonist

alpha adrenoreceptor
alpha-2-adrenoreceptor agonist
alpha-loop maneuver
alpha-sympatholytic agent
Alport syndrome
ALT
> alanine amino transaminase
> alanine aminotransferase
> serum ALT

Altemeier repair of rectal prolapse
alteration
> dentin crystal a.

alterative inflammation
altercursive intubation
altered gene product
altering route of administration
alternate-day therapy
alternating suture technique
alternation
alternative
> cost-effective a.
> a. introduction site
> a. medicine
> a. practitioner
> a. surgical approach
> therapeutic a.
> a. therapy
> a. treatment

altitude simulation study
ALTK
> automated lamellar therapeutic keratoplasty

aluminum
> a. cranioplasty
> implant alloy a.

alveodental suppuration
alveolar
> a. adenocarcinoma
> a. artery
> a. body
> a. canal
> a. carbon dioxide pressure
> a. cavity

a. cell carcinoma
a. dead space
a. dead-space fraction
a. diffusion measurement
a. ectasia
a. end-capillary difference
a. fistula
a. fluid transport
a. gas equation
a. hemorrhage
a. hyperventilation
a. hypoventilation
a. index
a. nerve
a. partial pressure
a. plateau
a. plate fenestration
a. point
a. point-meatus plane
a. point-nasal point line
a. point-nasion line
a. process
a. process fracture
a. rhabdomyosarcoma
a. sac
a. socket wall fracture
a. tumor
a. ventilation
a. ventilation per minute
a. yoke

alveolar-arterial
a.-a. oxygen gradient
a.-a. pressure difference

alveolarization

alveolectomy
partial a.

alveoli (*pl. of* alveolus)

alveolitis
acute allergic extrinsic a.
chronic extrinsic a.
extrinsic allergic a.

alveolobasilar line

alveolocapillary
a. membrane
a. partial pressure gradient

alveolodental membrane

alveololabial groove

alveolomerotomy

alveolonasal line

alveoloplasty
interradicular a.
intraseptal a.

alveolotomy

alveolus, pl. **alveoli**

alveoplasty

alvine calculus

alvinolith

Alvis operation

AM
anterior midpapillary
AM segment

amalgam
a. condensation
a. restoration

Amato body

amaurosis
intoxication a.
pressure a.

Amberg lateral sinus line

ambient
a. cisterna
a. oxygen concentration
a. temperature

ambiguous external genitalia

amblyopia
deprivation a.
eclipse a.
ex a.
exertional a.

ambulatory
a. anesthesia
a. blood pressure monitoring
a. gynecologic laparoscopy
a. hemorrhoidectomy
a. pneumoperitoneum
a. setup
a. surgery
a. surgery center

amebic
a. colitis
a. cyst
a. hepatic abscess
a. infection
a. perforation
a. peritonitis

ameboma

ameliorating myocardial stunning liposomal coenzyme

amelioration

ameloblastic
a. carcinoma
a. fibroma

ameloblastoma

NOTES

American
    A. Association of Nurse
      Anesthetists (AANA)
    A. Association for the Surgery of
      Trauma (AAST)
    A. Association for Surgery of
      Trauma Organ Injury Scale
      classification
    A. Board of Anesthesiology (ABA)
    A. Board of Pain Medicine
      (ABPM)
    A. Board of Surgery (ABS)
    A. College of Surgeons (ACS)
    A. Heart Association classification
    A. Joint Committee on Cancer
      (AJCC)
    A. laryngectomy technique
    A. Pediatric Surgical Association
      (APSA)
    A. Rheumatism Association index
    A. Society of Anesthesiologists
      (ASA)
    A. Society of Anesthesiologists
      classification
    A. Society of Anesthesiology score
    A. Society for Colon and Rectal
      Surgeons (ASCRS)
    A. Society for Gastrointestinal
      Endoscopy (ASGE)
    A. Society of Regional Anesthesia
      (ASRA)
    A. Urological Association symptom
      index

AMES
    age, distant metastases, extent of local
    size
    AMES criteria

ametropia
    position a.

amidation

amino acid

aminoglycoside
    a. toxicity
    a. tubular necrosis

aminotransferase
    alanine a. (ALT)

AML
    angiomyolipoma

AMLR
    auditory middle lateral response

Ammon
    A. canthoplasty
    A. operation

amnesia
    patch a.

amnestic effect

amnioinfusion

amnioma

amnion
    a. ring
    a. rupture

amnioscopy

amniotic
    a. band amputation
    a. cavity
    a. fluid embolism
    a. fold
    a. hernia
    a. infection syndrome
    a. membrane
    a. sac

amniotomy

amobarbital

ampere (A)

amphibolic fistula

amphibolous fistula

amphoric respiration

Amplatz technique

amplitude
    a. of fusion
    a. modulation

amplitude-summation
    a.-s. interferential current
    a.-s. interferential current therapy

ampulla, pl. ampullae
    duodenal a.
    hepatopancreatic a.
    rectal a.
    Thoma a.
    Vater a.

ampullaris

ampullary
    a. adenocarcinoma
    a. aneurysm
    a. cancer
    a. carcinoma
    a. granulation tissue
    a. sulcus
    a. tumor

ampullectomy

ampulloma

amputation
    above-elbow a. (AEA)
    above-knee a. (AKA)
    Alanson a.
    amniotic band a.
    Béclard a.
    below-elbow a. (BEA)
    below-knee a. (BKA)
    Berger interscapular a.
    Bier a.
    bilateral a.
    birth a.
    bloodless a.
    border ray a.
    Boyd ankle a.
    Bunge a.

A

Burgess below-knee a.
Callander a.
central ray a.
cervical a.
chop a.
Chopart a.
circular open a.
closed flap a.
congenital above-elbow a.
congenital below-elbow a.
consecutive a.
corporectomy a.
disarticular a.
dry a.
extremity a.
Farabeuf a.
fingertip a.
fishmouth a.
forearm a.
forequarter a.
Gordon-Taylor hindquarter a.
Gritti-Stokes a.
guillotine a.
hand a.
hindfoot a.
hindquarter a.
immediate a.
incomplete a.
index ray a.
interilioabdominal a.
interinnominoabdominal a.
intermediate a.
interpelviabdominal a.
interphalangeal a.
interscapular a.
intrapyretic a.
intrauterine a.
Jaboulay a.
Kendrick method below-knee a.
King-Steelquist hindquarter a.
Lisfranc a.
major a.
minor a.
multiple ray a.
open a.
pathologic a.
penile a.
Pirogoff a.
primary a.
pulp a.
quadruple a.
ray a.

rectangular a.
root a.
secondary a.
shoulder a.
Sorondo-Ferré hindquarter a.
spontaneous a.
1-stage a.
2-stage Syme a.
supracondylar a.
Syme ankle disarticulation a.
tarsal a.
tarsometatarsal a.
tendinomyoplastic a.
tertiary a.
through-knee a.
transcarpal a.
transiliac a.
transmetatarsal a.
transpelvic a.
traumatic a.
Wagner modification of Syme a.
Wagner 2-stage Syme a.
Wilms a.
amputee
unilateral a.
Amreich vaginal extirpation
Amsler operation
Amspacher-Messenbaugh
A.-M. closing wedge osteotomy
A.-M. technique
Amstutz-Wilson osteotomy
Amussat
A. incision
A. operation
A. valvula
amygdaline
amygdalohippocampectomy
amygdalotomy
amyloid
a. angiopathy
a. kidney
a. oral cavity disease
anabolic response
anaclitic therapy
anacrotic notch
anadidymus
anaerobe
anaerobic
a. ocular infection
a. respiration
anaeroplasty
anagenesis

NOTES

Anagnostakis operation
anal
- a. abscess
- a. anastomosis
- a. canal
- a. canal artery
- a. canal rhythmic contraction
- a. canal staining
- a. cleft
- a. column
- a. condyloma
- a. continence
- a. crypt
- a. dilation
- a. electrical stimulation
- a. endoscopy
- a. fascia
- a. fissure
- a. fistula
- a. fistulotomy
- a. foreign body
- a. HPZ
- a. incontinence
- a. manometry
- a. orifice
- a. pecten
- a. pouch
- a. region
- a. resting pressure
- a. sinus
- a. sphincter injury
- a. sphincter reconstruction
- a. sphincter repair
- a. sphincter squeeze pressure
- a. squamous intraepithelial lesion
- a. stretch
- a. transition zone (ATZ)
- a. triangle
- a. ulceration
- a. verge

analgesia
- ceiling a.
- conduction a.
- dermatomal level of a.
- fixed-dose patient-controlled a. (FDPCA)
- inhalation a.
- interpleural a.
- intrathecal opioid labor a.
- multimodal a.
- opioid a.
- parenteral a.
- patient-controlled a. (PCA)
- patient-controlled epidural a. (PCEA, PEA)
- patient-controlled epidural with intravenous a.
- patient-controlled intranasal a. (PCINA)

patient-controlled regional a. (PCRA)
- perineal a.
- perioperative a.
- a. permeation
- pinprick a.
- postoperative a.
- preemptive a.
- preoperative a.
- rescue a.
- spinal a.
- supplementary a.
- thoracic epidural a.
- tracheal topical a.

analgesia-induced PGID
analgesic
- a. abuse headache
- a. effect
- a. index
- a. infusion
- intranasal a.
- intrathecal a.
- intravenous a.
- narcotic a.
- NSAID a.
- opioid a.
- oral a.
- parenteral a.
- pediatric a.
- postoperative a.
- spinal a.
- transdermal a.

analgetic
analogous
analogue
- somatostatin a.

analysis, pl. **analyses**
- activity pattern a.
- advanced hyperspectral a.
- antinociception a.
- blood gas a.
- body composition a.
- combined a.
- deformity a.
- displacement a.
- failure a. (FA)
- fixed-dose a.
- frozen section a.
- histopathologic a.
- hyperspectral a.
- image a.
- immunohistochemical a.
- isobologram a.
- isobolographic a.
- Kruskal-Wallis nonparametric a.
- mutation a.
- neutron activation a.
- peak pressure a.
- power spectral a.

pressure-volume a.
p53 tumor suppressor gene a.
restriction endonuclease a.
retrospective a.
saturation a.
single strand conformation
    polymorphism a.
slot-blot hybridization a.
sound a.
total space a.
Vindelov method flow cytometry a.
visual a.
volumetric a.

analytic
    a. method
    a. reconstruction

analyzer
    oxygen a.
    patient state a.
    thromboelastograph hemostasis a.
        (TEG)

anaphylactoid-type reaction

anaphylaxis
    eosinophilic chemotactic factor
        of a. (ECF-A)

anaplastic
    a. adenocarcinoma
    a. astrocytoma
    a. carcinoma
    a. ependymoma

anapophysis

anastole

anastomose

anastomosed graft

anastomosis, pl. **anastomoses**
    anal a.
    antecolic a.
    antiperistaltic a.
    aortic a.
    arterial a.
    arteriolovenular a.
    arteriovenous a.
    Baffe a.
    Béclard a.
    beveled a.
    bidirectional superior
        cavopulmonary a.
    biliary-enteric a.
    biliary intestinal a.
    biliodigestive a.
    Billroth I, II gastrointestinal a.
    bladder neck-to-urethra a.

bowel a.
Brackin ureterointestinal a.
Braun a.
carotid-basilar a.
carotid-vertebral a.
cavopulmonary a.
cervical a.
choledochocholedochostomy side-to-
    side a.
circular a.
Clado a.
cobra-head a.
Coffey ureterointestinal a.
coloanal a.
colocolic a.
colocolonic a.
coloendoanal a.
colonic pouch anal a.
colorectal a.
conjoined a.
cornual a.
Couvelaire ileourethral a.
cross-facial nerve graft a.
crucial a.
cruciate a.
crunch-stick a.
crushing a.
curved end-to-end a.
D-D a.
delayed direct coloanal a.
delta-shaped a.
dismembered a.
distal a.
duct-to-duct a.
duct-to-mucosa a.
elliptical a.
endoanal a.
end-to-back bowel a.
end-to-end ileoanal a.
end-to-end splenoadrenal a.
end-to-side a.
end-weave a.
esophageal-jejunal a.
esophagocolic a.
esophagogastric a.
extended end-to-end a.
extraabdominal a.
extracorporeal a.
extrapleural a.
extravesical a.
fishmouth a.
flexor tendon a.

NOTES

anastomosis *(continued)*

Fontan atriopulmonary a.
Furniss a.
Galen a.
gastroduodenal a.
gastrointestinal a. (GIA)
gastrojejunal a.
genicular a.
Glenn a.
graft a.
Haight a.
handmade a.
handsewn a.
hand-sutured ileoanal a.
heel-toe a.
hepatojejunal a.
Hofmeister a.
Hofmeister-Pólya a.
Horsley a.
Hoyer a.
H-shaped ileal pouch-anal a.
hypoglossal facial nerve a.
Hyrtl a.
ileal pouch-anal a. (IPAA)
ileal pouch-distal rectal a.
ileal-sigmoid a.
ileoanal a.
ileorectal a. (IRA)
ileosigmoid a.
ileotransverse colon a.
ileovesical a.
intercoronary a.
intermesenteric arterial a.
intestinal a.
intracorporeal a.
intragastric a.
intrathoracic a.
intravesical a.
invaginating a.
isoperistaltic a.
jejunoileal a.
jejunojejunal a.
J-shaped ileal pouch-anal a.
Kocher a.
Kugel a.
laparoscopic bilioenteric a.
2-layer a.
LeDuc a.
leptomeningeal a.
Lich-Gregoir a.
longitudinal side-to-side a.
lymphaticovenous a.
Martin-Gruber a.
mechanical a.
mesocaval a.
microneurovascular a.
microsurgical tubocornual a.
microvascular surgical a.
mucosa-to-mucosa a.

Nakayama a.
nerve a.
nondismembered a.
onlay patch a.
pancreatic a.
pancreaticogastric a.
pancreaticogastrointestinal a.
pancreaticogastrostomy a. (PGA)
pancreaticojejunal a.
pancreaticojejunostomy a. (PJA)
Parks ileoanal a.
percutaneous portocaval a.
Politano-Leadbetter a.
Pólya a.
portacaval a.
portal-systemic a.
portoportal a.
portopulmonary venous a.
portosystemic a.
Potts a.
Potts-Smith a.
precapillary a.
primary end-to-end a.
rectosigmoid a.
Riche-Cannieu a.
right-angled end-to-side a.
Riolan a.
Roux-en-Y hepaticojejunal a.
Schmidel a.
Schoemaker a.
side-to-side a.
spinal accessory nerve-facial
  nerve a.
splenoadrenal a.
splenorenal venous a.
S-shaped ileal pouch-anal a.
STA-MCA a.
stapled coloanal a.
stapled ileal pouch-anal a.
stapled ileoanal a.
State end-to-end a.
stenotic esophagogastric a.
subcutaneous a.
Sucquet a.
Sucquet-Hoyer a.
supraoptic a.
suture a.
sutureless bowel a.
temporal-cerebral arterial a.
tension-free a.
terminoterminal a.
transanal mucosectomy with
  handsewn a.
transureteroureteral a.
triple a.
ureterocolonic a.
ureteroileal a.
ureterosigmoid a.
ureterotubal a.

ureteroureteral a.
valved conduit a.
vascular a.
venous a.
venous-to-venous a.
vesicourethral a.
Von Haberer-Finney a.
Waterston extrapericardial a.
wide elliptical a.
wide-open a.
W-shaped ileal pouch-anal a.
Z-shaped a.

anastomotic
a. abscess
a. area
a. branch
a. breakdown
a. complication
a. complication rate
a. dehiscence
a. edge
a. failure
a. fiber
a. fistula
a. flow
a. healing
a. leakage
a. operation
a. stoma
a. stricture
a. stricture formation
a. stricture rate
a. stump
a. stump leak
a. ulceration
a. vein

anatomic
a. abnormality
a. airway
a. barrier
a. dead space
a. diagnosis
a. equator
a. event
a. fracture
a. fracture reduction principle
a. imaging
a. imaging information
a. insertion
a. integrity
a. landmark
a. localization

a. pathology
a. plane
a. porous replacement (APR)
a. position
a. repair
a. site
a. structure
a. variation

anatomical
a. airway
a. landmark
a. position
a. radical retropubic prostatectomy
a. root
a. site
a. situation
a. snuffbox
a. sphincter
a. tooth
a. tubercle
a. variation

anatomicosurgical
anatomist
anatomy
anomalous a.
biliary a.
Billroth II a.
cervicothoracic pedicle a.
congenitally altered a.
coronary vessel a.
dental a.
designed after natural a. (DANA)
fetal intracranial a.
gingival a.
immune system a.
intracranial a.
intrahepatic a.
knee a.
Lowsley lobar a.
native coronary a.
neurovascular a.
normal planar MR a.
pathological a.
pedicle a.
peritoneal a.
plantar compartmental a.
surgical a.
vascular a.
zonal a.

anatrophic
a. nephrolithotomy

NOTES

anatrophic *(continued)*
    a. nephroscopy
    a. nephrotomy
anchor
    a. mastopexy
    a. molar
anchorage
    extramaxillary a.
    extraoral a.
    gastrophrenic a.
anchoring point
anchovy procedure
ancillary circuit
ancipital
anconeal
anconeus
    a. arthroplasty
    a. muscle
    a. muscle flap
Andersch
    A. ganglion
    A. nerve
Anderson
    A. ankle fusion
    A. modification of Berndt-Harty
      classification
    A. procedure
**Anderson-D'Alonzo odontoid fracture
  classification**
Anderson-Fowler
    A.-F. calcaneal displacement
      osteotomy
    A.-F. procedure
Anderson-Hutchins
    A.-H. technique
    A.-H. unstable tibial shaft fracture
Anderson-Hynes pyeloplasty
Anderson-Keys method
Andrews
    A. iliotibial band reconstruction
    A. technique
**Andrews-type nonorthodontic normal
  crown angulation**
androblastoma
androgen
    a. ablation
    adrenal a.
    excess a.
androgenic obesity
androgenization
android pelvis
Andy Gump deformity
anecdotal procedure
anechoic tissue
Anel
    A. method
    A. operation
anemia
    acute severe isovolemic a.

Fanconi a.
a. of hemodialysis
anergia
anesthesia
    a. action
    acupuncture a.
    a. adjuvant
    ambulatory a.
    American Society of Regional A.
     (ASRA)
    ankle block a.
    axillary block a.
    balanced a.
    barbiturate burst-suppression a.
    basal a.
    Bier block a.
    block a.
    bolus intravenous a.
    brachial a.
    a. breathing circuit
    bypass a.
    cardiac a.
    cardiovascular a.
    caudal a.
    centroneuroaxis a.
    cervical a.
    circle absorption a.
    closed circuit a.
    cocaine a.
    coinduction of a.
    combined epidural/general a.
    combined spinal/epidural a. (CSEA)
    come-and-go a.
    compression a.
    computer-assisted a.
    conduction a.
    continuous epidural a.
    continuous lumbar peridural a.
    continuous spinal a.
    controlled hypotensive a. (CHA)
    corneal a.
    crossed a.
    deep volatile a.
    dental a.
    depth of a.
    diagnostic a.
    differential spinal a.
    digital block a.
    direct vein a.
    dissociated a.
    dissociative a.
    a. dolorosa
    ear a.
    electric a.
    endotracheal a.
    epidural a. (EA)
    examination under a.
    extradural a.
    failed a.

A

fast-track cardiac a.
field block a.
fitness for general a.
fractional epidural a.
fractional spinal a.
general a. (GA)
general endotracheal a.
geriatric a.
girdle a.
glove a.
graded spinal a.
gustatory a.
gynecologic a.
high spinal a.
hydrate microcrystal theory of a.
hyperbaric spinal a.
hypnosis a.
hypobaric spinal a.
hypotensive a.
hypothermic a.
hysterical a.
induction of a.
infiltration a.
infraorbital a.
inhalant a.
inhalational a.
inhalation mask a.
insufflation a.
intercostal a.
interpleural a.
intracavitary a.
intraligamentary a.
intramedullary a.
intranasal a.
intraoral a.
intraorbital a.
intraosseous a.
intraperitoneal a.
intrapulpal a.
intraspinal a.
intrathecal a.
intratracheal a.
intravenous block a.
intravenous regional a. (IVRA)
intravenous sedation a.
isobaric spinal a.
laryngeal a.
laryngotracheal a. (LTA)
ligamental a.
local a.
low central venous pressure a.
low spinal a.

low thoracic level epidural a.
lumbar epidural a.
1-lung a.
MAC a.
management of a.
maternal a.
modified Van Lint a.
monitored anesthesia care a.
muscular a.
neonatal a.
nerve block a.
nerve compression a.
neuroleptanalgesia a.
neurosurgical a.
newborn a.
nonrebreathing a.
nose a.
O'Brien a.
obstetric a.
ocular microtremor during
  general a.
olfactory a.
open drop a.
ophthalmic a.
ophthalmologic a.
opioid a.
orbital a.
oropharyngeal a.
orthopaedic a.
outpatient a.
painful a.
paracervical block a.
paravertebral a.
parenteral a.
pediatric radiotherapy a.
peribulbar a.
peridural a.
perineal a.
perineural a.
periodontal ligament a.
peripheral nerve block a.
pharyngeal a.
Ponka technique for local a.
postcesarean a.
postoperative a.
preemptive a.
pregnancy-induced a.
preperitoneal a.
presacral a.
pressure a.
pudendal a.
rapid-sequence induction of a.

NOTES

anesthesia *(continued)*
    rebreathing a.
    a. record
    rectal a.
    refrigeration a.
    retrobulbar a.
    risk management of a.
    sacral a.
    saddle block a.
    segmental epidural a.
    segmental peridural spinal a.
    selective a.
    semiclosed a.
    semiopen a.
    single-breath induction of a.
    single-shot spinal a.
    spinal a. (SA)
    splanchnic a.
    stellate ganglion block a.
    stocking a.
    stocking-glove a.
    subarachnoid a.
    supraclavicular brachial block a.
    surgical a.
    tactile a.
    therapeutic a.
    thermal a.
    thermic a.
    thoracic a.
    throat a.
    a. time
    to-and-fro a.
    toe-block a.
    topical oropharyngeal a.
    total intravenous a. (TIVA)
    total spinal a.
    transdermal a.
    traumatic a.
    unilateral a.
    unmonitored local a.
    urologic a.
    Van Lint a.
    variable-dose patient-controlled a.
     (VDPCA)
    visceral a.
    volatile a.
anesthesia-induced PGID
anesthesiologist
    American Society of A.'s (ASA)
anesthesiology
    American Board of A. (ABA)
    critical care a.
    a. critical care medicine
anesthetic
    action of a.
    a. approach
    a. block
    a. blockade
    cardiac a.

    a. circuit
    a. consideration
    a. cutoff
    a. depth
    a. emergence
    EMLA a.
    epidural a.
    eutectic mixture of local a.'s
     (EMLA)
    flammable a.
    a. and fluid management
    gas a.
    a. gas
    a. gas exposure
    a. gas mixture
    general a.
    halogenated volatile a.
    a. hepatitis
    a. hepatotoxicity
    hyperbaric local a.
    a. immediate recovery
    a. index
    a. induction
    a. induction agent
    inhaled a.
    injection of local a.
    instillation of a.
    intradermal a.
    intramuscular a.
    intraperitoneal a.
    intrathecal a.
    intravenous a.
    a. leprosy
    local a.
    low-dose a.
    a. management
    a. monitoring
    multiple-mechanism inhaled a.
    multiple-site inhaled a.
    opioid a.
    oral a.
    pediatric a.
    polymer a.
    a. potency
    a. preconditioning
    preoperative a.
    primary a.
    a. reaction
    a. record
    rectal a.
    regional a.
    ring block digital a.
    a. risk
    secondary a.
    a. shock
    single-mechanism inhaled a.
    single-site inhaled a.
    spinal a.
    a. system

a. technique
a. time
a. tolerance
topical a.
trace a.
a. vapor
volatile a.
walking epidural a.
anesthetic/hypnotic
anesthetist
American Association of
Nurse A.'s (AANA)
certified registered nurse a.
(CRNA)
nurse a.
anesthetization
anesthetize
aneuploid cell line
aneurysm
abdominal aortic a. (AAA)
ampullary a.
anterior circulation a.
aortic a.
aortoiliac a.
arterial a.
arteriosclerotic a.
arteriovenous a.
atherosclerotic a.
axial a.
axillary artery a.
basilar artery a.
basilar bifurcation a.
basilar tip a.
Bérard a.
berry a.
bifurcation a.
celiac artery a.
circulation a.
clavicular fracture a.
a. clip ligation
coiled intracranial a.
complex intracranial a.
compound a.
congenital cerebral a.
consecutive a.
cylindroid a.
descending aortic a.
diffuse a.
dissecting a.
ectatic a.
endogenous a.
endovascular a.

exogenous a.
false a.
femoral artery a.
fusiform a.
hernial a.
iliac artery a.
inflammatory abdominal aortic a.
(IAAA)
infraclinoid a.
intracranial a.
isolated iliac artery a.
juxtarenal a.
a. management
miliary a.
mitral valve a.
mycotic a.
peripheral a.
phantom a.
posterior circulation a.
Pott a.
a. repair
ruptured abdominal aortic a.
saccular a.
serpentine a.
splenic artery a. (SAA)
staged repair of extensive aortic a.
subclavian artery a.
supraclinoid a.
thoracic a.
thoracoabdominal a.
thoracoabdominal aortic a. (TAA)
a. tissue
traction a.
traumatic false a.
true a.
tubular a.
varicose a.
aneurysmal
a. dilatation
a. dilation
a. disease
a. hematoma
a. hemorrhage
a. rupture
a. sac
a. tissue
a. varix
aneurysmectomy
aortic a.
conventional aortic a.
elective a.

NOTES

aneurysmectomy *(continued)*
    laparoscopic-assisted a.
    Matas a.
aneurysmoplasty
aneurysmorrhaphy
aneurysmotomy
ANF
    atrial natriuretic factor
Angelucci operation
angel-wing deformity
angiectasia
angiectatic
angiectopia
angiitis
    hypersensitivity a.
    necrotizing a.
angina
    abdominal a.
    intestinal a.
    unstable a.
angina-guided therapy
angioblastoma
angiocentric
    a. immunoproliferative lesion
    a. lymphoproliferative lesion
angiodysplastic lesion
angioembolization
angioendothelioma
angiofibrolipoma
angiofibroma, pl. **angiofibromata**
    facial a.
    juvenile a.
angiogenesis
    therapeutic a.
    tumor a.
angiogram
    mesenteric a.
    multigated a.
angiographic
    a. demonstration
    a. embolization
    a. evaluation
    a. intervention
    a. result
    a. road-mapping technique
    a. study
angiographically occult intracranial vascular malformation (AOIVM)
angiography
    abdominal a.
    fluorescein a.
    magnetic resonance a. (MRA)
    mesenteric a.
    selective a.
angioinvasive lesion
angiokeratoma
angioleiomyoma
angiolipofibroma
angiolipoma

angiolith
angiolithic
angiolysis
angioma
    arterial a.
    bleeding a.
    capillary a.
    cavernous a.
    cerebral a.
    cherry a.
    conjunctival a.
    gastric a.
    orbital a.
    pulmonary a.
    spider a.
    spinal a.
    strawberry a.
    superficial a.
    telangiectatic a.
    venous a.
angiomatosis
    skeletal-extraskeletal a.
angiomatous neoplastic tissue
angiomyofibroma
angiomyolipoma (AML)
    aggressive renal a.
    asymptomatic a.
    hemorrhagic a.
    malignant a.
    renal a.
    uncomplicated a.
    visceral a.
angiomyoma
angiomyoneuroma
angiomyxoma
angioneurectomy
angioneuromyoma
angioneurotomy
angio-osteohypertrophy syndrome
angiopathy
    amyloid a.
    radiation a.
angioplany
angioplasty
    ablative laser a.
    adjunctive balloon a.
    aortoiliac a.
    balloon catheter a.
    balloon coarctation a.
    balloon coronary a.
    balloon dilation a.
    balloon laser a.
    bootstrap 2-vessel a.
    brachiocephalic vessel a.
    carotid a.
    complementary balloon a.
    coronary artery a.
    coronary balloon a.
    culprit lesion a.

excimer laser coronary a.
facilitated a.
high-risk a.
Ho:YAG laser a.
iliac artery a.
infrapopliteal transluminal a.
Kinsey rotation atherectomy
 extrusion a.
kissing balloon a.
laser-assisted balloon a.
low-speed rotational a.
Osypka rotational a.
patch-graft a.
percutaneous balloon a.
percutaneous low-stress a.
percutaneous transluminal
 coronary a. (PTCA)
percutaneous transluminal renal a.
peripheral balloon a.
peripheral laser a.
postcoronary a.
renal a.
rescue a.
rotational a.
salvage balloon a.
subclavian vein patch a.
Tactilaze a.
thermal/perfusion balloon a.
tibioperoneal trunk a.
tibioperoneal vessel a.
transluminal coronary a.
vein patch a.
vibrational a.

angioplasty-related vessel occlusion
angioproliferative lesion
angioreticuloma
angiorrhaphy
angiorrhexis
angiosarcoma
angioscopy
fluorescein fundus a.
percutaneous transluminal a.

angioscotoma
angiostomy
angiotelectasis
angiotensin-converting enzyme (ACE)
angiotensinogen
angiotomy
angle
a. of aberration
anomaly a.
anorectal a.

anterior angulation a.
axial line a.
biorbital a.
a. bisection technique
Böhler calcaneal a.
Broca basilar a.
Broca facial a.
buccoocclusal line a.
calcaneal inclination a.
calcaneal-second metatarsal angle
 inclination a.
cardiohepatic a.
cavity line a.
costal a.
Daubenton a.
declination a.
deformity a.
distobuccal line a.
distobuccoocclusal point a.
distolabial line a.
distolabioincisal point a.
distolingual line a.
distolinguoincisal point a.
distoocclusal point a.
duodenojejunal a.
elevation a.
epigastric a.
facial a.
a. of femoral torsion
filtration a.
Frankfort mandibular incisor a.
Frankfort mandibular plane a.
hepatic-renal a.
hepatorenal a.
a. of His
hypsiloid a.
incisal mandibular plane a.
infrasternal a.
iridocorneal a.
Jacquart facial a.
labioincisal line a.
line a.
linguoincisal line a.
linguoocclusal line a.
Louis a.
Ludwig a.
lumbosacral a.
magnetization precession a.
A. malocclusion classification
mandibular incisor a.
mandibular plane a.
mesiobuccal line a.

NOTES

31

angle *(continued)*
    mesiobuccoocclusal point a.
    mesiolabial line a.
    mesiolabioincisal point a.
    mesiolingual line a.
    mesiolinguoincisal point a.
    mesiolinguo-occlusal point line a.
    mesioocclusal line a.
    metafacial a.
    nail-to-nail bed a.
    occipital a.
    occlusal plane a.
    ophryospinal a.
    a. of orientation
    parietal a.
    pelvivertebral a.
    Pirogoff a.
    point a.
    pubic a.
    Quatrefages a.
    a. of reflection
    Serres a.
    sharp a.
    sphenoidal a.
    splenorenal a.
    sternal a.
    sternoclavicular a.
    subpubic a.
    substernal a.
    superior a.
    a. suture technique
    talocalcaneal a.
    tip a.
    Topinard facial a.
    tracheal bifurcation a.
    venous a.
    y a.

angled blade plate fixation
Anglo-Saxon nomenclature
angular
    a. acceleration
    a. artery
    a. deformity
    a. incision
    a. line
    a. notch
    a. osteotomy
    a. phenolization
    a. position
    a. spine
    a. vein
angularis
angulated
    a. fracture
    a. lesion
angulation
    Andrews-type nonorthodontic normal
      crown a.
    anterior a.

    apex dorsal a.
    bracket slot a.
    built-in a.
    caudal a.
    coronal a.
    crown a.
    a. deformity
    a. fracture
    horizontal a.
    kyphotic a.
    limb length a.
    lower incisor a.
    a. motion
    a. osteotomy
    palmar a.
    plantar a.
    radius of a.
    RAO a.
    rectoanal a.
    right anterior oblique a.
    screw a.
    upper incisor a.
    valgus a.
    vertical a.
    volar a.

ANH
    acute normovolemic hemodilution
anhepatic
    a. phase
    a. stage of liver transplantation
anhydration
anhydrous facial foundation
ani (*pl. of* anus)
animation
    suspended a.
anisocoria
    postoperative a.
anisotropic
    a. rotation
    a. tissue
ankle
    a. block
    a. block anesthesia
    a. dislocation
    dorsiflexion of a.
    a. fusion
    lateral joint of a.
    a. mortise diastasis
    a. mortise fracture
    a. region
ankle-brachial
    a.-b. blood pressure ratio
    a.-b. pressure index (ABPI)
    a.-b. pressure measurement
ankyloglossia superior syndrome
ankylosing spondylitis
ankylosis
    extraarticular a.
    extracapsular a.

Ann
  A. Arbor classification
  A. Arbor classification of Hodgkin disease staging
  A. Arbor Hodgkin lymphoma (stage I, IE, II, IIE, IIIE, IIIS, IIISE, IV)
  A. Arbor (stage IE, IIE)
annexectomy
annexopexy
annular (*var. of* anular)
annuloplasty (*var. of* anuloplasty)
annulorrhaphy
annulotomy
annulus (*var. of* anulus) (*See* anulus)
ano
  fistula in a.
anociassociation
anococcygeal
  a. body
  a. ligament
anocutaneous
  a. line
  a. stimulation
anoderm
anoderm-preserving hemorrhoidectomy
anodyne
anogenital raphe
anomalad
  Pierre Robin a.
anomalous
  a. anatomy
  a. fixation
  a. innominate artery compression syndrome
  a. insertion
  a. junction of pancreatobiliary duct (AJPBD)
  a. mesenteric adhesion
  a. position
  a. rectification
  a. vertebral artery
anomaly
  Alder-Reilly a.
  a. angle
  anorectal a.
  arterial a.
  atrioventricular connection a.
  atrioventricular junction a.
  Axenfeld a.
  branchial a.
  cardiac a.

cervical a.
chest a.
Chiari a.
coloboma a.
congenital conotruncal a.
conjoined nerve-root a.
conotruncal a.
coronary artery a.
craniofacial a.
Cruveilhier-Baumgarten a.
dental a.
dentofacial a.
double-inlet ventricle a.
Duane a.
duplication a.
dysgnathic a.
Ebstein cardiac a.
eugnathic a.
facet a.
fetal cardiac a.
fetal chest a.
fetal gastrointestinal a.
fetal vascular a.
fixation a.
Freund a.
gastrointestinal a.
genetic a.
genitourinary a.
gestant a.
hand a.
heart a.
intracranial dural vascular a.
jugular bulb a.
kidney a.
Kimerle a.
Klippel-Feil a.
lacrimal angle duct a.
laryngeal a.
limb reduction a.
maxillofacial a.
megadolichovertebrobasilar a.
Michel a.
Moebius a.
Mondini a.
morning glory optic disc a.
motor a.
müllerian duct a.
nevoid a.
numerary renal a.
occipitoatlantoaxial a.
oculocephalic vascular a.
oral a.

NOTES

anomaly *(continued)*
    orthopaedic a.
    osseous a.
    Peters a.
    Poland a.
    postsurgical motor a.
    presacral a.
    pulmonary valve a.
    pulmonary venous connection a.
    pulmonary venous return a.
    renal a.
    reticulate pigmented a.
    root a.
    segmentation a.
    Shone a.
    Sprengel a.
    structural a.
    Taussig-Bing a.
    tracheobronchial a.
    Uhl a.
    umbilical cord a.
    Undritz a.
    urinary tract a.
    urogenital a.
    uterine a.
    VACTERL a.
    vaginal a.
    vascular a.
    ventricular inflow a.
    viscerobronchial cardiovascular a.
    vitelline duct a.
    a. of Zahn
anopia
anoplasty
    cutback a.
    House advancement a.
    House flap a.
    Martin a.
    a. treatment
    Y-V a.
anopsia
anorchia
anorchism
anorectal
    a. abscess
    a. angle
    a. anomaly
    a. carcinoma
    a. disorder
    a. fistula
    a. flexure
    a. foreign body
    a. function test
    a. impalement
    a. junction
    a. line
    a. malformation
    a. manometry
    a. melanoma

    a. mucosal prolapse
    a. myectomy
    a. outlet obstruction
    a. ring
    a. sepsis
    a. septum
    a. space
    a. sphincter
    a. surgery
    a. variceal bleeding
anorectoplasty
    Laird-McMahon a.
anorectovaginoplasty
anorectum
anorexigenic effect
anoscopy
anosigmoidoscopy
anosmia
anosmic
anospinal
anotia
anovesical
anovulation
    persistent a.
anoxemia
anoxia
    anoxic a.
    diffusion a.
    histotoxic a.
    stagnant a.
anoxic
    a. anoxia
    a. preconditioning phenomenon
ANP
    atrial natriuretic peptide
    autonomic nerve preservation
ansa, pl. **ansae**
    a. cervicalis
    a. cervicalis nerve
    a. cervicalis root
    Haller a.
    Vieussens a.
anserina
anserine bursa
anserinus
Anson-McVay
    A.-M. hernia repair
    A.-M. operation
ansotomy
antagonist
    alpha-adrenergic a.
    alpha-1-adrenergic a.
    alpha-2-adrenergic receptor a.
    antimuscarinic a.
    beta-receptor a.
    nonselective opioid receptor a.
antagonistic muscle
antagonize
antalgesia

antalgic medication
antebrachial
   a. fascia
   a. flexor retinaculum
   a. region
antecolic
   a. anastomosis
   a. long-loop isoperistaltic
     gastrojejunostomy
   a. position
antecubital
   a. approach
   a. arteriovenous fistula
   a. space
antegrade
   a. approach
   a. catheterization
   a. continence enema (ACE)
   a. continence enema procedure
   a. double balloon-double wire
     technique
   a. method
   a. nailing
   a. puncture
   a. transcystic sphincterotomy
antegrade/retrograde cardioplegia
  technique
antemortem clot
antenatal dislocation
antenna procedure
antepartum hemorrhage
anteposition
anteprostate
anterior
   a. abdominal injury
   a. abdominal wall
   a. and posterior (A & P)
   a. acromioplasty
   a. acromioplasty approach
   a. angulation
   a. angulation angle
   a. antebrachial region
   a. aortic wall
   a. apical (AA)
   a. aspiration
   a. auricular artery
   a. auricular groove
   a. auricular muscle
   a. auricular nerve
   a. axillary approach
   a. axillary fold
   a. axillary line
   a. basal (AB)

   a. basal branch
   a. basal segment
   a. brachial region
   a. calcaneal osteotomy
   a. capsulolabral reconstruction
   a. capsulotomy
   a. carotid artery
   a. cavernous sinus syndrome
   a. cecal artery
   a. cerebral artery
   a. cervical discectomy and fusion
   a. cervical intertransverse muscle
   a. cervical spine surgery
   a. cervical surgery vocal cord
     damage
   a. cervicothoracic junction surgery
   a. chest wall syndrome
   a. choroidal artery
   a. ciliary artery
   a. circulation aneurysm
   a. circumflex humeral artery
   a. clear space
   a. clinoid process
   a. column
   a. column fracture
   a. column osteosynthesis
   a. commissure-posterior commissure
     (AC-PC)
   a. commissure-posterior commissure
     line
   a. communicating artery
   a. complete dislocation
   a. condylar canal
   a. condyloid foramen
   a. cord
   a. cord compression
   a. cornea
   a. corneal curvature
   a. corpectomy
   a. correction
   a. cortex
   a. costotransverse ligament
   a. cranial base
   a. cranial fossa
   a. cruciate ligament (ACL)
   a. cruciate ligament reconstruction
     (ACLR)
   a. cutaneous branch
   a. cutaneous nerve
   a. cyst
   a. descending artery
   a. discectomy

NOTES

anterior *(continued)*
a. displacement
a. epineurotomy
a. esophagus
a. ethmoidal nerve
a. ethmoidectomy
a. extensile approach
a. extradural clinoidectomy
a. extraperitoneal approach
a. extremity
a. facial height (AFH)
a. focal point
a. fontanelle
a. fundoplasty
a. gastropexy
a. gastrotomy
a. great vessel
a. ground bundle
a. helical rim free flap
a. hip dislocation
a. humeral circumflex artery
a. incision
a. inferior cerebellar artery
a. inferior iliac spine
a. inferior segment
a. inguinal herniorrhaphy
a. innominate osteotomy
a. innominate rotation
a. intercostal artery
a. intermuscular septum
a. internal fixation
a. internal stabilization
a. intraoccipital joint
a. knee region
a. labial artery
a. labial commissure
a. labial nerve
a. labrum periosteum shoulder arthroscopic lesion
a. limiting ring
a. lingual gland
a. lip
a. lower cervical spine surgery
a. lumbar vertebral interbody fusion
a. mediastinal artery
a. mediastinal mass
a. mediastinum
a. meningeal artery
a. metallic fixation
a. midpapillary (AM)
a. midpapillary level
a. nasal meatus
a. nephrectomy
a. oblique position
a. oblique projection
a. parietal artery
a. partial laryngectomy
a. pelvic exenteration

a. plate fixation
a. Pólya procedure
a. and posterior (A&P)
a. and posterior repair
a. primary division
a. puncture
a. quadriceps musculocutaneous flap technique
a. radicular artery
a. rectopexy
a. rectus fascia
a. rectus muscle
a. rectus sheath
a. rectus sheath wall
a. resection
a. retroperitoneal decompression
a. retroperitoneal flank approach
a. rhizotomy
a. root
a. sandwich patch technique
a. scalene muscle
a. sclerotomy
a. screw fixation
a. scrotal nerve
a. semicircular canal
a. seromyotomy
a. serratus muscle
a. sheath
a. short-segment stabilization
a. shoulder dislocation
a. spinal artery
a. spinal artery syndrome
a. spinal fixation
a. spinal fusion
a. stabilization procedure
a. sternoclavicular ligament
a. sternomastoid approach
a. superior alveolar artery
a. superior iliac spine
a. superior segment
a. supraclavicular nerve
a. surgical exposure
a. synechia formation
a. talofibular ligament rupture
a. temporal artery
a. thoracic wall
a. thoracotomy
a. tibial bursa
a. tibialis tendon
a. tibial muscle
a. tibial recurrent artery
a. tibiotalar ligament
a. transabdominal approach
a. transhepatic approach
a. translation
a. transoral approach
a. transperitoneal approach
a. transthoracic approach
a. tubercle

a. ulnar recurrent artery
a. urethra
a. uveitis
a. vaginal fornix
a. vaginal trunk
a. vertical canal
a. view
a. vitrectomy
a. wound
anterior-inferior dislocation
anterior-posterior
a.-p. compression
a.-p. fusion with SSI
anteriro cervical approach
anterocrural celiac plexus block
anterograde
a. direction
a. transseptal technique
anterolateral
a. approach
a. compression fracture
a. cordotomy
a. dislocation
a. fontanelle
a. neck
a. thalamostriate artery
a. thoracotomy
a. thoracotomy incision
a. tractotomy
anterolisthesis
anteromedial
a. arm
a. bundle
a. incision
a. retropharyngeal approach
a. thalamostriate artery
anteroposterior (AP)
a. chest x-ray
a. compression
a. correction
a. nail
a. projection
a. translation
anterosuperior external ilium movement
antevesical hernia
anthelix (*var. of* antihelix)
anthracosis
anthrone method
anthropoid pelvis
anthropometric evaluation
antiadhesion agent
antianalgesia

antiangiogenic effect
antiantibody formation
antiarrhythmic therapy
antibacterial agent
antibasement membrane
antibiotic
a. bead pouch
broad-spectrum a.
perioperative a.
postoperative a.
prophylactic a. (PA)
prophylactic intravenous a.
a. prophylaxis
systemic a.
a. therapy
topical a.
antibody
Bipolaris specific IgE, IgG a.
a. formation
fungal a.
HCV a.
human monoclonal a.
a. linkage method
monoclonal a. (MAb)
unfractionated heparin a.
anticalculous
anticholinergic medication
anticipated blood loss
anticipatory coarticulation
anticoagulant
a. effect
lupus a.
a. monitoring
oral a.
a. therapy
anticoagulation
a. monitoring
a. monitoring requirement
oral a.
prophylactic a.
systemic a.
a. therapy
anticus
antidote
antidromic stimulation
antiembolic position
antiemetic
prophylactic a.
a. prophylaxis
rescue a.
a. therapy
antiepileptic medication

NOTES

antifibrinolytic agent
antifungal
    a. agent
    a. esophageal infection
    a. prophylaxis
    a. regimen
    a. therapy
    a. treatment
antifungal-resistant opportunistic
  infection
antigen
    cancer a. 19-9 (CA19-9)
    carcinoembryonic a. (CEA)
    CTL-inducing peptide a.
    hepatitis B surface a. (HB$_s$)
    human leukocyte a. (HLA)
    human leukocyte class II DR a.
    proliferating cell nuclear a.
      (PCNA)
    serum carcinoembryonic a.
    tumor a.
antigen-extracted allogeneic bone
antigenic modulation
antiglaucoma surgery
antiglomerular
    a. basement membrane
    a. basement membrane antibody
      disease
antigravity muscle
antihelix, anthelix
antihemophilic
antihemorrhagic
antihormonal therapy
antiincontinence procedure
antiinflammatory medication
antilymphoid therapy
antimesenteric
    a. enterotomy
    a. fat pad
    a. incision
    a. side
antimetabolite
antimotility agent
antimuscarinic antagonist
antimycotic
antineoplastic agent
antinephritic
antiniad
antinial
antinion
antinociception
    a. analysis
    intrathecal a.
antinociceptive
antioxidant
antiperistaltic
    a. anastomosis
    a. operation
antiphospholipid antibody assay

antiplatelet regimen
antipyogenic
antireflux
    a. flap-valve mechanism
    a. operation
    a. procedure
    a. surgery
    a. therapy
    a. ureteral implantation technique
antirefluxing colonic conduit
antisaccade
antisense
antisialagogue
antitension line
antithrombin III (ATIII)
    a. III plasma level
antithromboembolic prophylaxis
antithrombotic
    a. activity
    a. therapy
antitragicus muscle
antitragus
antitubular basement membrane
antra (*pl. of* antrum)
antral
    a. biopsy
    a. edema
    a. exclusion
    a. irrigation
    a. membrane
    a. sphincter
    a. stenting
    a. tumor
    a. web
antrectomy
    Roux-en-Y biliary bypass with a.
antroduodenectomy
antropyloric canal
antroscopy
antrostomy
    inferior meatal a.
    intraoral a.
    nasal a.
antrotomy
antrum, pl. antra
    gastric a.
    a. of Highmore
    mastoid a.
    maxillary a.
    pyloric a.
    Willis a.
Antyllus method
anular, annular
    a. adenocarcinoma
    a. cartilage
    a. constricting lesion
    a. corneal graft operation
    a. pancreas
    a. sphincter

anuloplasty, annuloplasty
  a. band insertion
  Carpentier a.
  DeVega tricuspid valve a.
  Gerbode a.
  isolated a.
  prosthetic ring a.
  reduction a.
  tricuspid valve a.
  Wooler-type a.
anulus, annulus, pl. **anuli**
  Haller a.
  mitral valve a.
  tricuspid valve a.
anum
  per a.
anuria
anuric
anus, pl. **ani**
  artificial a.
  ectopic a.
  imperforate a.
  vaginal ectopic a.
anusitis
AO
  Arbeitsgemeinschaft für
  Osteosynthesefragen
    AO classification
    AO dynamic compression plate
    construct
    AO external fixation
    AO procedure
    AO rigid fixation
    AO spinal internal fixation
    AO technique
AOD
  aortic occlusive disease
  arterial occlusive disease
AOIVM
  angiographically occult intracranial
  vascular malformation
aorta, pl. **aortae**
  abdominal a.
  appendicular a.
  arcuate a.
  coarctation of a.
  deep articular a.
  dissection of a.
  infrarenal a.
  posterior articular a.
  proximal a.
  pseudocoarctation of a.

  recoarctation of a.
  thoracic a.
aortectomy
aortic
  a. anastomosis
  a. aneurysm
  a. aneurysmal disease
  a. aneurysmectomy
  a. aneurysm tissue
  a. arch
  a. arch disease
  a. atheromatous disease
  a. bifurcation
  a. blood pressure
  a. body
  a. body tumor
  a. clamping
  a. conduit
  a. cross-clamping
  a. cuff
  a. dicrotic notch pressure
  a. dissection
  a. foramen
  a. graft placement
  a. hiatus
  a. hypoplasia
  a. intramural hematoma
  a. knob
  a. laceration
  a. neck
  a. nipple
  a. node metastasis
  a. occlusion
  a. occlusive disease (AOD)
  a. patch
  a. perfusion
  a. pressure gradient
  a. pullback pressure
  a. reconstructive surgery
  a. regurgitation murmur
  a. ring
  a. root reconstruction
  a. root replacement
  a. root velocity waveform
  a. rupture
  a. sac
  a. stump blow-out
  a. transection
  a. valve area
  a. valve atresia
  a. valve disease
  a. valve gradient

NOTES

aortic *(continued)*
  a. valve insufficiency
  a. valve leaflet
  a. valve repair
  a. valve replacement
  a. valve resistance
  a. valve restenosis
  a. valve velocity profile
  a. valvotomy
  a. valvuloplasty
  a. wall
  a. wall deterioration
aorticorenal ganglion
aortic-pulmonic window
aortoannular ectasia
aortocaval fistula
aortocoronary
aortoduodenal fistula
aortoenteric fistula
aortoesophageal fistula
aortofemoral
  a. bypass
  a. bypass graft (AFBG)
aortogastric fistula
aortograft duodenal fistula
aortogram
  flush a.
aortoiliac
  a. aneurysm
  a. angioplasty
  a. bypass
  a. occlusive disease
aortoplasty
  patch a.
aortopulmonary
  a. fenestration
  a. window
aortorenal
  a. bypass
  a. reconstruction
  a. reimplantation
aortorrhaphy
aortosigmoid fistula
aortotomy
AP
  acute pancreatitis
  airway pressure
  anteroposterior
A&P
  anterior and posterior
  A&P projection
  A&P repair
APACHE
  acute physiology and chronic health
    evaluation
APACHE-II
  APACHE-II point
  APACHE-II score
  APACHE-II system

apatite calculus
A-P-C
  adenoidal-pharyngeal-conjunctival
APC
  adenomatous polyposis coli
apellous
aperta
Apert syndrome
aperture
  a.'s of abdomen
  inferior pelvic a.
  inferior thoracic a.
  laryngeal a.
  lateral cerebral a.
  superior pelvic a.
  superior thoracic a.
  upper thorax a.
apex, pl. **apices (A)**
  corneal a.
  a. dorsal angulation
  a. fracture
  lateral a.
Apgar score
aphakia
  extracapsular a.
aphakic correction
aphthous
  a. ulcer
  a. ulceration
aphthous-type lesion
apical
  anterior a. (AA)
  a. canal
  a. fenestration
  a. gland
  a. infection
  inferior a. (IA)
  lateral a. (LA)
  a. left ventricular puncture
  a. lordotic projection
  a. lordotic view
  a. polar nephrectomy
  a. ramification
  a. segment
  septal a. (SA)
  a. space
  a. suture
  a. transverse (AP-T)
apically
  a. repositioned flap
  a. repositioned flap in
    mucogingival surgery
apically repositioned flap
apiceotomy
apices (*pl. of* apex)
apicoectomy
apicolysis
  extrapleural a.
  Semb a.

apicoposterior segment
apicoposterius
apicostomy
apicotomy
Apley
- A. compression test
- A. maneuver
- A. sign

apnea
- induced a.
- obstructive a.
- posthyperventilation a.
- postoperative a.

apnea-induced hemoglobin desaturation
apneic
- a. arrest
- a. oxygenation
- a. threshold

apneustic
- a. breathing
- a. respiration

apocrine
- a. carcinoma
- a. gland
- a. metaplasia

APOLT
- auxiliary partial orthotopic liver transplantation
- APOLT technique

aponeurectomy
aponeurorrhaphy
aponeurosis, pl. **aponeuroses**
- abdominal a.
- Denonvilliers a.
- epicranial a.
- external oblique a.
- internal oblique a.
- Petit a.
- temporal a.
- thoracolumbar a.
- transversus abdominis a.
- triangular a.

aponeurotic
- a. abscess
- a. closure
- a. defect
- a. flap
- a. layer

aponeurotica
aponeurotomy
apophysary point

apophysial, apophyseal
- a. fracture
- a. point

apophysis, pl. **apophyses**
- iliac a.
- ring a.
- slipped vertebral a.
- temporal a.
- vertebral ring a.

apophysitis
- calcaneal a.

apoplectic coma
apoplexy
apoptosis
- pulmonary a.
- resuscitation-induced pulmonary a.
- selective lectin-triggered a.

apostaxis
apotreptic therapy
apparatus
- alimentary a.
- digestive a.
- genitourinary a.
- hyoid a.
- lacrimal a.
- temperature exchange a.
- urinary a.
- urogenital a.

appearance
- batwing a.
- beads-on-a-string a.
- beefy a.
- cobblestone a.
- coiled spring a.
- collar-bone a.
- corkscrew a.
- dewy a.
- gland a.
- granular a.
- ground-glass a.
- hobnailed a.
- honeycombed a.
- lead-pipe a.
- macroscopic a.
- mammographic a.
- meaty a.
- moth-eaten a.
- mottled a.
- nutmeg a.
- onion peel a.
- sausage-shaped a.
- signet-ring a.

NOTES

appearance *(continued)*
    speckled a.
    spoke-wheel a.
    steamy a.
    string-of-beads a.
    tigroid a.
    whorled a.
appendage
    epiploic a.
    omental a.
    testicular a.
    vermiform a.
    vesicular a.
appendectomy, appendicectomy
    auricular a.
    colonoscopic a.
    emergency a.
    emergent a.
    incidental a.
    a. incision
    interval a.
    inversion a.
    inversion-ligation a.
    laparoscopic a. (LA)
    laser-assisted a.
    McBurney a.
    negative a.
    open a. (OA)
    percutaneous a.
appendiceal
    a. abscess
    a. adenocarcinoma
    a. cancer
    a. colic
    a. CT
    a. fecalith
    a. gangrene
    a. intussusception
    a. mass
    a. opening
    a. orifice
    a. perforation
appendices *(pl. of* appendix)
appendicitis
    chronic a.
    epiploic a.
    gangrenous a.
appendicocele
appendicocystostomy
    continent cutaneous a.
    dismembered reimplanted a.
    nonplicated a.
    orthotopic a.
    plicated a.
    reversed reimplanted a.
appendicoenterostomy
appendicolithiasis
appendicolysis
appendicostomy

appendicovesicostomy
    Mitrofanoff a.
appendicular
    a. aorta
    a. artery
    a. colic
    a. muscle
    a. skeleton
    a. vein
appendix, pl. **appendices**
    cecal a.
    ensiform a.
    epiploic a.
    a. mucocele
    pelvic a.
    smoldering a.
    vermiform a.
apperceptive mass
applanation
    a. pressure
    tension by a.
    a. tonometry
apple
    Adam's a.
apple-core lesion
appliance modification
application
    arch bar a.
    cast a.
    clip a.
    cold a.
    force a.
    frame a.
    heat a.
    ice a.
    interpleural a.
    Kumar a.
    laparoscopic clip a.
    paraspinal rod a.
    pilot a.
    topical iodine a.
    traction a.
    transverse fixator a.
Appolito
    A. operation
    A. suture technique
apponensplasty
appose
apposition
    stent a.
    a. suture technique
approach
    Abbott-Carpenter posterior a.
    Abbott knee a.
    abdominal a.
    acetabular extensile a.
    acromiothoracic a.
    adaptational a.
    Adson anterior transperitoneal a.

aggressive surgical a.
Alken a.
alternative surgical a.
anesthetic a.
antecubital a.
antegrade a.
anterior acromioplasty a.
anterior axillary a.
anterior extensile a.
anterior extraperitoneal a.
anterior retroperitoneal flank a.
anterior sternomastoid a.
anterior transabdominal a.
anterior transhepatic a.
anterior transoral a.
anterior transperitoneal a.
anterior transthoracic a.
anteriro cervical a.
anterolateral a.
anteromedial retropharyngeal a.
Atkin a.
axillary a.
Bailey-Badgley anterior cervical a.
Banks-Laufman a.
basal subfrontal a.
Bennett posterior shoulder a.
Berger-Bookwalter posterior a.
Berke a.
bilateral ilioinguinal a.
bilateral sacroiliac a.
Bosworth a.
Boyd a.
Boyd-Sisk a.
brachial artery a.
Brackett-Osgood posterior a.
Brodsky-Tullos-Gartsman a.
Broomhead medial a.
Brown knee a.
Brown lateral a.
Bruner a.
Bruser knee a.
Bruser lateral a.
Bryan-Morrey elbow a.
Bryan-Morrey extensive posterior a.
buccopharyngeal a.
buttonhole a.
Caldwell-Luc a.
Callahan a.
Campbell posterior shoulder a.
Campbell posterolateral a.
Carnesale acetabular extensile a.
Carnesale hip a.

case-by-case a.
Cave hip a.
Cave knee a.
central a.
cerebellopontine angle a.
cervical a.
cervicothoracic a.
closed a.
Cloward cervical disc a.
cochleovestibular a.
Codman saber-cut shoulder a.
Colonna-Ralston ankle a.
Colonna-Ralston medial a.
combined anterior and posterior a.
combined laparoscopic and
  thoracoscopic a.
combined low cervical and
  transthoracic a.
combined neurosurgical-external
  sinus a.
combined presigmoid-
  transtransversarium intradural a.
combined transsylvian and middle
  fossa a.
consortial a.
Coonse-Adams knee a.
costotransversectomy a.
Cubbins shoulder a.
curved a.
deltoid-splitting shoulder a.
deltopectoral a.
Dickinson a.
distal interphalangeal joint a.
dorsal finger a.
dorsal midline a.
dorsalward a.
dorsolateral a.
dorsomedial a.
dorsoplantar a.
dorsoradial a.
dorsorostral a.
dorsoulnar a.
double-doughnut a.
double-seton modified surgical a.
Duran a.
DuVries a.
elbow a.
Endius a.
endoscopic a.
endovascular a.
ethmoidal a.
extended iliofemoral a.

NOTES

approach *(continued)*
    extended subfrontal a.
    extensive a.
    extensive posterior a.
    extrabursal a.
    extracapsular a.
    extracavitary a.
    extralaryngeal a.
    extraperitoneal a.
    extrapharyngeal a.
    extrapleural a.
    extravesical Lich a.
    extreme lateral transcondylar a.
    Fahey a.
    far lateral inferior suboccipital a.
    fascial sling a.
    femoral artery a.
    Fernandez extensile anterior a.
    flank a.
    foraminal a.
    fornix a.
    Fowler-Philip a.
    frontal cortical a.
    frontotemporal a.
    gasless laparoscopic a.
    Gatellier-Chastang ankle a.
    Gatellier-Chastang posterolateral a.
    genetic a.
    Gibson a.
    Gordon a.
    Guleke-Stookey a.
    Hardinge lateral a.
    Harmon cervical a.
    Harmon modified posterolateral a.
    Harmon shoulder a.
    Harris anterolateral a.
    Harris lateral a.
    Hay lateral a.
    Henderson posterolateral a.
    Henderson posteromedial a.
    Henry anterior strap a.
    Henry anterolateral a.
    Henry extensile a.
    Henry posterior interosseous
     nerve a.
    Henry radial a.
    high cervical anterior
     retropharyngeal a.
    Hoffmann a.
    Hoppenfeld-Deboer a.
    Howorth a.
    humeral a.
    idiographic a.
    Iliff a.
    iliofemoral a.
    ilioinguinal acetabular a.
    immunocytochemical a.
    inferior extradural a.

    inferior-lateral endonasal
     transsphenoidal a.
    inferior transvermian a.
    infralabyrinthine a.
    inframammary a.
    infratemporal fossa a.
    infratentorial supracerebellar a.
    inguinal a.
    interfascial a.
    interforniceal a.
    interhemispheric a.
    interscalene a.
    intracapsular a.
    intradural a.
    intranasal a.
    intrapleural a.
    intratentorial supracerebellar a.
    inverted-U a.
    Ivor Lewis a.
    Japanese a.
    keyhole a.
    Kikuchi-MacNap-Moreau a.
    Kocher curved L a.
    Kocher-Gibson posterolateral a.
    Kocher-Langenbeck a.
    Kocher lateral J a.
    Koenig-Schaefer medial a.
    Kraske parasacral a.
    Kugel a.
    labioglossomandibular a.
    labiomandibular a.
    laparoscopic common bile duct
     exploration transcystic a.
    lateral deltoid splitting a.
    lateral extracavitary a.
    lateral Gatellier-Chastang a.
    lateral J a.
    lateral Kocher a.
    Lazepen-Gamidov anteromedial a.
    Leslie-Ryan anterior axillary a.
    lesser sac a.
    Letournel-Judet a.
    limbal a.
    lingual a.
    Lortat-Jacob a.
    low cervical a.
    Ludloff medial a.
    lumbar a.
    Mason a.
    Mayo a.
    McConnell extensile a.
    McConnell median and ulnar
     nerve a.
    McFarland-Osborne lateral a.
    McLaughlin a.
    McWhorter posterior shoulder a.
    Mears-Rubash a.
    medial extradural a.
    medial parapatellar capsular a.

midlateral a.
midline medial a.
midline spinal a.
minimally invasive a.
Minkoff-Jaffe-Menendez posterior a.
Mize-Bucholz-Grogen a.
modified surgical a.
Molesworth-Campbell elbow a.
Moore posterior a.
multidisciplinary a.
multiple-stage a.
neurosurgical a.
nonoperative a.
occipitocervical a.
Ollier arthrodesis a.
Ollier lateral a.
open laparoscopic a.
operative a.
orbitozygomatic temporopolar a.
oropharyngeal a.
Osborne posterior a.
osteoplastic flap a.
otomicrosurgical transtemporal a.
palatal a.
palmar a.
paramedian a.
pararectus a.
parasacral a.
paraspinal a.
parietooccipital a.
patella turndown a.
percutaneous transhepatic a.
peroral a.
Perry extensile anterior a.
petrosal a.
Pfannenstiel transverse a.
Phemister medial a.
piggyback a.
plantar a.
Pogrund lateral a.
portal vein a.
posterior costotransversectomy a.
posterior extraperitoneal a.
posterior inverted-U a.
posterior laparoscopic a.
posterior lumbar a.
posterior midline a.
posterior occipitocervical a.
posterior radial a.
posterior shoulder a.
posterior transolecranon a.
posterolateral a.

posteromedial a.
preperitoneal a.
presigmoid-transtransversarium
  intradural a.
proprioceptive neuromuscular
  facilitation a.
proximal interphalangeal joint a.
pterional a.
pulp a.
Putti posterior a.
rapid-volume a.
Redman a.
regressive-reconstructive a.
Reinert acetabular extensile a.
retrocrural a.
retrograde endoscopic a.
retrograde femoral a.
retrolabyrinthine presigmoid a.
retroperitoneal a.
retropharyngeal a.
retrosigmoid a.
retrosternal a.
rhinoseptal a.
Risdon a.
Roberts a.
robotic a.
Roos a.
Rowe posterior shoulder a.
Royle posterior a.
saber-cut a.
sacral-foraminal a.
sacroiliac a.
sacroperineal a.
screw-plate a.
sensorimotor stimulation a.
skull base a.
Smith-Petersen a.
Smith-Petersen-Cave-Van Gorder
  anterolateral a.
Smith-Robinson cervical disc a.
somatic gene-transfer a.
Somerville anterior a.
Southwick-Robinson anterior
  cervical a.
Spetzler anterior transoral a.
split-heel a.
split-patellar a.
stabilization a.
standard open a.
sternum-splitting a.
subchoroidal a.
subclavicular a.

NOTES

approach *(continued)*
  subfrontal a.
  subfrontal-transbasal a.
  sublabial midline rhinoseptal a.
  suboccipital-subtemporal a.
  suboccipital-transmeatal a.
  subtemporal-intradural a.
  superior-intradural a.
  supine-oblique a.
  supracerebellar a.
  supraclavicular a.
  supraduodenal a.
  supraorbital-pterional a.
  supratentorial a.
  surgical a.
  suspended-pedicle a.
  Swedish a.
  sylvian a.
  takedown abdominal a.
  Taylor a.
  therapeutic a.
  Thompson anterolateral a.
  Thompson anteromedial a.
  Thompson posterior radial a.
  thoracic a.
  thoracoabdominal extrapleural a.
  thoracoabdominal intrapleural a.
  thoracolumbar retroperitoneal a.
  thoracolumbar transdiaphragmatic a.
  thoracoscopic a.
  thoracotomy a.
  thumb metacarpophalangeal joint a.
  tongue-splitting transmandibular a.
  transabdominal a.
  transacromial a.
  transanal a.
  transantral a.
  transantral ethmoidal a.
  transaxillary a.
  transbrachioradialis a.
  transcallosal transventricular a.
  transcanine a.
  transcavernous transpetrous apex a.
  transcerebellar hemispheric a.
  transcervical a.
  transclavicular a.
  transcoccygeal a.
  transcochlear a.
  transcortical transventricular a.
  transcranial frontal-temporal-
    orbital a.
  transcranial-supraorbital a.
  transcubital a.
  transcystic a.
  transdiaphragmatic a.
  transduodenal a.
  transfibular a.
  transfrontal a.
  transgluteal a.

  transhepatic a.
  transhiatal esophagectomy a.
  translabyrinthine and suboccipital a.
  transmandibular-glossopharyngeal a.
  transmastoid a.
  transmeatal a.
  transmural a.
  transolecranon a.
  transoral a.
  transpalatal a.
  transpapillary a.
  transpedicular a.
  transperitoneal a.
  transpleural a.
  transradial a.
  transrectal a.
  transseptal a.
  transsinus a.
  transsphenoidal a.
  transsphincteric a.
  transsternal a.
  transsylvian a.
  transtentorial a.
  transthoracic a.
  transtorcular a.
  transtrochanteric a.
  transvaginal a.
  transvenous a.
  transventricular a.
  transverse a.
  transxiphoid a.
  trapdoor a.
  triradiate acetabular extensile a.
  triradiate transtrochanteric a.
  unilateral sacroiliac a.
  vaginal wall a.
  volar finger a.
  volar midline a.
  volar radial a.
  volar ulnar a.
  volarward a.
  Wadsworth elbow a.
  Wadsworth posterolateral a.
  Wagoner posterior a.
  Watson-Jones anterior a.
  Watson-Jones lateral a.
  Wiltberger anterior cervical a.
  Wiltse-Spencer paraspinal a.
  Yee posterior shoulder a.
  zig-zag a.
  Z-plasty a.
approximate
  a. entropy
  a. lethal concentration
approximation
  Friedewald a.
  skin a.
  successive a.
  a. suture technique

tissue a.
vocal fold a.
wound a.

APR
abdominoperineal resection
anatomic porous replacement
APR cement fixation

aproctia

apron
abdominal a.
fatty a.
a. flap
a. flap incision
a. skin incision

APRV
airway pressure release ventilation

APSA
American Pediatric Surgical Association

AP-T
apical transverse

aquapuncture

aquatic stabilization program

aqueduct
Cotunnius a.
sylvian a.
a. veil

aqueductal intubation

aqueductus

aqueous
a. extract
a. exudation
a. humor
a. solution
a. vein

arachnoid
a. cyst
a. granulation
a. hemorrhage
a. membrane
a. retrocerebellar pouch
a. space
a. villus

arachnoiditis
adhesive a.

Araki-Sako technique

Arantius
A. body
canal of A.
A. duct
A. ligament
plate of A.

Arbeitsgemeinschaft für Osteosynthesefragen (AO)

Arbor
Ann A. (stage IE, IIE)

arborization
a. block
pattern a.
pulmonary a.

Arbuthnot Lane disease

arc
bregmatolambdoid a.
flexion-extension a.
mobile a.
nasobregmatic a.
nasooccipital a.
Riolan a.

arcade
gastroepiploic a.
intestinal arterial a.
pancreaticoduodenal arterial a.
Riolan a.

arch
abdominothoracic a.
aortic a.
arterial a.
axillary a.
a. bar application
crural a.
deep crural a.
deep palmar a.
double aortic a.
expansion of the a.
extramedullary alignment a.
femoral a.
a. fracture
hemal a.
iliopectineal a.
interrupted aortic a.
jugular venous a.
Langer a.
neural a.
posterior a.
prepancreatic a.
pubic a.
Simon expansion a.
superciliary a.
superficial palmar a.
supraorbital a.
tendinous a.
transverse aponeurotic a.
Treitz a.
vertebral a.

NOTES

arch *(continued)*
    wire a.
    zygomatic a.
arch-and-slouch position
archenteronoma
archicerebellum
architectural pattern
architecture
    lesion a.
    tissue a.
arch-loop-whorl
arciform vein of kidney
arctation
arcuata
arcuate
    a. aorta
    a. artery
    a. eminence
    a. incision
    a. line
    a. nerve fiber bundle
    a. pubic ligament
    a. suture technique
    a. transverse keratotomy
    a. vein
    a. zone
arcuation
arcuatum
arcus
    corneal a.
ARDS
    acute respiratory distress syndrome
    adult respiratory distress syndrome
area
    anastomotic a.
    aortic valve a.
    articulation a.
    bare a.
    body surface a. (BSA)
    cortical a.
    cribriform a.
    cross-sectional a.
    crural a.
    denture foundation a.
    end-diastolic cross-sectional a.
      (EDA)
    end-systolic a. (ESA)
    end-systolic cross-sectional a.
    fusion a.
    gastric a.
    graft a.
    jejunal puncture a.
    Kiesselbach a.
    Killian-Jamieson a.
    Laimer a.
    laser controlled a.
    left ventricular end-diastolic a.
      (LVEDa)

    left ventricular end-systolic a.
      (LVESa)
    Little a.
    mitral valve a.
    Panum fusion a.
    paraglottic a.
    periaqueductal gray a.
    pericolostomy a.
    pressure a.
    pressure-sensitive a.
    proliferation a.
    pulmonary valve a.
    right crural a.
    skip a.
    Stroud pectinated a.
    tissue-bearing a.
    total body surface a. (TBSA)
    total graft a.
    tricuspid valve a.
    a. under curve (AUC)
    valve orifice a.
    visual association a.
    voluntary a.
area-length method
areflexia
    detrusor a.
areola, pl. **areolae**
areolar
    a. complex
    a. connective tissue
    a. gland
    a. incision
    a. mastopexy
argatroban
argon
    a. beam coagulation
    a. beam plasma coagulation
      (ABPC)
    a. laser endophotocoagulation
    a. laser iridectomy
    a. laser photocoagulation
    a. laser therapy
    a. laser trabeculopexy
    a. laser trabeculoplasty
Argyll-Robertson
    A.-R. operation
    A.-R. suture technique
argyrophilic
    a. nucleolar organizer region
    a. nucleolar organizer region
      staining
Aria coronary bypass
Aries-Pitanguy
    A.-P. breast reduction
    A.-P. mammaplasty
    A.-P. operation
Arion operation
aristotelian method

Arlt
>A. epicanthus repair
>A. eyelid repair
>A. line
>A. operation
>A. suture technique

Arlt-Jaesche
>A.-J. excision
>A.-J. operation

arm
>anteromedial a.
>batwing a.
>brawny a.
>dissected tissue a.
>endosteal implant a.
>a. flap
>a. position
>posterior a.

Armaly-Drance technique
armamentarium
>endodontic a.

arm-extension position
Armistead
>A. technique
>A. ulnar lengthening operation

Armstrong acromionectomy
Arneth classification
Arnold
>A. body
>A. bundle
>A. canal
>A. ganglion
>A. nerve
>A. tract

Arnold-Chiari
>A.-C. deformity
>A.-C. malformation
>A.-C. syndrome

Aronson-Prager technique
around the clock (ATC)
around-the-clock
>a.-t.-c. dosing
>a.-t.-c. oral maintenance bronchodilator therapy

arrangement
>lesion a.

array
>epidural electrode a.
>subdural electrode a.

arrector, pl. **arrectores**
>arrectores pilorum
>a. pilus

arrest
>apneic a.
>cardiac a.
>circulatory a.
>deep hypothermic circulatory a. (DHCA)
>hypothermic circulatory a.
>hypothermic hypokalemic cardioplegic a. (HHCA)
>imminent cardiac a.
>profoundly hypothermic circulatory a. (PHCA)
>secondary a.
>traumatic cardiac a.
>vagal a.

arrested-heart
>a.-h. revascularization
>a.-h. revascularization technique

arrhenoblastoma
Arrhigi
>point of A.

arrhythmia
>atrial a.
>exercise-induced a.
>supraventricular a.

arrhythmogenic
Arrowhead operation
Arroyo
>A. cataract extraction
>A. dacryostomy
>A. keratoplasty
>A. operation
>A. tenotomy

Arruga
>A. cataract extraction
>A. dacryostomy
>A. keratoplasty
>A. operation
>A. tenotomy

Arruga-Berens operation
arsenal
>therapeutic a.

arteria, pl. **arteriae**
arterial
>a. adaptation
>a. anastomosis
>a. aneurysm
>a. angioma
>a. anomaly
>a. arch
>a. bleeding
>a. bleeding site

NOTES

arterial *(continued)*
a. blood
a. blood collection
a. blood gas
a. blood pressure
a. branch
a. cannulation
a. cannulation anesthetic technique
a. carbon dioxide
a. carbon dioxide pressure
a. catheterization
a. cerebral circle
a. chemoembolization
a. circulation
CT with hepatic a. (CTHA)
a. decortication
a. dicrotic notch pressure
a. disorder
a. embolectomy
a. embolization
a. entry site
a. flap
a. groove
a. hemorrhage
a. hypertension
a. inflow
a. injury
a. lactate level
a. mean line
a. occlusion
a. occlusive disease (AOD)
a. oxygen desaturation
a. oxygen saturation (SaO_2)
a. oxyhemoglobin saturation (SpO_2)
a. partial pressure
a. partial pressure of CO_2
a. reconstructive procedure
a. reconstructive surgery
a. revascularization
a. ring
a. stenosis
a. supply
a. switch operation
a. switch procedure
a. system
a. thrombosis
a. transfusion
umbilical a. (UA)
a. vein
a. wall dissection
a. web
a. wedge
arterial-arterial fistula
arterial-enteric fistula
arterialization
arterialized flap
arterial-portal fistula
arterial-selective intravenous vasodilator
arteriectomy

arteriobiliary fistula
arteriocapillary
arteriococcygeal gland
arteriogram
arteriographic presence
arteriography
arteriola, pl. **arteriolae**
arteriolar attenuation
arteriole
afferent glomerular a.
capillary a.
copper-wire a.
efferent glomerular a.
silver-wire a.
arteriolith
arteriolovenular anastomosis
arterionephrosclerosis
arterioplasty
arterioportal fistula
arterioportobiliary fistula
arteriorrhaphy
arteriorrhexis
arteriosa
arteriosclerosis obliterans (ASO)
arteriosclerotic
a. aneurysm
a. gangrene
a. kidney
arteriosinusoidal penile fistula
arteriostenosis
arteriosum
arteriosus
ductus a.
patent ductus a. (PDA)
arteriotomy
brachial a.
end-to-side a.
arteriovenosa
arteriovenous (A-V, AV)
a. anastomosis
a. aneurysm
a. dialysis
a. fistula (AVF)
a. hemofiltration
a. malformation (AVM)
a. subclavian fistula
arteritis
giant cell a.
inflammatory a.
Takayasu a.
temporal a.
artery
abdominal aortic a.
aberrant obturator a.
accessory obturator a.
acetabular a.
acromial a.
acromiothoracic a.
alveolar a.

A

anal canal a.
angular a.
anomalous vertebral a.
anterior auricular a.
anterior carotid a.
anterior cecal a.
anterior cerebral a.
anterior choroidal a.
anterior ciliary a.
anterior circumflex humeral a.
anterior communicating a.
anterior descending a.
anterior humeral circumflex a.
anterior inferior cerebellar a.
anterior intercostal a.
anterior labial a.
anterior mediastinal a.
anterior meningeal a.
anterior parietal a.
anterior radicular a.
anterior spinal a.
anterior superior alveolar a.
anterior temporal a.
anterior tibial recurrent a.
anterior ulnar recurrent a.
anterolateral thalamostriate a.
anteromedial thalamostriate a.
appendicular a.
arcuate a.
ascending cervical a.
ascending pharyngeal a.
atherosclerotic carotid a.
axillary a.
basilar a.
blood supply a.
brachial a.
brachiocephalic trunk a.
bronchial a.
buccal a.
buccinator a.
calcaneal a.
calcareous a.
calcarine a.
callosomarginal a.
caroticotympanic a.
carpal a.
caudal pancreatic a.
cecal a.
celiac a.
celiacomesenteric a.
central retinal a.
central sulcal a.

cerebellar a.
cerebral a.
cervicovaginal a.
choroidal a.
ciliary a.
cilioretinal a.
circumflex femoral a.
circumflex humeral a.
circumflex iliac a.
circumflex scapular a.
coarctation of pulmonary a.
coeliac a.
colic a.
collateral digital a.
colli a.
common femoral a. (CFA)
common femoral artery-superficial
  femoral a. (CFA-SFA)
common hepatic a.
common iliac a.
common interosseous a.
common palmar digital a.
common peroneal a.
common plantar digital a.
communicating a.
companion a.
copper-wire a.
cortical a.
costocervical a.
cricothyroid a.
cystic a.
deep auricular a.
deep brachial a.
deep cervical a.
deep circumflex inguinal a.
deep epigastric a.
deep femoral a.
deep profunda brachial a.
deep temporal a.
deferential a.
descending genicular a.
descending palatine a.
descending scapular a.
digital collateral a.
diploic a.
D-loop transposition of great a.
dolichoectatic a.
dorsal digital a.
dorsal interosseous a.
dorsal pancreatic a.
dorsal scapular a.
dorsal thoracic a.

NOTES

artery *(continued)*
   a. ectasia
   ectatic carotid a.
   endometrial spiral a.
   epigastric a.
   esophageal a.
   ethmoidal a.
   external acoustic meatus a.
   external carotid a. (ECA)
   external iliac a.
   external mammary a.
   external maxillary a.
   external pudendal a.
   external spermatic a.
   extradural vertebral a.
   facial a.
   femoral a.
   first metacarpal a.
   frontal a.
   gastric a.
   gastroduodenal a. (GDA)
   gastroepiploic a.
   gastroomental a.
   genicular a.
   gingival a.
   gonadal a.
   great anastomotic a.
   greater palatine a.
   great pancreatic a.
   great radicular a.
   great superior pancreatic a.
   hepatic a.
   Huebner recurrent a.
   humeral a.
   hyaloid a.
   hypogastric a.
   hypoglossal a.
   hypophysial a.
   ileal a.
   ileocolic a.
   iliac a.
   iliofemoral flap a.
   iliolumbar a.
   inferior alveolar a.
   inferior carotid a.
   inferior cerebral a.
   inferior epigastric a. (IEA)
   inferior gluteal a.
   inferior hemorrhoidal a.
   inferior hypophysial a.
   inferior internal parietal a.
   inferior labial a.
   inferior laryngeal a.
   inferior lateral genicular a.
   inferior medial genicular a.
   inferior mesenteric a.
   inferior pancreatic a.
   inferior pancreaticoduodenal a.
   inferior phrenic a.

inferior rectal a.
inferior suprarenal a.
inferior thoracic a.
inferior thyroid a.
inferior ulnar collateral a.
inferior vesical a.
infragenicular popliteal a. (IGPA)
infraorbital a.
infrascapular a.
innominate a.
insular a.
intercostal a.
interlobular a.
intermediate temporal a.
internal auditory a.
internal carotid a. (ICA)
internal iliac a.
internal mammary a. (IMA)
internal maxillary a.
internal pudendal a.
internal rectal a.
internal spermatic a.
internal thoracic a.
intestinal a.
intramural a.
a. island flap
jejunal a.
labyrinthine a.
lacrimal a.
left carotid a. (LCA)
left coronary a. (LCA)
left vertebral a.
lenticulostriate a.
lesser palatine a.
lienal a.
a. ligation
lingual a.
long thoracic a.
lower thyroid a.
lowest lumbar a.
lowest thyroid a.
lumbar a.
major a.
marginal a.
masseteric a.
mediastinal a.
medium-sized a.
medullary spinal a.
mental a.
mesenteric a.
metacarpal a.
metatarsal a.
middle cerebral a. (MCA)
muscular a.
musculophrenic a.
mylohyoid a.
Neubauer a.
nutrient a.
obturator a.

A

occipital a.
a. occlusion
ophthalmic a.
orbitofrontal a.
ovarian a.
palmar interosseous a.
palpebral a.
pancreatic a.
pancreaticoduodenal a.
a. of pancreatic tail
parathyroid a.
parietal a.
parietooccipital a.
pericallosal a.
pericardiacophrenic a.
perineal a.
peroneal a.
persistent sciatic a. (PSA)
petrosal a.
pontine a.
popliteal a.
postcentral sulcal a.
posterior alveolar a.
posterior auricular a.
posterior cecal a.
posterior cerebral a.
posterior choroidal a.
posterior circumflex humeral a.
posterior communicating a.
posterior humeral circumflex a.
posterior inferior cerebellar a.
posterior interosseous a.
posterior labial a.
posterior mediastinal a.
posterior meningeal a.
posterior pancreaticoduodenal a.
posterior parietal a.
posterior radicular a.
posterior spinal a.
posterior superior alveolar a.
posterior temporal a.
posterior tibial recurrent a.
posterior ulnar recurrent a.
posterolateral central a.
posteromedial central a.
precentral sulcal a.
precuneal a.
pre-rolandic a.
princeps cervicis a.
princeps pollicis a.
profunda brachii a.
profunda cervicalis a.

proper hepatic a.
proper palmar digital a.
proper plantar digital a.
pterygoid a.
pubic a.
pulmonary a. (PA)
pyloric a.
radial collateral a.
radial index a.
radial recurrent a.
radicular a.
a. reconstruction
recurrent interosseous a.
recurrent radial a.
recurrent ulnar a.
renal a.
retroduodenal a.
retroesophageal a.
retrograde vascularization of
  superior mesenteric a.
right colic a.
right femoral a.
right middle suprarenal a.
right obturator a.
right replaced hepatic a.
right subclavian a.
right testicular a.
rolandic a.
scrotal a.
second lumbar a.
sheathed a.
short central a.
short gastric a.
sigmoid a.
sphenopalatine a.
spinal a.
splenic a. (SA)
a. stenosis
sternal a.
sternocleidomastoid a.
sternomastoid a.
striate a.
stylomastoid a.
subclavian a.
subcostal a.
sublingual a.
submental a.
subscapular a.
sulcal a.
superficial brachial a.
superficial cervical a.
superficial circumflex iliac a.

NOTES

artery *(continued)*
    superficial epigastric a.
    superficial external pudendal a.
    superficial palmar a.
    superficial perineal a.
    superficial temporal a.
    superficial temporal artery/middle
      cerebral a. (STA-MCA)
    superficial temporalis a.
    superficial volar a.
    superior alveolar a.
    superior cerebellar a.
    superior epigastric a.
    superior gluteal a.
    superior hemorrhoidal a.
    superior hypophysial a.
    superior intercostal a.
    superior internal parietal a.
    superior labial a.
    superior lateral genicular a.
    superior medial genicular a.
    superior mesenteric a. (SMA)
    superior pancreaticoduodenal a.
    superior phrenic a.
    superior rectal a.
    superior suprarenal a.
    superior thoracic a.
    superior thyroid a.
    superior ulnar collateral a.
    superior vesical a.
    supraduodenal a.
    supragenicular popliteal a. (SGPA)
    supraorbital a.
    suprascapular a.
    supratrochlear a.
    supreme intercostal a.
    sural a.
    temporal a.
    testicular a.
    thoracoacromial a.
    thoracodorsal a.
    thymic a.
    thyrocervical a.
    tortuous intercostal a.
    transverse cervical a.
    transverse facial a.
    transverse pancreatic a.
    transverse scapular a.
    ulnar a.
    umbilical a.
    urethral a.
    uterine a.
    vaginal a.
    vertebral a.
    volar interosseous a.
    Wilkie a.
    a. of Willis
    zygomaticofacial a.
    zygomaticoorbital a.

arthralgia
    asymmetrical a.
    recurrent a.
arthrifluent abscess
arthritis, pl. **arthritides**
    gonococcal a.
    A. Helplessness Index (AHI)
    hemophilic a.
    juvenile rheumatoid a.
    Lyme a.
    pisotriquetral a.
    psoriatic a.
    pyogenic a.
    reactive a.
    rheumatoid a.
    scaphotrapezial trapezoid a.
    septic a.
    tuberculous a.
arthrocele
arthrodesis
    Adkins technique spinal a.
    atlantoaxial a.
    Batchelor-Brown extraarticular
     subtalar a.
    beak modification with triple a.
    Brockman-Nissen wrist a.
    Charnley compression a.
    compression a.
    excisional a.
    extension injury posterior
     atlantoaxial a.
    extraarticular a.
    resection a.
    tarsometatarsal truncated-wedge a.
    tibiocalcaneal a.
    tibiotalocalcaneal a.
    triple a.
    truncated tarsometatarsal wedge a.
    truncated-wedge a.
arthrodial
    a. articulation
    a. cartilage
    a. joint
**arthrographic capsular distention and
rupture technique**
arthrogryposis multiplex congenita
arthrology
arthropathy
    cuff tear a.
    hemophilic a.
    hydroxyapatite a.
    osteopulmonary a.
    rotator cuff a.
arthrophyte
arthroplasty
    abrasion a.
    acetabular cup a.
    Albright-Chase a.
    anconeus a.

Ashworth hand a.
Ashworth implant a.
Aufranc cup a.
Austin-Moore a.
autogenous interpositional
  shoulder a.
Bechtol a.
bipolar hip a.
Bryan a.
Campbell interpositional a.
Campbell resection a.
capitellocondylar total elbow a.
capsular interposition a.
carpometacarpal a.
Carroll a.
cemented total hip a.
cementless total hip a.
Charnley total hip a.
Clayton forefoot a.
Colonna trochanteric a.
condylar implant a.
constrained ankle a.
constrained shoulder a.
convex condylar implant a.
Coonrad-Morrey total elbow a.
Coonrad total elbow a.
Cracchiolo forefoot a.
Crawford-Adams cup a.
Cubbins a.
cuff tear a.
débridement a.
Dewar-Barrington a.
distraction a.
duToit-Roux a.
Eaton implant a.
Eaton volar plate a.
Eden-Hybbinette a.
elbow a.
Ewald capitellocondylar total
  elbow a.
Ewald-Walker kinematic knee a.
excision a.
fascial a.
finger joint a.
forefoot a.
Girdlestone resection a.
Gristina-Webb total shoulder a.
Gunston a.
Harrington total hip a.
Head hip a.
Helal flap a.
hemiresection interposition a.

hip a.
Hungerford-Krackow-Kenna knee a.
ICLH double-cup a.
implant a.
Inglis triaxial total elbow a.
Insall-Burstein-Freeman knee a.
interpositional elbow a.
interpositional shoulder a.
intracapsular temporomandibular
  joint a.
Jones resection a.
Keller resection a.
knee a.
Kocher-McFarland hip a.
Larmon forefoot a.
Mann-DuVries a.
Matchett-Brown hip a.
Mayo modified total elbow a.
Mayo resection a.
metacarpophalangeal joint a.
Meuli a.
Millender a.
Miller-Galante knee a.
modified mold and surface
  replacement a.
mold acetabular a.
monospherical total shoulder a.
Morrey-Bryan total elbow a.
Mould a.
Mueller hip a.
Mumford-Gurd a.
NEB hip a.
Neer unconstrained shoulder a.
Niebauer trapeziometacarpal a.
noncemented total hip a.
Post total shoulder a.
prosthetic a.
Putti-Platt a.
resection a.
revision hip a.
rotator cuff tear a.
Schlein elbow a.
semiconstrained total elbow a.
shoulder a.
Silastic lunate a.
silicone implant a.
silicone rubber a.
silicone wrist a.
Smith-Petersen cup a.
Speed a.
Stanmore shoulder a.
Steffee thumb a.

NOTES

arthroplasty *(continued)*
  Suave-Kapandji a.
  surface replacement hip a.
  Swanson Convex condylar a.
  Swanson radial head implant a.
  Swanson silicone wrist a.
  tendon interposition a.
  total ankle a.
  total articular replacement a.
  total articular resurfacing a.
  total elbow a.
  total hip a.
  total knee a.
  total patellofemoral joint a.
  total shoulder a.
  total wrist a.
  trapeziometacarpal silicone a.
  triaxial total elbow a.
  Tupper a.
  ulnar hemiresection interposition a.
  unconstrained shoulder a.
  unicompartmental knee a.
  Vaino MP a.
  volar plate a.
  Volz a.
  Wilson-McKeever a.

arthroscopic
  a. abrasion chondroplasty
  a. anterior cruciate ligament
    reconstruction (AACLR)
  a. augmentation
  a. entry portal
  a. examination
  a. laser surgery
  a. meniscectomy
  a. microdiscectomy
  a. synovectomy

arthroscopy
  a. and débridement
  diagnostic and operative a.
  laser a.
  midcarpal a.
  needle a.
  operative a.
  radiocarpal a.
  Ringer a.
  total knee a. (TKA)

arthrosia

arthrotomy
  diagnostic arthroscopy, operative
    arthroscopy, and possible
    operative a.
  Magnuson-Stack shoulder a.
  operative a.
  parapatellar a.

articular
  a. bone loss
  a. branch
  a. capsule

  a. cartilage
  a. cartilage lesion
  a. cavity
  a. crescent
  a. crest
  a. facet
  a. fragment
  a. manifestation
  a. mass separation fracture
  a. pillar fracture
  a. process
  a. recurrent nerve
  a. surface
  a. vascular circle
  a. vascular network

articulate

articulated

articulatio

articulation
  acromioclavicular a.
  a. area
  arthrodial a.
  articulator a.
  atlantoaxial a.
  atlantooccipital a.
  balanced a.
  bicondylar a.
  calcaneocuboid a.
  carpometacarpal a.
  Chopart a.
  condylar a.
  coracoclavicular a.
  coxofemoral a.
  cricothyroid a.
  a. curve
  dental a.
  deviant a.
  a. disorder
  glenohumeral a.
  humeral a.
  humeroradial a.
  humeroulnar a.
  incudomalleolar a.
  a. index
  infantile a.
  intercarpal a.
  interchondral a.
  intermetacarpal a.
  interphalangeal a.
  Lisfranc a.
  mandibular a.
  metacarpophalangeal a.
  metatarsocuneiform a.
  metatarsophalangeal a.
  patellofemoral a.
  peg-and-socket a.
  a. of pisiform bone
  place of a.
  proximal radioulnar a.

radiocapitellar a.
radiocarpal a.
radioulnar a.
sacroiliac a.
scapuloclavicular a.
secondary a.
spheroid a.
sternocostal a.
subtalar a.
superior tibial a.
talocalcaneal a.
talocalcaneonavicular a.
tarsometatarsal a.
temporomandibular joint a.
a. test
tibiofemoral a.
tibiofibular a.
triquetropisiform a.
trochoid a.
Vermont spinal fixator a.
articulator articulation
articulatory procedure
artifact
pacemaker a.
artificial
a. anus
a. classification cavity
a. endocrine pancreas
a. erection test
a. fat pad
a. fistulation
a. intravaginal insemination
a. kidney
a. method
a. nose
a. respiration
a. sphincter
a. ventilation
a. vertebral body
Arvidsson dimension-length method
arycorniculata
aryepiglottic (AE)
a. fold
a. muscle
arytenoid
a. cartilage
a. gland
a. muscle
arytenoidal
arytenoidectomy
arytenoidopexy

aryvocalis
ASA
American Society of Anesthesiologists
ASA physical status
ASA-induced gastric ulceration
ascendens
ascending
a. anterior branch
a. aortic pressure
a. cervical artery
a. colon
a. lumbar vein
a. mesocolon
a. pathway
a. pathway of pain projection
a. pharyngeal artery
a. pharyngeal plexus
a. posterior branch
a. technique
Ascher
A. glass-rod phenomenon
A. syndrome
Aschoff body
ascites
bile a.
blood-tinged a.
chyliform a.
chylous a.
cloudy a.
exudative a.
fatty a.
gelatinous a.
hemorrhagic a.
marked a.
massive a.
milky a.
mucinous a.
mucoid a.
myxedema a.
progressive a.
pseudochylous a.
recurrent a.
refractory a.
straw-colored a.
transudative a.
tumor a.
ascitic fluid
ascitogenous
ASCRS
American Society for Colon and Rectal
Surgeons

NOTES

ASCUS
> atypical squamous cell of undetermined significance

Aselli pancreas

asepsis

aseptic
> a. peritonitis
> a. surgery
> a. technique

asepticism

ASGE
> American Society for Gastrointestinal Endoscopy

Ashby differential agglutination method

Ashford retracted nipple operation

Ashhurst-Bromer ankle fracture classification

ash-leaf
> a.-l. patch
> a.-l. spot

Ashworth
> A. hand arthroplasty
> A. implant arthroplasty

ASI
> active specific immunotherapy

ASIF
> Association for the Study of Internal Fixation
> ASIF screw fixation technique

Ask-Upmark kidney

ASM
> airway smooth muscle

Asnis technique

ASO
> arteriosclerosis obliterans

aspect
> buccal a.
> dorsal a.
> inferomedial a.
> laminar cortex posterior a.
> medial a.
> medicolegal a.
> paraspinous a.
> physiologic a.
> plantar a.
> posterior a.
> posterolateral a.
> puriform a.
> spinous a.
> volar a.

aspergilloma formation

aspergillosis
> allergic bronchopulmonary a. (ABA)
> a. infection

Aspergillus **infection**

aspermatogenic

aspermia

asphyxia

asphyxial

asphyxiant

asphyxiate

asphyxiating thoracic dysplasia

asphyxiation
> intrapartum a.

aspirate
> endotracheal a.
> percutaneous a.
> transtracheal a.

aspirated foreign body

aspiration
> acid a.
> Alcon a.
> anterior a.
> a. biopsy cytology
> bone marrow a.
> breast cyst a.
> cataract a.
> cervical a.
> cold knife cone a.
> corporeal a.
> a. of cortex
> CT-directed needle a.
> CT-guided fine-needle a.
> CT scan-guided needle a.
> cyst a.
> endoscopic transesophageal fine-needle a.
> epididymal sperm a.
> EUS-guided fine-needle a.
> fine-needle a. (FNA)
> fluid a.
> foreign body a.
> full-thickness rectal a.
> gastric fluid a.
> guided fine-needle a.
> hematoma a.
> iliac crest bone a.
> image-guided pancreatic core a.
> irrigation and a.
> joint a.
> lateral a.
> Mammotest Plus breast a.
> meconium a.
> medial a.
> menstrual a.
> Michele vertebral a.
> microscopic epididymal sperm a.
> microsurgical epididymal sperm a.
> mineral oil a.
> mucosal needle a.
> myringotomy with a.
> needle a.
> a. needle biopsy
> negative a.
> percutaneous balloon a.
> percutaneous CT-guided a.
> percutaneous epididymal sperm a.

percutaneous fine-needle a.
peritoneal a.
pleural fluid a.
a. pneumonia
a. pneumonitis
a. portal
preoperative percutaneous a.
a. prophylaxis
pulmonary a.
real-time endoscopic ultrasound-
  guided fine-needle a.
recurrent a.
seminal vesicle a.
silent a.
sonography-guided a.
sperm a.
stereotactic a.
suction a.
suprapubic needle a.
tracheal a.
transbronchial needle a.
transthoracic needle a.
transtracheal a.
ultrasonic a.
ultrasound-guided fine-needle a.
uterine a.
vacuum a.
vertebral a.
vitreous a.

aspirator
handgun a.

asplenia
ASRA
American Society of Regional Anesthesia

assay
antiphospholipid antibody a.
coagulation factor a.
hydrophobicity a.
immunoreactive parathyroid
  hormone a.
intact parathyroid hormone a.
intraoperative iPTH a.
iPTH a.
a. normalization
parathyroid hormone
  chemiluminescent a.
PTH chemiluminescent a.
rapid intraoperative parathormone a.
rapid intraoperative parathormone
  immunoradiometric a.
a. technique

assessment
awake neurological a.
computer-assisted a.
cytological a.
echocardiographic a.
endoscopic color Doppler a.
extrapyramidal function a.
histologic a.
histological a.
intraoperative a.
jugular bulb catheter placement a.
noninvasive a.
nutritional a.
peritoneal cytological a.
weight estimation and a.

Assézat triangle
assimilation
a. pelvis
a. sacrum

assist
certified surgical technologist,
  first a. (CSTFA)
hand a.
registered nurse, first a. (RNFA)

assistance
laparoscopic a.

assist-control mode ventilation
assisted
a. circulation
a. expiration
a. medical procreation
a. reproduction technology
a. reproductive technique
a. respiration
a. ventilation

associated
a. injury
a. myofascial trigger point

association
American Pediatric Surgical A.
  (APSA)
auditory-vocal a.
a. cortex
a. fiber
law of a.
a. mechanism
megacystis-megaureter a.
noncausal a.
A. for the Study of Internal
  Fixation (ASIF)
a. time

NOTES

association *(continued)*
    a. tract
    VATER a.
asterion
asternal
asteroid body
asthma
    exercise-induced a.
    extrinsic a.
asthmatic
    steroid-dependent a.
asthmoid respiration
astigmatic keratotomy
astigmatism
    corneal a.
    a. correction
Astler-Coller
    A.-C. classification (A, B1, B2,
    C1, C2)
    A.-C. modification
    A.-C. modification of Dukes
    classification
astragalar
astragalocalcanean
astragaloscaphoid
astragalotibial
Astrand
    A. 30-beat stopwatch method
    A. 6-minute submaximal cycle
    ergometer test
astriction
astringent
astroblastoma
astrocyte
    fibrillary a.
astrocytoma
    adulthood a.
    anaplastic a.
    giant cell a.
    high-grade a.
    subependymal giant cell a.
Astwood-Coller staging
asymmetric
    a. hyperplasia
    a. parathyroid enlargement
    a. surgery
    a. unit membrane
asymmetrical
    a. arthralgia
    a. gradient coil
asymmetry
asymptomatic
    a. angiomyolipoma
    A. Carotid Atherosclerosis Study
    (ACAS)
    a. cholecystitis
    a. infection
    a. mass

    a. neoplasm
    a. patient
asynchronism
asynclitic position
ataractic
Atasoy
    A. palmar flap
    A. triangular advancement flap
    A. volar V-Y flap
    A. V-Y technique
Atasoy-Kleinert flap
Atasoy-type flap
atavistic epiphysis
ataxia
    respiratory a.
ATC
    around the clock
    ATC dosing
atelectasis
atherectomy
    Auth a.
    coronary angioplasty versus
    excisional a.
    coronary rotational a.
    directional coronary a.
    excisional a.
    high-speed rotational a.
    a. index
    Kinsey a.
    percutaneous coronary rotational a.
    rotational coronary a.
    Simpson a.
    transluminal extraction a.
atheroma embolism
atheromatous plaque
atherosclerosis
    carotid a.
atherosclerotic
    a. aneurysm
    a. carotid artery
    a. carotid artery disease (ACAD)
    a. carotid artery lesion
    a. heart disease
    a. plaque
    a. renal artery stenosis
ATI
    Abdominal Trauma Index
ATIII
    antithrombin III
Atkin
    A. approach
    A. epiphysial fracture
Atkinson
    A. lid block
    A. technique
atlantad
atlantal fracture
atlantica
atlantis

atlantoaxial
>a. arthrodesis
>a. articulation
>a. dislocation
>a. fracture-dislocation
>a. fusion
>a. instability
>a. joint
>a. lesion
>a. rotatory fixation
>a. stabilization

atlantoepistrophic
atlantooccipital
>a. articulation
>a. extension
>a. fusion
>a. joint
>a. joint dislocation
>a. ligament
>a. membrane
>a. stabilization
>a. transection

atlantoodontoid
atlas
atlas-axis combination fracture
atloaxoid
atloid
ATLS
>acute tumor lysis syndrome
>advanced trauma life support

atmosphere
>oxygen-enriched a.
>a.'s of pressure

ATN
>acute tubular necrosis

atomic mass
atomizer
atonic bladder
atony
>gastric a.

atopic line
ATP
>adenosine triphosphate
>ATP hydrolysis

atrabiliaris
atrabiliary capsule
atraumatic suture technique
atresia
>aortic valve a.
>biliary a.
>extrahepatic biliary a.

>pulmonary a.
>urethral a.

atretocystia
atretogastria
atria (*pl. of* atrium)
atrial
>a. activation mapping
>a. activity (AA)
>a. arrhythmia
>a. baffle operation
>a. balloon septostomy
>a. defibrillation threshold
>a. dissociation
>a. ectopic tachycardia
>a. extrastimulus method
>a. fibrillation
>a. fibrillation-flutter
>a. filling pressure
>a. natriuretic factor (ANF)
>a. natriuretic peptide (ANP)
>a. ring
>a. septal defect
>a. septal resection
>a. septectomy
>a. stasis index

atrial-well technique
atriocaval shunt
atriocommissuropexy
atriodextrofascicular tract
atriofascicular tract
atrionodal bypass tract
atriopulmonary connection
atriotomy
>pursestring a.

atrioventricular
>a. bundle
>a. canal
>a. canal defect
>a. conduction tissue
>a. connection anomaly
>a. dissociation
>a. junctional ablation
>a. junction anomaly
>a. malformation
>a. nodal function
>a. node
>a. reentry tachycardia
>a. ring
>a. septal defect
>a. sulcus
>a. valve insufficiency

atrium, pl. **atria**

NOTES

atrophic
- a. excavation
- a. fenestration
- a. fracture
- a. inflammation
- a. kidney
- a. skin

atrophy
- brown a.
- cortical a.
- crypt a.
- endometrial a.
- exhaustion a.
- gastric a.
- graft a.
- healed yellow a.
- intestinal villous a.
- mammary a.
- mucosal a.
- multiple system a.
- muscular a.
- optic nerve a.
- peroneal muscle a.
- pressure a.
- scapular peroneal a.
- skeletal muscle a.
- traction a.
- villous a.
- vocal cord a.
- yellow a.

attached
- a. cranial section
- a. craniotomy
- a. gingiva extension

attack
- recurrent a.
- transient ischemic a. (TIA)

attenuating tissue

attenuation
- arteriolar a.
- beam a.
- broadband a.
- a. correction
- digital beam a.
- heterogeneous a.
- high a.
- interaural a.
- a. level
- signal a.
- a. of tendon
- ultrasonic a.

attic adhesion

attorney
- power of a.

Attwood staining method

atypia
- nuclear a.

atypical
- a. dislocation

- a. hyperplasia (AH)
- a. junction
- a. mycobacterial infection
- a. regeneration
- a. squamous cell of undetermined significance (ASCUS)

ATZ
- anal transition zone

AUC
- area under curve
- postprandial AUC

Auchincloss
- A. modified radical mastectomy
- A. operation

audioanalgesia

audiological evaluation

auditory
- a. canal
- a. closure
- a. method
- a. middle lateral response (AMLR)
- a. tract
- a. tube
- a. tube nerve

auditory-vocal association

auditus

Auerbach
- A. ganglion
- A. plexus

Aufranc cup arthroplasty

Aufrecht sign

augmentation
- alloplastic chin a.
- arthroscopic a.
- bladder a.
- bone marrow a.
- breast a.
- chin a.
- connective tissue a.
- a. cystoplasty
- demucosalized a.
- donor-specific bone marrow a.
- endoscopic breast a.
- extraarticular a.
- gastroileac a.
- a. genioplasty
- gingival a.
- a. graft
- hamstring ligament a.
- ileocecocystoplasty bladder a.
- iliotibial band graft a.
- Leach-Schepsis-Paul a.
- Mainz pouch a.
- a. mammaplasty
- a. plaque
- reverse a.
- simultaneous areolar mastopexy and breast a. (SAMBA)
- slotted acetabular a.

A

submucosal urethral a.
synthetic a.
a. therapy
thiol a.
transumbilical breast a. (TUBA)
ureteral bladder a.
augmentor nerve
aural fistula
auricle
auricular
a. acupuncture
a. appendectomy
a. branch
a. canaliculus
a. cartilage
a. fibrillation
a. fissure
a. ganglion
a. index
a. ligament
a. muscle
a. nerve
a. notch
a. point
a. surface
a. triangle
a. tubercle
a. vein
auriculocranial
auriculoinfraorbital plane
auriculomastoid
auriculotemporal nerve
auriculoventricular groove
auscultation
Austin
A. bunionectomy
A. Flint murmur
A. Flint respiration
A. osteotomy
Austin-Moore arthroplasty
Autenrieth and Funk method
Auth atherectomy
autoamputation
autoaugmentation
bladder a.
autocastration
autocatheterization
autocystoplasty
autocytolysis
autodilation
Frank nonsurgical perineal a.
autodrainage

autogeneic graft
autogenous
a. bone graft
a. fascial heterograft
a. interpositional shoulder
arthroplasty
a. keratoplasty
a. strip
a. tooth transplantation
a. vein
autograft
cultured epithelial a.
a. fusion
a. harvesting
parathyroid a.
pulmonary a. (PA)
Russell fibular head a.
autografting
autoimmune
a. connective tissue disorder
a. demyelination
a. hepatitis
autoimmunization
surgical a.
autoinflation
autoinfusion
autokeratoplasty
autolesion
autologous
a. blood
a. blood clot pulmonary embolism
a. blood donation
a. blood stem cell transplantation
a. blood unit
a. bone marrow transplant (ABMT)
a. bone marrow transplantation
(ABMT)
A. Bone and Marrow Transplant
Registry (ABMTR)
a. clot
a. internal jugular vein
a. melanoma system
a. osteochondral allograft
transplantation
a. osteochondral mosaicplasty
a. ovarian transplantation
a. pericardial patch
a. RBC unit
autolytic débridement
automated
a. anesthesia record
a. boundary protection

NOTES

automated *(continued)*
    a. computerized axial tomography
    a. endoscopic system for optimal positioning (AESOP)
    a. lamellar therapeutic keratoplasty (ALTK)
    a. large-core breast biopsy
    a. percutaneous discectomy
automatic ectopic tachycardia
autonephrectomy
    silent a.
autonomic
    a. blockade
    a. dysreflexia
    a. dysregulation
    a. ganglion block
    a. modulation
    a. nerve
    a. nerve block
    a. nerve preservation (ANP)
    a. neurogenic bladder
autonomicorum
autonomous function
auto-PEEP
autoplasty
autopod
autopodium
autopsy
    laparoscopic a.
autoreinfection
autorrhaphy
autoscopy
autosomal
    a. dominant polycystic kidney disease
    a. recessive
autosuture technique
autotransfusion
    massive a.
autotransplant
autotransplantation
    colostomy pyloric a.
    pancreatic a.
    posttraumatic a.
    pyloric a.
    renal a.
autotrophic fixation
autovaccination
Auvray incision
auxiliary
    a. canal
    a. partial orthotopic liver transplantation (APOLT)
    a. transplant
A-V, AV
    arteriovenous
    A-V bundle
    A-V dissociation
    A-V fistula

    A-V malformation
    A-V nodal modification
avascular
    a. fragment
    a. necrosis
avascularization
average
    a. extubation time
    a. flow rate
    a. mean pressure
    moving time a. (MTA)
AVF
    arteriovenous fistula
avidin-biotin-peroxidase complex method
Avila technique
avium-intracellulare
    Mycobacterium a.-i. (MAI)
AVM
    arteriovenous malformation
avoidance maneuver
avulse
avulsed
    a. fragment
    a. wound
avulsion
    a. stress fracture
    a. technique
    a. trauma
awake
    a. craniotomy
    a. fiberoptic intubation
    a. intraoperative electrocorticography
    a. neurological assessment
awaken
    failure to a.
awakening
    planned a.
awareness
    body a.
AXBF
    axillobifemoral
Axenfeld
    A. anomaly
    A. suture technique
Axer
    A. lateral opening wedge osteotomy
    A. varus derotational osteotomy
Axer-Clark procedure
axes *(pl. of* axis)
axial
    a. aneurysm
    a. calcaneal projection
    a. compression
    a. compression injury
    a. compression principle
    a. compression test
    a. fixation
    a. flag flap

a. hiatal hernia
a. illumination
a. inclination
a. lesion
a. line angle
a. loading fracture
a. melanoma
a. muscle
a. pattern scalp flap
a. plane
a. point
a. rotation
a. rotation joint
a. section
a. sesamoid projection
a. skeleton
a. spin-echo image
a. surface cavity
axifugal
axilla, pl. **axillae**
hot a.
a. temperature
axillary
a. abscess
a. adenopathy
a. approach
a. arch
a. artery
a. artery aneurysm
a. bed
a. block
a. block anesthesia
a. block anesthetic technique
a. endoscopic reduction
a. envelope
a. fascia
a. fat pad
a. flap
a. fold
a. fossa
a. hematoma
a. incision
a. insertion
a. line
a. lymphadenectomy
a. lymphadenopathy
a. lymph node dissection (ALND)
a. nerve
a. node dissection
a. node dissection mastectomy
a. node metastasis
a. node negative

a. perivascular technique
a. plexus
a. region
a. relapse
a. sheath
a. skin lesion
a. space
a. sweat gland
a. tail
a. thoracotomy
a. triangle
a. vascular injury
a. vein
axilloaxillary bypass
axillobifemoral (AXBF)
a. bypass
a. bypass graft
axillofemoral bypass
axillounifemoral (AXUF)
a. bypass
axiobuccolingual plane
axiolabiolingual plane
axiomesiodistal plane
axis, pl. **axes**
basibregmatic a.
basicranial a.
basifacial a.
celiac a.
cephalocaudal a.
coeliac a.
conjugate a.
craniofacial a.
facial a.
a. fixation
flexion-extension a.
a. fracture
hypothalamic-hypophysial-ovarian-
endometrial a.
long a.
mesentericoportal a.
pelvic a.
a. of rotation
thoracic a.
thyroid a.
axis-atlas combination fracture
axofugal
axon
corticospinal a.
axonal
a. demyelination
a. injury
a. regeneration

NOTES

axotomy
AXR
    abdominal x-ray
AXUF
    axillounifemoral
Aylett operation
Ayoub-Shklar method
Ayre spatula-Zelsmyr cytobrush technique
azeotrope
azeotropic solution

azotemia
    transient a.
azure lunula
azygoesophageal
    a. line
    a. recess
azygos
    a. artery of vagina
    a. fissure
    a. vein
azygous

β (*var. of* beta)
B
    B cell line
    B point
    B ring
    B, T phenotypic lymphocyte
Babcock
    B. operation
    B. suture technique
Babinski sign
Bachmann
    B. bundle
    internodal tract of B.
back
    b. gunshot wound
    b. pain
    b. projection
back-and-forth suture technique
backbone
backcut incision
backfire fracture
backflow
    b. bleeding
    pyelovenous b.
background illumination
back-knee deformity
back-propagation neural network program
back-up position
backward
    b. coarticulation
    b. position
    b., upward, rightward pressure (BURP)
Bacon-Babcock operation
bacteremia
    perioperative b.
bacteremic donor
bacteria (*pl. of* bacterium)
bacterial
    b. agar method
    b. complication
    b. contamination
    b. endotoxin
    b. flora
    b. infection
    b. mucosal infiltration
    b. overgrowth
    b. synergistic gangrene
    b. translocation
bactericidal concentration
bacteriologic data
bacteriolysis
bacteriopexy
bacteriospermia

bacteriostasis
bacteriostatic barrier
bacterium, pl. bacteria
    probiotic bacteria
bacteriuria
BAD
    bipolar affective disorder
Badal operation
Badenoch urethroplasty
Badgley
    B. combination procedure
    B. iliac wing resection
    B. technique
Bado classification
Baehr-Lohlein lesion
Baffe anastomosis
baffle fenestration
bag-and-mask ventilation
bag extraction
bagged mask ventilation
bag-of-bones technique
bag-valve-mask
bag-valve-mask-assisted ventilation
Bailey-Badgley
    B.-B. anterior cervical approach
    B.-B. cervical spine fusion
    B.-B. technique
Bailey-Dubow
    B.-D. osteotomy
    B.-D. technique
bailout valvuloplasty
Bailyn classification
Bain circle
Baker
    B. cyst
    B. patellar advancement operation
    B. pyridine extraction
    B. Sudan black method
    B. technique
    B. translocation operation
Baker-Hill osteotomy
Balacescu closing wedge osteotomy
Balacescu-Golden technique
balance
    acid-base b.
    extravascular fluid b.
    heat b.
    thermal b.
balanced
    b. anesthesia
    b. anesthetic technique
    b. articulation
    b. salt solution volume diuresis
balanic
balanitis

B

balanocele
balanoplasty
balanoposthitis
balanus
Balbiani body
Baldy operation
Baldy-Webster
    B.-W. operation
    B.-W. procedure
    B.-W. uterine suspension
Balfour gastroenterostomy
Balkan nephrectomy
ball
    8-b. hemorrhage
    B. operation
    b. valve action
    b. wedge
ball-and-socket
    b.-a.-s. epiphysis
    b.-a.-s. joint
    b.-a.-s. trochanteric osteotomy
Ballard examination
Ball-Hoffman operation
ballistics
balloon
    b. aortic valvotomy
    b. aortic valvuloplasty
    b. atrial septostomy
    b. bronchoplasty
    b. catheter angioplasty
    b. catheter technique
    b. cell formation
    b. coarctation angioplasty
    b. coronary angioplasty
    b. counterpulsation
    b. dilatation
    b. dilation
    b. dilation angioplasty
    b. dilation valvuloplasty
    b. dissection
    b. embolectomy
    b. epiphysis
    b. esophagoplasty
    b. expulsion test
    b. fenestration procedure
    b. inflation
    b. laser angioplasty
    b. mitral commissurotomy
    b. mitral valvotomy
    b. mitral valvuloplasty
    b. occlusive intravascular lysis
      enhanced recanalization
    b. photodynamic therapy
    b. pulmonary valvotomy
    b. pulmonary valvuloplasty
    b. rupture
    b. septectomy
    b. tamponade technique
    b. tricuspid valvotomy

    b. tube tamponade
    b. tuboplasty
    B. Valvuloplasty Registry
    b. valvulotomy
balloon-catheter and basket-retrieval
    technique
balloon-occluded retrograde transvenous
    obliteration (B-RTO)
ball-valve obstruction
bamboo spine
banana
    b. fracture
    b. sign
band
    adhesive b.
    ciliary body b.
    Clado b.
    fracture b.
    gastric b.
    iliotibial b.
    b. keratopathy
    Ladd b.
    Lane b.
    b. ligation
    Maissiat b.
    Meckel b.
    moderator b.
    pecten b.
    peritoneal b.
    b. placement
    b. sigmoidopexy
    Simonart b.
    zonular b.
bandage
    adhesive b.
    compression b.
    b. method
Band-Aid operation
band-assist device
bandeau defect
banded gastroplasty
banding
    adjustable gastric b.
    Kuzmak gastric b.
    laparoscopic adjustable silicone
      gastric b.
    laparoscopic gastric b.
    open adjustable silicone gastric b.
Bandi procedure
bandy leg
Banff classification
Bangerter
    B. method
    B. method of pleoptics
    B. pterygium operation
banjo-string adhesion
bank
    blood b.
    shoulder dislocation bone b.

staple capsulorraphy bone b.
tissue b.
Traumatic Coma Data B.

Bankart
B. fracture
B. operation
B. procedure
B. reconstruction
B. shoulder dislocation
B. shoulder lesion
B. shoulder repair

Bankart-Putti-Platt operation
banking
cryopreserved tissue b.

Banks-Laufman
B.-L. approach
B.-L. incision
B.-L. technique

Bannayan-Riley-Ruvalcaba syndrome
Baptist
New England B. (NEB)

bar
b. bolt fixation
Mercier b.
Passavant b.
b. resection
b. section

barber
b. chair position
b. pole stripe transfer

barbiturate
b. burst-suppression anesthesia
b. coma

barbiturate-related hyperalgesia
barbotage
Barcat technique
Bard endoscopic suturing
bare
b. area
b. area diaphragm
b. scleral technique

bariatric
b. operation
b. patient
b. surgery

barium
b. contrast x-ray
b. enema
b. enema examination
b. enema finding
b. esophagogram
b. peritonitis

b. swallow
b. swallow study

Barkan
B. double cyclodialysis operation
B. goniotomy operation
B. membrane
B. technique

Barkan-Cordes linear cataract operation
Barlow maneuver
Barnard operation
Barnett-Bourne acetic alcohol-silver
nitrate method
barogenic esophageal perforation
barometric pressure
baroreceptor
b. nerve
b. test

baroreflex
b. activation
b. response
b. responsiveness

barostat method
barotrauma
Barr
B. body
B. open reduction and internal
fixation
B. tendon transfer operation
B. tibial fracture fixation

barrage cryopexy
Barraquer
B. enzymatic zonulolysis operation
B. keratomileusis operation
B. method
B. suture technique
B. zonulolysis

barrel-shaped lesion
barrel staving
Barrett
B. epithelium
B. esophagus
B. metaplasia

Barrie-Jones canaliculodacryorhinostomy
operation
barrier
ABO b.
adhesion b.
anatomic b.
bacteriostatic b.
blood-air b.
blood-brain b. (BBB)
blood-cerebral b.

NOTES

barrier *(continued)*
    blood-cerebrospinal fluid b.
    blood-liquor b.
    blood-ocular b.
    blood-optic nerve b.
    blood-retinal b.
    blood-thymus b.
    blood-urine b.
    cerebrospinal fluid-brain b.
    elastic b.
    endothelial b.
    epithelial b.
    gastric mucosal b.
    integumentary b.
    b. layer
    b. method
    motion b.
    mucosal b.
    ocular b.
    B.'s Pain Questionnaire
    pathologic b.
    physical b.
    physiologic b.
    placental b.
    posterior capsular zonular b.
    b. protection
    side-bending b.
    sterile field b.
    b. technique
    b. zone
Barrio operation
Barrnett-Seligman
    B.-S. dihydroxydinaphthyl disulfide
      method
    B.-S. indoxyl esterase method
Barron
    B. hemorrhoidal banding technique
    B. ligation
Barroso-Moguel and Costero silver method
Barsky
    B. cleft closure
    B. macrodactyly reduction
    B. procedure
    B. technique
Barth hernia
Bartholin
    B. cystectomy
    B. duct
    B. gland
Bartlett
    B. nail fold
    B. nail fold excision
    B. procedure
Barton fracture
Barton-Smith fracture
basad
basal
    b. anal canal pressure

    b. anal sphincter pressure
    b. anesthesia
    anterior b. (AB)
    b. body temperature
    b. cell carcinoma
    b. cell hyperplasia
    b. cell membrane
    b. cistern
    b. ganglia hematoma
    b. ganglion
    b. ganglionic lesion
    inferior b. (IB)
    b. iridectomy
    b. lamina
    lateral b. (LB)
    b. line
    b. neck fracture
    septal b. (SB)
    b. skull fracture
    b. sphincter
    b. subfrontal approach
    b. tentorial branch
    b. vein
    b. vein of Rosenthal
basaloid
bascule
    cecal b.
base
    anterior cranial b.
    b. of bladder
    cavity preparation b.
    cement b.
    cranial b.
    b. deficit (BD)
    extension b.
    fixation b.
    b. line
    b. medication
    National Cancer Data B. (NCDB)
    b. plane
    b. projection
    saddle connector b.
    tissue-supported b.
    tissue-tissue-supported b.
    b. wedge osteotomy
baseball
    b. finger fracture
    b. stitch
    b. suture technique
baseline capacity evaluation
basement
    b. membrane
    b. membrane zone
base-of-neck osteotomy
base-ring tilt
bas-fond
basialis
basialveolar
basibregmatic axis

basicranial axis
basic technique
basifacial axis
basihyal
basihyoid
basilar
    b. artery
    b. artery aneurysm
    b. artery migraine
    b. bifurcation
    b. bifurcation aneurysm
    b. bone
    b. cartilage
    b. femoral neck fracture
    b. fibrocartilage
    b. index
    b. invagination
    b. lamina
    b. membrane
    b. osteotomy
    b. process
    b. skull fracture
    b. suture
    b. suture technique
    b. tip aneurysm
    b. venous plexus
    b. venous sinus
    b. vertebra
basilateral
basilic vein
basin
    lymph node b.
    nonclassic nodal b.
    portal lymph node b.
    regional lymph node b.
    retropancreatic lymph node b.
basinasal line
basioccipital bone
basiocciput
basioglossus
basion
basipetal
basipharyngeal canal
basis
basisphenoid bone
basitemporal
basivertebral vein
basket
    b. extraction technique
    b. fragmentation technique
    b. impaction
basketing technique

basket-weave vacuolization
basolateral membrane
basosquamous cell carcinoma
Bass
    B. method
    B. technique
Basset radical vulvectomy
Bassini
    B. inguinal hernia repair
    B. inguinal herniorrhaphy
    B. method
    B. operation
    B. procedure
    B. technique
Bassini-Stetten hernia repair
bastard suture technique
Batchelor-Brown extraarticular subtalar
    arthrodesis
Batch least-squares method
Batch-Spittler-McFaddin
    B.-S.-M. knee disarticulation
    B.-S.-M. technique
bat ear surgery
Bateman
    B. hemiarthroplasty
    B. modification
    B. modification of Mayer transfer
      operation
bath
    contrast b.
bathing trunk nevus
Batista procedure
batrachian position
Batson plexus
Battle
    B. incision
    B. operation
    B. sign
battledore incision
Battle-Jalaguier-Kammerer incision
batwing
    b. appearance
    b. arm
    b. deformity
Baudelocque operation
Bauer-Jackson classification
Bauer-Tondra-Trusler
    B.-T.-T. operation
    B.-T.-T. technique
Bauhin
    B. gland
    valve of B.

B

NOTES

Baume classification
Baumgard-Schwartz tennis elbow technique
Baumgartner method
BAVM
  brain arteriovenous malformation treatment
Baxter
  B. VAMP
  B. venous/arterial management protection
Baxter-D'Astous procedure
Bayne-Klug centralization
Baynton operation
bayonet
  b. canal
  b. dislocation
  b. fracture position
bayonet-curved canal
bayonet-type incision
BBB
  blood-brain barrier
  bundle branch block
BCSS
  breast cancer-specific survival
BCT
  breast conservation therapy
BD
  base deficit
BEA
  below-elbow amputation
beach chair position
bead
  b. bed
  b. chain study
  b. pouch
  b. technique filling
beads-on-a-string appearance
beak
  b. fracture
  b. modification
  b. modification with triple arthrodesis
  b. nail
Beall-Webel-Bailey technique
beam
  b. attenuation
  fluoroscopy b.
Beard-Cutler operation
Beard operation
beating-heart bypass surgery
Beatson ovariotomy
beat-to-beat variation of fetal heart rate
Beau line
Beaver direct smear method
Bechterew (*var. of* Bekhterev)
Bechtol arthroplasty

Beck
  B. cardiopericardiopexy
  B. gastrostomy
  B. I, II operation
  B. method
  B. triad
Beckenbaugh
  B. correction
  B. technique
Becker
  B. muscular dystrophy
  B. technique
Béclard
  B. amputation
  B. anastomosis
  B. hernia
  B. suture technique
  B. triangle
Becton
  B. open reduction
  B. technique
bed
  axillary b.
  bead b.
  bone graft b.
  fracture b.
  gastric b.
  graft b.
  hot axillary b.
  liver b.
  mud b.
  nail b.
  parotid b.
  tumor b.
  vascular b.
bedroom fracture
bedside laparoscopy
beefy appearance
Beer operation
Begg light wire differential force technique
behavior
  pain b.
behavioral
  b. inhibition system (BIS)
  b. technique
Behçet
  B. disease
  B. skin puncture test
  B. syndrome
behind-sternum column esophagoplasty
Bekhterev, Bechterew
  line of B.
bell
  B. muscle
  B. palsy
  B. respiratory nerve
bell-clapper deformity
Bell-Dally cervical dislocation

Bellemore-Barrett closing wedge osteotomy
bellied
  2-b. muscle
Bell-Tawse
  B.-T. open reduction technique
  B.-T. procedure
belly
  b. bath therapy
  occipital b.
  posterior b.
bellybutton augmentation mammaplasty
below-elbow amputation (BEA)
below-knee amputation (BKA)
Belsey
  B. esophagoplasty
  B. fundoplication method
  B. fundoplication procedure
  B. fundoplication technique
  B. IV fundoplasty
  B. Mark II, IV fundoplication
  B. Mark IV antireflux operation
  B. Mark IV cardioplasty
  B. Mark IV 240-degree
    fundoplication
  B. Mark IV gastropexy
  B. Mark IV repair
  B. partial fundoplication
  B. two-thirds wrap fundoplication
belt
  b. loop gastropexy
  b. muscle
  B. technique
Belt-Fuqua hypospadias repair
Bence Jones body
bench
  b. examination
  b. surgery
  b. surgical technique
Benchekroun stoma
Benedict orbit operation
Benedict-Talbot body surface area method
Benelli lollipop mastopexy
Bengston method
benign
  b. bone lesion
  b. bone tumor
  b. duodenocolic fistula
  b. dysphagia
  b. esophageal disorder
  b. fasciculation

  b. germ cell tumor
  b. giant cell synovioma
  b. inflammatory disease
  b. liver cyst
  b. lymphoepithelial lesion
  b. lymphoproliferative lesion
  b. mass
  b. mesothelioma
  b. nature
  b. papillomavirus infection
  b. paroxysmal positional vertigo
    (BPPV)
  b. pneumatic colonoscopy
    complication
  b. process
  b. prostatic hyperplasia (BPH)
  b. prostatic hypertrophy (BPH)
  b. reading
  b. stricture
  b. subcutaneous cyst
  b. vascular lesion
benign-acting renal cell carcinoma
Bennett
  B. classification
  B. comminuted fracture
  B. dislocation
  B. fracture-dislocation
  B. lesion
  B. nail biopsy
  B. posterior shoulder approach
  B. sulfhydryl method
Bennhold Congo red method
Bensley aniline-acid fuchsin-methyl green method
Bentall
  B. composite graft technique
  B. inclusion technique
  B. procedure
bent-nail syndrome
bentonite flocculation test
benzodiazepine-induced hypoventilation
benzo sky blue method
Bérard aneurysm
Berci-Shore choledochoscopy
Berens
  B. graft
  B. pterygium transplant operation
  B. sclerectomy operation
Berens-Smith
  B.-S. cul-de-sac restoration
  B.-S. operation
Berg chelate removal method

B

NOTES

Berger
B. disease
B. interscapular amputation
B. operation
B. space
Berger-Bookwalter posterior approach
Bergey classification
Bergmann incision
Bergmann-Israel incision
Berke
B. approach
B. operation
Berke-Krönlein orbitotomy
Berke-Motais operation
Berman-Gartland
B.-G. metatarsal osteotomy
B.-G. procedure
Bernard
B. canal
B. duct
B. lip reconstruction procedure
B. operation
B. puncture
Berndt-Harty classification
Bernese periacetabular osteotomy
Bernoulli effect
berry
b. aneurysm
B. ligament
Bertel position
Bertin column
Bertrandi suture technique
beta, β
b. adrenoreceptor
b. hemolytic streptococci infection
beta-2-adrenergic receptor
beta-adrenergic
b.-a. agonist
b.-a. blockade
b.-a. receptor
beta-blocker medication
beta-oxidation pathway
beta-receptor
b.-r. agonist
b.-r. antagonist
beta-sympathomimetic agent
betel carcinoma
Bethke
B. iridectomy
B. operation
Bevan
B. abdominal incision
B. orchiopexy
beveled anastomosis
bevel preparation
Beverly-Douglas lip-tongue adhesion technique
BeWo choriocarcinoma cell line

bezoar
medication b.
Bezold abscess
Bezold-Jarisch reflex
B.H. Moore procedure
biarticular
biasterionic
biaxial joint
BIB
biliointestinal bypass
bicameral abscess
bicanalicular sphincter
biceps
b. interval lesion
b. tendon
Bichat
B. canal
B. fat pad
B. fossa
B. membrane
bicipital
b. groove
b. rib
b. ridge
bicipitoradial bursa
bicipitoradialis
bursa b.
Bickel-Moe procedure
bicondylar
b. articulation
b. joint
b. T-shaped fracture
b. Y-shaped fracture
bicoronal
b. incision
b. scalp flap
bicortical screw fixation
bicycle spoke fracture
BID
bilateral interfacetal dislocation
bidirectional
b. Glenn shunt
b. ligation
b. superior cavopulmonary anastomosis
Biebl loop
Bielschowsky
B. maneuver
B. method
B. operation
B. 3-step, head-tilt test
Bielschowsky-Parks head-tilt, 3-step test
Bier
B. amputation
B. block
B. block anesthesia
B. method
Biesiadecki fossa

B

bifid
- b. penis
- b. rib
- b. thumb deformity

bifida
- spina b.

bifocal fixation

bifoveal fixation

bifrontal
- b. craniotomy
- b. incision

bifurcated vascular graft

bifurcation
- b. aneurysm
- aortic b.
- basilar b.
- carotid artery b.
- coronary b.
- b. graft
- b. involvement
- b. lesion
- b. osteotomy
- portal b.
- b. of root

Bigelow
- B. litholapaxy
- B. maneuver
- B. septum

BIH
- bilateral inguinal hernia

bikini skin incision

bilabe

bilaminar membrane

bilateral
- b. adrenal hemorrhage
- b. amputation
- b. anterior thoracotomy
- b. bundle branch block
- b. ilioinguinal approach
- b. inguinal hernia (BIH)
- b. inguinal hernia repair
- b. inguinal hernia repair method
- b. inguinal hernia repair procedure
- b. inguinal hernia repair technique
- b. interfacetal dislocation (BID)
- b. lithotomy
- b. lymphadenectomy
- b. myocutaneous graft
- b. neck dissection
- b. neck exploration
- b. nephroureterectomy
- b. resection

- b. sacroiliac approach
- b. salpingo-oophorectomy (BSO)
- b. sequential lung transplant
- b. subcostal incision
- b. subcutaneous mastectomy
- b. temporary tarsorrhaphy
- b. torsion
- b. total adrenalectomy
- b. transabdominal incision
- b. ureterostomy takedown
- b. vagotomy
- b. ventral rhizotomy
- b. V-Y Kutler flap

bilayered cellular matrix

bilayer patch hernia repair

bile
- b. acid circulation
- b. ascites
- b. duct
- b. duct adenocarcinoma
- b. duct adenoma
- b. duct calculus
- b. duct cannulation
- b. duct carcinoma
- b. duct catheterization
- b. duct colic
- b. duct cystadenocarcinoma
- b. duct dilatation
- b. duct epithelium
- b. duct exploration
- b. duct injury
- b. duct ligation
- b. duct lumen
- b. duct manipulation
- b. duct pressure
- b. duct stricture
- b. duct wall
- b. encrustation
- b. fluid examination
- b. leak
- b. leakage
- b. papilla
- b. plug syndrome
- b. sample
- b. stained cyst content
- b. tract
- b. tract drainage

bilevel positive airway pressure (BiPAP)

bilharzial carcinoma

Bilhaut-Cloquet procedure

biliaris

NOTES

biliary
- b. anatomic variation
- b. anatomy
- b. atresia
- b. calculus
- b. canaliculus
- b. cannulation
- b. carcinoma
- b. colic
- b. conduit
- b. dilation
- b. drainage
- b. duct
- b. ductule
- b. endoprosthesis insertion
- b. endoscopy
- b. enteric bypass
- b. fistula
- b. intestinal anastomosis
- b. leakage
- b. lithiasis
- b. lithotripsy
- b. pancreatitis
- b. problem
- b. reconstruction
- b. saturation index
- b. secretion
- b. sludge
- b. sphincterotomy
- b. sphincterotomy and stent placement
- b. stenting
- b. stent patency
- b. stricture
- b. sump syndrome
- b. system
- b. tract
- b. tract cancer
- b. tract disease
- b. tract infection
- b. tract obstruction
- b. tract pressure
- b. tract stone
- b. tract torsion
- b. tract tumor
- b. tree

biliary-bronchial fistula
biliary-cutaneous fistula
biliary-duodenal
- b.-d. fistula
- b.-d. pressure gradient

biliary-enteric
- b.-e. anastomosis
- b.-e. anastomosis operation
- b.-e. fistula

biliocystic fistula

biliodigestive
- b. anastomosis
- b. origin

biliointestinal bypass (BIB)
biliopancreatic
- b. bypass (BPB)
- b. diversion
- b. diversion with duodenal switch
- b. limb

biliopleural fistula
bilious
- b. colic
- b. empyema
- b. vomit

bilirubin
- b. concentration
- b. level
- serum b.

Billings method
Bill maneuver
billowing mitral valve syndrome
Billroth
- B. I gastroduodenostomy
- B. II anatomy
- B. II gastrojejunostomy
- B. I, II gastrectomy
- B. I, II gastroenterostomy
- B. I, II gastrointestinal anastomosis
- B. I, II operation
- B. I, II procedure
- B. I, II reconstruction
- B. I, II technique
- B. II pancreatoduodenectomy
- B. I method
- B. I partial gastrectomy
- splenic cord of B.

bilobar
- b. disease
- b. liver metastasis
- b. resection

bilobate
bilobectomy
bilobed
- b. polypoid lesion
- b. skin flap
- b. transposition flap

bilobular
bilocular
- b. femoral hernia
- b. joint
- b. stomach

biloma
bimalleolar ankle fracture
bimanual
- b. palpation
- b. pelvic examination

bimastoid line
bimodal method
bimucosa

B

binaural
> b. fusion
> b. integration

Binet system of classification
Bing-Siebenmann malformation
Bing-Taussig heart procedure
binocular
> b. fixation
> b. fusion
> b. indirect ophthalmoscopy
> b. microscopy

bioartificial
> b. liver device
> b. liver support system

bioavailability
> nitric oxide b.

biobehavioral response
biochemical
> b. evidence
> b. metastasis
> b. modulation

biocompatibility
> implant b.

bioelectric treatment
biofeedback
biofilm production
bioimpedance
> thoracic b.

biologic
> b. fixation
> b. liver support
> b. marker

biological effect
biology
> cellular b.
> molecular b.

biomagnetic therapy
biomechanical preparation
bioprogressive technique
bioprosthesis
biopsy
> abdominal lymph node b.
> abrasive brush b.
> adrenal gland b.
> alcohol-fixed gastric b.
> Allis-Abramson breast b.
> antral b.
> aspiration needle b.
> automated large-core breast b.
> Bennett nail b.
> bite b.
> blind percutaneous liver b.

bone marrow aspiration and b.
brain b.
breast b.
bronchial brush b.
bronchoscopic needle b.
brush b.
Campylobacter-like organism b.
catheter-guided b.
b. cavity
cervical cone b.
channel and core b.
chorionic villus b.
CLO b.
coin b.
cold cone b.
cold cup b.
colonoscopic b.
colorectal b.
computed tomography-guided b.
cone b.
core needle b.
corporal b.
cortical b.
Crosby-Kugler capsule for b.
CT-guided liver b.
CT-guided needle-aspiration b.
cutting needle b.
cytobrush b.
cytologic b.
diagnostic b.
diathermic loop b.
digitally guided b.
direct-vision liver b.
Dunn b.
elliptical b.
embryo b.
endometrial b.
endomyocardial b.
endoscopic small bowel b.
endoscopic sphenoidal b.
ERCP-guided b.
esophageal b.
excision b.
excisional b.
fetal liver b.
fetal skin b.
fine-needle aspiration b.
FNA b.
forage core b.
Fosnaugh nail b.
guided transcutaneous b.
guillotine needle b.

NOTES

biopsy *(continued)*

hilar b.
hot b.
ileal b.
iliac crest b.
image-guided breast b. (IGBB)
image-guided fine-needle
  aspiration b.
image-guided stereotactic brain b.
incisional b.
internal mammary node b.
intestinal b.
intramedullary tumor b.
intraoperative b.
jejunal b.
jumbo b.
Kevorkian punch b.
Keyes punch b.
kidney b.
laparoscopic liver b.
large-core needle aspiration b.
large-particle b.
lift-and-cut b.
liver b.
lumbar spine b.
lung b.
lymph node b.
mammary node b.
mediastinal lymph node b.
Menghini technique for
  percutaneous liver b.
minimally invasive b.
mirror-image breast b.
mucosal b.
multiple core b.
muscle b.
nasopharyngeal b.
native renal b.
needle core b.
needle-localized open b. (NLOB)
negative breast b.
nerve b.
node b.
onion-bulb changes on b.
open brain b.
open liver b.
open lung b.
open surgical b.
optical b.
out-of-phase endometrial b.
outpatient b.
pancreatic b.
paracollicular b.
parathyroid b.
pelvic aspiration b.
percutaneous excisional breast b.
  (PEBB)
percutaneous fine needle
  aspiration b.

percutaneous fine-needle
  pancreatic b.
percutaneous native renal b.
percutaneous needle liver b.
percutaneous pancreas b.
pericardial b.
peritoneal b.
peroral intestinal b.
PET-guided b.
pinch b.
Pipelle b.
pleural b.
4-point b.
point-in-space stereotactic b.
positron emission tomography-
  guided b.
pouch b.
preoperative b.
punch b.
random bladder b.
rectal suction b.
renal b.
b. sample
saucerized b.
scalene fat pad b.
scalene lymph node b.
scalene node b. (SNB)
scan-directed b.
Scher nail b.
secondary diagnostic b.
sentinel lymph node b.
sentinel node b. (SNB)
serial percutaneous liver b.
shave b.
single b.
b. site
skeletal b.
skin b.
skinny-needle b.
SLN b.
snap-frozen b.
snare excision b.
snare loop b.
sonoguided b.
b. specimen
spinal infection b.
sponge b.
StereoGuide stereotactic needle
  core b.
stereotactic aspiration b.
stereotactic brain b.
stereotactic core breast b.
stereotactic-guided b.
stereotactic needle core b.
stereotactic percutaneous needle b.
strip b.
suction b.
supraclavicular lymph node b.
sural nerve b.

surface b.
surgical excision b.
synovial b.
systematic sextant b.
tangential b.
targeted brain b.
b. technique
temporal artery b.
testicular b.
thin-needle b.
thoracic spine b.
thyroid needle b.
total b.
transbronchial lung b.
transcutaneous b.
transfemoral liver b.
transgastric fine-needle aspiration b.
transitional zone b.
transjugular hepatic b.
transjugular liver b.
transnasal b.
transpapillary b.
transrectal ultrasound-guided
  sextant b.
transthoracic needle aspiration b.
transthoracic percutaneous fine-
  needle aspiration b.
transvenous liver b.
trephine needle b.
trophectoderm b.
Tru-Cut needle b. (TCNB)
ultrasonography-guided fine-needle
  aspiration b.
ultrasound-guided anterior subcostal
  liver b.
ultrasound-guided automated large-
  core breast b.
ultrasound-guided core breast b.
ultrasound-guided core needle b.
  (US-CNB)
ultrasound-guided echo b.
ultrasound-guided fine-needle
  aspiration b. (US-FNAB)
ultrasound-guided needle b.
ultrasound-guided stereotactic b.
vaginal cone b.
Valls-Ottolenghim-Schajowicz
  needle b.
ventricular endomyocardial b.
vertical lip b.
video-assisted excisional b.

Vim-Silverman technique for
  liver b.
b. volume
vulvar b.
Watson capsule b.
wedge hepatic b.
wedge liver b.
wire-guided breast b.
wound b.
Zaias nail b.
biopsy-proven metastasis
biorbital angle
biospectroscopy
biosurfactant
Biot
  B. breathing
  B. respiration
biotransformation
BiPAP
  bilevel positive airway pressure
    BiPAP nasal continuous positive
    airway pressure
biparietal
  b. diameter (BPD)
  b. suture technique
bipartition
  facial b.
bipedicle dorsal flap
bipennate muscle
bipennatus
biperforate
biphase pin fixation
biplanar fluoroscopy
biplane
  b. cineangiography
  b. fluoroscopy
  b. scan
  b. trochanteric osteotomy
bipolar
  b. affective disorder (BAD)
  b. cauterization
  b. coagulation
  b. electrocautery
  b. electrocoagulation
  b. hip arthroplasty
Bipolaris specific IgE, IgG antibody
BI-RADS
  Breast Imaging Reporting and Data
  System
    BI-RADS classification
    BI-RADS score
biramous

NOTES

Bircher operation
Bircher-Weber technique
Birch-Hirschfeld entropion operation
bird-beak deformity
bird's nest lesion
Birkett hernia
birth
  b. amputation
  b. canal
  b. canal laceration
  b. fracture
birthing position
BIS
  behavioral inhibition system
  bispectral index
bis
  central b.
bisacromial
bisaxillary
Bischof myelotomy
bisecting
  b. angle cone position
  b. angle technique
bisecting-the-angle technique
bisection
bisector line
bisegmentectomy
bisensory method
bisexual
Bishop classification
Bishop-Koop ileostomy
bismuth
  b. benign bile duct stricture
  classification
  b. bile duct stricture (type I-V)
  classification
  b. line
  b. type IV stricture
bispectral
  b. index (BIS)
  b. index monitoring
bissac
  hernia en b.
bisubcostal incision
bite
  b. biopsy
  b. plane
  b. plane therapy
  b. sign
bitemporal
biterminal
bitewing technique
biting pressure
bitrochanteric
biventral
bizygomatic
Björk method of Fontan procedure
Björk-Shiley graft

BKA
  below-knee amputation
BL
  blood lactate
  buccolingual
black
  b. blood clot
  B. classification
  b. epidermoidoma
  b. line
  b. patch syndrome
  b. periodic acid method
  B. repair
  B. technique
Black-Broström staple technique
Blackburn technique
bladder
  atonic b.
  b. augmentation
  b. autoaugmentation
  autonomic neurogenic b.
  base of b.
  b. calculus
  b. carcinoma
  b. carcinoma classification
  b. catheterization
  b. chimney procedure
  b. distention
  b. diverticulectomy
  b. drainage
  b. fistula
  b. flap
  b. flap hematoma
  b. hemorrhage
  b. hernia
  hyperreflexic b.
  hypertonic b.
  ileal b.
  b. laceration
  b. neck elevation test
  b. neck preserving technique
  b. neck suspension
  b. neck-to-urethra anastomosis
  neurogenic b.
  neuropathic b.
  orthotopic b.
  b. outlet reconstruction
  b. perforation
  poorly compliant b.
  b. pressure
  pseudoneurogenic b.
  reflex neurogenic b.
  b. replacement urinary pouch
  b. stone
  b. temperature
  trabeculated b.
  uninhibited neurogenic b.
  unstable b.

urinary b.
valve b.

blade
   b. atrial septostomy
   b. bone
   inferior turbinate b.
   b. plate fixation
   shoulder b.

Blair
   B. epicanthus repair
   B. fusion
   B. incision
   B. operation
   B. technique

Blair-Brown
   B.-B. procedure
   B.-B. skin graft

Blair-Byars hypospadias technique
Blaivas classification of urinary
  incontinence
Blalock-Hanlon
   B.-H. atrial septectomy
   B.-H. operation
   B.-H. procedure

Blalock-Taussig
   B.-T. operation
   B.-T. procedure
   B.-T. shunt
   B.-T. shunt ligation

blanchable red lesion
blanched cutaneous elevation
Bland-Altman method
Blandin gland
Blandin-Nuhn gland
Bland onlay flap
blanket suture technique
Blaschko line
Blasius
   B. duct
   B. lid flap operation

Blaskovics
   B. canthoplasty operation
   B. dacryostomy operation
   B. flap
   B. lid operation
   B. tarsectomy

blast
   b. gut injury
   b. lung injury

blastic
   b. lesion
   b. metastasis

blastocele
blastocytoma
blastolysis
blastoma
   pulmonary b.
blastotomy
Blatt
   B. operation
   B. procedure
Blatt-Ashworth procedure
bleb
   endothelial b.
   b. resection
Bleck
   B. method
   B. recession technique
bleed
   postgastrectomy b.
   postpolypectomy b.
   trocar wound b.
bleeding
   abnormal b.
   b. abnormality
   active source of b.
   acute digestive b.
   b. angioma
   anorectal variceal b.
   arterial b.
   backflow b.
   chronic digestive b.
   colorectal b.
   concomitant b.
   b. controlled with direct pressure
   b. controlled with electrocautery
   digestive b.
   distal b.
   b. duodenal ulcer
   b. episode
   esophageal variceal b.
   esophagogastric variceal b.
   excessive b.
   external b.
   gastric variceal b.
   gastrointestinal b.
   implantation b.
   intraabdominal b.
   intracranial b.
   intraoperative b.
   intrathoracic b.
   b. lesion
   massive lower gastrointestinal b.
   occult b.

B

NOTES

bleeding *(continued)*
    painless rectal b.
    pinpoint gastric mucosal defect b.
    placentation b.
    b. point
    portal hypertensive b.
    postcoital b.
    postmenopausal b.
    postoperative b.
    retroperitoneal b.
    b. risk
    b. site
    b. site ligation
    b. site localization
    b. time
    b. time coagulation panel
    b. tumor
    upper gastrointestinal b.
    variceal b.
    b. vessel
Blenderm patch technique
blenorrhagic inflammation
blepharal
blepharectomy
blepharochalasis repair
blepharon
blepharoplasty
    Davis-Geck b.
    reoperative b.
blepharoptosis repair
blepharorrhaphy
    Elschnig b.
blepharospasm
blepharosphincterectomy
blepharotomy
blind
    b. abscess
    b. clamping
    b. dilatation
    b. end
    b. fistula
    b. foramen
    b. gut
    b. insertion
    b. lithotripsy
    b. loop syndrome
    b. nasal intubation anesthetic
     technique
    b. nasotracheal intubation
    b. nasotracheal intubation anesthetic
     technique
    b. osteotomy
    b. percutaneous liver biopsy
    b. pouch syndrome
    b. rectal pouch
    b. upper esophageal pouch
blind-spot projection technique
blister
    fracture b.

    pressure b.
    subcorneal b.
bloc
    en b.
Bloch-Paul-Mikulicz operation
block
    b. anesthesia
    anesthetic b.
    ankle b.
    anterocrural celiac plexus b.
    arborization b.
    Atkinson lid b.
    autonomic ganglion b.
    autonomic nerve b.
    axillary b.
    Bier b.
    bilateral bundle branch b.
    brachial plexus b. (BPB)
    bundle branch b. (BBB)
    caudal b.
    celiac plexus b.
    central b.
    cervical plexus b.
    ciliovitrectomy b.
    complete left bundle branch b.
    complete right bundle branch b.
    continuous peripheral nerve b.
    continuous popliteal sciatic
     nerve b.
    controlled diagnostic b.
    coracoid infraclavicular brachial
     plexus b.
    depolarization b.
    depolarizing b.
    differential nerve b.
    differential spinal b.
    direct obturator nerve b.
    epidural b.
    exit b.
    extradural b.
    fascia iliaca b.
    femoral nerve b.
    field b.
    ganglion impar b.
    gasserian ganglion b.
    glossopharyngeal nerve b.
    greater occipital nerve b.
    Hara infiltration b.
    hepatic outflow b.
    His bundle heart b.
    iliohypogastric nerve b.
    ilioinguinal-iliohypogastric nerve b.
     (IINB)
    ilioinguinal nerve b. (IINB)
    3-in-1 b.
    incomplete right bundle branch b.
    indirect obturator nerve b.
    infiltration b.
    infraclavicular brachial plexus b.

infraorbital nerve b.
inguinal field b.
inguinal perivascular b.
b. injection
intercostal fossa b.
intercostal nerve b.
interpleural b.
interscalene brachial plexus b.
intrapleural b.
intravenous b.
Labat sciatic nerve b.
laparoscopic celiac plexus pain b.
left bundle branch b.
lower extremity nerve b.
lumbar plexus b.
lumbar sympathetic b.
mandibular nerve b.
maxillary nerve b.
mental nerve b.
modified coracoid approach
 infraclavicular brachial plexus b.
motor point b.
nerve b.
neuraxial neurolytic b.
neurolytic celiac plexus b. (NCPB)
neuromuscular b.
nondepolarizing b.
obturator nerve b.
b. osteotomy
paracervical b.
paravertebral lumbar sympathetic b.
penile b.
percutaneous neurolytic
 intercostal b.
peribulbar b.
peripheral nerve b.
phase I, II b.
phrenic nerve b.
2-point nerve b.
preganglionic sympathetic b.
prognostic b.
psoas sheath b.
regional b.
retrobulbar nerve b.
retrocrural celiac plexus b.
right bundle branch b.
ring b.
saddle b.
sciatic-femoral nerve b.
sciatic nerve b.
selective obturator nerve b.
sensory b.

single injection ultrasound-assisted
 femoral nerve b.
single-shot caudal b.
single-shot subarachnoid b.
sinoatrial exit b.
sinus exit b.
skull b.
spinal b.
Steinberg infiltration b.
stellate ganglion b.
subarachnoid b.
subclavian perivascular b.
subdural b.
supine sciatic b.
supraclavicular brachial b.
sympathetic nerve b.
therapeutic nerve b.
tibial augmentation b.
tracheal b.
ultrasound-guided lumbar facet
 nerve b.
upper extremity nerve b.
uterosacral b.
Van Lint lid b.
wrist b.
yoke b.

3-in-1 block
blockade
afferent b.
anesthetic b.
autonomic b.
beta-adrenergic b.
cholinergic b.
epidural neural b.
flickering b.
ganglionic b.
gasserian ganglion b.
interscalene b.
intervertebral disc b.
intravenous regional b.
local anesthetic sympathetic b.
lytic b.
myoneural b.
neurolytic b.
neuromuscular b. (NMB)
nondepolarizing b.
onset of b.
paravertebral somatic nerve b.
preganglionic cardiac sympathetic b.
pulmonary sympathetic b.
residual neuromuscular b.
segmental neural b.

NOTES

blockade *(continued)*
    sensory b.
    sphenopalantine ganglion b.
    stellate ganglion b.
    sympathetic b.
    temporary nerve b.
blockage
    complete b.
    ganglion b.
    shunt b.
blocker
    calcium entry b.
    dihydropyridine calcium channel b.
    ganglion b.
    H_2 b.
    use-dependent sodium channel b.
    wire-guided endobronchial b.
blocking
    b. procedure
    tissue b.
    vecuronium neuromuscular b.
Blom-Singer tracheoesophageal fistula
blood
    b. alcohol concentration
    allogenic b.
    arterial b.
    autologous b.
    b. bank
    b. calculus
    b. cell count
    cerebral b.
    circulating b.
    b. clot
    b. coagulation
    b. coagulation disorder
    b. donation
    b. flow
    b. flow rate
    b. gas
    b. gas analysis
    b. gas exchange
    intraoperatively donated
      autologous b.
    intravenous b.
    b. lactate (BL)
    b. loss
    b. marker
    mediastinal shed b. (MSB)
    MV b.
    occult b.
    b. oxygenation level-dependent
    b. oxygenation level-dependent
      contrast
    oxygen concentration in pulmonary
      capillary b.
    oxygen saturation of hemoglobin of
      arterial b.
    b. patch
    b. patch injection

    b. perfusion
    preoperatively donated
      autologous b.
    b. pressure
    b. pressure monitoring
    b. pressure support
    b. product
    b. product transfusion
    pulmonary capillary b.
    b. substitute
    b. substitute resuscitation
    b. supply
    b. supply artery
    b. transfusion volume
    b. tumor
    UA b.
    umbilical artery b.
    umbilical vein b.
    UV b.
    b. vessel
    b. vessel formation
    b. vessel invasion (BVI)
    b. vessel tumor
blood-air barrier
blood-borne
    b.-b. infection
    b.-b. metastasis
blood-brain
    b.-b. barrier (BBB)
    b.-b. equilibration time
blood-cerebral barrier
blood-cerebrospinal fluid barrier
Bloodgood syndrome
bloodless
    b. amputation
    b. decerebration
    b. field
    b. operation
    b. phlebotomy
    b. zone of necrosis
bloodletting
    general b.
    local b.
blood-liquor barrier
blood-ocular barrier
blood-optic nerve barrier
blood-retinal barrier
bloodstream infection
blood-thymus barrier
blood-tinged
    b.-t. ascites
    b.-t. CSF
blood-urine barrier
bloody peritoneal fluid
Bloom-Raney
    B.-R. modification
    B.-R. modification of Smith-
      Robinson technique
blot hemorrhage

Blount
- B. displacement osteotomy
- B. technique for osteoclasis
- B. tracing technique

blowhole
- b. decompressing colostomy
- b. ileostomy

blow-in fracture

blow-out
- aortic stump b.-o.
- b.-o. fracture

blue
- b. dome breast cyst
- b. dot sign
- b. line
- b. staining
- b. toe syndrome

blue-gray lesion

Blumberg sign

Blumenbach clivus

Blumensaat line

Blumenthal lesion

Blumer shelf

Blundell-Jones technique

blunderbuss apical canal

blunt
- b. carotid injury
- b. eversion carotid endarterectomy
- b. hepatic trauma
- b. liver injury
- b. and sharp dissection
- b. torso injury

blur point

blush
- tumor b.

BMI
- body mass index

B-mode imaging

BNP
- brain natriuretic peptide

boardlike rigidity

Boari
- B. bladder flap
- B. bladder flap procedure
- B. ureteral flap repair

Boari-Ockerblad flap

Boas
- B. point
- B. sign

boatlike abdomen

boat nail

boat-shaped abdomen

Bobath method

bobby-pin abrasion

Bochdalek
- B. gap
- B. hernia

Bock
- B. ganglion
- B. nerve

Boden-Gibb tumor staging

Bodian method

body
- adipose b.
- adrenal b.
- alveolar b.
- Amato b.
- anal foreign b.
- anococcygeal b.
- anorectal foreign b.
- aortic b.
- Arantius b.
- Arnold b.
- artificial vertebral b.
- Aschoff b.
- aspirated foreign b.
- asteroid b.
- b. awareness
- Balbiani b.
- Barr b.
- Bence Jones b.
- Bracht-Wachter b.
- brassy b.
- cancer b.
- carotid b.
- cartilaginous loose b.
- b. cast syndrome
- caudate b.
- cavernous b.
- b. cavity
- b. cell mass
- central fibrous b.
- chromaffin b.
- chromatinic b.
- ciliary b.
- coccidian b.
- coccygeal b.
- colloid b.
- colonic foreign b.
- b. composition analysis
- compressed b.
- compressible cavernous b.
- corneal foreign b.
- Creola b.

NOTES

body *(continued)*
crescent b.
cystoid b.
cytoid b.
dense b.
duodenal foreign b.
Dutcher b.
Ehrlich inner b.
Elschnig b.
esophageal foreign b.
esophageal Lewy b.
external geniculate b.
fat b.
b. fat
fibrous loose b.
foreign b.
b. of gallbladder
Gamna-Gandy b.
gastric foreign b.
gelatin compression b.
geniculate b.
glomus b.
Goldmann-Larson foreign b.
Gordon elementary b.
b. habitus
Hamazaki-Wesenberg b.
Harting b.
Hassall b.
Heinz b.
Heinz-Ehrlich b.
b. hematocrit-venous hematocrit
    ratio
hematoxylin b.
Henle b.
Hensen b.
Highmore b.
Hirano b.
Howell-Jolly b.
hyaline b.
hyaloid b.
b. image
inclusion b.
infrapatellar fat b.
ingested foreign b.
intraarticular loose b.
intraluminal foreign b.
intraocular foreign b.
intraorbital foreign b.
intrauterine foreign b.
intravascular foreign b.
Jaworski b.
juxtaglomerular b.
juxtarestiform b.
Kelvin b.
Lallemand b.
Lallemand-Trousseau b.
Landolt b.
lateral geniculate b.
Lewy b.

Lieutaud b.
loose intraarticular b.
lower gastrointestinal tract
    foreign b.
Luys b.
malpighian b.
mamillary b.
Maragiliano b.
b. mass index (BMI)
Maxwell b.
May-Hegglin b.
melon seed b.
metallic foreign b.
mineral oil foreign b.
Mott b.
Müller duct b.
multilamellar b.
Neill-Mooser b.
newtonian b.
nigroid b.
olivary b.
osteocartilaginous loose b.
osteochondral loose b.
owl's eye inclusion b.
pampiniform b.
pancreatic b.
paranephric b.
paraterminal b.
pectinate b.
pedunculated loose b.
perineal b.
pineal b.
pituitary b.
b. position
Prowazek-Greeff b.
psammoma b.
pubic b.
pyknotic b.
radiopaque foreign b.
rectal foreign b.
refractile b.
Reilly b.
removal of foreign b.
residual b.
restiform b.
retained foreign b.
rice b.
b. righting reflex
rigid b.
Rosenmüller b.
Ross b.
round b.
Rucker b.
sand b.
Sandström b.
Savage perineal b.
b. scanning
Schaumann b.
b. schema

Schiller-Duvall b.
Seidelin b.
selenoid b.
b. side integration
spongy b.
S-shaped b.
b. stalk
striate b.
suprarenal b.
b. surface area (BSA)
b. surface burned
b. surface Laplacian mapping
Symington anococcygeal b.
b. temperature
thoracic vertebral b.
thrombogenic foreign b.
thyroid b.
tracheobronchial foreign b.
trapezoid b.
b. tumor
upper gastrointestinal tract
  foreign b.
vagal b.
vaginal foreign b.
vermiform b.
vertebral b.
vitreous foreign b.
wall of b.
3-b. wear
b. weight
Wesenberg-Hamazaki b.
Winkler b.
wolffian b.
X b.
Y b.
yellow b.

Boehler
  B. calcaneal view
  B. lumbosacral view
Boerema
  B. anterior gastropexy
  B. hernia repair
Boerhaave
  B. gland
  B. syndrome
Bogorad syndrome
Bogros space
Böhler calcaneal angle
Bohlman
  B. anterior cervical vertebrectomy
  B. cervical fusion technique
  B. triple-wire technique

Böhm operation
Bohr
  B. effect
  B. equation
  B. isopleth method
Boitzy open reduction
bolster suture technique
bolt fixation
Bolton-nasion line
Bolton point
bolus
  fluid b.
  b. injection
  b. intravenous anesthesia
  b. intravenous anesthetic technique
  b. thermodilution (BTD)
Bonaccolto-Flieringa vitreous operation
bonded cast restoration
bonding
  adhesive b.
bone
  b. abscess
  Albrecht b.
  allogeneic b.
  antigen-extracted allogeneic b.
  articulation of pisiform b.
  b. autogenous graft
  basilar b.
  basioccipital b.
  basisphenoid b.
  blade b.
  b. block procedure
  breast b.
  Breschet b.
  b. bruise sign
  bundle b.
  calcaneal b.
  calf b.
  capitate b.
  central b.
  cheek b.
  b. chip
  b. chip graft
  collar b.
  compact b.
  3-cornered b.
  cornua of hyoid b.
  cortical b.
  coxal b.
  cranial b.
  cuboid b.
  cuneiform b.

B

NOTES

bone (*continued*)
    b. cyst excision
    b. cyst fracture probability
    b. destruction
    b. disease
    b. dissection
    dorsal talonavicular b.
    ear b.
    ectopic b.
    enchondroma of b.
    endochondral b.
    epactal b.
    epipteric b.
    episternal b.
    ethmoid b.
    exoccipital b.
    b. exposure
    facial b.
    first cuneiform b.
    flank b.
    b. flap
    b. flap osteitis
    flower b.
    b. formation
    b. fragment
    frontal b.
    Goethe b.
    b. graft bed
    b. graft collapse
    b. graft decompression
    b. graft extrusion
    b. graft incorporation
    b. graft placement
    b. graft repair
    b. graft substitute
    b. graft substitute graft
    greater multangular b.
    hamate b.
    heel b.
    hip b.
    hollow b.
    hooked b.
    b. hunger
    hyoid b.
    iliac b.
    incarial b.
    b. ingrowth fixation
    innominate b.
    intermediate cuneiform b.
    interparietal b.
    irregular b.
    ischial b.
    jaw b.
    jugal b.
    Krause b.
    lacrimal b.
    lamellar b.
    lentiform b.
    lingual b.

long b.
b. loss
lower jaw b.
lunate b.
lyophilization of b.
b. marrow aspiration
b. marrow aspiration and biopsy
b. marrow augmentation
b. marrow dysfunction
b. marrow examination
b. marrow failure
b. marrow graft
b. marrow infiltration
b. marrow lesion
b. marrow pressure
b. marrow puncture
b. marrow transplantation
b. mass
b. matrix
mesethmoid b.
metacarpal b.
b. metastasis
metatarsal b.
multangular b.
navicular b.
occipital b.
osteonal lamellar b.
osteoporotic b.
b. pain
palatine b.
parietal b.
b. peg graft
periotic b.
petrosal b.
pipe b.
Pirie b.
pisiform b.
pneumatic b.
postsphenoid b.
preinterparietal b.
presphenoid b.
pubic b.
pyramidal b.
b. regeneration
b. resection
Riolan b.
sacred b.
scaphoid b.
second cuneiform b.
semilunar b.
sesamoid b.
shank b.
shin b.
short b.
sieve b.
sphenoid b.
sphenoidal turbinated b.
suprainterparietal b.
suprasternal b.

sutural b.
tail b.
talonavicular b.
b. tamp
b. technique
temporal b.
thigh b.
tongue b.
triangular b.
triquetral b.
b. tumor
turbinated b.
tympanic b.
tympanohyal b.
unciform b.
upper jaw b.
Vesalius b.
b. wedge
wedge b.
wormian b.
yoke b.
zygomatic b.
bone-cement interface
bone-holding clamp
bone-implant interface
bone-ligament dissection
bone-patellar tendon-bone preparation
bone-retinaculum-bone autograft graft
bone-screw interface strength
bone-tendon-bone graft
bone-to-bone graft
Bonferroni correction
Bonfiglio
B. bone graft
B. modification
B. modification of Phemister
technique
Bonfiglio-Bardenstein technique
Bonnaire method
Bonner position
Bonnet
B. capsule
B. enucleation operation
Bonney
B. abdominal hysterectomy
B. test
Bonola technique
bony
b. bridge resection
b. deformity
b. demineralization
b. dissection

b. element destruction
b. excrescence
b. exposure
b. fragment
b. labyrinth
b. landmark
b. lesion
b. mass
b. metastasis
b. necrosis
b. necrosis and destruction
b. procedure
b. projection
b. semicircular canal
b. structure
Bonzel operation
book thoracotomy
boomerang-shaped lesion
boost technique
bootstrap
b. dilation
b. 2-vessel angioplasty
b. 2-vessel technique
boot-top fracture
Boplant graft
Bora
B. centralization
B. operation
B. technique
Borchgrevink method
border
frontal b.
interosseous b.
b. involvement
mesenteric b.
nasal b.
occipital b.
parietal b.
b. ray amputation
squamous b.
b. tissue
b. tissue of Jacoby
b. tissue movement
vermilion b.
Borggreve
B. limb rotation
B. method
Borggreve-Hall technique
Borg treadmill exertion scale
boron neutron-capture therapy
Borrmann
B. carcinoma (type I–IV)

NOTES

Borrmann *(continued)*
    B. gastric cancer classification
    B. gastric cancer typing systems
      classification (type I–IV)
Bose
    B. nail fold excision
    B. operation
    B. procedure
Bosniak classification
boss
    carpal b.
Bossalino blepharoplasty operation
bosselation
Bosworth
    B. approach
    B. femoroischial transplantation
    B. fracture
    B. spinal fusion
    B. tendo calcaneus repair
both-bone fracture
both-column fracture
Böttcher
    B. canal
    B. space
botulinum A toxin
Bouchut respiration
bougienage technique
bounce point
boundary
    air-bone-tissue b.
    inferior b.
    superior b.
boutonnière
    b. deformity
    b. hand dislocation
    b. incision
Bovero muscle
Bovie
    B. cauterization
    B. coagulation
bowel
    b. abscess
    b. anastomosis
    b. bypass
    b. bypass syndrome
    b. cleansing
    compliant b.
    b. continuity
    denuded b.
    dilated loop of b.
    b. dilation
    edematous b.
    b. fistula
    b. function
    b. habits
    b. injury
    b. lavage
    b. length
    b. loop

    b. loop air
    b. movement
    Noble surgical plication of b.
    obstructed b.
    b. obstruction
    b. perforation
    b. plication
    b. preparation
    prepared large b.
    b. refashioning procedure
    b. resection
    b. sounds
    b. stoma
    supple b.
    b. wall
    b. wall hematoma
    weakened b.
Bowen cavity primer
Bowers technique
bowing
    b. deformity
    b. fracture
bowleg deformity
Bowles technique
Bowman
    B. gland
    B. membrane
    B. operation
    B. space
bow-tie
    b.-t. knot
    b.-t. sign
    b.-t. stitch
boxer fracture
Box technique
Boyce
    longitudinal nephrotomy of B.
    B. position
Boyce-Vest procedure
Boyd
    B. ankle amputation
    B. approach
    B. classification
    B. hip disarticulation
    B. operation
    B. point
Boyd-Anderson
    B.-A. biceps tendon repair
    B.-A. technique
Boyd-Bosworth procedure
Boyden
    B. chamber technique
    B. sphincter
Boyd-Griffin trochanteric fracture
    classification
Boyd-Ingram-Bourkhard treatment
Boyd-McLeod
    B.-M. procedure
    B.-M. tennis elbow technique

Boyd-Sisk
>B.-S. approach
>B.-S. posterior capsulorrhaphy

Boyer bursa
Boyes brachioradialis transfer technique
Boytchev procedure
Bozeman
>B. operation
>B. position
>B. suture technique

BP
>bronchopleural

BPB
>biliopancreatic bypass
>brachial plexus block

BPCF
>bronchopleurocutaneous fistula

BPD
>biparietal diameter
>bronchopulmonary dysplasia

BP fistula
BPH
>benign prostatic hyperplasia
>benign prostatic hypertrophy

BPI
>Brief Pain Inventory

BPPV
>benign paroxysmal positional vertigo

BPTT
>brachial plexus tension test

Braasch bulb technique
brachia (*pl. of* brachium)
brachial
>b. anesthesia
>b. arteriotomy
>b. artery
>b. artery approach
>b. cleft cyst
>b. fascia
>b. gland
>b. muscle
>b. plexopathy
>b. plexus
>b. plexus block (BPB)
>b. plexus block anesthetic
> technique
>b. plexus infiltration
>b. plexus nerve
>b. plexus repair
>b. plexus tension test (BPTT)
>b. plexus traction injury
>b. region

brachialis
brachioaxillary
>b. bridge
>b. bridge graft fistula

brachiocephalic
>b. trunk
>b. trunk artery
>b. vein
>b. vessel angioplasty

brachiocephalicus
brachiodxillary bridge
brachioplasty
brachioradialis flap
brachioradial muscle
brachiosubclavian
>b. bridge
>b. bridge graft
>b. bridge graft fistula

brachiosubclavian bridge
brachium, pl. **brachia**
Bracht maneuver
Bracht-Wachter
>B.-W. body
>B.-W. lesion

brachybasocamptodactyly
brachybasophalangia
brachycheilia
brachydactyly
brachyfacial
brachygnathia
brachymorphic
brachypellic pelvis
brachyprosopic
brachyrhinia
brachyrhynchus
brachystaphyline
brachysyndactyly
brachytherapy
>endobronchial b.
>interstitial b.

bracing
>external b.
>fracture b.

bracket
>b. modification
>b. slot angulation

Brackett-Osgood posterior approach
Brackett-Osgood-Putti-Abbott technique
Brackett osteotomy
Brackin
>B. incision

NOTES

B

Brackin *(continued)*
   B. technique
   B. ureterointestinal anastomosis
Bradford fusion
Bradley
   B. method
   B. method of prepared childbirth
Brady-Jewett technique
bradykinesia
Bragg peak proton-beam therapy
Brahms procedure
braidlike lesion
Brailey operation
brain
   b. abscess
   b. arteriovenous malformation
      treatment (BAVM)
   b. biopsy
   b. concussion
   b. congestion
   b. contusion
   b. death
   b. edema
   b. herniation
   b. infection
   b. injury
   b. laceration
   b. mass
   b. metastasis
   b. natriuretic peptide (BNP)
   b. neoplasm
   b. puncture
   b. region
   respirator b.
   b. revascularization
   b. stimulation
   b. temperature
   b. transplantation
   b. tumor
   b. tumor headache
   B. Tumor Registry
brain-dead patient
brainstem
   b. compression
   b. evoked response
   b. hemorrhage
   b. hypoperfusion
   b. lesion
braking radiation
branch
   acetabular b.
   acromial b.
   adrenal b.
   anastomotic b.
   anterior basal b.
   anterior cutaneous b.
   arterial b.
   articular b.
   ascending anterior b.

ascending posterior b.
auricular b.
basal tentorial b.
buccal b.
capsular b.
carotid sinus b.
caudate b.
celiac b.
cervical b.
clavicular b.
communicating b.
deep palmar b.
deep plantar b.
deltoid b.
descending anterior b.
descending posterior b.
digastric b.
dorsal b.
epiploic b.
esophageal b.
external b.
faucial b.
frontal b.
ganglionic b.
gastric b.
genital b.
glandular b.
gonadal b.
hepatic b.
iliac b.
inferior temporal b.
inguinal b.
internal b.
joint b.
lateral calcaneal b.
lateral nasal b.
b. lesion
lingual b.
lingular b.
lumbar b.
major sinistral b.
mammary b.
marginal mandibular b.
marginal tentorial b.
mastoid b.
medial cutaneous b.
medial mammary b.
mediastinal b.
meningeal b.
mental b.
occipital b.
omental b.
orbital b.
ovarian b.
b. pad
palmar b.
palpebral b.
pancreatic b.
parietal b.

parotid b.
pectoral b.
perforating b.
pericardial b.
petrosal b.
pharyngeal b.
phrenicoabdominal b.
posterior basal b.
pterygoid b.
pubic b.
recurrent meningeal b.
renal b.
right b.
saphenous b.
sectorial b.
sinoatrial nodal b.
splenic b.
sternal b.
stylohyoid b.
subscapular b.
superficial b.
superior cervical cardiac b.
superior labial b.
superior laryngeal nerve external b.
suprahyoid b.
sympathetic b.
temporal b.
thoracic cardiac b.
thymic b.
tonsillar b.
tracheal b.
tubal b.
ulnar b.
ureteral b.
ureteric b.
zygomatic b.
zygomaticofacial b.
zygomaticotemporal b.
branched
    b. calculus
    b. vascular graft
branchial
    b. anomaly
    b. cartilage
    b. cyst
    b. fistula
    b. sinus
branching
    b. canal
    b. morphogenesis
    b. tubule formation
branchiogenous cyst

branchiomeric muscle
Brandt-Andrews maneuver
Brand tendon transfer technique
Brantigan procedure
Brantigan-Voshell procedure
Brasdor method
brassy body
Braun
    B. anastomosis
    B. procedure
    B. shoulder tenotomy
Braune
    B. canal
    B. muscle
Braun-Jaboulay gastroenterostomy
Braun-Wangensteen graft
brawny
    b. arm
    b. induration
breach
    serosal b.
breakdown
    anastomotic b.
    epithelial b.
    muscle b.
    sepsis-induced muscle b.
break point
breast
    b. abscess
    accessory b.
    adenoma of b.
    b. approach thyroidectomy
    b. augmentation
    b. biopsy
    b. biopsy tissue
    b. bone
    b. calcification
    b. cancer
    B. Cancer Detection Demonstration
      Project
    b. cancer-related mutation
    b. cancer risk
    b. cancer risk prediction
    b. cancer-specific survival (BCSS)
    b. carcinoma
    comedocarcinoma of b.
    b. conservation therapy (BCT)
    b. contour
    b. cyst
    b. cyst aspiration
    b. discharge
    b. flap

NOTES

breast *(continued)*
 B. Imaging Reporting and Data System (BI-RADS)
 b. implant
 b. incision
 b. irradiation
 b. lymphatic mapping
 male b.
 b. mctastasis
 b. mucocele
 b. parenchyma
 b. preservation
 b. reconstruction
 b. reduction
 b. reduction technique
 b. resection
 b. size
 b. skin envelope
 b. stimulation contraction test
 supernumerary b.
breast-conserving
 b.-c. method
 b.-c. procedure
 b.-c. surgery
 b.-c. technique
 b.-c. therapy
breast-lift mastopexy
breast-milk jaundice
breast-preservation therapy
breast-sparing mastectomy
breath
 b. excretion test
 b. stacking
breathing
 apneustic b.
 Biot b.
 b. circuit
 continuous positive pressure b. (CPPB)
 intermittent positive pressure b. (IPPB)
 b. lung
 b. method
 negative inspiratory b.
 pattern of b.
 positive-negative pressure b. (PNPB)
 sign mechanism for ventilator b.
 spontaneous b.
 ventilator b.
 work of b. (WOB)
Brecher-Cronkite
 B.-C. method
 B.-C. technique
Brecher new methylene blue technique
breech
 b. extraction
 b. head
bregma

bregma-mentum projection
bregmatic fontanelle
bregmatolambdoid arc
bregmatomastoid
 b. suture
 b. suture technique
Brenner
 B. gastrojejunostomy technique
 B. operation
brephoplastic graft
Breschet
 B. bone
 B. canal
 B. hiatus
Brescia-Cimino
 B.-C. A-V fistula
 B.-C. graft
Breslow
 B. classification
 B. thickness
Brett-Campbell tibial osteotomy
Breuer-Hering inflation reflex
Breuerton view
brevis
 extensor carpi radialis b. (ECRB)
 extensor digitorum b.
 extensor pollicis b.
Bricker
 B. conduit
 B. operation
 B. procedure
 B. ureteroileostomy
Brickner position
bridge
 adhesive resin-bonded b.
 brachioaxillary b.
 brachiosubclavian b.
 colostomy b.
 conjugation b.
 extension b.
 fascial b.
 Gaskell b.
 b. graft
 loop ostomy b.
 membrane b.
 mucosal b.
 mylohyoid b.
 B. operation
 b. organ transplantation
 b. pedicle flap
 b. pedicle flap operation
 b. plate fixation
 retention suture b.
 suture b.
bridgelike
 b. lesion
 b. septum
bridging syndesmophyte

bridle
>   B. procedure
>   b. suture technique

Brief Pain Inventory (BPI)
Briggs strabismus operation
Bright disease
brightness modulation
brim
>   pelvic b.
>   b. sign

brine flotation method
Brinell hardness indenter point
Brisbane method
brisement therapy
Bristow-Helfet procedure
Bristow-May procedure
Bristow operation
brittle
>   b. nail
>   b. nail syndrome

broad
>   b. fascia
>   b. ligament hernia
>   b. uterine ligament

broadband attenuation
Broadbent registration point
Broadbent-Woolf 4-limb Z-plasty
broadest muscle
broad-spectrum antibiotic
Broca
>   B. basilar angle
>   B. facial angle
>   B. pouch
>   B. visual plane

Brock
>   B. incision
>   B. infundibulectomy
>   B. operation
>   B. procedure

Brockenbrough
>   B. technique
>   B. transseptal commissurotomy

Brockhurst technique
Brockman incision
Brockman-Nissen wrist arthrodesis
Brödel bloodless line
Broders
>   B. index
>   B. index of malignant tumor
>   classification

Brodie
>   B. bursa
>   B. metaphysial abscess

Brodie-Trendelenburg tourniquet test
Brodsky-Tullos-Gartsman approach
Broesike fossa
Bromage scale
bromide
bromination
Bromley foreign body operation
Brom repair
bronchi (*pl. of* bronchus)
bronchia (*pl. of* bronchium)
bronchial
>   b. adenocarcinoma
>   b. adenoma
>   b. artery
>   b. brush biopsy
>   b. brushing
>   b. carcinoma
>   b. fracture
>   b. gland
>   b. inflammation
>   b. inhalation challenge test
>   b. respiration
>   b. sleeve procedure
>   b. sleeve resection
>   b. tract
>   b. tree
>   b. vein

bronchial-associated lymphoid tissue
bronchiogenic
bronchiolar adenocarcinoma
bronchiole
>   respiratory b.
>   terminal b.

bronchioli (*pl. of* bronchiolus)
bronchiolitis
>   obliterative b.

bronchioloalveolar
>   b. adenocarcinoma
>   b. carcinoma

bronchiolopulmonary
bronchiolus, pl. **bronchioli**
bronchiomediastinalis
bronchitis
bronchium, pl. **bronchia**
bronchoalveolar carcinoma
bronchobiliary fistula
bronchocavernous respiration
bronchoconstriction

B

NOTES

bronchoesophageal
  b. fistula
  b. muscle
bronchoesophageus
bronchoesophagoscopy
bronchogenic adenocarcinoma
bronchomediastinal trunk
bronchoplasty
  balloon b.
bronchopleural (BP)
  b. fistula
  b. leak squeak
bronchopleurocutaneous fistula (BPCF)
bronchopneumonia
  sequestration b.
bronchoprovocation test
bronchopulmonary
  b. dysplasia (BPD)
  b. fistula
  b. foregut malformation
  b. segment
bronchorrhaphy
bronchoscope-guided intubation
bronchoscopic
  b. needle biopsy
  b. photodynamic therapy
bronchoscopy
  b. anesthetic technique
  fiberoptic b.
  flexible fiberoptic b.
  laser b.
  rigid b.
  ultrasound-guided b.
bronchospasm
  exercise-induced b.
  induced b.
bronchospirography
bronchospirometry
bronchostomy
bronchotomy
bronchotracheal
bronchovesicular respiration
bronchus, pl. **bronchi**
  ectatic b.
  intermediate b.
  lobar b.
  right main b.
  segmental b.
  stem b.
Bronson foreign body removal operation
Brooke ileostomy
Brooks-Jenkins atlantoaxial fusion technique
Brooks-Seddon transfer technique
Brooks technique
Brooks-type fusion
Broomhead medial approach
Brophy operation

Broström
  B. injection technique
  B. procedure
Broström-Gould foot procedure
brow
  b. fixation
  b. position
brow-anterior position
brow-down position
browlift
brown
  b. adipose tissue
  b. atrophy
  B. dietary method
  B. dietary method for colon preparation
  b. fat tumor
  B. knee approach
  B. knee joint reconstruction
  B. lateral approach
  B. technique
  B. and Wickham pressure profile method
Brown-Beard technique
brown-black lesion
Brown-Brenn technique
Brown-Dodge method
Browning vein
Brown-McHardy pneumatic mercury bougie dilation
Brown-Wickham technique
brow-posterior position
brow-up position
B-RTO
  balloon-occluded retrograde transvenous obliteration
Bruce bundle
Bruch membrane
Brudzinski sign
Bruger
  cul-de-sac of B.
Bruhat
  B. laser fimbrioplasty
  B. technique
Bruhn method
bruit
  peripheral b.
Bruner approach
Brunner
  B. gland
  B. modified incision
  B. palmar incision
Brunn nest
Brunschwig operation
Bruser
  B. knee approach
  B. lateral approach
  B. skin incision
  B. technique

brush
 b. biopsy
 b. cytology
 b. technique filling
brush-border
 b.-b. membrane
 b.-b. membrane vesicle
brushing
 bronchial b.
bruxism
Bryan
 B. arthroplasty
 B. procedure
Bryan-Morrey
 B.-M. elbow approach
 B.-M. extensive posterior approach
 B.-M. technique
Bryant operation
BSA
 body surface area
BSO
 bilateral salpingo-oophorectomy
BTD
 bolus thermodilution
bubble
 b. oxygenation
 b. ventriculography
bubbly bone lesion
bucca, pl. **buccae**
buccal
 b. artery
 b. aspect
 b. branch
 b. cavity
 b. drug administration
 b. fat pad
 b. mucosal flap
 b. nerve
 b. ostectomy
 b. restoration
 b. smear
 b. space
 b. space abscess
 b. space infection
 b. surface
 b. transmucosal delivery
 b. vein
buccinator
 b. artery
 b. crest
 b. muscle
 b. nerve

 b. node
 b. plication
 b. space
buccolingual (BL)
 b. plane
 b. relation
bucconeural duct
buccoocclusal line angle
buccopharyngeal
 b. approach
 b. fascia
 b. space
Buck
 B. fascia
 B. method
bucket-handle
 b.-h. fracture
 b.-h. incision
 b.-h. tear
Buck-Gramcko
 B.-G. pollicization
 B.-G. technique
bucking
 coughing and b.
buckle
 b. fracture
 scleral b.
Budd-Chiari
 B.-C. syndrome
 B.-C. syndrome with Behçet disease
 B.-C. syndrome without Behçet disease
Budin-Chandler method
Budinger blepharoplasty operation
Bugg-Boyd technique
Buie position
built-in angulation
Buist method
bulb
 b. deformity
 duodenal b.
 jugular venous b.
 olfactory b.
 Rouget b.
 b. suction
bulbar
 b. cephalic pain tractotomy
 b. sheath fascia
bulbocavernosus
 b. fat flap

NOTES

bulbocavernosus *(continued)*
>   b. fat pad
>   b. muscle

bulboid
bulbospongiosus muscle
bulbourethral gland
bulbourethralis
bulbous internal auditory canal
bulb-tip retrograde study
bulge
>   gastric b.

bulk
>   b. pack technique
>   tumor b.

bulkhead method
bulla, pl. **bullae**
>   ethmoid b.

bulldog head
bullectomy
>   transaxillary apical b.

bullet
>   b. trajectory
>   b. wound

bullous
>   b. edema
>   b. granulomatous inflammation
>   b. skin lesion

bull's eye macular lesion
bumper fracture
bunching
>   b. maneuver
>   b. suture technique

Buncke technique
bundle
>   anterior ground b.
>   anteromedial b.
>   arcuate nerve fiber b.
>   Arnold b.
>   atrioventricular b.
>   A-V b.
>   Bachmann b.
>   b. bone
>   b. branch block (BBB)
>   b. branch reentrant tachycardia
>   b. branch reentry
>   Bruce b.
>   cingulum b.
>   coherent b.
>   commissural b.
>   fiber b.
>   b. fiber
>   fiberoptic b.
>   Gierke respiratory b.
>   Held b.
>   Helweg b.
>   His b.
>   Hoche b.
>   IG b.
>   image guide b.

>   inferior arcuate b.
>   intercostal b.
>   intermediate b.
>   b. of Itis
>   James b.
>   Keith b.
>   Kent b.
>   Kent-His b.
>   Killian b.
>   Krause respiratory b.
>   lateral ground b.
>   LG b.
>   light guide b.
>   Lissauer b.
>   Loewenthal b.
>   maculopapillary b.
>   Mahaim b.
>   main b.
>   master IG b.
>   Meynert retroflex b.
>   microfilament b.
>   Monakow b.
>   neovascular b.
>   nerve fiber b.
>   neurovascular b.
>   olfactory b.
>   olivocochlear b.
>   papillomacular nerve fiber b.
>   paracentral nerve fiber b.
>   Pick b.
>   posterior longitudinal b.
>   posterolateral b.
>   precommissural b.
>   predorsal b.
>   principal fiber b.
>   Rathke b.
>   respiratory b.
>   Schütz b.
>   sensory nerve fiber b.
>   solitary b.
>   b. of Stanley Kent
>   superior arcuate b.
>   superior gluteal neurovascular b.
>   Thorel b.
>   Türck b.
>   vascular b.
>   Vicq d'Azyr b.

Bunge amputation
bunion
>   b. deformity
>   b. formation

bunionectomy
>   Akin b.
>   Austin b.
>   chevron b.
>   DuVries-Mann modified b.
>   Hauser b.
>   Joplin b.
>   Keller b.

Kreuscher b.
Lapidus b.
Ludloff b.
Mayo-Heuter b.
McBride b.
Peabody-Mitchell b.
Reverdin b.
Reverdin-Laird b.
Reverdin-McBride b.
Silver b.
tailor b.
tricorrectional b.
Wilson b.

bunk-bed fracture
Bunnell
B. atraumatic technique
B. modification
B. modification of Steindler
flexorplasty
B. opponensplasty
B. stitch
B. suture technique
B. tendon repair
B. tendon transfer technique

Bunnell-Williams procedure
Bunyavirus infection
**buprenorphine narcotic analgesic
therapy**
bur
b. hole
b. hole placement
Burch
B. bladder suspension
B. bladder suspension method
B. bladder suspension procedure
B. bladder suspension technique
B. colposuspension
B. colpourethropexy
B. eye evisceration operation
B. iliopectineal ligament
urethrovesical suspension
B. modification

Burdach tract
burden
tumor b.
**Burger technique for scapulothoracic
disarticulation**
Burgess
B. below-knee amputation
B. method
B. technique
Burhenne biliary duct stone extraction

buried
b. flap
b. mass far-and-near suture
technique
b. penis
Burkhalter
B. modification of Stiles-Bunnell
technique
B. transfer technique
burn
b. boutonnière deformity
b. classification
corneal alkali b.
b. débridement
first-degree b.
full-thickness b.
b. injury
irrigation b.
b. pain
partial-thickness b.
plaster cast application b.
radiation b.
b. scar carcinoma
second-degree b.
superficial b.
third-degree b.
burned
body surface b.
**Burnet-Talmadge-Lederberg theory of
antibody formation**
Burnett syndrome
burn-induced muscle proteolysis
burning
b. dysesthesia
b. feet syndrome
b. pain
burn-out procedure
Burns-Haney incision
Burns space
Burow
B. flap operation
B. quantitative method
B. triangle
B. vein
BURP
backward, upward, rightward pressure
BURP maneuver
Burrows technique
bursa, pl. **bursae**
Achilles b.
b. Achillis
acromial b.

NOTES

bursa *(continued)*
    anserine b.
    anterior tibial b.
    bicipitoradial b.
    b. bicipitoradialis
    Boyer b.
    Brodie b.
    calcaneal b.
    Calori b.
    coracobrachial b.
    deep infrapatellar b.
    Fleischmann b.
    gluteofemoral b.
    iliac b.
    iliopectineal b.
    infrahyoid b.
    infrapatellar b.
    infraspinatus b.
    intermuscular gluteal b.
    intertendinous b.
    intrapatellar b.
    ischial b.
    laryngeal b.
    medial malleolar subcutaneous b.
    b. of Monro
    b. mucosa
    olecranon b.
    omental b.
    ovarian b.
    pharyngeal b.
    prepatellar b.
    radial b.
    retrocalcaneal b.
    retrohyoid b.
    subacromial b.
    subcoracoid b.
    subcutaneous acromial b.
    subcutaneous calcaneal b.
    subcutaneous infrapatellar b.
    subcutaneous olecranon b.
    subdeltoid b.
    subfascial prepatellar b.
    subhyoid b.
    sublingual b.
    subscapular b.
    subtendinous iliac b.
    subtendinous prepatellar b.
    suprapatellar b.
    synovial b.
    tibial intertendinous b.
    triceps b.
    trochanteric b.
    trochlear synovial b.
    ulnar b.
bursa-equivalent tissue
bursal
    b. flap
    b. projection
    b. sac
    b. tissue
bursectomy
burst
    b. fracture
    b. spike button
bursting dislocation
burst-type laceration
Burton line
Burwell-Scott modification of Watson-Jones incision
Buschke-Löwenstein tumor
Butchart staging classification
Butler
    B. fifth toe operation
    B. procedure
    B. procedure to correct overlapping toes
butterfly
    b. flap
    b. fracture
    b. fracture fragment
    b. patch
    b. pattern
buttocks pad
button
    b. abscess
    burst spike b.
    b. 1-step gastrostomy
    stoma b.
    b. suture technique
buttonhole
    b. approach
    b. deformity
    b. fracture
    b. iridectomy
    b. operation
    b. puncture technique for hemodialysis needle insertion
    b. skin incision
    b. suture technique
Buxton bolus suture technique
Buzzard maneuver
Buzzi operation
BVI
    blood vessel invasion
Byers flap
bypass
    Alden loop gastric b.
    b. anesthesia
    aortofemoral b.
    aortoiliac b.
    aortorenal b.
    Aria coronary b.
    axilloaxillary b.
    axillobifemoral b.
    axillofemoral b.
    axillounifemoral b.
    biliary enteric b.

biliointestinal b. (BIB)
biliopancreatic b. (BPB)
bowel b.
cardiac b. (CBP)
cardiopulmonary b. (CPB)
carotid artery b.
carotid-subclavian artery b.
cervical-to-MCA b.
CFA-SFA b.
coronary artery b.
dual-temperature cardiopulmonary b.
end-to-end jejunoileal b.
end-to-side jejunoileal b.
exclusion b.
extraanatomic b.
extracorporeal venous b.
extracranial-intracranial b.
b. failure
femoral-popliteal artery b.
femoral-tibial-peroneal b.
femorodistal b.
femoropopliteal b.
full cardiopulmonary b.
gastric b.
gastric loop b.
b. graft catheterization
Greenville gastric b.
Griffen Roux-en-Y b.
Hallberg biliointestinal b.
hand-assisted laparoscopic gastric b.
hepatorenal b.
ileojejunal b.
infrainguinal b.
infrapopliteal b.
in situ b.
jejunoileal b. (JIB)
laparoscopic gastric b.
left atrium-to-femoral artery
  circulatory b.
Litwak aortic b.
long-limb gastric artery b.
loop gastric b.
lower extremity b.

lymphaticovenous b.
b. method
minimally invasive direct coronary
  artery b. (MIDCAB)
nonanatomic renal b.
obturator b.
off-pump coronary artery b.
  (OPCAB)
b. operation
operative biliary b.
palliative b.
pancreatic b.
partial cardiopulmonary b.
partial ileal b.
Payne-DeWind jejunoileal b.
petrous-to-supraclinoid b.
primary antecubital jump b. (PAJB)
b. procedure
Roux-en-Y biliary b.
Roux-en-Y gastric b. (RYGB)
saphenous ICA b.
saphenous vein b.
Scopinaro pancreaticobiliary b.
Scott jejunoileal b.
Silastic ring vertical-banded
  gastric b. (SRVGB)
simple b.
subclavian-subclavian b.
superficial temporal artery-to-
  MCA b.
b. surgery
b. technique
thoracofemoral b.
b. tract
transected vertical gastric b.
venovenous b. (VVB)
venovenous extracorporeal b.
vertical gastric b.
Byron
  B. Smith ectropion operation
  B. Smith lazy-T correction
Bywaters lesion
Byzantine arch palate

NOTES

C

C graft
C sliding osteotomy
CA19-9
cancer antigen 19-9
CABG
coronary artery bypass graft
redo CABG
cable wire suture technique
Cabot-Nesbit orchiopexy
Cabot trumpet valve
cachexia
cancer c.
muscle c.
CACI
computer-assisted controlled infusion
CACT
celite-activated clotting time
CAD
cadaver donor
cadaver
c. donor (CAD)
c. renal preservation
cadaveric
c. donor
c. donor hepatectomy
c. hand transplant
c. whole organ transplant
CAF
coronary artery fistula
caffeine and halothane contracture test (CHCT)
cage
thoracic c.
Cairns
C. maneuver
C. operation
C. trabeculectomy
Cajal
C. gold-sublimate method
C. uranium silver method
cake kidney
Calandriello procedure
calcaneal
c. apophysitis
c. arterial network
c. artery
c. avulsion fracture
c. bone
c. bursa
c. displaced fracture
c. fracture reduction
c. inclination angle
c. L osteotomy
c. process

c. region
c. spur syndrome
c. stance position
c. sulcus
c. tendon
c. tenodesis
c. tuber
c. tubercle
calcaneal-second metatarsal angle inclination angle
calcanean tendon
calcanei (*pl. of* calcaneus)
calcaneoastragaloid
calcaneocavovarus deformity
calcaneocavus deformity
calcaneocuboid articulation
calcaneofibular
calcaneonavicular bar resection
calcaneoscaphoid
calcaneotibial fusion
calcaneovalgus deformity
calcaneovarus deformity
calcaneum
calcaneus, pl. calcanei
calcar
calcareous
c. artery
c. infiltration
c. metastasis
calcarina
calcarine artery
calces (*pl. of* calx)
calcific aortic stenosis
calcification
breast c.
clustered c.
focal c.
intratumoral c.
c. line
linear c.
multiple c.
subependymal brain c.
c. zone
calcified
c. gallbladder
c. granulomatous inflammation
c. lesion
c. liver metastasis
c. renal mass
calcifying metastasis
calciotraumatic line
calcipexy
calcitonin
calcitriol supplementation

C

calcium
    c. carbonate supplementation
    c. entry blocker
    c. pyrophosphate deposition disease
    c. sensor
calcium-sensing receptor
calculous
    c. cholecystitis
    c. formation
    c. gallbladder
calculus, pl. calculi
    alvine c.
    apatite c.
    bile duct c.
    biliary c.
    bladder c.
    blood c.
    branched c.
    caliceal diverticular c.
    cat's eye c.
    cerebral c.
    cholesterol c.
    combination c.
    common duct c.
    coral c.
    cystine c.
    decubitus c.
    dendritic c.
    ductal c.
    encysted c.
    fibrin c.
    gallbladder c.
    gastric c.
    hard c.
    hemic c.
    hepatic duct c.
    impacted c.
    infection c.
    intestinal c.
    matrix c.
    c. migration
    mulberry c.
    nephritic c.
    oxalate c.
    pancreatic c.
    pleural c.
    pocketed c.
    preputial c.
    primary renal c.
    prostatic c.
    renal c.
    secondary renal c.
    staghorn c.
    struvite c.
    urethral c.
    urinary c.
    vesical c.
    weddellite c.
    whewellite c.

Caldwell-Coleman flatfoot technique
Caldwell-Luc
    C.-L. approach
    C.-L. incision
    C.-L. operation
    C.-L. window procedure
Caldwell-Moloy
    C.-M. classification
    C.-M. method
Caldwell projection
calf, pl. calves
    c. bone
Calhoun-Hagler lens extraction operation
caliber
    airway c.
calibrated electrical stimulation
calibration
    c. curve
    oscillometric c.
    c. overshoot
caliceal, calyceal
    c. abnormality
    c. diverticular calculus
    c. diverticulum
    c. extension
    c. fistula
    c. fornix
    c. infundibulum
    c. nephrostolithotomy
calicectasis
calicectomy
calices (*pl. of* calix)
caliciform, calyciform
calicine, calycine
calicoplasty, calycoplasty (*var. of* calioplasty)
calicotomy, calycotomy (*var. of* caliotomy)
caliectasis
caliectomy
caligation
calioplasty, calicoplasty, calyoplasty
caliorrhaphy, calyorrhaphy
caliotomy, calicotomy, calyotomy
calix, pl. calices
    major c.
    minor c.
    c. puncture
Callahan
    C. approach
    C. extension
    C. extension of cervical injury
    C. fusion technique
    C. operation
    C. root canal filling method
Callander amputation
Callender cell-type classification
callosal disconnection syndrome

callosomarginal artery
callosotomy
    corpus c.
callus
    c. formation
    fracture c.
    irritation c.
    c. response
Calori bursa
caloric
    c. expenditure
    c. irrigation
calorimetry
Calot triangle
calvaria, pl. **calvariae**
calvarial free bone graft
calves (*pl. of* calf)
calx, pl. **calces**
calyceal (*var. of* caliceal)
calycectomy
calyciform (*var. of* caliciform)
calycine (*var. of* calicine)
calycle
calycoplasty (*var. of* calicoplasty)
calycotomy (*var. of* caliotomy)
calyoplasty (*var. of* calioplasty)
calyorrhaphy (*var. of* caliorrhaphy)
calyotomy (*var. of* caliotomy)
calyx, pl. **calyces**
CAM
    cystic adenomatoid malformation
Cambridge classification
cameral fistula
Cameron femoral component removal
Camey
    C. enterocystoplasty
    C. enterocystoplasty urinary
      diversion
    C. I, II operation
    C. ileocystoplasty
    C. procedure
Camino catheter technique
Camitz technique
Campbell
    C. interpositional arthroplasty
    C. onlay bone graft
    C. osteotomy
    C. posterior shoulder approach
    C. posterolateral approach
    C. resection arthroplasty
    C. technique
    C. triceps reflection

Campbell-Akbarnia procedure
Campbell-Goldthwait procedure
Camper
    C. chiasm
    C. fascia
    C. ligament
    C. line
    C. plane
Camp-Gianturco method
Campodonico
    C. canal
    C. operation
campotomy
camptomelic syndrome
Campylobacter **infection**
Campylobacter-**like**
    C.-l. organism (CLO)
    C.-l. organism biopsy
    C.-l. organism test (CLOtest)
Canadian Cardiovascular Society
   classification
canal
    abdominal c.
    accessory palatine c.
    accessory root c.
    acoustic c.
    additional c.
    adductor c.
    Alcock c.
    alimentary c.
    alveolar c.
    anal c.
    anterior condylar c.
    anterior semicircular c.
    anterior vertical c.
    antropyloric c.
    apical c.
    c. of Arantius
    Arnold c.
    atrioventricular c.
    auditory c.
    auxiliary c.
    basipharyngeal c.
    bayonet c.
    bayonet-curved c.
    Bernard c.
    Bichat c.
    birth c.
    blunderbuss apical c.
    bony semicircular c.
    Böttcher c.
    branching c.

C

NOTES

canal *(continued)*
  Braune c.
  Breschet c.
  bulbous internal auditory c.
  Campodonico c.
  caroticoclinoid c.
  caroticotympanic c.
  carotid c.
  cartilage c.
  caudal c.
  central c.
  cervical c.
  cervicoaxillary c.
  ciliary c.
  Cloquet c.
  collateral pulp c.
  common c.
  condylar c.
  cortical bone primary c.
  Cotunnius c.
  cranial c.
  craniopharyngeal c.
  crural c.
  C-shaped c.
  c. curvature
  curved c.
  c. of Cuvier
  c. débridement
  defalcated root c.
  deferent c.
  dehiscent mandibular c.
  dental c.
  dentinal c.
  dilacerated c.
  diploic c.
  Dorello c.
  Dupuytren c.
  ear c.
  endocervical c.
  ethmoid c.
  external auditory c.
  facial c.
  fallopian c.
  femoral c.
  Ferrein c.
  filling c.
  Fontana c.
  furcation c.
  galactophorous c.
  Gartner c.
  gastric c.
  gubernacular c.
  Guyon c.
  Hannover c.
  haversian c.
  Hensen c.
  c. of Hering
  Hirschfeld c.
  His c.

  horizontal c.
  Hovius c.
  Hoyer c.
  Huguier c.
  humeral c.
  Hunter c.
  hyaloid c.
  hypoglossal c.
  identifying c.
  incisal c.
  incisive c.
  infraorbital c.
  inguinal c.
  c. innominate osteotomy
  inoperable c.
  interdental c.
  interfacial c.
  internal auditory c.
  intramedullary c.
  c. irrigation
  Kovalevsky c.
  lacrimal c.
  Lambert c.
  large c.
  lateral c.
  Lauth c.
  locating c.
  longitudinal c.
  Löwenberg c.
  lumbar c.
  lumbosacral c.
  lymphatic c.
  mandibular c.
  maxillary c.
  medullary c.
  mental c.
  mesiobuccal c.
  musculotubal c.
  nasal c.
  nasolacrimal c.
  neural c.
  neurenteric c.
  Nuck c.
  nutrient c.
  c. obturation
  obturator c.
  optic c.
  orbital c.
  overfilled c.
  palatine c.
  palatomaxillary c.
  palatovaginal c.
  pancreatobiliary c.
  partial atrioventricular c.
  parturient c.
  pelvic c.
  perforating c.
  perivascular c.

persistent common
  atrioventricular c.
Petit c.
pharyngeal c.
pleuroperitoneal c.
posterior vertical c.
pterygoid c.
pterygopalatine c.
pudendal c.
pulmoaortic c.
pulp c.
pyloric c.
radicular c.
c. resonance response
Rivinus c.
root c.
ruffed c.
sacral c.
Santorini c.
Schlemm c.
scleral c.
semicircular c.
sickle-shaped c.
Sondermann c.
sphenopalatine c.
spinal c.
Stensen c.
c. of Stilling
straight c.
subsartorial c.
Sucquet c.
Sucquet-Hoyer c.
supplementary c.
supraciliary c.
supraoptic c.
supraorbital c.
talar c.
tarsal c.
temporal c.
tensor tympani c.
Tourtual c.
tympanic c.
type I–IV c.
uniting c.
urogenital c.
uterovaginal c.
Van Hoorne c.
Velpeau c.
ventricular c.
Verneuil c.
vertebral c.
c. of Vesalius

vesicourethral c.
vestibular c.
vidian c.
Volkmann c.
vomerine c.
vomerobasilar c.
vomerorostral c.
vomerovaginal c.
c. wall-up technique
Walther c.
Wirsung c.
zipped c.
Zuckerkandl perforating c.
zygomaticofacial c.
zygomaticotemporal c.
Canale
  C. osteotomy
  C. technique
canales (*pl. of* canalis)
canalicular
  c. duct
  c. laceration
  c. sphincter
canaliculi (*pl. of* canaliculus)
canaliculodacryocystostomy
canaliculodacryorhinostomy
canaliculorhinostomy
canaliculus, pl. **canaliculi**
  auricular c.
  biliary c.
  lacrimal c.
  mastoid c.
  tympanic c.
  c. vein
  vestibular c.
canalis, pl. **canales**
canalith
  free-floating c.
  c. repositioning procedure
canalization
canaloplasty
cancellectomy
cancellous
  c. chip bone graft
  c. and cortical bone graft
  c. insert graft
  c. tissue
Cancell therapy
cancer
  American Joint Committee on C.
  (AJCC)
  ampullary c.

C

NOTES

cancer *(continued)*
    c. antigen 19-9 (CA19-9)
    appendiceal c.
    biliary tract c.
    c. body
    breast c.
    c. cachexia
    clinically node-negative breast c.
    colloid c.
    colon c.
    colorectal c. (CRC)
    digestive glandular c.
    ductal c.
    early gastric c.
    endobronchial c.
    endometrial c.
    esophageal c.
    esophagogastric c.
    European Organization for Research
      and Treatment of C. (EORTC)
    extrahepatic bile duct c.
    familial breast c.
    familial colon c. (FCC)
    gallbladder c.
    gastric c.
    c. genetics
    C. Genetics Network
    glandular c.
    hard palate c.
    hepatocellular c.
    hereditary breast c.
    hereditary nonpolyposis colon c.
      (HNPCC)
    hereditary nonpolyposis colorectal c.
      (HNPCC)
    high-risk papillary c.
    intraductal c.
    c. invasion
    invasive breast c.
    invasive ductal c.
    islet cell c.
    c. juice
    c. lesion
    life-threatening c.
    localized prostate c.
    low rectal c.
    low-risk papillary c.
    lung c.
    Merkel cell c.
    metastatic colorectal c.
    nasal cavity c.
    neuroendocrine c.
    node-positive breast c.
    nonpalpable invasive breast c.
    obstructing colorectal c.
    obstructive esophagogastric c.
    ovarian c.
    c. pain
    pancreas c.

    pancreatic head c.
    papillary c.
    penile c.
    perforated c.
    periampullary c.
    peritoneal c.
    postgastrectomy c.
    primary c.
    prostate c.
    proximal gastric c.
    QUART procedure for breast c.
    rectal c.
    rectum c.
    resectable periampullary c.
    soft palate c.
    c. status
    c. Surveillance Program
    c. susceptibility syndrome
    suture line c.
    thyroid c.
    Union Internationale Contre le C.
      (UICC)
    unresectable periampullary c.
    urologic system c.
    Whitmore-Jewett classification for
      staging of prostate c.
    W-J classification for staging of
      prostate c.
    young onset c.
cancer-causing gene
cancerization
    field c.
candela lithotripsy
Candida **infection**
candidal infection
candidemia
canine
    c. fossa
    c. teeth
Cannon point
cannulated nail
cannulation
    arterial c.
    bile duct c.
    biliary c.
    c. of biliary tree
    ductal c.
    endoscopic retrograde c.
    endoscopic transpapillary c.
    ERCP c.
    ex vivo c.
    intravenous c.
    pedicle c.
    percutaneous arterial c.
    peripheral venous c.
    postsphincterotomy ERCP c.
    retrograde c.
    selective ductal c.
    transpapillary c.

tubal c.
unilateral pedicle c.
vascular c.
venous c.
cannulization
canonical
c. correlation
c. univariate parameter
canthal
canthectomy
canthi (*pl. of* canthus)
cantholysis
canthomeatal line
canthopexy
canthoplasty
Agnew c.
Ammon c.
canthorrhaphy
Elschnig c.
canthotomy
external c.
lateral c.
canthus, pl. **canthi**
external c.
internal c.
lateral c.
medial c.
cantilevered bone graft
Cantlie line
Cantwell-Ransley
C.-R. epispadias repair
C.-R. urethroplasty
cap
corneal c.
duodenal c.
fibrous c.
metanephric c.
phrygian c.
capacity
demand minimum functional c.
(DMFC)
exercise c.
forced expiratory c.
functional residual c. (FRC)
knot holding c. (KHC)
maximum breathing c. (MBC)
single-breath diffusing c.
treadmill exercise c.
vital c.
CAPD
continuous ambulatory peritoneal dialysis
Capello technique

Capener lateral rhachotomy
Cape Town technique
capillaroscopy
nail fold c.
capillary
c. angioma
c. arteriole
c. dilation
c. drainage
c. endothelium
c. fracture
c. hemangioma
c. hyperfiltration
c. leak syndrome
c. malformation
c. permeability
c. vein
c. wedge pressure
capillus, pl. **capilli**
capita (*pl. of* caput)
capital
c. femoral epiphysis
c. fragment
c. operation
capitate
c. bone
c. fracture
capitation
capitatum
capitellar fracture
capitellocondylar total elbow arthroplasty
capitellum
capitis
capitonnage suture technique
capitopedal
capitular
c. epiphysis
c. joint
capitulum, pl. **capitula**
capnograph
capnography
spectral edge frequency c.
capnometry
volumetric c.
capping technique
capstan knot
capsula, pl. **capsulae**
capsular
c. branch
c. dissection
c. exfoliation syndrome

NOTES

capsular *(continued)*
   c. fixation
   c. flap pyeloplasty
   c. imbrication
   c. incision
   c. interposition arthroplasty
   c. invasion
   c. ligament
   c. shift procedure
   c. space
   c. support tissue
capsule
   adipose c.
   adrenal c.
   articular c.
   atrabiliary c.
   Bonnet c.
   cricothyroid articular c.
   Crosby c.
   Crosby-Kugler biopsy c.
   external c.
   extreme c.
   fatty renal c.
   fibrous articular c.
   c. flap technique
   c. forceps technique
   Gerota c.
   Glisson c.
   glissonian c.
   glomerular c.
   hepatic c.
   joint c.
   liver c.
   Müller c.
   pancreatic c.
   renal c.
   suprarenal c.
   Tenon c.
   tumor c.
   Watson c.
capsulectomy
capsulitis
   adhesive c.
   glenohumeral adhesive c.
capsuloplasty
   Zancolli c.
capsulorrhaphy
   Boyd-Sisk posterior c.
   duToit-Roux staple c.
   medial c.
   pants-over-vest c.
   posterior c.
   Rockwood posterior c.
   Roux-duToit staple c.
   staple c.
capsulotomy
   anterior c.
   Castroviejo c.
   Curtis PIP joint c.

   Darling c.
   dorsal transverse c.
   dorsolateral and medial c.
   posterior c.
   renal c.
   triangular c.
   T-shaped c.
   Vannas c.
   Verhoeff-Chandler c.
capture
   c. cross-section
   pacemaker c.
Capuron point
caput, pl. **capita**
   c. medusa
carbon
   c. dioxide (CO_2)
   c. dioxide concentration
   c. dioxide dissociation curve
   c. dioxide elimination ($VECO_2$)
   c. dioxide fixation
   c. dioxide laser plaque ablation
   c. dioxide pressure
   c. dioxide response
   c. gelatin mass
   c. monoxide (CO)
   c. tetrachloride-induced liver
      regeneration
carbonate
carbonization
carbuncle
   kidney c.
carcinoembryonic antigen (CEA)
carcinogenesis
   foreign body c.
carcinoid
   nonappendiceal c.
   c. tumor
   c. valve disease
carcinoma
   abdominal c.
   acinous cell c.
   adenocystic c.
   adenoid cystic c.
   adenoid squamous cell c.
   adenosquamous c.
   adnexal c.
   adrenal c.
   adrenocortical c.
   aldosterone-producing c.
   alveolar cell c.
   ameloblastic c.
   ampullary c.
   anaplastic c.
   anorectal c.
   apocrine c.
   basal cell c.
   basosquamous cell c.
   benign-acting renal cell c.

betel c.
bile duct c.
bilharzial c.
biliary c.
bladder c.
Borrmann c. (type I–IV)
breast c.
bronchial c.
bronchioloalveolar c.
bronchoalveolar c.
burn scar c.
cecal c.
cerebriform c.
cervical c.
chimney sweep's c.
cholangitis c.
choroid plexus c.
clay pipe c.
clear cell hepatocellular c.
colloid c.
colon c.
colonic c.
colorectal c.
columnar cuff c.
corpus c.
cortisol-producing c.
cribriform c.
cutaneous metastatic breast c.
cylindrical c.
dendritic c.
differentiated thyroid c.
disseminated c.
ductal c.
Dukes classification of c.
dye worker's c.
eccrine c.
Edmondson grading system for
  hepatocellular c.
embryonal cell c.
encephaloid gastric c.
c. en cuirasse
endometrial c.
epidermoid c.
esophageal c.
ethmoid sinus c.
excavated gastric c.
exophytic c.
extrahepatic abdominal c.
fallopian tube c.
false cord c.
follicular c.
gallbladder c.

gastric stump c.
gastrointestinal c.
gelatinous c.
genital c.
glandular c.
glottic c.
granulosa cell c.
gynecological c.
hepatic cell c.
hepatocellular c. (HCC)
hereditary nonpolyposis colon c.
  (HNPCC)
hilar c.
hypernephroid c.
infantile embryonal c.
infiltrating ductal c.
infiltrating lobular c.
infiltrative c.
inflammatory breast c.
insular c.
intraductal c.
intraepidermal c.
intraepithelial nonkeratinizing c.
invasive breast c.
invasive ductal c.
invasive lobular c.
Japanese Classification for
  Gastric C. (JCGC)
juvenile embryonal c.
Kulchitsky cell c.
large cell c.
laryngeal c.
leptomeningeal c.
lobular c.
lung c.
maxillary sinus c.
medullary c.
meibomian gland c.
melanotic c.
meningeal c.
Merkel cell c.
metastatic colorectal c.
metastatic prostatic c.
metastatic renal cell c.
microinvasive c.
micropapillary c.
microscopic multifocal medullary c.
microtrabecular hepatocellular c.
morpheaform basal cell c.
mucoepidermal c.
mucoepidermoid c.
napkin-ring c.

NOTES

111

carcinoma *(continued)*
  nasopharyngeal c. (NPC)
  neuroendocrine skin c.
  oat cell c.
  orofacial c.
  oropharyngeal c.
  ovarian c.
  Paget c.
  pancreatic c.
  papillary gastric c.
  parathyroid c.
  parotid c.
  penile c.
  periampullary c.
  pharyngeal wall c.
  polypoid superficial gastric c.
  prickle cell c.
  primary bile duct c.
  primary intraosseous c.
  prostatic c.
  pure insular c.
  radiation-induced c.
  rectal c.
  rectosigmoid c.
  renal cell c.
  renal pelvis c.
  resectable c.
  salivary duct c.
  salivary gland c.
  scar c.
  schistosomal bladder c.
  schneiderian c.
  sigmoid colon c.
  signet-ring cell c.
  sinonasal c.
  c. in situ (CIS)
  small cell lung c.
  small round cell c.
  spindle cell c.
  splenic flexure c.
  sporadic renal cell c.
  squamous cell c.
  stage B, C c.
  c. stage irresectable
  string cell c.
  swamp c.
  terminal duct c.
  testicular c.
  thymic c.
  thyroid c.
  transitional cell c.
  tuberous sclerosis-associated renal
    cell c.
  tubular c.
  c. of uncertain primary site
  undifferentiated squamous cell c.
  urachal c.
  ureteral c.
  urethral c.

  urothelial c.
  uterine papillary serous c.
  vaginal c.
  vulvar c.
  vulvovaginal c.
  wolffian duct c.
  yolk sac c.
carcinomatosis
  diffuse c.
  peritoneal c.
carcinosarcoma
card
  Memorial Pain Assessment C.
    (MPAC)
cardia
  gastric c.
cardiac
  c. anesthesia
  c. anesthetic
  c. anomaly
  c. arrest
  c. bypass (CBP)
  c. catheterization
  c. compression
  c. decompression
  c. defibrillation
  c. dilatation
  c. dilation
  c. edema
  c. event
  c. examination
  c. fibrillation
  c. fibrous skeleton
  c. herniation
  c. impression
  c. index (CI)
  c. irradiation
  c. lymphatic ring
  c. mass
  c. massage
  c. metastasis
  c. muscle wrap
  c. nerve
  c. output (CO)
  c. patch
  c. perforation
  c. plexus
  c. position
  c. resuscitation
  c. retransplantation
  c. rhabdomyoma
  c. rupture
  c. segment
  c. surgery
  c. symphysis
  c. transplantation
  c. tumor
  c. tumor plop

c. valvular malformation
c. vein
cardiacum
cardiacus
cardiae
achalasia c.
cardiectomy
cardinal
c. ligament
c. point
c. position
cardioesophageal relaxation
cardiogenic shock
cardiohepatic angle
cardiologist
interventional c.
cardiomyopathy
ischemic c.
underlying c.
cardiomyoplasty
dynamic c.
cardiomyotomy
Heller c.
laparoscopic c.
stomach c.
videolaparoscopic c.
cardioomentopexy
cardiopericardiopexy
Beck c.
cardiopexy
cardiophrenic angle mass
cardioplasty
Belsey Mark IV c.
cardioplegia
cardioplegic solution
cardiopressor reflex
cardioprotective effect
cardiopulmonary
c. bypass (CPB)
c. complication
c. manifestation
C. Research Institute
c. resuscitation (CPR)
cardiorespiratory
c. complication
c. endurance (CRE)
cardiorrhaphy
cardiothoracic surgery
cardiotomy
cardiotoxic
c. effect
c. myolysis

cardiovalvotomy
cardiovalvulotomy
cardiovascular
c. adverse effect
c. anesthesia
c. complication
c. disease
c. imaging technique
c. malformation
c. patch graft
c. pressure
c. stability
c. surgery
cardiovasculorenal
cardioversion
cardiovert
care
dedicated intercostals c.
medical c.
monitored anesthesia c. (MAC)
palliative c.
respiratory c.
tertiary c.
trauma c.
Carey Ranvier technique
caries classification
carina, pl. **carinae**
splayed c.
carinate abdomen
carinatum
carious
c. pulp exposure
c. restoration margin
Carlo Traverso maneuver
C-arm fluoroscopy
Carmody-Batson operation
Carnesale
C. acetabular extensile approach
C. hip approach
C. technique
Carnesale-Stewart-Barnes hip dislocation classification
Caroli
C. syndrome
C. type I distal bile duct stricture
Carolinas
C. Laparoscopic Advanced Surgery Program (CLASP)
C. Laparoscopic Advanced Surgery Program procedure
Caroli-Sarles classification

NOTES

caroticoclinoid
- c. canal
- c. foramen
- c. ligament

caroticotympanic
- c. artery
- c. canal
- c. nerve

caroticum

caroticus

carotid
- c. ablative procedure
- c. angioplasty
- c. angioplasty with stenting
- c. arterial blood flow
- c. artery atherosclerotic stenosis
- c. artery bifurcation
- c. artery bypass
- c. artery compression
- c. artery disease
- c. artery dissection
- c. artery occlusion
- c. artery stump pressure
- c. atherosclerosis
- c. body
- c. body tumor
- c. canal
- c. circulation
- c. clamping
- c. duplex ultrasonography
- c. ejection time
- c. endarterectomy (CEA)
- external c.
- c. foramen
- c. ganglion
- c. groove
- c. injury
- c. plaque
- c. preservation
- c. preservation technique
- c. sheath
- c. sinus
- c. sinus branch
- c. siphon
- c. space
- c. stenting
- c. sulcus
- c. surgery
- c. transposition
- c. triangle
- c. tubercle
- c. venous plexus

carotid-basilar anastomosis

carotid-cavernous sinus fistula

carotid-dural fistula

carotid-subclavian artery bypass

carotid-vertebral
- c.-v. anastomosis
- c.-v. vein bypass graft

carotidynia

carpal
- c. artery
- c. bone stress fracture
- c. boss
- c. compression test
- c. region
- c. synovectomy
- c. tunnel syndrome

carpectomy
- distal-row c.
- Omer-Capen c.
- proximal-row c.

Carpentier
- C. anuloplasty
- C. tricuspid valvuloplasty

Carpentier-Edwards
- C.-E. stented bovine pericardial valve
- C.-E. stented porcine xenograft valve

carpet lesion

carpetlike polyposis

carpi (*pl. of* carpus)

carpocarpal

carpometacarpal
- c. arthroplasty
- c. articulation
- c. fracture-dislocation
- c. joint dislocation
- c. joint fracture

carpometacarpeae

carpopedal

Carpue method

carpus, pl. **carpi**

Carrel
- C. operation
- C. suture technique
- C. treatment

Carrell
- C. fibular substitution technique
- C. resection

carrier
- c. flap
- c. fluid
- mutation c.
- c. status

Carroll arthroplasty

CARS
- compensatory antiinflammatory response syndrome

Carstan reverse wedge osteotomy

Cartam-Treander reverse wedge osteotomy

Carter operation

cartilage
- alar c.
- anular c.
- arthrodial c.

articular c.
arytenoid c.
auricular c.
basilar c.
branchial c.
c. canal
connecting c.
corniculate c.
costal c.
cricoid c.
cuneiform c.
diarthrodial c.
ensiform c.
epiglottic c.
falciform c.
c. flap
c. graft
hypsiloid c.
c. inflammation
interosseous c.
intervertebral c.
intraarticular c.
intrathyroid c.
investing c.
Jacobson c.
Luschka c.
mandibular c.
c. matrix
meatal c.
Meckel c.
Meyer c.
Morgagni c.
c. overgrowth
quadrangular c.
Reichert c.
Santorini c.
Seiler c.
semilunar c.
sesamoid c.
sternal c.
sternum c.
supraarytenoid c.
thyroid c.
tracheal c.
triangular c.
triquetrous c.
triticeal c.
uniting c.
vomeronasal c.
Weitbrecht c.
Wrisberg c.

xiphoid c.
Y c.
cartilagines (*pl. of* cartilago)
cartilagineus
cartilaginous
   c. growth plate disorder
   c. loose body
   c. part of skeletal system
   c. septum
   c. tissue
cartilago, pl. **cartilagines**
cartwheel fracture
caruncle
   Morgagni c.
   Santorini major c.
   Santorini minor c.
   urethral c.
caruncula, pl. **carunculae**
   hymenal c.
   sublingual c.
caryothecae
CAS
   computer-assisted surgery
Casanellas lacrimal operation
cascade
   coagulation c.
caseated tissue
caseating granulomatous inflammation
caseation
   c. necrosis
   tuberculous c.
case-by-case approach
caseous
   c. abscess
   c. inflammation
Casey operation
CaSki cell line
Casoni test
Caspari repair
CASS
   coronary artery surgery study
Casselberry position
Casser perforated muscle
cast
   c. application
   c. immobilization
   c. removal
Castaneda procedure
Castellani point
Castle procedure
castrate

NOTES

castration
  female c.
  functional c.
  male c.
  parasitic c.
Castroviejo
  C. capsulotomy
  C. iridectomy
  C. keratectomy
  C. minikeratoplasty
  C. operation
  C. radial iridotomy
Castroviejo-Scheie cyclodiathermy operation
catabolic condition
cataract
  c. aspiration
  congenital c.
  c. extraction
  c. extraction operation
  flap operation c.
  c. formation
  hard c.
  irradiation c.
  c. irradiation
  c. mask ring
  c. procedure
  radiation c.
  reduplication c.
  ring-form congenital c.
  ring-shaped c.
  Soemmerring ring c.
  soft c.
  c. surgery
catarrhal
  c. inflammation
  c. marginal ulceration
catastrophe
  intraabdominal c.
catastrophic
  c. event
  c. illness
catastrophizing subscale
catecholamine-resistant hypotension
caterpillar flap
catheter
  c. ablation
  c. balloon valvuloplasty
  c. dilation
  c. drainage
  c. embolectomy
  c. embolism
  end-hole c.
  c. exchange
  c. fixation
  c. fragment
  c. insertion
  c. instability
  c. introduction method

c. kinking
c. knotting
c. knotting and entrapment
c. malposition
c. manipulation
c. mapping
c. obstruction
c. patency
c. position
pulmonary artery c.
c. sepsis
c. site
c. specimen
c. tip placement
c. toe
torque tube c.
c. tunnel
c. tunnel infection
c. whip
catheter-directed
  c.-d. fenestration
  c.-d. interventional procedure
  c.-d. thrombolysis
catheter-guided
  c.-g. biopsy
  c.-g. endoscopic intubation
catheter-induced pulmonary artery hemorrhage
catheterizable stoma
catheterization
  antegrade c.
  arterial c.
  bile duct c.
  bladder c.
  bypass graft c.
  cardiac c.
  central venous c.
  chronic c.
  clean intermittent c.
  combined heart c.
  coronary sinus c.
  cystic duct c.
  diagnostic cardiac c.
  fallopian tube c.
  in-and-out c.
  intermittent c.
  interventional cardiac c.
  Judkins-Sones technique of cardiac c.
  left heart c.
  long-term epidural c.
  percutaneous transhepatic cardiac c.
  portal vein c.
  pulmonary artery c.
  retrograde c.
  right heart c.
  Seldinger cystic duct c.
  selective c.
  subclavian vein c.

c. technique
thoracic epidural c.
transfemoral venous c.
transhepatic c.
transnasal bile duct c.
transpapillary c.
transseptal left heart c.
transvaginal fallopian tube c.
transvaginal tubal c.
umbilical artery c.
umbilical vein c.
ureteral c.
urinary c.
catheterize
catheter-related infection
catheter-securing technique
catholysis
cation exchange
cat's eye calculus
Cattell operation
Cattell-Warren pancreaticojejunostomy
Catterall classification
cauda, pl. **caudae**
c. epididymis
c. equina compression
c. equina syndrome
caudad
caudal
c. anesthesia
c. angulation
c. block
c. canal
c. corner
c. direction
c. dysplasia sequence
c. epidural anesthetic technique
c. fragment
c. lamina resection
c. ligament
c. pancreatic artery
c. pancreaticojejunostomy
c. retinaculum
c. sac
c. translation
c. transtentorial herniation
c. transverse fissure
c. vertebra
caudal-cranial rotation
caudate
c. body
c. branch

c. lobe
c. process
caudocephalad
causalgia
genitofemoral c.
cause
cholestatic c.
definitive c.
idiopathic c.
pathologic c.
underlying c.
cause-effect relationship
cause-specific mortality
cauterant
cauterization
bipolar c.
Bovie c.
phenol c.
unipolar c.
cauterize
cautery
c. conization
hook c.
c. incision
insulated c.
looped c.
c. operation
pure cutting c.
snare c.
wet field c.
cava (*pl. of* cavum)
caval
c. drainage
c. fold
c. insertion
cave
C. hip approach
C. knee approach
Meckel c.
trigeminal c.
caverna, pl. **cavernae**
cavernosa
cavernosal alpha blockade technique
cavernous
c. angioma
c. body
c. groove
c. hemangioma
c. malformation
c. nerve
c. nerve-sparing prostatectomy
c. plexus

NOTES

cavernous (*continued*)
    c. respiration
    c. sinus fistula
    c. sinus syndrome
    c. venous sinus
Cave-Rowe shoulder dislocation technique
CAVH
    continuous arteriovenous hemofiltration
cavitary
    c. lung lesion
    c. small bowel lesion
cavitas, pl. **cavitates**
cavitating
    c. inflammation
    c. metastasis
cavitation
    collapse c.
    pulmonary c.
    stable c.
    transient c.
cavity
    abdominal c.
    abdominopelvic c.
    access c.
    c. access
    acetabular c.
    alveolar c.
    amniotic c.
    articular c.
    artificial classification c.
    axial surface c.
    biopsy c.
    body c.
    buccal c.
    chorionic c.
    c. classification
    complex c.
    compound c.
    cotyloid c.
    cranial c.
    cystic c.
    c. débridement
    dental c.
    distal c.
    DO c.
    endodontic c.
    endolymphatic c.
    endometrial c.
    epidural c.
    exocelomic c.
    fissure c.
    frontal sinus c.
    gingival c.
    glenoid c.
    greater peritoneal c.
    idiopathic bone c.
    incisal c.
    inferior laryngeal c.

inflammatory c.
infraglottic c.
intermediate laryngeal c.
intracranial c.
intraperitoneal c.
joint c.
labial c.
laryngeal c.
laser c.
lesser peritoneal c.
c. line angle
lingual c.
c. lining
c. lining agent
lung c.
c. margin
marrow c.
mastoid c.
maxillary sinus c.
Meckel c.
medullary c.
miniature uterine c.
nasal c.
nephrotomic c.
nonseptate c.
occlusal c.
open c.
optic papilla c.
oral c.
orbital c.
pelvic c.
perilymphatic c.
peritoneal c.
pharyngonasal c.
pit and fissure c.
pleural c.
postexcision c.
c. preparation
c. preparation base
prepared c.
c. primer
proximal c.
pulmonary c.
pulp c.
residual cystic c.
retroperitoneal c.
Retzius c.
saclike c.
c. seal
seroma c.
sinonasal c.
sinus c.
smooth surface c.
Stafne idiopathic bone c.
subarachnoid c.
subdural c.
subglottic c.
superior laryngeal c.
synovial c.

syringohydromyelic c.
c. test
thoracic c.
c. toilet
trigeminal c.
tympanic c.
uterine c.
vitreous c.
c. wall
wound c.
cavoatrial shunt
cavohepatic junction
cavopulmonary anastomosis
cavotomy
infrahepatic c.
cavovarus deformity
cavum, pl. **cava**
inferior vena c. (IVC)
inferior vena cava (IVC)
infrahepatic inferior vena cava
infrarenal cava
retrohepatic inferior vena cava
Spencer plication of vena cava
superior vena cava (SVC)
suprahepatic inferior vena cava
(SHVC)
suprahepatic vena cava
cavus deformity
Cawthorne
C. destruction
C. operation
Cawthorne-Day procedure
CBD
common bile duct
CBDS
common bile duct stone
CBF
cerebral blood flow
CBP
cardiac bypass
CBT
cognitive behavior treatment
CCAM
congenital cystic adenomatoid
malformation
CCD
central core disease
CCM
critical care medicine
CCS
celiac artery compression syndrome
Clinical Classification System

CCSG
Children's Cancer Study group
C-D
Cotrel-Dubousset
C-D screw modification
CDBR
computerized diaphragmatic breathing
retraining
CDH
congenital diaphragmatic hernia
CEA
carcinoembryonic antigen
carotid endarterectomy
CEA level
serum CEA
ceanothus extract
CEAP
clinical manifestations, etiologic factors,
anatomic involvement, pathophysiologic
features
CEAP classification
ceca (*pl. of* cecum)
cecal
c. appendix
c. artery
c. bascule
c. carcinoma
c. colonoscopy
c. deformity
c. distention
c. diverticulitis
c. flap
c. fold
c. foramen
c. hernia
c. imbrication procedure
c. intussusception
c. ligation
c. ligation and puncture (CLP)
c. recess
c. serosa
c. volvulus
cecal flap
cecectomy
Cecil
C. procedure
C. urethroplasty
cecocolostomy
cecocystoplasty
cecofixation
cecoileostomy

NOTES

C

cecopexy
    laparoscopic c.
cecoplication
cecoproctostomy
cecorrhaphy
cecosigmoidostomy
cecostomy
    percutaneous catheter c. (PCC)
    tube c.
cecotomy
cecoureterocele
cecum, pl. **ceca**
Cedars-Sinai classification
ceiling analgesia
Celermajer method
Celestin procedure
celiac
    c. alcohol ablation
    c. arterial system
    c. artery
    c. artery aneurysm
    c. artery compression syndrome
    (CCS)
    c. axis
    c. axis compression syndrome
    c. band syndrome
    c. branch
    c. dimple
    c. ganglion
    c. gland
    c. infantilism
    c. lymph node metastasis
    c. nervous plexus
    c. nodal involvement
    c. ostium
    c. plexus block
    c. plexus block anesthetic
    technique
    c. plexus reflex
    c. rickets
    c. trunk
    c. tumor
    c. vessel
celiacography
celiacomesenteric artery
celiectomy
celiocentesis
celioenterotomy
celiogastrostomy
celiogastrotomy
celiohysterectomy
celiohysterotomy
celioma
celiomyomectomy
celiomyomotomy
celioparacentesis
celiorrhaphy
celiosalpingectomy
celiosalpingotomy

celioscopy
celiotomy
    damage-control c.
    exploratory c.
    formal c.
    c. incision
    mandatory c.
    negative c.
    staging c.
    vaginal c.
celite-activated clotting time (CACT)
cell
    Claudius c.
    c. collection
    Deiters c.
    ependymal c.
    epithelial c.
    epitympanic c.
    ethmoid c.
    follicular c.
    gut epithelial c.
    Hensen c.
    hypotympanic c.
    inflammation c.
    inflammatory c.
    irradiated melanoma c.
    islet c.
    Kirchner c.
    c. line
    lymphocyte c.
    malignant c.
    mastoid c.
    c. membrane
    mesothelial c.
    c. migration
    multipotential stem c.
    c. oxygenation
    packed red blood c.'s (PRBC)
    paranasal c.
    parenchymal c.
    petrous apex c.
    pharyngeal c.
    photosensitive c.
    pituitary tumor c.
    pulmonary epithelial c.
    retinal pigment epithelial c.
    rod c.
    Schwann c.
    c. separation technique
    stem c.
    T c.
    tumor c.
    c. web
    white c.
cell-cell adhesion
cell-extracellular matrix adhesion
cellophane tape method
cellula, pl. **cellulae**

cellular
- c. biology
- c. cooperation
- c. damage
- c. debris
- c. immunity
- c. infiltration
- c. migration
- c. nidus
- c. polyp
- c. xenograft rejection
- c. xenotransplantation

cellularity
- high c.

cellulocutaneous flap
cellulose-based membrane
celotomy
Celsus-Hotz operation
Celsus spasmodic entropion operation
cement
- c. base
- c. disease
- c. interface
- c. line
- c. removal
- c. substance
- c. technique

cemental
- c. lesion
- c. line
- c. repair

cementation
- final c.
- trial c.

cement-bone interface
cemented total hip arthroplasty
cementification
cementing line
cementless
- c. technique
- c. total hip arthroplasty

cementoid tissue
cementoma
cementum
- c. fracture
- c. pain

center
- ambulatory surgery c.
- C.'s for Disease Control HIV infection classification
- limbic c.
- tertiary trauma c.

trauma c.
urban trauma c.

centesis
centra (*pl. of* centrum)
central
- c. anesthetic technique
- c. anticholinergic syndrome
- c. approach
- c. bearing point
- c. bis
- c. block
- c. bone
- c. canal
- c. carbon dioxide ventilatory response
- c. chemoreflex loop
- c. cone technique reduction
- c. cord syndrome
- c. core disease (CCD)
- c. dislocation
- c. excitatory state
- c. extensor mechanism
- c. fibroelastic core
- c. fibrous body
- c. fixation
- c. fracture
- c. fusion
- c. heel pad syndrome
- c. hepatectomy
- c. hepatic gunshot wound
- c. herniation
- c. hyperalimentation
- c. illumination
- c. incisor teeth
- c. iridectomy
- c. lesion
- c. line infection
- c. nervous system
- c. nervous system disease
- c. nervous system malformation
- c. nervous system manifestation
- c. nervous system tuberculosis
- c. obesity
- c. pain
- c. palmar space
- c. perineum tendon
- c. physiolysis
- c. pontine myelinolysis
- c. posterior-anterior pressure
- c. poststroke pain (CPSP)
- c. ray amputation
- c. respiration

NOTES

121

central *(continued)*
   c. retinal artery
   c. sensitization
   c. slip sparing technique
   c. stellate laceration
   c. sulcal artery
   c. systemic-to-pulmonary shunt
   c. tegmental tract
   c. tendon
   c. tendon diaphragm
   c. vein
   c. venous access
   c. venous alimentation
   c. venous cannulation anesthetic
     technique
   c. venous catheterization
   c. venous hypercarbia
   c. venous pressure (CVP)
   c. venous pressure monitoring
   c. vision
   c. yellow point
   c. zone inflammation
centrales
centralis
centralization
   Bayne-Klug c.
   Bora c.
   Manske-McCarroll-Swanson c.
   tendon c.
centration
centric
   c. fusion
   c. jaw relation
   c. occluding relation
   c. occluding relation record
   point c.
   c. position
   c. relation occlusion
centriciput
centrifugalization
centrifugal nerve
centrifugation
centrifuged
centrilobular
   c. lesion
   c. necrosis
   c. pancreatitis
centriole
   distal c.
   proximal c.
centripetal nerve
centroneuroaxis anesthesia
centrum, pl. **centra**
cephalad
   c. corner
   c. direction
   c. fragment
   c. translation

cephalalgia
   coital c.
cephalic
   c. index
   c. tetanus
   c. triangle
   c. vein
   c. vein graft
cephalin-cholesterol flocculation
cephalization
cephalocaudal axis
cephalocele
   occipital c.
   oral c.
cephalocentesis
cephalodactyly
cephalomedullary nail fracture
cephalometric
   c. correction
   c. landmark
cephalopelvic disproportion
cephalopharyngeus
cephalorrhachidian index
cephalothoracic
cephalotrigonal technique
ceramic restoration
ceramometal restoration
ceratectomy
ceratocricoid
   c. ligament
   c. muscle
ceratocricoideum
ceratocricoideus
ceratopharyngeus
cerclage
   elective c.
   emergent c.
   McDonald c.
   c. operation
   Shirodkar cervical c.
   c. wire fixation
cerebellar
   c. artery
   c. ectopia
   c. hematoma
   c. hemisphere
   c. hemorrhage
   c. vein
cerebellomedullary
   c. cistern
   c. malformation syndrome
cerebellopontine
   c. angle approach
   c. angle cistern
   c. angle syndrome
cerebellorubral tract
cerebellothalamic tract
cerebra (*pl. of* cerebrum)

cerebral
    c. abscess
    c. angioma
    c. aqueduct compression
    c. arteriovenous malformation
    c. artery
    c. blood
    c. blood flow (CBF)
    c. calculus
    c. circulation
    c. circulation time
    c. death
    c. decompression
    c. decortication
    c. edema
    c. event
    c. fornix
    c. hemicorticectomy
    c. hemisphere
    c. hemorrhage
    c. hernia
    c. herniation
    c. index
    c. injury
    c. lesion
    c. metabolic rate (CMR)
    c. metastasis
    c. palsy pathological fracture
    c. perfusion
    c. perfusion pressure (CPP)
    c. protection
    c. protective therapy
    c. radiation necrosis (CRN)
    c. respiration
    c. revascularization
    c. sinus
    c. spinal fluid drainage
    c. sulcus
    c. vascular malformation
    c. vein
cerebral-sacral loop
cerebration
cerebriform carcinoma
cerebrospinal
    c. fluid (CSF)
    c. fluid-brain barrier
    c. fluid fistula
    c. fluid outflow
    c. fluid pressure (CSFP)
    c. index
cerebrotendinous xanthomatosis
cerebrotomy

cerebrovascular
    c. accident
    c. complication
    c. disease
    c. event
    c. malformation
    c. resistance (CVR)
cerebrum, pl. **cerebra**
cerecloth
cereolus, pl. **cereoli**
certified
    c. registered nurse anesthetist (CRNA)
    c. surgical technologist (CST)
    c. surgical technologist, first assist (CSTFA)
cervical
    c. acceleration-deceleration syndrome
    c. adenocarcinoma
    c. adenopathy
    c. amputation
    c. anastomosis
    c. anesthesia
    c. anomaly
    c. approach
    c. aspiration
    c. branch
    c. canal
    c. carcinoma
    c. carcinoma stimulation
    c. compression syndrome
    c. condyloma
    c. cone biopsy
    c. conization
    c. corpectomy
    c. decompression surgery
    c. dilation
    c. discectomy
    c. disc excision
    c. disc surgery
    c. diverticulum
    c. dystonia
    c. esophagogastrostomy
    c. esophagoplasty
    c. esophagostomy
    c. esophagotomy
    c. esophagus
    c. extension strength
    c. fascia
    c. fistula
    c. flap

NOTES

cervical (*continued*)
   c. fusion syndrome
   c. ganglion
   c. ganglionectomy
   c. general rotation
   c. gland
   c. immobilization
   c. incision
   c. infection
   c. inflammation
   c. injury
   c. insemination
   c. instability
   c. interbody fusion
   c. laceration
   c. leakage
   c. lesion
   c. ligament
   c. line
   c. loop
   c. manipulation
   c. metastasis
   c. midline disc herniation
   c. nerve root injection
   c. node dissection
   c. osteotomy
   c. perivascular sympathectomy
   c. pleura
   c. plexus
   c. plexus block
   c. plexus block anesthetic
     technique
   c. position
   c. rib
   c. rotator muscle
   c. screw fixation
   c. screw insertion technique
   c. segment
   c. sinus
   c. soft tissue
   c. space
   c. spine fracture
   c. spine internal fixation
   c. spine kyphotic deformity
   c. spine laminectomy
   c. spine posterior fusion
   c. spine screw-plate fixation
   c. spine stabilization
   c. spine stabilization procedure
   c. splanchnic nerve
   c. spondylitic myelopathy
   c. spondylotic myelopathy fusion
     technique
   c. spondylotic myelopathy
     vertebrectomy
   c. stenosis
   c. stump
   c. suture
   c. thymectomy

   c. transformation zone
   c. triangle
   c. tumor
   c. ulcer
   c. ultrasound
   c. vein
   c. vertebra
   c. vessel compression
cervicalis
   ansa c.
cervicalium
cervical-to-MCA bypass
cervicectomy
cervices (*pl. of* cervix)
cervicis
   semispinalis c.
cervicoaxillary canal
cervicobrachial
cervicofacial
cervicogenic headache
cervicomedullary
   c. deformity
   c. junction compression
cervicooccipital
cervicoplasty
cervicothoracic
   c. approach
   c. ganglion
   c. junction stabilization
   c. junction surgery
   c. orthosis (CTO)
   c. pedicle anatomy
   c. sympathectomy
   c. transition
cervicothoracicum
cervicotomy
cervicotrochanteric displaced fracture
cervicovaginal
   c. artery
   c. fistula
   c. infection
cervicovaginalis
cervicovesical
cervix, pl. **cervices**
   implant c.
cesarean
   c. delivery
   c. hysterectomy
   c. operation
   c. resection
   c. section (C-section)
   c. section incision
cesium irradiation
CFA
   common femoral artery
CFA-SFA
   common femoral artery-superficial
   femoral artery
     CFA-SFA bypass

C-form osteotomy
CGS
   clinical grading scale
CHA
   controlled hypotensive anesthesia
CHADD
   controlled heat-aided drug delivery
Chadwick-Bentley classification
Chadwick sign
chain
   lymphatic c.
   obturator lymphatic c.
   recurrent nerve lymphatic c.
   c. suture technique
chain-of-lakes
   c.-o.-l. deformity
   c.-o.-l. filling defect
   c.-o.-l. sign
challenge
   methacholine bronchoprovocation c.
chamber
   2-c. longitudinal (2C-L)
   c. rupture
   4-c. transverse (4C-T)
   5-c. transverse (5C-T)
Chamberlain
   C. mediastinoscopy
   C. procedure
Chambers
   C. osteotomy
   C. procedure
chamfer preparation
Chance
   C. fracture thoracolumbar spine
   C. vertebral fracture
chancre
   hard c.
   mixed c.
   monorecidive c.
   c. redux
   soft c.
chancriform
chancroid
chandelier sign
Chandler
   C. hip fusion
   C. iridectomy
   C. vitreous operation
Chandler-Verhoeff
   C.-V. lens extraction
   C.-V. operation
Chang aniline-acid fuchsin method

change
   aging degenerative c.
   degenerative c.
   diffuse c.
   fibrocystic c.
   fractional area c. (FAC)
   hemodynamic c.
   Hürthle cell c.
   ischemic mesenteric c.
   metabolic c.
   mitral valve prolapse, aortic anomalies, skeletal changes, skin c.'s (MASS)
   motor c.
   multifocal c.
   muscular c.
   nail c.
   neurocognitive c.
   onion-bulb c.'s
   parenchymal c.
   physiologic c.
   c. point
   postradiation c.
   postsurgical motor c.
   postthoracotomy c.
   sepsis-induced metabolic c.
   supraesophageal reflux c.'s
   surgical c.
Chang-Miltner incision
channel
   c. activity
   c. and core biopsy
   open venous c.
   c. shoulder pin technique
   venous c.
Chaput
   C. anal operation
   C. fracture
   C. operation
characteristic
   clinical c.
   heterogeneity c.
   histologic c.
   pathologic c.
   c. radiation
Charcot
   C. triad
   C. triangle
charged-particle irradiation
Charles
   C. lensectomy

NOTES

Charles *(continued)*
    C. operation
    C. procedure
Charnley
    C. compression
    C. compression arthrodesis
    C. compression-type knee fusion
    C. incision
    C. total hip arthroplasty
Charrière scale
CHART
    continuous hyperfractionated accelerated
    radiotherapy
Charters
    C. method
    C. technique
char-zone depth
chasm
Chassaignac
    C. space
    C. tubercle
Chassar
    C. Moir-Sims procedure
    C. Moir sling procedure
Chauffard point
chauffeur fracture
Chaussier line
Chaves-Rapp muscle transfer technique
Chayes method
CHCT
    caffeine and halothane contracture test
Cheatle
    C. slit
    C. syndrome
Cheatle-Henry hernia
checklist
    Rotterdam Symptom C.
checkrein deformity
cheek
    c. advancement flap
    c. bone
    c. muscle
    c. rotation flap
cheesy necrosis
cheilectomy
    Garceau c.
    Mann-Coughlin-DuVries c.
    Sage-Clark c.
cheilion
cheiloangioscopy
cheiloplasty
cheilorrhaphy
cheilostomatoplasty
cheilotomy
cheiroplasty
chemexfoliation
chemical
    c. disinfection
    c. exchange

    c. exposure
    c. hemostasis
    c. litholysis
    c. matrixectomy
    c. peritonitis
    c. rhizolysis
    c. sedation
    c. shift imaging
    c. shift misregistration
    c. splanchnicectomy
    c. sympathectomy
    c. thrombectomy
    c. tourniquet
    c. vapor sterilization
chemical shift imaging
chemicocautery
chemiluminescence
chemiluminescent
chemoactivation
chemoattraction
    fibroblast c.
chemocautery
chemocoagulation
chemodectoma
chemoembolization
    arterial c.
    intraarterial c.
    transarterial c.
chemolysis
    intrarenal c.
chemoneurolysis
    glycerol c.
    percutaneous retrogasserian
    glycerol c.
chemonucleolysis
    chymopapain c.
    double-needle c.
chemopallidectomy
chemopallidothalamectomy
chemopallidotomy
chemoprevention
    c. agent
    medical c.
chemopreventive agent
chemoprophylaxis
chemoradiation
chemoradiotherapy
    c. effect
    preoperative c.
chemoreceptor trigger zone
chemoreflex
chemosensitive
chemosterilization
chemostimulation
chemosurgery
chemosurgical gingivectomy
chemotactic property
chemothalamectomy
chemothalamotomy

chemotherapeutic
    c. scheme
    c. treatment
chemotherapist
chemotherapy
    adjunctive c.
    adjuvant c.
    combination c.
    concurrent c.
    induction c.
    infusional c.
    initial systemic c.
    intraarterial c. (IAC)
    intraperitoneal hyperthermic c.
      (IPHC)
    intravesical c.
    postoperative systemic c.
    preoperative induction c.
    preoperative systemic c.
    c. protocol
    second-line c.
    systemic c.
Cherney
    C. lower transverse abdominal
      incision
    C. suture technique
cherry angioma
Cherry-Crandall procedure
cherry-picking procedure
chessboard graft
chest
    c. anomaly
    c. compression
    c. deformity
    c. examination
    flail c.
    flat c.
    c. index
    c. lesion
    c. physical therapy
    pneumonectomy c.
    c. port
    stove-in c.
    c. tube drainage (CTD)
    c. tube output (CTO)
    c. wall
    c. wall compliance
    c. wall fixation
    c. wall invasion
    c. wall stabilization
    c. x-ray
Chester-Winter procedure

chevron
    c. bunionectomy
    c. hallux valgus correction
    c. incision
    c. laceration
    c. osteotomy
    c. technique
chevron-shaped incision
chevron-type transmalleolar osteotomy
chewing method
chew-in technique
Cheyne operation
Cheyne-Stokes respiration
Chiari
    C. anomaly
    C. I–III malformation
    C. II syndrome
    C. innominate osteotomy
    C. technique
Chiari-Salter-Steel pelvic osteotomy
chiasm
    Camper c.
chiasma, pl. chiasmata
    c. formation
chiasmal
    c. compression
    c. lesion
    c. metastasis
chiasmapexy
chiasmata (*pl. of* chiasma)
chiasmatic
    c. cistern
    c. cisterna
    c. groove
    c. sulcus
chiasmatis
Chicago classification
chicken fat clot
Chiene incision
Chiffelle and Putt method
child
    C. classification of cirrhosis
    C. esophageal varix classification
    C. hepatic dysfunction classification
    C. hepatic risk criteria
      classification
    C. liver disease classification
    C. operation
    C. pancreaticoduodenostomy
    C. radical pancreatectomy
childbirth
    Bradley method of prepared c.

NOTES

childbirth (*continued*)
Kitzinger method of c.
Lamaze method of c.
childhood thyroid irradiation
Child-Phillips bowel plication
Child-Pugh classification
children
C.'s Cancer Study group (CCSG)
c. coma scale
faces rating scale for c.
Childress ankle fixation technique
Child-Turcotte hepatic surgery classification
chiloplasty
chilostomatoplasty
chimera
radiation c.
chimerism
chimney sweep's carcinoma
chin
c. augmentation
double c.
c. elevation
c. muscle
c. position
Chinese flap
CHIP
Coping with Health, Injuries, and Problems
chip
bone c.
c. fracture
c. graft
chiroplasty
chiropractic treatment of fracture
chisel fracture
chlamydial infection
Chlamydia trachomatis **infection**
chloramine T technique
chloranilate method
chlormerodrin accumulation test
2-chloroprocaine
Cho
C. anterior cruciate ligament reconstruction
C. tendon technique
choana, pl. **choanae**
chocolate cyst
cholangiectasis
cholangiocarcinoma
hilar c.
cholangioenterostomy
cholangiofibroma
cholangiofibrosis
cholangiogastrostomy
cholangiogram
common duct c.
false-negative c.
intraoperative c. (IOC)

preoperative retrograde c.
retrograde c.
cholangiographic
c. interpretation
c. technique
cholangiography
completion c.
drip infusion c.
endoscopic retrograde c.
infusion c.
intraoperative dynamic c.
magnetic resonance imaging c.
MRI c.
operative c. (OC)
percutaneous transhepatic c. (PTC)
cholangiohepatitis
Oriental c.
recurrent pyogenic c. (RPC)
cholangiole
cholangioma
cholangiopancreatography
endoscopic retrograde c. (ERCP)
magnetic resonance c. (MRCP)
cholangiopancreatoscopy
peroral c.
cholangioplasty
cholangioscopy
3-dimensional virtual c.
intraductal c.
percutaneous transhepatic c.
peroral c.
cholangiostomy
cholangiotomy
cholangitis
c. carcinoma
primary sclerosing c.
cholecyst
cholecystectasia
cholecystectomy
combined laparoscopic splenectomy and c.
laparoscopic c. (LC)
laparoscopic laser c. (LLC)
laser laparoscopic c. (LLC)
microlaparoscopic c.
minilaparoscopic c.
needlescopic laparoscopic c.
open c.
percutaneous c.
prophylactic c.
retrograde c.
surgical c.
transcylindrical c.
c. treatment
2-trocar laparoscopic c.
3-trocar technique c.
cholecystenteric fistula
cholecystenteroanastomosis
cholecystenterorrhaphy

cholecystenterostomy
cholecystenterotomy
cholecystic
cholecystis
cholecystitis
    acalculous c.
    acute acalculous c. (AAC)
    acute calculous c.
    asymptomatic c.
    calculous c.
    chronic c.
    emphysematous c.
    erythromycin-induced c.
    follicular c.
    gangrenous c.
    gaseous c.
    perforated c.
    scleroatrophic c.
    suppurative c.
    typhoidal c.
    uncomplicated acute c.
    xanthogranulomatous c.
cholecystobiliary fistulization
cholecystocholangiography
cholecystocholedochal fistula
cholecystocholedocholithiasis
cholecystocolic fistula
cholecystocolonic fistula
cholecystocolostomy
cholecystoduodenal
    c. fistula
    c. ligament
cholecystoduodenocolic
    c. fistula
    c. fold
cholecystoduodenostomy
cholecystoendoprosthesis
    endoscopic retrograde c.
cholecystoenterostomy
    direct c.
cholecystogastrostomy
cholecystoileostomy
cholecystojejunostomy
cholecystokinin secretion
cholecystolithiasis
cholecystolithotomy
    percutaneous c.
cholecystolithotripsy
cholecystomy
cholecystopaque
cholecystopexy
cholecystorrhaphy

cholecystoscopy
    percutaneous transhepatic c.
cholecystostomy
    percutaneous c.
    surgical c.
    c. tube
cholecystotomy
    laparoscopic c.
    transpapillary endoscopic c.
choledochal
    c. basal pressure
    c. cyst
    c. cyst disease
    c. region
    c. sphincter
choledochal-colonic fistula
choledochectomy
choledochendysis
choledochocele
choledochocholedochostomy side-to-side
    anastomosis
choledochocolonic fistula
choledochoduodenal
    c. fistula
    c. fistulotomy
    c. junction
    c. junctional stenosis
choledochoduodenostomy
choledochoenteric fistula
choledochoenterostomy
choledochofiberoscopy
    T-tube tract c.
choledochogastrostomy
choledochohepatostomy
choledochoileostomy
choledochojejunostomy
    end-to-side c.
    laparoscopic Roux-en-Y c.
    loop c.
    retrocolic end-to-side c.
    Roux-en-Y c.
choledocholith
choledocholithiasis
choledocholithotomy
choledocholithotripsy
choledochopancreatic ductal junction
choledochoplasty
choledochorrhaphy
choledochoscopy
    Berci-Shore c.
    cystic duct c.
    jejunostomy tract c.

NOTES

C

choledochoscopy *(continued)*
    operative c.
    postoperative c.
    transcystic c.
    T-tube tract c.
choledochostomy
choledochotomy
    c. incision
    laparoscopic common bile duct
      exploration c.
    longitudinal c.
choledochous
choledochus
cholelith
cholelithiasis
cholelitholysis
cholelithotomy
cholelithotripsy
cholelithotrity
cholescintigraphy
cholestasis
cholestatic
    c. cause
    c. cirrhosis
    c. jaundice
cholesteatoma
    pars flaccida c.
    c. pearl
cholesterol
    c. calculus
    c. saturation index
    c. solitaire
    c. stone
cholicele
cholinergic
    c. blockade
    c. mechanism
    c. tract
chondral
    c. edge
    c. fracture
    c. fragment
chondrectomy
chondrification
chondritis
    xiphisternal junction c.
chondrocostal
chondrodermatitis
    nodular c.
chondroepiphysis
chondroglossus muscle
chondrolysis
    posttraumatic c.
chondromalacia
chondromyofibroma
chondromyxofibroma
chondromyxoma
chondroosseous
chondroosteodystrophy

chondropharyngeus
chondrophyte
chondroplasty
    abrasion c.
    arthroscopic abrasion c.
chondroporosis
chondrosarcoma
chondrosteoma
chondrosternal
chondrosternoplasty
chondrotomy
chondroxiphoid ligament
chop amputation
Chopart
    C. amputation
    C. ankle dislocation
    C. articulation
chorda, pl. **chordae**
    chordae tendineae rupture
    c. tympani
    c. tympani nerve
chordal
    c. rupture
    c. shortening
chordee removal
chord incision
chordoblastoma
chordotomy
chorioadenoma
chorioallantoic membrane
chorioamnionic infection
chorioangioma
chorioblastoma
choriocapillaris
choriocarcinoma
choriocele
chorioepithelioma
chorioma
chorion
chorionic
    c. cavity
    c. sac
    c. villus biopsy
chorioretinitis
choristoblastoma
choristoma nest
choroid
    c. plexus
    c. plexus carcinoma
    c. plexus papilloma
    c. point
    c. vein
choroidal
    c. artery
    c. hemangioma
    c. hemorrhage
    c. infiltration
    c. lesion
    c. metastasis

c. neovascularization
c. neovascular membrane
c. ring
c. rupture
choroidectomy
choroiditis
choroidocapillaris
Chow technique
Chrisman-Snook
C.-S. ankle technique
C.-S. procedure
C.-S. reconstruction
chromaffin
c. body
c. tissue
chromate method
chromatic lens aberration
chromatin
c. condensation
c. pattern
chromatinic body
chromatography
gas c.
chrome alum hematoxylin-phloxine method
chromocystoscopy
chromogenic method
chromohydrotubation
chromolytic method
chromopertubation
chromoscopy
chromotubation
chronic
c. allograft rejection
c. anoplasty treatment
c. appendicitis
c. atrial fibrillation
c. catheterization
c. cholecystitis
c. course
c. digestive bleeding
c. Epstein-Barr virus infection
c. extrinsic alveolitis
c. graft-versus-host disease
c. granular myringitis
c. hemolysis
c. hyperparathyroid state
c. hyperventilation syndrome
c. inflammatory demyelinating polyradiculoneuropathy (CIDP)
c. intestinal failure

c. intestinal pseudoobstruction syndrome
c. jejunal inflammation
c. liver disease
c. mesenteric ischemia
c. motor disturbance
c. multisystem disorder
c. nonmalignant
c. nonmalignant pain
c. obstructive airways disease (COAD)
c. obstructive pulmonary dysfunction
c. opioid analgesic therapy (COAT)
c. pancreatitis
c. paroxysmal hemicrania (CPH)
c. presentation
c. reflux symptom
c. renal failure (CRF)
c. sinusitis
c. subareolar abscess
c. subcutaneous infusion
c. subdural hematoma
c. thrombosis
c. transplant rejection
c. ulcerative colitis (CUC)
c. venous insufficiency (CVI)
chronicity
Chuinard-Peterson ankle fusion
chylangioma
chyle
c. cistern
c. cyst
c. fistula
c. vessel
chylifera
chyliform ascites
chylocyst
chyloma
chyloperitoneum
chylothorax
chylous
c. ascites
c. ascitic fluid
c. effusion
c. hydrotherapy
c. leak
c. leakage
chyme
chymopapain chemonucleolysis
CI
cardiac index

NOTES

CI *(continued)*
  normal CI
  supranormal CI
Ciaccio method
Cibis
  C. liquid silicone procedure
  C. operation
cicatrectomy
cicatrices (*pl. of* cicatrix)
cicatriceum
cicatricial
  c. entropion
  c. kidney
  c. mass
  c. stricture
  c. tissue
cicatricotomy
cicatrix, pl. cicatrices
cicatrizant
cicatrization
CIDP
  chronic inflammatory demyelinating
  polyradiculoneuropathy
Cierny-Mader technique
ciliarotomy
ciliary
  c. artery
  c. beat frequency
  c. body
  c. body band
  c. canal
  c. ganglion
  c. ganglion root
  c. injection
  c. ligament
  c. nerve
  c. procedure
  c. process
  c. ring
  c. vein
  c. zone
  c. zonule
ciliectomy
ciliodestructive surgery
cilioretinal artery
ciliotomy
ciliovitrectomy block
Cimino-Brescia arteriovenous fistula
Cimino fistula
cinching operation
Cincinnati
  C. incision
  C. technique
cineangiography
  biplane c.
cinedefecography
cine-esophagoscopy
cinefluoroscopic method

cinefluoroscopy
  valve c.
cinegastroscopy
cinereum
cine view
cingula (*pl. of* cingulum)
cingulate
  c. cortex
  c. herniation
  c. sulcus
cingulectomy
cingulotomy
  rostral c.
cingulum, pl. cingula
  c. bundle
cingulumotomy
circinate exudate
circle
  c. absorption anesthesia
  arterial cerebral c.
  articular vascular c.
  Bain c.
  closed c.
  c. dissipation
  Huguier c.
  c. loop biliary drainage
  Pagenstecher c.
  pediatric c.
  semiclosed c.
  c. straight cutting
  c. system
  vascular c.
  c. wire nephrostomy
circuit
  ancillary c.
  anesthesia breathing c.
  anesthetic c.
  breathing c.
  extracorporeal cardiopulmonary c.
  feedback reduction c.
  low-flow c.
  ventilation c.
circuitry
  intrinsic c.
circular
  c. anastomosis
  c. cherry-red lesion
  c. fold
  c. griseotomy
  c. incision
  c. myotomy
  c. open amputation
  c. pharyngeal muscle
  c. suture technique
  c. venous sinus
circulating
  c. air pocket
  c. blood

c. hormone
c. MEN I-specific growth factor

circulation
abdominal c.
airway, breathing, c. (ABC)
allantoic c.
c. aneurysm
arterial c.
assisted c.
bile acid c.
carotid c.
cerebral c.
collateral abdominal c.
collateral arterial c.
collateral mesenteric c.
compensatory c.
conjunctival c.
coronary collateral c.
cutaneous collateral c.
derivative c.
ductal-dependent pulmonary c.
enterohepatic c.
episcleral c.
extracorporeal c. (ECC)
extracranial carotid c.
femoral c.
fetal c.
fetoplacental c.
hepatic c.
hyperdynamic c.
hypophysial portal c.
hypothalamic-hypophysial portal c.
intracranial c.
left dominant coronary c.
mesenteric c.
perichondral c.
peripheral c.
persistent fetal c.
placental c.
portal-collateral c.
portal-hypophysial c.
portosystemic collateral c.
posterior fossa c.
pulmonary c.
c. rate
retinal c.
sludging of c.
spinal cord c.
splanchnic c.
systemic venous c.
thalamic c.
thebesian c.

c. time
umbilical c.
uteroplacental c.
venous c.
c. volume

circulator fold
circulatory
c. arrest
c. arrest anesthetic technique
c. arrest procedure
c. decompensation
c. overload
c. steal

circulus, pl. circuli
circumalveolar fixation
circumanal gland
circumareolar
c. incision
c. mastopexy
c. quadrant

circumaxillary
circumbulbar
circumcise
circumcision
pharaonic c.
Sunna c.
c. suture technique

circumcorneal injection
circumcostal gastropexy
circumduction maneuver
circumference
fetal head c.
lung-to-head c.

circumferentia
circumferential
c. esophageal reconstruction
c. esophagomyotomy
c. fibrocartilage
c. fracture
c. implantation
c. incision
c. mesorectal excision
c. mobilization
c. mucosal dissection
c. strip
c. venolysis
c. wire-loop fixation

circumferentially ligated
circumflex
c. femoral artery
c. humeral artery
c. iliac artery

NOTES

circumflex *(continued)*
   c. nerve
   c. scapular artery
   c. vein
circumintestinal
circumlental space
circumlimbal incision
circumlinear incision
circummandibular fixation
circummesencephalic cistern
circumocular
circumorbital
circumrenal
circumscribed
   c. inflammation
   c. mass
circumscribing incision
circumumbilical
   c. incision
   c. pyloromyotomy
circumvallate papilla
circumvascular
circumzygomatic fixation
cirrhosis
   Child classification of c.
   cholestatic c.
   end-stage c.
   primary biliary c.
cirrhotic
   c. liver
   c. liver parenchyma
   c. liver remnant
cirsectomy
cirsodesis
cirsotomy
CIS
   carcinoma in situ
cisatracurium
cistern
   basal c.
   cerebellomedullary c.
   cerebellopontine angle c.
   chiasmatic c.
   chyle c.
   circummesencephalic c.
   interpeduncular c.
   lumbar c.
   mesencephalic c.
   Pecquet c.
   perimesencephalic c.
   pontine c.
   prepontine c.
   quadrigeminal c.
   subarachnoid c.
   suprasellar subarachnoid c.
   sylvian c.
cisterna, pl. **cisternae**
   ambient c.

   chiasmatic c.
   cylindrical confronting c.
   perinuclear c.
   subsarcolemma c.
   terminal c.
cisternal
   c. herniation
   c. puncture
citrate
   c. intoxication
   oral transmucosal fentanyl c.
Civinini
   C. ligament
   C. process
CKC
   cold knife cone
2C-L
   2-chamber longitudinal
   2C-L image
Clado
   C. anastomosis
   C. band
   C. ligament
   C. point
Clagett
   C. closure
   C. operation
Clagett-Barrett esophagogastrostomy
clam
   c. enterocystoplasty
   c. ileocystoplasty
clamp
   bone-holding c.
clamp-and-sew technique
clamping
   aortic c.
   blind c.
   carotid c.
   portal triad c.
   selective vascular c. (SVC)
clamshell
   c. closure
   c. incision
   c. technique
   c. thoracotomy
Clancy
   C. cruciate ligament reconstruction
   C. ligament technique
   C. patellar tendon graft
CLAP
   contact laser ablation of prostate
Clapton line
Clark
   C. level
   C. transfer technique
Clark-Collip method
Clark-Southwick-Odgen modification

CLASP
    Carolinas Laparoscopic Advanced
    Surgery Program
    CLASP procedure
clasped thumb deformity
classic
    c. abdominal Semm hysterectomy
    c. DSRS technique
    c. multiple organ failure syndrome
classical
    c. cesarean section
    c. Judd-Mayo overlap midline
    incisional hernioplasty
    c. subtotal resection
    c. transverse incision
classification
    Ackerman-Proffitt c. of
    malocclusion
    Acosta c.
    acromioclavicular injury c.
    Aitken epiphysial fracture c.
    AJCC TNM tumor c.
    Allman acromioclavicular injury c.
    Alonso-Lej c.
    American Association for Surgery
    of Trauma Organ Injury Scale c.
    American Heart Association c.
    American Society of
    Anesthesiologists c.
    Anderson-D'Alonzo odontoid
    fracture c.
    Anderson modification of Berndt-
    Harty c.
    Angle malocclusion c.
    Ann Arbor c.
    AO c.
    Arneth c.
    Ashhurst-Bromer ankle fracture c.
    Astler-Coller c. (A, B1, B2, C1,
    C2)
    Astler-Coller modification of
    Dukes c.
    Bado c.
    Bailyn c.
    Banff c.
    Bauer-Jackson c.
    Baume c.
    Bennett c.
    Bergey c.
    Berndt-Harty c.
    Binet system of c.
    BI-RADS c.

Bishop c.
bismuth benign bile duct
    stricture c.
bismuth bile duct stricture (type I-
    V) c.
Black c.
bladder carcinoma c.
Borrmann gastric cancer c.
Borrmann gastric cancer typing
    systems c. (type I–IV)
Bosniak c.
Boyd c.
Boyd-Griffin trochanteric fracture c.
Breslow c.
Broders index of malignant
    tumor c.
burn c.
Butchart staging c.
Caldwell-Moloy c.
Callender cell-type c.
Cambridge c.
Canadian Cardiovascular Society c.
caries c.
Carnesale-Stewart-Barnes hip
    dislocation c.
Caroli-Sarles c.
Catterall c.
cavity c.
CEAP c.
Cedars-Sinai c.
Centers for Disease Control HIV
    infection c.
Chadwick-Bentley c.
Chicago c.
Child esophageal varix c.
Child hepatic dysfunction c.
Child hepatic risk criteria c.
Child liver disease c.
Child-Pugh c.
Child-Turcotte hepatic surgery c.
clean-contaminated operative
    wound c.
clean operative wound c.
cleft palate c.
clinical pathologic c.
Codman c.
Cohen-Rentrop c.
Colonna hip fracture c.
Colton c.
contaminated operative wound c.
Cori c.
Correa c.

C

NOTES

classification (*continued*)

Couinaud c.
Croften c.
Crowe c.
Cummer c.
Dagradi esophageal variceal c.
Danis-Weber ankle injury c.
DeBakey c.
DeLee c.
Denis Browne spinal fracture c.
denture c.
Denver c.
Dexter-Grossman c.
Diamond c.
Dias-Tachdijian physical injury c.
dichotomous c.
Dickhaut-DeLee discoid meniscus c.
dirty operative wound c.
Dripps c.
Duane c.
Dubin-Amelar varicocele c.
Dukes c.
Eckert-Davis c.
Edmondson-Steiner c.
Efron jackknife c.
Ellis c.
Enneking c.
Epstein hip dislocation c.
Epstein-Thomas c.
Essex-Lopresti calcaneal fracture c.
Evans intertrochanteric fracture c.
FAB c.
Federation of Gynecology and
  Obstetrics c.
Fielding femoral fracture c.
Fielding-Magliato subtrochanteric
  fracture c.
Flatt c.
Foucher epiphysial injury c.
fracture c.
Fränkel neurologic deficit c.
Franz-O'Rahilly c.
Fredrickson hyperlipoproteinemia c.
Fredrickson-Levy-Lees c.
Freeman calcaneal fracture c.
French-American-British c.
Frykman distal radius fracture c.
Frykman radial fracture c.
Fukunaga-Hayes unbiased
  jackknife c.
functional capacity c.
Garden femoral neck fracture c.
Gartland humeral supracondylar
  fracture c.
Gartland Universal radial
  fracture c.
gastric mucosal pattern c.
Gell and Coombs c.
Goldman c.

Grantham femur fracture c.
Greenfield spinocerebellar ataxia c.
Gustilo-Anderson open fracture c.
Gustilo puncture wound c.
Haggitt c.
Hannover c.
Hansen fracture c.
Hara gallbladder inflammation c.
Hardcastle tarsometatarsal joint
  injury c.
Hawkins talar fracture c.
Henderson c.
Hepatitis Activity Index c.
Herring lateral pillar c.
Hinchey diverticulitis grade c.
HIV c.
Hoaglund-States c.
Hohl-Luck tibial plateau fracture c.
Hohl-Moore c.
Hohl tibial condylar fracture c.
Holdsworth spinal fracture c.
House-Brackmann c.
Hughston c.
human immunodeficiency virus c.
Hunt and Kosnik c.
Ideberg glenoid fracture c.
immunologic c.
Insall patellar injury c.
International Cancer of Cervix C.
International Federation of
  Gynecology and Obstetrics c.
international stage c.
Isaacson c. (IC)
Jackson and Parker c.
Jansky c.
Japanese cancer c.
Jeffery radial fracture c.
Jensen c.
Jewett and Whitmore c.
Johner-Wruhs tibial fracture c.
Jones-Barnes-Lloyd-Roberts c.
Kajava c.
Kalamchi c.
Karnofsky rating scale c.
Kasugai c.
Kauffman-White c.
Keil tumor cell c.
Keith-Wagener c.
Keith-Wagener-Barker c.
Kelami c.
Kellam-Waddel c.
Kennedy c.
Kernohan system of glioma c.
KESS constipation scoring
  system c.
Key-Conwell pelvic fracture c.
Kiel c.
Kilfoyle humeral medial condylar
  fracture c.

Killip c.
Killip-Kimball heart failure c.
Kocher c.
KWB c.
Kyle-Gustilo c.
Kyle-Gustilo-Premer c.
Lancefield c.
Lanza scale for drug-induced
  mucosal damage c.
Lauge-Hansen ankle fracture c.
Lauren gastric carcinoma c.
Le Fort c.
Leishman c.
Lennert c.
Letournel-Judet acetabular
  fracture c.
Leung thumb loss c.
Levine-Harvey c.
Lindell c.
Linell-Ljungberg c.
Lloyd-Roberts-Catteral-Salamon c.
Loesche c.
Lown c.
Lukes and Butler Hodgkin
  disease c.
Lukes-Collins c.
MacCallan c.
Macewen c.
MacNichol-Voutsinas c.
malignant tumor c.
Mallampati oropharyngeal c.
Mallampati pharyngeal visibility c.
Marseille pancreatitis c.
Mason radial head fracture c.
Mast-Spieghel-Pappas c.
Mathews olecranon fracture c.
Mayo carpal instability c.
Mayo rheumatoid elbow c.
McNeer c.
Melone distal radius fracture c.
Meyers-McKeever tibial fracture c.
microinvasive carcinoma c.
Milch condylar fracture c.
Milch elbow fracture c.
Milch humeral fracture c.
Ming gastric carcinoma c.
Minnesota EKG c.
Moore tibial plateau fracture c.
morphologic c.
Moss c.
Mueller femoral supracondylar
  fracture c.

Mueller tibial fracture c.
multiaxial c.
Munro and Parker laparoscopic
  hysterectomy c.
Nalebuff c.
Neer femur fracture c.
Neer shoulder fracture c.
Newman radial neck and head
  fracture c.
New York Heart Association heart
  disease c.
Nicoll c.
Niemeier c.
Nyhus c.
Ogden epiphysial fracture c.
Ogden knee dislocation c.
O'Rahilly limb deficiency c.
ordinal c.
Orthopaedic Trauma Association c.
Outerbridge c.
Paley c.
Papavasiliou olecranon fracture c.
Pap smear c.
Paris c.
Pauwels femoral neck fracture c.
Pell and Gregory c.
Pennal c.
Pipkin femoral fracture c.
Pipkin posterior hip dislocation c.
Pipkin subclassification of Epstein-
  Thomas c.
Poland epiphysial fracture c.
Poland physical injury c.
Potter c.
Pugh c.
Pugh-Child bleeding esophageal
  varices grading scale c.
Pulec and Freedman c.
Quénu-Küss tarsometatarsal
  injury c.
Quinby pelvic fracture c.
Rai c.
Ranawat c.
Ranson acute pancreatitis c.
Rappaport c.
Rastelli c.
Rentrop c.
Riseborough-Radin intercondylar
  fracture c.
Rockwood acromioclavicular
  injury c.
Rockwood clavicular fracture c.

C

NOTES

classification *(continued)*
    Rosenthal nail injury c.
    round-robin c.
    Rowe calcaneal fracture c.
    Rowe-Lowell hip dislocation c.
    Rowe-Lowell system for fracture-
        dislocation c.
    Ruedi-Allgower c.
    Runyon c.
    Russe c.
    Russell-Taylor c.
    Rüter c.
    Rutkow-Robbins-Gilbert c.
    Rutledge extended hysterectomy c.
    Rye Hodgkin disease c.
    Sage-Salvatore acromioclavicular
        joint injury c.
    Saha shoulder muscle c.
    Sakellarides calcaneal fracture c.
    Salter epiphysial fracture c.
    Salter-Harris epiphysial fracture c.
    Santiani-Stone c.
    Sassouni c.
    Savary-Mille grading scale c.
    scalar c.
    Schatzker tibial plateau fracture c.
    Scheie c.
    Schuknecht c.
    Seattle c.
    Seddon c.
    Seinsheimer femoral fracture c.
    sentence c.
    Severin c.
    Shaffer-Weiss c.
    Shaher-Puddu c.
    Shelton femoral fracture c.
    Singh osteoporosis c.
    Siurala c.
    Skinner c.
    Snyder c.
    Solcia c.
    Sonnenberg c.
    Sorbie calcaneal fracture c.
    Spaulding c.
    Speed radial head fracture c.
    Spetzler-Martin c.
    Stark c.
    Steinbrocker c.
    Stulberg c.
    Suda papilla c. (type I–III)
    Sunderland nerve injury c.
    Swanson c.
    Sydney system gastritis c.
    Tachdjian c.
    Tessier c.
    Thomas c.
    Thompson-Epstein femoral
        fracture c.
    Three Color Concept of wound c.
    Thrombolysis in Myocardial
        Infarction c.
    Tile c.
    TIMI c.
    TNM carcinoma c.
    tongue thrust c.
    Torg c.
    Torode-Zieg c.
    Toronto pelvic fracture c.
    Tronzo intertrochanteric fracture c.
    Tscherne c.
    Tscherne-Gotzen tibial fracture c.
    tumor, node, metastasis
        carcinoma c.
    UICC tumor c.
    Vaughan Williams antiarrhythmic
        drug c.
    Veau c.
    Venn-Watson c.
    Visick dysphagia c.
    Vostal radial fracture c.
    Wagener-Clay-Gipner c.
    Wagner c.
    Walter Reed c.
    Warren-Marshall c.
    Wassel thumb duplication c.
    Watanabe discoid meniscus c.
    Watson-Jones tibial tubercle
        avulsion fracture c.
    Weber-Danis ankle injury c.
    Weber physical injury c.
    Weiland c.
    Weissman c.
    White c.
    Whitehead c.
    Whitmore-Jewett c.
    WHO gastric carcinoma c.
    Wiberg patellar c.
    Wiley-Galey c.
    Wilkins radial fracture c.
    Winquist femoral shaft fracture c.
    Winquist-Hansen femoral fracture c.
    Winter c.
    Wolfe breast carcinoma c.
    Woofry-Chandler c.
    World Health Organization c.
    Yacoub and Radley-Smith c.
    Young pelvic fracture c.
    Zickel c.
    Zlotsky-Ballard acromioclavicular
        injury c.
    Zollinger c.
claudication
Claudius
    C. cell
    C. fossa
Clausen method
claustra

claustral
claustrum, pl. claustra
clavi (*pl. of* clavus)
clavicectomy
clavicle excision
clavicula, pl. claviculae
clavicular
    c. birth fracture
    c. branch
    c. epiphysis
    c. facet
    c. fracture aneurysm
    c. incision
claviculectomy
clavipectoral fascia
clavipectoralis
clavus, pl. clavi
clawfoot deformity
clawhand deformity
clawing deformity
clawtoe deformity
clay pipe carcinoma
clayshoveler's fracture
Clayton
    C. forefoot arthroplasty
    C. procedure
    C. procedure with panmetatarsal
    head resection
Clayton-Fowler technique
C-LDP
    complete laparoscopic distal
    pancreatectomy
CLE
    continuous lumbar epidural
clean
    c. intermittent catheterization
    c. intermittent self-catheterization
    c. operation
    c. operative wound classification
clean-catch collection method
clean-contaminated
    c.-c. operation
    c.-c. operative wound classification
    c.-c. surgery
cleaning solution
cleansing
    bowel c.
clear
    c. cell hepatocellular carcinoma
    c. cell hidradenoma
    c. effluent
    c. fluid

    c. liquid diet
    c. otorrhea
clearance
    elimination c.
    lactate c.
    mucociliary c.
    oncologic c.
    c. technique
Cleasby iridectomy operation
cleavage
    c. fracture
    c. lesion
    c. line
    c. plane
cleft
    anal c.
    c. closure
    corneal c.
    facial c.
    c. hand deformity
    Larrey c.
    c. lip
    c. lip deformity
    natal c.
    c. nose
    oblique facial c.
    c. palate
    c. palate classification
    pudendal c.
    residual c.
    soft palate c.
    subdural c.
    urogenital c.
cleidocostal
cleidocranial
cleidoepitrochlearis
cleidomastoideus
cleido-occipitalis
cleidotomy
Cleveland
    C. Clinic weighted scale
    C. procedure
Cleveland-Bosworth-Thompson technique
clidal
clidocostal
clidocranial
clinch knot
clinic
    dialysis c.
    outpatient dialysis c.
clinical
    c. acute pancreatitis

C

NOTES

clinical *(continued)*
    c. characteristic
    C. Classification System (CCS)
    c. correlation
    c. defect
    c. deterioration
    c. diagnosis
    c. encephalopathy
    c. evaluation
    c. evidence
    c. examination
    c. followup
    c. geneticist
    c. grading scale (CGS)
    c. implication
    c. improvement
    c. indication
    c. intestinal transplantation
    c. manifestation
    c. manifestations, etiologic factors, anatomic involvement, pathophysiologic features (CEAP)
    c. outcome
    c. parameter
    c. pathologic classification
    c. pathology
    c. picture
    c. presentation
    c. principle
    c. problem
    c. response
    c. spectroscopy
    c. suspicion
    c. syndrome
clinically
    c. node-negative breast cancer
    c. severe obesity (CSO)
    c. silent rhabdomyoma
clinician
    nonsurgical c.
    surgical c.
clinicopathologic
    c. correlation
    c. data
    c. feature
Clinitron air-fluidized therapy
clinoidectomy
    anterior extradural c.
    extradural c.
clinoideus
clinoid process
clip
    c. application
    c. graft
    c. occlusion
    c. placement
    c. technique
clip-induced bile duct stricture
clitoral recession

clitoridectomy
clitoridis
clitoris, pl. **clitorides**
clitoroplasty
clitorovaginoplasty
clival
clivus, pl. **clivi**
    Blumenbach c.
    c. canal line
    c. metastasis
    c. syndrome
CLO
    Campylobacter-like organism
    CLO biopsy
cloaca, pl. **cloacae**
cloacal
    c. formation
    c. malformation
    c. membrane
clock
    around the c. (ATC)
clockwise
    c. direction
    c. rotation
clomiphene fetal malformation
clonal
    c. deletion
    c. expansion
C-loop intraocular lens
Cloquet
    C. canal
    C. canal remnant
    C. fascia
    C. hernia
    C. ligament
    C. node
    C. pseudoganglion
    C. septum
close
    c. margin
    c. monitoring
    c. proximity
closed
    c. anesthesia system
    c. approach
    c. break fracture
    c. chest commissurotomy
    c. chest thoracostomy
    c. circle
    c. circuit anesthesia
    c. circuit anesthetic technique
    c. circuit method
    c. dislocation
    c. flap amputation
    c. gloving technique
    c. head injury
    c. hemorrhoidectomy
    c. intramedullary osteotomy
    c. irrigation

c. laparoscopy
c. loop automated delivery
c. loop intestinal obstruction
c. manipulative maneuver
c. nail
c. patch test
c. pinning
c. reduction
c. reduction/chemical splinting
c. reduction and percutaneous fixation (CRPF)
c. skull fracture
c. soft tissue injury
c. space infection
c. suction drainage
c. surgery
c. system pars plana vitrectomy
c. transventricular mitral commissurotomy
c. tubule fixation technique
c. wedge osteotomy

closed-loop
c.-l. control
c.-l. system

closing
c. abductory wedge osteotomy
c. base wedge
c. base wedge osteotomy
c. pressure
c. ring of Winkler-Waldeyer

clostridial
c. infection
c. myonecrosis

closure
abdominal wall c.
abdominal wound c.
aponeurotic c.
auditory c.
Barsky cleft c.
Clagett c.
clamshell c.
cleft c.
colostomy c.
compression skull-cap c.
crowfoot c.
crural c.
delayed primary c.
direct c.
double-umbrella c.
end stoma c.
epiphysial c.
exstrophy c.

fascial c.
c. of fistula
flask c.
floor-of-mouth c.
Fontan fenestration c.
forced eye c.
general c.
glottic c.
Graham c.
Hartmann c.
ileostomy c.
incision c.
King ASD umbrella c.
latex c.
layered c.
2-layer latex c.
Marlex c.
mastectomy c.
maxillary antrum c.
midline aponeurotic c.
muscularis tunnel c.
nonoperative c.
nonprosthetic c.
palatopharyngeal c.
pancreatic stump c.
percutaneous patent ductus arteriosus c.
premature airway c.
premature ductus arteriosis c.
c. pressure
primary c.
c. principle
retainer c.
scalloped c.
scalp c.
secondary c.
shoelace fasciotomy c.
single-layer continuous c.
sinus c.
skin c.
Smead-Jones c.
stoma c.
suture c.
sutureless colostomy c.
transcatheter c.
transmural c.
umbrella c.
vacuum-assisted c. (VAC)
velopharyngeal c.
ventricular septal defect c.
visual c.
Von Langenbeck palatal c.

C

NOTES

closure *(continued)*
    V-to-Y c.
    watertight c.
    wound c.
clot
    afferent c.
    agonal c.
    antemortem c.
    autologous c.
    black blood c.
    blood c.
    chicken fat c.
    c. colic
    currant jelly c.
    distal c.
    evacuating c.
    exogenous fibrin c.
    c. extension
    external c.
    c. formation
    fresh blood c.
    friable c.
    heart c.
    internal c.
    laminated c.
    marantic c.
    organized c.
    passive c.
    plastic c.
    postmortem c.
    c. propagation
    proximal c.
    c. regression
    retraction of c.
    c. retraction coagulation panel
    Schede c.
    sentinel blood c.
    c. size
    spider-web c.
    stratified c.
    washed c.
CLOtest
    Campylobacter-like organism test
clothespin H spinal fusion
clot-induced urinary tract obstruction
clotting
    abnormal c.
    c. abnormality
    c. factor
    graft c.
    c. mechanism
    c. parameter
    c. time coagulation panel
cloudy
    c. ascites
    c. fluid
cloverleaf
    c. condylar plate fixation
    c. skull

    c. skull deformity
    c. skull syndrome
Cloward
    C. anterior spinal fusion
    C. back fusion
    C. cervical disc approach
    C. fusion discectomy
    C. operation
    C. procedure
    C. technique
CLP
    cecal ligation and puncture
clubbed
    c. nail
    c. penis
clubbing
    nail c.
clubfoot deformity
cluneal
clunium
cluster
    c. headache
    c. operation
    c. reduction
    repetitive c.
    c. tic syndrome
clustered calcification
CMAP
    compound muscle action potential
CMR
    cerebral metabolic rate
CMV
    controlled mechanical ventilation
    cytomegalovirus
        CMV colitis
        CMV infection
        CMV prophylaxis
CMV-associated ulceration
CMV-induced esophageal ulceration
CMV-positive donor
cnemial
cnemis
CO
    carbon monoxide
    cardiac output
CO$_2$
    carbon dioxide
    arterial partial pressure of CO$_2$
    CO$_2$ elimination
    CO$_2$ inhalation test
    CO$_2$ pneumoperitoneum
COAD
    chronic obstructive airways disease
coagula (*pl. of* coagulum)
coagulate
coagulating
    c. diathermy
    c. factor

coagulation
- argon beam c.
- argon beam plasma c. (ABPC)
- bipolar c.
- blood c.
- Bovie c.
- c. cascade
- cold c.
- c. defect
- diffuse intravascular c.
- c. disorder
- disseminated intravascular c. (DIC)
- electric c.
- endoscopic microwave c.
- endovascular c.
- exogenous anticoagulant c.
- c. factor
- c. factor assay
- c. factor transfusion
- fibrinolysin c.
- free-beam c.
- heater-probe c.
- infrared c.
- laser c.
- light c.
- low-current monopolar c.
- Meyer-Schwickerath light c.
- microwave c.
- monopolar c.
- multipolar c.
- c. necrosis
- plasmin c.
- c. profile
- c. screen
- sepsis-induced disseminated intravascular c.
- tissue c.

coagulative
- c. laser therapy
- c. myocytolysis

coagulator
- suction c.

coagulopathic disorder

coagulopathy
- hypothermia-induced c.
- hypothermia-related c.
- uremia-related c.

coagulum, pl. **coagula**
- c. formation
- c. pyelolithotomy

Coakley suture technique

coalesce

coal-mining lensectomy

coapt

coaptation
- end-to-side nerve c.
- nerve c.
- c. site
- c. suture technique
- urethral c.

coarct

coarctate

coarctation
- c. of aorta
- postductal c.
- c. of pulmonary artery
- c. repair
- c. syndrome

coarctectomy

coarctotomy

coarticulation
- anticipatory c.
- backward c.
- forward c.

COAT
- chronic opioid analgesic therapy

coat
- muscular c.
- seromuscular c.

Coats white ring

coaxial
- c. illumination
- c. pressure

cobalt-60 moving strip technique

cobaltinitrite method

cobalt therapy

cobbler's suture technique

cobblestone appearance

Cobb scoliosis measuring technique

cobra-head anastomosis

cocaine anesthesia

cocaine-induced respiratory failure

cocainization

coccidian body

Coccidioides **infection**

coccygeal
- c. body
- c. cornua
- c. dimple
- c. fistula
- c. foveola
- c. ganglion
- c. gland
- c. horn

NOTES

C

coccygeal (*continued*)
  c. joint
  c. muscle
  c. nerve
  c. plexus
  c. vertebra
  c. whorl
coccygectomy
  Lougheed-White c.
coccyges (*pl. of* coccyx)
coccygeum
coccygeus muscle
coccygotomy
coccyx, pl. coccyges
  c. fracture
cochlea, pl. cochleae
cochlear
  c. duct
  c. ganglion
  c. lesion
  c. nerve
  c. stimulator
cochleariform process
cochleosacculotomy
cochleostomy
cochleovestibular
  c. approach
  c. neurectomy
cocked-half flap
Cocke maxillectomy
Cockett procedure
Cockroft method
cocktail
  lytic c.
cock-up deformity
codfish deformity
Codivilla tendon lengthening technique
Codman
  C. classification
  C. incision
  C. saber-cut shoulder approach
coefficient
  intraclass correlation c.'s
  octanol/water c.
coeliac
  c. artery
  c. axis
co-eluted
coenzyme
  ameliorating myocardial stunning
    liposomal c.
coexistence
coffee-ground
  c.-g. emesis
  c.-g. vomitus
Coffey
  C. incision
  C. suspension

  C. technique
  C. ureterointestinal anastomosis
Coffey-Witzel jejunostomy technique
Cofield technique
Cogan syndrome
cognitive
  c. anxiety subscale
  c. behavior treatment (CBT)
  c. dysfunction
  C. Errors Questionnaire
cognitive-attitudinal factor inquiry
cognitive-behavioral therapy
cogwheel respiration
Cohen
  C. antireflux procedure
  C. cross-trigonal reimplantation
  C. cross-trigonal technique
Cohen-Rentrop classification
coherent bundle
coil
  asymmetrical gradient c.
coiled
  c. intracranial aneurysm
  c. spring appearance
  c. spring sign
coiling
  endovascular c.
coil-shaped varix
coin
  c. biopsy
  fracture en c.
  c. lesion
coincidence correction
coinduction of anesthesia
coital cephalalgia
Coiter muscle
Colcher-Sussman method
cold
  c. abscess
  c. application
  c. coagulation
  c. cone biopsy
  c. conization
  c. cup biopsy
  c. defect
  c. erythema
  c. exposure
  c. forceps ablation
  c. gangrene
  c. gas sterilization
  c. gas sterilized
  c. ischemia time
  c. knife cone aspiration
  c. knife conization
  c. knife endoureterotomy
  c. knife method
  c. lesion
  c. nodule
  c. pressor test (CPT)

c. pressor testing maneuver
c. restraint stress
c. saline-induced paresthesia technique
c. snare ablation
c. snare excision
c. soak solution
c. spot

cold-cup resection

Cole
C. intubation procedure
C. osteotomy
C. sign
C. technique
C. tendon fixation

colectasia

colectomy
abdominal c.
hand-assisted laparoscopic c.
laparoscopic c.
left c.
open c.
partial c.
prophylactic c.
restorative c.
1-stage left c.
subtotal c. (SC)
total c. (TC)
total abdominal c. (TAC)
transverse c.

Coleman
C. flatfoot technique
C. plasty

coleocele

coleoptosis

coleotomy

coli
adenomatous polyposis c. (APC)

colic
abdominal c.
appendiceal c.
appendicular c.
c. artery
bile duct c.
biliary c.
bilious c.
clot c.
common duct c.
Devonshire c.
episodic c.
c. epithelium
esophageal c.

flatulent c.
c. flexure
gallbladder c.
gallstone c.
hepatic c.
hysterical c.
c. impression
infantile c.
intestinal c.
kidney c.
lead c.
mucous c.
nephritic c.
c. omentum
Painter c.
pancreatic c.
c. patch
c. patch esophagoplasty
c. plexus
psychogenic c.
renal c.
saturnine c.
spasmodic c.
c. sphincter
ureteral c.
c. vein
vermicular c.

colicky pain

coliform urinary infection

coliplication

colipuncture

colitis
amebic c.
chronic ulcerative c. (CUC)
CMV c.
c. cystica profunda
cytomegalovirus c.
granulomatous c.
ischemic c.
c. perineal complication
radiation-induced c.
ulcerative c. (UC)

colla (*pl. of* collum)

collagen
c. accumulation
c. injection
c. production
c. staining method
c. synthesis

collagenase level

collagenous
c. sprue

NOTES

collagenous *(continued)*
  c. tissue
  c. trabecular ring
collapse
  abrupt hemodynamic c.
  bone graft c.
  c. cavitation
  hemodynamic c.
  lobar c.
collar
  c. bone
  c. incision
collar-bone appearance
collar-button
  c.-b. abscess
  c.-b. ulceration
collar-button-like ulcer
collateral
  c. abdominal circulation
  c. arterial circulation
  c. digital artery
  c. ligament
  c. ligament rupture
  c. mesenteric circulation
  portal c.
  portal-systemic c.
  pulmonary c.
  c. pulp canal
  c. respiration
  c. vein
  venous c.
  c. vessel
collateralization
  ventilation c.
collecting duct
collection
  abdominal air c.
  abdominal fluid c.
  air c.
  arterial blood c.
  cell c.
  duodenal fluid c.
  encysted intraabdominal c.
  expired air c.
  extraaxial fluid c.
  extracerebral fluid c.
  fluid c.
  gas c.
  globular c.
  gravitational particle c.
  infected c.
  intraglandular fluid c.
  isokinetic c.
  pancreatic fluid c.
  periarticular fluid c.
  pericholecystic fluid c.
  perinephric fluid c.
  pleural fluid c.

  posttraumatic subcapsular hepatic
    fluid c.
  pus c.
  quantitative stool c.
  saccular c.
  urine specimen c.
Colles
  C. fascia
  C. fracture
  C. ligament
  C. space
colli artery
colliculectomy
colliculitis
colliculus, pl. **colliculi**
  facial c.
  seminal c.
Collier tract
collimator
  high-resolution parallel hole c.
Collin-Beard operation
Collis
  C. antireflux operation
  C. broken femoral stem technique
  C. gastroplasty
  C. gastroplasty procedure
  C. repair
Collis-Dubrul femoral stem removal
Collis-Nissen
  C.-N. esophageal lengthening
    procedure
  C.-N. fundoplication
  C.-N. fundoplication method
  C.-N. fundoplication procedure
  C.-N. fundoplication technique
  C.-N. gastroplasty
collodion
  flexible c.
  hemostatic c.
  c. membrane
  styptic c.
collodium
colloid
  c. body
  c. cancer
  c. carcinoma
  c. cyst
  c. formation
  c. goiter
  c. material
  c. osmotic pressure (COP)
  c. solution
  c. theory of narcosis
colloidal osmotic pressure
collum, pl. **colla**
coloanal
  c. anastomosis
  c. resection
coloboma anomaly

colobronchial fistula
colocentesis
colocholecystostomy
colocolic
    c. anastomosis
    c. intussusception
colocolonic anastomosis
colocolostomy
colocutaneous fistula
colocystoplasty
    seromuscular c.
coloendoanal anastomosis
cologastrocutaneous fistula
colohepatopexy
coloileal fistula
cololysis
colon
    ascending c.
    c. cancer
    c. carcinoma
    c. conduit
    descending c.
    distended c.
    c. epithelium
    c. flexure
    giant c.
    haustration of c.
    iliac c.
    c. incarceration
    lead-pipe c.
    normal c.
    c. obstruction
    c. perforation
    c. polyp
    c. preparation
    c. problem
    c. procedure
    pulled-down c.
    c. and rectal surgery
    c. resection
    sigmoid c.
    spastic c.
    spike burst on electromyogram
     of c.
    transverse c.
    c. tumor
colonic
    c. abscess
    c. adenocarcinoma
    c. adenoma
    c. air
    c. carcinoma

    c. dilation
    c. distention
    c. diverticular hemorrhage
    c. esophagoplasty
    c. explosion
    c. fistula
    c. foreign body
    c. inertia
    c. infiltration
    c. intussusception
    c. J-pouch
    c. lavage
    c. lavage solution
    c. lesion identification
    c. loop
    c. mass
    c. mesenteric plexus
    c. metastasis
    c. mobilization
    c. mucosal line
    c. neoplasm
    c. obstruction
    c. patch
    c. perforation
    c. pouch
    c. pouch anal anastomosis
    c. pseudoobstruction
    c. resection
    c. tattooing
    c. vascular lesion
colonization
    concomitant c.
    c. infection
colonizing organism
Colonna
    C. hip fracture classification
    C. trochanteric arthroplasty
Colonna-Ralston
    C.-R. ankle approach
    C.-R. incision
    C.-R. medial approach
colonoscopic
    c. appendectomy
    c. biopsy
    c. examination
    c. polypectomy
    c. removal
colonoscopy
    cecal c.
    complete c.
    c. complication
    diagnostic c.

C

NOTES

colonoscopy *(continued)*
    emergency c.
    high-magnification c.
    incomplete c.
    pediatric c.
    c. per rectum
    c. per stoma
    real-time c.
    c. screening
    splenic flexure c.
    stomal c.
    tandem c.
    therapeutic c.
    total c.
    upper endoscopy and c.
    virtual c.
colonoscopy-related
    c.-r. emphysema
    c.-r. incarceration
colony
    c. culture
    c. formation
colopexostomy
colopexotomy
colopexy
coloplasty
    c. pouch
    c. procedure
coloplication
coloproctostomy
coloptosis
colopuncture
color
    c. aberration
    c. duplex ultrasonography
    c. fusion
    c. imaging
    c. saturation
colorectal
    c. adenocarcinoma
    c. adenoma
    c. anastomosis
    c. biopsy
    c. bleeding
    c. cancer (CRC)
    c. cancer endoscopy
    c. cancer resection
    c. carcinoma
    c. disease
    c. disorder
    c. distention pain
    c. fistula
    c. hemorrhage
    c. metastasis
    c. mucosa
    c. operation
    c. pathology
    c. physiology
    c. polyp

    c. primary
    c. primary tumor
    c. segment
    c. septum
    c. specimen
    c. surgeon
    c. surgery
colorectostomy
Colored Visual Analogue Scale (CVAS)
colorrhaphy
colosigmoidostomy
colosigmoid resection
colostomy
    blowhole decompressing c.
    c. bridge
    c. closure
    continent c.
    decompression c.
    descending loop c.
    Devine c.
    diverting loop c.
    diverting proximal c.
    divided-stoma c.
    double-barrel c.
    dry c.
    end c.
    end-loop c.
    end-sigmoid c.
    exteriorization c.
    fecal diversion c.
    Hartmann c.
    ileoascending c.
    ileosigmoid c.
    ileotransverse c.
    initial c.
    juxta-anal c.
    Lazaro da Silva technique c.
    loop transverse c.
    Mikulicz c.
    permanent end c.
    c. pyloric autotransplantation
    resective c.
    sigmoid end c.
    sigmoid loop rod c.
    c. soiling
    c. takedown
    temporary diverting c.
    temporary end c.
    terminal c.
    transverse c.
    transverse-loop rod c.
    Turnbull c.
    wet c.
colotomy
colovaginal fistula
colovesical fistula
colpectomy
    skinning c.

colpocleisis
Latzko partial c.
Le Fort partial c.
colpocystoplasty
colpocystotomy
colpocystoureterotomy
colpocystourethropexy
colpohysterectomy
colpohysteropexy
colpohysterotomy
colpomicroscopy
colpomyomectomy
colpoperineopexy
abdominal-sacral c.
colpoperineoplasty
colpoperineorrhaphy
colpopexy
colpoplasty
colpopoiesis
colporectopexy
colporrhaphy
Goffe c.
posterior c.
colposcopic diagnosis
colposcopy
digital imaging c.
estrogen-assisted c.
colpostenotomy
colposuspension
Burch c.
laparoscopic needle c.
laparoscopic retropubic c.
colpotomy incision
colpoureterotomy
colpourethrocystopexy
retropubic c.
colpourethropexy
Burch c.
Coltart
C. calcaneotibial fusion
C. fracture technique
Colton classification
columellar
c. reconstruction
c. repair
column
anal c.
anterior c.
Bertin c.
lateral c.
posterior c.
rectal c.

renal c.
rugal c.
spinal c.
vaginal c.
variceal c.
vertebral c.
columnar
c. cuff carcinoma
c. epithelium
c. metaplasia
columnar-lined esophagus
coma
c. aberration
acute hepatic c.
alcoholic c.
apoplectic c.
barbiturate c.
c. dé passé
diabetic c.
electrolyte imbalance c.
c. grade
hepatic c.
hyperosmolar diabetic c.
hyperosmolar hyperglycemic
nonketotic c. (HHNKC)
hyperosmolar hyperglycemic
nonketotic c. (HHNKC)
insulin c.
irreversible c.
Kussmaul c.
metabolic c.
myxedema c.
c. scale
thyrotoxic c.
trance c.
uremic c.
c. vigil
Comberg foreign body operation
combination
c. calculus
c. chemotherapy
c. fracture
c. of isotonics technique
c. restoration
c. skin
c. surgery
combination fracture
combined
c. analysis
c. anterior and posterior approach
c. cavus deformity
c. chemoradiation therapy

NOTES

combined *(continued)*
    c. defect
    c. epidural/general anesthesia
    c. flexion-distraction injury and burst fracture
    c. gastrointestinal resection
    c. heart catheterization
    c. hiatal hernia
    c. injuries
    c. laparoscopic splenectomy and cholecystectomy
    c. laparoscopic and thoracoscopic approach
    c. low cervical and transthoracic approach
    c. method
    c. neurosurgical-external sinus approach
    c. organ resection
    c. presigmoid-transtransversarium intradural approach
    c. radial-ulnar-humeral fracture
    c. spinal/epidural (CSE)
    c. spinal/epidural anesthesia (CSEA)
    c. spinal/epidural anesthetic technique
    c. spinal/epidural technique
    c. system disease
    c. transsylvian and middle fossa approach
    c. ureterolysis
comblike septum
comb sign
combustion
    surgical drape c.
come-and-go anesthesia
comedo, pl. **comedos, comedones**
    c. extraction
    c. subtype
comedocarcinoma of breast
comitans vein
commando
    c. operation
    c. procedure
    C. radical glossectomy
commensal organism
comminuted
    c. intraarticular fracture
    c. orbital fracture
    c. skull fracture
comminution
commissura, pl. **commissurae**
commissural
    c. bundle
    c. fusion
    c. lip pit
    c. myelorrhaphy
    c. myelotomy

commissure
    anterior commissure-posterior c. (AC-PC)
    anterior labial c.
    posterior labial c.
commissurotomy
    balloon mitral c.
    Brockenbrough transseptal c.
    closed chest c.
    closed transventricular mitral c.
    mitral balloon c.
    percutaneous mitral balloon c.
    percutaneous transatrial mitral c.
    percutaneous transvenous mitral c.
    transventricular mitral valve c.
common
    c. annular ring
    c. annular tendon
    c. basal vein
    c. bile duct (CBD)
    c. bile duct exploration
    c. bile duct ligation
    c. bile duct stone (CBDS)
    c. canal
    c. carotid plexus
    c. cavity phenomenon
    c. duct calculus
    c. duct cholangiogram
    c. duct colic
    c. duct obstruction
    c. dural sac
    c. extensor tendon
    c. facial vein
    c. femoral artery (CFA)
    c. femoral artery-superficial femoral artery (CFA-SFA)
    c. flexor sheath
    c. hepatic artery
    c. hepatic duct
    c. iliac artery
    c. interosseous artery
    c. mode rejection ratio
    c. palmar digital artery
    c. peroneal artery
    c. peroneal nerve
    c. peroneal nerve syndrome
    c. plantar digital artery
    c. tendinous ring
communicating
    c. artery
    c. branch
    c. fistula
    c. hematoma
    c. nerve
communication
    microfistulous c.
communis
community-acquired infection
commutator

comorbid medical problem
compact
    c. bone
    c. substance
companion
    c. artery
    c. lymph node
comparative radiographic examination
comparison operation
compartment
    c. compression syndrome
    extraaxial c.
    extracellular c.
    extravascular c.
    4-c. fascial decompression
    c. procedure
compartmental
    c. pressure
    c. radioimmunoglobulin therapy
    c. volume
compartmentalization
compensation
    c. reaction
    c. technique
compensatory
    c. antiinflammatory response
      syndrome (CARS)
    c. basilar osteotomy
    c. blood supply
    c. circulation
    c. deformity
    c. head posture
    c. regeneration
    c. wedge
competency
    valvular c.
competing messages integration
compilation autogenous vein graft
complementary
    c. and alternative medicine
    c. balloon angioplasty
    c. therapy
    c. treatment
complement fixation
complement-induced lung injury
complete
    c. adrenalectomy
    c. anterior dislocation
    c. atrioventricular dissociation
    c. A-V dissociation
    c. axillary dissection
    c. bilateral deformity

    c. blockage
    c. circumferential mesorectal
      excision
    c. colonoscopy
    c. common peroneal nerve lesion
    c. duplication
    c. fistula
    c. fracture
    c. hemostasis
    c. hernia
    c. inferior dislocation
    c. integration
    c. internal hemipelvectomy
    c. iridectomy
    c. laparoscopic distal
      pancreatectomy (C-LDP)
    c. lateral hemilaminectomy
    c. left bundle branch block
    c. mesh excision
    c. motor paraplegia
    c. obstruction
    c. posterior dislocation
    c. pulpectomy
    c. pulpotomy
    c. resection
    c. right bundle branch block
    c. rupture
    c. skin-sparing mastectomy
    c. sphincter relaxation
    c. sternotomy
    c. superior dislocation
    c. surgical exploration
    c. thymectomy
    c. thyroidectomy
    c. wrap Nissen operation
completion
    c. cholangiography
    c. thyroidectomy
complex
    c. adrenal endocrine disorder
    c. anorectal fistula
    c. aortic disease
    areolar c.
    c. cavity
    c. chest mass
    disordered hip c.
    c. dissection
    epispadias-exstrophy c.
    exstrophy-epispadias c.
    fibrocystic c.
    c. fracture
    fusion c.

C

NOTES

complex *(continued)*
    Ghon c.
    c. gonadal endocrine disorder
    growth plate c.
    c. hepatojejunostomy
    internal hemorrhoidal c.
    c. intracranial aneurysm
    juxtaglomerular c.
    c. left ventricular outflow tract
      obstruction
    limb-body wall c.
    major histocompatibility c. (MHC)
    c. pituitary endocrine disorder
    plasmin-inhibitor c. (PIC)
    c. regional pain syndrome (I, II)
      (CRPS)
    c. signal transduction
    sling-ring c.
    c. syndactyly repair
    c. thyroid endocrine disorder
    triangular fibrocartilage c. (TFCC)
    triarticular c.
    tuberous sclerosis c.
    vertebral subluxation c.
    Xase c.
compliance
    chest wall c.
    dynamic c.
    pulmonary c.
    c., rate, oxygenation, pressure
      (CROP)
    static c.
compliant bowel
complicated
    c. diverticular disease
    c. fracture
complication
    abdominal c.
    anastomotic c.
    bacterial c.
    benign pneumatic colonoscopy c.
    cardiopulmonary c.
    cardiorespiratory c.
    cardiovascular c.
    cerebrovascular c.
    colitis perineal c.
    colonoscopy c.
    concomitant obesity c.
    deep abdominal c. (DAC)
    delayed c.
    diabetic c.
    disease-related c.
    endoscopy c.
    extraabdominal infective c.
    extraintestinal c.
    feeding c.
    gastroduodenal c.
    gastrointestinal c.
    gonadal c.

    hematologic c.
    hemorrhagic c.
    hepatic c.
    immunologic c.
    infectious c.
    infective extraabdominal c.
    intraoperative c.
    late c.
    life-threatening c.
    metabolic c.
    neurologic c.
    neurovascular c.
    nonfatal c.
    nonimmunologic c.
    noninfective extraabdominal c.
    obstetrical c.
    operative site c.
    opportunistic c.
    oral c.
    pancreatic c.
    perioperative c.
    postbiopsy vascular c.
    postoperative respiratory c.
    postsplenectomy c.
    pregnancy c.
    pulmonary c.
    c. rate
    recurrent thromboembolic c.
    renal c.
    respiratory c.
    sclerotherapy c.
    septic c.
    stomal c.
    surgery c.
    thromboembolic c.
    thrombotic c.
    trocar wound site c.
    urologic c.
    vascular c.
    venous-related c.
    wound c.
component
    allogenic blood c.
    dominant c.
    extensive intraductal c. (EIC)
    intraductal c.
    monoclonal c.
    nonseminomatous c.
    trabecular arachnoid c.
composite
    c. addition technique
    c. flap
    c. free tissue transfer
    c. joint
    c. pelvic resection
    c. pelvic resection method
    c. pelvic resection procedure
    c. pelvic resection technique
    c. resin restoration

c. rib graft
c. skin graft
c. tissue transplantation

compound
c. aneurysm
c. cavity
c. comminuted fracture
c. cyst
c. dislocation
c. flap
c. joint
c. muscle action potential (CMAP)
c. restoration
c. skull fracture
c. suture technique

compressed
c. body
c. fracture

compressible cavernous body

compression
c. anesthesia
anterior cord c.
anterior-posterior c.
anteroposterior c.
c. arthrodesis
axial c.
c. bandage
c. bone conduction
brainstem c.
c. button gastrojejunostomy
cardiac c.
carotid artery c.
cauda equina c.
cerebral aqueduct c.
cervical vessel c.
cervicomedullary junction c.
Charnley c.
chest c.
chiasmal c.
continuous c.
cord c.
c. cough
c. cyanosis
direct c.
disc c.
duodenal c.
duplex-guided c.
dynamic c.
early supraclavicular c.
elastic c.
esophageal c.
c. extension

external pneumatic calf c.
extrinsic bladder c.
c. fracture
gastric c.
gentle c.
head c.
image c.
c. injury
c. instrumentation posterior construct
interfragmentary c.
intermittent pneumatic calf c.
intrinsic c.
ischemic c.
lateral c.
limbal c.
lower plexus c.
mechanical variceal c.
median nerve c.
c. molding
napkin-ring c.
nerve root c.
neurovascular cross c.
optic chiasm c.
optic tract c.
c. overload
c. paralysis
percutaneous balloon c.
c. plate fixation
c. plating
pneumatic c.
prechiasmal c.
progressive c.
c. rod treatment
root c.
c. skull-cap closure
spinal cord c.
spot c.
static c.
c. strain
supraclavicular c.
suprascapular nerve c.
c. switch
c. syndrome
c. technique
c. test
c. testing
thecal sac c.
thoracic outlet c.
tissue c.
tracheal c.
ultrasound-guided c.

C

NOTES

compression *(continued)*
uterine c.
variable-release c.
vascular c.
venous c.
vertebral c.
vertical c.
c. wiring
compression-evoked allodynia
compressor naris muscle
compromise
airway c.
organ c.
renal c.
respiratory c.
visual c.
computed
c. tomography (CT)
c. tomography arterial portography (CTAP)
c. tomography-guided biopsy
c. tomography-guided localization using platinum microcoil
c. tomography-guided selective drainage
c. tomography scan
c. tomography severity index (CTSI)
computer-assisted
c.-a. anesthesia
c.-a. assessment
c.-a. continuous infusion anesthetic technique
c.-a. controlled infusion (CACI)
c.-a. design-controlled alignment method
c.-a. stereotactic surgery
c.-a. surgery (CAS)
c.-a. treatment
computer-controlled
c.-c. drug administration anesthetic technique
c.-c. infusion anesthetic technique
computerized
c. diaphragmatic breathing retraining (CDBR)
c. electronic endoscopy
c. image guidance
concatenation
concave abdomen
concealed
c. bypass tract
c. hemorrhage
c. hernia
c. penis
c. umbilical stoma
concentrate
platelet c.

concentration
ambient oxygen c.
approximate lethal c.
bactericidal c.
bilirubin c.
blood alcohol c.
carbon dioxide c.
end-tidal nitrogen c.
hazardous c.
hydrogen ion c. (pH)
inspiratory vapor c.
lethal c.
mass c.
maximal drug c.
maximum permissible c.
minimal alveolar c.
minimal anesthetic c. (MAC)
minimal bactericidal c.
minimum alveolar c. (MAC)
1-minimum alveolar c. (1-MAC)
minimum alveolar anesthetic c. (MAC)
minimum bactericidal c.
minimum detectable c.
minimum effective c. (MEC)
minimum effective analgesic c.
minimum lethal c.
minimum local analgesic c. (MLAC)
nitrogen c.
oxygen c.
c. performance test
plasma endotoxin c.
plasma gastrin c.
plasma iron c.
plasma norepinephrine c.
plasma renin c.
plasma urea c.
predialysis plasma phosphate c.
prick-test c.
c. procedure
radioactive c.
renal vein renin c.
serum bactericidal c.
serum bilirubin c.
serum calcium c.
serum lithium c.
steroid c.
subanesthetic c.
substance c.
target plasma c. (TPC)
thyroid hormone serum c.
time of maximum c.
c. times time
total L-chain c.
total protein c.
concentration-effect relation
concentric
c. exercise

c. hernia
c. lesion
c. mastopexy
c. reduction

concept
C. ablation
c. formation
Three Color C.

concertina-like fashion

concha, pl. **conchae**
nasal c.
sphenoidal c.

conchoidal

concomitant
c. acidosis
c. administration
c. antireflux surgery
c. bleeding
c. colonization
c. hepatectomy
c. median sternotomy
c. medication
c. obesity complication
c. spinal cord injury
c. therapy

concordance
ventriculoarterial c.

Concorde position

concurrent
c. chemotherapy
c. DVT
c. hepatic laceration
c. medical condition

concussion
brain c.
spinal cord c.

condensation
amalgam c.
chromatin c.
filling material c.
gold foil c.
heavy c.
lateral c.
porcelain c.
pressure c.
resin c.
spatulation c.
vibration c.
warm c.
whipping c.

condenser point

condition
catabolic c.
concurrent medical c.
fibrocystic c.
gastrointestinal c.
genetic c.
medical systemic c.
predisposing c.
premalignant c.
systemic c.
tumorlike bone c.

conditioning
interceptive c.
operant c.
c. program
semantic c.
c. therapy

conductance
skin c.

conduction
c. analgesia
c. anesthesia
compression bone c.
osteotympanic bone c.

conductivity
tissue c.

conduit
antirefluxing colonic c.
aortic c.
biliary c.
Bricker c.
colon c.
cutaneous appendiceal c.
ileal c.
ileocolic c.
intestinal c.
Koch c.
Mitrofanoff c.
Rastelli c.
respiratory syncytial virus c.
urinary c.

condylar
c. articulation
c. canal
c. emissary vein
c. femoral fracture
c. guidance inclination
c. hinge position
c. implant arthroplasty
c. process
c. process fracture
c. screw fixation

NOTES

condylarthrosis
condyle
 c. cord
 c. dissection
 c. head
 lateral c.
 mandibular c.
 medial c.
 occipital c.
 c. resection
condylectomy
 DuVries plantar c.
 mandibular c.
 plantar c.
condylion
condylocephalic nail
condyloideum
condyloid process
condyloma, pl. **condylomata**
 c. acuminatum
 anal c.
 cervical c.
 flat c.
 genital c.
 giant c.
 perianal c.
 c. planus
 pointed c.
 vaginal c.
 venereal c.
condylomatous
condylotomy
condylus
cone
 c. biopsy
 cold knife c. (CKC)
coned-down view
configuration
 stellate c.
confirmation
 histopathologic c.
 intraoperative c.
 tissue c.
confirmatory
 c. axillary dissection
 c. incision
confluence
 hepatic venous c.
 vein c.
 venous c.
confluent inflammation
conformal radiation therapy
confrontation
 c. method
 c. testing
 c. visual field test
congenita
 arthrogryposis multiplex c.

congenital
 c. above-elbow amputation
 c. adrenal hyperplasia
 c. aspiration pneumonia
 c. below-elbow amputation
 c. brain malformation
 c. cataract
 c. central hypoventilation syndrome
 c. cerebral aneurysm
 c. cervical instability
 c. choledochal cyst
 c. conotruncal anomaly
 c. cystic adenomatoid malformation
  (CCAM)
 c. cystic dilatation
 c. depigmentation
 c. diaphragmatic hernia (CDH)
 c. diverticulum
 c. duplication
 c. esotropia
 c. fracture
 c. goiter
 c. heart malformation
 c. hip dislocation
 c. HIV infection
 c. lens dislocation
 c. lesion
 c. long QT syndrome
 c. nasal mass
 c. postural deformity
 c. pulmonary arteriovenous fistula
 c. pyloric membrane
 c. pyloric stenosis
 c. renal mass
 c. ring
 c. ring syndrome
 c. scapular elevation
 c. splenomegaly
 c. stippled epiphysis
 c. tracheobiliary fistula
 c. urethroperineal fistula
 c. vascular malformation
congenitally altered anatomy
congestion
 brain c.
 flap c.
 hepatic c.
 sinusoidal c.
 splanchnic c.
congestive
 c. heart disease
 c. heart failure
 c. hepatomegaly
conglomerate mass
conglutinant
conglutination
congruent affect
coni (*pl. of* conus)
coniotomy

conization
 cautery c.
 cervical c.
 cold c.
 cold knife c.
 hot knife c.
 laser cervical c.
 LEEP c.
 loop diathermy cervical c.
 loop electrosurgical excision
  procedure c.
conjoined
 c. anastomosis
 c. nerve-root anomaly
 c. tendon
conjoint tendon
conjugate
 c. axis
 c. foramen
 c. point
conjugation bridge
conjunctiva, pl. **conjunctivae**
conjunctiva-associated lymphoid tissue
conjunctival
 c. angioma
 c. circulation
 c. cul-de-sac
 c. exudate
 c. flap
 c. fornix
 c. hemorrhage
 c. incision
 c. injection
 c. laceration
 c. limbus
 c. melanotic lesion
 c. membrane
 c. patch graft
 c. ring
 c. sac
conjunctiva-Müller muscle excision
conjunctiviplasty
conjunctivitis
conjunctivodacryocystorhinostomy
conjunctivodacryocystostomy
conjunctivoplasty
conjunctivorhinostomy
conjunctivo-Tenon flap
conjunctivus
Con-Lish polishing method
connecting cartilage

connection
 atriopulmonary c.
connective
 c. tissue
 c. tissue activating peptide
 c. tissue augmentation
 c. tissue disease
 c. tissue disorder
 c. tissue graft
 c. tissue massage
 c. tissue membrane
 c. tissue plasticity
Connell
 C. incision
 C. stitch
 C. suture technique
Connolly
 C. procedure
 C. technique
Conn operation
conoid
 c. process
 c. tubercle
conotruncal anomaly
Conradi line
Conrad orbital blowout fracture
 operation
consciousness
conscious sedation
consecutive
 c. amputation
 c. aneurysm
 c. dislocation
consent
 informed c.
consequence
 familial c.
 psychologic c.
 social c.
conservation
 splenic c.
 c. surgery
conservative
 c. resection
 c. surgery
 c. surgical treatment
 c. therapy
consideration
 anesthetic c.
 oncologic c.
 technical c.
consonant-injection method

C

NOTES

consonant position
consortial approach
constant
    c. flow insufflation
    c. vacuum
constipation
    idiopathic c.
constitutive heterochromatin method
constrained
    c. ankle arthroplasty
    c. reconstruction
    c. shoulder arthroplasty
constricting lesion
constriction
    duodenopyloric c.
    esophageal c.
    pyloric c.
    c. ring
constrictive pericarditis
construct
    AO dynamic compression plate c.
    compression instrumentation
     posterior c.
    double-rod c.
    hook-rod c.
    pedicle screw c.
    segmental compression c.
    TSRH double-rod c.
    Wiltse system double-rod c.
    Wiltse system H c.
    Wiltse system single-rod c.
construction
    Abbe vaginal c.
    absolute c.
    exocentric c.
    ileal reservoir c.
    ileostomy c.
    loop ileostomy c.
    McIndoe-Hayes c.
    pelvic ileal reservoir c.
    single denture c.
    sphincteric c.
    stent c.
    tandem c.
    Thiersch-Duplay urethral c.
    U-pouch c.
    vaginal c.
consumption
    oxygen c.
    peak exercise oxygen c.
    splanchnic oxygen c.
contact
    c. activation product
    c. area point
    c. diode laser tonsillectomy
    c. dissolution therapy
    grid c.
    c. illumination
    c. laser ablation

    c. laser ablation of prostate
     (CLAP)
    c. laser vaporization
    c. manipulation
    c. metastasis
    c. method
contained rupture
contaminated operative wound
    classification
contamination
    bacterial c.
    fecal c.
    gas c.
    graft c.
    gross fecal c.
    hub c.
    intraoperative c.
    metastatic c.
content
    abdominal c.
    bile stained cyst c.
    cyst c.
    gastrointestinal c.
    intestinal c.
    luminal c.
    mixed venous oxygen c.
    platelet nucleotide c.
    protein c.
    tissue water c.
context-sensitive half-time
contiguity
    solution of c.
contiguous loop
contiguum
    per c.
continence
    anal c.
    short-term total c.
    sphincteric c.
    total c.
continent
    c. colostomy
    c. cutaneous appendicocystostomy
    c. ileal pouch
    c. ileostomy
    c. urinary pouch
continuity
    bowel c.
    digestive c.
    gastrointestinal c.
    gut c.
    solution of c.
continuous
    c. ambulatory peritoneal dialysis
     (CAPD)
    c. arteriovenous hemofiltration
     (CAVH)
    c. arteriovenous ultrafiltration
    c. atrial fibrillation

c. bladder irrigation
c. catheter drainage
c. compression
c. distending airway pressure
c. endothelium
c. epidural anesthesia
c. flow ventilation
c. gastric decompression
c. gum technique
c. hyperfractionated accelerated radiotherapy (CHART)
c. hyperthermic peritoneal perfusion
c. infusion anesthetic technique
c. intramucosal PCO_2 measurement
c. loop wiring
c. lumbar epidural (CLE)
c. lumbar peridural anesthesia
c. mandatory ventilation
c. medical treatment
c. negative airway pressure
c. NG suction
c. on-line recording
c. peripheral nerve block
c. popliteal sciatic nerve block
c. positive airway pressure (CPAP)
c. positive pressure breathing (CPPB)
c. positive pressure ventilation (CPPV)
c. postoperative closed lavage
c. pull-through technique
c. renal replacement therapy
c. sanguineous perfusion
c. spinal anesthesia
c. spinal anesthetic technique
c. subcutaneous insulin injection
c. suture technique
c. venovenous hemodialysis (CVVHD)
c. venovenous hemofiltration
c. wave laser ablation
c. wave technique

continuum
per c.

contour
breast c.
corneal c.
intonation c.
c. line
lobulated c.
restoration c.

c. restoration
rounded c.

contoured
c. adduction trochanteric-controlled alignment method
c. anterior spinal plate technique

contouring
3-dimensional c.

contraangle

contraaperture

contraceptive
c. method
c. technique

contracted
c. kidney
c. pelvis

contractile
c. motility
c. ring
c. ring dysphagia

contractility

contraction
anal canal rhythmic c.
c. fasciculation
muscular c.
propagating clustered c. (PCC)
c. wave

contract-relax technique

contracture
Dupuytren c.
functional c.
Volkmann ischemic c.

contraindication

contralateral
c. axillary metastasis
c. carotid artery occlusion
c. groin exploration
c. ischemia
c. mobile cord
c. parathyroid gland
c. side
c. site
c. weakness

contralaterally

contrast
c. bath
blood oxygenation level-dependent c.
c. enema
c. injection
intravenous c.
I.V. c.

NOTES

contrast *(continued)*
    c. material
    c. material instillation
    c. medium
    c. study
    c. venography
    c. visualization
contrast-enhanced
    c.-e. computed tomography
    c.-e. CT
    c.-e. CT scan
    c.-e. CT scanning
    c.-e. ultrasonography
contrecoup fracture
control
    closed-loop c.
    endoscopic c.
    exsanguination tourniquet c.
    extrahepatic c.
    fluoroscopic c.
    hemorrhage c.
    inflow c.
    intrahepatic c.
    monitored anesthesia c.
    outflow c.
    Pringle vascular c.
    pronation c.
    proximal vascular c.
    tourniquet c.
    transcriptional c.
    vascular c.
    c. of ventilation
    x-ray c.
controlled
    c. diagnostic block
    c. diaphragmatic respiration
    c. expansion
    c. fistula
    c. heat-aided drug delivery
    (CHADD)
    c. hypotension
    c. hypotensive anesthesia (CHA)
    c. mechanical ventilation (CMV)
    c. release anesthetic technique
    c. release silver technology
    c. rotational osteotomy
    c. ventilation
    c. water-added technique
controller
    oxygen-ratio monitoring c.
control-mode ventilation
contusion
    brain c.
    corneal c.
    myocardial c.
    pulmonary c.
conus, pl. **coni**
convalescence
    short-term c.

convection
    hemodiafiltration c.
convenience
    c. jaw relation
    c. point
conventional
    c. aortic aneurysmectomy
    c. distal pancreatectomy
    c. endarterectomy
    c. method
    c. operation
    c. pancreatoduodenectomy
    c. parameter
    c. procedure
    c. surgery
    c. suturing
    c. technique
    c. thoracoplasty
convergence
    c. facilitation
    c. point
    c. position
    c. projection
convergent beam irradiation
converse
    scalping flap of C.
conversion
    above-knee amputation c.
    extraglandular c.
    pressure c.
converter
convex
    c. condylar implant arthroplasty
    c. fusion
    c. nail
convexoconcave
convoluted seminiferous tubule
convulsion
    ether c.
convulsive therapy
Conyers technique
cooled-knife method
cooling
    active core c.
    external c.
    passive tissue c.
    topical c.
    whole-body c.
Coomassie brilliant blue technique
Coonrad-Morrey total elbow
    arthroplasty
Coonrad total elbow arthroplasty
Coonse-Adams
    C.-A. knee approach
    C.-A. technique
Cooper
    C. fascia
    C. hernia
    C. ligament

C. operation
C. reduction
C. syndrome

cooperation
cellular c.

coordination
hand-eye c.

co-oximetry

COP
colloid osmotic pressure

Cope
C. method
C. technique

Copeland
C. retinoscopy
C. technique

Copeland-Howard scapulothoracic fusion

coping
C. Strategies Questionnaire (CSQ)
C. with Health, Injuries, and
Problems (CHIP)

copious
c. irrigation
c. peritoneal lavage

copper sulfate method

copper-wire
c.-w. arteriole
c.-w. artery
c.-w. reflex

coproporphyria
hereditary c.

copular point

copulating pouch

coracoacromial ligament

coracobrachial
c. bursa
c. muscle

coracobrachialis
c. muscle

coracoclavicular
c. articulation
c. ligament
c. screw fixation
c. space
c. suture fixation
c. technique

coracoclaviculare

coracohumeral ligament

coracoid
c. fracture

c. infraclavicular brachial plexus
block
c. process

coral calculus

Corbin technique

cord
anterior c.
c. compression
condyle c.
contralateral mobile c.
false vocal c.
Ferrein c.
gangliated c.
genital c.
germinal c.
gonadal c.
lateral c.
nephrogenic c.
oblique c.
c. paralysis
presentation of c.
rete c.
spermatic c.
spinal c.
splenic c.
c. structure
tendinous c.
testicular c.
testis c.
c. traction syndrome
true vocal c.
umbilical c.
vocal c.
Weitbrecht c.
Willis c.

cordate pelvis

cordectomy

cordis

cordopexy

cordotomy
anterolateral c.
dorsal c.
open surgical c.
percutaneous c.
posterior column c.
spinothalamic c.
stereotactic c.

core
c. body temperature
central fibroelastic c.
c. drilling procedure
c. hypothermia

NOTES

161

core *(continued)*
    c. needle biopsy
    c. vitrectomy
corectomy
coreoplasty
corepexy
Cori classification
corium, pl. **coria**
corkscrew
    c. appearance
    c. maneuver
corn
    hard c.
    soft c.
    web c.
cornea, pl. **corneae**
    anterior c.
    c. guttate lesion
corneal
    c. abrasion
    c. abscess
    c. abscission
    c. alkali burn
    c. anesthesia
    c. apex
    c. arcus
    c. astigmatism
    c. blood staining
    c. cap
    c. cleft
    c. contour
    c. contusion
    c. curvature
    c. dendrite
    c. diameter
    c. distortion
    c. dystrophy
    c. ectasia
    c. edema
    c. endothelium
    c. epithelium
    c. erosion
    c. erysiphake
    c. facet
    c. filament
    c. fissure
    c. fistula
    c. flap
    c. foreign body
    c. full-thickness
    c. graft operation
    c. graft step
    c. guttering
    c. incision
    c. inlay
    c. iron line
    c. laceration
    c. lamella
    c. lamellar groove

    c. leakage
    c. lens
    c. light reflex
    c. limbus
    c. luster
    c. marginal furrow
    c. meridian
    c. mushroom
    c. nebula
    c. neovascularization
    c. nerve
    c. perforation
    c. protrusion
    c. punctate lesion
    c. reflection
    c. rejection
    c. scarring
    c. scarring
    c. spot
    c. staining test
    c. stria
    c. substance
    c. surgery
    c. thinning
    c. tissue
    c. transplant
    c. transplantation
    c. trauma
    c. trepanation
    c. ulceration
    c. velum
corneoscleral
    c. incision
    c. laceration
corner
    caudal c.
    cephalad c.
    c. fracture
    4-c. midcarpal fusion
cornered
3-cornered
    3-c. bone
    3-c. therapy
corniculate
    c. cartilage
    c. process
    c. tubercle
corniculum laryngis
cornification disorder
Corning method
cornu, pl. **cornua**
    coccygeal cornua
    cornua of hyoid bone
    styloid c.
cornual anastomosis
cornucopia
    sinusoidal endothelium c.
corona, pl. **coronae**

coronal
  c. angulation
  c. oblique projection
  c. plane
  c. plane correction
  c. plane deformity
  c. plane deformity sagittal translation
  c. pulp tissue
  c. reconstruction
  c. section
  c. split fracture
  c. suture
coronalis
coronary
  c. angioplasty versus excisional atherectomy
  c. artery angioplasty
  c. artery anomaly
  c. artery bypass
  c. artery bypass graft (CABG)
  c. artery disease
  c. artery dissection
  c. artery ectasia
  c. artery fistula (CAF)
  c. artery revascularization procedure
  c. artery-right ventricular fistula
  c. artery surgery study (CASS)
  c. balloon angioplasty
  c. bifurcation
  c. bypass procedure
  c. collateral circulation
  c. endarterectomy
  c. flow reserve technique
  c. node
  c. perfusion pressure
  c. plexus
  c. revascularization
  c. ring
  c. rotational ablation
  c. rotational atherectomy
  c. sinus
  c. sinus catheterization
  c. sinus perfusion system
  c. sulcus
  c. syndrome
  c. thrombolysis
  c. vein
  c. vein ligation
  c. venous pressure
  c. vessel anatomy

coronoid
  c. line
  c. process
  c. process fracture
coronoidectomy
coronoideus
coronoradicular stabilization
coroplasty
coroscopy
corotomy
corpectomy
  anterior c.
  cervical c.
  median c.
  c. model
  vertebral body c.
corpora (*pl. of* corpus)
corporal biopsy
corporeal
  c. aspiration
  c. reconstruction
  c. rotation procedure
  c. sacrospinous suspension
corporectomy amputation
corporoplasty
  Essed-Schroeder c.
  incisional c.
  modified Essed-Schroeder c.
corporotomy
corpus, pl. **corpora**
  c. callosotomy
  c. carcinoma
  c. epididymis
  c. luteum cyst
  c. luteum hematoma
Correa classification
corrected sternal position
correction
  adaptive c.
  Allen c.
  Allison GE reflux c.
  anterior c.
  anteroposterior c.
  aphakic c.
  astigmatism c.
  attenuation c.
  Beckenbaugh c.
  Bonferroni c.
  Byron Smith lazy-T c.
  cephalometric c.
  chevron hallux valgus c.
  coincidence c.

NOTES

correction *(continued)*
    coronal plane c.
    cubitus varus c.
    dioptric c.
    epicanthal c.
    frontal plane c.
    hallux varus c.
    heparinase c.
    Johnson-Spiegl hallux varus c.
    King curve posterior c. (type IV)
    Küstner uterine inversion c.
    kyphosis c.
    occlusal c.
    oligosegmental c.
    operative c.
    optical c.
    phalangeal malunion c.
    protamine c.
    rotational c.
    Ruiz-Mora c.
    scatter c.
    scoliosis c.
    secondary ptosis c.
    skeletal c.
    spectacle c.
    speech c.
    Steel c.
    surgical c.
    Tukey post-hoc c.
    Yates c.
corrective therapy
correlation
    canonical c.
    clinical c.
    clinicopathologic c.
    negative c.
    positive c.
    semilinear canonical c.
    c. time
correlational method
Correrra line
corresponding point
corridor
    c. incision
    c. procedure
Corrigan respiration
corrin ring
corrosion preparation
corrugator
    c. cutis muscle
    c. supercilii muscle
corset suspension
cortex, pl. **cortices**
    adrenal c.
    anterior c.
    aspiration of c.
    association c.
    cingulate c.

    ovarian c.
    renal c.
    suprarenal c.
    vertebral body anterior c.
cortical
    c. activation
    c. arch of kidney
    c. area
    c. artery
    c. atrophy
    c. biopsy
    c. bone
    c. bone graft
    c. bone primary canal
    c. destruction
    c. dysplasia
    c. fracture
    c. fragment
    c. hamartoma
    c. implantation
    c. incision
    c. lateralization
    c. lesion
    c. mass
    c. perforation
    c. respiration
    c. ring sign
    c. stimulation
    c. strut graft
    c. substance
    c. tuber
corticalosteotomy
corticectomy
cortices (*pl. of* cortex)
corticoadenoma
corticobulbar tract
corticocancellous bone graft
corticoid injection
corticomedullary demarcation
corticopontine tract
corticospinal
    c. axon
    c. tract
corticosteroid
    depot c.
corticotomy
    DeBastiani c.
    percutaneous c.
Corti organ
cortisol-producing carcinoma
Cortrosyn stimulation test
Cosgrove mitral valve replacement
cosmesis
cosmetic
    c. evaluation
    c. outcome
    c. problem
    c. result

c. score
c. surgery
costa, pl. **costae**
costal
c. angle
c. cartilage
c. facet
c. groove
c. margin
c. notch
c. pit
c. pleura
c. process
c. respiration
c. surface
c. tuberosity
costectomy
cost-effective alternative
Costen syndrome
costicartilage
costiform
costoaxillary vein
costocentral
costocervical
c. artery
c. trunk
costochondral
c. articulation
c. joint
c. junction
costoclavicular
c. ligament
c. line
c. maneuver
c. space
costocolic ligament
costocoracoid
costodiaphragmatic recess
costoinferior
costomediastinal
c. recess
c. sinus
costophrenic septal line
costoscapular
costoscapularis
costosternal
costosternoplasty
costosuperior
costotomy
costotransversaria
costotransversarium

costotransverse
c. foramen
c. joint
c. ligament
costotransversectomy
c. approach
Seddon dorsal spine c.
c. technique
costoversion thoracoplasty
costovertebral joint
costoxiphoid ligament
cot
finger c.
cotransplantation
Cotrel-Dubousset (C-D)
C.-D. fixation
Cotte
C. operation
C. presacral neurectomy
Cotting toenail operation
Cotton
C. ankle fracture
C. cartilage graft
C. reduction
cottonloader position
cotton-wool
c.-w. exudate
c.-w. patch
c.-w. separation
c.-w. sign
Cotunnius
C. aqueduct
C. canal
C. space
cotyloid
c. cavity
c. joint
c. ligament
cough
compression c.
c. CPR technique
extrapulmonary c.
c. fracture
c. trick
coughing
c. and bucking
expulsive c.
cough-pressure transmission ratio
Couinaud
C. classification
C. nomenclature
coulometric titration

NOTES

coumadinization
Councilman lesion
Counsellor-Davis artificial vagina operation
Counsellor-Flor
    C.-F. modification
    C.-F. modification of McIndoe technique
count
    blood cell c.
    ex vivo c.
    posttetanic c.
counterbalance
counterclockwise
    c. direction
    c. rotation
countercurrent
    c. extraction
    c. heat exchanger
    c. mechanism
counterincision
counterirritation
counteropening
counterpulsation
    balloon c.
    enhanced external c.
    intraaortic balloon c.
    intraarterial c.
    percutaneous intraaortic balloon c.
counterpuncture
countersinking osteotomy
countersink screw head
counterstimulation
countertraction
coup injury
coupling head
course
    chronic c.
    intrahepatic c.
    postoperative c.
Courvoisier
    C. gastroenterostomy
    C. incision
    C. sign
Couvelaire
    C. ileourethral anastomosis
    C. incision
Coventry
    C. distal femoral osteotomy
    C. vagal osteotomy
cove plane
Cowen-Loftus toe-phalanx transplantation
cow face
cowl muscle
Cowper
    C. gland
    C. ligament

COX-2
    cyclooxygenase-2
    COX-2 inhibitor
coxa, pl. **coxae**
coxal bone
Cox Maze III procedure
coxofemoral articulation
coxsackievirus A, B virus
Cozen-Brockway
    C.-B. technique
    C.-B. Z-plasty
CPAP
    continuous positive airway pressure
CPB
    cardiopulmonary bypass
CPH
    chronic paroxysmal hemicrania
C-plasty
CPP
    cerebral perfusion pressure
CPPB
    continuous positive pressure breathing
CPPV
    continuous positive pressure ventilation
CPR
    cardiopulmonary resuscitation
        simultaneous compression-ventilation CPR
CPS
    cumulative pain score
CPSP
    central poststroke pain
CPT
    cold pressor test
    current perception threshold
Cracchiolo
    C. forefoot arthroplasty
    C. procedure
Cragg endoluminal graft
Craigie tube method
cramp
    abdominal c.
Crampton
    C. line
    C. test
crania (*pl. of* cranium)
craniad
cranial
    c. base
    c. bone
    c. canal
    c. cavity
    c. duplication
    c. epidural space
    c. extension
    c. fontanelle
    c. fossa
    c. fracture
    c. index

c. insufflation
c. irradiation
c. nerve dissection
c. nerve (I–XII)
c. nerve manipulation
c. nerve rhizotomy
c. osteopetrosis
c. osteosynthesis
c. pin
c. section
c. suture
c. vault
c. venous sinus
craniamphitomy
craniectomy
    endoscopic strip c.
    keyhole-shaped c.
    linear c.
    partial-thickness c.
    retromastoid suboccipital c.
    strip c.
cranio-aural
craniocele
craniocerebral
craniofacial
c. anomaly
c. axis
c. deformity
c. en bloc resection
c. fixation
c. malformation
c. notch
c. osteotomy
c. reconstruction
c. reconstructive surgery
c. suspension wiring
craniomeningocele
craniometric point
cranio-orbital surgery
craniopathy
craniopharyngeal
c. canal
c. duct
craniopharyngioma
    ectopic c.
cranioplasty
    aluminum c.
    hydroxyapatite cement c.
    metallic c.
    tantalum c.
craniopuncture
craniorrhachidian

craniosacral outflow
cranioscopy
craniosinus fistula
craniospinal
c. irradiation
c. space
craniosynostosis
craniotomy
    attached c.
    awake c.
    bifrontal c.
    c. defect
    detached c.
    endoscopic frontal c.
    frontal c.
    frontotemporal c.
    left frontal c. (LFC)
    open stereotactic c.
    osteoplastic c.
    pterional c.
    right temporoparietal c.
    stereotactic c.
    subtemporal c.
    supratentorial c.
    Yasargil c.
craniotonoscopy
craniotrypesis
craniotympanic
cranium, pl. crania
crash technique
crassum
crater formation
Crawford
    C. graft inclusion technique
    C. incision
    C. method
    C. sling operation
Crawford-Adams cup arthroplasty
Crawford-Marxen-Osterfeld technique
craze line
CRC
    colorectal cancer
    CRC resection
    sporadic CRC
CRE
    cardiorespiratory endurance
crease
    digital flexion c.
    flexion c.
    inframammary c.
    midline abdominal c.
    palmar c.

NOTES

crease *(continued)*
 skin c.
 torso c.
 c. wound
creation
 kyphosis c.
 lordosis c.
 McIndoe vaginal c.
 Politano-Leadbetter tunnel c.
 tunnel c.
Credé
 C. maneuver
 C. method
Creech
 C. aortoiliac graft
 C. technique
creeping fat
Crego
 C. femoral osteotomy
 C. tendon transfer technique
cremasteric
 c. fascia
 c. muscle
 c. reflex
 c. vein
crena, pl. **crenae**
Creola body
crescent
 articular c.
 c. body
 C. corneal graft
 glomerular c.
 c. mastopexy
 c. operation
 sublingual c.
crescentic
 c. calcaneal osteotomy
 c. osteotomy
 c. rupture
Crespo operation
crest
 articular c.
 buccinator c.
 deltoid c.
 endoalveolar c.
 ethmoidal c.
 external occipital c.
 falciform c.
 frontal c.
 iliac c.
 infratemporal c.
 inguinal c.
 intermediate sacral c.
 internal occipital c.
 interosseous c.
 intertrochanteric c.
 lacrimal c.
 nasal c.
 obturator c.

 pubic c.
 sacral c.
 supinator c.
 supraventricular c.
 terminal c.
 tibial c.
 trochanteric c.
 urethral c.
 vestibular c.
CRF
 chronic renal failure
Cribier method
cribra (*pl. of* cribrum)
cribriform
 c. area
 c. carcinoma
 c. fascia
 c. plate
 status c.
 c. subtype
cribrous lamina
cribrum, pl. **cribra**
cricoarytenoid
 c. ligament
 c. muscle
cricoesophageal tendon
cricohyoidepiglottopexy
cricoid
 c. cartilage
 c. myotomy
 c. pressure
 c. pressure anesthetic technique
 c. ring
 stenotic c.
 c. yoke
cricomyotomy
cricopharyngeal
 c. dilatation
 c. myotomy
cricopharyngeus muscle
cricothyroid
 c. artery
 c. articular capsule
 c. articulation
 c. joint
 c. ligament
 c. membrane
 c. muscle
cricothyroidotomy
cricothyrotomy
 scalpel c.
cricotracheal
 c. ligament
 c. membrane
 c. resection
cricotracheotomy
cricovocal membrane
Crile-Matas operation

Crippa lead tetraacetate method
crisis, pl. **crises**
    pheochromocytoma c.
crisscrossing abdominal wall incisions
Critchett operation
criterion, pl. **criteria**
    AMES criteria
    Dawson criteria
    Light criteria
    MACIS criteria
    observer-dependent criteria
    organ failure criteria
    Ranson pancreatitis criteria
    standard organ failure criteria
critical
    c. care anesthesiology
    c. care medicine (CCM)
    c. closing pressure
    c. illumination
    c. mass
CRN
    cerebral radiation necrosis
CRNA
    certified registered nurse anesthetist
Crock encircling operation
Croften classification
Crohn disease
Cronkhite-Canada syndrome
CROP
    compliance, rate, oxygenation, pressure
Crosby
    C. capsule
    C. reduction
Crosby-Kugler
    C.-K. biopsy capsule
    C.-K. capsule for biopsy
cross
    c. flap
    c. infection
    c. section
cross-arch fulcrum line
crossarm flap
crossbar stomach deformity
cross-bracing, crossbracing
cross-clamping, crossclamping
    aortic c.-c.
    infrarenal aortic c.-c.
    thoracic aortic c.-c. (TACC)
cross-consonant injection method
crossed
    c. anesthesia
    c. extension reflex

    c. extensor reflex
    c. fixation
    c. pyramidal tract
cross-facial, crossfacial
    c.-f. nerve graft
    c.-f. nerve graft anastomosis
    c.-f. technique
cross-finger flap
crosshatch incision
cross-leg flap
crosslink plate size
cross-lip pedicle flap
cross-modality matching
crossover
    femorofemoral c.
    FF c.
    c. toe deformity
crosspin
cross-polarization photography
crossreact
crossreactivity
cross-section
    capture c.-s.
cross-sectional
    c.-s. area
    c.-s. method
    c.-s. projection
cross-table lateral projection
cross-tolerance
cross-trigonal repair
cross-tunneling incision
cross-vector A scan
crotaphion
croup
    postextubation c.
croupous
    c. inflammation
    c. membrane
Crouzon
    C. disease
    C. syndrome
crowded carpal sign
Crowe
    C. classification
    C. pilot point
crowfoot closure
crowing inspiration
crown
    c. angulation
    c. fracture
    c. inclination

C

NOTES

crown *(continued)*
    c. restoration
    C. suture technique
crown-contouring method
crown-root fracture
Crozat therapy
CRPF
    closed reduction and percutaneous
    fixation
CRPS
    complex regional pain syndrome (I, II)
crucial
    c. anastomosis
    c. incision
cruciate
    c. anastomosis
    c. eminence
    c. incision
    c. ligament reconstruction
    c. muscle
cruciform
    c. eminence
    c. ligament
    c. suture technique
crunch-stick anastomosis
cruor
crura (*pl. of* crus)
crural
    c. arch
    c. area
    c. canal
    c. closure
    c. fascia
    c. fossa
    c. hernia
    c. repair
    c. ring
    c. septum
    c. sheath
cruris
crurotomy
crus, pl. **crura**
    lateral c.
    medial c.
    c. muscle
crush
    c. fracture
    c. injury
    c. preparation
    c. syndrome
crushed
    c. eggshell fracture
    c. tissue
crushing
    c. anastomosis
    oval-shaped c.
    c. technique
crusotomy

Crutchfield reduction technique
Cruveilhier
    C. fascia
    C. fossa
    C. plexus
    C. ulcer
Cruveilhier-Baumgarten anomaly
cryoablation
    encircling c.
    laparoscopically guided c.
    c. probe
cryoanalgesia
cryoanesthesia
cryoapplication
cryo-assisted resection
cryocautery
cryocoagulation
cryoconization
cryoelectron microscopy
cryoextraction operation
cryogenic
    c. ablation
    c. neuroablation
cryohypophysectomy
CryoLife Single Step dilution method
cryolysis
cryopallidectomy
cryopexy
    barrage c.
    double freeze-stalk c.
    double freeze-thaw c.
cryopreserved
    c. aortic homograft
    c. extrapelvic ovarian
    transplantation
    c. heart-valve allograft
    c. tissue banking
cryoprostatectomy
cryopulvinectomy
cryoretinopexy
cryoscopy
cryostat
    c. section
    c. tissue
cryosurgery
cryosurgical
    c. ablation
    c. technique
cryothalamectomy
cryotherapy operation
crypt
    c. abscess
    anal c.
    c. atrophy
    enamel c.
    c. epithelium
    ileal c.
    Lieberkühn c.

Morgagni c.
tonsillar c.
crypta, pl. **cryptae**
cryptectomy
cryptococcal infection
Cryptococcus **infection**
cryptogenic infection
cryptoglandular infection
cryptorchidectomy
cryptorchidopexy
cryptorchid testis
cryptorchism
cryptosis
cryptosporidial infection
crystalline lens equator
crystallized trypsin
crystalloid
c. cardioplegic solution
Reinke c.
Csapody orbital repair operation
CSE
combined spinal/epidural
CSEA
combined spinal/epidural anesthesia
C-section
cesarean section
lower uterine segment transverse C-section
LUST C-section
CSF
cerebrospinal fluid
blood-tinged CSF
CSF pressure
CSFP
cerebrospinal fluid pressure
C-shaped
C-s. canal
C-s. scalp flap
CSO
clinically severe obesity
CSQ
Coping Strategies Questionnaire
CST
certified surgical technologist
CSTFA
certified surgical technologist, first assist
CT
computed tomography
appendiceal CT
CT arterial portography (CTAP)
contrast-enhanced CT
helical CT

CT portography
CT scan
CT scan-guided needle aspiration
CT scanning
CT volumetry
CT with hepatic arterial (CTHA)
CT with hepatic arterial injection
4C-T
4-chamber transverse
4C-T image
5C-T
5-chamber transverse
5C-T image
CTAP
computed tomography arterial portography
CT arterial portography
CTD
chest tube drainage
mediastinal CTD
CT-directed needle aspiration
CT-guided
CT-g. fine-needle aspiration
CT-g. liver biopsy
CT-g. needle-aspiration biopsy
CT-g. selective drainage
CT-g. stereotactic evacuation
CTHA
CT with hepatic arterial
CTL
cytolytic T-lymphocyte
cytotoxic T-lymphocyte
CTL immunity
CTL immunity against melanoma
CTL-inducing peptide antigen
CTO
cervicothoracic orthosis
chest tube output
CTSI
computed tomography severity index
Cubbins
C. arthroplasty
C. incision
C. open reduction
C. shoulder approach
C. shoulder dislocation technique
cubital tunnel syndrome
cubitus
c. valgus deformity
c. varus correction
cuboid bone

NOTES

C

CUC
chronic ulcerative colitis
cue exposure
cuff
c. abscess
aortic c.
denuded rectal c.
distal vein c.
gastric c.
c. malfunction
musculotendinous c.
rectal muscle c.
c. resection
rotator c.
suprahepatic c.
c. suspension
c. tear arthropathy
c. tear arthroplasty
4-c. technique segmental pressure measurement
vaginal c.
vein c.
Cuignet method
cuirasse
carcinoma en c.
cuirass ventilation
Culcher-Sussman technique
cul-de-sac
c.-d.-s. of Bruger
conjunctival c.-d.-s.
c.-d.-s. of Douglas
c.-d.-s. fluid
glaucomatous c.-d.-s.
greater c.-d.-s.
Gruber c.-d.-s.
lesser c.-d.-s.
c.-d.-s. mass
ocular c.-d.-s.
ophthalmic c.-d.-s.
optic c.-d.-s.
rectouterine c.-d.-s.
c.-d.-s. restoration
culdoplasty
Halban c.
Marion-Moschcowitz c.
McCall c.
culdoscopy
culdotomy
Cullen sign
culprit
c. lesion
c. lesion angioplasty
Culp spiral flap pyeloplasty
culture
colony c.
fibroblast c.
c. medium

cultured
c. epithelial autograft
c. human skin equivalent
culturing technique
cumarin necrosis
Cummer classification
cumulative
c. operative morbidity
c. operative mortality
c. pain score (CPS)
c. score
c. trauma disorder
cuneiform
c. bone
c. cartilage
c. osteotomy
c. tubercle
cuneocerebellar tract
cuneonavicular
cunnus
cup
c. insemination
optic c.
cup-and-ball osteotomy
cup-and-cone method
cup-cement interface
cup-patch technique
Cüppers
C. method
C. method of pleoptics
cuprophane membrane
cup-to-disc ratio
cupula, pl. **cupulae**
pleural c.
cupular blind sac
cupulolithiasis
curability
curage
curare
curarization
curative
c. intent
c. potential
c. procedure
c. radical total gastrectomy
c. resection
c. sphincter-saving operation
curative-intent
c.-i. operation
c.-i. procedure
c.-i. surgery
curb tenotomy
curettage
dilatation and c. (D&C)
dilation and c. (D&C)
endocervical c. (ECC)
endometrial c.
fractional dilation and c.
periapical c.

soft tissue c.
suction c.

curettement
curioscopy
curlicue ureter
currant jelly clot
current

amplitude-summation interferential c.
demarcation c.
Limoge c.
membrane c.
c. perception threshold (CPT)
saturation c.

curse

Ondine c.

Curth-Maklin cornification disorder
Curtin

C. incision
C. plantar fibromatosis excision

Curtis

C. PIP joint capsulotomy
C. technique

Curtis-Fisher knee technique
curvatura, pl. **curvaturae**
curvature

c. aberration
anterior corneal c.
canal c.
corneal c.
greater c.
lesser c.

curve

accommodation c.
area under c. (AUC)
articulation c.
calibration c.
carbon dioxide dissociation c.
discrimination c.
displacement c.
dissociation c.
dose-effect c.
dose-response c.
elimination c.
hemoglobin-oxygen dissociation c.
indicator-dilution c.
interpolated c.
intracardiac pressure c.
load-deflection c.
load-deformation c.
load-displacement c.
oxygen dissociation c.
oxygen-hemoglobin dissociation c.

oxyhemoglobin dissociation c.
pressure-natriuresis c.
pressure-volume c.
strength-duration c.
survival c.
time-concentration c.
Traube-Hering c.
whole-body titration c.

curved

c. approach
c. canal
c. end-to-end anastomosis
c. flank position
c. incision
c. radiolucent line

curved-needle surgeon's knot
curvilinear incision
Cushing

C. operation
C. pressure response
C. reflex
C. suture technique

cushioning suture technique
Cusick operation
Cusick-Sarrail ptosis operation
cusp

c. fenestration
c. plane
c. restoration
valve c.

cusp-fossa relation
cuspid-molar position
Custodis nondraining procedure
cut

c. end
c. point
sector c.
semilunate c.
c. surface

cutaneobiliary fistula
cutaneomucosal
cutaneomucous muscle
cutaneomucouveal syndrome
cutaneous

c. appendiceal conduit
c. bacterial infection
c. burn injury
c. cervical nerve
c. collateral circulation
c. examination
c. forearm flap
c. gangrene

NOTES

173

cutaneous *(continued)*
    c. gland
    c. graft-versus-host disease
    c. graft-versus-host reaction
    c. heat loss
    c. hemorrhoid
    c. ileocystostomy
    c. innervation
    c. lesion
    c. loop ureterostomy
    c. malformation
    c. manifestation
    c. melanoma
    c. metastasis
    c. metastatic breast carcinoma
    c. muscle
    c. suture technique
    c. tissue
    c. vesicostomy
    c. viral infection
cutaneus
    nodulus c.
cutback anoplasty
cutback-type vaginoplasty
cutdown
    c. access
    c. incision
    c. technique
    venous c.
cuticular
    c. membrane
    c. stitch
    c. suture technique
cuticularization
cutin
cutis graft
Cutler-Beard
    C.-B. bridge flap
    C.-B. operation
Cutler-Ederer method
Cutler operation
cutoff
    anesthetic c.
cutting
    circle straight c.
    c. needle biopsy
    section c.
    ultrasonic c.
Cuvier
    canal of C.
CVAS
    Colored Visual Analogue Scale
CVI
    chronic venous insufficiency
CVP
    central venous pressure
    intraoperative CVP
    CVP line

CVR
    cerebrovascular resistance
CVVHD
    continuous venovenous hemodialysis
cyanogen bromide method
cyanosis
    compression c.
    shunt c.
cyanotic induration
cyclarthrodial
cyclarthrosis
cycle
    healing c.
cyclectomy
cyclic
    c. fasting motility
    c. pain
    c. respiration
    c. vertigo
cyclicotomy
cyclitic membrane
cyclocryopexy
cyclodestructive procedure
cyclodiathermy operation
cycloelectrolysis
cyclooxygenase-2 (COX-2)
cyclophotocoagulation
    Nd:YAG c.
    transpupillary c.
cyclopropane
cyclops
    c. formation
    c. procedure
cycloscopy
cyclotomy
cylicotomy
cylinder
    hilar c.
    c. retinoscopy
cylindrical
    c. carcinoma
    c. confronting cisterna
    c. osteotomy
cylindroadenoma
cylindroid aneurysm
cylindroma
cylindromatous lesion
cylindrosarcoma
cyma line
cyst
    air c.
    amebic c.
    anterior c.
    arachnoid c.
    c. aspiration
    Baker c.
    benign liver c.
    benign subcutaneous c.
    blue dome breast c.

brachial cleft c.
branchial c.
branchiogenous c.
breast c.
chocolate c.
choledochal c.
chyle c.
colloid c.
compound c.
congenital choledochal c.
c. content
corpus luteum c.
daughter c.
dermoid c.
double unilateral c.'s
duplication c.
echinococcal liver c.
echinococcus c.
enteric c.
enterogenous c.
epidermal inclusion c.
epidermoid c.
epithelial c.
c. fenestration
follicular c.
ganglion c.
gastric duplication c.
granddaughter c.
hepatic parasitic c.
hydatid liver c.
hyperplastic c.
inclusion c.
intraluminal c.
involution c.
laryngeal c.
liver c.
mesenteric c.
milk-filled c.
mother c.
multilocular c.
myoid c.
nabothian c.
old posterior c.
omental c.
ovarian dermoid c.
pancreatic c.
parasitic c.
pilonidal c.
posterior c.
preauricular c.
primordial c.
Rathke pouch c.

renal c.
residual c.
retention c.
sacrococcygeal c.
Sampson c.
sebaceous c.
splenic c.
subcutaneous c.
sublingual c.
theca-lutein c.
thymic c.
thyroglossal duct c.
Tornwaldt c.
unilateral c.
unilocular c.
vitellointestinal c.
c. wall
wolffian c.
young c.
cystadenocarcinoma
bile duct c.
mucinous c.
papillary c.
pseudomucinous c.
serous c.
cystadenofibroma
cystadenoma
ductal c.
ductectatic mucinous c.
hyperplastic c.
thyroid c.
cystauchenotomy
cystectomy
Bartholin c.
ovarian c.
partial c.
pilonidal c.
radical c.
salvage c.
total c.
vulvovaginal c.
cysteic acid method
cystenterostomy
direct c.
endoscopic c.
cystgastrostomy
endoscopic c.
surgical c.
cystic
c. acute inflammation
c. adenocarcinoma

NOTES

cystic (*continued*)
    c. adenomatoid malformation (CAM)
    c. artery
    c. bone lesion
    c. cavity
    c. chronic inflammation
    c. dilatation
    c. dilation
    c. duct
    c. duct catheterization
    c. duct choledochoscopy
    c. duct-infundibulum junction
    c. duct stump leak
    c. granulomatous inflammation
    c. hidradenoma
    c. kidney
    c. kidney disease
    c. lymphoepithelial AIDS-related lesion
    c. mass
    c. medial necrosis
    c. metastasis
    c. node
    c. polyp
    c. puncture
    c. structure

cystica
cysticercal infection
cystici
cysticolithectomy
cysticolithotripsy
cysticorrhaphy
cysticotomy
cysticus
cystides (*pl. of* cystis)
cystidoceliotomy
cystidolaparotomy
cystidotrachelotomy
cystine calculus
cystis, pl. **cystides**
cystitis
    interstitial c.
    schistosomal c.
cystoadenoma
cystocarcinoma
cystocele repair
cystochromoscopy
cystocolostomy
cystodiaphanoscopy
cystoduodenal ligament
cystoduodenostomy
    endoscopic c.
    pancreatic c.
cystoenterocele
cystoenterostomy
cystoepithelioma
cystofibroma
cystogastric fistula

cystogastrostomy
    endoscopic c.
cystography
cystoid body
cystojejunostomy
    Roux-en-Y c.
cystolith
cystolithectomy
cystolithiasis
cystolithic
cystolitholapaxy
cystolithotomy
cystolysis
cystoma
cystometrography
cystometry
cystopanendoscopy
cystopericystectomy
cystopexy
cystoplasty
    augmentation c.
    Gil-Vernet ileocecal c.
    human lyophilized dura c.
    ileocecal c.
    nonsecretory sigmoid c.
    sigmoid c.
cystoproctostomy
cystoprostatectomy
cystoprostatourethrectomy
cystoprostatovesiculectomy
cystorectostomy
cystorrhaphy
cystosarcoma phyllodes
cystoscopic electrohydraulic lithotripsy
cystoscopy
    percutaneous fetal c.
    steerable c.
    virtual c.
cystostomy
    trocar c.
cystotomy
    suprapubic c.
cystotrachelotomy
cystourethrocele
cystourethrography
cystourethropexy
    obturator shelf c.
    Pereyra-Raz c.
    vaginal c.
cystourethroplasty
    Kropp c.
    Leadbetter c.
cystourethroscopy
    dynamic c.
cytobrush biopsy
cytochrome
    myocardial c.
cytoid body
cytokeratin immunostain

cytokine
  inflammatory c.
  c. network
  c. receptor inhibitor
cytologic
  c. abnormality
  c. biopsy
  c. diagnosis
  c. evaluation
  c. examination
  c. feature
  c. result
  c. specimen
  c. study
  c. washing
cytological assessment
cytology
  abnormal c.
  aspiration biopsy c.
  brush c.
  endometrial c.
  endoscopic brush c.
  endoscopic fine-needle aspiration c.
  endoscopic ultrasonography-
    guided c.
  equivocal pancreatic c.
  EUS-guided c.
  c. examination
  exfoliative c.
  fine-needle aspiration c.
  gastric c.
  guided-needle aspiration c.

  intraoperative touch prep c.
  needle aspiration c.
  negative c.
  negative peritoneal c. (NPC)
  nipple aspiration c.
  oral cavity c.
  peritoneal c.
  positive c.
  positive peritoneal c. (PPC)
  salvage c.
  c. sample
  c. specimen
cytolytic T-lymphocyte (CTL)
cytomegalovirus (CMV)
  c. colitis
  c. infection
  c. prophylaxis
cytomegalovirus-positive donor
cytoplasm
cytoplasmic membrane
cytopreparation
cytoreduction
cytoreductive surgery
cytospin collection fluid
cytotoxicity
cytotoxic T-lymphocyte (CTL)
Czermak pterygium operation
Czerny
  C. operation
  C. suture technique
Czerny-Lembert suture technique

NOTES

δ (*var. of* delta)

D
- D chromosome ring syndrome
- D line
- D point

D2
- D2 dissection
- D2 lymphadenectomy
- D2 resection

2D
- 2-dimensional

3D
- 3-dimensional
  - 3D computer reconstruction
  - 3D transesophageal echocardiography

DAC
- deep abdominal complication

dacryoadenectomy operation
dacryocyst
dacryocystectomy operation
dacryocystocele
dacryocystoethmoidostomy
dacryocystorhinostomy
dacryocystorhinotomy operation
dacryocystostomy operation
dacryon
dacryorhinocystostomy
dacryorhinocystotomy
dacryostenosis
dacryostomy
- Arroyo d.
- Arruga d.
- Dupuy-Dutemps d.
- Rowinski d.

dactyledema
dactylitis
dactylomegaly
dactyloscopy
dactylospasm
dacuronium
dagger sign
Dagradi esophageal variceal classification
Dailey operation
Dakin-Carrel treatment
Dale-Laidlaw clotting time method
Dalgleish operation
Dallas operation
Dalrymple sign
damage
- anterior cervical surgery vocal cord d.
- cellular d.
- end-organ d.
- endothelial d.
- irradiation d.
- liver d.
- nervous d.
- obturator nerve d.
- postsurgical nervous d.
- projection fiber d.
- radiation d.
- soft tissue d.
- subretinal d.
- sun and chemical combination d.
- tourniquet-related nerve d.
- vocal cord d.

damage-control celiotomy
damaged parenchyma
Damian graft procedure
Damus-Kaye-Stansel (DKS)
- D.-K.-S. operation
- D.-K.-S. procedure

Damus-Stansel-Kaye procedure
DANA
- designed after natural anatomy

Dana
- D. operation
- D. posterior rhizotomy

Dana-Farber Cancer Institute
Dance sign
Dandy
- D. maneuver
- D. myocutaneous scalp flap
- D. operation

Dandy-Walker
- D.-W. deformity
- D.-W. malformation
- D.-W. syndrome

Dane method
Danforth fetal operation
danger space
Daniel iliac bone graft
Danielson method
Danis-Weber
- D.-W. ankle injury classification
- D.-W. fracture

Danus-Fontan procedure
Danus-Stanzel repair
Dardik umbilical graft
dark-field
- d.-f. examination
- d.-f. illumination
- d.-f. microscopy

dark-ground illumination
Darling capsulotomy
Darrach
- D. procedure
- D. resection

D

Darrach-McLaughlin shoulder technique
darting incision
dartos
    d. fascia
    d. muscle
    d. pouch procedure
Das
    D. Gupta procedure
    D. Gupta scapular excision
    D. Gupta scapulectomy
dashboard
    d. dislocation
    d. fracture
datum, pl. **data**
    bacteriologic data
    clinicopathologic data
    followup data
    histopathologic data
    manometric data
    on-line data
    d. plane
    ultrasonographic data
Daubenton
    D. angle
    D. line
    D. plane
d'Aubigné
    d. femoral reconstruction
    d. resection reconstruction
daughter cyst
Davey-Rorabeck-Fowler decompression
  technique
David Letterman sign
Daviel operation
Davis
    D. drainage technique
    D. fusion
    D. intubated ureterostomy
    D. intubated ureterotomy
    D. muscle-pedicle graft
Davis-Geck blepharoplasty
Davis-Kitlowski procedure
Davydov procedure
DAWG
    demucosalized augmentation with gastric
    segment
    DAWG procedure
Dawson criteria
day
    d. care surgical unit (DCSU)
    postoperative d. (POD)
    posttransplant d.
day-case operation
DBP
    diastolic blood pressure
D&C
    dilatation and curettage
    dilation and curettage

DCIS
    ductal carcinoma in situ
        focal DCIS
        multifocal extensive DCIS
        residual DCIS
DCS
    dorsal column stimulation
DCSU
    day care surgical unit
DCT
    deceleration time
D-D
    duct-to-duct
        D-D anastomosis
D-dimer
D&E
    dilatation and evacuation
    dilation and evacuation
de
    de Grandmont operation
    de Mussy point
    de novo lesion
    de novo needle-knife technique
    de Quervain fracture
    de Quervain stenosing tenosynovitis
     release
    de Quervain syndrome
    de Quervain tenosynovitis
    de Vincentiis operation
deactivation
    trigger point d.
dead
    d. space
    d. space:tidal volume ratio
    d. tract
deafferentation
    d. pain
    d. pain syndrome
de-airing procedure
Dean and Webb titration
dearterialization
    hepatic d.
death
    brain d.
    cerebral d.
    intraoperative d.
    noncancer d.
    perioperative d.
    postoperative d.
    trauma-related d.
    tumor-related d.
    vascular disease d.
Deaver incision
DeBakey
    D. classification
    D. graft
DeBakey-Creech aneurysm repair
DeBakey-type aortic dissection
DeBastiani corticotomy

debility
debouch
débouchement
Debove membrane
débridement
    d. arthroplasty
    arthroscopy and d.
    autolytic d.
    burn d.
    canal d.
    cavity d.
    diagnostic arthroscopy and d.
    enzymatic d.
    exploration and d.
    operative d.
    root canal d.
    surgical d.
    tangential d.
debris
    cellular d.
    valve d.
debt
    oxygen d.
debubbling procedure
debulking
    d. operation
    ovarian carcinoma d.
    d. procedure
    d. surgery
    surgical d.
    d. of tumor
decalcification
decannulation
decayed, extracted, filled
deceleration time (DCT)
deception
    pain d.
decerebration
    bloodless d.
decerebrize
dechondrification
decidua
decidual membrane
deciduous
decimal reduction time
declamping
    d. phenomenon
    d. shock
declination angle
décollement
    d. hemicolectomy
    d. maneuver

decompensated liver disease
decompensation
    circulatory d.
    hepatic d.
    d. injury
    vascular d.
decompress
decompression
    anterior retroperitoneal d.
    bone graft d.
    cardiac d.
    cerebral d.
    d. colostomy
    4-compartment fascial d.
    continuous gastric d.
    endoscopic biliary d.
    extensive posterior d.
    fascial d.
    d. fasciotomy
    gaseous d.
    gastric d.
    d. incision
    internal d.
    d. jejunostomy
    d. laminectomy
    microvascular d. (MVD)
    nerve d.
    orbital d.
    paraclavicular thoracic outlet d.
    pericardial d.
    portal d.
    posterior fossa d.
    retroperitoneal d.
    d. rhachotomy
    Rowbotham orbital d.
    selective portal d.
    spinal d.
    suboccipital d.
    subtemporal d.
    surgical portal d.
    d. technique
    thoracic outlet d.
    transduodenal endoscopic d.
    trigeminal d.
    tube d.
    variceal d.
    vein d.
    vertebral body d.
decompressive
    d. laminectomy
    d. surgery
deconditioned exercise response

NOTES

D

decontamination
    selective bowel d.
deconvolution
decortication
    arterial d.
    cerebral d.
    laparoscopic cyst d.
    renal cyst d.
    reversible d.
    d. technique
decrease
    hypoxic ventilatory d.
decreased
    d. afterload
    d. preload
    d. respiration
decubital gangrene
decubitus
    d. calculus
    d. position
    d. view
decussation
    dorsal tegmental d.
    Forel d.
    fountain d.
    Held d.
    Meynert d.
    motor d.
    oculomotor d.
    optic d.
    pyramidal d.
    rubrospinal d.
    tectospinal d.
    ventral tegmental d.
    Wernekinck d.
dedicated intercostals care
dedolation
deendothelialization
deendothelialized
deep
    d. abdominal complication (DAC)
    d. anal sphincter
    d. anterior neck
    d. anterior wall
    d. articular aorta
    d. articulation test
    d. auricular artery
    d. brachial artery
    d. cardiac plexus
    d. cervical artery
    d. cervical fascia
    d. cervical vein
    d. chest therapy
    d. circumflex iliac artery-iliac crest
      flap
    d. circumflex inguinal artery
    d. crural arch
    d. delayed infection
    d. Doppler velocity interrogation

    d. epigastric artery
    d. extubation in tonsil position
    d. femoral artery
    d. forearm
    d. gastric-longitudinal (DG-L)
    d. gastric-transverse (DG-T)
    d. hypothermia
    d. hypothermic circulatory arrest
      (DHCA)
    d. iliac dissection
    d. infrapatellar bursa
    d. inguinal ring
    d. interloop abscess
    d. lamina
    d. liver tract
    d. lymphatic vessel
    d. orbit
    d. palmar arch
    d. palmar branch
    d. penis
    d. perineal pouch
    d. perineal space
    d. peroneal nerve
    d. petrosal nerve
    d. plantar branch
    d. postanal anorectal space
    d. profunda brachial artery
    d. temporal artery
    d. temporal nerve
    d. tumor
    d. vein thrombosis
    d. venous thrombosis (DVT)
    d. venous thrombosis prophylaxis
    d. venous thrombus
    d. volatile anesthesia
    d. wound infection
deepicardialization
deepithelialization
deepithelialized
    d. rectus abdominis muscle
      (DRAM)
    d. rectus abdominis muscle flap
deep-seated fungal infection
defalcated root canal
Defares rebreathing method
defasciculating dose
defecation
    d. score
    sense of d.
defecography
defect
    aponeurotic d.
    atrial septal d.
    atrioventricular canal d.
    atrioventricular septal d.
    bandeau d.
    chain-of-lakes filling d.
    clinical d.
    coagulation d.

cold d.
combined d.
craniotomy d.
dentinoenamel d.
diaphragmatic d.
direct d.
fascial d.
filling d.
frondlike filling d.
hernia d.
hot d.
iatrogenic hernia d.
indirect d.
mass d.
napkin-ring d.
neural tube d.
oromandibular d.
osteoarticular d.
osteochondral d.
parietal d.
perineal d.
peritoneal d.
pinpoint gastric mucosal d.
postinjury immunologic d.
postresection d.
Rastelli classification of atrioventricular septal d. (type A–C)
repairable parietal d.
septal d.
slitlike d.
surgical d.
tumor d.
ventilation d.
ventilation/perfusion d.
ventricular septal wound d.

deferens
vas d.

deferent
d. canal
d. duct

deferentectomy

deferential
d. artery
d. plexus

deferentialis

deferentis

deferred shock

defibrillation
cardiac d.
d. shock
d. threshold

defibrillatory shock

deficiency
protein C d.

deficit
base d. (BD)
neurologic d.
neuropsychological d.
normal base d.
transient neurologic d.
transient profound neurologic d.

defined sterilization

definitive
d. cause
d. local therapy
d. method
d. resection
d. stabilization
d. surgery
d. tracheostomy
d. treatment

deflation
targeted lobar d.

deformation

deformity
abduction d.
acetabular protrusio d.
acquired d.
adduction d.
adduction-internal rotation d.
adductovarus d.
Åkerlund d.
d. analysis
Andy Gump d.
angel-wing d.
d. angle
angular d.
angulation d.
Arnold-Chiari d.
back-knee d.
batwing d.
bell-clapper d.
bifid thumb d.
bird-beak d.
bony d.
boutonnière d.
bowing d.
bowleg d.
bulb d.
bunion d.
burn boutonnière d.
buttonhole d.
calcaneocavovarus d.

D

NOTES

183

deformity *(continued)*
 calcaneocavus d.
 calcaneovalgus d.
 calcaneovarus d.
 cavovarus d.
 cavus d.
 cecal d.
 cervical spine kyphotic d.
 cervicomedullary d.
 chain-of-lakes d.
 checkrein d.
 chest d.
 clasped thumb d.
 clawfoot d.
 clawhand d.
 clawing d.
 clawtoe d.
 cleft hand d.
 cleft lip d.
 cloverleaf skull d.
 clubfoot d.
 cock-up d.
 codfish d.
 combined cavus d.
 compensatory d.
 complete bilateral d.
 congenital postural d.
 coronal plane d.
 craniofacial d.
 crossbar stomach d.
 crossover toe d.
 cubitus valgus d.
 Dandy-Walker d.
 dentofacial d.
 duodenal bulb d.
 elevatus d.
 equinovalgus d.
 equinus d.
 Erlenmeyer flask d.
 eversion-external rotation d.
 extension d.
 facial d.
 finger d.
 fishtail d.
 fixed d.
 flat back d.
 flexion d.
 flexion-internal rotation d.
 foot d.
 funnel chest d.
 garden spade d.
 genu valgum d.
 genu varum d.
 gibbous d.
 gingival d.
 gooseneck d.
 gross d.
 Haglund d.
 hallux valgus d.

 hammertoe d.
 hand d.
 hatchet-head d.
 Hill-Sachs d.
 hindbrain d.
 hindfoot d.
 hip d.
 hockey-stick d.
 hook-nail d.
 hourglass d.
 humpback d.
 hyperextension d.
 internal rotation d.
 intrinsic minus d.
 intrinsic plus d.
 joint d.
 J-sella d.
 keyhole d.
 Kirner d.
 kleeblatschädel d.
 Klippel-Feil d.
 knock-knee d.
 kyphotic d.
 lanceolate d.
 limb d.
 lobster-claw d.
 lumbar spine kyphotic d.
 Madelung d.
 mallet finger d.
 mallet toe d.
 Michel d.
 Mondini d.
 nasal d.
 opera-glass d.
 parachute d.
 pectus carinatum d.
 pectus excavatum d.
 pencil-in-cup d.
 penile d.
 percutaneous compression device-
  tow d.
 pes planus d.
 phrygian cap d.
 pigeon-breast d.
 ping-pong ball d.
 1-plane d.
 2-plane d.
 3-plane d.
 plantar flexion-inversion d.
 posttraumatic spinal d.
 postural d.
 protrusio d.
 pseudoboutonnière d.
 rat-tail d.
 recurvatum angulation d.
 rotational d.
 round back d.
 round shoulder d.
 sabre-shin d.

saddle-nose d.
sagittal d.
scoliotic d.
segmental wall motion d. (SWMA)
shepherd's crook d.
shoulder d.
silver-fork d.
skeletal d.
skull d.
spastic thumb-in-palm d.
spinal coronal plane d.
spine d.
spinning-top d.
splayfoot d.
splenic vein d.
split-hand d.
split-nail d.
spondylitic d.
Sprengel d.
S-shaped d.
stomach d.
subcondylar d.
supination d.
swan-neck finger d.
talipes cavus d.
thoracic spine kyphotic d.
thoracic spine scoliotic d.
thumb d.
thumb-in-palm d.
trefoil d.
triphalangeal thumb d.
turned-up pulp d.
ulnar deviation d.
ulnar drift d.
valgus d.
varus hindfoot d.
Velpeau d.
volar angulation d.
Volkmann clawhand d.
whistling d.
Whitehead d.
windblown d.
windsock d.
windswept d.
wrist d.
Zancolli procedure for clawhand d.
zig-zag compensatory d.
Z-type d.
deformity-instability
spinal d.-i.

DEFT
driven equilibrium Fourier transform DEFT technique
defunctionalization
defunctioning loop ileostomy
Dega pelvic osteotomy
degasified distilled water
degenerated fibroadenolipoma
degenerating otoconia
degeneration
aberrant third nerve d.
age-related macular d.
malignant d.
degenerative
d. change
d. discogenic end-plate disease
d. encephalopathy
d. inflammation
d. mitral valve insufficiency
degloving procedure
degradation
intracellular protein d.
d. product
protein d.
degrade
degree
d. of inspiration
270-d. laparoscopic posterior fundoplasty
dehiscence
abdominal incision d.
anastomotic d.
Roux limb stump d.
scar d.
staple line d.
stump d.
suture line d.
total d.
wound d.
dehiscent mandibular canal
dehydration fever
dehydrogenation
Deisting prostatic dilation technique
Deiter operation
deiterospinal tract
Deiters cell
Dejerine-Roussy syndrome
delay
fixation d.
d. line
delayed
d. complication

D

NOTES

delayed *(continued)*
    d. direct coloanal anastomosis
    d. expansion
    d. femoral osteotomy
    d. flap
    d. fracture union
    d. gastric emptying
    d. graft
    d. hyperacute transplant rejection
    d. onset muscle soreness (DOMS)
    d. open reduction
    d. pneumothorax
    d. primary closure
    d. primary repair
    d. primary suture technique
    d. pulmonary toxicity syndrome
    d. resuscitation
    d. urination
DeLee
    D. classification
    D. maneuver
deletion
    clonal d.
deliberate
    d. hypotension (DH)
    d. hypotension anesthetic technique
delimiting keratotomy
delineating
delirium
    emergence d.
delivery
    buccal transmucosal d.
    cesarean d.
    closed loop automated d.
    controlled heat-aided drug d.
     (CHADD)
    epidural d.
    spinal d.
    transmucosal d.
    vacuum extractor d.
    vaginal birth after cesarean d.
Dellepiane hysterectomy
Deller modification
Delorme
    D. procedure
    D. rectal prolapse operation
    D. thoracoplasty
delta, δ
    portal d.
delta-shaped anastomosis
deltoid
    d. branch
    d. crest
    d. eminence
    d. flap
    d. muscle
deltoid-splitting
    d.-s. incision
    d.-s. shoulder approach

deltopectoral
    d. approach
    d. fascia
    d. flap
    d. groove
    d. incision
    d. sulcus
Del Toro operation
deltoscapular flap
demand-adapted administration
    anesthetic technique
demand minimum functional capacity
    (DMFC)
demarcation
    corticomedullary d.
    d. current
    d. potential
demineralization
    bony d.
demonstration
    angiographic d.
Demours membrane
demucosalized
    d. augmentation
    d. augmentation with gastric
     segment (DAWG)
demyelinating lesion
demyelination
    autoimmune d.
    axonal d.
    intramedullary d.
DeMyer system of cerebral
    malformation
dendriform
dendrite
    corneal d.
dendritic
    d. calculus
    d. carcinoma
    d. lesion
dendrocytoma
denervate
denervation
    d. disease
    d. dysesthesia
    extrinsic d.
    facet d.
    d. hypersensitivity
    Krause d.
    law of d.
    d. potential
    preganglionic sympathetic d.
    sinoaortic d.
    sympathetic d.
dengue hemorrhagic fever infection
Denham external fixation

Denis
> D. Browne spinal fracture
> classification
> D. Browne urethroplasty technique

denitrogenation
Denker sinus operation
Dennie line
Dennie-Morgan line
Dennis-Brooke ileostomy
Dennis technique
Dennis-Varco pancreaticoduodenostomy
Denonvilliers
> D. aponeurosis
> D. fascia
> D. ligament

dens
> d. anterior screw fixation
> d. fracture
> pit of atlas for d.

dense
> d. adhesion
> d. body
> d. brain mass
> d. nature

density
> functional capillary d.
> lymphatic microvessel d. (LMVD)
> raspberry-like d.
> vapor d.

density-dependent repair
dental
> d. anatomy
> d. anesthesia
> d. anomaly
> d. arch expansion
> d. articulation
> d. canal
> d. cavity
> d. fenestration
> d. fistula
> d. implant
> d. index
> d. infection
> d. nerve
> d. polyp
> d. prosthetic laboratory procedure
> d. psychosedation
> d. pulp extirpation
> d. puncture
> d. restoration
> d. sac
> d. sinus tract

> d. surgery
> d. trepanation
> d. trephination
> d. tubercle
> d. wedge

dentate
> d. fracture
> d. line
> d. margin
> d. suture

dentatectomy
dentatothalamic tract
denticulate ligament
dentin
> d. crystal alteration
> d. pain

dentinal canal
dentinoenamel
> d. defect
> d. membrane

dentoalveolar joint
dentofacial
> d. anomaly
> d. deformity
> d. surgery

denture
> d. classification
> d. foundation
> d. foundation area
> d. foundation surface
> d. space

denudation
> endothelial d.
> interdental d.

denuded
> d. bowel
> d. connective tissue
> d. furcation
> d. rectal cuff

Denver classification
Depage incision
Depage-Janeway
> D.-J. gastrostomy
> D.-J. gastrotomy

DePalma modified patellar technique
dependency
> ventilator d.

dependent drainage
depigmentation
> congenital d.

depigmented lesion
depilation

D

NOTES

deplasmolysis
deployment
   stent d.
DepoDur
depolarization
   d. block
   primary afferent d.
depolarizing
   d. block
   d. relaxant
deposition
   abdominal iron d.
depot corticosteroid
depressant
depressed
   d. lesion
   d. side
   d. skull fracture
   d. type
depression
   d. fracture
   Hamilton Rating Scale for D.
   inspiratory rib cage d.
   respiratory d.
   twitch d.
   ventilatory d.
deprivation amblyopia
depth
   d. of anesthesia
   d. of anesthesia monitoring
   anesthetic d.
   d. caliper-meter stick method
   char-zone d.
   d. electrode
   indicator of anesthetic d.
   d. of insertion (DOI)
   d. pulse technique
derby
   d. hat fracture
   D. operation
derivation
derivative circulation
dermabrasion
dermal
   d. fasciectomy
   d. fat free flap
   d. fat free tissue transfer
   d. fat graft
   d. fat pedicle flap
   d. fibroblast
   d. injection
   d. lesion
   d. loss
   d. lymphatics
   d. pouch
   d. pouch reconstruction
   d. route of injection
   d. sinus tract
   d. suture technique

dermatoalloplasty
dermatoautoplasty
dermatocele
dermatofibroma
dermatofibrosarcoma
dermatoheteroplasty
dermatohomoplasty
dermatologic
   d. disorder
   d. problem
dermatolysis
dermatomal
   d. level of analgesia
   d. mapping
dermatome
   d. mapping
   trigeminal d.
dermatomyoma
dermatophyte fungal infection
dermatoplasty
dermatoscopy
dermatosis
dermatoxenoplasty
dermis
   human fibroblast-derived d. (HFDD)
   d. patch graft
dermodesis
   resection d.
dermoid cyst
dermoidectomy
dermolipoma
dermolysis
dermoplasty
dermovascular
derotation
derotational osteotomy
DES
   diffuse esophageal spasm
desaturation
   apnea-induced hemoglobin d.
   arterial oxygen d.
   jugular bulb oxyhemoglobin d.
   oxygen d.
   red d.
Desault wrist dislocation
Descemet
   D. membrane
   D. membrane detachment
descending
   d. anterior branch
   d. aortic aneurysm
   d. artery of knee
   d. colon
   d. genicular artery
   d. genicular vein
   d. loop colostomy
   d. mesocolon
   d. nerve
   d. palatine artery

d. posterior branch
d. scapular artery
d. technique
Descot fracture
Descriptor Differential Scale of Pain Intensity
desensitization with towel rubbing
desflurane
desiccation
electrosurgical d.
mucous d.
designated blood donation
designed after natural anatomy (DANA)
Desjardins point
Desmarres operation
desmocytoma
desmoid lesion
desmoplastic
d. medulloblastoma
d. trichilemmoma
desmopressin
desmotomy
destruction
bone d.
bony element d.
bony necrosis and d.
Cawthorne d.
cortical d.
moth-eaten bone d.
mucosal d.
parenchymal d.
progressive parenchymal d.
destructive
d. bone lesion
d. interference technique
desyndactylization
Weinstock d.
detached
d. cranial section
d. craniotomy
detachment
Descemet membrane d.
exudative retinal d.
traction d.
detection
pancreatic fungal d.
sentinel lymph node d. (SLND)
d. threshold
detector response
deterioration
aortic wall d.
clinical d.

determinant
prognostic d.
detritus
tissue d.
detrusor
d. areflexia
d. instability
d. muscle
d. pressure
d. stability
devascularization
gastric d.
paraesophagogastric d.
devascularized parathyroid remnant
DeVega tricuspid valve anuloplasty
development
discontinuation-emergent symptom d.
pouch d.
sternal d.
developmental
d. coordination disorder
d. landmark
d. line
d. retardation
Deventer pelvis
Devereux-Reichek method
Deverle fixation
deviant articulation
deviated septum
deviation to the right
device
band-assist d.
bioartificial liver d.
intrauterine d. (IUD)
plate-guided distraction d.
d. therapy
Devine
D. antral exclusion
D. colostomy
D. hypospadias repair
devitalization
pulp d.
devitalized
d. bone graft
d. tissue
devitalize the tracheal mucosa
devolvulization
endoscopic d.
Devonshire
D. colic
D. technique

D

NOTES

189

Dewar
  D. posterior cervical fixation procedure
  D. posterior cervical fusion
  D. posterior cervical fusion technique
Dewar-Barrington
  D.-B. arthroplasty
  D.-B. clavicular dislocation technique
Dewar-Harris shoulder technique
DeWecker operation
dewy appearance
Dexter-Grossman classification
dextran reaction
dextrocardia
dextrogyration
dextromethorphan
dextrorotation
dextrotorsion
dextroversion
Deyerle femoral fracture technique
DFI
  disease-free interval
DFS
  disease-free survival
DG-L
  deep gastric-longitudinal
    DG-L image
DG-T
  deep gastric-transverse
    DG-T image
DH
  deliberate hypotension
DHCA
  deep hypothermic circulatory arrest
diabetes mellitus
diabetic
  d. coma
  d. complication
  d. gangrene
  d. ketoacidosis (DKA)
  d. patient
  d. pseudotabes
  d. puncture
  d. retinal treatment
  d. retinopathy
diacele
diacetylcholine
diacondylar fracture
diagnosis, pl. **diagnoses**
  anatomic d.
  clinical d.
  colposcopic d.
  cytologic d.
  frozen section d.
  genetic d.
  histologic d.
  histopathologic d.

  microscopic d.
  noninvasive d.
  nonoperative d.
  operative d.
  pathologic d.
  postoperative d.
  preoperative d.
  presumptive d.
  surgical d.
diagnostic
  d. accuracy
  d. anesthesia
  d. arthroscopy and débridement
  d. arthroscopy, operative arthroscopy, and possible operative arthrotomy
  d. articulation test
  d. biopsy
  d. cardiac catheterization
  d. colonoscopy
  d. dilemma
  d. endoscopy
  d. fiberoptic stomatoscopy
  d. finding
  d. IGBB
  d. imaging evaluation
  d. investigation
  d. laparoscopy
  d. modality
  d. and operative arthroscopy
  d. peritoneal lavage (DPL)
  d. procedure
  d. program
  d. radiation
  d. small bowel series
  d. step
  d. study
  d. surgical therapy
  d. technique
  d. tube
  d. value
  d. workup
diagonal section
dial
  d. pelvic osteotomy
  d. periacetabular osteotomy
dialysate preparation module
dialysis
  d. access surgery
  arteriovenous d.
  d. clinic
  continuous ambulatory peritoneal d. (CAPD)
  d. disequilibrium syndrome
  d. encephalopathy syndrome
  extracorporeal d.
  d. fistula
  inpatient d.
  maintenance d.

d. membrane
outpatient d.
peritoneal d.
postoperative d.
d. treatment
dialysis-dependent patient
dialytic ultrafiltration
dialyzer membrane
diameter
biparietal d. (BPD)
corneal d.
end-diastolic d. (EDD)
end-systolic d. (ESD)
maximal rectal d.
rectal d.
diametric pelvic fracture
diamond
D. classification
d. ejection murmur
d. inlay bone graft
Diamond-Gould
D.-G. reduction syndactyly
D.-G. syndactyly operation
diamond-shaped incision
Dianoux operation
diaphragm
bare area d.
central tendon d.
d. eventration
d. injury
d. laceration
laryngeal d.
pelvic d.
d. perforation
sternal part of d.
urogenital d.
diaphragma, pl. **diaphragmata**
diaphragmatic
d. crural repair
d. defect
d. elevation
d. eventration
d. hernia
d. herniation
d. injury
d. laceration
d. node
d. pleura
d. reflection
d. respiration
d. rupture
d. surface

diaphragmatic-abdominal respiration
diaphysial, diaphyseal
d. fracture
d. osteotomy
diaphysis, pl. **diaphyses**
femoral d.
diarthric
diarthrodial
d. cartilage
d. joint
diarthrosis
diarticular
Dias-Giegerich
D.-G. fracture technique
D.-G. open reduction
Dias-Tachdijian physical injury
classification
diastasis
ankle mortise d.
d. fibula
iris d.
palpable rib d.
pubic d.
rectus d.
rib d.
sutural d.
tibiofibular d.
diastatic skull fracture
diastolic
d. blood pressure (DBP)
d. filling pressure
d. hypertension
d. pressure-time index
d. pressure-volume relation
d. relaxation
d. suction
diathermic
d. fistulotomy
d. loop biopsy
d. resection
d. therapy
diathermocoagulation
diathermy
coagulating d.
d. dissection
electrocoagulation d.
d. hemorrhoidectomy
medical d.
d. operation
d. puncture
short wave d.
surgical d.

D

NOTES

diazo staining method
Dibbell cleft lip-nasal reconstruction
DIC
    disseminated intravascular coagulation
dichotomization
dichotomous classification
dichotomy
Dickey-Fox operation
Dickey operation
Dickhaut-DeLee
    D.-D. classification of discoid
      meniscus
    D.-D. discoid meniscus
      classification
Dickinson
    D. approach
    D. calcaneal bursitis technique
Dickinson-Coutts-Woodward-Handler
  osteotomy
Dick method
Dickson
    D. geometric osteotomy
    D. transplant technique
Dickson-Diveley procedure
Dickson-Wright operation
dicondylar fracture
Didiee projection
Dieffenbach
    D. method
    D. operation
Dieffenbach-Duplay hypospadias
  technique
die punch fracture
dieresis
dieretic
diet
    advance to regular d.
    clear liquid d.
    regular d.
Dieterle method
Dieulafoy
    D. lesion
    D. vascular malformation
    D. vascular malformation of
      stomach
Dieulafoy-like lesion
difference
    alveolar-arterial pressure d.
    alveolar end-capillary d.
    morphological d.
differential
    d. blood pressure
    d. force technique
    d. nerve block
    d. relaxation
    d. spinal anesthesia
    d. spinal block
    d. spinal block anesthetic technique

    d. ureteral catheterization test
    d. variable reluctance transducer
differentiated thyroid carcinoma
differentiation failure
difficult ventilation
diffuse
    d. abdominal pain
    d. abdominal tenderness
    d. abscess
    d. acute inflammation
    d. air space disease
    d. aneurysm
    d. breast involvement
    d. carcinomatosis
    d. change
    d. chronic inflammation
    d. colloid goiter
    d. esophageal spasm (DES)
    d. fatty infiltration
    d. fibroma
    d. fusiform dilatation
    d. GI hamartoma polyp
    d. hemorrhagic pancreatitis
    d. idiopathic skeletal hyperostosis
    (DISH)
    d. illumination
    d. intravascular coagulation
    d. lobular fibrosis
    d. lymphatic tissue
    d. metastasis
    d. microcalcification
    d. microvascular thrombosis
    d. mucosal polyposis
    d. multinodular goiter
    d. necrosis
    d. papillomatosis
    d. peritonitis
    d. plane
    d. pulmonary alveolar hemorrhage
    d. reflection
    d. toxic nonnodular goiter
    d. transmural ganglioneuromatosis
    d. tumor
    d. ulceration
    d. ulcerative lesion
    d. variety
    d. vasculitis
diffusely tender abdomen
diffusion
    d. anoxia
    exchange d.
    d. hypoxia
    d. respiration
    d. root canal filling method
digastric
    d. branch
    d. fossa
    d. groove
    d. line

d. muscle
d. muscle flap
d. space
d. triangle
digestive
d. apparatus
d. bleeding
d. continuity
d. glandular cancer
d. manifestation
d. system
d. system vascular disease
d. tract
d. tract malignancy
d. tube
digital
d. artery protection
d. beam attenuation
d. block anesthesia
d. collateral artery
d. dilation
d. dissection
d. divulsion
d. extensor mechanism
d. extensor tendon
d. flap
d. flexion crease
d. furrow
d. imaging colposcopy
d. mammography
d. manipulation
d. nail
d. pad
d. pressure
d. pulp
d. rectal evacuation
d. rectal examination
d. retinacular ligament
d. subtraction echocardiography
 (DSE)
d. subtraction technique
d. templating
d. vein
digitalization
digitally guided biopsy
digitate impression
digitation
digiti (*pl. of* digitus)
digitization
digitonin method
digitorum

Digit Symbol Substitution Test
digitus, pl. **digiti**
dihydropyridine calcium channel blocker
dilacerated canal
dilaceration
sharp d.
dilatable lesion
dilatation (*See also* dilation)
aneurysmal d.
balloon d.
bile duct d.
blind d.
cardiac d.
congenital cystic d.
cricopharyngeal d.
d. and curettage (D&C)
cystic d.
diffuse fusiform d.
ductal d.
endoscopic retrograde balloon d.
esophageal d.
d. and evacuation (D&E)
ex vacuo d.
fusiform d.
gaseous d.
homatropine d.
junctional d.
pancreatic duct d.
percutaneous stricture d. (PSD)
percutaneous transhepatic balloon d.
 (PTBD)
periportal sinusoidal d.
pneumatic d.
poststenotic d.
pouch d.
prestenotic d.
pupillary d.
secondary arrest of d.
segmental d.
transurethral balloon d.
Virchow-Robin space d.
dilatator
dilated loop of bowel
dilating window
dilation (*See also* dilatation)
achalasia balloon d.
anal d.
aneurysmal d.
balloon d.
biliary d.
bootstrap d.
bowel d.

D

NOTES

dilation (*continued*)
  Brown-McHardy pneumatic mercury bougie d.
  capillary d.
  cardiac d.
  catheter d.
  cervical d.
  colonic d.
  d. and curettage (D&C)
  cystic d.
  digital d.
  ductal d.
  ectatic d.
  Eder-Puestow d.
  endoscopic papillary balloon d.
  episcleral vascular d.
  esophageal d.
  d. and evacuation (D&E)
  extrahepatic biliary cystic d.
  finger d.
  Frank technique of d.
  gastric d.
  Grüntzig balloon d.
  hepatic web d.
  hydrostatic balloon d.
  idiopathic d.
  inadequate d.
  intrahepatic biliary cystic d.
  intrahepatic ductal d.
  junctional d.
  d. lag
  lag d.
  Lord d.
  mechanical ureteral d.
  medical d.
  mucosal vascular d.
  percutaneous balloon d.
  periportal sinusoidal d.
  peroral esophageal d.
  pneumatic bag esophageal d.
  pneumatic balloon catheter d.
  pneumostatic d.
  postoperative ductal d.
  poststenotic d.
  progressive d.
  pupil d.
  pyloric d.
  reactive d.
  rectal d.
  serial d.
  submucosal vascular d.
  d. therapy
  through-the-scope balloon d.
  tract d.
  transurethral balloon d.
  TTS balloon d.
  urethral d.
  Uromat d.
  ventricular d.

  wire-guided d.
  Wirsung d.
dilator
  d. muscle
  d. placement
  d. placement failure
dilator-and-sheath technique
dilemma
  diagnostic d.
Dillwyn-Evans
  D.-E. osteotomy
  D.-E. resection
dilution
  tracer d.
dilution-filtration technique
dimension
  X, Y d.
2-dimensional (2D)
  2-d. Fourier transformation imaging
  2-d. Fourier transform gradient-echo imaging
  2-d. monitoring
3-dimensional (3D)
  3-d. conformal radiation therapy
  3-d. contouring
  3-d. FATS method
  3-d. Fourier transform gradient-echo imaging
  3-d. grid electrode
  3-d. projection reconstruction imaging
  3-d. reconstruction
  3-d. stereography
  3-d. videoscopy
  3-d. virtual cholangioscopy
Dimon-Hughston
  D.-H. fracture fixation
  D.-H. intertrochanteric osteotomy
  D.-H. technique
dimorphism
  gender d.
dimple
  celiac d.
  coccygeal d.
dinitrogen monoxide
dioptric
  d. aberration
  d. correction
dioxide
  arterial carbon d.
  carbon d. (CO_2)
  end-tidal carbon d.
  intraabdominally insufflated carbon d.
  partial pressure of arterial carbon d. ($PaCO_2$)
  partial pressure of carbon d. (PCO_2)

partial pressure of intramuscular
  carbon d. ($PiCO_2$)
partial pressure of mesenteric
  venous carbon d. ($PmvCO_2$)
DIP
  distal interphalangeal
  DIP fusion
diphtheritic membrane
diploë
diploic
  d. artery
  d. canal
  d. vein
dipolë-dipolë
  d.-d. relaxation
  d.-d. relaxation rate
Diprivan technique
direct
  d. acrylic restoration
  d. brain stimulation
  d. cardiac puncture
  d. cautery puncture
  d. cholecystoenterostomy
  d. closure
  d. composite resin restoration
  d. compression
  d. current electrocoagulation
  d. current shock ablation
  d. cystenterostomy
  d. defect
  d. electrical nerve stimulation
  d. embolectomy
  d. flap
  d. fluoroscopic visualization
  d. Fourier transformation imaging
  d. fracture
  d. gold restoration
  d. hemoperfusion
  d. histologic investigation
  d. illumination
  d. immunofluorescence test
  d. inguinal hernia
  d. insertion technique
  d. intraperitoneal insemination
  d. laparoscopic vision
  d. laryngoscopy
  d. ligation
  d. manipulation
  d. mechanical ventricular actuation
  d. method
  d. method for making inlays
  d. muscle lysis

d. needle puncture
d. neural stimulation
d. obturator nerve block
d. ophthalmoscopy
d. pressure
d. pyramidal tract
d. respiration
d. SSPCS
d. suturing
d. thrombin inhibitor
d. transfusion
d. vein anesthesia
direct/indirect technique
direction
  aboral d.
  anterograde d.
  caudal d.
  cephalad d.
  clockwise d.
  counterclockwise d.
  flow d.
  line of d.
  pelvic d.
  phase-encoding d.
  principal visual d.
  retrograde d.
  visual d.
  Z d.
directional coronary atherectomy
directive
  advance d.
direct-vision
  d.-v. internal urethrotomy
  d.-v. liver biopsy
dirty
  d. operative wound classification
  d. surgery
disarticular amputation
disarticulation
  Batch-Spittler-McFaddin knee d.
  Boyd hip d.
  Burger technique for
    scapulothoracic d.
  elbow d.
  hip d.
  joint d.
  Lisfranc d.
  Mazet d.
  metatarsophalangeal joint d.
  sacroiliac d.
  scapulothoracic d.

D

NOTES

195

disarticulation *(continued)*
    shoulder d.
    wrist d.
disassociation
disc, disk
    acromioclavicular d.
    d. compression
    d. diffusion method
    d. drusen hemorrhage
    d. excision
    extruded d.
    d. extrusion
    d. fragment
    free fragment d.
    herniated d.
    d. herniation
    intercalated d.
    interpubic d.
    d. lesion
    mandibular d.
    d. neovascularization
    optic d.
    d. oxygenation
    d. plication
    d. pressure
    protruded d.
    ruptured d.
    sacrococcygeal d.
    d. sensitivity method
    d. space
    d. space infection
    d. space narrowing
    d. space saline acceptance test
    sternoclavicular d.
    temporomandibular articular d.
discectomy, diskectomy
    anterior d.
    automated percutaneous d.
    cervical d.
    Cloward fusion d.
    laminotomy and d.
    lumbar d.
    microlumbar d.
    microsurgical d.
    partial d.
    percutaneous lumbar d.
    Robinson anterior cervical d.
    Smith-Robinson anterior cervical d.
    thoracic d.
    thoracoscopic d.
    transthoracic d.
    Williams d.
discharge
    breast d.
    pathologic breast d.
    physiologic breast d.
    same-day d.
disci (*pl. of* discus)
discission

disclosing solution
discography, diskography
    provocative d.
discoid skin lesion
disconnection syndrome
disconnect wedge
discontinuation-emergent symptom development
discontinuous
    d. endothelium
    d. neck dissection
    d. sterilization
discotomy
discrete
    d. bleeding source
    d. lesion
    d. mass
    d. stenosis
    d. tumor
discrimination
    d. curve
    d. loss
    d. score
discus, pl. **disci**
disease
    abdominal hydatid d.
    Abrami d.
    acute graft-versus-host d.
    adaptation d.
    adhesive d.
    adult familial hyaline membrane d.
    adult polycystic liver d.
    advanced d.
    air space d.
    amyloid oral cavity d.
    aneurysmal d.
    antiglomerular basement membrane antibody d.
    aortic aneurysmal d.
    aortic arch d.
    aortic atheromatous d.
    aortic occlusive d. (AOD)
    aortic valve d.
    aortoiliac occlusive d.
    Arbuthnot Lane d.
    arterial occlusive d. (AOD)
    atherosclerotic carotid artery d. (ACAD)
    atherosclerotic heart d.
    autosomal dominant polycystic kidney d.
    Behçet d.
    benign inflammatory d.
    Berger d.
    biliary tract d.
    bilobar d.
    bone d.
    Bright d.

Budd-Chiari syndrome with
  Behçet d.
Budd-Chiari syndrome without
  Behçet d.
calcium pyrophosphate deposition d.
carcinoid valve d.
cardiovascular d.
carotid artery d.
cement d.
central core d. (CCD)
central nervous system d.
cerebrovascular d.
choledochal cyst d.
chronic graft-versus-host d.
chronic liver d.
chronic obstructive airways d.
  (COAD)
colorectal d.
combined system d.
complex aortic d.
complicated diverticular d.
congestive heart d.
connective tissue d.
coronary artery d.
Crohn d.
Crouzon d.
cutaneous graft-versus-host d.
cystic kidney d.
decompensated liver d.
degenerative discogenic end-plate d.
denervation d.
diffuse air space d.
digestive system vascular d.
distant nodal d.
diverticular d.
early-onset graft-versus-host d.
echinococcal cyst d.
Economo d.
elevator d.
endogenous d.
endomyocardial d.
end-stage renal d. (ESRD)
eosinophilic endomyocardial d.
eventration d.
exanthematous d.
exogenous d.
exophytic joint d.
extensive-stage d.
extraabdominal d.
extracapsular d.
extracranial carotid artery d.
extracranial carotid occlusive d.

extracranial occlusive vascular d.
extrahepatic nodal d.
extramammary Paget d.
extranodal d.
extraorbital d.
extrapyramidal d.
exudative papulosquamous d.
eye d.
familial multigland d.
femoropopliteal occlusive d.
fibrocystic d.
Fournier d.
fracture d.
gallstone d.
gastroesophageal reflux d. (GERD)
glomerular basement membrane d.
graft-versus-host d. (GVHD)
gross cystic d.
hard metal d.
hard pad d.
hepatic venous web d.
heritable connective tissue d.
Hirschsprung d.
Hodgkin d.
humeroperoneal neuromuscular d.
Huntington d.
hyaline membrane d.
hydatid d.
hyperacute graft-versus-host d.
idiopathic eczematous d.
idiopathic peptic ulcer d.
immunoproliferative small
  intestine d. (IPSID)
inclusion body d.
inflammatory bowel d.
interfacetal d.
intraabdominal d.
in-transit d.
intraperitoneal endometrial
  metastatic d.
intrathoracic d.
irresectable d.
ischemic aortic d.
ischemic heart d.
Jackson and Parker classification of
  Hodgkin d.
Kashin-Beck d.
Killip classification of heart d.
Lafora body d.
late-onset d.
late-stage d.
Leri-Weill d.

D

NOTES

disease *(continued)*
    lichenoid graft-versus-host d.
    liver d.
    localization of d.
    locally advanced d.
    lower extremity occlusive d.
    lung d.
    lupus-associated valve d.
    lysosomal storage d.
    malignant pancreatic d.
    Marion d.
    Ménière d.
    mesenteric nodal d.
    metastatic d.
    microcystic d.
    micrometastatic peritoneal d.
    microscopic d.
    minimal change d.
    mixed connective tissue d.
    Mondor d.
    multifocal extensive d.
    multigland d.
    multiglandular d.
    multilevel atherosclerotic arterial occlusive d.
    multiple hydatid d.
    neurologic d.
    nil d.
    nodal d.
    node-negative d.
    node-positive d.
    noncirrhotic metabolic liver d.
    nonfamilial multiglandular d.
    nonmalignant d.
    obstructive lung d. (OLD)
    occlusive carotid artery d.
    occlusive coronary artery d.
    occult extrahepatic d.
    occult hepatic d.
    occult irresectable d.
    occult systemic d.
    omental nodal d.
    Ormond d.
    osteoarthritis d.
    Paget extramammary d.
    pancreatic d.
    Parkinson d.
    pelvic adhesive d.
    peptic ulcer d.
    periodontal d.
    peripheral arterial aneurysmal d.
    peripheral vascular d.
    peritoneal d.
    Peyronie d.
    Plummer d.
    polycystic kidney d. (PKD)
    popliteal artery occlusive d. (PAOD)

    posttransplant lymphoproliferative d. (PTLD)
    preeclamptic liver d.
    Preiser d.
    progressive d.
    pulmonary valve d.
    radiation-induced d.
    radiation lung d.
    Recklinghausen d. type I
    d. recurrence rate
    recurrent thromboembolic d.
    reflux d.
    Reiter d.
    renal artery occlusive d.
    renal artery stenotic d.
    renal vascular d.
    resectable hepatic d.
    residual d.
    sclerodermoid graft-versus-host d.
    short-segment d.
    single hydatid d.
    sinonasal d.
    sixth venereal d.
    space-occupying d.
    sporadic multigland d.
    d. stage
    Steinert d.
    stenotic d.
    supraesophageal reflux d.
    surgical pancreatic d.
    systemic d.
    Takayasu d.
    thin basement membrane d.
    thoracic aortic d.
    thromboembolic d.
    thrombotic d.
    tricuspid valve d.
    unanticipated hepatic d.
    undifferentiated connective tissue d.
    unilobar d.
    unresectable extrahepatic d.
    upper tract d.
    urinary tract d.
    valvular aortic d.
    valvular heart d.
    van Buren d.
    vascular d.
    vasculo-Behçet d.
    venereal d.
    venous stasis d.
    venous web d.
    vertebral artery d.
    vibration d.
    von Economo d.
    von Hippel-Lindau d.
    Winiwarter-Buerger d.
disease-associated mortality
disease-free
    d.-f. interval (DFI)

d.-f. patient
d.-f. survival (DFS)
disease-related complication
DISH
    diffuse idiopathic skeletal hyperostosis
    DISH syndrome
dish face
dishpan fracture
disinfecting solution
disinfection
    chemical d.
    high-level d.
    root canal d.
    spray-wipe-spray d.
    surface d.
    thermal d.
disintegration
    endoscopic stone d.
    d. rate
disinvagination
disjoined pyeloplasty
disk (*var. of* disc)
diskectomy (*var. of* discectomy)
diskography (*var. of* discography)
dislocation
    acromioclavicular joint d.
    ankle d.
    antenatal d.
    anterior complete d.
    anterior hip d.
    anterior-inferior d.
    anterior shoulder d.
    anterolateral d.
    atlantoaxial d.
    atlantooccipital joint d.
    atypical d.
    Bankart shoulder d.
    bayonet d.
    Bell-Dally cervical d.
    Bennett d.
    bilateral interfacetal d. (BID)
    boutonnière hand d.
    bursting d.
    carpometacarpal joint d.
    central d.
    Chopart ankle d.
    closed d.
    complete anterior d.
    complete inferior d.
    complete posterior d.
    complete superior d.
    compound d.

congenital hip d.
congenital lens d.
consecutive d.
d. contour abnormality
dashboard d.
Desault wrist d.
divergent elbow d.
dorsal perilunate d.
dorsal transscaphoid perilunar d.
dysplasia d.
elbow d.
facet d.
fracture d.
d. fracture
frank d.
gamekeeper thumb d.
glenohumeral joint d.
habitual d.
Hill-Sachs shoulder d.
hip d.
incomplete d.
inferior complete closed d.
inferior complete compound d.
interphalangeal joint d.
intraocular lens d.
isolated d.
Kienböck d.
knee d.
lens d.
Lisfranc d.
lumbosacral d.
lunate d.
luxatio erecta shoulder d.
mandibular d.
metatarsophalangeal joint d.
midcarpal d.
milkmaid elbow d.
Monteggia d.
Nélaton ankle d.
occipitoatlantal d.
Otto pelvis d.
Palmer transscaphoid perilunar d.
panclavicular d.
parachute jumper d.
partial d.
patellar intraarticular d.
pathologic d.
perilunar transscaphoid d.
perilunate carpal d.
peroneal d.
phalangeal d.
posterior hip d.

D

NOTES

dislocation *(continued)*
  posterior shoulder d.
  posteromedial d.
  prenatal d.
  primitive d.
  proximal tibiofibular joint d.
  radial head d.
  radiocarpal d.
  recent d.
  recurrent patellar d.
  retrosternal d.
  rotational d.
  sacroiliac d.
  scapholunate d.
  shoulder d.
  Smith d.
  spontaneous hyperemic d.
  sternoclavicular joint d.
  subastragalar d.
  subcoracoid shoulder d.
  subglenoid shoulder d.
  subtalar d.
  superior d.
  swivel d.
  talar d.
  tarsal d.
  tarsometatarsal d.
  temporomandibular joint d.
  teratologic d.
  tibialis posterior d.
  tibiofibular joint d.
  transscaphoid perilunate d.
  traumatic atlantooccipital d.
  triquetrolunate d.
  unilateral interfacetal d. (UID)
  unreduced d.
  volar semilunar wrist d.
  wrist d.
dismembered
  d. anastomosis
  d. pyeloplasty
  d. reimplanted appendicocystostomy
disobliteration
disorder
  accommodation d.
  acquired cornification d.
  anorectal d.
  arterial d.
  articulation d.
  autoimmune connective tissue d.
  benign esophageal d.
  bipolar affective d. (BAD)
  blood coagulation d.
  cartilaginous growth plate d.
  chronic multisystem d.
  coagulation d.
  coagulopathic d.
  colorectal d.
  complex adrenal endocrine d.

complex gonadal endocrine d.
complex pituitary endocrine d.
complex thyroid endocrine d.
connective tissue d.
cornification d.
cumulative trauma d.
Curth-Maklin cornification d.
dermatologic d.
developmental coordination d.
ejaculation d.
elimination d.
endocrine d.
endonasal d.
esophageal d.
evacuation d.
experimental d.
gamma loop d.
gonadal endocrine d.
gynecologic d.
hematologic d.
hemidysplasia cornification d.
immune-mediated coagulation d.
intestinal ischemic d.
keratitis-deafness cornification d.
lymphoproliferative d.
lysosomal enzyme d.
mastication d.
metabolic d.
mitral valve d.
mixed connective tissue d.
movement d.
multisystem d.
musculoskeletal d.
nail d.
neurologic d.
ocular motility d.
organic articulation d.
pituitary endocrine d.
posttransplant lymphoproliferative d.
  (PTLD)
posttraumatic stress d. (PTSD)
somatization d.
thrombogenic d.
thyroid endocrine d.
unilateral hemidysplasia
  cornification d.
urinary tract d.
voice d.
disordered hip complex
disparate point
displaced fracture
displacement
  d. analysis
  anterior d.
  d. curve
  d. implantation
  d. osteotomy
  port d.

d. threshold
water d.

display
graphical anesthesia drug d.

disproportion
cephalopelvic d.

disruption
wound d.

dissected tissue arm

dissecting
d. aneurysm
d. intramural hematoma

dissection
acute aortic d.
d. of aorta
aortic d.
arterial wall d.
axillary lymph node d. (ALND)
axillary node d.
balloon d.
bilateral neck d.
blunt and sharp d.
bone d.
bone-ligament d.
bony d.
capsular d.
carotid artery d.
cervical node d.
circumferential mucosal d.
complete axillary d.
complex d.
condyle d.
confirmatory axillary d.
coronary artery d.
cranial nerve d.
D2 d.
DeBakey-type aortic d.
deep iliac d.
diathermy d.
digital d.
discontinuous neck d.
elective lymph node d. (ELND)
elective neck d.
en bloc d.
endoscopic d.
epiphenomena of d.
esophageal d.
extensive lymph node d.
extracapsular d.
extrahepatic d.
extraperitoneal endoscopic pelvic
lymph node d.

field of d.
2-field d.
3-field d.
finger fracture d.
fingertip d.
flank d.
Freer d.
full axillary d.
functional lymph node d.
functional neck d.
gauze d.
groin d.
hard palate d.
hydraulic d.
in situ d.
incisural d.
inguinal canal d.
inguinal-femoral node d.
intracapsular d.
intradural d.
intramural air d.
intraparenchymal digital d.
jugular vein d.
laparoscopic pelvic lymph node d.
lateral cervical node d.
lateroaortic lymph node d.
limited obturator node d.
lymphatic d.
lymph node d.
d. margin
medial d.
mediastinal lymph node d.
mesoesophageal d.
modified radical neck d.
muscle d.
nasal d.
neck d.
nerve-sparing d.
node d.
Pack-Ehrlich deep iliac d.
paraaortic lymph node d.
parenchymal d.
parotid d.
partial zonal d.
pelvic lymph node d. (PLND)
pelvic node d.
periadventitial d.
periesophageal lymph node d.
perirectal pelvic d.
plane of d.
postradical neck d.
precise d.

D

NOTES

dissection *(continued)*
    radical axillary d.
    radical lymph node d.
    radical mediastinal d.
    radical neck d.
    retrogastric d.
    retroperitoneal lymph node d.
    (RPLND)
    retroperitoneal pelvic lymph
    node d. (RPLND)
    scissors d.
    selective inguinal node d.
    sharp and blunt d.
    soft tissue d.
    spiral d.
    sponge d.
    spontaneous coronary artery d.
    Stanford aortic d. (type A, B)
    Stanford-type aortic d.
    subligamentous d.
    submucosal d.
    subperiosteal d.
    subtemporal d.
    suction d.
    suprahyoid neck d.
    supraomohyoid neck d.
    sylvian d.
    symptomatic traumatic d.
    systemic d.
    Taussig-Morton node d.
    2-team d.
    therapeutic d.
    therapeutic lymph node d. (TLND)
    thoracic aortic d.
    tissue d.
    tongue-jaw-neck d.
    transthoracic d.
    traumatic internal carotid artery d.
    d. tubercle
    ultrasonic d.
    vertebral d.
    water d.
disseminated
    d. asymptomatic unilateral
    neovascularization
    d. carcinoma
    d. CMV infection
    d. gonococcal infection
    d. inflammation
    d. intravascular coagulation (DIC)
dissemination
    hematologic d.
    intraperitoneal d.
    neoplastic d.
    peritoneal d.
Disse space
dissipation
    circle d.
dissociable tetrameric hemoglobin

dissociated
    d. anesthesia
    d. position
dissociation
    d., analgesia, immobility, and
    tension scale
    atrial d.
    atrioventricular d.
    A-V d.
    complete atrioventricular d.
    complete A-V d.
    d. curve
    electromechanical d.
    electromyocardial d.
    hypnotic d.
    incomplete atrioventricular d.
    incomplete A-V d.
    interference d.
    intracavitary pressure-electrogram d.
    isorhythmic d.
    longitudinal d.
    lunotriquetral d.
    microbic d.
    d. movement
    radioulnar d.
    scapholunate d.
    scapulothoracic d.
    sleep d.
    syringomyelic d.
    tabetic d.
dissociative anesthesia
distal
    d. anastomosis
    d. aortic perfusion
    d. biceps brachii tendon rupture
    d. bile duct
    d. bile duct stricture
    d. bleeding
    d. catheter lengthening
    d. cavity
    d. centriole
    d. clavicular excision
    d. clot
    d. ectasia
    d. esophageal diverticulum
    d. esophageal ring
    d. esophagectomy
    d. extension restoration
    d. femoral epiphysial fracture
    d. femoropopliteal bypass graft
    d. fragment
    d. humeral epiphysis
    d. humeral fracture
    d. interphalangeal (DIP)
    d. interphalangeal fusion
    d. interphalangeal joint approach
    d. laparoscopic pancreatectomy
    d. ligation
    d. limb

d. metaphysis
d. metastasis
d. nail matrix
d. nerve graft
d. neurolysis
d. pancreas
d. pancreatectomy (DP)
d. pancreaticojejunostomy
d. phalanx
d. portion
d. radial fracture
d. radioulnar joint stabilization
d. remnant
d. shave section
d. splenoadrenal shunting
d. splenorenal shunt (DSRS)
d. stump
d. tibiofibular fusion
d. tumor
d. ureterectomy
d. vein cuff
d. vertebral artery reconstruction
d. visceral perfusion
d. with excision of ulcer gastrectomy
distal-occlusal (DO)
distal-row carpectomy
distance
interincisor d.
skin-epidural d.
skin-to-tumor d.
thyromental d.
tube-carina d.
tube-patient d.
tube-to-film d.
distant
d. flap
d. metastasis
d. nodal disease
d. recurrence
d. recurrence-free survival (DRFS)
distantial aberration
distended
d. abdomen
d. afferent loop
d. colon
d. gallbladder
distention
abdominal d.
bladder d.
cecal d.
colonic d.

gallbladder d.
gaseous d.
gastric d.
liver d.
postprandial d.
progressive abdominal d.
proximal bowel d.
rectal d.
vessel d.
distilled water
distoangular position
distobuccal line angle
distobuccoocclusal point angle
distolabial line angle
distolabioincisal point angle
distolingual line angle
distolinguoincisal point angle
distoocclusal point angle
distortion
d. aberration
corneal d.
pin-cushion d.
distraction
d. arthroplasty
d. of fracture
muscle d.
d. osteogenesis
d. technique
distraction/compression scoliosis treatment
distractive extension
distractor
femur d.
hip d.
plate-guided d.
tibial d.
distress
D. Risk Assessment Method (DRAM)
D. Scale for Ventilated Newborn Infants (DSVNI)
distribution
lesion d.
loop d.
d. pattern
pattern of d.
stocking-glove pain d.
ventilation/perfusion d.
disturbance
acid-base d.
chronic motor d.
hemodynamic d.

D

NOTES

disturbance *(continued)*
    interdigestive motility d.
    microcirculatory d.
    motility d.
    motor d.
    postsurgical d.
    sensitive visceral postsurgical d.
    upper small bowel motor d.
    visceral postsurgical d.
diuresis
    balanced salt solution volume d.
diuretic therapy
diurnal
    d. enuresis
    d. intraocular pressure measurement
divergent
    d. elbow dislocation
    d. ray projection
diversion
    biliopancreatic d.
    Camey enterocystoplasty urinary d.
    Duke pouch cutaneous urinary d.
    fecal d.
    Gil-Vernet ileocecal cystoplasty
      urinary d.
    ileal conduit urinary d.
    ileocolonic pouch urinary d.
    Indiana continent reservoir
      urinary d.
    Koch pouch cutaneous urinary d.
    Mainz pouch cutaneous urinary d.
    orthotopic urinary d.
    simple d.
    Studer reservoir urinary d.
    temporary fecal d.
diversionary ileostomy
diverticula (*pl. of* diverticulum)
diverticular
    d. disease
    d. hemorrhage
    d. hernia
diverticularization
diverticulation abnormality
diverticulectomy
    bladder d.
    endocavitary bladder d.
    esophageal d.
    Harrington esophageal d.
    d. of hypopharynx
    Meckel d.
    open d.
    pharyngoesophageal d.
    urethral d.
    vesical d.
    d. with myotomy
diverticulitis
    cecal d.
diverticulopexy

diverticulotomy
    stapling d.
diverticulum, pl. **diverticula**
    acquired d.
    caliceal d.
    cervical d.
    congenital d.
    distal esophageal d.
    esophageal d.
    false d.
    Meckel d.
    midesophageal traction d.
    pulsion d.
    traction d.
    true d.
    Zenker d.
    Zuckerkandl d.
diverting
    d. loop colostomy
    d. loop ileostomy
    d. proximal colostomy
    d. stoma
divided
    doubly ligated and d.
    d. respiration
divided-stoma colostomy
division
    anterior primary d.
    d. I–IV lesion
    intrahepatic vascular d.
    maturation d.
    posterior primary d.
    reduction d.
    vascular ring d.
divulse
divulsion
    digital d.
Dix-Hallpike maneuver
Dixon
    D. fat suppression method
    D. method opposed imaging
    D. technique
DKA
    diabetic ketoacidosis
DKS
    Damus-Kaye-Stansel
    DKS operation
    DKS procedure
D-loop transposition of great artery
DMFC
    demand minimum functional capacity
DNAP
    dynamic negative airway pressure
DNA ploidy abnormality
DO
    distal-occlusal
    DO cavity
dobutamine subtraction
  echocardiography (DSE)

Döderlein
- D. method
- D. roll-flap operation

Dodge area-length method

dog-ear repair

dog-leg fracture

Dohlman
- D. operation
- D. procedure

DOI
- depth of insertion

dolasetron

Dolenc technique

dolichocephalic head

dolichoectatic artery

dolichopellic pelvis

doll
- d. eye maneuver
- d. head maneuver
- d. head phenomenon
- D. trochanteric reattachment technique

dolorosa
- anesthesia d.

domain
- abdominal d.

D'ombrain operation

dome
- d. excursion
- d. fracture
- d. osteotomy

dome-shaped osteotomy

dominant
- d. component
- d. gland
- d. mass

domino
- d. procedure
- d. transplant

DOMS
- delayed onset muscle soreness

Donald-Fothergill operation

Donald procedure

donation
- autologous blood d.
- blood d.
- designated blood d.
- organ d.

Donders
- D. line
- D. pressure

- D. procedure
- space of D.

donor
- bacteremic d.
- cadaver d. (CAD)
- cadaveric d.
- CMV-positive d.
- cytomegalovirus-positive d.
- extended criteria d. (ECD)
- d. hepatectomy
- d. iliac Y graft
- d. kidney
- living-related d. (LRD)
- living relative d.
- non-heart-beating d. (NHBD)
- organ d.
- d. pancreatectomy
- subhuman primate d.
- d. tissue

donor-specific bone marrow augmentation

donut (*var. of* doughnut)

dopamine receptor

dopaminergic
- d. medication
- d. tract

Doppler
- D. auto-correlation technique
- D. color flow
- D. color flow imaging
- D. duplex ultrasonography
- endoscopic color D.
- D. flow probe examination
- D. interrogation
- D. method
- D. pressure gradient
- D. pulse evaluation
- D. signal
- D. study
- D. tissue imaging (DTI)
- transcranial D. (TCD)
- D. ultrasound
- D. ultrasound segmental blood pressure testing

dopplergram

Doppler-guided artery ligation hemorrhoidectomy

Dor
- D. anterior fundoplication
- D. fundoplication method
- D. fundoplication procedure
- D. fundoplication technique

NOTES

D

Dorello canal
Dormia noose
Dorrance procedure
dorsa (*pl. of* dorsum)
dorsabdominal
dorsal
    d. aspect
    d. branch
    d. closing wedge osteotomy
    d. column stimulation (DCS)
    d. column tractotomy
    d. cordotomy
    d. cord stimulation
    d. cross-finger flap
    d. digital artery
    d. elevated position
    d. enteric fistula
    d. excision
    d. expansion
    d. finger approach
    d. fissure
    d. horn
    d. induction
    d. inertia position
    d. intercalary segmental instability
    d. interosseous artery
    d. interosseous nerve
    d. linear incision
    d. lithotomy
    d. lithotomy position
    d. longitudinal incision
    d. lumbotomy incision
    d. midline approach
    d. pancreatic artery
    d. penis
    d. perilunate dislocation
    d. plate
    d. point
    d. proximal metatarsal osteotomy
    d. radius tubercle
    d. rami nerve
    d. recumbent position
    d. rhizotomy
    d. rigid position
    d. root
    d. root entry zone (DREZ)
    d. root entry zone lesion
    d. root entry zone procedure
    d. root ganglion
    d. root ganglionectomy
    d. rotation flap
    d. sacrococcygeal muscle
    d. scapular artery
    d. scapular nerve
    d. spine
    d. supine position
    d. surface
    d. sympathectomy
    d. synovectomy

    d. talonavicular bone
    d. tegmental decussation
    d. tenosynovectomy
    d. thoracic artery
    d. thyroid mobilization
    d. tissue
    d. translation
    d. transposition flap
    d. transscaphoid perilunar dislocation
    d. transverse capsulotomy
    d. transverse incision
    d. vein patch graft
    d. vertebra
    d. V osteotomy
    d. wire-loop fixation
dorsalis pedis (DP)
dorsalward approach
dorsiflexion of ankle
dorsiflexory wedge osteotomy
dorsiscapular
dorsispinal vein
dorsocephalad
dorsolateral
    d. approach
    d. incision
    d. and medial capsulotomy
    d. tract
dorsolumbar
dorsomedial
    d. approach
    d. incision
dorsopancreaticus
dorsoplantar
    d. approach
    d. projection
dorsoradial approach
dorsorostral approach
dorsosacral position
dorsoulnar approach
dorsoventrad
dorsum, pl. **dorsa**
dose
    defasciculating d.
    d. escalation
    fixed d.
    fixed subcutaneous d.
    physiologic d.
    preoperative d.
    priming d.
    subcutaneous d.
    subparalyzing d.
    tissue tolerance d.
dose-effect curve
dose-related effect
dose-response curve
dosing
    around-the-clock d.
    ATC d.

dot-and-blot hemorrhage
dot-blot
    d.-b. procedure
    d.-b. technique
dot hemorrhage
Dotter-Judkins technique
Dotter technique
Doubilet sphincterotomy
double
    d. adenomas
    d. antibody method
    d. aortic arch
    d. bubble sign
    d. chin
    d. decidual sac
    d. enterostomy
    d. exposure
    d. extra stimulus
    d. fracture
    d. freeze-stalk cryopexy
    d. freeze-thaw cryopexy
    d. graft
    d. halo sign
    d. incision
    d. jaw surgery
    d. lateral advancement flap
    d. Maddox rod test
    d. osteotomy
    d. pedicle TRAM flap
    d. pyloroplasty
    d. ring
    d. simultaneous stimulation
    d. stapling technique (DST)
    d. unilateral cysts
double-armed suture technique
double-balloon
    d.-b. technique
    d.-b. valvotomy
    d.-b. valvuloplasty
double-barrel
    d.-b. colostomy
    d.-b. ileostomy
double-burst
    d.-b. stimulation
    d.-b. transmission
double-button suture technique
double-contrast
    d.-c. barium enema examination
    d.-c. enema
    d.-c. visualization
double-density sign
double-doughnut approach

double-dummy technique
double-exposed rib
double-folded cup-patch technique
double-freeze technique
double-incision fasciotomy
double-inlet ventricle anomaly
double lateral advancement flap
double-loop
    d.-l. hernia
    d.-l. pouch
double-looped semitendinosus technique
double-lumen
    d.-l. endotracheal tube
    d.-l. intubation
double-lung transplant
double-needle chemonucleolysis
double-papilla pedicle graft
double-point threshold
double-puncture laparoscopy
double-rod
    d.-r. construct
    d.-r. technique
double-sealant technique
double-seton modified surgical approach
double-skin mastopexy
double-stapled
    d.-s. ileoanal reservoir method
    d.-s. ileoanal reservoir procedure
    d.-s. ileoanal reservoir technique
double-staple technique
double-stick technique
double-tube technique
double-umbrella closure
double-volume exchange transfusion
double-wire technique
double-wrap graciloplasty
doubly
    d. ligated
    d. ligated and divided
    d. sutured
doughnut, donut
    d. mastopexy
    d. ring
doughy
    d. abdomen
    d. mass
Douglas
    D. abscess
    D. bag collection method
    D. bag technique
    cul-de-sac of D.
    D. fold

D

NOTES

Douglas *(continued)*
    D. graft
    D. line
    D. pouch
    D. procedure
douloureux
    tic d.
dowel
    d. bone graft
    d. spinal fusion
    d. technique
doweling spondylolisthesis technique
Dow method
Downey-McGlamery procedure
downregulate
downstream
    d. sampling method
    d. signaling
    d. venous pressure
downward
    d. drainage
    d. retraction
Doyen vaginal hysterectomy
Doyle operation
DP
    distal pancreatectomy
    dorsalis pedis
DPL
    diagnostic peritoneal lavage
DR-70 tumor marker test
dragon worm infection
drain
    d. site evisceration
    transcystic d.
    d. volume
drainable ostomy pouch
drainage
    abdominal d.
    bile tract d.
    biliary d.
    bladder d.
    capillary d.
    catheter d.
    caval d.
    cerebral spinal fluid d.
    chest tube d. (CTD)
    circle loop biliary d.
    closed suction d.
    computed tomography-guided
      selective d.
    continuous catheter d.
    CT-guided selective d.
    dependent d.
    downward d.
    endoscopic biliary d.
    endoscopic nasobiliary catheter d.
    endoscopic pancreatic d.
    endoscopic transpapillary cyst d.
    endosonography-guided d.

enteric d.
external bile d.
external bile tract d.
external biliary d.
external ventricular d.
extrapetrosal d.
fluid d.
d. gastrostomy
hematoma d.
d. implant
incision and d. (I&D)
internal d.
kinetic venous d.
lymphatic d.
lymphocele d.
Molteno d.
nephrostomy d.
open d.
operative d.
d. pattern
pattern of d.
percutaneous abscess d. (PAD)
percutaneous catheter d.
percutaneous external d. (PED)
percutaneous transhepatic biliary d.
  (PTBD)
peripancreatic abdominal d.
peritoneal d.
portal d.
postoperative irrigation-suction d.
postural d.
pseudocyst d.
sclerotomy with d.
simple external d.
spinal fluid d.
stereotactic catheter d.
suction d.
systemic d.
thorascopic d.
tidal d.
transcystic d.
T-tube d.
venous d.
video thoracoscopic d.
Wangensteen d.
wound d.
draining abscess
drain-trap stomach
Drake tandem clipping technique
DRAM
    deepithelialized rectus abdominis muscle
    Distress Risk Assessment Method
    DRAM flap
draped
    prepped and d.
draping
    preparation and d.
drawer sign
draw-over vaporizer

dressing
island wound d.
d. therapy
wound d.
DREZ
dorsal root entry zone
DREZ lesion
DREZ modification of Eriksson technique
DREZ procedure
DREZ surgery
DRFS
distant recurrence-free survival
drilling technique
drip
d. infusion
d. infusion cholangiography
intravenous d.
d. transfusion
Dripps-American Surgical Association score
Dripps classification
drip-tube feeding
drive
exploratory d.
hypercapnic d.
driven
d. equilibrium Fourier transform (DEFT)
d. equilibrium Fourier transform technique
drop
flow-dependent pressure d.
d. metastasis
droplet infection
drop-lock ring
drug
d. administration
gastroprotective d.
d. infusion
nonsteroidal antiinflammatory d. (NSAID)
d. resistance
second-line d.
d. synergy
drum membrane
Drummond
D. spinous wiring technique
D. wire technique
Drummond-Morison operation
drunken sailor effect
drusen

dry
d. abscess
d. amputation
d. colostomy
d. field technique
d. gangrene
d. heat oven sterilization
d. hernia
d. mucous membrane
d. needling
DSE
digital subtraction echocardiography
dobutamine subtraction echocardiography
DSRS
distal splenorenal shunt
DST
double stapling technique
DSVNI
Distress Scale for Ventilated Newborn Infants
DTI
Doppler tissue imaging
3D transesophageal echocardiography
dual
d. compression scoliosis treatment
d. impression technique
d. onlay cortical bone graft
d. percutaneous endoscopic gastrostomy
d. therapy
dual-delivery platform
dual-temperature cardiopulmonary bypass
Duane
D. anomaly
D. classification
Duane-Hunt relation
Dubin-Amelar varicocele classification
Dubowitz
D. evaluation
D. examination
Duckett procedure
duct
aberrant bile d.
accessory pancreatic d.
anomalous junction of pancreatobiliary d. (AJPBD)
Arantius d.
Bartholin d.
Bernard d.
bile d.
biliary d.

D

NOTES

duct (*continued*)
Blasius d.
bucconeural d.
canalicular d.
d. cell adenocarcinoma
cochlear d.
collecting d.
common bile d. (CBD)
common hepatic d.
craniopharyngeal d.
cystic d.
deferent d.
distal bile d.
d. ectasia
efferent d.
ejaculatory d.
endolymphatic d.
excretory d.
extrahepatic bile d.
frontonasal d.
galactophorous d.
gall d.
Gartner d.
genital d.
hemithoracic d.
Hensen d.
hepatic d.
hepatocystic d.
Hoffmann d.
hypophysial d.
incisive d.
inferior lacrimal d.
d. injury
intrahepatic bile d.
jugular d.
lactiferous d.
d. of Luschka
lymphatic d.
main pancreatic d. (MPD)
mamillary d.
mammary d.
mesonephric d.
metanephric d.
milk d.
minor sublingual d.
Müller d.
nasofrontal d.
pancreatic d.
papillary d.
paramesonephric d.
paraurethral d.
parotid d.
Pecquet d.
perilymphatic d.
periotic d.
pronephric d.
prostatic d.
right lymphatic d.
Rivinus d.

salivary d.
Santorini d.
Schüller d.
secretory d.
segmental d.
semicircular d.
seminal d.
spermatic d.
Stensen d.
d. stone
striated d.
subclavian d.
sublingual d.
submandibular d.
submaxillary d.
sudoriferous d.
superior lacrimal d.
sweat d.
d. system
testicular d.
thoracic d.
thymic d.
thyroglossal d.
thyrolingual d.
uniting d.
utriculosaccular d.
d. wall
Walther d.
Wharton d.
Wirsung d.
wolffian d.

ductal
d. adenoma
d. calculus
d. cancer
d. cannulation
d. carcinoma
d. carcinoma in situ (DCIS)
d. cystadenoma
d. dilatation
d. dilation
d. ectasia
d. hyperplasia
d. obstruction
d. proliferation
d. system
d. system perforation

ductal-dependent
d.-d. lesion
d.-d. pulmonary circulation

ductectasia
ductectatic mucinous cystadenoma
ductless gland
ductography
ductopenic rejection
ductoscopy
duct-to-duct (D-D)
d.-t.-d. anastomosis

duct-to-mucosa
> d.-t.-m. anastomosis
> d.-t.-m. pancreaticojejunostomy
> d.-t.-m. technique

ductule
> aberrant d.
> biliary d.
> efferent d.
> inferior aberrant d.
> interlobular d.
> prostatic d.
> superior aberrant d.
> transected d.

ductulus, pl. **ductuli**
ductus arteriosus
Duddell membrane
Dufourmentel technique
Duhamel
> D. colon operation
> D. laparoscopic pull-through
> D. procedure

Dührssen
> D. incision
> D. vaginofixation

Duke
> D. bleeding time
> D. pouch cutaneous urinary
>   diversion

Duke-Elder operation
Dukes
> D. classification
> D. classification of carcinoma
> D. procedure
> D. stage

dumbbell
> d. mass
> d. tumor

dumping
> d. stomach
> d. syndrome

Duncan-Lovell modification
Duncan position
dunk
dunked
dunking technique
Dunn
> D. biopsy
> D. osteotomy
> D. technique

Dunn-Brittain foot stabilization
  technique
Dunnett test

Dunn-Hess trochanteric osteotomy
Dunnington operation
duodenal
> d. adenocarcinoma
> d. adenoma
> d. ampulla
> d. bulb
> d. bulb deformity
> d. cap
> d. compression
> d. content examination
> d. duplication
> d. endoscopic polypectomy
> d. fistula
> d. flap
> d. fluid collection
> d. foreign body
> d. fossa
> d. gland
> d. hematoma
> d. hernia
> d. ileus
> d. impression
> d. loop
> d. mass
> d. metastasis
> d. migrating activity
> d. perforation
> d. recess
> d. scarring
> d. seromyectomy
> d. sphincter
> d. stump
> d. stump leak
> d. switch
> d. tumor
> d. ulcer
> d. ulceration
> d. web

duodenectomy
duodenobiliary pressure gradient
duodenocaval fistula
duodenocholecystostomy
duodenocholedochotomy
duodenocolic fistula
duodenocystostomy
duodenoduodenostomy
duodenoenterocutaneous fistula
duodenoenterostomy
duodenogastroscopy
> retrograde d.

duodenoileostomy ileoileostomy

D

NOTES

duodenojejunal
- d. angle
- d. flexure
- d. fold
- d. fossa
- d. hernia
- d. junction
- d. motor recording
- d. recess
- d. sphincter

duodenojejunostomy
- suprapapillary Roux-en-Y d.

duodenolysis

duodenomesocolic fold

duodenopyloric constriction

duodenorenal ligament

duodenorrhaphy

duodenoscopy

duodenostomy
- Witzel d.

duodenotomy
- transverse d.

duodenum

Duplay I, II technique

duplex-guided compression

duplex ultrasonography

duplication
- alimentary tract d.
- d. anomaly
- complete d.
- congenital d.
- cranial d.
- d. cyst
- duodenal d.
- esophageal d.
- fetal d.
- gallbladder d.
- gastric d.
- incomplete d.
- Marks-Bayne technique for thumb d.
- partial d.
- renal d.
- symmetric thumb d.
- thumb d.
- trunk d.
- tubular colonic d.
- ureteral d.
- Wassel thumb d.

Dupuy-Dutemps
- D.-D. dacryocystorhinostomy dye test
- D.-D. dacryostomy
- D.-D. operation

Dupuytren
- D. canal
- D. contracture
- D. fracture
- D. suture technique

dural
- d. arteriovenous fistula
- d. arteriovenous malformation
- d. cavernous sinus fistula
- d. ectasia
- d. incision
- d. nerve root
- d. patch reconstruction
- d. puncture
- d. rent
- d. repair
- d. ring
- d. shunt syndrome
- d. venous sinus

dura mater

Duran approach

duraplasty

duration
- d. tetany
- d. time

Duret
- D. hemorrhage
- D. lesion

Durham
- D. flatfoot operation
- D. plasty

Durkan carpal compression test

Durr
- D. nonpenetrating keratoplasty
- D. operation

dusky stoma

dust-borne infection

Dutcher body

duToit-Roux
- d.-R. arthroplasty
- d.-R. staple capsulorrhaphy

Duval
- D. pancreaticojejunostomy
- D. procedure

Duverger-Velter operation

Duverney
- D. fissure
- D. fracture
- D. gland
- D. muscle

DuVries
- D. approach
- D. deltoid ligament reconstruction technique
- D. hammertoe repair
- D. incision
- D. plantar condylectomy

DuVries-Mann modified bunionectomy

DVT
- deep venous thrombosis
- concurrent DVT
- DVT prevention
- DVT prophylaxis

dwarf pelvis

Dwyer
    D. clawfoot operation
    D. incision
    D. osteotomy
    D. procedure
Dyban technique
dye
    d. dilution method
    d. dilution technique
    d. exclusion test
    d. injection
    2-d. method
    d. reduction spot test
    d. scattering method
    d. sham intrarenal lesion
    d. worker's carcinoma
dyed starch method
dynamic
    d. bolus tracking technique
    d. cardiomyoplasty
    d. closure pressure
    d. compliance
    d. compression
    d. compression plate fixation
    d. condylar screw fixation
    d. cystourethroscopy
    d. end-tidal forcing
    d. fluorescence video endoscopy
    d. graciloplasty
    d. image
    d. lumbar stabilization
    d. negative airway pressure
      (DNAP)
    d. relation
    d. relaxation
    d. repair
    d. storage allocation
    d. traction method
dynamometry
    isometric force d.
dysarthric lesion
dysautonomia
    familial d.
dyscrasic fracture
dysesthesia
    burning d.
    denervation d.
dysesthetic pain
dysfunction
    bone marrow d.
    chronic obstructive pulmonary d.
    cognitive d.

    ejaculatory d.
    end-organ d.
    endothelial cell d.
    erectile d. (ED)
    esophageal body motor d.
    extensor mechanism d.
    gastrointestinal tract d.
    hepatic d.
    hepatocellular synthetic d.
    late graft d.
    multiorgan system d.
    multiple organ d. (MOD)
    myofascial d.
    neuromotor d.
    obstructive pulmonary d.
    organ d.
    pancreatitis d.
    pelvic floor d.
    postanesthetic central nervous
      system d.
    postgastrectomy d.
    postoperative cognitive d. (POCD)
    postoperative gastrointestinal tract d.
      (PGID)
    postoperative renal d.
    proximal myofascial d.
    pulmonary d.
    renal d.
    sphincter of Oddi d.
    superoxide-mediated endothelial
      cell d.
    vocal d.
dysgenesis
dysgnathic anomaly
dyskinesia
    extrapyramidal d.
    levodopa-induced d.
    retrolisthesis positional d.
dysmenorrheal membrane
dysmotility
    esophageal d.
dysmyelination
dysosteogenesis
dysostosis
dyspepsia
    flatulent d.
    postcholecystectomy flatulent d.
dysphagia
    benign d.
    contractile ring d.
    postoperative d.

D

NOTES

213

dysphagia *(continued)*
>   postvagotomy d.
>   recurrent d.

dysphasia
>   expressive d.

dysphoric mood state

dyspigmentation

dysplasia
>   asphyxiating thoracic d.
>   bronchopulmonary d. (BPD)
>   cortical d.
>   d. dislocation
>   fibromuscular d. (FMD)
>   focal cortical d.
>   high-grade d. (HGD)
>   low-grade d.
>   oculoauriculovertebral d.

dysplasia-associated
>   d.-a. lesion
>   d.-a. mass

dysplastic epithelium

dyspnea
>   exertional d.
>   expiratory d.
>   1-flight exertional d.
>   2-flight exertional d.
>   d. on exertion

dysraphic malformation

dysraphism
>   occult spinal d.

dysreflexia
>   autonomic d.

dysregulation
>   autonomic d.
>   microcirculatory d.

dysrhythmia
>   supraventricular d.
>   ventricular d.

dysrhythmogenicity

dystonia
>   cervical d.
>   muscle d.
>   posttraumatic cervical d.

dystonic
>   d. pain
>   d. tic

dystrophic nail

dystrophy
>   Becker muscular d.
>   corneal d.
>   Emery-Dreifuss muscular d.
>   facioscapulohumeral muscular d.
>   muscular d. (MD)
>   myotonic d.
>   oculopharyngeal muscular d.
>   reflex sympathetic d. (RSD)

dysuria

dysuric

EA
    epidural anesthesia
EAE
    external auditory exostosis
Eagle-Barrett syndrome
Eagle syndrome
Eagleton operation
ear
    e. anesthesia
    e. bone
    e. canal
    e. cartilage inflammation
    external e.
    surfer's e.
earlobe adipose tissue
early
    e. active treatment
    e. cancer lesion
    e. enteral feeding
    e. extubation
    e. gastric cancer
    e. graft thrombosis
    e. infection rate
    e. oversewing
    e. postoperative period
    e. supraclavicular compression
    e. thoracoscopic repair
    e. thrombectomy
    e. unequivocal shock
early-onset graft-versus-host disease
easily reducible hernia
EAST
    elevated arm stress test
**Eastern Cooperative Oncology Group
    (ECOG)**
Eastwood technique
Eaton
    E. closed reduction
    E. implant arthroplasty
    E. volar plate arthroplasty
Eaton-Littler
    E.-L. ligament reconstruction
    E.-L. technique
Eaton-Malerich
    E.-M. fracture-dislocation operation
    E.-M. fracture-dislocation technique
    E.-M. reduction
Ebbehoj procedure
Eberle contracture release technique
EBM
    evidence-based medicine
Ebner
    imbrication line of von E.
    E. line
    E. reticulum

ebonation
EBP
    epidural blood patch
ébranlement
Ebstein
    E. cardiac anomaly
    E. malformation
eburnation
EBV
    Epstein-Barr virus
    EBV infection
ECA
    external carotid artery
ECA-PCA bypass surgery
ECBP
    extracorporeal bypass pump
ECC
    endocervical curettage
    extracorporeal circulation
ECCE
    extracapsular cataract extraction
eccentric
    e. exercise
    e. fixation
    e. hypertrophy
    e. interocclusal record
    e. jaw position
    e. jaw relation
    e. ledge
    e. maxillomandibular record
    e. narrowing
    e. occlusion
eccentricity index
ecchondrosis
ecchymosed
ecchymosis, pl. **ecchymoses**
ecchymotic
    e. mark
    e. mask
eccrine
    e. carcinoma
    e. sweat gland
ECD
    extended criteria donor
ECF-A
    eosinophilic chemotactic factor of
    anaphylaxis
ECFV
    extracellular fluid volume
ECG signal-averaging technique
echinococcal
    e. cyst disease
    e. liver abscess
    e. liver cyst
echinococcotomy

E

echinococcus cyst
echo
    e. formation
    e. imaging
    inconsequential e.
    magnitude preparation-rapid
      acquisition gradient e. (MP-
      RAGE)
    e. rephasing
    e. reverberation
    e. score
    e. sign
    e. texture
    e. zone
echocardiogram
    intraoperative multiplane
      transesophageal e.
echocardiographic assessment
echocardiography
    digital subtraction e. (DSE)
    dobutamine subtraction e. (DSE)
    3D transesophageal e.
    3D transesophageal e.
    transesophageal e. (TEE)
    transesophageal color Doppler e.
    transthoracic e.
echodense
    e. mass
    e. structure
echodensity
echoduodenoscopy
echo-free space
echogenic
    e. liver
    e. plaque
    e. tissue
echographic layer
echolucency
echolucent plaque
echopenic liver metastasis
echoplanar magnetic resonance imaging
echo-poor layer
echovirus infection
Ecker fissure
Ecker-Lotke-Glazer
    E.-L.-G. patellar tendon repair
    E.-L.-G. tendon reconstruction
      technique
Eckert-Davis classification
Eck fistula
Eckhout vertical gastroplasty
eclipse
    e. amblyopia
    e. phase
ECLS
    extracorporeal life support
ECMO
    extracorporeal membrane oxygenation

ECOG
    Eastern Cooperative Oncology Group
ECoG
    electrocorticography
      ECoG monitoring
      ECoG performance status scale
Economo disease
ECOR
    extracorporeal CO_2 removal
ECPL
    endocavitary pelvic lymphadenectomy
ECRB
    extensor carpi radialis brevis
ECRL
    extensor carpi radialis longus
ECS
    elective cosmetic surgery
    electrocerebral silence
ECST
    European Carotid Surgery Trial
ectal origin
ectasia
    alveolar e.
    aortoannular e.
    artery e.
    corneal e.
    coronary artery e.
    distal e.
    duct e.
    ductal e.
    dural e.
    gastric antral vascular e. (GAVE)
    iris e.
    mammary duct e.
    papillary e.
    scleral e.
    senile e.
    vascular e.
ectasis
ectatic
    e. aneurysm
    e. bronchus
    e. carotid artery
    e. dilation
    e. emphysema
    e. vascular lesion
    e. vessel
ectocolostomy
ectoderm
ectodermal
ectopia
    cerebellar e.
    gallbladder e.
    macular e.
    renal e.
    testicular e.
    ureteral e.
ectopic
    e. ACTH syndrome

e. anus
e. atrial tachycardia
e. bone
e. craniopharyngioma
e. cutaneous schistosomiasis
e. endometrial tissue
e. eruption
e. eyelash
e. focus
e. gastric mucosa
e. hyperparathyroidism
e. impulse
e. kidney
e. pancreas
e. parathormone production
e. parathyroid adenoma
e. pregnancy
e. rhythm
e. sebaceous gland
e. spleen
e. ureter
e. ureterocele
e. varix

ectoscopy
ectosteal
ectostosis
ectothrix infection
ECTR
endoscopic carpal tunnel release
ectropion
ECU
extensor carpi ulnaris
eczematoid pruritic plaque
eczematous
e. lesion
e. patch
e. polymorphous light eruption
e. reaction
ED
erectile dysfunction
EDA
end-diastolic cross-sectional area
EDD
end-diastolic diameter
Edebohls
E. incision
E. position
edema
antral e.
brain e.
bullous e.
cardiac e.

cerebral e.
corneal e.
endothelial cell e.
hemorrhagic e.
ileocecal e.
laryngeal e.
lower extremity e.
lymphatic e.
massive pulmonary hemorrhagic e.
nephrotic e.
neurogenic pulmonary e. (NPE)
pericholecystic e.
peripheral extremity e.
pulmonary e.
reexpansion pulmonary e. (REPE)
retroarytenoidal e.
stasis e.
subglottic e.
supraglottic e.
transient e.
unilateral supraglottic e.
visceral e.

edematous
e. bowel
e. bowel wall
e. mesentery
Eden-Hybbinette
E.-H. arthroplasty
E.-H. procedure
Eden-Lange procedure
Eden-Lawson hysterectomy
edentulous space
Eder-Puestow dilation
edge
anastomotic e.
chondral e.
inferior e.
lateral e.
shelving e.
spectral e.
superior e.
edge-detection method
edge-to-edge suture technique
Edinburgh 2 Coma Scale
Edinger-Westphal nucleus
Edlan-Mejchar operation
Edmondson grading system for hepatocellular carcinoma
Edmondson-Steiner classification
Edmonton
E. Staging System for Cancer Pain
E. Symptom Assessment Schedule

E

NOTES

EDR
>   extreme drug resistance

EDT
>   emergency department thoracotomy

education
>>   Accreditation Council for Graduate Medical E. (ACGME)

Edwards
>>   E. procedure
>>   E. septectomy

Edwards-Tapp arterial graft

EEG
>   electroencephalography

EELV
>   end-expiratory lung volume

effect
>>   adverse e.
>>   amnestic e.
>>   analgesic e.
>>   anorexigenic e.
>>   antiangiogenic e.
>>   anticoagulant e.
>>   Bernoulli e.
>>   biological e.
>>   Bohr e.
>>   cardioprotective e.
>>   cardiotoxic e.
>>   cardiovascular adverse e.
>>   chemoradiotherapy e.
>>   dose-related e.
>>   drunken sailor e.
>>   esophageal e.
>>   Hawthorne e.
>>   hypnotic e.
>>   hypothermic e.
>>   immunomodulating e.
>>   motilin e.
>>   negative e.
>>   oxygen e.
>>   e. parameter
>>   pulmonary e.
>>   reverse steal e.
>>   second gas e.
>>   sedative e.
>>   stimulating e.
>>   synergistic e.
>>   therapeutic e.

effective
>>   e. function
>>   e. renal blood flow
>>   e. renal plasma flow
>>   e. setting expansion

effector
>>   e. operation
>>   e. organ
>>   e. pathway

efferens, efferentia

efferent
>>   e. duct
>>   e. ductule
>>   e. glomerular arteriole
>>   e. limb
>>   e. loop
>>   e. nerve activity
>>   PGA e.
>>   PJA e.
>>   e. vasodilation

efferentia

efficacy
>>   therapeutic e.

Effler-Groves
>>   E.-G. mode
>>   E.-G. mode of Allison procedure

Effler hiatal hernia repair

effluent
>>   clear e.

effort thrombosis

effusion
>>   chylous e.
>>   exudative pleural e.
>>   pleural e.
>>   subdural e.

Efron jackknife classification

Eftekhar broken femoral stem technique

EG/BUS
>>   external genitalia, Bartholin, urethral, and Skene

EGD
>>   esophagogastroduodenoscopy

EGF
>>   epidermal growth factor
>>   salivary EGF
>>   serum EGF
>>   urinary EGF

egg
>>   e. activation
>>   e. membrane

Egger line

Eggers
>>   E. neurectomy
>>   E. tendon transfer technique

Eggleston method

egg-shell nail

Eglis gland

EHL
>>   electrohydraulic lithotripsy
>>   extensor hallucis longus

EHPO
>>   extrahepatic portal vein obstruction

Ehrenritter ganglion

Ehrlich inner body

Ehrlich-Türck line

EIC
>>   extensive intraductal component

Eicken method

eighth cranial nerve

EIS
>>   endoscopic injection sclerotherapy

Eisenberger technique
ejaculation disorder
ejaculatorius
ejaculatory
    e. duct
    e. dysfunction
ejection
    e. murmur
    e. phase
    e. phase index
    e. rate
    e. shell image
    e. time
ejection-fraction image
Ejrup maneuver
Ekehorn
    E. operation
    E. rectopexy
Eklund technique
elastance
    airway e.
elastic
    e. band fixation
    e. band ligation
    e. barrier
    e. compression
    e. fiber fragmentation
    e. lamella
    e. recoil
    e. recoil pressure
    e. tissue
elastofibroma
elastolysis
    generalized e.
Elaut triangle
elbow
    e. approach
    e. arthroplasty
    e. disarticulation
    e. dislocation
    e. extensor tendon
    e. fracture
elective
    e. aneurysmectomy
    e. cerclage
    e. cosmetic surgery (ECS)
    e. dilatational tracheostomy
    e. hernia repair
    e. herniorrhaphy
    e. laparotomy
    e. lymphadenectomy

    e. lymph node dissection (ELND)
    e. neck dissection
    e. sigmoid resection
    e. surgery
    e. surgical procedure
electric
    e. anesthesia
    e. aversion therapy
    e. coagulation
    e. differential therapy
    e. induction
    e. stimulation
electrical
    e. activation abnormality
    e. catheter ablation
    e. fulguration
    e. heart position
    e. nerve stimulation
    e. stimulation therapy
    e. stimulator waveform
    e. surface stimulation
electro-acupoint stimulation
electroacupuncture
electroanalgesia
electroanesthesia
electrobioscopy
electrocardiogram
electrocardiography
electrocauterization
electrocautery
    bipolar e.
    bleeding controlled with e.
    hook e.
    low-current e.
    monopolar e.
    multipolar e.
    needlepoint e.
    e. resection
electrocerebral silence (ECS)
electrocholecystectomy
electrocoagulation
    bipolar e.
    e. diathermy
    direct current e.
    endoscopic e.
    monopolar e.
    multipolar e.
    e. necrosis
    pinpoint e.
    snare e.
    transendoscopic e.

E

NOTES

electroconvulsive therapy
electrocorticography (ECoG)
    awake intraoperative e.
electrode
    depth e.
    3-dimensional grid e.
    grid e.
    e. impedance
    e. migration
    e. placement
    e. potential
    e. response time
    surface e.
electrodesiccated bleeding point
electrodesiccation
electrode-skin interface
electrodiaphake
electrodispersive skin patch
electroejaculation
    rectal probe e.
electroencephalography (EEG)
electroepilation
electroexcision
electrofulguration
electrogalvanic stimulation
electrogastroenterostomy
electrogenesis
electrohemostasis
electrohydraulic
    e. fragmentation
    e. lithotripsy (EHL)
    e. shockwave lithotripsy (ESWL)
electrolaryngogram
electrolysis
    Faraday law of e.
electrolyte
    e. abnormality
    e. flush solution
    e. imbalance
    e. imbalance coma
electrolytic solution
electromagnetic
    e. field
    e. interference (EMI)
    e. radiation exposure
    e. signal
    e. system
    e. tracking
electromagnetic field
electromechanical dissociation
electromyocardial dissociation
electromyographic study
electromyography
    laryngeal e.
electronarcosis
electroneurolysis
electronic
    e. bone stimulation
    e. magnification

electron microscopy
electroparacentesis
electrophoresis
    hemoglobin e.
electrophrenic respiration
electrophysiologic
    e. function
    e. monitoring
electrophysiological stimulation
electrophysiology
    flickering blockade e.
    patch clamp e.
    e. study
electropuncture
electroresection
electroscission
electrosection
electrosterilization
    root canal e.
electrosurgery unit (ESU)
electrosurgical
    e. desiccation
    e. fulguration
    e. snare polypectomy
electrotherapeutic sleep therapy
electrotherm
electrotomy
element
    glandular e.
elementary
    e. fracture
    e. lesion
elephant trunk technique
elevated
    e. arm stress test (EAST)
    e. hemidiaphragm
    e. lesion
elevation
    e. angle
    blanched cutaneous e.
    chin e.
    congenital scapular e.
    diaphragmatic e.
    e. of extremity
    flap e.
    e. paresis
    periosteal e.
    scapular e.
    ST segment e.
    unilateral diaphragmatic e.
elevator
    e. disease
    e. esophagus
    e. extraction
    femoral e.
    e. muscle
elevatus deformity
eleventh
    e. cranial nerve

e. rib flank incision
e. rib transperitoneal incision
elimination
carbon dioxide e. ($VECO_2$)
e. clearance
CO_2 e.
e. curve
e. disorder
e. half-life
nonpulmonary route of e. (NPE)
e. pocket
e. procedure
e. reaction
Elizabethtown osteotomy
Elliot
E. operation
E. position
ellipsoid
e. joint
e. method
ellipsoidal joint
elliptical
e. anastomosis
e. biopsy
e. excision technique
e. recess
e. uterine incision
elliptocytosis
Ellis
E. classification
E. skin traction technique
Ellis-Jones peroneal tendon technique
Ellison
E. lateral knee reconstruction
E. technique
Elmslie procedure
Elmslie-Trillat
E.-T. patellar procedure
E.-T. patellar realignment method
ELND
elective lymph node dissection
Eloesser flap
Elsberg incision
Elschnig
E. blepharorrhaphy
E. body
E. canthorrhaphy
E. canthorrhaphy operation
E. central iridectomy
E. keratoplasty
Ely operation
embedded toenail

embolectomy
arterial e.
balloon e.
catheter e.
direct e.
femoral e.
pulmonary e.
emboli (*pl. of* embolus)
embolic gangrene
emboliform
embolism (*See also* embolus)
air e.
amniotic fluid e.
atheroma e.
autologous blood clot pulmonary e.
catheter e.
gas e.
paradoxical e.
pulmonary e. (PE)
transfusion-related air e.
tumor e.
venous air e. (VAE)
embolization
accelerated arteriolar gas e.
angiographic e.
arterial e.
hepatic artery e. (HAE)
pulmonary e.
renal arterial e.
selective arterial e.
subselective e.
superselective microcoil e.
venous e.
embolotherapy
embolus, pl. **emboli** (*See also* embolism)
air e.
fatal air e.
hemodynamically significant air e.
e. migration
paradoxical e.
embouchement
embrasure space
embryectomy
embryo
e. biopsy
e. encapsulation
e. reduction
embryonal
e. cell carcinoma
e. sarcoma
e. tumor

E

NOTES

embryonic
    e. fixation syndrome
    e. neural tube
    e. sac
embryotomy
emedullate
emergence
    e. agitation
    anesthetic e.
    e. delirium
    metachronous e.
    synchronous e.
emergency
    access e.
    e. airway management
    e. appendectomy
    e. colonoscopy
    e. department resuscitation
    e. department thoracotomy (EDT)
    e. indication
    e. laparotomy
    e. medicine
    e. operation
    e. procedure
    e. room (ER)
    e. room thoracotomy
    e. SSPCS
    e. surgery
    surgical e.
    e. tracheal intubation
    e. tracheostomy
    e. ventilation
emergent
    e. appendectomy
    e. cerclage
    e. endoscopic sclerotherapy
    e. herniorrhaphy
    e. intubation
    e. operation
    e. surgery
Emery-Dreifuss muscular dystrophy
emesis
    coffee-ground e.
EMI
    electromagnetic interference
    EMI scan
eminence
    arcuate e.
    cruciate e.
    cruciform e.
    deltoid e.
    frontal e.
    genital e.
    hypothenar e.
    ileocecal e.
    iliopectineal e.
    iliopubic e.
    intercondylar e.
    intertubercular e.

    orbital e.
    parietal e.
    pyramidal e.
    thenar e.
    thyroid e.
eminentia, pl. eminentiae
emissarium
emissary
    e. sphenoidal foramen
    e. vein
emission
    gas e.
    e. line
EMLA
    eutectic mixture of local anesthetics
    EMLA anesthetic
Emmet
    E. operation
    E. suture technique
Emmon osteotomy
EMMV
    extended mandatory minute ventilation
Emory Pain Estimate Model (EPEM)
emphysema
    colonoscopy-related e.
    ectatic e.
    endoscopy-related e.
    nonbullous e.
    subcutaneous e.
    subgaleal e.
    surgical e.
emphysematous
    e. cholecystitis
    e. gangrene
emprosthotonos position
empty
    e. gestational sac
    e. sella
emptying
    delayed gastric e.
    gastric e.
empyema
    bilious e.
    parapneumonic e.
    postpneumonectomy tuberculous e.
    tuberculous e.
empyemic
EMR
    endoscopic mucosal resection
en
    e. bloc
    e. bloc dissection
    e. bloc distal pancreatectomy
    e. bloc excision
    e. bloc lymphadenopathy
    e. bloc, no-touch technique
    e. bloc removal
    e. bloc vein resection
    e. face position

enamel
> e. crypt
> e. excrescence
> e. fracture
> e. knot
> e. membrane
> e. projection
> e. rod inclination
> e. sac

enameloplasty
enantiomer
enarthrodial joint
enarthrosis
encapsulated
> e. brain abscess
> e. breast implant

encapsulation
> embryo e.
> peritoneal e.
> tumor e.

encasement
encatarrhaphy
encephalemia
encephali
encephalitis
encephalization
encephalocele
encephaloid gastric carcinoma
encephaloma
encephalomeningocele
encephalomyelitis
> experimental allergic e.

encephalomyelocele
encephalopathy
> clinical e.
> degenerative e.
> hepatic e.
> ischemic e.
> portal-systemic e. (PSE)
> progressive e.
> refractory e.
> traumatic progressive e.

encephaloscopy
encephalotomy
enchondral
enchondroma of bone
enchondrosarcoma
encircling
> e. cryoablation
> e. endocardial ventriculotomy
> e. explant

encroachment

encrustation
> bile e.

encu method
encysted
> e. calculus
> e. hernia
> e. intraabdominal collection

end
> blind e.
> e. colostomy
> cut e.
> e. exhalation
> e. expiration
> e. expiratory
> e. ileostomy
> e. inspiration
> e. point
> proximal e.
> stapled blind e.
> e. stoma
> e. stoma closure
> e. tube
> upper e.

endarterectomy
endarterectomy
> blunt eversion carotid e.
> carotid e. (CEA)
> conventional e.
> coronary e.
> eversion carotid e.
> femoral e.
> gas e.
> open e.
> surgical e.

endaural mastoid incision
end-diastolic
> e.-d. cross-sectional area (EDA)
> e.-d. diameter (EDD)
> e.-d. left ventricular pressure

endemic fungal infection
Ender femoral fracture technique
end-expiratory
> e.-e. intragastric pressure
> e.-e. lung volume (EELV)
> e.-e. phase

endgut
end-hole catheter
end-inspiratory volume
Endius approach
endless-loop tachycardia
end-loop
> e.-l. colostomy

E

NOTES

end-loop (*continued*)
    e.-l. ileocolostomy
    e.-l. ileostomy
    e.-l. stoma
endoabdominal fascia
endoalveolar crest
endoanal
    e. anastomosis
    e. mucosectomy
    e. ultrasonography
endoaneurysmoplasty
endoaneurysmorrhaphy
    ventricular e.
endoauscultation
endobrachyesophagus
endobronchial
    e. brachytherapy
    e. cancer
    e. fistula
    e. intubation
    e. intubation anesthetic technique
    e. tree
    e. tuberculosis
endocapsular
endocardiac
endocardial
    e. flow
    e. mapping
    e. murmur
    e. resection
    e. stain
    e. thickening
endocarditic
endocarditis
    prosthetic valve e. (PVE)
endocardium
endocavitary
    e. bladder diverticulectomy
    e. pelvic lymphadenectomy (ECPL)
    e. radiation therapy
endoceliac
endocervical
    e. canal
    e. curettage (ECC)
    e. mucosa
    e. polyp
    e. sampling
endocervix
endochondral bone
endocolitis
endocolpitis
endocranial
endocranium
endocrine
    e. adenomatosis
    e. disorder
    e. fracture
    e. gland
    e. imaging

    e. pancreas
    e. screening
    e. surgeon
    e. surgery
    e. toxicity
    e. tumor
endocrinology
endocrinopathy
    multiple e.
endocryopexy
endocryoretinopexy
endocyst
endocytosis
endodermal sinus
endodiathermy
endodontia
endodontic
    e. armamentarium
    e. cavity
    e. irrigation
    e. surgery
    e. technique
endodontics
    pedodontic e.
    1-sitting e.
    surgical e.
endodontist
endodontium
endodontologist
endodontology
endofaradism
endofluoroscopic technique
endofluoroscopy
    flexible e.
    percutaneous e.
    rigid e.
endogalvanism
endogastric
endogenous
    e. algogenic agent
    e. aneurysm
    e. A-V fistula
    e. disease
    e. event-related potential
    e. fiber
    e. flora
    e. infection
    e. lipid pneumonia
    e. opiate receptor
    e. opioid
    e. opioid peptide
    e. opioid system
    e. protection
    e. pyrogen
    e. smile
    e. steroid
    e. uveitis
endoglobar
endoherniotomy

endoillumination
endolacrimal procedure
endolaryngeal
endoleak
> proximal e.
> retrograde collateral e.

endoligature
endolith
endoluminal
> e. excision
> e. repair
> e. stenting
> e. technology
> e. therapy

endolymph
endolymphatic
> e. cavity
> e. duct
> e. fluid
> e. hydrops
> e. sac
> e. space

endolymphaticus
endolymphic
endometria (*pl. of* endometrium)
endometrial
> e. ablation
> e. adenocarcinoma
> e. atrophy
> e. biopsy
> e. cancer
> e. carcinoma
> e. cavity
> e. chemical shift imaging
> e. curettage
> e. cytology
> e. island
> e. jet washing
> e. morphology
> e. polyp
> e. receptor
> e. resection
> e. sampling
> e. shedding
> e. spiral artery
> e. thickness
> e. tuberculosis

endometric epithelium
endometrioid
endometrioma
endometriosis
endometriotic focus

endometritis
endometrium, pl. **endometria**
endometropic
endomyocardial
> e. biopsy
> e. disease

endonasal disorder
endoneurium
endoneurolysis
endo-osseous (*var. of* endosseous)
endopelvic fascia
endophotocoagulation
> argon laser e.

endophytic
endoplasmic reticulum
endoprosthesis, pl. **endoprostheses**
endopyelotomy
endopyeloureterotomy
> percutaneous e.

endorectal
> e. coil magnetic resonance imaging
> e. flap
> e. ileal pouch
> e. ileal pull-through
> e. ileoanal pull-through
> e. ileoanal pull-through method
> e. ileoanal pull-through procedure
> e. ileoanal pull-through technique

end-organ
> e.-o. damage
> e.-o. dysfunction
> e.-o. failure

endoribonuclease
endorrhachis
endoscope-assisted technique
endoscope-body position relationship
endoscope impaction
endoscopic
> e. adrenalectomy
> e. ampullary stenting
> e. anterior cruciate ligament reconstruction
> e. approach
> e. aspiration lumpectomy
> e. band ligation
> e. biliary decompression
> e. biliary drainage
> e. biliary stent placement
> e. biopsy site
> e. bladder neck suspension
> e. breast augmentation
> e. brush cytology

E

NOTES

225

endoscopic *(continued)*
- e. cardiac surgery
- e. carpal tunnel release (ECTR)
- e. color Doppler
- e. color Doppler assessment
- e. condylectomy and costochondral graft reconstruction
- e. control
- e. cystenterostomy
- e. cystgastrostomy
- e. cystoduodenostomy
- e. cystogastrostomy
- e. devolvulization
- e. dissection
- e. electrocoagulation
- e. electrohydraulic lithotripsy
- e. esophageal ultrasound (EUS)
- e. esophagectomy
- e. esophagogastric variceal ligation
- e. ethmoidectomy
- e. examination
- e. extirpation cicatricial obliteration
- e. extraction
- e. extraction pancreatic duct stone
- e. finding
- e. fine-needle aspiration cytology
- e. fine-needle puncture
- e. fistulotomy
- e. frontal craniotomy
- e. fulguration
- e. fundoplication
- e. gastrocnemius release
- e. gastrostomy
- e. healing
- e. hemostasis
- e. hemostatic therapy
- e. incision
- e. India ink injection
- e. injection sclerotherapy (EIS)
- e. injection therapy
- e. jejunostomy
- e. laser therapy
- e. light source
- e. management
- e. mastopexy
- e. microwave coagulation
- e. mitral valve repair
- e. mucosal ablation
- e. mucosal resection (EMR)
- e. mucosal resection method
- e. mucosal resection procedure
- e. mucosal resection technique
- e. mucosectomy
- e. nasobiliary catheter drainage
- e. optical urethrotomy
- e. pancreatic drainage
- e. pancreatic duct sphincterotomy
- e. pancreatic stenting
- e. pancreatic therapy

- e. papillary balloon dilation
- e. papillotomy
- e. papillotomy and stenting
- e. parathyroidectomy
- e. photodynamic therapy
- e. photography
- e. plantar fasciotomy
- e. pulsed dye laser lithotripsy
- e. reflectance
- e. reflectance spectrophotometry
- e. removal
- e. retroflexion
- e. retrograde balloon dilatation
- e. retrograde biliary stenting
- e. retrograde cannulation
- e. retrograde cholangiography
- e. retrograde cholangiopancreatography (ERCP)
- e. retrograde cholecystoendoprosthesis
- e. retrograde sclerotherapy
- e. route
- e. sessile polypectomy
- e. sigmoidopexy
- e. sinus surgery
- e. small bowel biopsy
- e. snare resection
- e. sphenoidal biopsy
- e. sphincterectomy
- e. sphincterotomy (ES)
- e. spinal fusion
- e. stent exchange
- e. stone disintegration
- e. stricturotomy
- e. strip craniectomy
- e. surveillance
- e. sympathectomy
- e. technology
- e. transesophageal fine-needle aspiration
- e. transpapillary cannulation
- e. transpapillary cyst drainage
- e. treatment
- e. ultrasonographic imaging
- e. ultrasonography (EUS)
- e. ultrasonography-guided cytology
- e. ultrasound evaluation
- e. variceal sclerotherapy
- e. vertical ramus osteotomy
- e. video-assisted surgery
- e. video image
- e. visualization

endoscopically
- e. normal patient
- e. performed longitudinal incision

endoscopic-assisted
- e.-a. microsurgical technique
- e.-a. technique

endoscopic-controlled lithotripsy

endoscopist
endoscopy
    advanced therapeutic e.
    American Society for
      Gastrointestinal E. (ASGE)
    anal e.
    biliary e.
    colorectal cancer e.
    e. complication
    computerized electronic e.
    diagnostic e.
    dynamic fluorescence video e.
    fiberoptic intraosseous e.
    flexible fiberoptic e.
    fluorescent electronic e.
    gastrointestinal e.
    high-altitude e.
    high-magnification e.
    intestinal e.
    intragastric provocation under e.
    intralacrimal e.
    intraoperative biliary e.
    intraventricular e.
    laser-assisted spinal e.
    lumbar epidural e.
    lung-imaging fluorescent e.
    nasal e.
    outpatient e.
    pancreatic e.
    pancreaticobiliary e.
    pediatric e.
    percutaneous e.
    peripartum e.
    peroral e.
    postsurgical e.
    primary diagnostic e.
    e. procedure
    sinus e.
    small intestinal e.
    e. suite
    surveillance e.
    therapeutic upper e.
    transesophageal e.
    transnasal e.
    transoral e.
    UGI e.
    ultra-high-magnification e.
    upper alimentary e.
    upper gastrointestinal e.
    upper intestinal e.
    virtual e.
endoscopy-related emphysema

endosellar structure
endoskeleton
endosonography-guided drainage
endosonoscopy
endosseous, endo-osseous
endosteal
    e. implant arm
    e. surface
    e. vessel
endosteum
endostitis
endostoma
endothelia (*pl. of* endothelium)
endothelial
    e. barrier
    e. bleb
    e. cell basement membrane
    e. cell dysfunction
    e. cell edema
    e. damage
    e. denudation
    e. injury
    e. lysis
    e. tube
endothelial-dependent relaxation
endothelin
    e. A, B receptor
    e. plasma level
endotheliochorial placenta
endothelio-endothelial placenta
endothelioma
endotheliosis
endothelium, pl. endothelia
    capillary e.
    continuous e.
    corneal e.
    discontinuous e.
    fenestrated e.
    gastrointestinal e.
    sinusoidal e.
    vascular e.
endothelium-dependent fibrinolysis
endothelium-derived relaxing factor
endothelium-mediated relaxation
endothoracic fascia
endothorax
    tension e.
endothrix infection
endothyropexy
endotoxemia
    systemic e.

E

NOTES

endotoxic
- e. exposure
- e. shock

endotoxicosis

endotoxin
- bacterial e.
- e. shock

endotracheal
- e. anesthesia
- e. aspirate
- e. induction
- e. insufflation
- e. intubation
- e. suctioning
- e. tube placement

endotrachelitis

endoultrasonography

endoureterotomy
- cold knife e.

endourologic

endourological
- e. cold knife incision
- e. therapy

endourology

endovaginal
- e. finding
- e. imaging

endovascular
- e. aneurysm
- e. approach
- e. balloon occlusion
- e. coagulation
- e. coiling
- e. graft insertion
- e. graft treatment
- e. intervention
- e. repair
- e. stent graft
- e. stenting
- e. stenting technique
- e. surgery
- e. technology
- e. therapy

endovasculitis
- hemorrhagic e.

endovenous septum

endoventricular circular patch plasty

endplate compression fracture

endpoint
- e. measurement
- primary e.
- resuscitation e.
- resuscitative e.
- therapeutic e.

end-sigmoid colostomy

end-stage
- e.-s. cirrhosis
- e.-s. intestinal failure
- e.-s. lymphangiomyomatosis

- e.-s. reflux nephropathy
- e.-s. renal disease (ESRD)

end-systolic
- e.-s. area (ESA)
- e.-s. cross-sectional area
- e.-s. diameter (ESD)
- e.-s. left ventricular pressure
- e.-s. pressure-length relationship (ESPLR)
- e.-s. pressure-volume relation
- e.-s. stress-dimension relation
- e.-s. wall thickness (ESWT)

end-tidal
- e.-t. carbon dioxide
- e.-t. nitrogen concentration

end-to-back bowel anastomosis

end-to-end
- e.-t.-e. enterostomy
- e.-t.-e. esophagogastrostomy
- e.-t.-e. esophagojejunostomy
- e.-t.-e. ileoanal anastomosis
- e.-t.-e. ileoanal anastomosis without mucosal resection
- e.-t.-e. intussuscepted pancreaticojejunostomy
- e.-t.-e. invaginating
- e.-t.-e. inverting pancreaticojejunostomy
- e.-t.-e. jejunoileal bypass
- e.-t.-e. reconstruction
- e.-t.-e. reconstruction method
- e.-t.-e. reconstruction procedure
- e.-t.-e. reconstruction technique
- e.-t.-e. splenoadrenal anastomosis
- e.-t.-e. tendon repair

end-to-side
- e.-t.-s. anastomosis
- e.-t.-s. arteriotomy
- e.-t.-s. choledochojejunostomy
- e.-t.-s. esophagogastrostomy
- e.-t.-s. esophagojejunostomy
- e.-t.-s. jejunoileal bypass
- e.-t.-s. nerve coaptation
- e.-t.-s. portocaval shunt
- e.-t.-s. reimplantation
- e.-t.-s. repair
- e.-t.-s. splenorenal shunt
- e.-t.-s. vasoepididymostomy technique

endurance
- cardiorespiratory e. (CRE)

end-viewing sector

end-weave anastomosis

enema
- air e.
- air-contrast barium e.
- antegrade continence e. (ACE)
- barium e.
- contrast e.

double-contrast e.
water-soluble contrast e.
energy
e. expenditure
hepatic intracellular e.
enervation
engaged head
engineering
islet cell e.
Englisch sinus
English
E. position
E. rhinoplasty
engorged
engorgement
engraftment
engulf
enhanced external counterpulsation
enhancing
e. brain lesion
e. ring
enlarged
e. parathyroid gland
e. spleen
enlargement
asymmetric parathyroid e.
mediastinal e.
Enneking
E. classification
E. resection-arthrodesis
ensiform
e. appendix
e. cartilage
e. process
ensisternum
ensu method
entangling technique
enteral
e. alimentation
e. feeding
e. nutrition
enterelcosis
enteric
e. cyst
e. drainage
e. fistula
e. infection
e. intussusception
e. nervous system
e. organism
e. plexus
entericus

enteritis
radiation e.
enteroanastomosis
enterocele sac
enterocentesis
enterocholecystostomy
enterocholecystotomy
enterocleisis
omental e.
enterocolic fistula
enterocolitis
necrotizing e. (NEC)
enterocolostomy
enterocutaneous fistula
enterocystoplasty
Camey e.
clam e.
seromuscular e.
sigmoid e.
enteroenteral fistula
enteroenteric fistula
enteroenterostomy
2-layer e.
enterogenital fistula
enterogenous cyst
enterohepatic circulation
enterohepatopexy
enterolith
enterolithiasis
enterolithotomy
enterolysis
enteropathy
radiation e.
enteropeptidase
enteroperitoneal abscess
enteropexy
enteroplasty
enterorenal
enterorrhagia
enterorrhaphy
enteroscopy
intraoperative e.
push e.
push-type e.
Roux-en-Y limb e.
transgastrostomic e.
video small bowel e.
enterostomal therapy
enterostomy
double e.
end-to-end e.
percutaneous e.

E

NOTES

enterotomy
> antimesenteric e.
> inadvertent e.
> longitudinal e.
> occult e.

enterourethral fistula
enterourethrostomy
enterovaginal fistula
enterovesical fistula
enteroviral infection
enthesis
enthesitis
enthesopathy
entity
> pathologic e.

entocranial
entocranium
entomion
entoptoscopy
entrainment
> air e.

entrapment
> catheter knotting and e.
> lateral canal e.
> peroneal nerve e.
> popliteal artery e.
> e. syndrome

entrapped
> e. gland
> e. nerve

entropion
> cicatricial e.

entropionize
entropy
> approximate e.
> spectral e.

entry
> air e.
> implant e.
> e. phenomenon
> e. point
> e. site
> e. zone
> e. zone lesion

enucleate
enucleation
> eye e.
> Foix e.
> leiomyoma e.
> e. method
> e. procedure
> surgical e.
> e. technique

enuresis
> diurnal e.
> nocturnal e.

envelope
> axillary e.
> breast skin e.

> e. flap
> peritoneal e.
> soft tissue e.

enveloping scar tissue
environmental mycobacterial infection
environment modification
enzymatic
> e. débridement
> e. zonulolysis

enzyme
> angiotensin-converting e. (ACE)
> e. induction
> pancreatic e.

EORTC
> European Organization for Research and Treatment of Cancer

eosin
eosinophilic
> e. chemotactic factor of anaphylaxis (ECF-A)
> e. endomyocardial disease
> e. fibrohistiocytic lesion

epactal bone
epaulet flap
epauxesiectomy
epaxial
EPEM
> Emory Pain Estimate Model

ependymal cell
ependymoastrocytoma
ependymoblastoma
ependymoma
> anaplastic e.

EPH
> episodic paroxysmal hemicrania

ephaptic sprouting
ephippii
epiaortic imaging technique
epicanthal
> e. correction
> e. fold

epicardial
> e. fat pad
> e. monitoring

epicondylar avulsion fracture
epicondyle
epicondylectomy
epicondyli (*pl. of* epicondylus)
epicondylian
epicondylic
epicondylus, pl. **epicondyli**
epicoracoid
epicranial
> e. aponeurosis
> e. muscle

epicranium
epicranius muscle
epicystotomy
epidemiologic study

epidermal
- e. growth factor (EGF)
- e. inclusion cyst
- e. necrolysis
- e. ridge

epidermalization

epidermatoplasty

epidermic graft

epidermidis
- *Staphylococcus e.*

epidermization

epidermoid
- e. carcinoma
- e. cyst
- e. resection

epidermoidoma
- black e.
- incisural e.
- intradural e.
- prepontine white e.
- white e.

epidermolysis

epididymal
- e. sperm
- e. sperm aspiration

epididymectomy

epididymidectomy

epididymidis

epididymis, pl. **epididymides**
- cauda e.
- corpus e.
- e. lesion
- lobule of e.

epididymisoplasty

epididymitis

epididymoorchitis

epididymoplasty

epididymotomy

epididymovasectomy

epididymovasostomy

epidural
- e. abscess
- e. abscess evacuation
- e. administration
- e. anesthesia (EA)
- e. anesthetic
- e. block
- e. blood patch (EBP)
- e. blood patch anesthetic technique
- e. cavity
- continuous lumbar e. (CLE)
- e. delivery

- e. electrode array
- e. extramedullary lesion
- e. fibrosis
- e. hematoma
- e. hemorrhage
- e. neural blockade
- e. neuroplasty
- e. opioid
- e. opioid infusion
- e. pressure waveform (EPWF)
- e. space
- e. space infection
- e. steroid injection (ESI)
- e. top-up
- e. tumor evacuation
- walking e.

epidurogram

epidurography

epifascicular epineurotomy

epifluorescent microscopy

epigastric
- e. angle
- e. artery
- e. fold
- e. fossa
- e. fullness
- e. hernia
- e. incision
- e. pain
- e. region
- e. vein

epigastrium

epigastrius

epigastrocele

epigastrorrhaphy

epiglottic
- e. cartilage
- e. reconstruction

epiglottis

epiglottoplasty

epignathus teratoma

epihyal ligament

epihyoid

epi-illumination

epikeratophakic keratoplasty

epikeratoplasty
- tectonic e.

epilation

epilepidoma

epilepsy
- extratemporal e.

NOTES

epilepsy *(continued)*
    intractable e.
    e. surgery
epilepticus
    status e.
epileptogenic process
epimorphic regeneration
epimysiotomy
epinephrine-anesthetic mixture
epinephros
epineural
    e. repair
    e. suture technique
epineurectomy
    interfascicular e.
epineurial neurorrhaphy
epineurolysis
    volar e.
epineurotomy
    anterior e.
    epifascicular e.
    interfascicular e.
    local e.
epipapillary membrane
epipharynx
epiphenomena of dissection
epiphrenic
epiphyseolysis
epiphyses (*pl. of* epiphysis)
epiphysial, epiphyseal
    e. bar resection
    e. closure
    e. growth plate fracture
    e. line
    e. plate injury
    e. ring
    e. slip fracture
    e. tibial fracture
epiphysial-metaphysial osteotomy
epiphysiodesis
    open bone graft e.
    screw e.
epiphysiolysis
    femoral e.
    proximal femoral e.
epiphysis, pl. epiphyses
    atavistic e.
    ball-and-socket e.
    balloon e.
    capital femoral e.
    capitular e.
    clavicular e.
    congenital stippled e.
    distal humeral e.
    femoral e.
    humeral e.
    iliac e.
    ossifying e.
    pressure e.

    ring e.
    slipped capital femoral e.
    stippled e.
    tibial e.
    traction e.
epiphyte
epiplocele
epiploectomy
epiploic
    e. appendage
    e. appendicitis
    e. appendix
    e. branch
epiploica
epiplomerocele
epiplomphalocele
epiplopexy
epiplosarcomphalocele
epiploscheocele
epipteric bone
epiretinal membrane
episcleral
    e. circulation
    e. explant
    e. ganglion
    e. space
    e. tissue
    e. vascular dilation
episioperineoplasty
episioperineorrhaphy
episioplasty
episiorrhaphy
episiotomy
    median e.
    mediolateral e.
    e. repair
    ruptured e.
    e. scar
episode
    bleeding e.
    myopathy, encephapathy, lactic
        acidosis, stroke-like e.'s (MELAS)
    thrombotic e.
episodic
    e. colic
    e. hypoxemia
    e. paroxysmal hemicrania (EPH)
epispadias-exstrophy complex
epispadias repair
epispinal
epistasis
epistaxis
episternal bone
episternum
epistropheus
epitarsus
epithelia (*pl. of* epithelium)
epithelial
    e. barrier

e. basement membrane
e. breakdown
e. cell
e. cyst
e. hemangioendothelioma
e. inlay
e. invagination
e. migration
epithelialization technique
epithelioserosa
epithelium, pl. **epithelia**
Barrett e.
bile duct e.
colic e.
colon e.
columnar e.
corneal e.
crypt e.
dysplastic e.
endometric e.
esophageal e.
external dental e.
external enamel e.
follicular e.
gastric e.
germinal e.
glandular e.
gut e.
junctional e.
metaplastic e.
pseudostratified e.
pyramidal e.
regenerated esophageal e.
salivary e.
salmon-pink e.
squamous e.
stratified e.
surface e.
transitional e.
villous e.
epithelization
epithesis
epitrochlea
epitrochlear
epituberculous infiltration
epitympanic
e. cell
e. recess
Epley maneuver
épluchage
E point
epoophorectomy

epoophoron
Eppright dial osteotomy
Epstein
E. hip dislocation classification
E. method
Epstein-Barr
E.-B. viral infection
E.-B. virus (EBV)
Epstein-Thomas classification
eptifibatide
epulofibroma
EPWF
epidural pressure waveform
equal sagittal flap
equation
alveolar gas e.
Bohr e.
Henderson-Hasselbalch e.
equator
anatomic e.
crystalline lens e.
eyeball e.
geometric e.
lens e.
equatorial plane
equilibrating operation
equilibration
mandibular e.
occlusal e.
equilibrium
acid-base e.
sedimentation e.
equinovalgus deformity
equinovarus
talipes e.
equinus
e. deformity
e. position
equipotent
equipotential line
equivalence
e. point
e. relation
equivalent
cultured human skin e.
human skin e. (HSE)
e. refracting plane
ventilation e.
equivocal
e. finding
e. pancreatic cytology

E

NOTES

ER
> emergency room
>> ER thoracotomy
eradication therapy
Erb point
ERCP
> endoscopic retrograde
> cholangiopancreatography
>> ERCP cannulation
>> postoperative ERCP
>> preoperative ERCP
ERCP-guided biopsy
ERCP-induced splenic rupture
Erdheim cystic medial necrosis
erectile dysfunction (ED)
erect illumination
erection
> intraoperative penile e.
> penile e.
> pharmacologically induced e.
> reflex e.
> reflexogenic e.
erector
> e. spinae muscle
> e. spinae tendon
erector-spinal reflex
ergonovine provocation test
Erickson-Leider-Brown technique
erigentes
Eriksson
> E. brachial block technique
> E. ligament technique
Erlangen pull-type sphincterotomy
Erlenmeyer flask deformity
erosion
> corneal e.
> implant e.
> infraspinatus insertion e.
> limiting plate e.
> recurrent corneal e.
> tumor e.
> wedge-shaped e.
erosive inflammation
erroneous projection
eruption
> ectopic e.
> eczematous polymorphous light e.
> erythema nodosum-like e.
> surgical e.
erysipelas
> surgical e.
erysipelas-like skin lesion
erysipeloid
erysiphake
> corneal e.
> oval cup e.
> e. technique
erythema
> cold e.

> necrolytic migratory e.
> e. nodosum-like eruption
erythroblastoma
erythrocyte
> e. mass
> e. membrane
erythrocytolysis
erythrodermatous lesion
erythrolysis
erythromelalgia
erythromycin-induced cholecystitis
erythropoietin therapy
ES
> endoscopic sphincterotomy
ESA
> end-systolic area
escalation
> dose e.
Escapini cataract operation
escharectomy
eschar excision
escharotomy
ESD
> end-systolic diameter
ESI
> epidural steroid injection
esodic nerve
esophageal
> e. A, B ring
> e. achalasia
> e. adenocarcinoma
> e. artery
> e. banding technique
> e. band ligation
> e. biopsy
> e. body motor dysfunction
> e. branch
> e. cancer
> e. carcinoma
> e. colic
> e. compression
> e. constriction
> e. contractile ring
> e. contraction ring
> e. dilatation
> e. dilation
> e. dilation treatment
> e. disorder
> e. dissection
> e. diverticulectomy
> e. diverticulum
> e. duplication
> e. dysmotility
> e. ectopic sebaceous gland
> e. effect
> e. epithelium
> e. fistula
> e. foreign body
> e. fungal infection

e. gap
e. hernia
e. hiatus
e. impression
e. inflammation
e. intubation
e. Lewy body
e. manometry
e. mass
e. measurement
e. mobilization
e. mucosal ring
e. muscular ring
e. myotomy
e. obstruction
e. obturator airway
e. perforation
e. peristaltic pressure
e. pH
e. pH monitoring
e. photodynamic therapy
e. plexus
e. remnant
e. resection
e. rupture
e. shortening
e. sling procedure
e. spasm
e. sphincter
e. sphincter pressure
e. sphincter relaxation
e. stenosis
e. stricture
e. tear
e. transection
e. tumor
e. ulceration
e. variceal bleeding
e. variceal sclerotherapy
e. varix
e. vein
e. web
esophageal-jejunal anastomosis
esophageal lengthening
esophagectasis
esophagectomy
distal e.
endoscopic e.
3-incision e.
Ivor Lewis 2-stage subtotal e.
laparoscopic-assisted e.
laparoscopic transhiatal e.

mediastinoscopy-assisted
transhiatal e.
minimally invasive e.
near-total e.
open e.
subtotal e.
thoracoabdominal e.
thoracoscopic-assisted e.
total endoscopic e.
total laparoscopic e.
total thoracic e.
transhiatal e. (THE)
transhiatal blunt e.
transthoracic e.
video-assisted transsternal radical e.
e. with thoracotomy
esophageus
esophagi (*pl. of* esophagus)
esophagitis
pill-induced e.
reflux e.
esophagobronchial fistula
esophagocardiomyotomy
esophagocardioplasty
esophagocolic anastomosis
esophagocutaneous fistula
esophagodiverticulostomy
esophagoduodenostomy
esophagoenterostomy
esophagogastrectomy
Ivor Lewis e.
thoracoabdominal e.
esophagogastric
e. anastomosis
e. cancer
e. fat pad
e. fundoplasty
e. intubation
e. junction
e. orifice
e. resection
e. variceal bleeding
e. vestibule
esophagogastroanastomosis
esophagogastroduodenoscopy (EGD)
pediatric e.
esophagogastromyotomy
esophagogastroplasty
Grondahl-Finney e.
esophagogastroscopy
Abbott e.
intrathoracic e.

E

NOTES

esophagogastroscopy *(continued)*
   Johnson e.
   Thal e.
   Woodward e.
esophagogastrostomy
   Abbott e.
   cervical e.
   Clagett-Barrett e.
   end-to-end e.
   end-to-side e.
   intrathoracic e.
   Johnson e.
   Thal e.
   thoracic e.
   Woodward e.
esophagogram
   barium e.
   water-soluble contrast e.
esophagojejunostomy
   end-to-end e.
   end-to-side e.
   loop e.
   mechanical e.
   mediastinal e.
   Roux-en-Y e.
   stapled e.
   transhiatal e.
esophagomediastinal fistula
esophagomyotomy
   circumferential e.
   Heller e.
   laparoscopic e.
   modified Heller e.
   open e.
   thoracic short e.
   thoracoscopic e.
esophagoplasty
   balloon e.
   behind-sternum column e.
   Belsey e.
   cervical e.
   colic patch e.
   colonic e.
   gastric patch e.
   gastric tube e.
   Grondahl e.
   Grondahl-Finney e.
   intrathoracic e.
   laparoscopic e.
   patch e.
   pectoralis myocutaneous e.
   pediatric e.
   posterior mediastinal e.
   reverse gastric tube e.
   single-step e.
   subtotal e.
esophagoplication
esophagoproximal gastrectomy
esophagopulmonary fistula

esophagorespiratory fistula
esophagoscopy
   fiberoptic e.
esophagostomy
   cervical e.
   palliative e.
esophagotomy
   cervical e.
esophagotracheal fistula
esophagus, pl. **esophagi**
   anterior e.
   Barrett e.
   cervical e.
   columnar-lined e.
   elevator e.
   nutcracker e.
   proximal e.
   e. temperature
   thoracic e.
esotropia
   congenital e.
ESPLR
   end-systolic pressure-length relationship
ESRD
   end-stage renal disease
Essed-Schroeder corporoplasty
essential
   e. brown induration
   e. brown induration of lung
   e. hypertension
   e. tremor
Esser
   E. graft
   E. inlay operation
Essex-Lopresti
   E.-L. axial fixation technique
   E.-L. calcaneal fracture
      classification
   E.-L. calcaneal fracture technique
   E.-L. joint depression fracture
   E.-L. open reduction
established cell line
esterase-metabolized opioid
Estersohn osteotomy
Estes
   E. operation
   E. procedure
esthetic, aesthetic
   e. procedure
   e. restoration
   e. rhinoplasty
   e. septorhinoplasty
   e. surgery
esthetics, aesthetics
   gingival tissue e.
estimated
   e. Fick method
   e. time of ovulation (ETO)

Estlander
- E. flap
- E. operation

Estlander-Abbe flap
estrogen-assisted colposcopy
estrogen receptor localization
ESU
- electrosurgery unit

ESWL
- electrohydraulic shockwave lithotripsy

ESWT
- end-systolic wall thickness
- extracorporeal shock wave treatment

ethanol
- e. ablation
- e. injection
- e. injection therapy

ethanol-induced tumor necrosis
ether convulsion
etherization
ethmocranial
ethmofrontal
ethmoid
- e. bone
- e. bulla
- e. canal
- e. cell
- e. exenteration
- e. fistula
- e. registration point
- e. sinus carcinoma

ethmoidal
- e. approach
- e. artery
- e. crest
- e. foramen
- e. groove
- e. infundibulum
- e. labyrinth
- e. lacrimal fistula
- e. nerve
- e. notch
- e. osteotomy
- e. plate
- e. vein

ethmoidectomy
- anterior e.
- endoscopic e.
- external e.
- internal e.
- intranasal e.
- partial e.

- total e.
- transantral e.

ethmoidolacrimal suture
ethmoidomaxillary suture
ethmolacrimal
ethmomaxillary
ethmonasal
ethmopalatal
ethmosphenoid
ethmoturbinal
ethmovomerine
ethylene
- e. oxide (ETO)
- e. oxide sterilization

etiology
- infectious e.
- malignant e.

etiopathology
ETO
- estimated time of ovulation
- ethylene oxide
- ETO sterilization

etoricoxib
eucupine
eugnathic anomaly
EUPF
- extended uvulopalatal flap

euplastic
European
- E. Carotid Surgery Trial (ECST)
- E. Organization for Research and Treatment of Cancer (EORTC)

euryon
EUS
- endoscopic esophageal ultrasound
- endoscopic ultrasonography

EUS-guided
- EUS-g. cytology
- EUS-g. fine-needle aspiration

eustachian
- e. tube
- e. tube orifice

eutectic mixture of local anesthetics (EMLA)
euthyroid sick syndrome
euthyscopy
euvolemia
euvolemic
evacuating clot
evacuation
- CT-guided stereotactic e.
- digital rectal e.

E

NOTES

evacuation *(continued)*
    dilatation and e. (D&E)
    dilation and e. (D&E)
    e. disorder
    epidural abscess e.
    epidural tumor e.
    fimbrial e.
    fluid e.
    hematobilia e.
    hematoma e.
    e. procedure
    rectal e.
    e. score
    stool e.
    transsphenoidal e.

evagination
    optic e.

evaluation
    acute physiologic assessment and chronic health e.
    acute physiology and chronic health e. (APACHE)
    angiographic e.
    anthropometric e.
    audiological e.
    baseline capacity e.
    clinical e.
    cosmetic e.
    cytologic e.
    diagnostic imaging e.
    Doppler pulse e.
    Dubowitz e.
    endoscopic ultrasound e.
    followup e.
    functional capacity e.
    genitourinary e.
    hearing aid e.
    hormonal e.
    infertility e.
    job capacity e.
    laparoscopic e.
    mammographic e.
    manometric e.
    medical care e.
    mental status e.
    metabolic e.
    neurodiagnostic e.
    neurological e.
    neuroradiologic e.
    noninvasive e.
    pedicle e.
    physical capacity e.
    postoperative followup e.
    preoperative staging e.
    presurgical medical e.
    pretransplant e.
    pretreatment e.
    e. protocol
    quantitative e.
    radiographic e.
    radiologic e.
    roentgenographic e.
    serial radiographic e.
    sexual e.
    Smith physical capacity e.
    staging e.
    static e.
    status e.
    stent e.
    sudomotor e.
    urological e.
    uterine e.
    videoscopic e.
    videourodynamic e.
    visual function e.
    wake-up e.
    Wright-Giemsa e.

Evans
    E. ankle reconstruction technique
    E. anterior calcaneal osteotomy
    E. intertrochanteric fracture classification
    E. procedure
    E. reconstruction

Evans-Steptoe procedure
Eve method
even-echo rephasing
event
    acute cardiac e.
    adverse e.
    anatomic e.
    cardiac e.
    catastrophic e.
    cerebral e.
    cerebrovascular e.
    fatal cardiac e.
    neuroelectric e.
    noxious e.
    precipitating noxious e.
    soft e.
    thromboembolic e.

eventration
    diaphragm e.
    diaphragmatic e.
    e. disease

Everard Williams procedure
Eversbusch operation
eversion
    e. carotid endarterectomy
    e. operation
    e. orchiopexy
    e. osteotomy
    e. technique

eversion-external rotation deformity
evert
everting interrupted suture technique
evidement

evidence
> biochemical e.
> clinical e.
> macroscopic e.
> radiologic e.
> sonographic e.

evidence-based medicine (EBM)
eviration
evisceration
> abdominal e.
> drain site e.
> e. operation
> total abdominal e.
> upper abdominal e.

evisceroneurotomy
evoked
> e. external urethral sphincter
>   potential monitoring
> e. potential technique
> e. twitch

evolution
> lesion e.
> e. time

evolving myocardial infarction
evulsion
Ewald capitellocondylar total elbow arthroplasty
Ewald-Walker kinematic knee arthroplasty
Ewing operation
ex
> ex amblyopia
> ex situ
> ex situ bench surgery
> ex situ hepatectomy
> ex situ-in situ hepatectomy
> ex situ-in situ liver resection
> ex situ-in situ technique
> ex situ-in vivo procedure
> ex utero intrapartum treatment
>   (EXIT)
> ex utero intrapartum treatment
>   procedure
> ex vacuo dilatation
> ex vivo
> ex vivo cannulation
> ex vivo count
> ex vivo fertilization
> ex vivo gene therapy
> ex vivo marrow treatment
> ex vivo perfusion

> ex vivo resection
> ex vivo technique

exacerbated
exacerbation of pain
exaggerated sniffing position
examination, exam
> abdominal e.
> arthroscopic e.
> Ballard e.
> barium enema e.
> bench e.
> bile fluid e.
> bimanual pelvic e.
> bone marrow e.
> cardiac e.
> chest e.
> clinical e.
> colonoscopic e.
> comparative radiographic e.
> cutaneous e.
> cytologic e.
> cytology e.
> dark-field e.
> digital rectal e.
> Doppler flow probe e.
> double-contrast barium enema e.
> Dubowitz e.
> duodenal content e.
> endoscopic e.
> eye e.
> fiberoptic e.
> flashlight e.
> followup e.
> full-body cutaneous e.
> full-spine radiographic e.
> funduscopic e.
> gastric residue e.
> gray-scale e.
> hand-held Doppler flow probe e.
> histologic e.
> histopathologic e.
> history and physical e.
> immunofluorescent e.
> laparoscopic e.
> limited e.
> LUS e.
> mediastinoscopic e.
> mental status e.
> motor e.
> neonate e.
> nerve conduction velocity e.
> neurologic e.

E

NOTES

examination *(continued)*
    neuroophthalmologic e.
    neurophysiologic e.
    neurotologic e.
    newborn e.
    ophthalmic e.
    oral peripheral e.
    palpatory e.
    parasternal e.
    pathologic e.
    pathology e.
    pelvic e.
    pericardial fluid e.
    peripheral e.
    peritoneal fluid e.
    physical e.
    pleural fluid e.
    postmortem e.
    proctoscopic e.
    radiographic e.
    radiological e.
    rectal e.
    rectovaginal e.
    reflex e.
    retinal e.
    self-breast e.
    sensory e.
    serologic e.
    soft x-ray e.
    speculum e.
    sterile vaginal e.
    suboptimal e.
    supraclavicular e.
    suprasternal e.
    synovial fluid e.
    systemic e.
    tangent screen e.
    thermographic e.
    transvaginal ultrasonographic e.
    ultrasonographic e.
    ultrasound e.
    e. under anesthesia
    vaginal e.
    Wood light e.
exanthema
exanthematous
    e. disease
    e. fever
    e. inflammation
excavated
    e. gastric carcinoma
    e. lesion
excavatio
excavation
    atrophic e.
    glaucomatous e.
    physiologic e.
    retinal e.

excavatum
excementosis, pl. **excementoses**
    extension e.
    intraepithelial e.
    pronglike e.
    ultraterminal e.
excess
    e. androgen
    mandibular e.
    marginal e.
    maxillary e.
    morbidity e.
    e. mucus
    vertical maxillary e.
excessive
    e. bleeding
    e. blood loss
    e. callus formation
    e. fatigue
    e. heat production
    e. lacrimation
    e. lip support
    e. spacing
    e. straining
    e. tearing
    e. weight loss
exchange
    air e.
    air-fluid e.
    blood gas e.
    catheter e.
    cation e.
    chemical e.
    e. diffusion
    endoscopic stent e.
    fetal-maternal e.
    fiberoptic-assisted coaxial
      endotracheal tube e.
    fluid-gas e.
    gas e.
    gas-fluid e.
    lens e.
    multiple inert gas e.
    plasma e.
    pulmonary-gas e.
    respiratory e.
    e. technique
    e. transfusion
    wire-guided balloon-assisted
      endoscopic biliary stent e.
exchangeable mass
exchanger
    countercurrent heat e.
    thymocyte NA^+/H^+ e.
excimer
    e. laser ablation
    e. laser coronary angioplasty
    e. laser photorefractive keratectomy
    e. vascular recanalization

excipient
excised specimen
excision
    abdominoperineal e.
    alar wedge e.
    Arlt-Jaesche e.
    e. arthroplasty
    Bartlett nail fold e.
    e. biopsy
    bone cyst e.
    Bose nail fold e.
    cervical disc e.
    circumferential mesorectal e.
    clavicle e.
    cold snare e.
    complete circumferential
      mesorectal e.
    complete mesh e.
    conjunctiva-Müller muscle e.
    Curtin plantar fibromatosis e.
    Das Gupta scapular e.
    disc e.
    distal clavicular e.
    dorsal e.
    en bloc e.
    endoluminal e.
    eschar e.
    extended mesorectal e.
    extratemporal e.
    Ferciot e.
    Ferciot-Thomson e.
    Flatt e.
    funicular e.
    fusiform e.
    goiter e.
    hemivertebral e.
    hemorrhoid e.
    incomplete e.
    interdental e.
    intralesional e.
    laser hemorrhoid e.
    local e.
    marginal e.
    mass e.
    McKeever-Buck fragment e.
    meniscal e.
    mesorectal e.
    microlumbar disc e.
    operative e.
    partial mesh e.
    pentagonal block e.
    radical compartmental e.
    rectal e.
    retropulsed bone e.
    ruptured disc e.
    sentinel node e.
    sheet mesh e.
    Stewart distal clavicular e.
    subperichondrial e.
    superficial e.
    surgical e.
    tangential e.
    Thompson e.
    thymus gland e.
    total mesorectal e. (TME)
    transanal e.
    transoral odontoid e.
    ulnar head e.
    wedge e.
    wide local e.
    William microlumbar disc e.
excisional
    e. arthrodesis
    e. atherectomy
    e. biopsy
    e. biopsy method
    e. biopsy procedure
    e. biopsy site
    e. biopsy technique
    e. cardiac surgery
    e. removal
excision-curettage technique
excitability test
excitation
    nicotinic e.
excitatory
    e. junction potential
    e. postsynaptic potential
    e. synapse
excited skin syndrome
excitement phase
exciting eye
excitoreflex nerve
excitor nerve
exclave
exclusion
    antral e.
    e. bypass
    Devine antral e.
    hepatic vascular e. (HVE)
    intermittent vascular e.
    partial hepatic vascular e. (PHVE)
    subtotal gastric e.

NOTES

E

exclusion *(continued)*
    total vascular e.
    vascular e.
excoriate
excoriation
    neurotic e.
excrement
excrementitious
excrescence
    bony e.
    enamel e.
    Lambl e.
    wartlike e.
excrete
excretion
    urinary calcium e.
excretory duct
excursion
    dome e.
    insertional e.
    lateral e.
    protrusive e.
    range of e.
    respiratory e.
    retrusive e.
    tendon e.
excystation
execution time
exemia
exencephalia
exencephalic
exencephalocele
exencephalous
exencephaly
exenteration
    anterior pelvic e.
    ethmoid e.
    Iliff e.
    orbital e.
    pelvic e.
    petrous pyramid e.
    posterior pelvic e.
    supralevator pelvic e.
    total pelvic e.
exercise
    e. capacity
    concentric e.
    eccentric e.
    e. hyperemia blood flow
    e. imaging
    e. index
    e. ischemia
    e. physiology
    plyometric e.
    e. study
    treadmill e.
exercise-associated acute renal failure
exercise-induced
    e.-i. arrhythmia

    e.-i. asthma
    e.-i. bronchospasm
    e.-i. incontinence
    e.-i. silent myocardial ischemia
    e.-i. ventricular tachycardia
exeresis
    palliative e.
exergonic reaction
exertion
    dyspnea on e.
    perceived e.
    rated perceived e.
    rating of perceived e.
exertional
    e. amblyopia
    e. anterior compartment syndrome
    e. deep posterior compartment
      syndrome
    e. dyspnea
    e. rhabdomyolysis
Exeter bone lavage
exfoliant
exfoliate
exfoliation
    lamellar e.
    e. syndrome
    true e.
exfoliative cytology
exhalation
    end e.
exhaled oxygen tension
exhaustion
    e. atrophy
    nervous e.
    ovarian follicle e.
    postactivation e.
    e. state
exhilarant
existential pain
EXIT
    ex utero intrapartum treatment
      EXIT procedure
exit
    e. access
    e. block
    e. block murmur
    e. point
    e. pupil
    e. site
    e. site infection
    e. wound
exitatory reaction
Exner plexus
exocardia
exocardial murmur
exoccipital bone
exocelomic
    e. cavity
    e. membrane

exocentric construction
exocervix
exocranial orifice
exocrine
    e. pancreas
    e. pancreatic insufficiency
exocrinopathic process
exocytosis
exodic nerve
exodontia
exodontics
exodontist
exodontology
exogamy
exogenous
    e. aneurysm
    e. anticoagulant coagulation
    e. disease
    e. fiber
    e. fibrin clot
    e. flora
    e. hormone
    e. IGF-1
    e. infection
    e. reconstruction
    e. smile
    e. substance
exognathia
exognathion
exophoria
exophoric
exophthalmic
exophthalmogenic
exophthalmometric
exophthalmometry
exophthalmos, exophthalmus
    recurrent e.
exophthalmos-producing substance
exophytic
    e. carcinoma
    e. growth
    e. gut mass
    e. joint disease
exoplant
    scleral e.
exopneumopexy
exoserosis
exoskeletal
exoskeleton
exosmosis
exostectomy

exostosectomy
exostosis, pl. **exostoses**
    external auditory e. (EAE)
    hereditary multiple exostoses
    multiple exostoses
exothermic
exotropia
exotropic
expandable
expanded plasma
expanding retroperitoneal hematoma
expansible
expansile
    e. abdominal mass
    e. unilocular well-demarcated bone lesion
expansion
    e. and activator therapy
    e. of the arch
    clonal e.
    controlled e.
    delayed e.
    dental arch e.
    dorsal e.
    effective setting e.
    field e.
    hygroscopic e.
    infarct e.
    intravascular volume e.
    investment e.
    lateral extensor e.
    linear thermal e.
    maxillary e.
    mercuroscopic e.
    mesangial matrix e.
    monoclonal e.
    palatal e.
    perceptual e.
    plasma volume e.
    rapid maxillary e.
    repeated tissue e.
    secondary e.
    setting e.
    slow maxillary e.
    stent e.
    thermal coefficient e.
    tissue e.
    volume e.
    wax e.
expansive laminaplasty
expectancy
    life e.

E

NOTES

expectant management
expectorate
expectoration
    prune-juice e.
expenditure
    caloric e.
    energy e.
    resting energy e.
experimental
    e. allergic encephalomyelitis
    e. disorder
    e. method
    e. neurasthenia
    e. pain
    e. pathology
    e. threshold
expiration
    assisted e.
    end e.
expiratory
    e. computed tomography
    e. dyspnea
    end e.
    e. flow rate
    e. grunt
    e. murmur
    e. nitrogen
    e. positive airway pressure
    e. prolongation
    e. reserve volume
    e. residual volume
    e. retard
    e. rhonchi
    e. valve
    e. wheezing
expired
    e. air
    e. air collection
explant
    encircling e.
    episcleral e.
    Molteno episcleral e.
    posterior e.
    segmental e.
    sponge e.
explantation
explanted heart
explicit memory
exploding head syndrome
exploration
    abdominal e.
    bilateral neck e.
    bile duct e.
    common bile duct e.
    complete surgical e.
    contralateral groin e.
    e. and débridement
    formal surgical e.
    groin e.

laparoscopically guided
    transcystic e.
laparoscopic common bile duct e.
laparoscopic transcystic common
    bile duct e. (LTCBDE)
laparoscopic transcystic duct e.
neck e.
open common bile duct e.
petrous pyramid air cell e.
remedial inguinal e.
routine bilateral neck e.
routine unilateral e.
sclerotomy with e.
standard neck e.
unilateral neck e.
exploratory
    e. celiotomy
    e. drive
    e. laparotomy
    e. operation
    e. puncture
    e. stroke
    e. surgery
explosion
    colonic e.
    e. fracture
    e. injury
explosive doubling time
exponential phase
exposed pulp
exposure
    Abbott-Gill epiphysial plate e.
    accidental pulp e.
    aerosolized pollutant e.
    allergen e.
    anesthetic gas e.
    anterior surgical e.
    bone e.
    bony e.
    carious pulp e.
    chemical e.
    cold e.
    cue e.
    double e.
    electromagnetic radiation e.
    endotoxic e.
    extradural e.
    extrapharyngeal e.
    fast film e.
    graded e.
    heat e.
    Henry posterior interosseous
      nerve e.
    imaginal e.
    incident e.
    industrial e.
    e. keratopathy
    Kocher-Langenbeck e.
    light e.

log relative e.
magnetic radiation e.
maternal mercury e.
mechanical pulp e.
methamphetamine e.
midline e.
noise e.
occupational toxin e.
operative e.
operator e.
prenatal diethylstilbestrol e.
prior drug e.
radiation e.
repeated e.
subclavian vessel e.
subperiosteal e.
sun e.
surgical pulp e.
thoracolumbar junction surgical e.
thoracolumbar spine anterior e.
toxin e.
transpalatal e.
transperitoneal e.
upper cervical spine anterior e.
in utero e.
vertebral e.
vessel e.
vinyl chloride e.
expressed skull fracture
expression
facial e.
intragraft e.
pain e.
expressive dysphasia
expressivity
expressor loop
expulsion
graft e.
expulsive
e. coughing
e. hemorrhage
e. pain
exquisitely tender abdomen
exquisite pain
exsanguinate
exsanguinating hemorrhage
exsanguination
fetal e.
e. protocol
e. tourniquet control
e. transfusion
exsanguine

exsanguinotransfusion
exsect
exsection
exsiccant
exsiccate
exsiccation fever
exstrophy closure
exstrophy-epispadias complex
extended
e. criteria donor (ECD)
e. end-to-end anastomosis
e. field irradiation therapy
e. iliofemoral approach
e. jargon paraphasia
e. left hepatectomy
e. left subcostal incision
e. mandatory minute ventilation (EMMV)
e. maxillotomy
e. mesorectal excision
e. myotomy
e. pancreatoduodenectomy
e. pelvic lymphadenectomy
e. pyelotomy
e. radical mastectomy
e. resection
e. right hemicolectomy
e. right hepatectomy
e. Ross procedure
e. shoulder flap
e. subfrontal approach
e. uvulopalatal flap (EUPF)
extensibility
penile e.
extensible
extension
atlantooccipital e.
attached gingiva e.
e. base
e. block splinting method
e. bridge
caliceal e.
Callahan e.
clot e.
compression e.
cranial e.
e. deformity
distractive e.
e. excementosis
extranodal tumor e.
extrapancreatic e.
extrascleral e.

NOTES

extension (*continued*)
    femoral-trunk e.
    e. fiber
    fingerlike e.
    flexion and e.
    flexion, abduction, external
      rotation, e. (fabere)
    e. form
    full e.
    groove e.
    hip e.
    infarct e.
    e. injury
    e. injury posterior atlantoaxial
      arthrodesis
    e. instability
    internal rotation in e.
    intrasellar e.
    knee e.
    local tumor e.
    lumbar e.
    e. malposition
    orbital e.
    e. osteotomy
    paraplegia in e.
    e. for prevention
    radiolucent operating room table e.
    e. restriction
    ridge e.
    e. stent graft
    subependymal e.
    e. teardrop fracture
    thrombus e.
extension-type cervical spine injury
extensive
    e. approach
    e. bilateral pneumonia
    e. intraductal component (EIC)
    e. lymph node dissection
    e. posterior approach
    e. posterior decompression
extensive-stage disease
extensor
    e. carpi radialis brevis (ECRB)
    e. carpi radialis brevis muscle
    e. carpi radialis brevis tendon
    e. carpi radialis longus (ECRL)
    e. carpi radialis longus flap
    e. carpi radialis longus muscle
    e. carpi radialis longus tendon
    e. carpi ulnaris (ECU)
    e. carpi ulnaris muscle
    e. carpi ulnaris tendon
    e. digiti minimi muscle
    e. digiti minimi tendon
    e. digiti quinti
    e. digiti quinti muscle
    e. digiti quinti tendon
    e. digitorum brevis

    e. digitorum brevis muscle
    e. digitorum brevis tendon
    e. digitorum communis muscle
    e. digitorum communis tendon
    e. digitorum longus
    e. digitorum longus muscle
    e. digitorum longus tendon
    e. digitorum tendon
    e. hallucis
    e. hallucis brevis muscle
    e. hallucis longus (EHL)
    e. hallucis longus muscle
    e. hallucis longus strength
    e. hallucis longus tendon
    e. hood mechanism
    e. indicis proprius muscle
    e. indicis proprius tendon
    knee e.
    e. lengthening
    e. mechanism dysfunction
    e. pollicis brevis
    e. pollicis brevis muscle
    e. pollicis brevis tendon
    e. pollicis longus
    e. pollicis longus muscle
    e. pollicis longus tendon
    e. quinti tendon
    radial wrist e.
    e. retinaculum
    e. surface
    e. tendon injury
    e. tendon repair
    e. tenodesis
    e. tenotomy
    e. tetanus
    e. thrust reflex
    toe e.
    wrist e.
exteriorization colostomy
exteriorize
exteriorized
    e. stuttering
    e. uterine repair
externa
    otitis e.
external
    e. absorption
    e. acoustic foramen
    e. acoustic meatus artery
    e. arcuate fiber
    e. auditory canal
    e. auditory exostosis (EAE)
    e. auditory larynx
    e. auditory meatus
    e. beam irradiation
    e. beam radiation therapy
    e. bevel incision
    e. bile drainage
    e. bile tract drainage

e. biliary drainage
e. biliary fistula
e. biliary lavage
e. bleeding
e. bracing
e. branch
e. canthotomy
e. canthus
e. capsule
e. cardiac massage
e. carotid
e. carotid artery (ECA)
e. carotid plexus
e. clot
e. cooling
e. cuneate nucleus
e. dental epithelium
e. direct pressure
e. ear
e. elastic lamina
e. enamel epithelium
e. ethmoidectomy
e. female genital organ
e. fetal monitoring
e. geniculate body
e. genitalia
e. genitalia, Bartholin, urethral, and
Skene (EG/BUS)
e. genitalia, Bartholin, urethral, and
Skene glands
e. grid
e. hemipelvectomy
e. hemorrhage
e. hemorrhoid
e. hordeolum
e. iliac artery
e. iliac plexus
e. ilium
e. ilium movement
e. inguinal ring
e. ligament
e. male genital organ
e. mammary artery
e. maxillary artery
e. maxillary plexus
e. nasal nerve
e. nose
e. oblique
e. oblique aponeurosis
e. oblique fascia
e. oblique line
e. oblique reflex

e. oblique ridge
e. occipital crest
e. orbital fracture
e. orthovoltage irradiation
e. os
e. pancreatic fistula
e. pin fixation
e. pneumatic calf compression
posteroinferior e.
e. pudendal artery
e. rectal sphincter
e. respiration
e. rotation
e. rotation-abduction stress test
e. rotation-recurvatum test
e. rotator
e. route
e. saphenous nerve
e. scanning
e. shockwave lithotripsy
e. spermatic artery
e. spermatic fascia
e. spermatic nerve
e. sphincterotomy
e. spinal fixation
e. stimulus
e. support
e. surface
e. swelling
e. transcutaneous pacing
e. trauma
e. urethral orifice
e. urethral sphincter
e. urethrotomy
e. vacuum therapy
e. ventricular drainage
e. x-ray therapy
external-coil electrical stimulation
external/internal
e./i. rotation
e./i. rotation ratio
externalization
externally
e. releasable knot
e. rotated
externum
externus
extinction
e. phenomenon
sensory e.
visual e.
extinguishing

NOTES

extirpate
extirpation
    Amreich vaginal e.
    dental pulp e.
    nodal e.
    pulp e.
    Rubbrecht e.
    sac e.
    surgical e.
extorsion
extortor
extraabdominal
    e. anastomosis
    e. anastomotic healing
    e. disease
    e. infective complication
    e. injury
    e. operation
    e. position
    e. site
extraalveolar
extraanatomic
    e. bypass
    e. bypass method
    e. bypass procedure
    e. bypass technique
extraanatomical renal revascularization
  technique
extraarachnoid injection
extraarticular
    e. ankylosis
    e. arthrodesis
    e. augmentation
    e. graft
    e. hip fusion
    e. pain syndrome
    e. procedure
    e. reconstruction
    e. resection
    e. structure
    e. subtalar fusion
    e. subtalar joint
    e. technique
    e. tissue
    e. tuberculosis
extraaxial
    e. compartment
    e. fluid collection
extrabuccal
extrabursal approach
extracaliceal
extracanthic
extracapillary crescent formation
extracapsular
    e. ankylosis
    e. aphakia
    e. approach
    e. arterial ring
    e. cataract extraction (ECCE)

    e. cataract extraction operation
    e. disease
    e. dissection
    e. fracture
    e. metastasis
    e. tissue
extracardiac
    e. mass
    e. murmur
extracavitary approach
extracellular
    e. compartment
    e. fluid
    e. fluid volume (ECFV)
    e. granule
    e. ground substance
    e. matrix
    e. matrix remodeling
    e. matrix system
    e. plasma
    e. space
    e. toxin
extracellular-like, calcium-free solution
extracerebral fluid collection
extrachorial placenta
extrachromosomal
extraciliary fiber
extracolonic
extraconal fat reticulum
extracoronal
    e. retention
    e. splinting
extracoronary
extracorporeal
    e. anastomosis
    e. bypass pump (ECBP)
    e. cardiopulmonary circuit
    e. circulation (ECC)
    e. CO_2 removal (ECOR)
    e. dialysis
    e. exchange hypothermia
    e. heart
    e. irradiation
    e. jamming knot
    e. life support (ECLS)
    e. liver perfusion
    e. membrane oxygenation (ECMO)
    e. method
    e. partial nephrectomy
    e. piezoelectric shockwave
      lithotripsy
    e. procedure
    e. renal preservation
    e. repair
    e. shock wave lithotripsy
    e. shock wave treatment (ESWT)
    e. surgery
    e. technique

e. ultrafiltration
e. venous bypass

extracranial
e. carotid artery disease
e. carotid circulation
e. carotid occlusive disease
e. cerebral vasculature
e. mass lesion
e. occlusive vascular disease

extracranial-intracranial
e.-i. bypass
e.-i. bypass surgery

extract
adipose tissue e.
adrenocortical e.
aqueous e.
ceanothus e.
lyophilized e.
pancreatic e.
parathyroid e.
phenol-preserved e.
Rauwolfia e.
venom e.
whole-body e.

extraction
allograft e.
Arroyo cataract e.
Arruga cataract e.
bag e.
Baker pyridine e.
e. balloon technique
e. bile duct stone
breech e.
Burhenne biliary duct stone e.
cataract e.
Chandler-Verhoeff lens e.
comedo e.
countercurrent e.
elevator e.
endoscopic e.
extracapsular cataract e. (ECCE)
first-pass e.
e. flap
forceps e.
foreign body e.
harpoon e.
e. incision
intracapsular cataract e.
intraocular cataract e.
lactate e.
laparoscopic stone e.
liquid e.

magnetic e.
manual e.
Marshall-Taylor vacuum e.
menstrual e.
micro liquid e.
e. pancreatic stone
partial breech e.
planned extracapsular cataract e.
podalic e.
progressive e.
rubber-band e.
serial e.
e. site
solid phase e.
solvent e.
e. space
spontaneous breech e.
stone e.
systemic oxygen e.
tooth e.
total breech e.
vacuum e.

extractor
acetabular cup e.
intramedullary nail e.

extracystic
extradental projection
extradomain A positive
extradural
e. abscess
e. anesthesia
e. anesthetic technique
e. block
e. clinoidectomy
e. exposure
e. granulation
e. hematoma
e. hematorrhachis
e. hemorrhage
e. phase
e. space
e. vertebral artery

extraembryonic mesoderm
extraepiphysial
extrafascial hysterectomy
extragenital
extraglandular conversion
extraglomerular mesangium
extragonadal
extrahepatic
e. abdominal carcinoma
e. access

E

NOTES

extrahepatic *(continued)*
  e. bile duct
  e. bile duct cancer
  e. bile duct obstruction
  e. biliary atresia
  e. biliary cystic dilation
  e. biliary obstruction
  e. biliary tree
  e. binary obstruction
  e. control
  e. dissection
  e. lesion
  e. metastasis
  e. nodal disease
  e. portal vein obstruction (EHPO)
  e. portal venous hypertension
  e. stone
  e. tumor
  e. tumor site
extraintestinal complication
extrajection
extralaryngeal approach
extraligamentous
extralobar
extraluminal
  e. gas
  e. hemorrhage
extralymphatic metastasis
extramammary Paget disease
extramaxillary anchorage
extramedullary
  e. alignment
  e. alignment arch
  e. involvement
  e. mass
  e. myelopoiesis
  e. segment
  e. toxicity
extramucosal
  e. mass
  e. pyloromyotomy
  e. stitch
extramural
  e. lesion
  e. upper airway obstruction
extraneous movement
extranodal
  e. disease
  e. site
  e. tumor extension
extraoctave fracture
extraocular
  e. movement
  e. muscle
  e. muscle involvement
  e. muscles of Tillaux
extraoral
  e. anchorage
  e. radiographic examination profile

extraorbital disease
extraovular
extrapancreatic
  e. extension
  e. nerve plexus
extrapapillary
extraperineal
extraperiosteal
extraperitoneal
  e. approach
  e. carbon dioxide insufflation
  e. cesarean section
  e. CO_2 insufflation
  e. endoscopic hernia repair
  e. endoscopic pelvic lymph node
    dissection
  e. fascia
  e. ileostomy
  e. laparoscopic bladder neck
    suspension
  e. laparoscopic herniorrhaphy
  e. laparoscopic nephrectomy
  e. location
  e. space
  e. tissue
  totally e. (TEP)
extrapetrosal drainage
extrapharyngeal
  e. approach
  e. exposure
extraplacental
extrapleural
  e. air
  e. anastomosis
  e. apicolysis
  e. approach
  e. pneumothorax
  e. space
extrapolate
extrapolated end-tidal carbon dioxide
  tension (PETCO$_2$)
extrapolation
extraprostatic
extrapsychic
extrapulmonary
  e. cough
  e. *Pneumocystis carinii* infection
  e. site
  e. tuberculosis
extrapyramidal
  e. disease
  e. dyskinesia
  e. function assessment
  e. nucleus
  e. pathway
  e. reaction
  e. sign
  e. syndrome
  e. tract

extrarectus
extrarenal
    e. mass
    e. renal pelvis
extraretinal
extrasaccular hernia
extrascleral extension
extrasensory
extraskeletal
extrasphincteric anal fistula
extraspinal osteoid osteoma
extrastimulus test
extratemporal
    e. epilepsy
    e. excision
extratesticular lesion
extrathoracic
    e. metastasis
    e. position
    e. tuberculosis
extrathyroid
    e. invasion
    e. spread
extratracheal
extrauterine pelvic mass
extravaginal testicular torsion
extravasate
extravasation
    e. extremity
    e. extrusion
    e. feces
    fluid e.
    e. gas
    e. injury
    e. irrigation solution
    e. phenomenon
extravascular
    e. compartment
    e. fluid balance
    e. granulomatous feature
    e. lung water
    e. mass
    e. space
extraventricular
extraversion
    urinary e.
extravesical
    e. anastomosis
    e. infrasphincteric ectopic ureter
    e. Lich approach
    e. ureteral reimplantation technique
    e. ureterolysis

extreme
    e. capsule
    e. drug resistance (EDR)
    e. hearing loss
    e. lateral transcondylar approach
    e. somatosensory evoked potential
extremis
    in e.
extremital
extremitas
extremity
    e. abnormality
    acromial e.
    e. amputation
    anterior e.
    elevation of e.
    extravasation e.
    flaccid e.
    e. injury
    e. ischemia
    left lower e. (LLE)
    left upper e. (LUE)
    e. lesion
    lower e.
    e. malformation
    e. melanoma
    e. mobilization technique
    e. preservation
    right lower e. (RLE)
    right upper e. (RUE)
    upper e.
extrinsic
    e. allergic alveolitis
    e. asthma
    e. bladder compression
    e. denervation
    e. entrapment test
    e. environmental staining
    e. esophageal impression
    e. lesion
    e. mass
    e. mechanism
    e. muscle
    e. muscle strength
    e. nerve
    e. pathway
    e. semiconductor
    e. sphincter
extrodactyly
extrospection
extroversion

E

NOTES

extruded
- e. disc
- e. disc fragment
- e. teeth

extrusion
- bone graft e.
- disc e.
- extravasation e.
- implant e.
- oocyte e.
- placental e.
- sealer e.
- tube e.
- wire e.

extubate

extubation
- e. anesthetic technique
- early e.
- postoperative e.

exuberant granulation tissue

exudate
- acute inflammatory e.
- circinate e.
- conjunctival e.
- cotton-wool e.
- fatty e.
- fibrinous e.
- fluffy cotton-wool e.
- foaming e.
- gingival e.
- hard e.
- inflammatory e.
- mucopurulent e.
- pharyngeal e.
- purulent e.
- retinal e.
- sanguineous e.
- serous e.
- soft e.
- suppurative e.
- waxy e.

exudation
- aqueous e.
- fibrinous e.
- gingival e.
- proteinaceous aqueous e.
- purulent e.

exudative
- e. ascites
- e. eye
- e. granulomatous inflammation
- e. papulosquamous disease
- e. pleural effusion
- e. retinal detachment
- e. tuberculosis
- e. vitreoretinopathy
- e. zone

exude

exumbilication

eye
- e. disease
- e. enucleation
- e. examination
- exciting e.
- exudative e.
- e. irrigating solution
- e. muscle surgery
- pineal e.
- e. point
- e. rotation
- stony-hard e.
- e. tumor
- e. tumor localization
- web e.

eyeball
- e. compression reflex
- e. equator

eyebrow
- e. fixation
- e. laceration

eye-closure reflex

eye-ear plane

eyelash
- ectopic e.
- e. reflex

eyelid
- e. fusion
- e. molluscum contagiosum infection
- e. surgery
- e. tumor
- upper e.

eyelid-closure reflex

Eyler flexorplasty

F2 focal point
FA
    failure analysis
FAB
    French-American-British
        FAB classification
        FAB staging
fabere
    flexion, abduction, external rotation,
        extension
        fabere sign
Fabricius ship
FAC
    fractional area change
face
        cow f.
        dish f.
        f. form
        inferior f.
        f. line
        f.'s rating scale for children
        superior f.
face-down position
facelift
facet
        f. anomaly
        articular f.
        clavicular f.
        corneal f.
        costal f.
        f. denervation
        f. dislocation
        f. excision technique
        f. fracture stabilization wiring
        f. fusion
        f. imbrication
        inferior costal f.
        f. joint
        f. joint injection
        f. joint preparation
        f. joint syndrome
        perched f.
        f. plane
        f. rhizotomy
        f. subluxation stabilization wiring
        superior costal f.
        transverse costal f.
        f. tropism
facetectomy
        O'Donoghue f.
        partial f.
face-to-face venacavaplasty
face-to-pubes position
facetted corneal scar

facial
        F. Action Coding System
        f. angiofibroma
        f. angle
        f. artery
        f. axis
        f. bipartition
        f. bone
        f. butt joint preparation
        f. canal
        f. cleft
        f. colliculus
        f. deformity
        f. excursion measurement
        f. expression
        f. foundation
        f. fracture
        f. height
        f. index
        f. laser resurfacing
        f. muscle
        f. nerve
        f. nerve-preserving parotidectomy
        f. nerve root
        f. osteosynthesis
        f. pain
        f. plane
        f. plexus
        f. profile
        f. reanimation
        f. restoration
        f. root
        transverse f.
        f. triangle
        f. vein
facies
        acromial articular f.
        Potter f.
facilitated angioplasty
facilitating restoration
facilitation
        convergence f.
        neuromuscular f.
        postactivation f.
        posttetanic f.
        proprioceptive neuromuscular f.
        Wedensky f.
facioplasty
facioscapulohumeral muscular dystrophy
faciotelencephalic malformation
FACS
        Fellow of American College of Surgeons
        fluorescence-activated cell sorter
factitious hyperthyroidism

F

factor
- acidic fibroblast growth f.
- atrial natriuretic f. (ANF)
- circulating MEN I-specific growth f.
- clotting f.
- coagulating f.
- coagulation f.
- endothelium-derived relaxing f.
- epidermal growth f. (EGF)
- fibroblast growth f. (FGF)
- growth f.
- gut proliferative f.
- hepatocyte growth f. (HGF)
- human epidermal growth f. (hEGF)
- inflammatory transcription f.
- insulin-like growth f. I (IGF-1)
- luminal f.
- orexigenic f.
- pathophysiologic f.
- patient-dependent f.
- perioperative risk f.
- polypeptide growth f.
- predisposing f.
- preoperative f.
- prognostic f.
- proliferative f.
- f. replacement therapy
- risk f.
- technical f.
- thromboembolic risk f.
- transforming growth f. (TGF)
- tumor necrosis f. (TNF)
- vascular endothelial growth f. (VEGF)
- f. V Leiden mutation
- von Willebrand f.

factor-alpha
- tumor necrosis f.-a. (TNF-alpha)

faculty
- fusion f.

fade
- tetanic f.

Faden
- F. operation
- F. procedure

Fahey
- F. approach
- F. technique

Fahey-O'Brien technique
Fahraeus method
failed
- f. anesthesia
- f. back surgery syndrome
- f. femoral osteotomy
- f. intubation
- f. procedure
- f. spinal
- f. surgery

failure
- acute respiratory f.
- f. analysis (FA)
- anastomotic f.
- f. to awaken
- bone marrow f.
- bypass f.
- chronic intestinal f.
- chronic renal f. (CRF)
- cocaine-induced respiratory f.
- congestive heart f.
- differentiation f.
- dilator placement f.
- end-organ f.
- end-stage intestinal f.
- exercise-associated acute renal f.
- fulminant hepatic f. (FHF)
- functional intestinal f.
- graft f.
- Harrington rod instrumentation f.
- heart f.
- hepatic f.
- hepatorenal f.
- implant f.
- implantation f.
- instrumentation f.
- intestinal f.
- intubation f.
- irradiation f.
- late graft f.
- late-onset hepatic f. (LOHF)
- late wound f.
- liver f.
- microcirculatory f.
- multiorgan f. (MOF)
- multiorgan system f.
- multiple organ f. (MOF)
- multiple organ system f.
- multiple system organ f.
- multisystem f.
- multisystem organ f. (MSOF)
- pacemaker f.
- postburn bone marrow f.
- postoperative hepatic f.
- postoperative liver f.
- posttraumatic renal f.
- pouch f.
- progressive liver f.
- progressive respiratory f.
- renal f.
- f. to rescue
- respiratory f.
- sclerotherapy f.
- surgeon-dependent technique f.
- surgical f.
- suture f.
- technical f.
- wound f.

Fairbanks-Sever procedure

Fairbanks technique
falcate
falces (*pl. of* falx)
falciform
    f. cartilage
    f. crest
    f. ligament
    f. margin
    f. process
    f. retinal fold
Falconer lobectomy
Falk-Shukuris operation
Falk vesicovaginal fistula technique
Fallat-Buckholz method
falling hematocrit
fallopian
    f. canal
    f. hiatus
    f. ligament
    f. tube
    f. tube carcinoma
    f. tube catheterization
    f. tube mass
    f. tube metastasis
Fallot
    tetralogy of F.
false
    f. aneurysm
    f. channel formation
    f. cord carcinoma
    f. diverticulum
    f. knot
    f. membrane
    f. negative
    f. pelvis
    f. positive
    f. projection
    f. rib
    f. suture
    f. vertebra
    f. vocal cord
false-negative
    f.-n. cholangiogram
    f.-n. result
false-positive
    f.-p. interpretation
    f.-p. result
falx, pl. **falces**
familial
    f. adenomatous polyposis (FAP)
    f. aortic ectasia syndrome
    f. atypical mole and melanoma (FAM-M)
    f. atypical multiple mole melanoma syndrome
    f. breast cancer
    f. cardiac myxoma syndrome
    f. cholestasis syndrome
    f. colon cancer (FCC)
    f. consequence
    f. dysautonomia
    f. exudative vitreoretinopathy
    f. hemiplegic migraine
    f. HPT
    f. hypocalciuric hypercalcemia
    f. indication
    f. Mediterranean fever
    f. multigland disease
    f. osteochondrodystrophy
    f. paroxysmal rhabdomyolysis
    f. polyposis syndrome
FAM-M
    familial atypical mole and melanoma
    FAM-M syndrome
fan beam projection
Fanconi anemia
Fanta cataract operation
fan-type retractor
FAP
    familial adenomatous polyposis
far
    f. lateral inferior suboccipital approach
    f. point
Farabeuf
    F. amputation
    F. ischiopubiotomy
    F. triangle
Faraday
    F. law of electrolysis
    F. law of induction
far-and-near suture technique
Farmer
    F. operation
    F. technique
Farre white line
Fasanella operation
Fasanella-Servat
    F.-S. procedure
    F.-S. ptosis operation
fascia, pl. **fasciae**
    f. of abdomen
    Abernethy f.

NOTES

255

fascia *(continued)*
    alar f.
    anal f.
    antebrachial f.
    anterior rectus f.
    axillary f.
    brachial f.
    broad f.
    buccopharyngeal f.
    Buck f.
    bulbar sheath f.
    Camper f.
    cervical f.
    clavipectoral f.
    Cloquet f.
    Colles f.
    Cooper f.
    cremasteric f.
    cribriform f.
    crural f.
    Cruveilhier f.
    dartos f.
    deep cervical f.
    deltopectoral f.
    Denonvilliers f.
    endoabdominal f.
    endopelvic f.
    endothoracic f.
    external oblique f.
    external spermatic f.
    extraperitoneal f.
    fusion f.
    geniohyoid f.
    Gerota f.
    gluteal f.
    Godman f.
    Hesselbach f.
    iliac f.
    f. iliaca block
    iliopectineal f.
    incised f.
    infundibuliform f.
    intercolumnar f.
    internal spermatic f.
    investing f.
    lacrimal f.
    f. lata
    lumbodorsal f.
    masseteric f.
    muscular f.
    nuchal f.
    obturator f.
    orbital f.
    palpebral f.
    pancreatic f.
    parietal pelvic f.
    parotid f.
    parotideomasseteric f.
    pectineal f.

    pectoral f.
    pectoralis f.
    pelvic f.
    perirenal f.
    pharyngobasilar f.
    phrenicopleural f.
    popliteal f.
    Porter f.
    prepubic f.
    presacral f.
    pretracheal f.
    prevertebral f.
    psoas f.
    rectal f.
    rectovesical f.
    renal f.
    retrosacral f.
    retrovisceral f.
    salpingopharyngeal f.
    scalene f.
    Scarpa f.
    Sibson f.
    subcutaneous f.
    subperitoneal f.
    superficial inguinal f.
    superior f.
    temporal f.
    thoracolumbar f.
    Toldt f.
    transversalis f.
    transverse f.
    Treitz f.
    triangular f.
    Tyrrell f.
    umbilical prevesical f.
    umbilicovesical f.
    visceral pelvic f.
    Zuckerkandl f.

fascial
    f. arthroplasty
    f. bridge
    f. closure
    f. decompression
    f. defect
    f. flap
    f. graft
    f. hernia
    f. layer
    f. plane
    f. shutter mechanism
    f. sling approach
    f. sling procedure
    f. space
    f. space infection
    f. stranding
    f. wrapping
    f. zipper
fasciaplasty
fascia-splitting incision

fascicular
    f. graft
    f. repair
fasciculata
fasciculation
    benign f.
    contraction f.
    malignant f.
    f. potential
    tongue f.
fasciculus, pl. fasciculi
    wedge-shaped f.
fasciectomy
    dermal f.
    limited f.
    partial f.
    radical palmar f.
fasciitis
fasciocutaneous
    f. free flap
    f. island flap
fasciodesis
fasciola
fascioplasty
fasciorrhaphy
fascioscapulohumeral
fasciotomy
    decompression f.
    double-incision f.
    endoscopic plantar f.
    percutaneous plantar f.
    plantar f.
    prophylactic f.
    Rorabeck f.
    single-incision f.
    Skoog f.
    subcutaneous f.
    Yount f.
fashion
    concertina-like f.
    isolated f.
    perpendicular f.
    standard f.
    Z f.
FAST
    fluorescent antibody staining technique
    Fourier-acquired steady-state technique
fast
    f. exposure technique
    f. film exposure
    f. neutron radiation therapy
    f. spin-echo sequence

fast-flush test
fastigiobulbar tract
fasting
    preoperative f.
    f. recording
fast-pathway radiofrequency ablation
fast-track cardiac anesthesia
fat
    abdominal f.
    f. body
    body f.
    f. cell space
    creeping f.
    f. flap
    f. globule
    f. graft
    herniated preperitoneal f.
    f. herniation
    f. line
    f. necrosis
    f. pad
    f. pad sign
    periesophageal f.
    f. plane
    preperitoneal f.
    properitoneal f.
    total body f.
fatal
    F. Accident Reporting System
    f. air embolus
    f. cardiac event
fat-density line
fat-free mass
fatigue
    excessive f.
    f. fracture
    implant f.
    postoperative f.
    suture f.
fat-suppression technique
fatty
    f. apron
    f. ascites
    f. exudate
    f. hernia
    f. infiltration
    f. prostatic tissue
    f. renal capsule
fauces
faucial branch
faucium

NOTES

F

faulty
    f. contact point
    f. restoration
Favaloro saphenous vein bypass graft
FBS
    fetal bovine serum
FCC
    familial colon cancer
FDA Anesthesia Apparatus Checkout Recommendations
FDPCA
    fixed-dose patient-controlled analgesia
FDT
    forced duction test
Feagin shoulder dislocation test
fear subscale
feather-edged proximal finishing line
featural surgery
feature
    clinical manifestations, etiologic factors, anatomic involvement, pathophysiologic f.'s (CEAP)
    clinicopathologic f.
    cytologic f.
    extravascular granulomatous f.
    histopathologic f.
    immunohistochemical f.
    preoperative f.
    tumor f.
febrile morbidity
fecal
    f. abscess
    f. contamination
    f. diversion
    f. diversion colostomy
    f. fistula
    f. impaction
    f. incontinence
    f. load
    f. loading
    f. occult blood testing (FOBT)
    f. soiling
    f. stream
fecalith
    appendiceal f.
fecaloma
    stercoral f.
fecaluria
feces
    extravasation f.
Federation of Gynecology and Obstetrics classification
feedback reduction circuit
feeder-frond technique
feeding
    f. complication
    drip-tube f.
    early enteral f.
    enteral f.

    gastrostomy f.
    f. gastrostomy
    jejunostomy elemental diet f.
    jejunostomy tube f.
    oral f.
    postoperative regimen for oral early f. (PROEF)
    tube f.
    f. tube placement
Feiss line
Feist-Mankin position
Fellow of American College of Surgeons (FACS)
felon infection
Felson
    silhouette sign of F.
feltwork
female
    f. castration
    f. gonad
    f. prostate
    f. urethra
    f. urethral syndrome
feminization syndrome
feminizing genitoplasty
femoral
    f. arch
    f. artery
    f. artery aneurysm
    f. artery approach
    f. canal
    f. circulation
    f. cortical ring allograft
    f. diaphysial fracture
    f. diaphysis
    f. elevator
    f. embolectomy
    f. endarterectomy
    f. epiphysial fracture
    f. epiphysiolysis
    f. epiphysis
    f. fossa
    f. head
    f. head line
    f. hernia
    f. intertrochanteric fracture
    f. metaphysis
    f. muscle
    f. nailing
    f. neck fracture
    f. neck fracture reduction
    f. nerve
    f. nerve block
    f. nerve traction test
    f. osteotomy
    f. plexus
    f. prosthesis
    f. prosthesis fixation
    f. puncture

f. region
f. resection
f. ring
f. septum
f. shaft
f. shaft fracture
f. sheath
f. stem removal
f. supracondylar fracture
f. 3-in-1 technique
f. triangle
f. vein

femoral-popliteal artery bypass
femoral-tibial-peroneal bypass
femoral-trunk extension
femoris
femorodistal

f. bypass
f. reconstructive surgery

femorofemoral (FF)

f. crossover

femoroischial transplantation
femoropopliteal

f. bypass
f. bypass graft
f. occlusive disease

femorotibial
femur distractor
fender fracture
fenestra, pl. **fenestrae**
fenestrated

f. endothelium
f. Fontan operation
f. membrane
f. sheath

fenestration

alveolar plate f.
aortopulmonary f.
apical f.
atrophic f.
baffle f.
catheter-directed f.
cusp f.
cyst f.
dental f.
intercellular f.
laparoscopic f.
Lempert f.
f. operation
tracheal f.

Fenton vaginoplasty
Ferciot excision

Ferciot-Thomson excision
Ferguson

F. hemorrhoidectomy
F. scoliosis measuring method

Fergus operation
Fergusson incision
Ferkel torticollis technique
fermentation

mixed acid f.

Fernandez

F. extensile anterior approach
F. osteotomy

ferning technique
Ferrein

F. canal
F. cord
F. foramen
F. ligament
F. pyramid

ferromagnetic microembolization treatment
Ferry line
fertility
fertilization

f. age
ex vivo f.
in vitro f.
in vivo f.

FESS

functional endoscopic sinus surgery

festination
fetal

f. acoustic stimulation test
f. aspiration syndrome
f. body movement
f. bone fracture
f. bovine serum (FBS)
f. cardiac anomaly
f. cell transplantation
f. chest anomaly
f. circulation
f. cystic adenomatoid malformation
f. drug therapy
f. duplication
f. exsanguination
f. gastrointestinal anomaly
f. growth acceleration
f. growth retardation
f. head
f. head:abdominal circumference ratio
f. head circumference

F

NOTES

fetal *(continued)*
    f. head position
    f. heart rate
    f. heart rate acceleration
    f. heart rate monitoring
    f. hemorrhage
    f. infection
    f. intracranial anatomy
    f. intrahepatic vein
    f. liver biopsy
    f. liver transplantation
    f. lymphoid tissue
    f. malpresentation
    f. medicine
    f. membrane
    f. reduction
    f. rejection
    f. scalp oxygenation
    f. skin biopsy
    f. surgery
    f. thymus transplantation
    f. tissue sampling
    f. tissue transplant
    f. urogenital tract
    f. vascular anomaly

fetal-maternal
    f.-m. exchange
    f.-m. hemorrhage

fetation

fetoplacental circulation

fetoscopy

FEV₁
    forced expiratory volume in 1 second

fever
    dehydration f.
    exanthematous f.
    exsiccation f.
    familial Mediterranean f.
    fracture f.
    inundation f.
    Mediterranean exanthematous f.
    syphilitic f.

FF
    femorofemoral
    FF crossover

FFP
    fresh frozen plasma

FGF
    fibroblast growth factor
    fresh gas flow

FHF
    fulminant hepatic failure

fiber
    accelerator f.
    anastomotic f.
    association f.
    bundle f.
    f. bundle
    f. bundle volume

    endogenous f.
    exogenous f.
    extension f.
    external arcuate f.
    extraciliary f.
    Gerdy f.
    intercolumnar f.
    intercrural f.
    Nélaton f.
    f. optic laryngoscopy
    osteogenetic f.
    parasympathetic f.
    postganglionic parasympathetic f.
    postganglionic sympathetic f.
    preganglionic parasympathetic f.
    preganglionic sympathetic f.
    projection f.
    pupillodilator f.
    rod f.
    Rosenthal f.
    Sappey f.
    Sharpey f.
    skinned muscle f.
    sympathetic f.
    f. tip modification
    zonular f.

fiberglass graft

fiberoptic
    f. bronchoscopy
    f. bronchoscopy anesthetic technique
    f. bundle
    f. endoscopy anesthetic technique
    f. esophagoscopy
    f. examination
    f. injection sclerotherapy
    f. intraosseous endoscopy
    f. intubation method
    f. intubation procedure
    f. panendoscopy
    f. sigmoidoscopy
    f. tracheal intubation anesthetic technique

fiberoptic-assisted coaxial endotracheal tube exchange

fiberotomy

fiber-splitting incision

fibra, pl. **fibrae**

fibrillary astrocyte

fibrillation
    atrial f.
    auricular f.
    cardiac f.
    chronic atrial f.
    continuous atrial f.
    idiopathic ventricular f.
    lone atrial f.
    paroxysmal atrial f. (PAF)
    f. potential

f. rhythm
synchronized f.
f. threshold
ventricular tachycardia/ventricular f.
fibrillation-flutter
atrial f.-f.
fibrillogranuloma
fibrin
f. calculus
f. degradation product
f. peel
f. plate method
postvitrectomy f.
fibrinogen
f. degradation product
f. method
fibrinogen-fibrin degradation product
fibrinogenolysis
fibrinoid necrotizing inflammation
fibrinolysin coagulation
fibrinolysis
endothelium-dependent f.
primary f.
fibrinopeptide A
fibrinopurulent inflammation
fibrinoscopy
fibrinous
f. adhesion
f. exudate
f. exudation
f. inflammation
fibroadenolipoma
degenerated f.
fibroadenoma
giant f.
fibroadipose tissue
fibroangioma
fibroblast
f. chemoattraction
f. culture
dermal f.
f. growth factor (FGF)
harvested f.
human lung f. (HLF)
keloid f.
f. migration
f. proliferation
fibroblastic tissue
fibroblastoma
fibrocalcification
fibrocalcific lesion
fibrocarcinoma

fibrocartilage
basilar f.
circumferential f.
interarticular f.
semilunar f.
stratiform f.
fibrocartilaginous
fibrocaseous inflammation
fibrocementoma
fibrochondroma
fibrocystic
f. breast syndrome
f. change
f. complex
f. condition
f. disease
fibrocystoma
fibrodentinoma
fibroelastic tissue
fibroelastoma
fibroenchondroma
fibroepithelioma
fibrofascial compartment syndrome
fibrofatty breast tissue
fibrofolliculoma
fibrogliosis
fibrogranuloma
fibrohemangioma
fibrohistiocytic lesion
fibrohistiocytoma
fibroid
f. adenoma
f. inflammation
fibroidectomy
fibrokeratoma
fibroleiomyoma
fibrolipoma
fibroliposarcoma
fibroma
ameloblastic f.
diffuse f.
ossifying f.
psammomatoid ossifying f.
ungual f.
fibromectomy
fibromus
fibromuscular dysplasia (FMD)
fibromusculoelastic lesion
fibromyalgia trigger point
fibromyectomy
fibromyoma
uterine f.

F

NOTES

fibroneuroma
fibroosseous
    f. lesion
    f. ring of Lacroix
fibroplate
fibroproliferative membrane
fibrosa
fibrosarcoma
fibroscopy
fibrosis
    diffuse lobular f.
    epidural f.
    hepatic f.
    idiopathic pulmonary f. (IPF)
    interstitial pulmonary f. (IPF)
    periductal f.
    pulmonary f.
fibrosum
fibrothorax
fibrotic
    f. nub
    f. tissue
    f. wall
fibrotomy
fibrous
    f. adhesion
    f. articular capsule
    f. bone lesion
    f. cap
    f. connective tissue
    f. ingrowth
    f. integration
    f. joint
    f. loose body
    f. obliteration
    f. polypoid lesion
    f. repair
    f. ring
    f. scar tissue
    f. skeleton
    f. tendon sheath
    f. union
fibula
    diastasis f.
fibular
    f. flap
    f. fracture
    f. head
    f. metaphysis
    f. ostectomy
    f. sesamoidectomy
    f. strut graft
fibularis
    f. brevis muscle
    f. longus muscle
    f. longus tendon
    f. tertius muscle
    f. tertius tendon

fibulectomy
    partial f.
fibulocalcaneal ligament
Ficat procedure
Fick
    F. cardiac output measurement
    F. oxygen extraction method
    F. position
    F. principle
    F. technique
Ficoll-Hypaque technique
field
    f. block
    f. block anesthesia
    bloodless f.
    f. cancerization
    f. dissection
    f. of dissection
    2-f. dissection
    electromagnetic f.
    f. expansion
    f. lymphadenectomy
    f. method
    operative f.
    pulsed electromagnetic f. (PEMF)
    surgical f.
3-field
    3-f. dissection
    3-f. lymphanedectomy
field-echo
    f.-e. image
    f.-e. imaging
Fielding
    F. femoral fracture classification
    F. membrane
    F. modification
    F. modification of Gallie technique
Fielding-Magliato subtrochanteric
  fracture classification
fierce cellular rejection
fifth
    f. cranial nerve
    f. metatarsal base fracture
fighter fracture
FIGO
  International Federation of Gynecology
    and Obstetrics
    FIGO classification staging
figure-of-8
    f.-o.-8 preparation
    f.-o.-8 stitch
    f.-o.-8 suture technique
figure-of-4 position
fila (*pl. of* filum)
filament
    corneal f.
filar mass
Filatov
    F. flap

F. keratoplasty
F. operation
Filatov-Gillies
F.-G. flap
F.-G. tubed pedicle
Filatov-Marzinkowsky operation
fill breast implant
filled
decayed, extracted, f.
filler graft
filleted graft
fillet local flap graft
filling
bead technique f.
brush technique f.
f. canal
f. defect
f. first technique
flow technique f.
f. material condensation
nature root canal f.
postresection f.
pressure technique f.
f. procedure
root canal f.
film
abdominal f.
f. identification
f. oxygenation
plain abdominal f.
filmy adhesion
filopressure
filter
f. placement
f. tilt
filtered-back projection
filtered radioisotope
filtering
f. operation
f. procedure
filtration
f. angle
fluid f.
gel f.
glass-wool f.
glomerular f.
f. method
rate of fluid f.
spontaneous ascites f.
f. surgery
filtration-slit membrane

filtrum
filum, pl. **fila**
fimbria, pl. **fimbriae**
ovarian f.
fimbrial evacuation
fimbriated fold
fimbriectomy
fimbrioplasty
Bruhat laser f.
final
f. cementation
f. cone position
f. consonant position
f. growth
f. outcome
finding
barium enema f.
diagnostic f.
endoscopic f.
endovaginal f.
equivocal f.
histologic liver biopsy f.
intraoperative ultrasound f.
irresectable f.
mammographic f.
manometric f.
operative f.
physical f.
prognostic f.
suspicious f.
ultrasonic endovaginal f.
fine manipulation
fine-needle
f.-n. aspiration (FNA)
f.-n. aspiration biopsy
f.-n. aspiration cytology
finger
f. cot
f. deformity
f. dilation
f. flap
f. fracture
f. fracture dissection
f. fracture technique
f. indicator
f. joint arthroplasty
F. Oscillation Test
ring f.
f. web
finger-fillet flap
fingerlike extension
fingerprint line

NOTES

F

263

fingertip
    f. amputation
    f. dissection
fingertrap suspension
Finkelstein maneuver
Fink operation
Finney
    F. gastroenterostomy
    F. operation
    F. pyloroplasty
    F. stricturoplasty
Finochietto-Billroth I gastrectomy
  technique
fire
    nosocomial f.
Fired-Hendel procedure
firm
    f. lesion
    f. mass
    f. texture
first
    f. arch syndrome
    f. carpometacarpal joint fracture
    f. cone position
    f. cranial nerve
    f. cuneiform bone
    f. intention
    f. metacarpal artery
    f. parallel pelvic plane
    f. ray surgery
    f. rib resection via subclavicular
      approach technique
    f. twitch height (T1)
    f. web space
first-degree
    f.-d. burn
    f.-d. hemorrhoid
    f.-d. radiation injury
    f.-d. tuberculum
first-grade fusion
first-line screening technique
first-pass
    f.-p. extraction
    f.-p. technique
first-set graft rejection
first-stage repair
first-strand cDNA synthesis
Fischer projection
Fish cuneiform osteotomy technique
Fisher advancement flap
fisherman's knot
Fishgold line
fishmouth
    f. amputation
    f. anastomosis
    f. fracture
    f. incision
fishtail deformity
fissura, pl. **fissurae**

fissure
    abdominal f.
    anal f.
    auricular f.
    azygos f.
    caudal transverse f.
    f. cavity
    corneal f.
    dorsal f.
    Duverney f.
    Ecker f.
    glaserian f.
    horizontal f.
    inferior accessory f.
    inferior orbital f.
    major f.
    minor f.
    oral f.
    orbital f.
    palpebral f.
    petrooccipital f.
    petrosquamous f.
    petrotympanic f.
    portal f.
    pterygoid f.
    pterygomaxillary f.
    rectal f.
    right sagittal f.
    Rolando f.
    sagittal f.
    Santorini f.
    sphenoidal f.
    sphenomaxillary f.
    sphenopetrosal f.
    squamotympanic f.
    superior orbital f.
    sylvian f.
    tympanomastoid f.
    tympanosquamous f.
    umbilical f.
    vestibular f.
fissured fracture
fistula, pl. **fistulae**
    abdominal wall f.
    alveolar f.
    amphibolic f.
    amphibolous f.
    anal f.
    anastomotic f.
    f. in ano
    anorectal f.
    antecubital arteriovenous f.
    aortocaval f.
    aortoduodenal f.
    aortoenteric f.
    aortoesophageal f.
    aortogastric f.
    aortograft duodenal f.
    aortosigmoid f.

arterial-arterial f.
arterial-enteric f.
arterial-portal f.
arteriobiliary f.
arterioportal f.
arterioportobiliary f.
arteriosinusoidal penile f.
arteriovenous f. (AVF)
arteriovenous subclavian f.
aural f.
A-V f.
benign duodenocolic f.
biliary f.
biliary-bronchial f.
biliary-cutaneous f.
biliary-duodenal f.
biliary-enteric f.
biliocystic f.
biliopleural f.
bladder f.
blind f.
Blom-Singer tracheoesophageal f.
bowel f.
BP f.
brachioaxillary bridge graft f.
brachiosubclavian bridge graft f.
branchial f.
Brescia-Cimino A-V f.
bronchobiliary f.
bronchoesophageal f.
bronchopleural f.
bronchopleurocutaneous f. (BPCF)
bronchopulmonary f.
caliceal f.
cameral f.
carotid-cavernous sinus f.
carotid-dural f.
cavernous sinus f.
cerebrospinal fluid f.
cervical f.
cervicovaginal f.
cholecystenteric f.
cholecystocholedochal f.
cholecystocolic f.
cholecystocolonic f.
cholecystoduodenal f.
cholecystoduodenocolic f.
choledochal-colonic f.
choledochocolonic f.
choledochoduodenal f.
choledochoenteric f.
chyle f.

Cimino f.
Cimino-Brescia arteriovenous f.
closure of f.
coccygeal f.
colobronchial f.
colocutaneous f.
cologastrocutaneous f.
coloileal f.
colonic f.
colorectal f.
colovaginal f.
colovesical f.
communicating f.
complete f.
complex anorectal f.
congenital pulmonary
  arteriovenous f.
congenital tracheobiliary f.
congenital urethroperineal f.
controlled f.
corneal f.
coronary artery f. (CAF)
coronary artery-right ventricular f.
craniosinus f.
cutaneobiliary f.
cystogastric f.
dental f.
dialysis f.
dorsal enteric f.
duodenal f.
duodenocaval f.
duodenocolic f.
duodenoenterocutaneous f.
dural arteriovenous f.
dural cavernous sinus f.
Eck f.
endobronchial f.
endogenous A-V f.
enteric f.
enterocolic f.
enterocutaneous f.
enteroenteral f.
enteroenteric f.
enterogenital f.
enterourethral f.
enterovaginal f.
enterovesical f.
esophageal f.
esophagobronchial f.
esophagocutaneous f.
esophagomediastinal f.
esophagopulmonary f.

F

NOTES

fistula *(continued)*

esophagorespiratory f.
esophagotracheal f.
ethmoid f.
ethmoidal lacrimal f.
external biliary f.
external pancreatic f.
extrasphincteric anal f.
fecal f.
forearm graft arteriovenous f.
gastric f.
gastrocolic f.
gastrocutaneous f.
gastroduodenal f.
gastroenteric f.
gastrointestinal f.
gastrointestinal-cutaneous f.
gastrojejunocolic f.
gastropleural f.
genitourinary f.
gingival f.
graft-enteric f.
Gross tracheoesophageal f.
hepatic artery-portal vein f.
hepatopleural f.
hepatoportal biliary f.
horseshoe f.
H-type tracheoesophageal f.
iatrogenic arteriovenous f.
ileoduodenal f.
ileosigmoid f.
ileovesical f.
incomplete f.
inflammatory f.
internal lacrimal f.
intersphincteric anal f.
intestinal f.
intracranial arteriovenous f.
intrahepatic arterioportal f.
intrahepatic A-V f.
intrahepatic spontaneous
  arterioportal f.
intralabyrinthine f.
intraocular f.
jejunocolic f.
labyrinthine f.
lacrimal f.
lacteal f.
mammary f.
Mann-Bollman f.
mesenteric arteriovenous f.
metroperitoneal f.
mucous f.
oroantral f.
orocutaneous f.
orofacial f.
oronasal f.
pancreatic-cutaneous f.
pancreaticopleural f.

pararectal f.
parietal f.
perianal f.
perilymph f.
perilymphatic f.
perineal urinary f.
perineovaginal f.
pharyngocutaneous f.
pilonidal f.
pleurobiliary f.
pleuroesophageal f.
postbiopsy renal A-V f.
postoperative pleurobiliary f.
postradiation f.
posttraumatic pancreatic-cutaneous f.
preauricular f.
primary arteriovenous f.
pseudocystobiliary f.
pulmonary arteriovenous f. (PAF)
radiculomedullary f.
rectal f.
rectolabial f.
rectourethral f.
rectourinary f.
rectovaginal f.
rectovesical f.
rectovestibular f.
rectovulvar f.
renal f.
renogastric f.
respiratory-esophageal f.
retroperitoneal f.
reverse Eck f.
salivary f.
scleral f.
sigmoid cutaneous f.
sigmoidovesical f.
solitary pulmonary arteriovenous f.
spermatic f.
spinal dural arteriovenous f.
splanchnic A-V f.
splenic A-V f.
splenobronchial f.
stercoral f.
subclavian arteriovenous f.
submental f.
suprasphincteric f.
sylvian f.
synovial f.
systemic arteriovenous f.
TE f.
f. test
thigh graft arteriovenous f.
Thiry f.
Thiry-Vella f.
thoracic duct f.
thromboembolic f.
thyroglossal f.
tracheobiliary f.

tracheobronchoesophageal f.
tracheocutaneous f.
tracheoesophageal f. (TEF)
transsphincteric anal f.
traumatic f.
ulcerogenic f.
umbilical f.
urachal f.
ureteral f.
ureterocolic f.
ureterocutaneous f.
ureteroperitoneal f.
ureterouterine f.
ureterovaginal f.
urethrocavernous f.
urethroperineal f.
urethrorectal f.
urethrovaginal f.
urinary f.
urinary-umbilical f.
urinary-vaginal f.
urogenital f.
uteroperitoneal f.
vaginal f.
vasocutaneous f.
Vella f.
venobiliary f.
vesical f.
vesicoacetabular f.
vesicocolic f.
vesicocutaneous f.
vesicoenteric f.
vesicointestinal f.
vesicoovarian f.
vesicorectal f.
vesicosalpingovaginal f.
vesicouterine f.
vesicovaginal f.
vesicovaginorectal f.
vitelline f.
fistular formation
fistulation
artificial f.
spreading f.
fistulectomy
fistulization
cholecystobiliary f.
fistulizing surgery
fistuloenterostomy
fistulography
fistulotomy
anal f.

choledochoduodenal f.
diathermic f.
endoscopic f.
laying-open f.
Parks method of anal f.
Parks staged f.
fistulous tract
Fite method
fitness for general anesthesia
fitting
fixation
acromioclavicular pin f.
adjunctive screw f.
alcohol f.
angled blade plate f.
anomalous f.
f. anomaly
anterior internal f.
anterior metallic f.
anterior plate f.
anterior screw f.
anterior spinal f.
AO external f.
AO rigid f.
AO spinal internal f.
APR cement f.
Association for the Study of
Internal F. (ASIF)
atlantoaxial rotatory f.
autotrophic f.
axial f.
axis f.
bar bolt f.
Barr open reduction and internal f.
Barr tibial fracture f.
f. base
bicortical screw f.
bifocal f.
bifoveal f.
binocular f.
biologic f.
biphase pin f.
blade plate f.
bolt f.
bone ingrowth f.
bridge plate f.
brow f.
capsular f.
carbon dioxide f.
catheter f.
central f.
cerclage wire f.

F

NOTES

fixation *(continued)*
  cervical screw f.
  cervical spine internal f.
  cervical spine screw-plate f.
  chest wall f.
  circumalveolar f.
  circumferential wire-loop f.
  circummandibular f.
  circumzygomatic f.
  closed reduction and
    percutaneous f. (CRPF)
  cloverleaf condylar plate f.
  Cole tendon f.
  complement f.
  compression plate f.
  condylar screw f.
  coracoclavicular screw f.
  coracoclavicular suture f.
  Cotrel-Dubousset f.
  craniofacial f.
  crossed f.
  f. delay
  Denham external f.
  dens anterior screw f.
  Deverle f.
  Dimon-Hughston fracture f.
  dorsal wire-loop f.
  dynamic compression plate f.
  dynamic condylar screw f.
  eccentric f.
  elastic band f.
  external pin f.
  external spinal f.
  eyebrow f.
  femoral prosthesis f.
  flexion f.
  formalin f.
  fracture f.
  Galveston pelvic f.
  Gouffon pin f.
  graft f.
  greenstick f.
  Guyton-Noyes f.
  Hackethal intramedullary bouquet f.
  half-pin f.
  hook f.
  hook-plate f.
  iliac f.
  Ilizarov external f.
  ingrowth f.
  interference fit f.
  intermaxillary f.
  internal spinal f.
  interosseous wire f.
  intestinal f.
  intramedullary bouquet f.
  intramedullary rod f.
  intraosseous f.
  Kavanaugh-Brower-Mann f.

  Kirschner pin f.
  Kirschner wire f.
  Kronner external f.
  Kyle internal f.
  lag screw f.
  line of f.
  loop f.
  lumbar pedicle f.
  lumbar spine segmental f.
  lumbar spine transpedicular f.
  Luque-Galveston f.
  Luque loop f.
  Luque rod f.
  Magerl posterior cervical screw f.
  mandibular f.
  mandibulomaxillary f.
  Matta-Saucedo f.
  maxillomandibular f. (MMF)
  McKeever medullary clavicle f.
  medial malleolus f.
  medullary clavicle f.
  medullary nail f.
  metallic rod f.
  microwave f.
  monocular f.
  multiple-point sacral f.
  nail plate f.
  nasomandibular f.
  near f.
  neutralization plate f.
  Nichols sacrospinous f.
  f. object
  occipitocervical f.
  odontoid fracture internal f.
  odontoid screw f.
  open reduction and internal f.
    (ORIF)
  Orthofix large-pin f.
  osseous f.
  pedicle screw-rod f.
  pedicular f.
  pelvic f.
  percutaneous f.
  phalangeal fracture f.
  Phemister acromioclavicular pin f.
  pin f.
  pin-and-plaster f.
  plate f.
  plate-screw f.
  f. point
  4-point f.
  porous ingrowth f.
  posterior cervical f.
  posterior screw f.
  posterior segmental f.
  prophylactic skeletal f.
  provisional f.
  pubic f.
  f. reflex

restorative f.
rigid internal f.
rigid plate f.
rod sleeve f.
role f.
rotatory f.
sacral pedicle screw f.
sacral spine f.
sacroiliac extension f.
sacroiliac flexion f.
sacrospinous ligament vaginal f.
sacrum fusion screw f.
Schneider f.
scoliotic curve f.
screw f.
screw-and-plate f.
screw-and-wire f.
secondary f.
segmental f.
skeletal f.
spinal f.
split f.
spring f.
standard formalin f.
staple f.
static f.
Steinmann pin f.
strut plate f.
sublaminar f.
sulcus f.
suture f.
f. suture technique
f. target
f. technique
tension band f.
tibial fracture f.
transarticular wire f.
transcapitellar wire f.
transiliac rod f.
transodontoid screw f.
transpedicular screw-rod f.
transverse f.
TSRH rod f.
tunnel and sling f.
vaginal f.
visual f.
white f.
wire-loop f.

fixator
f. interne
f. muscle

fixed
f. deformity
f. dose
f. drain pipe urethra
f. lung
f. maintainer space
f. point
f. sediment method
f. subcutaneous dose

fixed-dose
f.-d. analysis
f.-d. patient-controlled analgesia
(FDPCA)

fixture
implant f.

flabby abdomen

flaccida
pars f.

flaccid extremity

flag flap

flail
f. chest
f. knee

FLAIR
fluid-attenuated inversion recovery
FLAIR image
FLAIR sequence

Flajani operation

FLAK
flow artifact killer
FLAK technique

flame hemorrhage

flame-shaped hemorrhage

flammable anesthetic

flank
f. approach
f. bone
f. dissection
f. gunshot wound
f. incision
f. incisional hernia
f. mass
f. position

flap
Abbe f.
Abbe-Estlander f.
abdominal fasciocutaneous f.
access f.
advancement f.
advancement of rectal f.
anconeus muscle f.
anterior helical rim free f.

F

NOTES

flap *(continued)*

apically repositioned f.
aponeurotic f.
apron f.
arm f.
arterial f.
arterialized f.
artery island f.
Atasoy-Kleinert f.
Atasoy palmar f.
Atasoy triangular advancement f.
Atasoy volar V-Y f.
axial flag f.
axial pattern scalp f.
axillary f.
bicoronal scalp f.
bilateral V-Y Kutler f.
bilobed skin f.
bilobed transposition f.
bipedicle dorsal f.
bladder f.
Bland onlay f.
Blaskovics f.
Boari bladder f.
Boari-Ockerblad f.
bone f.
brachioradialis f.
breast f.
bridge pedicle f.
buccal mucosal f.
bulbocavernosus fat f.
buried f.
bursal f.
butterfly f.
Byers f.
carrier f.
cartilage f.
caterpillar f.
cecal f.
cellulocutaneous f.
cervical f.
cheek advancement f.
cheek rotation f.
Chinese f.
cocked-half f.
composite f.
compound f.
f. congestion
conjunctival f.
conjunctivo-Tenon f.
corneal f.
cross f.
crossarm f.
cross-finger f.
cross-leg f.
cross-lip pedicle f.
C-shaped scalp f.
cutaneous forearm f.
Cutler-Beard bridge f.

Dandy myocutaneous scalp f.
deep circumflex iliac artery-iliac crest f.
deepithelialized rectus abdominis muscle f.
delayed f.
deltoid f.
deltopectoral f.
deltoscapular f.
dermal fat free f.
dermal fat pedicle f.
digastric muscle f.
digital f.
direct f.
distant f.
dorsal cross-finger f.
dorsal rotation f.
dorsal transposition f.
double lateral advancement f.
double pedicle TRAM f.
DRAM f.
duodenal f.
f. elevation
Eloesser f.
endorectal f.
envelope f.
epaulet f.
equal sagittal f.
Estlander f.
Estlander-Abbe f.
extended shoulder f.
extended uvulopalatal f. (EUPF)
extensor carpi radialis longus f.
extraction f.
fascial f.
fasciocutaneous free f.
fasciocutaneous island f.
fat f.
fibular f.
Filatov f.
Filatov-Gillies f.
finger f.
finger-fillet f.
Fisher advancement f.
flag f.
flat f.
foot first-web f.
foramen ovale f.
forearm f.
forehead f.
foreskin f.
forked f.
fornix-based f.
free bone f.
free fasciocutaneous f.
free fibular harvest f.
free latissimus dorsi f.
free microsurgical f.
free radial forearm f.

free skin f.
free temporal f.
French f.
full-thickness periodontal f.
fusiform f.
galeal f.
gastrocnemius sliding f.
Gilbert scapular f.
gingival f.
glabellar bilobed f.
glabellar rotation f.
gluteus maximus f.
gracilis muscle f.
gracilis myocutaneous f.
f. graft
groin f.
Gunderson conjunctival f.
hemipulp f.
hemitongue f.
hinged corneal f.
horizontal f.
horseshoe-shaped f.
Hughes tarsoconjunctival f.
hypogastric f.
ideal f.
iliac crest free f.
iliac crest osseous f.
iliac crest osteocutaneous f.
iliac crest osteomuscular f.
iliac osteocutaneous free f.
iliofemoral pedicle f.
immediate f.
Indian f.
inferior f.
intercostal f.
interdigitating skin f.
internal oblique osteomuscular f.
interpolated f.
interpolation f.
intimal f.
intraoral f.
inverted skin f.
I-shaped scalp f.
island pedicle scalp f.
island skin f.
Italian f.
jejunal free f.
jump f.
Karapandzic f.
Karydakis f.
Koerner f.
Kutler digital f.

Kutler double lateral
  advancement f.
Kutler V-Y f.
lateral cartilage f.
latissimus dorsi island f.
latissimus dorsi muscle f.
latissimus dorsi musculocutaneous f.
latissimus dorsi myocutaneous f.
latissimus-scapular muscle f.
latissimus-serratus muscle f.
limbal-based f.
Limberg f.
lined f.
lingual tongue f.
Linton f.
lip switch f.
liver f.
local muscle f.
local skin f.
lower trapezius f.
lumbrical muscle f.
major myocutaneous f.
maple leaf f.
Martius bulbocavernosus fat f.
masseter muscle f.
Mathieu island onlay f.
McCraw gracilis myocutaneous f.
McFarlane skin f.
medial f.
melolabial f.
f. meniscal tear
mesiolabial bilobed transposition f.
microsurgical free f.
microvascular free f.
midline forehead f.
Moberg advancement f.
modified dorsalis pedis
  myofascial f.
Morrison neurovascular free f.
mucoperichondrial f.
mucoperiosteal periodontal f.
mucoperiosteal sliding f.
mucosal periodontal f.
multistaged carrier f.
muscle f.
muscle-periosteal f.
musculocutaneous free f.
musculotendinous f.
Mustardé rotational cheek f.
myocutaneous f.
myodermal f.
myofascial f.

F

NOTES

flap *(continued)*
  nasolabial rotation f.
  neck f.
  f. necrosis
  necrotic f.
  neurocutaneous island f.
  neurovascular free f.
  neurovascular island pedicle f.
  nutrient f.
  oblique f.
  Ockerblad-Boari f.
  omental f.
  omocervical f.
  onlay island f.
  open f.
  opening f.
  f. operation
  f. operation cataract
  Oriental V-Y f.
  osseous f.
  osteocutaneous f.
  osteomuscular f.
  osteomusculocutaneous f.
  osteomyocutaneous f.
  osteoperiosteal f.
  osteoplastic f.
  osteoplastic bone f.
  palatal f.
  palatine f.
  palmar advancement f.
  palmar cross-finger f.
  parabiotic f.
  paraexstrophy skin f.
  parascapular f.
  parasitic f.
  partial-thickness f.
  pectoralis major myocutaneous f.
  pectoralis myocutaneous f.
  pectoralis myofascial f.
  pedicled myocutaneous f.
  pedicle groin f.
  peg f.
  penile island f.
  pericardial f.
  pericoronal f.
  pericranial temporalis f.
  perineal f.
  periodontal f.
  periosteal f.
  permanent pedicle f.
  peroneal island f.
  pharyngeal f.
  f. physiology
  platysma myocutaneous f.
  Pontén fasciocutaneous f.
  postangioplasty intimal f.
  posterior f.
  pulp f.
  racket-shaped f.

radial-based f.
radial forearm f.
random cutaneous f.
random pattern f.
rectal f.
rectus abdominis free f.
rectus abdominis muscle f.
rectus abdominis
  musculocutaneous f.
rectus abdominis myocutaneous f.
rectus femoris f.
regional f.
remote pedicle f.
retinal f.
retroauricular free f.
reversal pedicle f.
reverse cross-finger f.
reverse forearm island f.
rhomboid transposition f.
rope f.
rotation f.
rotational f.
rotator f.
Rubens breast f.
saphenous f.
scalping f.
scalp sickle f.
scapular f.
Scardino f.
scleral f.
segmented f.
semilunar f.
serratus anterior muscle f.
shoulder f.
sickle f.
simple periodontal f.
single pedicle TRAM f.
skew f.
skin f.
sliding f.
soft tissue f.
split-thickness periodontal f.
3-square f.
Steichen neurovascular free f.
subcutaneous f.
superior f.
supramalleolar f.
supraorbital pericranial f.
supraperiosteal f.
surgical f.
Tait f.
tarsoconjunctival f.
f. technique
temporal f.
temporalis fascia f.
temporalis fascial f.
temporalis muscle f.
temporoparietal fascial f.
tendon f.

tensor fascia femoris f.
tensor fascia lata muscle f.
Tenzel rotational cheek f.
thenar f.
thoracoacromial f.
thoracoepigastric f.
tongue f.
f. tracheostomy
TRAM f.
transposition f.
transverse rectus abdominis
  muscle f.
trapezius f.
triangular advancement f.
triceps f.
Truc f.
tubed groin f.
tubed pedicle f.
tubularized cecal f.
tumbler f.
tummy tuck f.
turned-down tendon f.
turnover f.
tympanomeatal f.
umbilical f.
unipedicled f.
unrepositioned f.
upper trapezius f.
Urbaniak neurovascular free f.
Urbaniak scapular f.
U-shaped scalp f.
uvulopalatal f.
Van Lint f.
vascularized free f.
vascularized pericranial f.
ventrum penis f.
vertical f.
vesical f.
f. viability
visor f.
volar V-Y f.
Von Langenbeck bipedicle
  mucoperiosteal f.
Von Langenbeck pedicle f.
V-Y advancement f.
V-Y Kutler f.
waltzed f.
Warren f.
web space f.
Widman f.
winged V double f.
wraparound neurovascular free f.

Zimany bilobed f.
4-f. Z-plasty
flapping valve syndrome
flap-valve mechanism
flashback protocol
flashlight examination
flash photolysis
flash-point temperature
flask closure
flat
  f. abdomen
  f. back deformity
  f. chest
  f. condyloma
  f. depressed lesion
  f. elevated lesion
  f. flap
  f. pelvis
  f. substrate method
flatfoot
  peroneal spastic f.
Flatt
  F. classification
  F. excision
  F. technique
flattened duodenal fold
flatulence
flatulent
  f. colic
  f. dyspepsia
flatus tube insertion
Flechsig tract
Fleischmann bursa
Fleischner line
Fletcher rule of irradiation tolerance
flexed
  f. incision
  f. position
flexibility
flexible
  f. collodion
  f. endofluoroscopy
  f. endoscopic surgery
  f. fiberoptic bronchoscopy
  f. fiberoptic endoscopy
  f. fiberoptic myeloscopy
  f. hinge suspension
  f. laparoscopy
  f. lightwand-guided intubation
  f. nephroscopy
  f. sigmoidoscopy
  f. ureteropyeloscopy

F

NOTES

flexion
f. in abduction and external rotation
f., abduction, external rotation, extension (fabere)
f. in adduction and internal rotation
f. compression spine injury stabilization
f. crease
f. deformity
f. and extension
f. fixation
f. osteotomy
f. teardrop fracture
flexion-extension
f.-e. arc
f.-e. axis
f.-e. injury
f.-e. maneuver
f.-e. plane
f.-e. reflex
flexion-internal rotation deformity
flexion-rotation-drawer knee instability test
flexor
f. carpi radialis tendon
f. digitorum longus tendon
f. digitorum profundus tendon
f. digitorum superficialis tendon
f. hallucis brevis muscle
f. hallucis brevis tendon
f. hallucis longus tendon
f. pollicis longus abductorplasty
f. pollicis longus tendon
f. sheath
f. tendon anastomosis
f. tendon laceration
f. tendon repair
f. tendon rupture
f. tenosynovectomy
flexorplasty
Bunnell modification of Steindler f.
Eyler f.
Steindler f.
flexor-pronator
f.-p. origin
f.-p. origin release
flexura, pl. **flexurae**
flexural
flexure
anorectal f.
colic f.
colon f.
duodenojejunal f.
fluctuant f.
hepatic f.
iliac f.
inferior f.

lumbar f.
perineal f.
sigmoid f.
splenic f.
superior f.
flicker-fusion
f.-f. frequency technique
f.-f. stimulus
f.-f. threshold
flicker fusion
flickering
f. blockade
f. blockade electrophysiology
Flick-Gould technique
flight
1-f. exertional dyspnea
2-f. exertional dyspnea
flip-flap
Mathieu-Horton-Devine f.-f.
f.-f. procedure
f.-f. technique
floating
f. forehead operation
f. gallbladder
f. kidney
f. liver
f. organ
f. rib
f. spleen
floccillation
floccular fossa
flocculation
cephalin-cholesterol f.
limit of f.
Ramon f.
thymol f.
flocculonodular arteriovenous malformation
floor
f. fracture
rectal f.
floor-of-mouth
f.-o.-m. closure
f.-o.-m. lesion
floppy
f. Nissen fundoplication
f. Nissen fundoplication method
f. Nissen fundoplication procedure
f. Nissen fundoplication technique
f. valve syndrome
floppy-type Nissen fundoplication
flora
aerobic f.
bacterial f.
endogenous f.
exogenous f.
GI tract f.
intestinal f.

florid
f. duct lesion
f. hyperplasia
flotation rate
flow
anastomotic f.
f. artifact killer (FLAK)
blood f.
carotid arterial blood f.
cerebral blood f. (CBF)
f. convergence method
f. detection technique
f. direction
Doppler color f.
effective renal blood f.
effective renal plasma f.
endocardial f.
exercise hyperemia blood f.
free f.
fresh gas f. (FGF)
hepatofugal f.
hepatopetal f.
f. interruption technique
intraluminal f.
f. mapping technique
microcirculatory f.
f. misregistration
f. pattern
peak expiratory f.
plug f.
regional cerebral blood f. (rCBF)
f. technique filling
tracheal blood f. (TBF)
tricuspid valve f.
xenon-enhanced cerebral blood f.
flow-dependent
f.-d. oxygen
f.-d. pressure drop
flower
f. bone
F. dental index
flowmetry
fluorescein f.
laser Doppler f. (LDF)
scanning laser Doppler f.
flow-on gradient-echo image
flow-over vaporizer
floxuridine in hepatic metastasis
fluctuans
myotonia f.
fluctuant
f. abscess

f. flexure
f. mass
fluctuantes
fluctuation test
fluffy cotton-wool exudate
fluid
ascitic f.
f. aspiration
bloody peritoneal f.
f. bolus
carrier f.
cerebrospinal f. (CSF)
chylous ascitic f.
clear f.
cloudy f.
f. collection
cul-de-sac f.
cytospin collection f.
f. drainage
endolymphatic f.
f. evacuation
extracellular f.
f. extravasation
f. filtration
free peritoneal f.
infused f.
f. loading anesthetic technique
loculation of f.
maintenance f.
f. management
motor oil peritoneal f.
oxygen-carrying resuscitative f.
pancreatic f.
perilymphatic f.
peritoneal cavity f.
pleural f.
prostatic f.
prune-juice peritoneal f.
Rees-Ecker f.
f. replacement
respiratory tract f.
f. resuscitation
resuscitative f.
scolicidal f.
seminal f.
serosal f.
f. shift
subphrenic f.
supraphysiologic f.
synovial f.
turbid peritoneal f.

F

NOTES

fluid *(continued)*
- f. warmer
- wound f.

fluid-attenuated
- f.-a. inversion recovery (FLAIR)
- f.-a. inversion recovery image

fluid-filled sac

fluid-gas exchange

fluke
- tissue f.

fluorescein
- f. angiography
- f. flowmetry
- f. fundus angioscopy
- f. instillation test
- f. string test

fluorescence
- f. intensity
- f. microscopy
- f. polarization method
- f. spectrophotometry

fluorescence-activated cell sorter (FACS)

fluorescent
- f. antibody staining technique (FAST)
- f. electronic endoscopy
- f. optode technology

fluorodeoxyglucose-positron
- f.-p. emission tomography
- f.-p. emission tomography scanning

fluoroscopic
- f. control
- f. guidance
- f. insertion
- f. method
- f. placement
- f. pushing technique
- f. visualization

fluoroscopically
- f. guided corticosteroid injection
- f. guided low-volume peritendinous corticosteroid injection

fluoroscopy
- f. beam
- biplanar f.
- biplane f.
- C-arm f.
- lateral f.
- 2-plane f.
- portable C-arm image intensifier f.
- rapid scan f.

flush
- f. aortogram
- f. method

flush-and-bathe technique

flushing technique

fluxmetry
- laser Doppler f.

Flynn
- F. femoral neck fracture reduction
- F. technique

FMD
- fibromuscular dysplasia

fMRI
- functional magnetic resonance imaging

FNA
- fine-needle aspiration
- FNA biopsy
- follicular FNA
- Hürthle FNA
- indeterminate FNA
- nondiagnostic FNA
- percutaneous FNA
- FNA sample
- FNA specimen
- suspicious FNA

FNH
- focal nodular hyperplasia

foaming exudate

FOBT
- fecal occult blood testing

focal
- f. bleeding point
- f. calcification
- f. cortical dysplasia
- f. DCIS
- f. fatty infiltration
- f. granulomatous inflammation
- f. hemorrhage
- f. illumination
- f. image point
- f. infection
- f. nodular hyperplasia (FNH)
- f. parenchymal brain lesion
- f. peritonitis
- f. plane
- f. segmental glomerulosclerosis (FSGS)
- f. splenic lesion
- f. tumor

focus, pl. **foci**
- ectopic f.
- endometriotic f.
- hemorrhage f.
- image-space f.
- f. localization
- necrotic f.
- object-space f.
- residual f.
- septic f.
- f. of tumor

focused
- f. abdominal sonography
- f. radiation therapy

Foerster operation

fogging retinoscopy

Foix enucleation

folate-targeted imaging
fold

adipose f.
alar f.
amniotic f.
anterior axillary f.
aryepiglottic f.
axillary f.
Bartlett nail f.
caval f.
cecal f.
cholecystoduodenocolic f.
circular f.
circulator f.
Douglas f.
duodenojejunal f.
duodenomesocolic f.
epicanthal f.
epigastric f.
falciform retinal f.
fimbriated f.
flattened duodenal f.
gastric f.
gastropancreatic f.
glossoepiglottic f.
glossopalatine f.
Guérin f.
Hasner f.
haustral f.
hepatopancreatic f.
Houston f.
ileocecal f.
incudal f.
inferior duodenal f.
inferior rectal f.
inferior transverse rectal f.
inguinal aponeurotic f.
interureteric f.
Kerckring f.
labioscrotal f.
lacrimal f.
f. of laryngeal nerve
lateral glossoepiglottic f.
lateral nail f.
longitudinal f.
malar f.
mallear f.
median glossoepiglottic f.
mucobuccal f.
nail f.
nasojugal f.
Nélaton f.

palatoglossal f.
palatopharyngeal f.
palmate f.
palpebronasal f.
Passavant f.
pharyngoepiglottic f.
pleuroperitoneal f.
presplenic f.
rectal f.
rectouterine f.
rectovesical f.
retinal f.
right umbilical f.
sacrogenital f.
sacrouterine f.
sacrovaginal f.
sacrovesical f.
salpingopalatine f.
salpingopharyngeal f.
sigmoid f.
spiral f.
sublingual f.
superior duodenal f.
superior rectal f.
synovial f.
tarsal f.
tonsillar f.
transverse palatine f.
transverse rectal f.
transverse vesical f.
Treves f.
triangular f.
urachal f.
ureteric f.
uterosacral f.
uterovesical f.
vascular f.
Vater f.
ventricular f.
vestibular f.
vocal f.

folding

f. larynx
skin f.

Foley

F. operation
F. Y-plasty pyeloplasty
F. Y-V plasty

foliate papilla
Folin and Wu method
follicle maturation stimulation

NOTES

F

follicular
    f. carcinoma
    f. cell
    f. cholecystitis
    f. cyst
    f. epithelium
    f. FNA
    f. hematoma
    f. inflammation
    f. lesion
    f. neoplasm
    f. proliferation
folliculoma
folliculus, pl. **folliculi**
followup, follow-up
    clinical f.
    f. data
    f. evaluation
    f. examination
    long-term f.
    f. time
Fones
    F. method
    F. technique
Fontan
    F. atriopulmonary anastomosis
    F. fenestration closure
    F. modification of Norwood
      procedure
    F. operation
    F. repair
Fontana
    F. canal
    F. space
    space of F.
Fontana-Masson staining method
Fontan-Baudet procedure
fontanelle
    anterior f.
    anterolateral f.
    bregmatic f.
    cranial f.
    occipital f.
    posterior f.
Fontan-Kreutzer procedure
fonticulus, pl. **fonticuli**
foot
    f. deformity
    f. first-web flap
    goose f.
    F. reticulin method
    f. rotation
forage
    f. core biopsy
    f. procedure
foramen, pl. **foramina**
    acoustic f.
    anterior condyloid f.
    aortic f.

blind f.
caroticoclinoid f.
carotid f.
cecal f.
f. compression test
conjugate f.
costotransverse f.
emissary sphenoidal f.
ethmoidal f.
external acoustic f.
Ferrein f.
frontal f.
great f.
Huschke f.
Hyrtl f.
incisive f.
inferior dental f.
infraorbital f.
internal auditory f.
internal neurocranial f.
intervertebral f.
jugular f.
lacerated f.
Luschka and Magendie f.
f. magnum
f. magnum line
malar f.
mandibular f.
mastoid f.
mental f.
Monro f.
Morgagni f.
nasal f.
foramina nervosa
nutrient f.
obturator f.
oculomotor f.
optic f.
f. ovale flap
palatine f.
papillary f.
parietal f.
petrosal f.
pleuroperitoneal f.
posterior condyloid f.
round f.
sacral f.
solitary f.
sphenoid emissary f.
sphenopalatine f.
sphenotic f.
stylomastoid f.
supraorbital f.
transverse f.
venous f.
vertebral f.
vertebroarterial f.
Vesalius f.
zygomaticofacial f.

zygomaticoorbital f.
zygomaticotemporal f.
foraminal
f. approach
f. compression test
f. herniation
f. node
foraminalis
foraminotomy
Forbes modification of Phemister graft technique
force
f. application
f. feedback system
f. translation (FTR)
forcé
redressement f.
force-couple splint reduction
forced
f. air warming
f. alimentation
f. duction test (FDT)
f. expiratory capacity
f. expiratory spirogram
f. expiratory time
f. expiratory volume
f. expiratory volume in 1 second (FEV_1)
f. eye closure
f. generation test
f. mandatory intermittent ventilation
f. respiration
force-frequency relation
force-length relation
forceps
f. extraction
f. maneuver
f. removal
f. rotation
force-velocity-length relation
force-velocity relation
force-velocity-volume relation
forcing
dynamic end-tidal f.
forcipate
forcipressure
Ford triangulation technique
fore-and-aft suture technique
forearm
f. amputation
deep f.
f. flap

f. fracture
f. graft
f. graft arteriovenous fistula
f. ischemic exercise test
f. plethysmography
superficial f.
f. supination test
forebrain
forefoot arthroplasty
foregut malformation
forehead
f. flap
f. reflectance oximetry
forehead-nose position
foreign
f. body
f. body aspiration
f. body carcinogenesis
f. body extraction
f. body loop
f. body management
f. body reaction
f. body removal
f. body response
f. body retrieval
f. body sclerotomy
f. body trauma
f. body tumorigenesis
forekidney
Forel decussation
forequarter amputation
foreskin
f. flap
f. restoration
Forest-Hastings technique
Forest I, II lesion
forestomach
forked flap
form
extension f.
face f.
IPPS Pelvic Pain Assessment F.
QWB-SA f.
formal
f. celiotomy
f. hemipelvectomy
f. hepatic resection
f. laparotomy
f. method
f. surgical exploration
formaldehyde-induced fluorescence method

F

NOTES

formalin-ether sedimentation method
formalin fixation
formatio, pl. **formationes**
formation
- abscess f.
- adhesion f.
- anastomotic stricture f.
- anterior synechia f.
- antiantibody f.
- antibody f.
- aspergilloma f.
- balloon cell f.
- blood vessel f.
- bone f.
- branching tubule f.
- bunion f.
- Burnet-Talmadge-Lederberg theory of antibody f.
- calculous f.
- callus f.
- cataract f.
- chiasma f.
- cloacal f.
- clot f.
- coagulum f.
- colloid f.
- colony f.
- concept f.
- crater f.
- cyclops f.
- echo f.
- excessive callus f.
- extracapillary crescent f.
- false channel f.
- fistular f.
- gallstone f.
- gender identity f.
- germinal center f.
- Gothic arch f.
- granuloma f.
- hemostatic plug f.
- heterotopic bone f.
- identity f.
- ileostomy f.
- image f.
- impulse f.
- inflammatory pseudotumor f.
- intramembranous f.
- keloid f.
- kerion f.
- ketone body f.
- lappet f.
- localized plaque f.
- mesencephalic reticular f.
- micelle f.
- midbrain reticular f.
- neocartilage f.
- neointima f.
- osteophyte f.

- pannus f.
- paramedian pontine reticular f.
- periosteal new bone f.
- plaque f.
- pontine paramedian reticular f.
- posterior synechia f.
- procallus f.
- pseudoaneurysm f.
- pseudopod f.
- pseudotumor f.
- reaction f.
- reticular f.
- root f.
- rouleaux f.
- sac f.
- scar f.
- somite f.
- spur f.
- star f.
- stone granuloma f.
- stricture f.
- struvite crystal f.
- symptom f.
- synechia f.
- trellis f.
- twin f.
- web f.

formocresol pulpotomy
fornix, pl. **fornices**
- anterior vaginal f.
- f. approach
- caliceal f.
- cerebral f.
- conjunctival f.
- pharyngeal f.
- posterior vaginal f.
- f. reformation
- vaginal f.

fornix-based flap
fortification
fortified topical preparation
forward
- f. coarticulation
- f. head posture
- f. traction test
- f. triangle method
- f. triangle technique

Fosnaugh nail biopsy
fossa, pl. **fossae**
- anterior cranial f.
- axillary f.
- Bichat f.
- Biesiadecki f.
- Broesike f.
- canine f.
- Claudius f.
- cranial f.
- crural f.
- Cruveilhier f.

digastric f.
duodenal f.
duodenojejunal f.
epigastric f.
femoral f.
floccular f.
gallbladder f.
Gerdy hyoid f.
glenoid f.
greater supraclavicular f.
Gruber-Landzert f.
hyoid f.
hypophysial f.
iliac f.
iliacosubfascial f.
iliopectineal f.
incisive f.
inferior duodenal f.
infraclavicular f.
infraduodenal f.
infraspinous f.
infratemporal f.
inguinal f.
intercondylar f.
intercondyloid f.
intrabulbar f.
ischioanal f.
ischiorectal f.
Jobert de Lamballe f.
Jonnesco f.
jugular f.
juxta-auricular f.
lacrimal sac f.
Landzert f.
lesser supraclavicular f.
Malgaigne f.
mandibular f.
mastoid f.
Merkel f.
mesentericoparietal f.
Mohrenheim f.
Morgagni f.
mylohyoid f.
omoclavicular f.
paraduodenal f.
parajejunal f.
pararectal f.
paravesical f.
petrosal f.
piriform f.
pituitary f.
popliteal f.

posterior cranial f.
preauricular f.
pterygoid f.
pterygomaxillary f.
pterygopalatine f.
retroduodenal f.
retromandibular f.
retromolar f.
Rosenmüller f.
scaphoid f.
sigmoid f.
sphenomaxillary f.
splenic f.
subarcuate f.
subcecal f.
subinguinal f.
sublingual f.
submandibular f.
submaxillary f.
subscapular f.
superior duodenal f.
supramastoid f.
supraspinous f.
supratonsillar f.
supravesical f.
temporal f.
Treitz f.
triangular f.
trochlear f.
umbilical f.
Velpeau f.
vermian f.
Waldeyer f.
zygomatic f.
fossula, pl. **fossulae**
    petrosal f.
fossulate
Fothergill
    F. operation
    F. stitch
Fothergill-Donald operation
Fothergill-Hunter operation
Foucher epiphysial injury classification
foundation
    anhydrous facial f.
    denture f.
    facial f.
    level f.
    f. surface
fountain decussation
Fourier-acquired steady-state technique (FAST)

F

NOTES

Fournier
  F. disease
  F. gangrene
  syphiloma of F.
fourth
  f. carpometacarpal joint fracture
  f. cranial nerve
  f. lumbar nerve
  f. parallel pelvic plane
fourth-degree radiation injury
fovea, pl. **foveae**
  Morgagni f.
  pterygoid f.
  trochlear f.
foveola, pl. **foveolae**
  coccygeal f.
foveolar
Fowler-Philip
  F.-P. approach
  F.-P. incision
Fowler-Stephens
  F.-S. maneuver
  F.-S. orchiopexy
  F.-S. procedure
Fowles
  F. dislocation technique
  F. open reduction
Fox-Blazina procedure
Fox operation
fraction
  alveolar dead-space f.
fractional
  f. area change (FAC)
  f. dilation and curettage
  f. epidural anesthesia
  f. spinal anesthesia
  f. sterilization
fractionated
  f. external beam irradiation
  f. radiation therapy
fractionation
  indicator f.
  f. protocol
fracture
  abduction-external rotation f.
  acetabular rim f.
  acute f.
  agenetic f.
  alveolar process f.
  alveolar socket wall f.
  anatomic f.
  Anderson-Hutchins unstable tibial
    shaft f.
  angulated f.
  angulation f.
  ankle mortise f.
  anterior column f.
  anterolateral compression f.
  apex f.

apophysial f.
arch f.
articular mass separation f.
articular pillar f.
Atkin epiphysial f.
atlantal f.
atlas-axis combination f.
atrophic f.
avulsion stress f.
axial loading f.
axis f.
axis-atlas combination f.
backfire f.
banana f.
f. band
Bankart f.
Barton f.
Barton-Smith f.
basal neck f.
basal skull f.
baseball finger f.
basilar femoral neck f.
basilar skull f.
beak f.
f. bed
bedroom f.
Bennett comminuted f.
bicondylar T-shaped f.
bicondylar Y-shaped f.
bicycle spoke f.
bimalleolar ankle f.
birth f.
f. blister
blow-in f.
blow-out f.
boot-top f.
Bosworth f.
both-bone f.
both-column f.
bowing f.
boxer f.
f. bracing
bronchial f.
bucket-handle f.
buckle f.
bumper f.
bunk-bed f.
burst f.
butterfly f.
buttonhole f.
calcaneal avulsion f.
calcaneal displaced f.
f. callus
capillary f.
capitate f.
capitellar f.
carpal bone stress f.
carpometacarpal joint f.
cartwheel f.

cementum f.
central f.
cephalomedullary nail f.
cerebral palsy pathological f.
cervical spine f.
cervicotrochanteric displaced f.
Chance vertebral f.
Chaput f.
chauffeur f.
chip f.
chiropractic treatment of f.
chisel f.
chondral f.
circumferential f.
f. classification
clavicular birth f.
clayshoveler's f.
cleavage f.
closed break f.
closed skull f.
coccyx f.
Colles f.
combination f.
combined flexion-distraction injury and burst f.
combined radial-ulnar-humeral f.
comminuted intraarticular f.
comminuted orbital f.
comminuted skull f.
complete f.
complex f.
complicated f.
compound comminuted f.
compound skull f.
compressed f.
compression f.
condylar femoral f.
condylar process f.
congenital f.
contrecoup f.
coracoid f.
corner f.
coronal split f.
coronoid process f.
cortical f.
Cotton ankle f.
cough f.
cranial f.
crown f.
crown-root f.
crush f.
crushed eggshell f.

Danis-Weber f.
dashboard f.
dens f.
dentate f.
depressed skull f.
depression f.
de Quervain f.
derby hat f.
Descot f.
diacondylar f.
diametric pelvic f.
diaphysial f.
diastatic skull f.
dicondylar f.
die punch f.
direct f.
f. disease
dishpan f.
f. dislocation
dislocation f.
displaced f.
distal femoral epiphysial f.
distal humeral f.
distal radial f.
distraction of f.
dog-leg f.
dome f.
double f.
Dupuytren f.
Duverney f.
dyscrasic f.
elbow f.
elementary f.
enamel f.
f. en coin
endocrine f.
endplate compression f.
f. en rave
epicondylar avulsion f.
epiphysial growth plate f.
epiphysial slip f.
epiphysial tibial f.
Essex-Lopresti joint depression f.
explosion f.
expressed skull f.
extension teardrop f.
external orbital f.
extracapsular f.
extraoctave f.
facial f.
fatigue f.
femoral diaphysial f.

NOTES

F

fracture *(continued)*
    femoral epiphysial f.
    femoral intertrochanteric f.
    femoral neck f.
    femoral shaft f.
    femoral supracondylar f.
    fender f.
    fetal bone f.
    f. fever
    fibular f.
    fifth metatarsal base f.
    fighter f.
    finger f.
    first carpometacarpal joint f.
    fishmouth f.
    fissured f.
    f. fixation
    flexion teardrop f.
    floor f.
    forearm f.
    fourth carpometacarpal joint f.
    f. fragment
    frontal sinus f.
    Gaenslen f.
    Galeazzi f.
    f. gap
    Garden femoral neck f.
    glenoid rim f.
    Gosselin f.
    greater trochanteric femoral f.
    greater tuberosity f.
    greenstick f.
    growing f.
    growth plate f.
    Guérin f.
    gunshot f.
    Gustilo-Anderson open clavicular f.
    gutter f.
    Hahn-Steinthal f.
    hairline f.
    hamate tail f.
    hangman f.
    head-splitting humeral f.
    healed f.
    f. healing
    healing f.
    hemicondylar f.
    Henderson f.
    Hermodsson f.
    hickory-stick f.
    high-energy f.
    Hill-Sachs f.
    hip f.
    hockey-stick f.
    Hoffa f.
    Holstein-Lewis f.
    hoop stress f.
    horizontal maxillary f.
    humeral head-splitting f.

    humeral physial f.
    humeral shaft f.
    humeral supracondylar f.
    Hutchinson f.
    hyoid bone f.
    ice skater f.
    ileofemoral wing f.
    impacted f.
    implant f.
    impression f.
    incomplete compound f.
    indirect f.
    inflammatory f.
    infraction f.
    insufficiency f.
    intercondylar femoral f.
    intercondylar humeral f.
    intercondylar tibial f.
    internal fixation f.
    interperiosteal f.
    intertrochanteric femoral f.
    intertrochanteric 4-part f.
    intraarticular proximal tibial f.
    intracapsular f.
    intraoperative f.
    intrauterine f.
    inverted-Y f.
    ipsilateral acetabular f.
    ipsilateral femoral neck f.
    ipsilateral femoral shaft f.
    ipsilateral pelvic f.
    ipsilateral tibial f.
    irreducible f.
    Jefferson f.
    joint depression f.
    Jones f.
    juxtacortical f.
    knee f.
    Kocher f.
    Kocher-Lorenz f.
    laminar f.
    lap seatbelt f.
    laryngeal cartilage f.
    lateral condylar humeral f.
    lateral mass f.
    Laugier f.
    lead-pipe f.
    Le Fort I-III f.
    Le Fort fibular f.
    Le Fort mandibular f.
    Le Fort-Wagstaffe f.
    lesser trochanter f.
    f. line
    linear skull f.
    Lisfranc f.
    loading f.
    long bone f.
    longitudinal f.
    loose f.

lorry driver f.
low-energy f.
lower extremity f.
low lumbar spine f.
lumbar spine burst f.
lumbosacral junction f.
Maisonneuve fibular f.
malar f.
Malgaigne pelvic f.
malleolar f.
mallet f.
malunited calcaneus f.
malunited forearm f.
malunited radial f.
mandibular body f.
mandibular condyle f.
mandibular ramus f.
mandibular symphysis f.
March f.
marginal ridge f.
maternal f.
maxillary f.
maxillofacial f.
mesiodistal f.
metacarpal neck f.
metaphysial tibial f.
metatarsal f.
midface f.
midfoot f.
midshaft f.
milkman f.
minimally displaced f.
missed f.
Moberg-Gedda f.
molar tooth f.
monomalleolar ankle f.
Monteggia forearm f.
Montercaux f.
Moore f.
Mouchet f.
multangular ridge f.
multilevel f.
multiple f.
multiray f.
nasal f.
nasoorbital f.
navicular f.
naviculocapitate f.
neck f.
neoplastic f.
neurogenic f.
neuropathic f.

nightstick f.
nonarticular distal radial f.
noncontiguous f.
nondisplaced f.
nonphysial f.
nonrotational burst f.
nonunion f.
nonunited f.
nutcracker f.
oblique f.
obturator avulsion f.
occipital condyle f.
occult f.
odontoid condyle f.
odontoid neck f.
olecranon f.
open-book f.
open-break f.
open skull f.
orbital blow-out f.
orbital floor f.
orbital rim f.
orbital wall f.
osteochrondral slice f.
osteoporotic f.
outlet strut f.
pacemaker lead f.
Pais f.
paratrooper f.
1-part f.
2-part f.
3-part f.
4-part f.
patellar sleeve f.
pathological f.
Pauwels f.
pedicle f.
pelvic avulsion f.
pelvic ring f.
pelvic straddle f.
penetrating f.
periarticular f.
periprosthetic f.
peritrochanteric f.
petrous pyramid f.
phalangeal diaphysial f.
physial f.
Piedmont f.
pillion f.
pillow f.
pilon ankle f.
ping-pong f.

F

NOTES

fracture *(continued)*
pisiform f.
plafond f.
plaque f.
plastic bowing f.
pond f.
porcelain f.
Posada f.
posterior arch f.
posterior column f.
posterior element f.
posterior ring f.
posterior wall f.
postirradiation f.
postoperative f.
Pott f.
Pott ankle f.
pronation-abduction f.
pronation-eversion f.
proximal femoral f.
proximal humeral f.
proximal tibial metaphysial f.
pyramidal f.
radial head f.
radial neck f.
radial styloid f.
f. reduction
f. repair
reverse Barton f.
reverse Colles f.
reverse Monteggia f.
rib f.
ring f.
ring-disrupting f.
Rolando f.
roof f.
root f.
rotation f.
rotational burst f.
sacral f.
sacroiliac f.
sacrum f.
sagittal slice f.
Salter-Harris f.
Salter I-VI f.
scaphoid f.
scotty dog f.
seatbelt f.
secondary f.
segmental f.
Segond f.
sentinel spinous process f.
SER-IV f.
shaft f.
shear f.
Shepherd f.
short oblique f.
sideswipe elbow f.
simple skull f.

single f.
f. site
skier f.
Skillern f.
skull f.
sleeve f.
slice f.
slot f.
Smith f.
spinal compression f.
spine f.
spinous process f.
spiral oblique f.
splintered f.
split f.
split-heel f.
splitting f.
spontaneous f.
sprain f.
sprinter f.
f. stabilization
stable burst f.
stairstep f.
stellate skull f.
Stieda f.
straddle f.
stress f.
strut f.
subcapital f.
subperiosteal f.
subtrochanteric femoral f.
supination-adduction f.
supination-eversion f.
supination-external rotation IV f.
supraclavicular f.
supracondylar humeral f.
supracondylar Y-shaped f.
surgical neck f.
T f.
talar avulsion f.
talar neck f.
talar osteochondral f.
tarsal bone f.
T condylar f.
teacup f.
teardrop f.
temporal bone f.
tension f.
testis f.
thoracic spine f.
thoracolumbar burst f.
thoracolumbar spine f.
through-and-through f.
thrower f.
tibial bending f.
tibial condyle f.
tibial diaphysial f.
tibial open f.
tibial plafond f.

tibial plateau f.
tibial shaft f.
tibial triplane f.
tibial tuberosity f.
Tillaux-Chaput f.
Tillaux-Kleiger f.
toddler f.
tongue f.
tooth f.
torsional f.
torus f.
trabecular bone f.
tracheal f.
traction f.
trampoline f.
transcaphoid f.
transcapitate f.
transcervical femoral f.
transchondral f.
transcondylar f.
transepiphysial f.
transhamate f.
transiliac f.
translational f.
transsacral f.
transscaphoid dislocation f.
transtriquetral f.
transverse comminuted f.
transverse facial f.
transversely oriented endplate
  compression f.
transverse maxillary f.
transverse process f.
trapezium f.
traumatic f.
trimalleolar ankle f.
triplane tibial f.
tripod f.
triquetral f.
trophic f.
tuft f.
type I, II, III, IIIA, IIIB, IIIC
  open f.
type C pelvic ring f.
ulnar f.
uncinate process f.
uncomminuted f.
undisplaced f.
unicondylar f.
unimalleolar f.
unstable f.
ununited f.

Vancouver f.
vertebral body f.
vertebral stable burst f.
vertebral wedge compression f.
vertebra plana f.
vertical shear f.
vertical tooth f.
Volkmann f.
wagon-wheel f.
Wagstaffe f.
Walther f.
wedge compression f.
wedge-shaped uncomminuted tibial
  plateau f.
willow f.
Wilson f.
Y f.
Y-shaped f.
Y-T f.
zygomatic arch f.
zygomatic maxillary complex f.
zygomaticomaxillary f.

fracture-dislocation

atlantoaxial f.-d.
Bennett f.-d.
carpometacarpal f.-d.
Galeazzi f.-d.
Lisfranc f.-d.
pedicolaminar f.-d.
perilunate f.-d.
posterior f.-d.
f.-d. reduction
tarsometatarsal f.-d.
thoracolumbar spine f.-d.
tibial plateau f.-d.
transcapitate f.-d.
transhamate f.-d.
transtriquetral f.-d.
unstable f.-d.
volar plate arthroplasty
  technique f.-d.

fragment

articular f.
avascular f.
avulsed f.
bone f.
bony f.
butterfly fracture f.
capital f.
catheter f.
caudal f.
cephalad f.

NOTES

F

fragment *(continued)*
    chondral f.
    cortical f.
    disc f.
    distal f.
    f. E
    extruded disc f.
    fracture f.
    free disc f.
    free-floating cartilaginous f.
    hinged f.
    Hoskins razor blade f.
    hypervascular f.
    loose f.
    metallic f.
    osteochondral f.
    placental f.
    residual f.
    retained placental f.
    sternal f.
    trapdoor f.
    tuberosity f.
fragmentation
    elastic fiber f.
    electrohydraulic f.
    graft f.
    laser-induced f.
    stone f.
    ultrasonic f.
Fraley syndrome
frame application
frame-based stereotaxy
frameless
    f. stereotactic guidance
    f. stereotactic surgery
    f. stereotaxy
framework
    implant f.
Franceschetti
    F. coreoplasty operation
    F. corepraxy operation
    F. deviation operation
    F. keratoplasty operation
    F. pupil deviation operation
    F. syndrome
frank
    f. dislocation
    f. hemorrhage
    F. intrabiliary rupture
    f. necrosis
    F. nonsurgical perineal autodilation
    f. perforation
    F. permanent gastrotomy technique
    F. procedure
    f. pus
    f. rigors
    F. technique of dilation

Fränkel
    F. neurologic deficit classification
    F. white line
Frankenhäuser ganglion
Franke tabes operation
Frankfort
    F. horizontal light line
    F. horizontal plane
    F. mandibular incisor angle
    F. mandibular plane angle
Frank-Starling relation
Franz-O'Rahilly classification
frappage therapy
Fraser syndrome
Fraunfelder no-touch technique
Fraunhofer line
Frazier
    F. incision
    F. suction
Frazier-Spiller
    F.-S. operation
    F.-S. rhizotomy
FRC
    functional residual capacity
freckle
    Hutchinson f.
Fredet-Ramstedt
    F.-R. operation
    F.-R. procedure
    F.-R. pyloromyotomy
Fredrickson hyperlipoproteinemia
    classification
Fredrickson-Levy-Lees classification
free
    f. air
    f. bone flap
    f. disc fragment
    f. fasciocutaneous flap
    f. fat graft
    f. fibular harvest flap
    f. flap transfer
    f. flow
    f. fragment disc
    f. fragment herniation
    f. gastric margin
    f. hepatic venous pressure
    f. latissimus dorsi flap
    f. ligature suture technique
    f. microsurgical flap
    f. node
    f. peritoneal fluid
    f. radial forearm flap
    f. rupture
    f. skin flap
    f. temporal flap
    f. tenia
    f. tenotomy
    f. tissue transfer
free-beam coagulation

Freebody-Bendall-Taylor fusion technique
free-floating
    f.-f. canalith
    f.-f. cartilaginous fragment
    f.-f. particle
freehand
    f. method
    f. suturing technique
Freeman calcaneal fracture classification
Freer dissection
free-root insertion technique
freeway space
freeze-cleave method
freeze-etch method
freeze-fracture-etch method
freezing
    gastric f.
    f. point
frena (*pl. of* frenum)
frenal
French
    F. flap
    F. fracture technique
    F. lateral closing wedge osteotomy
    F. method
    F. plane
    F. position
    F. scale
    F. supracondylar fracture operation
French-American-British (FAB)
    F.-A.-B. classification
frenectomy
frenoplasty
frenotomy
frenula (*pl. of* frenulum)
frenulectomy
frenuloplasty
frenulum, pl. **frenula**
    lingual f.
    synovial frenula
frenum, pl. **frena**
    Morgagni f.
    synovial f.
Frenzel maneuver
frequency
    ciliary beat f.
    f. modulation
    respiratory f.
    spectral edge f. (SEF)
    wavelength f.

frequency-difference interferential current therapy
frequency-duration index
fresh
    f. blood clot
    f. extrapelvic ovarian transplantation
    f. frozen plasma (FFP)
    f. gas flow (FGF)
    f. tissue allocation
    f. wound
Fresnel membrane
fretum, pl. **freta**
Freund
    F. anomaly
    F. operation
Frey
    F. pancreaticojejunostomy
    F. syndrome
friable clot
Friberg microsurgical agglutination test
Fricke operation
friction
    intraabdominal f.
    f. knot
Friedenwald-Guyton operation
Friedenwald operation
Friede operation
Friedewald approximation
Fried-Green foot procedure
Fried-Hendel tendon technique
fringe
    Richard f.
    synovial f.
frogleg
    f. lateral projection
    f. position
Froimson
    F. procedure
    F. technique
Froimson-Oh repair
frondlike filling defect
frons
frontal
    f. abscess
    f. arteriovenous malformation
    f. artery
    f. bone
    f. border
    f. branch
    f. cortical approach
    f. craniotomy
    f. crest

F

NOTES

frontal *(continued)*
  f. eminence
  f. foramen
  f. gyrectomy
  f. lobotomy
  f. margin
  f. notch
  f. plane
  f. plane correction
  f. projection
  f. recess
  f. section
  f. sinus
  f. sinus cavity
  f. sinus fracture
  f. sinus mucocele
  f. sinus septoplasty
  f. squama
  f. suture
  f. triangle
  f. tuber
  f. vein
  f. x-ray
  f. x-ray view
frontalis
  f. muscle
  f. sling procedure
  f. sling technique
frontalium
frontoanterior position
frontoethmoidal
  f. mucocele
  f. suture
frontoethmoidalis
frontoethmoidectomy
frontolacrimalis
frontolateral laryngectomy
frontomalar
frontomaxillaris
frontomaxillary suture
frontonasal
  f. duct
  f. suture
frontonasalis
frontonasomaxillary osteotomy
frontooccipital
frontoorbital osteotomy
frontoparietal
  f. arteriovenous malformation
  f. suture
frontopontine tract
frontoposterior position
frontosphenoidal process
frontosphenoid suture
frontotemporal
  f. approach
  f. craniotomy
  f. tract
frontotransverse position

frontozygomatic suture
Froriep induration
Frost
  F. procedure
  F. stitch
  F. suture technique
frosted liver
Frost-Lang operation
Frouin
frown incision
frozen
  f. section (FS)
  f. section analysis
  f. section diagnosis
  f. section method
Frykman
  F. distal radius fracture
    classification
  F. radial fracture classification
FS
  frozen section
FSGS
  focal segmental glomerulosclerosis
FTR
  force translation
Fuchs
  F. canthorrhaphy operation
  F. iris bombe transfixation
    operation
  F. position
fugax
  proctalgia f.
Fukala operation
**Fukunaga-Hayes unbiased jackknife
  classification**
fulcrum line
Fulford procedure
fulgurant
fulgurating
fulguration
  electrical f.
  electrosurgical f.
  endoscopic f.
  nephroscopic f.
full
  f. axillary dissection
  f. cardiopulmonary bypass
  f. cast restoration
  f. diagnostic laparoscopy
  f. extension
  f. mastopexy
  f. shoulder preparation
full-body cutaneous examination
fullness
  epigastric f.
full-spine radiographic examination
full-stomach precautions
full-thickness
  f.-t. burn

corneal f.-t.
f.-t. periodontal flap
f.-t. rectal aspiration
fulminant
f. hepatic failure (FHF)
f. hepatitis
f. hyperpyrexia
function
atrioventricular nodal f.
autonomous f.
bowel f.
effective f.
electrophysiologic f.
gait f.
graft f.
hemodynamic f.
hepatocellular f.
liver f.
mucociliary f.
neorectal f.
neurologic f.
preoperative liver f.
pulmonary f.
renal f.
sinoatrial nodal f.
functional
f. activation PET scanning
f. capacity classification
f. capacity evaluation
f. capillary density
f. castration
f. contracture
f. electrical stimulation
f. endoscopic sinus surgery (FESS)
f. intestinal failure
f. lymph node dissection
f. magnetic resonance imaging
  (fMRI)
f. neck dissection
f. neuromuscular stimulation
f. orthodontic therapy
f. parenchyma
f. prepubertal castration syndrome
f. problem
f. renal tissue
f. repair
f. residual capacity (FRC)
f. sphincter
f. stereotactic neurosurgery
f. technique
f. veloplasty
functioning allograft

fundal plication
fundament
fundectomy
fundi (*pl. of* fundus)
fundiform ligament
fundoplasty
anterior f.
Belsey IV f.
270-degree laparoscopic posterior f.
esophagogastric f.
Gomez f.
Hill f.
laparoscopic esophagogastric f.
Nissen f.
posterior f.
Thal f.
Thal-Nissen f.
Toupet f.
fundoplication
Belsey Mark II, IV f.
Belsey Mark IV 240-degree f.
Belsey partial f.
Belsey two-thirds wrap f.
Collis-Nissen f.
Dor anterior f.
endoscopic f.
floppy Nissen f.
floppy-type Nissen f.
Guarner wrap f.
Heller myotomy with Dor f.
Heller plus Nissen f.
herniated f.
high-resistance f.
Hill gastropexy f.
Hunter technique for Toupet f.
intrathoracic Nissen f.
laparoscopic anterior partial f.
laparoscopic esophagogastroplasty
  with Nissen f.
laparoscopic Nissen f. (LNF)
laparoscopic Nissen and Toupet f.
low-resistance f.
microlaparoscopic Nissen f.
modified Belsey f.
Nissen 360-degree wrap f.
Nissen-Rossetti f.
open f.
open Nissen f. (ONF)
redo f.
Rossetti modification of Nissen f.
slipped Nissen f.
Thal f.

F

NOTES

fundoplication *(continued)*
    total f.
    Toupet hemifundoplication f.
    transthoracic Nissen f.
    twisted f.
    uncut Collis-Nissen f.
    videoscopic f.
fundus, pl. **fundi**
    f. gland
    f. microscopy
    f. rotation gastroplasty
funduscopic examination
fundusectomy
fungal
    f. antibody
    f. organism
    f. overgrowth
    f. pancreatic infection
    f. pathogen
    f. sinusitis
    f. species
    f. superinfection
fungating
    f. mass
    f. sore
    f. tumor
fungemia
fungous infection
fungus, pl. **fungi**
    pancreatic f.
funic reduction
funicular
    f. excision
    f. graft
    f. inguinal hernia
    f. process
funiculopexy
funiculus, pl. **funiculi**
funnel
    f. chest deformity
    f. stitch
funnelization of metaphysis
funnel-shaped pelvis
furcalis
furcal nerve
furcation
    f. canal
    denuded f.
    invaded f.
    root f.
Furlow-Fisher
    F.-F. modification
    F.-F. modification of Virag 1
      operation
Furlow procedure
Furniss anastomosis
furrier's suture technique
furrow
    corneal marginal f.

    digital f.
    mentolabial f.
furrowing
fusca lamina
fusiform
    f. aneurysm
    f. dilatation
    f. excision
    f. flap
fusing point
fusion
    Adkins spinal f.
    Albee spinal f.
    amplitude of f.
    Anderson ankle f.
    ankle f.
    anterior cervical discectomy and f.
    anterior lumbar vertebral
      interbody f.
    anterior spinal f.
    f. area
    atlantoaxial f.
    atlantooccipital f.
    autograft f.
    Bailey-Badgley cervical spine f.
    binaural f.
    binocular f.
    Blair f.
    Bosworth spinal f.
    Bradford f.
    Brooks-type f.
    calcaneotibial f.
    central f.
    centric f.
    cervical interbody f.
    cervical spine posterior f.
    Chandler hip f.
    Charnley compression-type knee f.
    Chuinard-Peterson ankle f.
    clothespin H spinal f.
    Cloward anterior spinal f.
    Cloward back f.
    color f.
    Coltart calcaneotibial f.
    commissural f.
    f. complex
    convex f.
    Copeland-Howard scapulothoracic f.
    4-corner midcarpal f.
    Davis f.
    Dewar posterior cervical f.
    DIP f.
    distal interphalangeal f.
    distal tibiofibular f.
    dowel spinal f.
    endoscopic spinal f.
    extraarticular hip f.
    extraarticular subtalar f.
    eyelid f.

facet f.
f. faculty
f. fascia
first-grade f.
flicker f.
Gallie spinal f.
Gallie subtalar ankle f.
Glissane ankle f.
f. grade
Hall facet f.
Harris-Smith cervical f.
Henry-Geist spinal f.
H-graft f.
Hibbs-Jones spinal f.
hip f.
Horwitz-Adams ankle f.
f. implantation
in situ spinal f.
interbody spinal f.
interfacet wiring and f.
intertransverse f.
intraarticular hip f.
intraarticular knee f.
joint f.
Kellogg-Speed lumbar spinal f.
King intraarticular hip f.
knee f.
labial f.
Langenskiöld f.
lateral f.
long-segment spinal f.
lower cervical spine f.
lumbar interbody f.
lumbar spinal f.
lumbar spine f.
lumbar vertebral interbody f.
lumbosacral f.
lunotriquetral f.
midcarpal f.
motor f.
müllerian duct f.
naviculocuneiform f.
f. nonunion rate
occipitocervical f.
pantalar f.
partial wrist f.
f. peptide
peripheral f.
posterior cervical f.
posterior-interbody lumbar spinal f.
posterior-lateral lumbar spinal f.

posterior lumbar interbody f.
  (PLIF)
posterior spinal f.
posterolateral interbody f.
posterolateral lumbosacral f.
radiolunate f.
radioscaphoid f.
f. reflex
robertsonian f.
Robinson cervical spine f.
root f.
sacral spine f.
scaphocapitate f.
scaphotrapeziotrapezoidal f.
scapulothoracic f.
second-grade f.
selective thoracic spine f.
sensory f.
short-segment spinal f.
Simmons cervical spine f.
single-level spinal f.
f. in situ
Smith-Petersen sacroiliac joint f.
Smith-Robinson anterior f.
Smith-Robinson cervical f.
Smith-Robinson interbody f.
Soren ankle f.
spinal f.
splenogonadal f.
2-stage hip f.
Stamm procedure for intraarticular
  hip f.
f. stiffness
symmetric vertebral f.
talocalcaneal f.
talonavicular f.
f. technique
third-grade f.
thoracic facet f.
thoracic spinal f.
tibiofibular f.
tibiotalar f.
tibiotalocalcaneal f.
tissue f.
total wrist f.
trapeziometacarpal f.
triscaphe f.
upper cervical spine f.
urethrohymenal f.
vertebral f.
vertebral interbody f.
Watson scaphotrapeziotrapezoidal f.

F

NOTES

fusion *(continued)*
    f. welding
    White posterior ankle f.
    whole-arm f.
    Wilson ankle f.

    Wiltberger f.
    Wiltse bilateral lateral f.
    Winter convex f.
fusion-free position
Futcher line

γ (*var. of* gamma)

GA
    general anesthesia

gabapentin

Gaenslen
    G. fracture
    G. split-heel incision
    G. split-heel technique

Gail
    G. model
    G. model of breast cancer risk
      prediction

gait function

galactocele

galactography

galactophorous
    g. canal
    g. duct

Galanti-Giusti colorimetric method

galea

galeal flap

Galeati gland

galeatomy

Galeazzi
    G. fracture
    G. fracture-dislocation
    G. patellar operation

Galen
    G. anastomosis
    G. nerve

galenic
    g. preparation
    g. venous malformation

gallamine triethiodide

gallbladder
    body of g.
    calcified g.
    calculous g.
    g. calculus
    g. cancer
    g. carcinoma
    g. colic
    distended g.
    g. distention
    g. duplication
    g. ectopia
    g. ejection rate
    floating g.
    g. fossa
    g. neck
    g. perforation
    g. plate
    porcelain g.
    g. removal

    stasis g.
    g. wall abscess

gallbladder-vena cava line

gall duct

Gallie
    G. atlantoaxial fusion technique
    G. operation
    G. procedure
    G. spinal fusion
    G. subtalar ankle fusion
    G. transplant
    G. wiring technique

gallstone
    g. colic
    g. disease
    g. formation
    g. ileus
    g. migration
    g. pancreatitis
    silent g.

GALT
    gastrointestinal-associated lymphoid
      tissue
    gut-associated lymphoid tissue

galvanic stimulation

galvanocautery

galvanosurgery

Galveston
    G. pelvic fixation
    G. technique

Gambee suture technique

gamekeeper thumb dislocation

gamete
    g. intrafallopian tube transfer
      (GIFT)
    g. manipulation
    g. micromanipulation

Gamgee tissue

gamma, γ
    g. irradiation
    g. loop disorder
    g. probe localization
    g. thalamotomy

gammagraphy

gamma-probe radiolocalization

Gamna-Gandy body

ganglia (*pl. of* ganglion)

ganglial tissue

gangliated
    g. cord
    g. nerve

gangliectomy

gangliocytoma

ganglioglioma

G

gangliolysis
    percutaneous radiofrequency g.
ganglioma
    intracerebral g.
ganglion, pl. **ganglia**
    aberrant g.
    Acrel g.
    Andersch g.
    aorticorenal g.
    Arnold g.
    Auerbach g.
    auricular g.
    basal g.
    g. blockage
    g. blocker
    Bock g.
    carotid g.
    celiac g.
    cervical g.
    cervicothoracic g.
    ciliary g.
    coccygeal g.
    cochlear g.
    g. cyst
    dorsal root g.
    Ehrenritter g.
    episcleral g.
    Frankenhäuser g.
    gasserian g.
    geniculate g.
    glossopharyngeal g.
    hypogastric g.
    g. impar block
    inferior cervical g.
    inferior mesenteric g.
    intermediate g.
    intervertebral g.
    intracranial g.
    jugular g.
    lacrimal g.
    Laumonier g.
    Lee g.
    Lobstein g.
    Ludwig g.
    lumbar g.
    Meckel g.
    mesenteric g.
    nasociliary g.
    nodose g.
    oculomotor g.
    optic g.
    otic g.
    parasympathetic g.
    paravertebral g.
    pelvic g.
    petrosal g.
    phrenic g.
    prevertebral g.
    pterygopalatine g.
    Remak g.
    renal g.
    Ribes g.
    sacral g.
    Scarpa g.
    Schacher g.
    semilunar g.
    solar g.
    sphenopalatine g.
    spinal g.
    spiral g.
    splanchnic g.
    stellate g.
    sublingual g.
    submandibular g.
    submaxillary g.
    superior cervical g.
    superior mesenteric g.
    thoracic g.
    trigeminal g.
    vertebral g.
    vestibular g.
    Vieussens g.
    Walther g.
ganglionated
ganglionectomy
    cervical g.
    dorsal root g.
    Meckel sphenopalatine g.
    sphenopalatine g.
    superior cervical g.
ganglioneuroblastoma
ganglioneuroma
ganglioneuromatosis
    diffuse transmural g.
ganglionic
    g. blockade
    g. branch
ganglionostomy
gangrene
    appendiceal g.
    arteriosclerotic g.
    bacterial synergistic g.
    cold g.
    cutaneous g.
    decubital g.
    diabetic g.
    dry g.
    embolic g.
    emphysematous g.
    Fournier g.
    gas g.
    hemorrhagic g.
    hot g.
    Meleney g.
    moist g.
    nosocomial g.
    Pott g.
    pressure g.

primary g.
progressive bacterial synergistic g.
secondary g.
static g.
thrombotic g.
traumatic g.
venous g.
wet g.
white g.
gangrenosum
gangrenous
    g. appendicitis
    g. cholecystitis
    g. granulomatous inflammation
    g. hernia
Ganley technique
gantry rotation
Ganzfeld stimulation
gap
    Bochdalek g.
    esophageal g.
    fracture g.
    interincisor g.
Garceau
    G. cheilectomy
    G. tendon technique
garden
    G. femoral neck fracture
    G. femoral neck fracture
      classification
    g. spade deformity
Gardner
    G. meningocele repair
    G. operation
Garré
    sclerosing osteomyelitis of G.
Garrett orientation line
Gartland
    G. humeral supracondylar fracture
      classification
    G. procedure
    G. Universal radial fracture
      classification
Gartner
    G. canal
    G. duct
Gärtner method
gas
    g. abscess
    anesthetic g.
    g. anesthetic
    arterial blood g.

    g. chromatography
    g. chromatography-mass
      spectrometry
    g. clearance method
    g. collection
    g. contamination
    g. density line
    g. embolism
    g. emission
    g. endarterectomy
    g. exchange
    extraluminal g.
    extravasation g.
    g. gangrene
    g. incontinence
    inspired g.
    g. insufflation
    g. isotope ratio mass spectrometry
    laparoscopic g.
    nonanesthetic g.
    partial pressure of CO_2 g.
    serial blood g.
    g. sterilization
    g. trapping
    venous blood g.
    xenon g.
gaseous
    g. cholecystitis
    g. decompression
    g. dilatation
    g. distention
    g. laparoscopy
    g. laparoscopy method
    g. laparoscopy procedure
    g. laparoscopy technique
gas-fluid exchange
gas-forming
    g.-f. liver abscess
    g.-f. pyogenic liver infection
Gaskell bridge
gasless
    g. endoscopic thyroidectomy
    g. laparoscopic approach
    g. laparoscopic hysterectomy
    g. laparoscopy
    g. laparoscopy method
    g. laparoscopy procedure
    g. laparoscopy technique
gas-producing streptococcal infection
gasserectomy
gasserian
    g. ganglion

G

NOTES

gasserian *(continued)*
    g. ganglion block
    g. ganglion blockade
gastrectasis
gastrectomy
    Billroth I, II g.
    Billroth I partial g.
    curative radical total g.
    distal with excision of ulcer g.
    esophagoproximal g.
    hand-assisted laparoscopic g.
    high subtotal g.
    Hofmeister g.
    Horsley g.
    Japanese-style g.
    laparoscopic-assisted subtotal g.
    laparoscopic total g.
    limited g.
    near-total g.
    palliative total g.
    pancreatic-preserving total g.
    partial g. (PG)
    Pólya g.
    proximal g.
    pylorus-preserving g. (PPG)
    radical total g.
    segmental g.
    sleeve g.
    g. specimen
    standard D1 g.
    standardized curative radical
      total g.
    subtotal g.
    total g. (TG)
    video-assisted g.
gastric
    g. accommodation test
    g. adenocarcinoma
    g. angioma
    g. antral vascular ectasia (GAVE)
    g. antrum
    g. area
    g. arteriovenous malformation
    g. artery
    g. atony
    g. atrophy
    g. balloon implantation
    g. band
    g. bed
    g. bed metastasis
    g. branch
    g. bulge
    g. bypass
    g. bypass procedure (GBP)
    g. bypass surgery
    g. calculus
    g. canal
    g. cancer
    g. cardia

g. chloric acid
g. coin removal
g. compression
g. cuff
g. cytology
g. decompression
g. devascularization
g. dilation
g. distention
g. duplication
g. duplication cyst
g. electrical stimulation
g. emptying
g. emptying procedure (GEP)
g. epithelial cell infiltration
g. epithelium
g. fistula
g. fluid aspiration
g. fold
g. foreign body
g. freezing
g. fundus wrap
g. gland
g. hemorrhage
g. hernia
g. impression
g. infection
g. insufflation
g. leiomyoma resection
g. loop bypass
g. malignancy
g. MALT lymphoma
g. margin
g. mass
g. mucosa
g. mucosal barrier
g. mucosal hypercarbia
g. mucosal pattern classification
g. mucosal pH
g. non-Hodgkin lymphoma
g. outlet obstruction (GOO)
g. pacemaker region
g. partitioning procedure
g. patch esophagoplasty
g. perforation
g. perforation peritonitis
g. pit
g. polypectomy
g. pouch
g. pressure
g. pull-through procedure
g. pull-up
g. pull-up procedure
g. reduction surgery
g. reflux
g. remnant
g. residue examination
g. rupture
g. segment

g. serosa
g. stapling
g. stromal tumor
g. stump carcinoma
g. tonometry
g. tube esophagoplasty
g. ulcer
g. ulceration
g. vagotomy
g. valve tightening
g. valve tightening method
g. valve tightening procedure
g. valve tightening technique
g. variceal bleeding
g. vein
g. vessel
g. volvulus
g. wall
g. wrap (GW)
gastric-longitudinal
deep g.-l. (DG-L)
gastric-transverse
deep g.-t. (DG-T)
gastrinoma
gastrin secretion
gastritis
phlegmonous g.
gastroanastomosis
gastrocardiac
gastrocele
gastrocnemius sliding flap
gastrocolic
g. fistula
g. ligament
g. omentum
gastrocolostomy
gastrocutaneous fistula
gastrocystoplasty
gastrodiaphragmatic ligament
gastroduodenal
g. anastomosis
g. artery (GDA)
g. complication
g. fistula
g. mucosa
g. mucosal protection
g. orifice
gastroduodenopancreatectomy
gastroduodenoscopy
gastroduodenostomy
Billroth I g.

Jaboulay g.
vagotomy and antrectomy with g.
gastroendoscopy
gastroenteric fistula
gastroenteroanastomosis
gastroenterocolostomy
gastroenterologist
gastroenteropancreatic (GEP)
gastroenteroplasty
gastroenteroptosis
gastroenterostomy
Balfour g.
Billroth I, II g.
Braun-Jaboulay g.
Courvoisier g.
Finney g.
Heineke-Mikulicz g.
Hofmeister g.
g. intussusception
laparoscopic g.
percutaneous g.
Pólya g.
prophylactic g.
Roux g.
Roux-en-Y g.
Schoemaker g.
short limb Roux-en-Y g.
side-to-side g.
g. stoma
truncal vagotomy and g.
Von Haberer g.
Wölfler g.
gastroenterotomy
gastroepiploic
g. arcade
g. artery
g. vein
g. vessel
gastroesophageal
g. hernia
g. junction
g. reflux disease (GERD)
g. variceal plexus
g. vestibule
gastroesophagostomy
gastrogastrostomy
gastrogavage
gastrohepatic
g. ligament
g. omentum
gastroileac augmentation

G

NOTES

gastroileostomy
gastrointestinal (GI)
    g. anastomosis (GIA)
    g. anomaly
    g. bleeding
    g. carcinoma
    g. complication
    g. condition
    g. content
    g. continuity
    g. endoscopy
    g. endothelium
    g. fistula
    g. infection
    g. lesion
    g. malignancy
    g. metastasis
    g. problem
    G. Quality of Life Index (GIQLI)
    g. resection
    g. stoma
    g. stromal tumor (GIST)
    g. surgery
    g. tract
    g. tract dysfunction
    g. ulceration
gastrointestinal-associated lymphoid tissue (GALT)
gastrointestinal-cutaneous fistula
gastrojejunal
    g. anastomosis
    g. loop obstruction syndrome
gastrojejunocolic fistula
gastrojejunostomy
    antecolic long-loop isoperistaltic g.
    Billroth II g.
    compression button g.
    loop g.
    partial inferior retrocolic end-to-side g.
    partial superior retrocolic end-to-side g.
    percutaneous endoscopic g.
    prophylactic g.
    retrocolic end-to-side g.
    Roux-en-Y g.
    total retrocolic end-to-side g.
gastrolavage
gastrolienal ligament
gastrolith
gastrolithiasis
gastrolysis
gastronesteostomy
gastroomental
    g. artery
    g. node
gastropancreatic
    g. fold
    g. vagovagal reflex

gastroparesis
    postvagotomy g.
gastropathy
    indomethacin-induced g.
gastropexy
    anterior g.
    Belsey Mark IV g.
    belt loop g.
    Boerema anterior g.
    circumcostal g.
    Hill posterior g.
    incisional g.
    laparoscopic-assisted g.
    percutaneous anterior g.
    posterior diaphragmatic g.
    T-fastener g.
    T-tack g.
gastrophrenic
    g. anchorage
    g. ligament
gastrophrenicum
gastroplasty
    adjustable ring g.
    Albert-Lembert g.
    banded g.
    Collis g.
    Collis-Nissen g.
    Eckhout vertical g.
    fundus rotation g.
    Gomez horizontal g.
    greater curvature banded g.
    hand-assisted laparoscopic vertical-banded g.
    horizontal g.
    Kuzmak g.
    laparoscopic g.
    layer-to-layer g.
    Mason vertical banded g.
    open vertical banded g.
    silicone elastomer ring vertical g.
    Stamm g.
    tubular vertical g.
    unbanded g.
    V-banded g.
    vertical adjustable banded g.
    vertical banded g. (VBG)
    vertical ring g. (VRG)
    vertical Silastic ring g.
    V-Y g.
gastropleural fistula
gastroplication
gastropneumonic
gastroprotective drug
gastroptosis
gastroptyxis
gastropulmonary
gastropylorectomy
gastropyloric
gastrorrhagia

gastrorrhaphy
gastrorrhexis
gastroschisis
gastroscopic
gastroscopy
    high-magnification g.
    infrared transillumination g.
gastrosphincteric pressure gradient
gastrosplenic
    g. ligament
    g. omentum
gastrosplenicum
gastrostaxis
gastrostenosis
gastrostogavage
gastrostolavage
gastrostomy
    Beck g.
    button 1-step g.
    Depage-Janeway g.
    drainage g.
    dual percutaneous endoscopic g.
    endoscopic g.
    g. feeding
    feeding g.
    Gauderer-Ponsky-Izant PEG g.
    Glassman g.
    Janeway g.
    Kader g.
    laparoscopic g.
    Olympus g.
    palliative g.
    Partipilo g.
    percutaneous endoscopic g. (PEG)
    Russell percutaneous endoscopic g.
    g. scarring
    Ssabanejew-Frank g.
    Stamm g.
    tube g.
    ultrasound-assisted percutaneous
      endoscopic g.
    venting percutaneous g.
    Witzel g.
gastrotomy
    anterior g.
    Depage-Janeway g.
gastrulation
gate
    spinal g.
gate-control
    g.-c. hypothesis
    g.-c. theory

gated technique
Gatellier-Chastang
    G.-C. ankle approach
    G.-C. incision
    G.-C. posterolateral approach
Gauderer-Ponsky-Izant PEG gastrostomy
Gauderer-Ponsky PEG operation
Gaur balloon distention technique
gaussian line
gauze dissection
gavage
Gavard muscle
GAVE
    gastric antral vascular ectasia
gay
    g. bowel infection
    G. gland
Gayet operation
Gaynor-Hart position
GBP
    gastric bypass procedure
GCS
    Glasgow Coma Scale
GD2
    melanoma-associated antigen GD2
GD3
    melanoma-associated antigen GD3
GDA
    gastroduodenal artery
GEA graft
Geenen sphincterotomy
gelatin compression body
gelatinous
    g. acute inflammation
    g. ascites
    g. carcinoma
    g. infiltration
gelation
gel filtration
**Gelfoam particles transarterial
    embolization treatment**
Gell and Coombs classification
gelling phenomenon
Gelman procedure
Gelpi-Lowry hysterectomy
Gély suture technique
gemination
gemistocyte
gemistocytoma
gender
    g. dimorphism
    g. identity formation

G

NOTES

gene
cancer-causing g.
g. induction
innate immunity g.
mutator g.
g. replacement therapy
susceptibility g.
tumor suppressor g.

general
g. adaptation reaction
g. anesthesia (GA)
g. anesthetic
g. anesthetic technique
g. bloodletting
g. closure
g. endotracheal anesthesia
g. laparoscopic surgical procedure
g. radiation
g. surgeon
g. thoracic surgery
g. thrust manipulation

generales

generalized
g. cortical hyperostosis
g. elastolysis
g. peritonitis

genetic
g. abnormality
g. anomaly
g. approach
g. condition
g. diagnosis
g. lesion
g. marker
g. testing

geneticist
clinical g.

genetics
cancer g.
molecular g.

gene-transfer therapy
genial tubercle
genicula (*pl. of* geniculum)
genicular
g. anastomosis
g. artery

geniculate
g. body
g. ganglion
g. neuralgia

geniculocalcarine
g. radiation
g. tract

geniculotemporal tract
geniculum, pl. genicula
genioglossal muscle
genioglossus
geniohyoglossus

geniohyoid
g. fascia
g. muscle
g. space

geniohyoideus
genion
genioplasty
augmentation g.

genital
g. branch
g. carcinoma
g. condyloma
g. cord
g. duct
g. eminence
g. gland
g. infection
g. organ
g. papulosquamous lesion
g. reconstruction
g. swelling
g. tract
g. tract trauma
g. tract tumor
g. tubercle
g. ulcer
g. ulceration

genitalia
ambiguous external g.
external g.
indifferent g.

genitocrural nerve
genitofemoral
g. causalgia
g. nerve
g. neurectomy

genitoinguinal ligament
genitoplasty
feminizing g.
masculinizing g.

genitourinary (GU)
g. anomaly
g. apparatus
g. evaluation
g. fistula
g. infection
g. tract

Gennari
line of G.

gentle
g. compression
g. traction

genu
g. valgum deformity
g. varum deformity

genual
genucubital position
genufacial position
genupectoral position

genus
geographic stippling
geometric
> g. equator
> g. supracondylar extension osteotomy

George
> G. Lewis technique
> G. line

GEP
> gastric emptying procedure
> gastroenteropancreatic

Gerbert-Mellilo method
Gerbert osteotomy
Gerbode anuloplasty
GERD
> gastroesophageal reflux disease

Gerdy
> G. fiber
> G. hyoid fossa
> G. tubercle

geriatric
> g. anesthesia
> g. injury

Gerlach
> G. tonsil
> G. valvula

germ
> g. line
> g. tube
> g. tube test

German method
germinal
> g. center formation
> g. cord
> g. epithelium
> g. matrix
> g. matrix hemorrhage
> g. membrane

germinoma
Gerota
> G. capsule
> G. fascia

Gesell test with Knobloch modification
gestant anomaly
gestational sac
GFR
> glomerular filtration rate

Ghon
> G. complex
> G. primary lesion

GI
> gastrointestinal
> GI oncology
> GI tract
> GI tract flora

GIA
> gastrointestinal anastomosis

Giannestras
> G. modification of Lapidus technique
> G. oblique metatarsal osteotomy

giant
> g. cell arteritis
> g. cell astrocytoma
> g. cell lesion
> g. colon
> g. condyloma
> g. fibroadenoma
> g. prosthetic reinforce
> g. prosthetic reinforcement of visceral sac (GPRVS)

Giardia **infection**
Gibbon hernia
gibbous deformity
Gibson
> G. approach
> G. long vertical relaxing incision
> G. suture technique

Gibson-Piggott osteotomy
Gibson-type incision
Giemsa-stained section
Gierke respiratory bundle
Gifford delimiting keratotomy operation
GIFT
> gamete intrafallopian tube transfer

gift wrap suture technique
Gigli operation
Gilbert scapular flap
Gilbert-Tamai-Weiland technique
Gilchrist procedure
Giliberty bipolar femoral head
Gill
> G. laminectomy
> G. lesion
> G. massive sliding graft
> G. procedure
> G. sliding graft technique

Gilles operation
Gilliam-Doleris
> G.-D. operation
> G.-D. uterine suspension

Gilliam operation

G

NOTES

Gillies
  G. bone graft
  G. scar correction operation
Gillies-Millard cocked-hat technique
**Gill-Jonas modification of Norwood
  procedure**
**Gill-Manning-White spondylolisthesis
  technique**
Gillquist procedure
Gil-Vernet
  G.-V. ileocecal cystoplasty
  G.-V. ileocecal cystoplasty urinary
    diversion
  G.-V. operation
  G.-V. procedure
  G.-V. technique
Gimbernat ligament
gingiva, pl. **gingivae**
gingival
  g. anatomy
  g. artery
  g. augmentation
  g. cavity
  g. cavity wall
  g. deformity
  g. exudate
  g. exudation
  g. finishing line
  g. fistula
  g. flap
  g. hemorrhage
  g. inflammation
  g. point
  g. position
  g. space
  g. stimulation
  g. tissue
  g. tissue esthetics
  g. zone
gingivectomy
  chemosurgical g.
  Ochsenbein g.
gingivolabial groove
gingivoplasty
ginglymoarthrodial
ginglymoid joint
ginglymus
  helicoid g.
  lateral g.
Giordano operation
GIQLI
  Gastrointestinal Quality of Life Index
  GIQLI score
Girard
  G. keratoprosthesis operation
  G. procedure
girdle
  g. anesthesia
  pelvic g.

shoulder g.
thoracic g.
Girdlestone
  G. hip procedure
  G. laminectomy
  G. resection
  G. resection arthroplasty
Girdlestone-Taylor procedure
Gironcoli hernia
girth
  abdominal g.
GIST
  gastrointestinal stromal tumor
Gittes
  G. operation
  G. procedure
  G. technique
  G. urethropexy
Gittes-Loughlin
  G.-L. bladder neck suspension
  G.-L. procedure
glabella
glabellar
  g. bilobed flap
  g. exposure osteotomy
  g. rotation flap
  g. tapping
gladiate
gladiolus
glancing wound
gland
  abnormally hyperplastic g.
  abnormal parathyroid g.
  accessory parotid g.
  accessory suprarenal g.
  accessory thyroid g.
  acid g.
  acinous g.
  admaxillary g.
  adrenal g.
  aggregate g.
  agminate g.
  Albarran g.
  anterior lingual g.
  apical g.
  apocrine g.
  g. appearance
  areolar g.
  arteriococcygeal g.
  arytenoid g.
  axillary sweat g.
  Bartholin g.
  Bauhin g.
  Blandin g.
  Blandin-Nuhn g.
  Boerhaave g.
  Bowman g.
  brachial g.
  bronchial g.

Brunner g.
bulbourethral g.
celiac g.
cervical g.
circumanal g.
coccygeal g.
contralateral parathyroid g.
Cowper g.
cutaneous g.
dominant g.
ductless g.
duodenal g.
Duverney g.
eccrine sweat g.
ectopic sebaceous g.
Eglis g.
endocrine g.
enlarged parathyroid g.
entrapped g.
esophageal ectopic sebaceous g.
external genitalia, Bartholin,
  urethral, and Skene g.'s
fundus g.
Galeati g.
gastric g.
Gay g.
genital g.
Gley g.
greater vestibular g.
Guérin g.
Havers g.
hematopoietic g.
hypercellular g.
hyperplastic g.
inferior g.
inguinal g.
intestinal g.
ipsilateral g.
Knoll g.
labial g.
lactiferous g.
laryngeal g.
lesser vestibular g.
Lieberkühn g.
lingual g.
Littré g.
Luschka g.
lymph g.
mammary g.
master g.
Meibom g.
meibomian g.

Méry g.
mesenteric g.
milk g.
Moll g.
Montgomery g.
mucilaginous g.
muciparous g.
mucous g.
nondominant g.
Nuhn g.
odoriferous g.
oil g.
palatine g.
parathyroid g.
paraurethral g.
parotid g.
peptic g.
perspiratory g.
Peyer g.
pharyngeal g.
pineal g.
pituitary g.
Poirier g.
prehyoid g.
preputial g.
prostate g.
pyloric g.
remnant g.
g. removal
retrosternal g.
Rivinus g.
Rosenmüller g.
salivary g.
sebaceous g.
seminal g.
seromucous g.
serous g.
sexual g.
g. size
Skene g.
solitary g.
sublingual g.
substernal g.
sudoriferous g.
supernumerary g.
suprahyoid g.
suprarenal g.
synovial g.
target g.
tarsal g.
thymus g.
thyroid g.

NOTES

G

gland *(continued)*
    tracheal g.
    trachoma g.
    Tyson g.
    urethral g.
    uterine g.
    vaginal g.
    vesical g.
    vestibular g.
    g. volume
    Von Ebner g.
    vulvovaginal g.
    Waldeyer g.
    Wasmann g.
    Wepfer g.
    Wölfler g.
    Zeis g.
4-gland
    4-g. hyperplasia
    4-g. visualization
glandes (*pl. of* glans)
glandis
glandular
    g. branch
    g. cancer
    g. carcinoma
    g. element
    g. epithelium
    g. substance
    g. tissue
glandulectomy
glandulopexy
glans, pl. **glandes**
    g. penis
glansplasty
    meatal advancement and g.
    (MAGPI)
glanuloplasty
glaserian fissure
Glasgow
    G. Coma Scale (GCS)
    G. Coma Score
    G. Outcome Scale
    G. Outcome Score (GOS)
glass-bead retention method
Glassman gastrostomy
glass-rod
    g.-r. negative phenomenon
    g.-r. positive phenomenon
glass-wool filtration
glassy membrane
glaucoma
    g. surgery
    uncontrollable g.
glaucomatous
    g. cul-de-sac
    g. excavation
    g. ring
Gleason score

Gleich osteotomy
Glen
    G. Anderson technique
    G. Anderson ureteroneocystostomy
Glenn
    G. anastomosis
    G. operation
    G. procedure
    G. shunt
glenohumeral
    g. adhesive capsulitis
    g. articulation
    g. dislocation repair
    g. joint
    g. joint dislocation
glenoid
    g. cavity
    g. fossa
    g. osteotomy
    g. point
    g. rim fracture
    g. surface
glenoplasty
    posterior g.
    Scott posterior g.
Gley gland
glial
    g. ring
    g. tumor
gliding-hole-first technique
gliding joint
glioblastoma
glioma
    low-grade g.
    malignant g.
    mixed malignant g.
    g. sarcomatosum
glioma-polyposis
gliomatous
glioneuroma
gliosarcoma
gliosis
gliotic membrane
Glissane ankle fusion
Glisson
    G. capsule
    G. sphincter
glissonian
    g. capsule
    g. pedicle
    g. sheath
global
    g. hemostasis
    g. hypoperfusion
globi (*pl. of* globus)
globular collection
globule
    fat g.
globus, pl. **globi**

glomangioma
glomangiomatous osseous malformation syndrome
glomangiosarcoma
glomangiosis
    pulmonary g.
glomectomy
glomerular
    g. basement membrane disease
    g. capillary pressure
    g. capsule
    g. crescent
    g. extracellular matrix
    g. filtration
    g. filtration rate (GFR)
    g. hyperfiltration
    g. macrophage infiltration
    g. neutrophil infiltration
    g. tip lesion
    g. ultrafiltration
glomerulation
glomeruli (*pl. of* glomerulus)
glomerulitis
glomerulonephritis
    membranoproliferative g.
glomerulosa
glomerulosclerosis
    focal segmental g. (FSGS)
glomerulus, pl. **glomeruli**
glomus
    g. arteriovenous malformation
    g. body
glossectomy
    Commando radical g.
    partial g.
    radical g.
    subtotal g.
    total g.
glossocinesthetic
glossodynia
glossoepiglottic fold
glossopalatine
    g. fold
    g. muscle
glossopharyngeal
    g. ganglion
    g. nerve
    g. nerve block
    g. nerve root
glossopharyngeus
glossoplasty
glossorrhaphy

glossoscopy
glossotomy
    labiomandibular g.
    median labiomandibular g.
glottic
    g. carcinoma
    g. closure
    g. insufficiency
glove anesthesia
gloved-fist technique
Glover suture technique
glucagonoma syndrome
Gluck incision
glucose oxidase method
glucuronidation
glue
    g. patch
    g. patch leak
glutamate toxicity
glutamic
    g. oxaloacetic transaminase
    g. pyruvic transaminase
glutaraldehyde sterilization
glutathione modification
gluteal
    g. fascia
    g. hernia
    g. line
    g. region
gluteofemoral bursa
gluteoinguinal
gluteus
    g. maximus flap
    g. maximus muscle
glycerin method
glycerol
    g. chemoneurolysis
    g. rhizotomy
glycogen infiltration
Glynn-Neibauer technique
GM2
    melanoma-associated antigen GM2
GMS
    Gomori methenamine silver
    GMS staining
gnathic index
gnathoplasty
gnathoschisis
goblet incision
Godman fascia
Goebel-Frangenheim-Stoeckel technique
Goebel procedure

G

NOTES

Goebel-Stoeckel-Frangenheim procedure
Goethe bone
Goffe colporrhaphy
Gohil-Cavolo method
goiter
    aberrant g.
    colloid g.
    congenital g.
    diffuse colloid g.
    diffuse multinodular g.
    diffuse toxic nonnodular g.
    g. excision
    multinodular g.
    g. recurrence
    toxic multinodular g.
goitrous thyroid
gold
    g. foil condensation
    g. plate technique
    g. ring
    g. seed implantation technique
    g. weight and wire spring
      operation
Goldberg technique
Goldblatt
    G. kidney
    G. phenomenon
Golden closing wedge osteotomy
Goldman
    G. classification
    G. classification operative risk
Goldmann
    G. coherent radiation
    G. kinetic technique
    G. static technique
Goldmann-Larson
    G.-L. foreign body
    G.-L. foreign body operation
Goldner-Clippinger technique
Goldner-Hayes procedure
Goldner reconstruction
Goldsmith operation
Goldstein spinal fusion technique
Goldthwait-Hauser procedure
golf-hole ureteral orifice
Golgi membrane
Goligher extraperitoneal ileostomy
Gomco
    G. suction
    G. technique
Gomez
    G. fundoplasty
    G. horizontal gastroplasty
Gomez-Marquez lacrimal operation
Gomori
    G. methenamine silver (GMS)
    G. methenamine silver staining
gomphosis

gonad
    female g.
    male g.
gonadal
    g. artery
    g. branch
    g. complication
    g. cord
    g. endocrine disorder
    g. vein
gonadectomy
gonadoblastoma
gonadopathy
gonadotrophic
gonaduct
gonangiectomy
gonatocele
gonecyst
gonecystolith
Gonin cautery operation
gonioma
goniometry
goniophotocoagulation
gonioplasty
gonioscopy
    indentation g.
goniotomy operation
gonocele
gonococcal
    g. arthritis
    g. infection
    g. perihepatitis
GOO
    gastric outlet obstruction
Goodall-Power operation
Goodwin
    G. cup-patch principle
    G. technique
Goodwin-Hohenfellner technique
Goodwin-Scott technique
goose foot
gooseneck deformity
Gordon
    G. approach
    G. elementary body
    G. joint injection technique
Gordon-Broström technique
Gordon-Taylor
    G.-T. hindquarter amputation
    G.-T. technique
Gorlin-Chaudhry-Moss syndrome
GOS
    Glasgow Outcome Score
Gosselin fracture
Gothic arch formation
Gouffon pin fixation
Gould
    G. procedure
    G. suture technique

Goulding procedure
Gowers tract
Goyrand hernia
GPRVS
  giant prosthetic reinforcement of visceral
  sac
    GPRVS hernioplasty
    Stoppa GPRVS
grabbing technique
gracilis
  g. flap technique
  g. muscle flap
  g. myocutaneous flap
  g. procedure
  g. tendon
graciloplasty
  double-wrap g.
  dynamic g.
gradation
  Levine g. 1–6
grade
  coma g.
  fusion g.
  g. I, II oscillation
  g. 1–5 mobilization
  nuclear g.
  tumor g.
graded
  g. exposure
  g. spinal anesthesia
gradient
  alveolar-arterial oxygen g.
  alveolocapillary partial pressure g.
  aortic pressure g.
  aortic valve g.
  biliary-duodenal pressure g.
  Doppler pressure g.
  duodenobiliary pressure g.
  gastrosphincteric pressure g.
  intracavitary pressure g.
  g. method
  mitral valve g.
  peak systolic g.
  peak transaortic valve g.
  pressure g.
  pullback pressure g.
  pulmonary valve g.
  temperature g.
  transaortic valve g.
  transcapillary hydrostatic pressure g.
  transmural hydrostatic pressure g.
  transvalvular g.

gradient-echo
  2DFT g.-e. imaging
  3DFT g.-e. MR imaging
  g.-e. method
  g.-e. MR image
  g.-e. MR imaging
gradient-recalled
  g.-r. echo image
  multiple planar g.-r. (MPGR)
gradient-reversal fat suppression method
grading
  tumor g.
Gradle keratoplasty operation
graduated tenotomy
Graefe operation
graft
  accordion g.
  acetabular augmentation g.
  adipodermal g.
  adipose g.
  adrenal medulla g.
  advancement flap g.
  allogenic bone g.
  allogenic fetal g.
  allogenous bone g.
  anastomosed g.
  g. anastomosis
  aortofemoral bypass g. (AFBG)
  g. area
  g. atrophy
  augmentation g.
  autogeneic g.
  autogenous bone g.
  axillobifemoral bypass g.
  g. bed
  Berens g.
  bifurcated vascular g.
  bifurcation g.
  bilateral myocutaneous g.
  Björk-Shiley g.
  Blair-Brown skin g.
  bone autogenous g.
  bone chip g.
  bone graft substitute g.
  bone marrow g.
  bone peg g.
  bone-retinaculum-bone autograft g.
  bone-tendon-bone g.
  bone-to-bone g.
  Bonfiglio bone g.
  Boplant g.
  brachiosubclavian bridge g.

G

NOTES

graft *(continued)*
branched vascular g.
Braun-Wangensteen g.
brephoplastic g.
Brescia-Cimino g.
bridge g.
C g.
calvarial free bone g.
Campbell onlay bone g.
cancellous chip bone g.
cancellous and cortical bone g.
cancellous insert g.
cantilevered bone g.
cardiovascular patch g.
carotid-vertebral vein bypass g.
cartilage g.
cephalic vein g.
chessboard g.
chip g.
Clancy patellar tendon g.
clip g.
g. clotting
compilation autogenous vein g.
composite rib g.
composite skin g.
conjunctival patch g.
connective tissue g.
g. contamination
coronary artery bypass g. (CABG)
cortical bone g.
cortical strut g.
corticocancellous bone g.
Cotton cartilage g.
Cragg endoluminal g.
Creech aortoiliac g.
Crescent corneal g.
cross-facial nerve g.
cutis g.
Daniel iliac bone g.
Dardik umbilical g.
Davis muscle-pedicle g.
DeBakey g.
delayed g.
dermal fat g.
dermis patch g.
devitalized bone g.
diamond inlay bone g.
distal femoropopliteal bypass g.
distal nerve g.
donor iliac Y g.
dorsal vein patch g.
double g.
double-papilla pedicle g.
Douglas g.
dowel bone g.
dual onlay cortical bone g.
Edwards-Tapp arterial g.
endovascular stent g.
epidermic g.

Esser g.
g. expulsion
extension stent g.
extraarticular g.
g. failure
fascial g.
fascicular g.
fat g.
Favaloro saphenous vein bypass g.
femoropopliteal bypass g.
fiberglass g.
fibular strut g.
filler g.
filleted g.
fillet local flap g.
g. fixation
flap g.
forearm g.
g. fragmentation
free fat g.
g. function
funicular g.
GEA g.
Gillies bone g.
Gill massive sliding g.
H g.
Haldeman bone g.
Hancock pericardial valve g.
Hancock vascular g.
Harris superior acetabular g.
g. harvest
Henderson onlay bone g.
Henry bone g.
heterodermic g.
heterogeneous g.
heterologous g.
heteroplastic g.
heterospecific g.
heterotopic g.
Hey-Groves-Kirk bone g.
H-graft bone g.
HLA identical kidney g.
Hoaglund bone g.
homogeneous g.
homogenous g.
homologous g.
homoplastic g.
Horton-Devine dermal g.
Huntington bone g.
HUV bypass g.
hyperplastic g.
IEA g.
IMA g.
g. impingement
implantation g.
g. infection
infusion g.
inlay bone g.
insert g.

interbody bone g.
intercalary g.
internal mammary g.
interposition saphenous vein g.
interspecific g.
g. interstice
intracranial-extracranial nerve g.
intracranial-intratemporal nerve g.
intramedullary g.
island g.
isogeneic g.
isologous g.
isoplastic g.
Judet g.
jump g.
Kebab g.
Keystone g.
Kiel g.
Kimura cartilage g.
Koenig g.
Krause-Wolfe g.
Kutler V-Y flap g.
Langenskiöld bone g.
Lee anterosuperior iliac spine g.
Lee bone g.
ligament g.
load-bearing g.
loop forearm g.
lyophilized bone g.
mandrel g.
Marquez-Gomez conjunctival g.
Massie sliding g.
matchstick g.
Matti-Russe bone g.
McFarland bone g.
McMaster bone g.
medullary bone g.
mesenteric bypass g.
Meyers quadratus muscle-pedicle
  bone g.
g. migration
Millesi interfascicular g.
Millesi nerve g.
mitral valve homograft g.
morcellized bone g.
mucoperiosteal periodontal g.
mucosal periodontal g.
mucous membrane g.
Mueller patellar tendon g.
Mules g.
multivisceral g.
murine g.

mushroom corneal g.
myocutaneous g.
neuromuscular pedicle g.
neurovascular island g.
Nicoll cancellous bone g.
Nicoll cancellous insert g.
nonisometric g.
g. occlusion
Ollier thick split free g.
Ollier-Thiersch g.
orthotopic g.
osteoarticular g.
osteocartilaginous g.
osteochondral g.
osteoperiosteal bone g.
Ostrup vascularized rib g.
Overton dowel g.
papillary pedicle g.
Papineau bone g.
paraffin g.
particulate cancellous bone g.
g. patency
pattern-cut corneal g.
pedicle fat g.
peg bone g.
Phemister onlay bone g.
pie-crusting skin g.
pigskin g.
pinch skin g.
g. placement
polytetrafluoroethylene g.
portacaval H g.
postage stamp skin g.
posterior cartilage g.
powdered bone g.
preclotted g.
g. preparation
prophylactic bone g.
prosthetic arterial g.
proud g.
punch g.
Rastelli g.
reduced-size g.
g. rejection
reoperative coronary artery
  bypass g. (rCABG)
Reverdin epidermal free g.
reversed left saphenous vein
  bypass g.
rigid g.
roof-patch g.
Ryerson bone g.

G

NOTES

graft *(continued)*
    sandwiched iliac bone g.
    saphenous vein bypass g.
    saphenous vein patch g.
    scotty dog g.
    seamless g.
    Seddon nerve g.
    segmental tendon g.
    Sheen tip g.
    sieve g.
    g. site
    skin g.
    skip g.
    sleeve g.
    sliding inlay bone g.
    Soto-Hall bone g.
    Sparks mandrel g.
    g. spatulation
    Speed osteotomy g.
    spiral vein g.
    split-thickness skin g.
    spreader g.
    Stark g.
    stent g.
    stentless composite g.
    straight g.
    g. strength
    g. structure
    strut g.
    g. surveillance
    g. survival
    syngeneic g.
    Taylor-Townsend-Corlett iliac crest bone g.
    tendon g.
    Thiersch-Duplay tube g.
    Thiersch medium split free g.
    Thiersch thin split free g.
    Thomas extrapolated bar g.
    thrombosed g.
    g. thrombosis
    transplanted stamp g.
    g. treatment
    tubed free skin g.
    tube flap g.
    Tudor-Thomas g.
    tumbler g.
    tunnel g.
    upper arm straight g.
    vascularized bone g.
    g. vasculopathy
    vein g.
    venous interposition g.
    g. versus host
    wedge g.
    g. weight
    Weiland iliac crest bone g.
    white g.
    Whitecloud-LaRocca fibular strut g.
    whole lobar g.
    Wilson bone g.
    Wilson-Jacobs patellar g.
    Windson-Insall-Vince bone g.
    Wolfe-Kawamoto bone g.
    Wolfe-Krause g.
    Wolf full-thickness free g.
    xenogeneic g.
    xenograft g.
    Y g.
    zooplastic g.
    Z-plasty local flap g.

graftectomy
graft-enteric fistula
graft-host interface
graft-versus-host
    g.-v.-h. disease (GVHD)
    g.-v.-h. disease reaction
Graham
    G. closure
    G. plication
grammatic method
Gram-negative
    G.-n. aerobe
    G.-n. aerobic organism
    G.-n. microorganism
    G.-n. pneumonia
    G.-n. sepsis
Gram-positive
    G.-p. bacterial infection
    G.-p. microorganism
    G.-p. sepsis
Gram stain morphology
granddaughter cyst
Granger
    G. line
    G. method
    G. projection
granisetron
granny knot
Grantham femur fracture classification
Grant-Small-Lehman supracondylar extension osteotomy
Grant-Ward operation
granular
    g. appearance
    g. kidney
    g. pit
    g. respiration
granulation
    arachnoid g.
    extradural g.
    pacchionian g.
    g. phase
    red g.
    g. stenosis
    g. tissue
    toxic g.

granule
> extracellular g.
> membrane-coating g.
> rod g.
> seminal g.

granuloma
> g. formation
> infectious g.
> inflammatory g.
> sterile g.
> Teflon g.

granulomatous
> g. bacterial infection
> g. colitis
> g. fungal infection
> g. inflammation
> g. mastitis
> g. tissue

granulosa cell carcinoma
graphical anesthesia drug display
grasping technique
grasp reflex
Gratiolet radiation
grattage
Gräupner method
Graves
> G. operation
> G. technique

gravidarum
> nasal granuloma g.

gravidity
gravimetric technique
gravitation abscess
gravitational
> g. line
> g. particle collection

gravity
> intensity-weighted center of g.
> g. line
> g. method
> g. method of Stimson

gray
> g. hepatization
> g. induration
> g. infiltration
> g. line
> g. patch

gray-line incision
gray-scale examination
gray-white corneal scar
great
> g. anastomotic artery

> g. auricular nerve
> g. foramen
> G. Ormond Street tracheostomy
> g. pancreatic artery
> g. radicular artery
> g. saphenous vein
> g. superior pancreatic artery
> g. toe

greater
> g. cul-de-sac
> g. curvature
> g. curvature banded gastroplasty
> g. curve position
> g. multangular bone
> g. occipital nerve block
> g. omentectomy
> g. omentum
> g. palatine artery
> g. pelvis
> g. peritoneal cavity
> g. peritoneal sac
> g. rhomboid muscle
> g. ring
> g. saphenous phlebectomy
> g. sciatic notch
> g. supraclavicular fossa
> g. trochanter
> g. trochanteric femoral fracture
> g. tuberosity fracture
> g. vestibular gland

Green-Banks technique
Greenfield
> G. osteotomy
> G. spinocerebellar ataxia
>   classification

Greenhow incision
Green procedure
Green-Reverdin osteotomy
greenstick
> g. dorsal proximal metatarsal
>   osteotomy
> g. fixation
> g. fracture

Greenville gastric bypass
Greenwald and Lewman method
Green-Watermann osteotomy
Gregoir-Lich procedure
grenz ray therapy
Greulich-Pyle technique
Grice-Green technique
Grice incision

G

NOTES

313

grid
> g. contact
> g. electrode
> external g.

gridiron incision
Griffen Roux-en-Y bypass
Griffith incision
Grimelius
> G. argyrophil method
> G. technique

Grimsdale operation
griseotomy
> circular g.

Gristina-Webb total shoulder arthroplasty
Gritti-Stokes
> G.-S. amputation
> G.-S. knee amputation technique

gritty tumor
Grocott-Gomori methenamine-silver method
groin
> g. dissection
> g. exploration
> g. flap
> g. hernia
> g. mass

Grondahl esophagoplasty
Grondahl-Finney
> G.-F. esophagogastroplasty
> G.-F. esophagoplasty
> G.-F. operation

groove
> alar g.
> alveololabial g.
> anterior auricular g.
> arterial g.
> auriculoventricular g.
> bicipital g.
> carotid g.
> cavernous g.
> chiasmatic g.
> corneal lamellar g.
> costal g.
> deltopectoral g.
> digastric g.
> ethmoidal g.
> g. extension
> gingivolabial g.
> inferior petrosal g.
> infraorbital g.
> intermuscular g.
> interosseous g.
> intertubercular g.
> intraorbital g.
> lateral bicipital g.
> Lucas g.
> median g.
> meningeal g.

> musculospiral g.
> mylohyoid g.
> nail g.
> nasolabial g.
> nasopharyngeal g.
> obturator g.
> occipital g.
> palatovaginal g.
> paraglenoid g.
> pectoral g.
> peroneal g.
> pharyngotympanic g.
> popliteal g.
> posterior auricular g.
> preauricular g.
> pterygopalatine g.
> Sibson g.
> skin g.
> spiral g.
> subclavian g.
> subcostal g.
> supraacetabular g.
> g. suture technique
> transverse anthelicine g.
> uncinate g.
> urethral g.
> venous g.
> vertebral g.
> vomerovaginal g.

grooved incision
gross
> g. cystic disease
> g. deformity
> g. fecal contamination
> g. lesion
> g. manipulation
> G. operation
> G. tracheoesophageal fistula
> g. tumor volume (GTV)

Grosse-Kempf tibial technique
Grossmann operation
ground
> lateral g. (LG)

ground-glass
> g.-g. appearance
> g.-g. lesion

group
> g. A beta-hemolytic streptococcal infection
> g. A streptococcus infection
> Children's Cancer Study g. (CCSG)
> Eastern Cooperative Oncology G. (ECOG)
> g. fascicular repair
> Pediatric Oncology G. (POG)

grouping
> tumor stage g.

Groves-Goldner technique

growing
    g. fracture
    g. point
growth
    g. acceleration
    g. arrest line
    exophytic g.
    g. factor
    final g.
    hamartomatous g.
    monoclonal g.
    oligoclonal g.
    g. plate abscess
    g. plate complex
    g. plate fracture
    polyclonal g.
    g. retardation
    tumor g.
Gruber
    G. cul-de-sac
    G. ligament
    G. suture technique
    G. test
Gruber-Landzert fossa
Gruca stabilization
grunt
    expiratory g.
grunting
    g. maneuver
    g. respiration
Grüntzig
    G. balloon dilation
    G. technique
Grynfelt hernia
Grynfeltt triangle
GSW
    gunshot wound
    single GSW
G syndrome
GTV
    gross tumor volume
GU
    genitourinary
guaiac-negative stool
guaiac-positive stool
guanethidine
    intravenous regional block with g.
guard
    hypoxic g.
guarding
    abdominal g.

    involuntary g.
    voluntary g.
Guarner wrap fundoplication
gubernacular canal
gubernaculum
    Hunter g.
Gubler line
Gudas
    G. scarf Z-plasty
    G. scarf Z-plasty osteotomy
Guéneau de Mussy point
Guérin
    G. fold
    G. fracture
    G. gland
    G. sinus
    valve of G.
Guhl technique
guidance
    computerized image g.
    fluoroscopic g.
    frameless stereotactic g.
    g. image
    laparoscopic g.
    magnetic imaging g.
    g. method
    stereotactic g.
    ultrasound g.
    videolaparoscopic g.
guidance-cooperation model
guide
    image g. (IG)
    g. plane
    g. wire exchange technique
    g. wire manipulation
    g. wire and mini-snare technique
    g. wire perforation
    g. wire reflection
guided
    g. fine-needle aspiration
    g. transcutaneous biopsy
guided-needle aspiration cytology
guiding plane
guillotine
    g. amputation
    g. needle biopsy
guinea worm infection
Guleke-Stookey approach
Guller resection
gullet
gullwing incision

G

NOTES

gum
>g. line
>g. resection

Gunderson conjunctival flap
Gunderson-Sosin modification
gunpowder lesion
gunshot
>g. fracture
>g. wound (GSW)

Gunston arthroplasty
Gurd
>G. procedure
>G. resection

Gussenbauer
>G. operation
>G. suture technique

gustation
gustatory
>g. anesthesia
>g. nerve

Gustilo-Anderson
>G.-A. open clavicular fracture
>G.-A. open fracture classification

Gustilo puncture wound classification
gut
>blind g.
>g. continuity
>g. epithelial cell
>g. epithelium
>g. lumen
>g. mucosal homeostasis
>g. mucosal weight
>g. proliferative factor

gut-associated lymphoid tissue (GALT)
gut-derived Gram-negative aerobic
>**organism**

Guthrie muscle
gutta-percha point
gutter
>abdominal g.
>g. fracture

>left g.
>paracolic g.
>paravertebral g.
>g. wound

guttering
>corneal g.

Guttmann technique
Gutzeit dacryostomy operation
Guyon
>G. ankle amputation technique
>G. canal

guy suture technique
Guyton-Friedenwald suture technique
Guyton-Noyes fixation
Guyton ptosis operation
GVHD
>graft-versus-host disease

GW
>gastric wrap

gynandroblastoma
gynecoid pelvis
gynecologic
>g. anesthesia
>g. disorder
>g. laparoscopy
>g. malignancy
>g. surgeon
>g. tumor

gynecological carcinoma
gynecomastia
>mastectomy for g.

gynoplasty
gyration
gyrectomy
>frontal g.
>postcentral g.
>precentral g.

gyrose
gyrus, pl. **gyri**
>precentral g.

H

H graft
H space

H₂

histamine 2
H_2 blocker

habena, pl. **habenae**
habenula, pl. **habenulae**
habenular trigone
habenulointerpeduncular tract
Haber-Kraft osteotomy
habit

bowel h.'s
parafunctional h.

habitual

h. dislocation
h. temporomandibular joint luxation

habitus

body h.

Hackethal

H. intramedullary bouquet fixation
H. stacked nailing technique

Haddad metatarsal osteotomy
Hadju-Cheney acroosteolysis syndrome
HAE

hepatic artery embolization

Hagedorn and Jansen method
Haggitt classification
Haglund deformity
Hahn-Steinthal fracture
HAI

hepatic arterial infusion

Haight anastomosis
hair bulb incubation test
hairline fracture
Hajek incision
Håkanson technique
Halban

H. culdoplasty
H. procedure

Haldeman bone graft
half-and-half nail
half-axial projection
half-body irradiation
half-hitch knot
half-life

elimination h.-l.
plasma h.-l.

half-mouth technique
half-pin fixation
half-time

context-sensitive h.-t.
h.-t. method

Hall

H. facet fusion

H. method
H. technique

Hallberg biliointestinal bypass
Halle point
Haller

H. ansa
H. anulus
H. insula
H. membrane
H. rete
H. tripod

Hallermann-Streiff-François syndrome
Hallermann-Streiff syndrome
Hallpike maneuver
hallucal
halluces (*pl. of* hallux)
hallucis

extensor h.
h. longus laceration

hallus
hallux, pl. **halluces**

h. valgus deformity
h. valgus procedure
h. varus correction

halogenated volatile anesthetic
halothane

h. hepatitis
1-MAC h.

HALS

hand-assisted laparoscopic surgery

Halsted

H. inguinal herniorrhaphy
H. maneuver
H. operation
H. radical mastectomy
H. suture technique

Halsted-Bassini

H.-B. hernia repair
H.-B. herniorrhaphy

hamartoblastoma
hamartoma

cortical h.
plaquelike h.
visceral h.

hamartomatous

h. growth
h. lesion

Hamas technique
hamate

h. bone
h. tail fracture

hamatum
Hamazaki-Wesenberg body

H

Hamilton
  H. method
  H. Rating Scale for Depression
Hammerschlag method
hammertoe deformity
hammock
  omental h.
Hammon procedure
Hamou technique
Hampton
  H. line
  H. maneuver
  H. operation
hamstring
  h. ligament augmentation
  h. muscle
  h. tendon
hamular procedure
hamulus, pl. **hamuli**
  pterygoid h.
Hancock
  H. pericardial valve graft
  H. procedure
  H. vascular graft
hand
  h. amputation
  h. anomaly
  h. assist
  h. deformity
  h. massage
  radial club h.
  h. ratio
  h. reconstruction
  h. ventilation
hand-assisted
  h.-a. laparoscopic colectomy
  h.-a. laparoscopic gastrectomy
  h.-a. laparoscopic gastric bypass
  h.-a. laparoscopic hemicolectomy
  h.-a. laparoscopic live-donor
    nephrectomy
  h.-a. laparoscopic surgery (HALS)
  h.-a. laparoscopic vertical-banded
    gastroplasty
  h.-a. laparoscopy
handed
  1-h. knot
hand-eye coordination
handgun aspirator
hand-held Doppler flow probe
  examination
Handley
  H. incision
  H. lymphangioplasty
  H. operation
handling
  rough tissue h.
handmade anastomosis
handsewn anastomosis

hand-sutured ileoanal anastomosis
hanger
  yoke h.
hanging
  h. chain method
  h. hip operation
  h. toe operation
hangman fracture
hangnail
Hanhart syndrome
Hankin reduction
Hanley-McNeil method
Hanley rectal bladder procedure
Hannover
  H. canal
  H. classification
Hansen fracture classification
Hantavirus infection
Hapsburg jaw
Hara
  H. gallbladder inflammation
    classification
  H. infiltration block
Harada-Ito procedure
hard
  h. adhesion
  h. calculus
  h. callus stage
  h. cataract
  h. chancre
  h. corn
  h. exudate
  h. mass
  h. metal disease
  h. pad disease
  h. palate
  h. palate cancer
  h. palate dissection
  h. percussion
  h. socket
  h. and soft tissue
  h. sore
  h. stool
  h. tubercle
Hardcastle tarsometatarsal joint injury
  classification
hard-copy image
hardening solution
Hardinge
  H. lateral approach
  H. technique
hardness
  indentation h.
hard-soft palate junction
harelip suture technique
Hark
  H. procedure
  H. technique

Harmon
    H. cervical approach
    H. hip reconstruction
    H. incision
    H. modified posterolateral approach
    H. operation
    H. procedure
    H. shoulder approach
    H. transfer technique
Harmonic hemorrhoidectomy
Harms-Dannheim trabeculotomy operation
Harper-Warren incision
harpoon extraction
Harriluque
    H. sublaminar wiring modification
    H. technique
Harrington
    H. esophageal diverticulectomy
    H. hernia repair
    H. rod instrumentation failure
    H. total hip arthroplasty
Harrington-Allison repair
Harris
    H. anterolateral approach
    H. femoral component removal
    H. growth arrest line
    H. lateral approach
    H. superior acetabular graft
    H. suture technique
    H. 4-wire trochanter reattachment
Harris-Beath projection
Harrison method
Harris-Smith cervical fusion
harsh respiration
Hartel technique
Harting body
Hartmann
    H. closure
    H. colostomy
    H. operation
    H. point
    H. pouch
    H. procedure
    H. reconstruction technique
    H. resection
    H. stump
harvest
    graft h.
    organ h.
harvested fibroblast

harvesting
    autograft h.
Hasner
    H. fold
    H. operation
    valve of H.
Hassab operation
Hassall body
Hassan
    H. method technique
    H. open technique
Hassmann-Brunn-Neer elbow technique
Hass procedure
Hastings
    H. bipolar hemiarthroplasty
    H. open reduction
Hatafuku fundus onlay patch esophageal repair
hatchet-head deformity
Hatle method
Haultain
    H. operation
    H. procedure
Hauri technique
Hauser
    H. bunionectomy
    H. patellar realignment technique
    H. patellar tendon procedure
haustra (*pl. of* haustrum)
haustral
    h. fold
    h. indentation
    h. pouch
haustration of colon
haustrum, pl. **haustra**
Havers gland
haversian canal
Hawkins
    H. inside-out nephrostomy technique
    H. line
    H. method
    H. procedure
    H. single-stick technique
    H. talar fracture classification
Hawthorne effect
Hayes Martin incision
Hay lateral approach
hazardous concentration
HB$_s$
    hepatitis B surface antigen

NOTES

H

HBO
 hyperbaric oxygen therapy
HCC
 hepatocellular carcinoma
HCV
 hepatitis C virus
  HCV antibody
HD
 hemodialysis
HDR
 high dose radiation
 high dose rate
  HDR intracavitary radiation therapy
head
 breech h.
 bulldog h.
 h. circumference:abdominal
  circumference ratio
 h. compression
 h. compression test
 condyle h.
 countersink screw h.
 coupling h.
 h. dependent position
 h. distraction test
 dolichocephalic h.
 engaged h.
 femoral h.
 fetal h.
 fibular h.
 Giliberty bipolar femoral h.
 H. hip arthroplasty
 hourglass h.
 humeral h.
 h. injury
 lateral h.
 H. line
 mandibular h.
 Matroc femoral h.
 Medusa h.
 metatarsal h.
 Morse h.
 h. movement
 oblique h.
 optic nerve h.
 pancreatic h.
 H. paradoxical reflex
 h. posture
 radial h.
 h. ring
 short h.
 sternocostal h.
 superficial h.
 terminal h.
 h. tetanus
 h. titubation
 transverse h.
 h. trauma
 h. turn technique

 ulnar h.
 h. weaving
 H. zone
headache
 analgesic abuse h.
 brain tumor h.
 cervicogenic h.
 cluster h.
 myogenic h.
 postdural puncture h. (PDPH)
 rebound h.
 spinal h.
 traction h.
 visually triggered h.
head-bobbing doll syndrome
head:body ratio
head-down
 h.-d. tilt
 h.-d. tilt test
head-dropping test
head-injured patient
headless bone screw
head-splitting humeral fracture
head-tilt
 h.-t. method
 h.-t. test
head-turning reflex
head-up
 h.-u. tilt
 h.-u. tilt position
 h.-u. tilt-table test
 h.-u. tilt test
healed
 h. fracture
 h. yellow atrophy
healing
 anastomotic h.
 h. cycle
 endoscopic h.
 extraabdominal anastomotic h.
 fracture h.
 h. fracture
 impaired h.
 intestinal anastomotic h.
 intestinal wound h.
 primary h.
 h. process
 h. retardation
 soft tissue h.
 tertiary h.
 wound h.
heal intubation
healthy tissue
Heaney
 H. operation
 H. technique
hearing aid evaluation
heart
 h. anomaly

h. clot
explanted h.
extracorporeal h.
h. failure
h. laser revascularization
h. and lung transplant
h. position
h. rate (HR)
h. rate variability (HRV)
h. sac
h. synchronized ventilation
h. transplant
h. transplantation
transverse section of h.
h. valve leaflet
h. valve replacement
heart-lung
h.-l. preparation
h.-l. resuscitation
h.-l. transplantation
heart-shaped pelvis
heat
h. application
h. balance
h. exposure
h. hyperalgesia
h. production temperature
h. shock
heater-probe coagulation
Heaton operation
heat-seal pouch
heavy
h. condensation
h. metal injection
heavy-ion irradiation
Hedley procedure
heel
h. bone
h. fat pad
h. pad thickening
h. tendon
heel-toe anastomosis
heel-to-ear maneuver
hEGF
human epidermal growth factor
Heifetz procedure
height
anterior facial h. (AFH)
facial h.
first twitch h. (T1)
nasal h.

orbital h.
twitch h.
height-length index
Heimlich maneuver
Heinecke method
Heineke-Mikulicz
H.-M. gastroenterostomy
H.-M. incision
H.-M. pyloroplasty
H.-M. stricturoplasty
Heineke operation
Heine operation
Heinz body
Heinz-Ehrlich body
Heisrath operation
Heister
valve of H.
Helal flap arthroplasty
helcoma
helcoplasty
Held
H. bundle
H. decussation
helical
h. axis of motion
h. CT
h. suture technique
helices (*pl. of* helix)
helicine artery
helicoid ginglymus
helicotrema
helium
h. dilution method
h. equilibration time
h. insufflation
helix, pl. **helices**
helix-loop-helix structure
Heller
H. cardiomyotomy
H. esophagomyotomy
H. myotomy
H. myotomy with Dor fundoplication
H. operation
H. plexus
H. plus Nissen fundoplication
Heller-Belsey operation
Heller-Dor operation
Heller-Nissen operation
Helmholtz line
helminthic infection
helminthoma

NOTES

H

heloma
helotomy
helplessness subscale
Helweg bundle
hemal
    h. arch
    h. spine
hemangiectasia
hemangiectasis
hemangiectatic hypertrophy
hemangioameloblastoma
hemangioblastoma
hemangioendothelioblastoma
hemangioendothelioma
    epithelial h.
hemangioendotheliosarcoma
hemangioepithelioma
hemangiofibroma
    juvenile h.
hemangiolipoma
hemangiolymphangioma
hemangioma
    capillary h.
    cavernous h.
    choroidal h.
    * port-wine h.
hemangioma-thrombocytopenia syndrome
hemangiomatous tissue
hemangiopericytoma
hemangiosarcoma
hematencephalon
hemathorax
hematobilia evacuation
hematocele
    pelvic h.
    pudendal h.
    scrotal h.
hematocrit
    falling h.
    h. measurement
hematocystis
hematogenic metastasis
hematogenous
    h. mechanism
    h. metastasis
    h. micrometastasis
hematologic
    h. complication
    h. disorder
    h. dissemination
    h. workup
hematolymphangioma
hematolysis
hematoma
    acute subdural h.
    aneurysmal h.
    aortic intramural h.
    h. aspiration
    axillary h.

    basal ganglia h.
    bladder flap h.
    bowel wall h.
    cerebellar h.
    chronic subdural h.
    communicating h.
    corpus luteum h.
    dissecting intramural h.
    h. drainage
    duodenal h.
    epidural h.
    h. evacuation
    expanding retroperitoneal h.
    extradural h.
    follicular h.
    interhemispheric subdural h.
    interstitial loculated h.
    intracerebral h.
    intracranial h.
    intrahepatic h.
    intramural h.
    intraparenchymal h.
    isodense subdural h.
    mediastinal h.
    mesenteric h.
    nasopharyngeal h.
    orbital h.
    organized h.
    paraaortic h.
    parenchymal h.
    perianal h.
    periaortic mediastinal h.
    pericardial h.
    peridiaphragmatic h.
    perigraft h.
    perinephric h.
    perirenal h.
    placental h.
    puerperal h.
    pulsatile h.
    rectus sheath h.
    renal h.
    retroperitoneal h.
    retropharyngeal h.
    retroplacental h.
    sciatic nerve palsy h.
    septal h.
    solid visceral h.
    spinal h.
    subcapsular renal h.
    subchorionic h.
    subcutaneous h.
    subdural h.
    subfascial h.
    subgaleal h.
    subgluteal h.
    sublingual h.
    submembranous placental h.
    submental h.

subperiosteal h.
subungual h.
sylvian h.
traumatic intracranial h.
umbilical cord h.
wound h.
wrap h.
hematomphalocele
hematomyelia
hematomyelopore
hematopoietic
h. gland
h. metastasis
h. tissue
hematorrhachis
extradural h.
subdural h.
hematospermatocele
hematospermia
hematoxylin body
hemendothelioma
heme-negative stool
heme-positive stool
hemiacidrin irrigation
hemiacrosomia
hemianopsia
homonymous h.
hemiarthroplasty
Bateman h.
Hastings bipolar h.
I-beam hip h.
large humeral head h.
McKeever and MacIntosh h.
Neer h.
prosthetic h.
Smith-Petersen h.
hemiazygos vein
hemibody irradiation
hemic calculus
hemicentrum
hemicircular incision
hemicolectomy
décollement h.
extended right h.
hand-assisted laparoscopic h.
laparoscopic-assisted h.
laparoscopic left h.
left h.
standard right h.
hemicondylar fracture
hemicorporectomy

hemicorticectomy
cerebral h.
hemicrania
chronic paroxysmal h. (CPH)
episodic paroxysmal h. (EPH)
hemicraniectomy
hemicraniosis
hemicraniotomy
hemidiaphragm
elevated h.
left h.
right h.
h. rupture
hemi-double stapling method
hemidysplasia cornification disorder
hemielliptica
hemifacial
hemi-Fontan
h.-F. operation
h.-F. procedure
hemifundoplication
laparoscopic posterior h.
Toupet h.
hemigastrectomy
hemiglossal
hemiglossectomy
hemihepatectomy
hemihepatic vascular occlusion
hemihydranencephaly
hemi-Koch procedure
hemilaminectomy
complete lateral h.
lumbar h.
partial h.
unilateral h.
hemilaryngectomy
hemilingual
hemiliver
hemimandible reconstruction
hemimandibulectomy
hemimaxillectomy
hemimyelocele
heminephroureterectomy
hemiorchiectomy
hemipancreatectomy
hemipancreaticosplenectomy
hemipelvectomy
complete internal h.
external h.
formal h.
internal h.
partial internal h.

NOTES

H

323

hemipelvis
hemipulp flap
hemiresection interposition arthroplasty
hemiscrotectomy
hemisection
 tooth h.
 triple h.
hemisectomy
hemisphere
 cerebellar h.
 cerebral h.
hemispherectomy
hemispherica
hemispheric disconnection syndrome
hemispherium
hemistrumectomy
hemithoracic duct
hemithoracicus
hemithorax
hemithyroidectomy
hemitongue flap
hemivertebral excision
hemivulvectomy
hemoaccess
hemobilia
hemocholecyst
hemocholecystitis
hemochromatosis
hemochromogen
hemocryoscopy
hemocytoblastoma
hemocytolysis
hemodiafiltration convection
hemodialysis (HD)
 anemia of h.
 continuous venovenous h.
 (CVVHD)
 h. treatment
hemodialysis-dependent patient
hemodilution
 acute isovolemic h.
 acute normovolemic h. (ANH)
 hypervolemic h.
 isovolemic h.
 normovolemic h.
hemodynamic
 h. change
 h. collapse
 h. disturbance
 h. function
 h. instability
 h. intolerance
 h. maneuver
 h. monitoring
 h. perturbation
 h. push
 h. response
 h. stability

hemodynamically
 h. significant air embolus
 h. stable
hemodynamics
hemofiltration
 arteriovenous h.
 continuous arteriovenous h.
 (CAVH)
 continuous venovenous h.
 h. therapy
hemoglobin
 dissociable tetrameric h.
 h. electrophoresis
hemoglobin-oxygen dissociation curve
hemoglobinuria
 paroxysmal nocturnal h.
Hemolink
hemolith
hemolymphangioma
hemolysis
 acid h.
 chronic h.
hemolytic
 h. mechanism
 h. uremic syndrome
hemomediastinum
hemonephrosis
hemoperfusion
 direct h.
 hepatic venous isolation by
  direct h. (HVI-DHP)
hemopericardium
hemoperitoneum
hemophilic
 h. arthritis
 h. arthropathy
hemoplasty
hemopneumopericardium
Hemopure
hemopyelectasis
hemorrhage
 abdominal h.
 accidental h.
 active h.
 adrenal h.
 alveolar h.
 aneurysmal h.
 antepartum h.
 arachnoid h.
 arterial h.
 8-ball h.
 bilateral adrenal h.
 bladder h.
 blot h.
 brainstem h.
 catheter-induced pulmonary
  artery h.
 cerebellar h.
 cerebral h.

choroidal h.
colonic diverticular h.
colorectal h.
concealed h.
conjunctival h.
h. control
diffuse pulmonary alveolar h.
disc drusen h.
diverticular h.
dot h.
dot-and-blot h.
Duret h.
epidural h.
expulsive h.
exsanguinating h.
external h.
extradural h.
extraluminal h.
fetal h.
fetal-maternal h.
flame h.
flame-shaped h.
focal h.
h. focus
frank h.
gastric h.
germinal matrix h.
gingival h.
hepatic h.
Icelandic form of intracranial h.
intermediate h.
internal h.
intestinal h.
intraabdominal arterial h.
intraalveolar h.
intracapsular h.
intracerebral h.
intracranial h. (ICH)
intraluminal h.
intramural intestinal h.
intraocular h.
intraoperative h.
intraparenchymal h.
intrapartum h.
intraperitoneal h.
intraplaque h.
intraventricular h.
laryngeal h.
lobar h.
lower gastrointestinal h.
massive h.
mediastinal h.

mesencephalic h.
nasal h.
nasopharyngeal h.
neonatal intracranial h.
neonatal intraventricular h.
nonaneurysmal perimesencephalic
   subarachnoid h.
oropharyngeal h.
pancreatitis-related h.
parenchymatous intracerebral h.
perianeurysmal h.
perinephric space h.
periventricular-intraventricular h.
h. per rhexis
petechial h.
placental h.
pontine h.
postextraction h.
postgastrectomy h.
postoperative h.
postpartum h.
postpolypectomy h.
posttraumatic h.
posttreatment h.
preplacental h.
preretinal h.
primary h.
punctate h.
refractory variceal h.
renal cyst h.
reperfusion-induced h.
retinal h.
retinopathy h.
retrobulbar h.
retroperitoneal h.
retropharyngeal h.
round h.
salmon-patch h.
scleral h.
secondary h.
signal h.
slit h.
splinter h.
spontaneous renal h.
sternocleidomastoid h.
stigmata of recent h.
stress ulcer h.
subarachnoid h.
subcapsular h.
subchorial h.
subchorionic h.
subconjunctival h.

NOTES

H

hemorrhage *(continued)*
- subcortical h.
- subdural h.
- subependymal h.
- subepithelial h.
- subgaleal h.
- subhyaloid h.
- subintimal h.
- submucosal gastric h.
- subperiosteal h.
- subretinal h.
- suprachoroidal h.
- syringomyelic h.
- thalamic-subthalamic h.
- torrential h.
- transplacental h.
- unavoidable h.
- upper gastrointestinal h.
- variceal h.
- venous h.
- vitreal h.
- vitreous breakthrough h.
- white-centered h.
- yellow-ochre h.

hemorrhagic
- h. angiomyolipoma
- h. ascites
- h. complication
- h. edema
- h. endovasculitis
- h. gangrene
- h. infarction
- h. inflammation
- h. lesion
- h. metastasis
- h. radiation injury
- h. shock
- h. stroke
- h. transformation

hemorrhoid
- cutaneous h.
- h. excision
- external h.
- first-degree h.
- internal h.
- ligation of h.
- Lord dilation of h.
- mixed h.
- mucocutaneous h.
- necrotic h.
- prolapsed h.
- rubber-band ligation of h.
- second-degree h.
- strangulated h.
- third-degree h.
- thrombosed internal and external h.

hemorrhoidal
- h. nerve
- h. plexus

- h. vein
- h. zone

hemorrhoidectomy
- ambulatory h.
- anoderm-preserving h.
- closed h.
- diathermy h.
- Doppler-guided artery ligation h.
- Ferguson h.
- Harmonic h.
- laser h.
- ligation h.
- limited h.
- Longo h.
- Lord h.
- Milligan-Morgan h.
- modified Whitehead h.
- nonmucosal h.
- open h.
- Parks h.
- 2-quadrant h.
- 3-quadrant h.
- 4-quadrant h.
- radical h.
- rubber-band h.
- scissors-excision h.
- semiopen h.
- stapled h.

hemospermia
hemostasia
hemostasis
- chemical h.
- complete h.
- endoscopic h.
- global h.
- immaculate h.
- meticulous h.
- proactive h.

hemostatic
- h. activation
- h. agent
- h. collodion
- h. plug formation
- h. staple line
- h. suture technique

hemostat technique
hemostyptic
hemotherapy
hemothorax, pl. **hemothoraces**
Henderson
- H. classification
- H. fracture
- H. onlay bone graft
- H. posterolateral approach
- H. posteromedial approach
- H. skin incision

Henderson-Hasselbalch equation
Hendler unitunnel technique

Henke
  H. space
  H. triangle
Henle
  H. body
  H. elastic membrane
  H. fenestrated membrane
  H. loop
  H. tubule
Henning inside-to-outside technique
Henry
  H. acromioclavicular technique
  H. anterior strap approach
  H. anterolateral approach
  H. bone graft
  H. extensile approach
  H. incision
  H. operation
  H. posterior interosseous nerve
    approach
  H. posterior interosseous nerve
    exposure
  H. radial, approach
  H. resection
  H. splenectomy
Henry-Geist spinal fusion
Hensen
  H. body
  H. canal
  H. cell
  H. duct
  H. plane
Hensing ligament
hepaplastin test
heparin
  h. cofactor II plasma level
  h. irrigation
  h. neutralized thrombin time
    (HnTT)
heparinase correction
heparin-binding protein
heparin-induced
  h.-i. lipolysis
  h.-i. thrombocytopenia (HIT)
heparinization procedure
hepar lobatum
hepatectomize
hepatectomy
  cadaveric donor h.
  central h.
  concomitant h.
  donor h.

ex situ h.
ex situ-in situ h.
extended left h.
extended right h.
laparoscopic h.
laparoscopic-assisted h. (LAH)
LCVP-aided h.
LCVP-assisted h.
left h.
limited h.
living donor partial h.
local h.
partial h.
recipient h.
regional h.
right lobe h.
segmental h.
simultaneous segmental h.
standardized h.
subsegmental h.
subtotal h.
total left h.
triple lobe h.
wedge h.
hepatic
  h. abscess
  h. adenoma
  h. allograft
  h. arterial buffer response
  h. arterial infusion (HAI)
  h. arterial therapy
  h. artery
  h. artery embolization (HAE)
  h. artery-portal vein fistula
  h. branch
  h. candidal infection
  h. capsule
  h. cell carcinoma
  h. circulation
  h. colic
  h. colorectal metastasis
  h. coma
  h. complication
  h. congestion
  h. dearterialization
  h. decompensation
  h. duct
  h. duct calculus
  h. dysfunction
  h. encephalopathy
  h. failure
  h. fibrosis

NOTES

H

327

hepatic *(continued)*
   h. flexure
   h. function reserve
   h. fungal infection
   h. gunshot wound
   h. hemorrhage
   h. hilum
   h. hydrothorax
   h. injury
   h. intraarterial yttrium-90
      microspheres treatment
   h. intracellular energy
   h. intracellular energy status
   h. ischemia
   h. ischemic time
   h. lobectomy
   h. lobule
   h. malignancy
   h. margin
   h. mass lesion
   h. necrosis
   h. neoplasm
   h. outflow block
   h. outflow tract
   h. parasitic cyst
   h. parenchyma
   h. parenchymal transection
   h. pedicle
   h. perfusion
   h. plexus
   h. portal vein
   h. portojejunostomy
   primary h.
   h. regeneration
   h. resection
   h. resectional surgery
   h. rupture
   h. scintigraphy
   h. segment
   h. sinusoid
   h. subsegmentectomy
   h. surface
   h. territory
   h. transplant
   h. transplantation
   h. trauma
   h. triad
   h. tumor
   h. vascular exclusion (HVE)
   h. vascular isolation (HVI)
   h. vascular isolation technique
   h. venous confluence
   h. venous insolation
   h. venous isolation by direct
      hemoperfusion (HVI-DHP)
   h. venous outflow obstruction
   h. venous trunk
   h. venous web disease

   h. web
   h. web dilation
hepaticocholangiojejunostomy
hepaticocutaneous jejunostomy
hepaticocystojejunostomy
hepaticodochotomy
hepaticoduodenostomy
hepaticoenterostomy
hepaticogastrostomy
hepaticojejunostomy
   Hepp-Couinaud h.
   mucosa-to-mucosa Roux-en-Y h.
   Roux-en-Y h.
   wide mucosa-to-mucosa Roux-en-
      Y h.
hepaticolithotomy
hepaticolithotripsy
hepaticoportoenterostomy
hepaticopulmonary
hepaticostomy
hepaticotomy
hepatic-renal angle
hepatis
hepatitis
   H. Activity Index classification
   h. A-E infection
   anesthetic h.
   autoimmune h.
   h. B surface antigen (HB$_s$)
   h. C virus (HCV)
   fulminant h.
   halothane h.
   peliosis h.
   radiation h.
   short incubation h.
hepatization
   gray h.
   red h.
   yellow h.
hepatobiliary
   h. imaging
   h. manifestation
   h. surgery
hepatoblastoma
   unresectable h.
hepatocarcinoma
hepatocele
hepatocellular
   h. acidosis
   h. cancer
   h. carcinoma (HCC)
   h. function
   h. synthetic dysfunction
hepatocholangioenterostomy
hepatocholangiojejunostomy
hepatocholangiostomy
hepatocolic ligament
hepatocolicum
hepatocystic duct

hepatocyte
  h. growth factor (HGF)
  h. transplantation
hepatoduodenal
  h. ligament
  h. reflection
hepatoduodenal-peritoneal reflection
hepatoduodenostomy
hepatoenteric
hepatoesophageal ligament
hepatoesophageum
hepatofugal flow
hepatogastric ligament
hepatogastricum
hepatojejunal anastomosis
hepatojejunostomy
  complex h.
  high h.
  hilar h.
  intracystic h.
  laparoscopic h.
  palliative h.
  pediatric h.
  peripheral h.
  Roux-en-Y h.
  side-to-side h.
  simple h.
hepatolith
hepatolithectomy
hepatolithiasis
  intrahepatic h.
hepatoma
hepatomegaly
  congestive h.
hepatomphalocele
hepatomphalos
hepatonephric
hepatonephromegaly
hepatopancreatic
  h. ampulla
  h. fold
  h. sphincter
hepatopathy
  radiation h.
hepatoperitonitis
hepatopetal flow
hepatopexy
hepatopleural fistula
hepatopneumonic
hepatoportal biliary fistula
hepatoportoenterostomy
  Kasai-type h.

hepatoptosis
hepatopulmonary
hepatorenal
  h. angle
  h. bypass
  h. failure
  h. ligament
  h. pouch
  h. recess
  h. syndrome
hepatorrhagia
hepatorrhaphy
hepatorrhexis
hepatoscopy
hepatostomy
hepatotomy
hepatotoxemia
hepatotoxicity
  anesthetic h.
hepatotrophic nutrient
Hepp-Couinaud
  H.-C. biliary tract procedure
  H.-C. hepaticojejunostomy
herald patch
herbal
  h. medicine
  h. therapy
Herbert operation
hereditary
  h. breast cancer
  h. cancer syndrome
  h. coproporphyria
  h. flat adenoma syndrome
  h. malignancy
  h. multiple exostoses
  h. nonpolyposis colon cancer
    (HNPCC)
  h. nonpolyposis colon carcinoma
    (HNPCC)
  h. nonpolyposis colorectal cancer
    (HNPCC)
  h. predisposition
Hering
  canal of H.
  H. nerve
Hering-Breuer reflex
heritable connective tissue disease
Herman-Gartland osteotomy
Hermodsson
  H. fracture
  H. internal rotation technique
  H. tangential projection

NOTES

H

hernia

abdominal incisional h.
abdominal wall h.
acquired h.
amniotic h.
antevesical h.
axial hiatal h.
Barth h.
Béclard h.
bilateral inguinal h. (BIH)
bilocular femoral h.
Birkett h.
bladder h.
Bochdalek h.
broad ligament h.
cecal h.
cerebral h.
Cheatle-Henry h.
Cloquet h.
combined hiatal h.
complete h.
concealed h.
concentric h.
congenital diaphragmatic h. (CDH)
Cooper h.
crural h.
h. defect
diaphragmatic h.
direct inguinal h.
diverticular h.
double-loop h.
dry h.
duodenal h.
duodenojejunal h.
easily reducible h.
h. en bissac
encysted h.
epigastric h.
esophageal h.
extrasaccular h.
fascial h.
fatty h.
femoral h.
flank incisional h.
funicular inguinal h.
gangrenous h.
gastric h.
gastroesophageal h.
Gibbon h.
Gironcoli h.
gluteal h.
Goyrand h.
groin h.
Grynfelt h.
Hesselbach h.
Hey h.
hiatal h.
Holthouse h.
iliacosubfascial h.

incarcerated h.
h. incarceration
h. incision
incisional h.
incomplete h.
indirect inguinal h.
infantile h.
inguinal h.
inguinocrural h.
inguinofemoral h.
inguinolabial h.
inguinoproperitoneal h.
inguinoscrotal h.
inguinosuperficial h.
intermuscular h.
internal h.
interparietal h.
intersigmoid h.
interstitial h.
intraepiploic h.
intrailiac h.
intrapelvic h.
irreducible h.
ischiatic h.
Krönlein h.
labial h.
laparoscopic repair of
  paraesophageal h. (LRPH)
Larrey h.
Laugier h.
left inguinal h. (LIH)
Lesgaft h.
lesser sac h.
levator h.
Littré h.
Littré-Richter h.
lower quadrant abdominal
  incisional h.
lumbar h.
Madden repair of incisional h.
Malgaigne h.
Maydl h.
meningeal h.
mesenteric h.
mesocolic h.
h. metastasis
midline incisional h.
Morgagni h.
Morgagni-Larrey type h.
mucosal h.
multiorgan h.
muscle h.
nontraumatic h.
oblique h.
obturator h.
omental h.
orbital h.
ovarian h.
pannicular h.

pantaloon h.
paraduodenal h.
paraesophageal diaphragmatic h.
paraesophageal hiatal h.
parahiatal h.
paraileostomal h.
h. paralysis
paraperitoneal h.
parapubic h.
parasaccular h.
parastomal h.
paraumbilical h.
parietal h.
pectineal h.
pediatric h.
pericolostomy h.
perineal h.
peritoneal h.
peritoneopericardial diaphragmatic h.
periumbilical h.
Petit h.
pleuroperitoneal h.
port site h.
posterior vaginal h.
postoperative h.
h. pouch
primary indirect inguinal h.
properitoneal inguinal h.
pudendal h.
pulsion h.
rectal h.
h. in recto
recurrent incisional h.
reducible h.
h. repair
retrocecal h.
retrocolic h.
retrograde h.
retroperitoneal h.
retropubic h.
retrosternal h.
Richter h.
Rieux h.
right inguinal h. (RIH)
Rokitansky h.
rolling hiatal h.
h. rupture
h. sac
sciatic h.
scrotal h.
secondary h.
Serafini h.

short esophagus type hiatal h.
sliding abdominal h.
sliding esophageal hiatal h.
slipped h.
spigelian h.
Spigelius h.
spontaneous lateral ventricle h.
spontaneous ventrolateral h.
stoma h.
strangulated incisional h.
strangulated paraesophageal h.
subpubic h.
suprapubic h.
synovial h.
thyroidal h.
tonsillar h.
transient hiatal h.
transmesenteric h.
traumatic diaphragmatic h.
Treitz h.
trocar site h.
true h.
tunicary h.
umbilical h.
unilateral h.
uterine h.
vaginal h.
vaginolabial h.
Velpeau h.
ventral h.
ventral incisional h.
ventrolateral h.
vesicle h.
vitreous h.
Von Bergman h.
W h.
wound h.

hernial aneurysm
herniated
    h. disc
    h. fundoplication
    h. preperitoneal fat
    h. presacral fat pad
    h. viscus
herniation
    brain h.
    cardiac h.
    caudal transtentorial h.
    central h.
    cerebral h.
    cervical midline disc h.
    cingulate h.

NOTES

H

herniation (*continued*)
    cisternal h.
    diaphragmatic h.
    disc h.
    fat h.
    foraminal h.
    free fragment h.
    intercervical disc h.
    intervertebral disc h.
    lumbar disc h.
    midline disc h.
    nucleus pulposus h.
    h. pit
    posterolateral h.
    rostral transtentorial h.
    sphenoidal h.
    subfalcial h.
    synovial h.
    tentorial h.
    thoracic disc h.
    tonsillar h.
    transtentorial h.
    traumatic cervical disc h.
    uncal h.
    ureteroneocystostomy h.
    visceral h.
    vitreous h.
hernioappendectomy
hernioenterotomy
hernioid
herniolaparotomy
hernioplasty
    abdominal midline incisional h.
    classical Judd-Mayo overlap midline
      incisional h.
    GPRVS h.
    incisional h.
    Judd-Mayo overlap midline
      incisional h.
    laparoscopic h.
    Lichtenstein tension-free h.
    massive incisional h.
    mesh plug h.
    midline incisional h.
    modified Shouldice h.
    modified TAPP h.
    overlap midline incisional h.
    prosthetic incisional h.
    Shouldice h.
    tension-free h.
    transabdominal preperitoneal h.
herniopuncture
herniorrhaphy
    anterior inguinal h.
    Bassini inguinal h.
    h. chronic inguinodynia
    elective h.
    emergent h.
    extraperitoneal laparoscopic h.

    Halsted-Bassini h.
    Halsted inguinal h.
    Hill-type hiatus h.
    inguinal h.
    laparoscopic total extraperitoneal h.
    Lichtenstein h.
    Macewen h.
    Madden incisional h.
    McVay h.
    mesh h.
    modified Bassini h.
    modified McVay h.
    open h.
    pants-over-vest h.
    polypropylene mesh h.
    Ponka h.
    primary inguinal h.
    Shouldice h.
    sutureless laparoscopic
      extraperitoneal inguinal h.
    totally extraperitoneal inguinal h.
    transabdominal laparoscopic h.
    umbilical h.
    ventral h.
    vest-over-pants h.
herniotomy
    Petit h.
herpes
    h. epithelial tropic ulceration
    h. simplex virus infection
    h. zoster infection
    h. zoster pain
herpetic infection
herpetoid lesion
Herring lateral pillar classification
hersage
hesitation phenomenon
Hess
    H. eyelid operation
    H. ptosis operation
Hesselbach
    H. fascia
    H. hernia
    H. ligament
    H. triangle
heteroautoplasty
heterocheiral
heterodermic graft
heterogeneity characteristic
heterogeneous
    h. attenuation
    h. gland size
    h. graft
    h. keratoplasty
heterograft
    autogenous fascial h.
heterokeratoplasty
heterolateral

heterologous
  h. graft
  h. insemination
heterolysis
heterophoric position
heteroplastic graft
heteroplastid
heteroplasty
heteroscopy
heterospecific graft
heterotopic
  h. bone formation
  h. graft
  h. ossification prevention
  h. transplantation
heterotransplantation
heterozygosity
heuristic method
Heuser membrane
hexametazime
hexokinase method
hex procedure
hexylcaine
Hey-Groves
  H.-G. fascia lata technique
  H.-G. ligament reconstruction
    technique
Hey-Groves-Kirk
  H.-G.-K. bone graft
  H.-G.-K. technique
Hey hernia
Heyman-Herndon clubfoot procedure
Heyman-Herndon-Strong technique
HFDD
  human fibroblast-derived dermis
HFJ
  high-frequency jet
  HFJ ventilation
H-flap incision
HFOV
  high-frequency oscillatory ventilation
HFPPV
  high-frequency positive-pressure
    ventilation
HFV
  high-frequency ventilation
HGD
  high-grade dysplasia
HGF
  hepatocyte growth factor
H-graft
  H-g. bone graft

H-g. fusion
  mesocaval H-g.
HHCA
  hypothermic hypokalemic cardioplegic
  arrest
HHNKC
  hyperosmolar hyperglycemic nonketotic
  coma
hiatal hernia
hiatopexy
hiatoplasty
  tension-free h.
hiatotomy
hiatus
  adductor h.
  aortic h.
  Breschet h.
  esophageal h.
  fallopian h.
  maxillary h.
  pleuroperitoneal h.
  sacral h.
  saphenous h.
  scalene h.
  Scarpa h.
  semilunar h.
Hibbs-Jones spinal fusion
Hibbs procedure
hibernal epidemic viral infection
hibernation
  myocardial h.
hibernoma
hickory-stick fracture
hidden
  h. layer
  h. nail skin
hidradenitis suppurativa
hidradenoma
  clear cell h.
  cystic h.
  nodular h.
  papillary h.
  poroid h.
  solid h.
hidrocystoma
Hiff operation
high
  h. attenuation
  h. blind tract
  h. blood pressure
  h. cellularity

NOTES

H

high *(continued)*
    h. cervical anterior retropharyngeal approach
    h. dose radiation (HDR)
    h. dose rate (HDR)
    h. endothelial venule
    h. hepatojejunostomy
    h. intraluminal pressure
    h. intrauterine insemination
    h. ligation
    h. lip line
    h. lithotomy
    h. neurological lesion
    h. output ileostomy
    h. predictive value
    h. pressure zone (HPZ)
    h. smile line
    h. spinal anesthesia
    h. subtotal gastrectomy
    h. threshold receptor
    h. tibial osteotomy
high-affinity progestin receptor
high-altitude
    h.-a. endoscopy
    h.-a. simulation test
high-amplitude sucking technique
high-attenuation mass
high-capacity fluid warmer
high-dose
    h.-d. radioiodine therapy
    h.-d. scan
    h.-d. thrombin time (HiTT)
high-energy fracture
high-flux dialysis membrane
high-frequency
    h.-f. jet (HFJ)
    h.-f. jet ventilation
    h.-f. jet ventilator
    h.-f. oscillation
    h.-f. oscillation ventilation
    h.-f. oscillatory ventilation (HFOV)
    h.-f. percussive ventilation
    h.-f. positive pressure
    h.-f. positive-pressure ventilation (HFPPV)
    h.-f. positive-pressure ventilator
    h.-f. ventilation (HFV)
high-grade
    h.-g. astrocytoma
    h.-g. dysplasia (HGD)
    h.-g. MALT lymphoma
    h.-g. primary extremity liposarcoma
    h.-g. squamous intraepithelial lesion
high-heat casting technique
high-intensity lesion
high-kV technique
high-level disinfection
high-loop cutaneous ureterostomy
highly selective vagotomy (HSV)

high-magnification
    h.-m. colonoscopy
    h.-m. endoscopy
    h.-m. gastroscopy
Highmore
    H. abscess
    antrum of H.
    H. body
high-resistance fundoplication
high-resolution
    h.-r. image
    h.-r. parallel hole collimator
    h.-r. ultrasonography
high-risk
    h.-r. angioplasty
    h.-r. papillary cancer
    h.-r. patient
high-speed rotational atherectomy
high-tension suturing technique
high-voltage
    h.-v. pulsed galvanic stimulation
    h.-v. therapy
hila (*pl. of* hilum)
hilar
    h. biopsy
    h. carcinoma
    h. cholangiocarcinoma
    h. cylinder
    h. hepatojejunostomy
    h. mass
    h. plate
    h. region
    h. release
    h. structure scar tissue
Hilgenreiner horizontal Y line
Hilgenreiner-Perkins line
Hill
    H. antireflux operation
    H. fundoplasty
    H. gastropexy fundoplication
    H. hiatus hernia repair
    H. median arcuate repair
    H. posterior gastropexy
    H. procedure
Hillis-Müller maneuver
Hill-Nahai-Vasconez-Mathes technique
hillock
    seminal h.
Hill-Sachs
    H.-S. deformity
    H.-S. fracture
    H.-S. shoulder dislocation
    H.-S. shoulder lesion
Hill-type hiatus herniorrhaphy
HILP
    hyperthermic isolated limb perfusion
Hilton
    H. law

H. method
H. white line
hilum, pl. **hila**
hepatic h.
splenic h.
h. stimulation
hilus
Hinchey diverticulitis grade classification
hindbrain deformity
hindfoot
h. amputation
h. deformity
hindgut
hindquarter amputation
hinge
h. joint
h. osteotomy
h. position
soft tissue h.
hinge-axis point
hinged
h. corneal flap
h. fragment
Hinman
H. procedure
H. syndrome
Hinsberg operation
hip
h. arthroplasty
h. bone
h. deformity
h. disarticulation
h. dislocation
h. distractor
h. extension
h. fracture
h. fusion
h. pinning
h. positioner
h. reduction
h. replacement
h. replacement surgery
h. rotation
transient osteoporosis of h.
Hippel operation
hippocampectomy
Hippocrates manipulation
Hippocratic maneuver
Hirano body
Hirayma osteotomy
Hirschberg method

Hirschfeld
H. canal
H. method
Hirschsprung disease
Hirst operation
hirudin
hirudinization
His
angle of H.
H. bundle
H. bundle ablation
H. bundle heart block
H. canal
H. line
H. perivascular space
H. plane
His-Purkinje tissue
histamine 2 (H$_2$)
histangic
histiocyte
histiocytic tissue
histiocytoma
histiocytosis
histioma
histoangic
histochemical method
histocompatibility
histologic
h. assessment
h. characteristic
h. diagnosis
h. examination
h. investigation
h. lesion
h. liver biopsy finding
h. marker
h. pattern
h. result
h. study
h. tolerance
h. tooth repair
h. type
histological assessment
histology
histolysis
histonectomy
histopathologic
h. analysis
h. confirmation
h. data
h. diagnosis
h. examination

NOTES

H

histopathologic *(continued)*
  h. feature
  h. information
  h. validation
Histoplasma **infection**
history and physical examination
histotoxic anoxia
HIT
  heparin-induced thrombocytopenia
    immune-mediated HIT
Hitchcock tendon technique
HiTT
  high-dose thrombin time
HIV
  human immunodeficiency virus
    HIV classification
HIV-1, -2 infection
HLA
  human leukocyte antigen
    HLA identical kidney graft
HLES
  hypertensive lower esophageal sphincter
HLF
  human lung fibroblast
HNPCC
  hereditary nonpolyposis colon cancer
  hereditary nonpolyposis colon carcinoma
  hereditary nonpolyposis colorectal cancer
    HNPCC syndrome
HnTT
  heparin neutralized thrombin time
Hoaglund bone graft
Hoaglund-States classification
hobnailed appearance
hobnail liver
Hoche
  H. bundle
  H. tract
Hochenegg operation
hockey-stick
  h.-s. deformity
  h.-s. fracture
  h.-s. incision
Hodge
  H. maneuver
  H. plane
Hodgkin disease
Hodgson technique
Hoechst dye method
Hoffa
  H. fat pad
  H. fracture
Hoffman jejunoplasty
Hoffmann
  H. approach
  H. duct
  H. panmetatarsal head resection
Hoffmann-Clayton procedure

Hofmeister
  H. anastomosis
  H. gastrectomy
  H. gastroenterostomy
  H. operation
  H. procedure
  H. technique
Hofmeister-Pólya anastomosis
Hogan operation
Hoguet
  H. maneuver
  H. operation
  H. pantaloon hernia repair
Hohl-Luck tibial plateau fracture classification
Hohl-Moore
  H.-M. classification
  H.-M. technique
Hohl tibial condylar fracture classification
Hohmann procedure
Hoke-Kite technique
Hoke-Miller procedure
Hoke procedure
Holdaway line
Holden line
holder
  needle h.
hold-relax
  h.-r. method
  h.-r. technique
Holdsworth spinal fracture classification
hole
  bur h.
  lag screw thread h.
  h. preparation method
hole-in-1 technique
Hollander test
Holl ligament
hollow
  h. bone
  Sebileau h.
  h. visceral injury
  h. viscus
  h. viscus injury
Holmes method
Holmgren method
holoacrania
holocord
hologastroschisis
holoprosencephaly
holorachischisis
Holstein-Lewis fracture
Holth
  H. iridencleisis
  H. operation
  H. sclerectomy
Holthouse hernia
Holzer method

Holzknecht space
Homans sign
homatropine dilatation
homeostasis
    gut mucosal h.
    mucosal h.
    operational h.
homocladic
homogeneity
    tissue h.
homogeneous
    h. ablation
    h. graft
homogenous
    h. graft
    h. keratoplasty
    h. radiation
    h. tooth transplantation
homograft
    h. aortic valve replacement
    cryopreserved aortic h.
    homovital h.
    pulmonary h.
    h. reaction
    h. rejection
homokeratoplasty
homolateral
homologous
    h. artificial insemination
    h. blood transfusion
    h. graft
homolysis
homomorphic
homonomous
homonomy
homonymous hemianopsia
homoplastic graft
homoplasty
homotopic transplantation
homotransplantation
homotype
homotypic
homovital homograft
homozygous achondroplasia
honeycombed appearance
honeycomb lesion
hood
    H. and Kirklin incision
    laminar flow h.
    H. procedure
    H. technique

hook
    h. cautery
    h. electrocautery
    h. fixation
hooked
    h. bone
    h. bundle of Russell
    h. intramedullary nail
    h. wire localization
hook-lying position
hook-nail deformity
hook-plate fixation
hook-rod construct
hoop stress fracture
Hopkins operation
Hoppenfeld-Deboer
    H.-D. approach
    H.-D. technique
Horay operation
hordeolum
    external h.
Hori technique
horizontal
    h. angulation
    h. canal
    h. external rotation
    h. fissure
    h. flap
    h. gastroplasty
    h. incision
    h. mattress suture technique
    h. maxillary fracture
    h. osteotomy
    h. plane
    h. position
    h. projection
    h. section
hormonal evaluation
hormone
    circulating h.
    exogenous h.
    intact parathyroid h. (iPTH)
    parathyroid h. (PTH)
    steroid h.
    syndrome of inappropriate antidiuretic h. (SIADH)
    tropic h.
horn
    coccygeal h.
    dorsal h.
    lesser h.
    nail h.

NOTES

H

horn (*continued*)
    sacral h.
    superior h.
Horner
    H. muscle
    H. syndrome
hornification
hornpipe position
horripilation
horseshoe
    h. abscess
    h. fistula
    h. incision
horseshoe-shaped
    h.-s. flap
    h.-s. incision
Horsley
    H. anastomosis
    H. gastrectomy
Horton-Devine
    H.-D. dermal graft
    H.-D. procedure
Horwitz-Adams ankle fusion
Hoskins razor blade fragment
hospital
    H. Anxiety and Depression Scale
    Imperial College London H.
      (ICLH)
    h. monitoring
    h. mortality
    h. pneumoperitoneum
    h. stay
    Texas Scottish Rite H. (TSRH)
hospital-acquired infection
host
    graft versus h.
    reservoir h.
hostile abdomen
hot
    h. abscess
    h. axilla
    h. axillary bed
    h. biopsy
    h. biopsy technique
    h. defect
    h. gangrene
    h. knife conization
    h. lesion
    h. line
    h. nodule
    h. sentinel node
Hotchkiss-McManus PAS technique
hot-dog technique
hottest spot
Hotz-Anagnostakis operation
Hotz entropion operation

Houghton-Akroyd
    H.-A. fracture technique
    H.-A. open reduction
Hounsfield unit (HU)
hour
    1-h. office pad test
    postoperative h.
    postprandial h.
hourglass
    h. deformity
    h. head
    h. membrane
    h. stomach
House
    H. advancement anoplasty
    H. flap anoplasty
    H. reconstruction
    H. stapedectomy
    H. technique
House-Brackmann classification
Houston
    H. fold
    H. muscle
    valve of H.
Hovius
    H. canal
    H. membrane
Howard
    H. method
    H. technique
    H. test
Howell-Jolly body
Howe silver precipitation method
Howland lock
Howorth
    H. approach
    H. procedure
Howorth-Keillor procedure
Ho:YAG laser angioplasty
Hoyer
    H. anastomosis
    H. canal
HPT
    hyperparathyroidism
      familial HPT
      nonfamilial untreated HPT
      primary untreated HPT
      secondary HPT
      sporadic primary HPT
      symptomatic primary HPT
      untreated HPT
HPV
    hypoxic pulmonary vasoconstriction
H.P. Wright method
HPZ
    high pressure zone
      anal HPZ
HR
    heart rate

HRV
　heart rate variability
HS
　hypertrophic scar
HSE
　human skin equivalent
H-shaped
　H-s. capsular incision
　H-s. ileal pouch-anal anastomosis
HSV
　highly selective vagotomy
H-type tracheoesophageal fistula
HU
　Hounsfield unit
hub contamination
Huber adductor digiti quinti
　opponensplasty
Hubscher maneuver
Hudson line
Hudson-Stähli line
hue
　salmon-patch h.
Huebner recurrent artery
Hueck ligament
Hueter
　H. incision
　H. line
　H. maneuver
Hugenholtz method
Huggins operation
Hughes
　H. modification
　H. modification of Burch technique
　H. operation
　H. tarsoconjunctival flap
Hughston
　H. classification
　H. external rotation recurvatum test
　H. procedure
Hughston-Degenhardt reconstruction
Hughston-Hauser procedure
Hughston-Jacobson
　H.-J. lateral compartment
　　reconstruction
　H.-J. technique
Huguier
　H. canal
　H. circle
　H. sinus
Hui-Linscheid procedure
human
　h. AML cell line

　h. bite infection
　h. epidermal growth factor (hEGF)
　h. fibroblast-derived dermis (HFDD)
　h. immunodeficiency virus (HIV)
　h. immunodeficiency virus
　　classification
　h. leukocyte antigen (HLA)
　h. leukocyte class II DR antigen
　h. lung
　h. lung fibroblast (HLF)
　h. lyophilized dura cystoplasty
　h. monoclonal antibody
　h. ovum fertilization test
　h. papillomavirus infection
　h. skin equivalent (HSE)
　h. subject
　h. thrombin
　h. umbilical vein (HUV)
humeral
　h. approach
　h. artery
　h. articulation
　h. canal
　h. epiphysis
　h. fracture malunion
　h. head
　h. head-splitting fracture
　h. line
　h. physial fracture
　h. shaft fracture
　h. supracondylar fracture
humeri (*pl. of* humerus)
humeroperoneal neuromuscular disease
humeroradial articulation
humeroscapular
humeroulnar articulation
humerus, pl. **humeri**
humidity
　absolute h.
　relative h.
Hummelsheim
　H. operation
　H. procedure
humor
　aqueous h.
　vitreous h.
humpback deformity
hump removal
hunger
　bone h.
Hungerford-Krackow-Kenna knee
　arthroplasty

NOTES

H

Hungerford technique
hungry bone syndrome
Hunt
    H. and Kosnik classification
    H. operation
Hunt-Early technique
Hunter
    H. canal
    H. gubernaculum
    H. line
    H. operation
    H. technique for Toupet
      fundoplication
hunterian ligation
Hunter-Schreger line
Huntington
    H. bone graft
    H. disease
    H. procedure
    H. tibial technique
Hunt-Transley operation
Hürthle
    H. cell change
    H. FNA
Huschke foramen
Hutchinson
    H. fracture
    H. freckle
    H. patch
Hutchison syndrome
Hutch ureteral reflux operation
HUV
    human umbilical vein
      HUV bypass graft
HVE
    hepatic vascular exclusion
HVI
    hepatic vascular isolation
HVI-DHP
    hepatic venous isolation by direct
      hemoperfusion
hyaline
    h. basement membrane
    h. body
    h. mass
    h. membrane disease
    h. membrane syndrome
hyalinization
hyalitis anterior membrane
hyalocapsular ligament
hyaloid
    h. artery
    h. body
    h. canal
    h. posterior membrane
hyaloidotomy
hybridization-subtraction technique
hybrid myocardial revascularization
hybridoma technique

hydatid
    h. cyst intrahepatic rupture
    h. disease
    h. liver cyst
    h. material
hydatidocele
hydatidoma
hydatidostomy
hydradenoma
hydranencephaly
hydrate microcrystal theory of
    anesthesia
hydration
    adequate h.
    intravenous h.
    h. layer water
    maternal h.
    h. status
    h. therapy
    vigorous h.
hydraulic dissection
hydrencephalocele
hydrencephalomeningocele
hydrencephalus
hydroappendix
hydrocalycosis
hydrocele
    postoperative h.
    h. sac
hydrocelectomy
hydrocephalic
hydrocephalocele
hydrocephaloid
hydrocephalus
    normal-pressure h.
    obstructive h.
    post-subarachnoid hemorrhage h.
hydrocephaly
hydrochloride
    intranasal hydromorphone h.
hydrocholecystis
hydrocirsocele
hydrocolpocele
hydrocystoma
hydrodelamination
hydrodelineation
hydrodissection
hydroencephalocele
hydroflotation
hydroflow technique
hydrogen
    h. inhalation technique
    h. ion concentration (pH)
    h. washout method
hydrogenation
hydrogenolysis
hydrolysis
    ATP h.
    intragastric h.

h. of solution
h. of surfactant
urea h.
hydroma
hydromeningocele
hydromyelia
hydromyelocele
hydromyelomeningocele
hydromyoma
hydronephrosis
hydronephrotic
hydroperitoneum
hydropertubation
hydrophobicity assay
hydropneumoperitoneum
hydrops
endolymphatic h.
hydropyonephrosis
hydrorchis
hydrosarca
hydrosarcocele
hydrostatic
h. balloon dilation
h. pressure
hydrosyringomyelia
hydrotherapy
chylous h.
hydrothorax
hepatic h.
hydrotomy
hydrotubation
hydroureter
hydroxyapatite
h. arthropathy
h. cement cranioplasty
hydroxyethyl starch
hyfrecation
hygroma
subdural h.
hygroscopic
h. expansion
h. technique
hyla
hyloma
hymenal
h. caruncula
h. membrane
h. ring
h. syndrome
hymenectomy
hymenoplasty
hymenorrhaphy

hymenotomy
Hynes pharyngoplasty
hyoepiglottic ligament
hyoepiglotticum
hyoepiglottidean
hyoglossal
h. membrane
h. muscle
Hyoglossus muscle
hyoid
h. apparatus
h. bone
h. bone fracture
h. bone resection
h. fossa
h. muscle
h. syndrome
hyoideus
hyopharyngeus
hyothyroid
hyothyroidea
hyparterial
hypaxial
hypencephalon
hyperacute
h. graft-versus-host disease
h. rejection
hyperaeration
hyperaldosteronism
hyperalgesia
barbiturate-related h.
heat h.
incision-induced h.
secondary h.
visceral h.
hyperalimentation
central h.
intravenous h.
parenteral h.
peripheral h.
hyperbaric
h. local anesthetic
h. oxygen
h. oxygenation
h. oxygen therapy (HBO)
h. pressure
h. spinal anesthesia
h. tetracaine
hyperbilirubinemia
hypercalcemia
familial hypocalciuric h.

NOTES

H

341

hypercalcemia *(continued)*
    persistent h.
    recurrent h.
hypercapnia
    permissive h. (PHC)
hypercapnic
    h. drive
    h. ventilatory response
hypercarbia
    central venous h.
    gastric mucosal h.
    venous h.
hypercellular gland
hypercoagulable state
hypercoagulation
hypercontractile external sphincter response
hyperdense brain lesion
hyperdeviation
hyperdistended abdomen
hyperdynamic
    h. circulation
    h. shock
hyperemia
hyperemic
hyperesthesia
hypereuryprosopic
hyperexplexia
hyperextension deformity
hyperextension-hyperflexion injury
hyperfibrinolysis
hyperfiltration
    capillary h.
    glomerular h.
    h. injury
    renal h.
hyperfractionated total body irradiation
hyperfractionation
hyperfunctioning nodule
hyperglycemia
hyperhydration
hyperhydropexy
hyperinfection
hyperinflation
hyperinsulinemia
    peripheral h.
hyperintense brain lesion
hyperkeratotic lesion
hyperlactation
hyperlactemia
hypermetabolic response
hypermetropia
hypernephroid carcinoma
hypernephroma
hyperorchidism
hyperosmolar
    h. diabetic coma
    h. hyperglycemic nonketotic coma (HHNKC)

    h. hyperglycemic nonketotic coma (HHNKC)
hyperostosis
    diffuse idiopathic skeletal h. (DISH)
    generalized cortical h.
hyperoxic ventilation
hyperparathyroidism (HPT)
    ectopic h.
    neonatal severe h.
    primary h.
    sporadic primary h.
    untreated h.
hyperpathia
hyperpigmented lesion
hyperplasia
    adenomatous h.
    asymmetric h.
    atypical h. (AH)
    basal cell h.
    benign prostatic h. (BPH)
    congenital adrenal h.
    ductal h.
    florid h.
    focal nodular h. (FNH)
    4-gland h.
    intimal h.
    intraductal h.
    lingual tonsil h. (LTH)
    lobular h.
    moderate h.
    multigland h.
    multiglandular parathyroid h.
    multiple gland h.
    papillary h.
    parathyroid h.
    polyclonal h.
    polypoid h.
    solid h.
    sporadic multigland h.
    sporadic multiple gland parathyroid h.
    squamous h.
    stent-induced intimal h.
    thyroid h.
hyperplastic
    h. cyst
    h. cystadenoma
    h. gland
    h. graft
    h. inflammation
    h. polyp
    h. tissue
    h. tumor
hyperpronation
hyperpyrexia
    fulminant h.
    malignant h.
hyperreflexic bladder

hyperresonant abdomen
hypersalivation
hypersensitive xiphoid syndrome
hypersensitivity
    h. angiitis
    denervation h.
hypersensitization
hyperspectral analysis
hypersplenism
hypertelorism
hypertension
    arterial h.
    diastolic h.
    essential h.
    extrahepatic portal venous h.
    idiopathic intracranial h.
    intraabdominal h.
    intrahepatic h.
    lithotripsy-induced h.
    malignant h. (MH)
    neurogenic h.
    pediatric portal h.
    portal h.
    primary pulmonary h. (PPH)
    pulmonary artery h. (PAH)
    renal h.
    renovascular h. (RVH)
    surgically corrected h.
    unshuntable portal h.
hypertensive lower esophageal sphincter (HLES)
hyperthermia
    malignant h. (MH)
    stress-induced h. (SIH)
    h. therapy
    whole-body h.
hyperthermic
    h. isolated limb perfusion (HILP)
    h. temperature
hyperthymization
hyperthyroidism
    factitious h.
hypertonic
    h. bladder
    h. lactated saline
hypertonic-hyperoncotic fluid resuscitation
hypertrophic
    h. granulation tissue
    h. scar (HS)
    h. scarring

hypertrophy
    benign prostatic h. (BPH)
    eccentric h.
    hemangiectatic h.
hypervalvular phonation
hypervascular fragment
hypervascularity
hyperventilation
    alveolar h.
    isocapnic h.
    h. maneuver
    h. syndrome
    h. test
    h. tetany
hypervolemia
hypervolemic hemodilution
hyphema
hypnosis anesthesia
hypnotic
    h. dissociation
    h. effect
    intravenous h.
    h. response
hypoactive bowel sounds
hypoaeration
hypoalgesia
    somatic h.
hypobaria
hypobaric spinal anesthesia
hypocalcemia
    postoperative h.
    transient h.
hypocapnia
hypocarbia
hypocellular fibrous tissue
hypochondriaca
hypochondriac region
hypochondrium
hypochordal
hypocystotomy
hypodense brain lesion
hypoderm
hypodermatomy
hypodermic implantation
hypodermoclysis
hypoeccrisis
hypoechoic lesion
hypoesthesia
hypogastric
    h. artery
    h. artery ligation
    h. flap

NOTES

H

hypogastric *(continued)*
    h. ganglion
    h. nerve
    h. plexus
    h. plexus block anesthetic
      technique
    h. region
    h. vein
hypogastricus
hypogastrium
hypogastrocele
hypogastroschisis
hypogenitalism
hypoglossal, hypoglossus
    h. artery
    h. canal
    h. canal venous plexus
    h. facial nerve anastomosis
    h. facial transfer procedure
hypoglottis, hypoglossis
hypoglycemia
hypognathous
hypogonadism
hypohyloma
hypolobulation
hypomelanotic macule
hyponatremia
    spurious h.
hyponychium
hypooncotic plasma substitute
hypoparathyroidism
    permanent h.
hypoperfusion
    brainstem h.
    global h.
    regional h.
    splanchnic h.
    spreading h.
    systemic h.
hypoperfusion-induced PGID
hypopharynx
    diverticulectomy of h.
hypophyseal *(var. of* hypophysial)
hypophysectomize
hypophysectomy
    partial central h.
    total h.
    transsphenoidal h.
    unilateral h.
hypophyseoportal vein
hypophysial, hypophyseal
    h. artery
    h. duct
    h. fossa
    h. portal circulation
hypophysis
hypopigmentation
    postinflammatory h.
hypopituitarism

hypoplasia
    aortic h.
    pulmonary h.
hypoplastic
    h. left heart repair
    h. left heart syndrome
hyposalivation
hyposcheotomy
hypospadiac
hypospadias
hyposplenism
hypostasis
    postmortem h.
    pulmonary h.
hypostatic abscess
hypostomia
hypotension
    catecholamine-resistant h.
    controlled h.
    deliberate h. (DH)
    induced h.
    intracranial h.
    systemic h.
hypotensive
    h. anesthesia
    h. resuscitation
    h. surgery
hypothalamic activation
hypothalamic-hypophysial-ovarian-endometrial axis
hypothalamic-hypophysial portal circulation
hypothalamohypophysial tract
hypothalamotomy
hypothenar
    h. eminence
    h. hammer syndrome
    h. muscle
    h. prominence
hypothermia
    accidental h.
    h. anesthetic technique
    core h.
    deep h.
    extracorporeal exchange h.
    intraoperative core h.
    moderate resuscitative h.
    pediatric h.
    profound h.
    redistribution h.
    regional h.
    total body h.
hypothermia-induced coagulopathy
hypothermia-related coagulopathy
hypothermic
    h. anesthesia
    h. circulatory arrest
    h. effect
    h. hepatic perfusion

h. hypokalemic cardioplegic arrest
(HHCA)
hypothesis, pl. **hypotheses**
gate-control h.
hypotonia
skeletal muscle h.
hypotonic solution
hypotympanic cell
hypotympanum
hypouresis
hypoventilation
alveolar h.
benzodiazepine-induced h.
sedation-induced h.
hypovolemia
hypovolemic shock
hypoxemia
episodic h.
stagnant h.
hypoxia
diffusion h.
hypoxic h.
ischemic h.
local h.
stagnant h.
tissue h.
tumor h.
hypoxia-induced rhabdomyolysis
hypoxic
h. guard
h. hypoxia
h. pulmonary vasoconstriction
(HPV)
h. ventilatory decrease
h. ventilatory response
hypsibrachycephalic
hypsiconchous
hypsiloid
h. angle
h. cartilage
hypsistaphylia
hypsistenocephalic
Hyrtl
H. anastomosis
H. foramen
H. loop
H. sphincter
hysterectomy
abdominal h.
abdominovaginal h.
Bonney abdominal h.
cesarean h.

classic abdominal Semm h.
Dellepiane h.
Doyen vaginal h.
Eden-Lawson h.
extrafascial h.
gasless laparoscopic h.
Gelpi-Lowry h.
laparoscopically assisted vaginal h.
(LAVH)
laparoscopic-assisted vaginal h.
laparoscopic Döderlein h.
laparoscopic radical h.
Latzko radical abdominal h.
Mayo h.
Meigs-Werthein h.
modified radical h.
obstetrical h.
paravaginal h.
pelviscopic intrafascial h.
radical abdominal h.
radical vaginal h.
Reis-Wertheim vaginal h.
supracervical h.
total abdominal h. (TAH)
vaginal h.
Ward-Mayo vaginal h.
hysterical
h. anesthesia
h. colic
hystericus
hysterocele
hysterocleisis
hysterocystopexy
hysterolysis
hysteromyoma
hysteromyomectomy
hysteromyotomy
hystero-oophorectomy
hysteropexy
abdominal h.
Alexander-Adams h.
hysteroplasty
hysterorrhaphy
hysterosacropexy
hysterosalpingectomy
laparoscopic h.
hysterosalpingo-oophorectomy
hysterosalpingostomy
hysteroscopic surgery
hysteroscopy
laparoscopic-assisted vaginal h.

NOTES

H

hysterotomy
    abdominal h.
    vaginal h.
hysterotrachelectomy

hysterotracheloplasty
hysterotrachelorrhaphy
hysterotrachelotomy

IA
> inferior apical
>> IA segment

IAAA
> inflammatory abdominal aortic aneurysm

IAC
> intraarterial chemotherapy

IAP
> intraabdominal pressure

IAR
> immediate asthmatic reaction

IAS
> internal anal sphincter

IASP
> International Association for the Study of Pain
>> IASP Classification of Chronic Pain

iatrogenic
> i. arteriovenous fistula
> i. bowel injury
> i. hernia defect
> i. infection
> i. tension pneumothorax
> i. transmission

iatrotechnique

IB
> inferior basal
>> IB segment

I-beam
> I-b. hip hemiarthroplasty
> I-b. hip operation

IBP
> invasive blood pressure

IC
> Isaacson classification

ICA
> internal carotid artery

ICDA
> International Classification of Diseases, Adapted for Use in the United States

ice
> i. application
> i. point
> i. skater fracture
> i. slush

ice-cold saline

Icelandic form of intracranial hemorrhage

ICH
> intracranial hemorrhage

icing liver

ICISS
> International Classification of Diseases-9 Version of Injury Severity Score

ICLH
> Imperial College London Hospital
>> ICLH double-cup arthroplasty

ICP
> intracranial pressure

ICSI
> intracytoplasmic sperm injection

ictal abnormality

ICU
> intensive care unit
>> ICU care priority
>> ICU sedation

I&D
> incision and drainage

ideal
> i. body weight
> i. flap
> i. solution

Ideberg glenoid fracture classification

identical point

identification
> colonic lesion i.
> film i.
> lesion i.
> nasal mucosal i.
> i. phenomenon

identifying canal

identity formation

IDET
> intradiscal electrothermal therapy

idiographic approach

idiopathic
> i. adult intussusception
> i. bone cavity
> i. brachial plexopathy
> i. brown induration
> i. cause
> i. constipation
> i. dilation
> i. eczematous disease
> i. hypertrophic subaortic stenosis
> i. ileocecal intussusception
> i. intracranial hypertension
> i. paroxysmal rhabdomyolysis
> i. peptic ulcer disease
> i. preretinal membrane
> i. pulmonary fibrosis (IPF)
> i. ventricular fibrillation

IEA
> inferior epigastric artery
>> IEA graft

IG
> image guide
>> IG bundle

IGBB
  image-guided breast biopsy
    diagnostic IGBB
IGF-1
  insulin-like growth factor I
    exogenous IGF-1
ignition point
IGPA
  infragenicular popliteal artery
IGS
  image-guided surgery
  implantable gastric stimulation
IINB
  ilioinguinal-iliohypogastric nerve block
  ilioinguinal nerve block
ileac
ileal
  i. artery
  i. biopsy
  i. bladder
  i. conduit
  i. conduit urinary diversion
  i. crypt
  i. inflammation
  i. inflow tract
  i. J-pouch
  i. loop
  i. neobladder urinary pouch
  i. outflow tract
  i. patch ureteroplasty
  i. perforation
  i. pouch-anal anastomosis (IPAA)
  i. pouch-distal rectal anastomosis
  i. pouch surgery
  i. resection
  i. reservoir construction
  i. sphincter
  i. vein
  i. W-pouch
ileal-sigmoid anastomosis
ileectomy
ileitis
  pouch i.
ileoanal
  i. anastomosis
  i. endorectal pull-through
  i. pouch
  i. pouch procedure
  i. pull-through procedure
ileoascending colostomy
ileocecal
  i. cystoplasty
  i. edema
  i. eminence
  i. fat pad
  i. fold
  i. junction
  i. opening
  i. orifice

  i. pouch
  i. recess
  i. region
  i. ureterosigmoidostomy
  i. valve
ileocecocolic sphincter
ileocecocystoplasty bladder augmentation
ileocecostomy
ileocecum
ileocolectomy
ileocolic
  i. artery
  i. conduit
  i. intussusception
  i. resection
  i. vein
ileocolonic
  i. pouch
  i. pouch urinary diversion
  i. resection
ileocolonoscopy
ileocolostomy
  end-loop i.
  LeDuc-Camey i.
ileocystoplasty
  Camey i.
  clam i.
  LeDuc-Camey i.
ileocystostomy
  cutaneous i.
ileoduodenal fistula
ileoentectropy
ileofemoral wing fracture
ileogastrostomy
ileoileostomy
  duodenoileostomy i.
  laparoscopic duodenoileostomy i.
ileojejunal bypass
ileopexy
ileoproctostomy
ileorectal anastomosis (IRA)
ileorectostomy
ileorrhaphy
ileoscopy
ileosigmoid
  i. anastomosis
  i. colostomy
  i. fistula
  i. knot
ileosigmoidostomy
ileostomy
  Bishop-Koop i.
  blowhole i.
  Brooke i.
  i. closure
  i. construction
  continent i.
  defunctioning loop i.
  Dennis-Brooke i.

diversionary i.
diverting loop i.
double-barrel i.
end i.
end-loop i.
extraperitoneal i.
i. formation
Goligher extraperitoneal i.
high output i.
incontinent i.
J-loop i.
Koch continent i.
Koch reservoir i.
loop i.
loop-end i.
permanent loop i.
pouched i.
i. reversal
split i.
i. spout
i. stenosis
i. stoma
temporary loop i.
terminal i.
Turnbull end-loop i.
ileotomy
ileotransverse
i. colon anastomosis
i. colostomy
ileotransversostomy
ileovesical
i. anastomosis
i. fistula
ileovesicostomy
incontinent i.
ileum
terminal i.
ileus
adhesive i.
duodenal i.
gallstone i.
occlusive i.
paralytic i.
postoperative i.
iliac
i. apophysis
i. arterial tree
i. artery
i. artery aneurysm
i. artery angioplasty
i. bone
i. branch

i. bursa
i. buttressing procedure
i. colon
i. compression test
i. crest
i. crest biopsy
i. crest bone aspiration
i. crest bone graft stabilization
i. crest free flap
i. crest osseous flap
i. crest osteocutaneous flap
i. crest osteomuscular flap
i. crest resection
i. epiphysis
i. fascia
i. fixation
i. flexure
i. fossa
i. muscle
i. osteocutaneous free flap
i. osteotomy
i. plexus
i. region
i. roll
i. spine
i. steal
i. tubercle
i. vein
i. wing resection
iliacosubfascial
i. fossa
i. hernia
iliacosubfascialis
Iliff
I. approach
I. exenteration
iliococcygeal muscle
iliococcygeus
iliocolotomy
iliocostalis
iliocostal muscle
iliofemoral
i. approach
i. flap artery
i. pedicle flap
iliohypogastric
i. muscle
i. nerve
i. nerve block
i. neurectomy
ilioinguinal
i. acetabular approach

NOTES

ilioinguinal *(continued)*
    i. incision
    i. nerve
    i. nerve block (IINB)
    i. neurectomy
    i. ring
ilioinguinal-iliohypogastric nerve block (IINB)
iliolumbar
    i. artery
    i. ligament
ilioneoureterocystotomy
iliopectineal
    i. arch
    i. bursa
    i. eminence
    i. fascia
    i. fossa
    i. line
iliopelvic sphincter
iliopsoas
    i. muscle
    i. ring
    i. tendon
iliopubic
    i. eminence
    i. tract
iliosacral and iliac fixation construct
iliosciatic
iliospinal
iliotibial
    i. band
    i. band graft augmentation
    i. tract
iliotrochanteric
ilium
    external i.
    internal-external i.
Ilizarov
    I. external fixation
    I. limb-lengthening technique
    I. method
ill-defined mass
illness
    catastrophic i.
    life-threatening i.
    medical i.
illumination
    axial i.
    background i.
    central i.
    coaxial i.
    contact i.
    critical i.
    dark-field i.
    dark-ground i.
    diffuse i.
    direct i.
    erect i.

    focal i.
    Köhler i.
    lateral i.
    narrow-slit i.
    oblique i.
    slit i.
    vertical i.
ILP
    isolated limb perfusion
IM
    intramuscular
IMA
    internal mammary artery
    IMA graft
image
    i. acquisition
    i. analysis
    axial spin-echo i.
    body i.
    2C-L i.
    i. compression
    4C-T i.
    5C-T i.
    DG-L i.
    DG-T i.
    dynamic i.
    ejection-fraction i.
    ejection shell i.
    endoscopic video i.
    field-echo i.
    FLAIR i.
    flow-on gradient-echo i.
    fluid-attenuated inversion
      recovery i.
    i. formation
    i. formation principle
    gradient-echo MR i.
    gradient-recalled echo i.
    guidance i.
    i. guide (IG)
    i. guide bundle
    hard-copy i.
    high-resolution i.
    i. intensification
    i. interpretation
    MP-L i.
    MP-T i.
    multiplanar i.
    MV-T i.
    i. point
    point-counting i.
    radiographic i.
    real-time echo-planar i.
    real-time multiplanar i.
    i. registration
    sagittal spin-echo i.
    second-echo i.
    short-pulse repetition time/echo
      time i.

I

single-slice gradient-echo i.
spin-echo i.
static i.
i. subtraction
surface-projection rendering i.
thin-section axial i.
transmission i.
T1-weighted spin-echo i.
T2-weighted spin-echo i.
ultrasound i.
video i.

image-guided
i.-g. breast biopsy (IGBB)
i.-g. fine-needle aspiration biopsy
i.-g. interactive neurosurgery
i.-g. navigation
i.-g. pancreatic core aspiration
i.-g. stereotactic brain biopsy
i.-g. surgery (IGS)

image-integrated surgery treatment planning
image-related screening technique
image-selected in vivo spectroscopy
image-space focus
imaginal exposure
imaging
abdominal i.
anatomic i.
B-mode i.
chemical shift i.
color i.
2DFT gradient-echo i.
3DFT gradient-echo MR i.
2-dimensional Fourier transformation i.
2-dimensional Fourier transform gradient-echo i.
3-dimensional Fourier transform gradient-echo i.
3-dimensional projection reconstruction i.
direct Fourier transformation i.
Dixon method opposed i.
Doppler color flow i.
Doppler tissue i. (DTI)
echo i.
echoplanar magnetic resonance i.
endocrine i.
endometrial chemical shift i.
endorectal coil magnetic resonance i.
endoscopic ultrasonographic i.

endovaginal i.
exercise i.
field-echo i.
folate-targeted i.
functional magnetic resonance i. (fMRI)
gradient-echo MR i.
hepatobiliary i.
intraoperative i.
intravenous digital subtraction i.
magnetic resonance i. (MRI)
magnetic source i. (MSI)
i. method
i. modality
multiple-echo i.
multiple line scan i.
multiple-plane i.
multiple spin-echo i.
oblique sagittal gradient-echo MR i.
pancreatic i.
paramagnetic enhancement accentuation by chemical shift i.
phase-sensitive gradient-echo MR i.
point i.
power Doppler i.
preoperative i.
projection-reconstruction i.
projection tract i.
rapid acquisition radiofrequency-echo-steady state i.
rapid bedside i.
rotating frame i.
sagittal plane i.
selective excitation projection reconstruction i.
sensitive plane projection reconstruction i.
sequential line i.
sequential plane i.
sequential point i.
serial i.
short inversion recovery i.
single-echo diffusion i.
spin-echo magnetic resonance i.
spoiled gradient-echo i.
steady-state gradient-echo i.
i. strategy
stress-redistribution-reinjection thallium-201 i.
i. study
i. technique

NOTES

351

imaging *(continued)*
    time-of-flight echoplanar i.
    tissue Doppler i.
    transverse section i.
    tumor i.
    ultrafast magnetic resonance i.
    (UMRI)
    ventilation/perfusion i.
    xenon lung ventilation i.
Imanaga method
imbalance
    electrolyte i.
imbricate
imbricated suture technique
imbrication
    capsular i.
    facet i.
    i. line of Pickerill
    i. line of von Ebner
    MacNab line for facet i.
    medial capsular i.
    medialis obliquus i.
    retinal i.
IML
    internal mammary lymphoscintigraphy
immaculate hemostasis
immediate
    i. amputation
    i. asthmatic reaction (IAR)
    i. breast reconstruction
    i. extension technique
    i. flap
    i. postoperative period
    i. transfusion
immersion
    i. method
    i. microscopy
    i. technique
imminent cardiac arrest
immobilization
    cast i.
    cervical i.
    i. method
    postoperative i.
    rigid cervical i.
    Rowe-Zarins shoulder i.
    sling i.
    spica cast i.
    sternal-occipital-mandibular i.
    tooth i.
    Treponema pallidum i.
    Webril i.
immotile cilia syndrome
immovable joint
ImmTher therapy
immune
    i. electron microscopy
    i. inflammation
    i. mechanism

    i. modulation
    i. response
    i. system anatomy
immune-mediated
    i.-m. coagulation disorder
    i.-m. HIT
    i.-m. unfractionated heparin-induced
    thrombocytopenia
immunity
    cellular i.
    CTL i.
immunocompetent tissue therapy
immunocytochemical approach
immunocytoma
immunodeficient
immunodepression
immunodiagnostic method
immunodiffusion test
immunofluorescence
    i. method
    i. microscopy
    i. test
immunofluorescent examination
immunohistochemical
    i. analysis
    i. feature
    i. marker
    i. method
    i. stain
    i. staining
    i. technique
immunohistochemistry
immunoincompetent
immunologic
    i. classification
    i. complication
    i. impairment
    i. method
    i. method of purging
immunometric sandwich method
immunomodulating
    i. effect
    i. infection
immunomodulation
immunonutrition
immunoperoxidase method
immunoproliferative
    i. lesion
    i. small intestine disease (IPSID)
immunoreactive parathyroid hormone
    assay
immunoreactivity
immunoscintigraphy
immunostain
    cytokeratin i.
immunostaining
immunostimulation
immunosuppression
    pharmacologic i.

short-term i.
tacrolimus-based i.
immunosympathectomy
immunotherapy
active specific i. (ASI)
systemic i.
impacted
i. calculus
i. fracture
impaction
basket i.
endoscope i.
fecal i.
i. lesion
i. point
stool i.
impaired
i. healing
i. mobility
i. oxygen utilization
i. regeneration syndrome
impairment
immunologic i.
impalement
abdominal i.
anorectal i.
impalpable testis
impatent
impedance
electrode i.
i. method
pacemaker i.
i. plethysmography
i. pneumography
imperfecta
lethal osteogenesis i.
osteogenesis i.
severe deforming osteogenesis i.
Sillence type II-IV osteogenesis i.
imperforate anus
imperforation
Imperial College London Hospital (ICLH)
impetiginization
impingement
graft i.
i. sign
implant
i. abutment
i. alloy aluminum
i. arthroplasty
i. biocompatibility

breast i.
i. cervix
dental i.
drainage i.
encapsulated breast i.
i. entry
i. erosion
i. extrusion
i. failure
i. fatigue
fill breast i.
i. fixture
i. fracture
i. framework
i. gingival sulcus
i. infrastructure
i. mesostructure
i. migration
i. model
i. neck
neoplastic port site i.
palatal i.
2-piece dental i.
i. placement
porous polyethylene i.
porous tantalum i.
i. reaction
i. removal
i. restoration
i. stage
i. structure
i. substructure interspace
i. superstructure neck
i. survival rate
titanium vocal fold medialization i.
implantable
i. cardioverter-defibrillator/atrial tachycardia pacing
i. gastric stimulation (IGS)
i. infusion port
i. pain modality
implantation
i. bleeding
circumferential i.
cortical i.
displacement i.
i. failure
fusion i.
gastric balloon i.
i. graft
hypodermic i.
interstitial i.

NOTES

implantation (*continued*)
    in-the-bag i.
    intracavitary i.
    intraocular lens i.
    intrusive i.
    mesh i.
    i. metastasis
    metastatic i.
    needle tract i.
    nerve i.
    periosteal i.
    i. phase
    placental i.
    radioactive seed i.
    radon seed i.
    real-time 3D biplanar transperineal prostate i.
    i. response
    screw i.
    i. site
    stent i.
    subcutaneous i.
    subdural grid i.
    submuscular i.
    subpectoral i.
    superficial i.
    tension-free mesh i.
    i. test
    tubouterine i.
    ureter i.
    virtual i.
implant-bearing surface
implant-cement interface
implanted suture technique
implication
    clinical i.
    psychologic i.
implicit memory
implosive therapy
impotence
impregnation
impressio, pl. **impressiones**
impression
    cardiac i.
    colic i.
    digitate i.
    duodenal i.
    esophageal i.
    extrinsic esophageal i.
    i. fracture
    gastric i.
    i. preparation
    prepared cavity i.
    renal i.
    suprarenal i.
    surgical bone i.
    i. technique
    trigeminal i.

imprint
    tissue i.
improvement
    clinical i.
impulse
    ectopic i.
    i. formation
    mobilization with i.
    point of maximum i.
Imre keratoplasty
Imrie prognostic scoring index
imus
IMV
    intermittent mandatory ventilation
in
    in extremis
    in situ bypass
    in situ dissection
    in situ hypothermic perfusion
    in situ photocoagulation
    in situ pinning
    in situ procedure
    in situ reconstruction
    in situ spinal fusion
    in situ split-liver procurement
    in situ uterine repair
    in vitro contracture test (IVCT)
    in vitro fertilization
    in vitro fertilization-embryo transfer
    in vivo
    in vivo duplex ultrasound
    in vivo fertilization
    in vivo optical spectroscopy
    opting in
    in situ
    in utero exposure
inactivation
    trigger-point i.
inadequate
    i. dilation
    i. surgery
    i. visualization
inadvertent
    i. enterotomy
    i. laceration
    i. serosal tear
    i. trauma
    i. venous injury
in-and-out catheterization
inapparent infection
in-between size
incarcerated hernia
incarceration
    colon i.
    colonoscopy-related i.
    hernia i.
    iris i.
    penile i.
    retrograde i.

incarial bone
incarnant
incarnative
incidence
incident
    i. exposure
    i. point
incidental
    i. appendectomy
    i. parathyroidectomy
    i. rupture
    i. splenectomy
incidentaloma
    adrenal i.
incineration
incisal
    i. canal
    i. cavity
    i. mandibular plane angle
    i. point
    i. preparation
incised
    i. fascia
    i. wound
incision
    abdominal wall i.
    abdominoinguinal i.
    abdominothoracic i.
    ab externo i.
    ab interno i.
    Agnew-Verhoeff i.
    alar i.
    Alexander i.
    i. aligner
    Amussat i.
    angular i.
    anterior i.
    anterolateral thoracotomy i.
    anteromedial i.
    antimesenteric i.
    appendectomy i.
    apron flap i.
    apron skin i.
    arcuate i.
    areolar i.
    Auvray i.
    axillary i.
    backcut i.
    Banks-Laufman i.
    Battle i.
    battledore i.
    Battle-Jalaguier-Kammerer i.

bayonet-type i.
Bergmann i.
Bergmann-Israel i.
Bevan abdominal i.
bicoronal i.
bifrontal i.
bikini skin i.
bilateral subcostal i.
bilateral transabdominal i.
bisubcostal i.
Blair i.
boutonnière i.
Brackin i.
breast i.
Brock i.
Brockman i.
Brunner modified i.
Brunner palmar i.
Bruser skin i.
bucket-handle i.
Burns-Haney i.
buttonhole skin i.
Caldwell-Luc i.
capsular i.
cautery i.
celiotomy i.
cervical i.
cesarean section i.
Chang-Miltner i.
Charnley i.
Cherney lower transverse
    abdominal i.
chevron i.
chevron-shaped i.
Chiene i.
choledochotomy i.
chord i.
Cincinnati i.
circular i.
circumareolar i.
circumferential i.
circumlimbal i.
circumlinear i.
circumscribing i.
circumumbilical i.
clamshell i.
classical transverse i.
clavicular i.
i. closure
Codman i.
Coffey i.
collar i.

NOTES

incision *(continued)*

Colonna-Ralston i.
colpotomy i.
confirmatory i.
conjunctival i.
Connell i.
corneal i.
corneoscleral i.
corridor i.
cortical i.
Courvoisier i.
Couvelaire i.
Crawford i.
crisscrossing abdominal wall i.'s
crosshatch i.
cross-tunneling i.
crucial i.
cruciate i.
Cubbins i.
Curtin i.
curved i.
curvilinear i.
cutdown i.
darting i.
Deaver i.
decompression i.
deltoid-splitting i.
deltopectoral i.
Depage i.
diamond-shaped i.
dorsal linear i.
dorsal longitudinal i.
dorsal lumbotomy i.
dorsal transverse i.
dorsolateral i.
dorsomedial i.
double i.
i. and drainage (I&D)
Dührssen i.
dural i.
DuVries i.
Dwyer i.
Edebohls i.
eleventh rib flank i.
eleventh rib transperitoneal i.
elliptical uterine i.
Elsberg i.
endaural mastoid i.
endoscopic i.
endoscopically performed
  longitudinal i.
endourological cold knife i.
epigastric i.
3-i. esophagectomy
extended left subcostal i.
external bevel i.
extraction i.
fascia-splitting i.
Fergusson i.

fiber-splitting i.
fishmouth i.
flank i.
flexed i.
Fowler-Philip i.
Frazier i.
frown i.
Gaenslen split-heel i.
Gatellier-Chastang i.
Gibson long vertical relaxing i.
Gibson-type i.
Gluck i.
goblet i.
gray-line i.
Greenhow i.
Grice i.
gridiron i.
Griffith i.
grooved i.
gullwing i.
Hajek i.
Handley i.
Harmon i.
Harper-Warren i.
Hayes Martin i.
Heineke-Mikulicz i.
hemicircular i.
Henderson skin i.
Henry i.
hernia i.
H-flap i.
hockey-stick i.
Hood and Kirklin i.
horizontal i.
horseshoe i.
horseshoe-shaped i.
H-shaped capsular i.
Hueter i.
ilioinguinal i.
infraclavicular i.
inframammary i.
infraumbilical i.
inguinal i.
inner bevel i.
intercartilaginous i.
internal bevel i.
intracapsular i.
intraoral i.
intraperitoneal i.
inverse bevel i.
inverted bevel i.
inverted-U abdominal i.
inverted-Y i.
Jackson i.
Jergesen i.
J-shaped skin i.
Kammerer-Battle i.
Kehr i.
keyhole i.

Killian i.
Koenig-Schaefer i.
Küstner i.
Lanz i.
laparotomy i.
LaRoque herniorrhaphy i.
lateral utility i.
lazy-C i.
lazy-H i.
lazy-S i.
lazy-Z i.
L-curved i.
Lempert i.
Lilienthal i.
limbal i.
i. line
linear i.
Linton i.
lip-splitting i.
Loeffler-Ballard i.
longitudinal i.
low-collar i.
lower uterine segment i.
low-segment transverse i.
low transverse i.
L-shaped capsular i.
Ludloff i.
Lynch i.
MacFee i.
Mackenrodt i.
Mallard i.
marginal i.
Martin i.
Mason i.
mastectomy i.
mastoid i.
Mayfield i.
Maylard i.
Mayo-Robson i.
McArthur i.
McBurney appendectomy i.
McLaughlin-Ryder i.
McVay i.
medial parapatellar i.
median sternotomy i.
Meyer i.
midabdominal transverse i.
midaxillary line i.
midline lower abdominal i.
midline oblique i.
midline upper abdominal i.
Mikulicz i.

minilaparotomy i.
modified Gibson i.
Morison i.
multiple-port i.
muscle-sparing i.
muscle-splitting i.
Nagamatsu i.
Nicola i.
non-rib-spreading thoracotomy i.
Ober i.
Ollier i.
omega-shaped i.
Orr i.
ovarian i.
overlapping i.
palmar i.
parainguinal i.
paramedial i.
paramedian i.
parapatellar i.
pararectus i.
parasagittal i.
parascapular i.
paraumbilical i.
paravaginal i.
Parker i.
Péan i.
perianal i.
periareolar i.
perilimbal i.
perineal i.
periscapular i.
peritoneal i.
periumbilical i.
Perthes i.
Pfannenstiel i.
Phemister i.
Picot i.
plantar longitudinal i.
plaque i.
popliteal i.
port i.
postauricular i.
posterior hemicircular i.
posterior transthoracic i.
posterolateral costotransversectomy i.
preauricular i.
precut i.
Pridie i.
4-i. procedure
5-i. procedure
proximal i.

NOTES

incision *(continued)*

Pulvertaft fishmouth i.
puncture i.
racquet i.
racquet-shaped i.
radial skin i.
recently healed surgical i.
rectus muscle-splitting i.
rectus sheath i.
recumbent i.
relaxing i.
relief i.
relieving i.
Rethi i.
retroauricular i.
reverse bevel i.
reverse-Y i.
right-sided submandibular
   transverse i.
rim i.
Robertson i.
Rodman i.
Rollet i.
Rosen i.
Roux-en-Y jejunal loop i.
Ruddy i.
S i.
saber-cut i.
salmon backcut i.
Sanders i.
Sanger i.
scalp i.
Schobinger i.
Schuchardt relaxing i.
scoring i.
scratch-type i.
Sellheim i.
semiflexed i.
semilunar i.
serpentine i.
S-flap i.
Shambaugh i.
shelving i.
shoulder strap i.
Simon i.
single midline extraperitoneal i.
Singleton i.
skin crease i.
skin knife i.
skived i.
Sloan i.
smiling i.
spindle-shaped i.
spiral i.
split i.
split-heel i.
S-shaped i.
stab wound i.
standard clavicular i.

standard Kocher i.
standard retroperitoneal flank i.
stellate i.
steri-stripped i.
sternal-splitting i.
sternotomy i.
Stewart i.
stocking-seam i.
straight i.
subciliary i.
subcostal flank i.
subcostal transperitoneal i.
subinguinal i.
sublabial i.
submammary i.
subtrochanteric i.
subumbilical i.
supracervical i.
suprapubic Pfannenstiel i.
supraumbilical i.
surgical i.
Sutherland-Rowe i.
Swan i.
T i.
tangential i.
temporal i.
Thomas-Warren i.
thoracoabdominal i.
thoracotomy i.
transection i.
transmeatal tympanoplasty i.
transpubic i.
transrectus i.
transurethral laser i.
transverse fundal i.
transverse mastectomy i.
transverse skin i.
trap i.
trapezoidal i.
T-shaped i.
umbilical skin-knife i.
unilateral subcostal i.
upper midline i.
upright-Y i.
U-shaped i.
uterine i.
vertical midline i.
vertical uterine i.
volar midline oblique i.
volar zig-zag finger i.
von Noorden i.
V-shaped i.
Wagner skin i.
Warren i.
watchband i.
Watson-Jones i.
Weber-Fergusson i.
web space i.
wedge i.

Weir i.
Westin-Hall i.
Whipple i.
Wigby-Taylor i.
Wilde i.
Willy Meyer mastectomy i.
W-shaped i.
xiphoid-to-pubis midline
abdominal i.
xiphoid-to-umbilicus i.
Y i.
York-Mason i.
Y-shaped i.
Y-V-plasty i.
Z-flap i.
zig-zag finger i.
Z-plasty i.
Z-shaped i.

incisional
i. biopsy
i. corporoplasty
i. gastropexy
i. hernia
i. hernioplasty
i. infiltration
i. metastasis
i. pain
i. scar

incision-induced hyperalgesia
incisive
i. canal
i. duct
i. foramen
i. fossa

incisor point
incisura
incisural
i. dissection
i. epidermoidoma
i. space

inciting pathology
inclination
axial i.
condylar guidance i.
crown i.
enamel rod i.
lateral condylar i.
lingual i.
pelvic i.

inclinatio pelvis

inclinometer
1-i. method
2-i. method

inclusion
i. body
i. body disease
i. cyst

inclusion cyst
incompetence
primary vascular i.
saphenofemoral i.

incompetent sphincter
incomplete
i. amputation
i. atrioventricular dissociation
i. A-V dissociation
i. colonoscopy
i. compound fracture
i. dislocation
i. duplication
i. excision
i. fistula
i. hernia
i. polypectomy
i. reduction
i. regeneration
i. relaxation
i. right bundle branch block
i. tumor resection

inconsequential echo
incontinence
anal i.
Blaivas classification of urinary i.
exercise-induced i.
fecal i.
gas i.
neurogenic i.
overflow i.
paradoxical i.
passive i.
postprostatectomy i.
reflex i.
stress urinary i.
urge i.
urinary exertional i.

incontinent
i. ileostomy
i. ileovesicostomy

incorporated
meatal advancement and
glansplasty i.

NOTES

incorporation
> bone graft i.

increased
> i. lateral joint space
> i. pressure
> i. systemic vascular resistance

incremental
> i. blood sampling
> i. therapy

incrustation
> stent i.

incudal fold
incudomalleolar
> i. articulation
> i. joint

incudostapedial
incus
indenization
indentation
> i. gonioscopy
> i. hardness
> haustral i.
> i. operation
> prominent i.
> i. tonometer
> i. tonometry

independent exercise program
indeterminate FNA
index, pl. **indices**
> Abdominal Trauma I. (ATI)
> acute physiology prognostic
>   scoring i.
> Addiction Severity I.
> alveolar i.
> American Rheumatism
>   Association i.
> American Urological Association
>   symptom i.
> analgesic i.
> anesthetic i.
> ankle-brachial pressure i. (ABPI)
> Arthritis Helplessness I. (AHI)
> articulation i.
> atherectomy i.
> atrial stasis i.
> auricular i.
> basilar i.
> biliary saturation i.
> bispectral i. (BIS)
> body mass i. (BMI)
> Broders i.
> cardiac i. (CI)
> cephalic i.
> cephalorrhachidian i.
> cerebral i.
> cerebrospinal i.
> chest i.
> cholesterol saturation i.

computed tomography severity i.
  (CTSI)
cranial i.
dental i.
diastolic pressure-time i.
eccentricity i.
ejection phase i.
exercise i.
facial i.
Flower dental i.
frequency-duration i.
Gastrointestinal Quality of Life I.
  (GIQLI)
gnathic i.
height-length i.
Imrie prognostic scoring i.
irritation i.
juxtaglomerular granulation i.
length-breadth i.
length-height i.
limb salvage i.
maturation i.
mean shunt i.
i. metacarpophalangeal joint
  reconstruction
mitral valve closure i.
nasal i.
Neck Disability I.
orbital i.
orbitonasal i.
oxygenation i. (OI)
oxygen saturation i.
palatal i.
palatomaxillary i.
patient state i. (PSI)
pectus i.
penetrating abdominal trauma i.
  (PATI)
penile-brachial pressure i.
phosphate excretion i.
physical therapy i.
i. pollicization
portal shunt i.
pressure-volume i.
PSE i.
pulmonary vascular resistance i.
  (PVRI)
Ranson prognostic scoring i.
i. ray amputation
relaxation time i.
Right Ventricular Stroke Work I.
  (RVSWI)
Röhrer i.
sacral i.
saturation i.
sedimentation i.
segmental pressure i.
Shoulder Pain and Disability I.
shunt i.

Singh osteoporosis i.
systolic pressure time i.
thoracic i.
transversovertical i.
i. of variability
ventilation i. (VI)
vertical i.
zygomaticoauricular i.
Indian
    I. flap
    I. method
    I. operation
    I. rhinoplasty
Indiana continent reservoir urinary diversion
indication
    clinical i.
    emergency i.
    familial i.
    surgical i.
indicator
    i. of anesthetic depth
    i. dilution technique
    finger i.
    i. fractionation
    prognostic i.
    redox i.
indicator-dilution curve
indices (*pl. of* index)
indifferent genitalia
indirect
    i. defect
    i. fracture
    i. hemagglutination test
    i. hernial sac
    i. inguinal hernia
    i. laryngoscopy
    i. manipulation
    i. memory
    i. obturator nerve block
    i. ophthalmoscopy
    i. portography
    i. pulpal therapy
    i. reduction
    i. restorative method
    i. technique
    i. transfusion
    i. triangulation
indiscriminate lesion
indocyanine
    i. green clearance result
    i. green indicator dilution technique

i. green method
i. green retention test
Indoklon therapy
indomethacin-induced gastropathy
indophenol method
induced
    i. apnea
    i. bronchospasm
    i. hypotension
    i. hypotension anesthetic technique
    i. tension pneumothorax
induction
    i. of anesthesia
    anesthetic i.
    i. anesthetic technique
    i. chemotherapy
    dorsal i.
    electric i.
    endotracheal i.
    enzyme i.
    Faraday law of i.
    gene i.
    labor augmentation i.
    lysogenic i.
    magnetic i.
    menstrual cycle i.
    negative control enzyme i.
    neuromuscular system electric i.
    ovulation i.
    pain i.
    positive control enzyme i.
    rapid-sequence i. (RSI)
    remission i.
    single-breath i.
    Spemann i.
    sputum i.
    superovulation i.
induration
    brawny i.
    cyanotic i.
    essential brown i.
    Froriep i.
    gray i.
    idiopathic brown i.
    plastic i.
    red i.
industrial exposure
ineffective esophageal motility
inequality
    ventilation/perfusion i.
inertia
    colonic i.

NOTES

inextensible
infant
> Distress Scale for Ventilated
> Newborn I.'s (DSVNI)
> i. respiratory distress syndrome
> (IRDS)

infantile
> i. articulation
> i. choriocarcinoma syndrome
> i. colic
> i. embryonal carcinoma
> i. hernia
> i. perseveration

infantilism
> celiac i.

infarct
> i. expansion
> i. extension

infarction
> evolving myocardial i.
> hemorrhagic i.
> myocardial i. (MI)
> renal i.
> Thrombolysis in Myocardial I.
> (TIMI)

infarctive lesion
infected
> i. collection
> i. necrosis
> i. tract

infection
> abortive i.
> *Absidia* i.
> active systemic bacterial i.
> adenoviral i.
> adenovirus i.
> adnexal i.
> aerobic i.
> airborne i.
> amebic i.
> anaerobic ocular i.
> antifungal esophageal i.
> antifungal-resistant opportunistic i.
> apical i.
> aspergillosis i.
> *Aspergillus* i.
> asymptomatic i.
> atypical mycobacterial i.
> bacterial i.
> benign papillomavirus i.
> beta hemolytic streptococci i.
> biliary tract i.
> blood-borne i.
> bloodstream i.
> brain i.
> buccal space i.
> Bunyavirus i.
> i. calculus
> *Campylobacter* i.

> *Candida* i.
> candidal i.
> catheter-related i.
> catheter tunnel i.
> central line i.
> cervical i.
> cervicovaginal i.
> chlamydial i.
> *Chlamydia trachomatis* i.
> chorioamnionic i.
> chronic Epstein-Barr virus i.
> closed space i.
> clostridial i.
> CMV i.
> *Coccidioides* i.
> coliform urinary i.
> colonization i.
> community-acquired i.
> congenital HIV i.
> cross i.
> cryptococcal i.
> *Cryptococcus* i.
> cryptogenic i.
> cryptoglandular i.
> cryptosporidial i.
> cutaneous bacterial i.
> cutaneous viral i.
> cysticercal i.
> cytomegalovirus i.
> deep delayed i.
> deep-seated fungal i.
> deep wound i.
> dengue hemorrhagic fever i.
> dental i.
> dermatophyte fungal i.
> disc space i.
> disseminated CMV i.
> disseminated gonococcal i.
> dragon worm i.
> droplet i.
> dust-borne i.
> EBV i.
> echovirus i.
> ectothrix i.
> endemic fungal i.
> endogenous i.
> endothrix i.
> enteric i.
> enteroviral i.
> environmental mycobacterial i.
> epidural space i.
> Epstein-Barr viral i.
> esophageal fungal i.
> exit site i.
> exogenous i.
> extrapulmonary *Pneumocystis*
> *carinii* i.
> eyelid molluscum contagiosum i.
> fascial space i.

felon i.
fetal i.
focal i.
fungal pancreatic i.
fungous i.
gas-forming pyogenic liver i.
gas-producing streptococcal i.
gastric i.
gastrointestinal i.
gay bowel i.
genital i.
genitourinary i.
Giardia i.
gonococcal i.
graft i.
Gram-positive bacterial i.
granulomatous bacterial i.
granulomatous fungal i.
group A beta-hemolytic
  streptococcal i.
group A streptococcus i.
guinea worm i.
Hantavirus i.
helminthic i.
hepatic candidal i.
hepatic fungal i.
hepatitis A-E i.
herpes simplex virus i.
herpes zoster i.
herpetic i.
hibernal epidemic viral i.
Histoplasma i.
HIV-1, -2 i.
hospital-acquired i.
human bite i.
human papillomavirus i.
iatrogenic i.
immunomodulating i.
inapparent i.
intestinal i.
intraabdominal i.
intraamniotic i.
intrauterine i.
IUD-related i.
kala-azar i.
laryngeal i.
latent herpes simplex virus i.
line i.
liver cyst i.
local i.
lower genital tract i.
lower respiratory tract i.

MAC i.
MAI i.
mass i.
masticator space i.
maternal i.
Meleney i.
metasynchronous bacterial urinary
  tract i.
middle ear i.
mixed fungal/bacterial i.
mixed nail i.
monilial i.
Mucor i.
multiple hepatitis virus i.
musculoskeletal i.
mycobacterial i.
Mycobacterium avium complex i.
*Mycobacterium avium-
  intracellulare* i.
Mycoplasma i.
mycotic i.
necrotizing i.
neisserial i.
nematode i.
neonatal i.
neutropenia-related bacterial i.
nondermatophyte fungal i.
nonopportunistic i.
nontuberculous mycobacterial i.
nosocomial fungal i.
odontogenic i.
opportunistic systemic fungal i.
oral i.
overwhelming postsplenectomy i.
pancreatic bacterial i.
papillomavirus i.
parainfluenza virus i.
parasitic i.
parastomal i.
paravaccinia virus i.
paronychial i.
pelvic i.
percutaneous bone marrow i.
perianal i.
periapical i.
perinatal i.
perineal i.
periorbital i.
peripancreatic i.
peristomal i.
peritoneal fungal i.
persistent tolerant i.

NOTES

infection *(continued)*
    pharyngeal gonococcal i.
    pin tract i.
    pneumococcal i.
    polymicrobial i.
    postoperative i.
    postpartum i.
    postsplenectomy i.
    i. prevention
    primary fungal i.
    primary herpes simplex i.
    protozoal i.
    Pseudomonas i.
    puerperal i.
    pulmonary bacterial i.
    pulmonary fungal i.
    pulmonary parenchymal i.
    pure fungal i.
    pyodermatous i.
    pyogenic spinal i.
    i. rate
    recurrent upper respiratory tract i.
    renal cyst i.
    renal fungal i.
    repeated respiratory i.
    reservoir of i.
    respiratory syncytial virus i.
    respiratory tract i.
    retroperitoneal i.
    retrovirus i.
    rhinocerebral i.
    Rhizopus i.
    rickettsial i.
    rotavirus i.
    Salinem i.
    salivary gland i.
    scalp i.
    secondary fungal i.
    serpent i.
    Shigella i.
    shunt i.
    skin i.
    spinal i.
    spirochetal i.
    spirochete i.
    staphylococcal i.
    streptococcal i.
    Streptococcus i.
    subclinical i.
    subcutaneous fungal i.
    subcutaneous necrotizing i.
    subperiosteal i.
    subumbilical i.
    superficial subumbilical i.
    suppurative i.
    surgical i.
    surgical site i. (SSI)
    sycosiform fungous i.
    symptomatic i.
    synchronous urinary tract i.
    systemic fungal i.
    tarsal joint i.
    temporal space i.
    terminal i.
    Torulopsis i.
    trematode i.
    Trichomonas i.
    tunnel i.
    ultralow anterior resection parastomal i.
    unusual opportunistic i.
    upper genital tract i.
    upper respiratory tract i.
    urinary tract i.
    uterine i.
    vaccinia i.
    vaginal i.
    varicella i.
    varicella-zoster virus i.
    vertically acquired i.
    vesicular viral i.
    Vibrio fetus i.
    Vincent i.
    viral respiratory i.
    vulvar i.
    vulvovaginal premenarchal i.
    Walter Reed classification for HIV i.
    web space i.
    Western blot i.
    whipworm i.
    wound i.
    xenogenic i.
    yeast i.
    zoonotic i.

infectious
    i. complication
    i. etiology
    i. granuloma

infective extraabdominal complication

inferior
    i. aberrant ductule
    i. accessory fissure
    i. alveolar artery
    i. alveolar nerve
    i. alveolar vein
    i. apical (IA)
    i. arcuate bundle
    i. articular pit
    i. articular process
    i. basal (IB)
    i. boundary
    i. carotid artery
    i. carotid triangle
    i. cerebral artery
    i. cervical ganglion
    i. complete closed dislocation
    i. complete compound dislocation

i. costal facet
i. costal pit
i. dental foramen
i. duodenal fold
i. duodenal fossa
i. duodenal recess
i. edge
i. epigastric artery (IEA)
i. extradural approach
i. face
i. flap
i. flexure
i. fornix reformation
i. gland
i. glenohumeral ligament
i. gluteal artery
i. hemorrhoidal artery
i. hemorrhoidal nerve
i. hemorrhoidal plexus
i. hypogastric plexus
i. hypophysial artery
i. ileocecal recess
i. iliac spine
i. internal parietal artery
i. interosseous vein
i. labial artery
i. lacrimal duct
i. lacrimal papilla
i. lacrimal punctum
i. laryngeal artery
i. laryngeal cavity
i. laryngotomy
i. lateral genicular artery
i. lateral genicular vein
i. lingular segment
i. longitudinal sinus
i. meatal antrostomy
i. meatus
i. medial genicular artery
i. medial genicular vein
i. mediastinum
i. mesenteric artery
i. mesenteric ganglion
i. mesenteric plexus
i. occipital triangle
i. omental recess
i. orbital fissure
i. palpebral nerve
i. pancreatic artery
i. pancreaticoduodenal artery
i. parietal lobe
i. pelvic aperture

i. petrosal groove
i. petrosal sinus
i. petrosal sulcus
i. phrenic artery
i. pole
i. pubic ligament
i. rectal artery
i. rectal fold
i. rectal nerve
i. rectal plexus
i. sagittal sinus
i. suprarenal artery
i. surface
i. tarsus
i. temporal branch
i. thoracic aperture
i. thoracic artery
i. thyroid artery
i. thyroid notch
i. thyroid plexus
i. thyroid tubercle
i. transvermian approach
i. transverse rectal fold
i. transverse scapular ligament
i. turbinate blade
i. ulnar collateral artery
i. vena cava (IVC)
i. vena cava balloon occlusion
   (IVCO)
i. vena cava ligation
i. vena cava pressure (IVCP)
i. vena cava reconstruction
i. vena cavum (IVC)
i. vertebral notch
i. vesical artery
i. vesical nerve
i. vesical plexus
inferior-lateral endonasal transsphenoidal
  approach
inferolateral
inferomedial aspect
infertility evaluation
infestation
   noninvasive i.
infiltrate
infiltrating
   i. duct adenocarcinoma
   i. ductal carcinoma
   i. lobular carcinoma
infiltration
   adipose i.
   i. anesthesia

NOTES

infiltration (*continued*)
    i. anesthetic technique
    bacterial mucosal i.
    i. block
    bone marrow i.
    brachial plexus i.
    calcareous i.
    cellular i.
    choroidal i.
    colonic i.
    diffuse fatty i.
    epituberculous i.
    fatty i.
    focal fatty i.
    gastric epithelial cell i.
    gelatinous i.
    glomerular macrophage i.
    glomerular neutrophil i.
    glycogen i.
    gray i.
    incisional i.
    leukemic i.
    leukocyte i.
    leukocytic i.
    lipomatous i.
    local tissue i.
    lymphocytic i.
    lymphoid i.
    massive malignant i.
    mononuclear cell i.
    neutrophilic i.
    panmucosal inflammatory cell i.
    paraneural i.
    patchy i.
    peribronchiolar lymphocyte i.
    pericapsular fat i.
    perineural i.
    plasma cell portal i.
    root i.
    sanguineous i.
    tuberculous i.
    tumor i.
infiltrative carcinoma
inflamed synovial pouch
inflammable
inflammation
    active chronic i.
    acute and chronic i.
    acute hemorrhagic i.
    adhesive i.
    allergic i.
    alterative i.
    atrophic i.
    blenorrhagic i.
    bronchial i.
    bullous granulomatous i.
    calcified granulomatous i.
    cartilage i.
    caseating granulomatous i.

caseous i.
catarrhal i.
cavitating i.
i. cell
central zone i.
cervical i.
chronic jejunal i.
circumscribed i.
confluent i.
croupous i.
cystic acute i.
cystic chronic i.
cystic granulomatous i.
degenerative i.
diffuse acute i.
diffuse chronic i.
disseminated i.
ear cartilage i.
erosive i.
esophageal i.
exanthematous i.
exudative granulomatous i.
fibrinoid necrotizing i.
fibrinopurulent i.
fibrinous i.
fibrocaseous i.
fibroid i.
focal granulomatous i.
follicular i.
gangrenous granulomatous i.
gelatinous acute i.
gingival i.
granulomatous i.
hemorrhagic i.
hyperplastic i.
ileal i.
immune i.
interstitial i.
intralobular i.
ischemic ocular i.
localized i.
membranous acute i.
microbiliary i.
miliary granulomatous i.
mucosal i.
multifocal i.
myocardial i.
necrotic i.
necrotizing granulomatous i.
neutrophilic i.
nonnecrotizing granulomatous i.
obliterative i.
ocular i.
organizing i.
ossifying i.
pelvic i.
periodontal i.
perirectal i.
portal eosinophilic i.

portal tract i.
prepatellar bursa i.
productive i.
proliferative i.
pseudomembranous acute i.
purulent i.
pustular i.
i. reaction
recurrent i.
retrodiscal temporomandibular joint
  pad i.
sanguineous i.
sclerosing i.
serofibrinous i.
serous acute i.
spinal i.
subacute i.
suppurative acute i.
suppurative chronic i.
suppurative granulomatous i.
transmural i.
transudative i.
traumatic i.
ulcerative i.
urate-associated i.
uremic i.
vaginal i.
vesicular acute i.
vesicular granulomatous i.
inflammation-induced PGID
inflammatory
  i. abdominal aortic aneurysm
    (IAAA)
  i. arteritis
  i. bowel disease
  i. breast carcinoma
  i. cavity
  i. cell
  i. cytokine
  i. exudate
  i. fistula
  i. fracture
  i. granuloma
  i. lesion
  i. membrane
  i. pain
  i. perforation
  i. problem
  i. pseudotumor formation
  i. response
  i. rupture

  i. sinus tract
  i. transcription factor
inflated lung
inflation
  balloon i.
  i. reflex
inflection, inflexion
  point of i.
inflow
  arterial i.
  i. control
  i. occlusion
  portal i.
  i. tract
  i. vessel
infold
informal method
information
  anatomic imaging i.
  histopathologic i.
  prognostic i.
informed consent
infraauricular mass
infraclavicular
  i. brachial plexus block
  i. fossa
  i. incision
  i. part of brachial plexus
  i. triangle
infraclinoid aneurysm
infracostal line
infracotyloid
infraction fracture
infradiaphragmatic
infraduodenal fossa
infragastric pancreoscopy
infragenicular popliteal artery (IGPA)
infraglenoid tubercle
infraglottic
  i. cavity
  i. space
infrahepatic
  i. cavotomy
  i. inferior vena cava
infrahyoid
  i. bursa
  i. muscle
infrainguinal bypass
infralabyrinthine approach
inframammary
  i. approach
  i. crease

NOTES

367

inframammary *(continued)*
  i. incision
  i. region
inframandibular
inframarginal
inframaxillary
inframesocolic space
infraorbital
  i. anesthesia
  i. artery
  i. canal
  i. foramen
  i. groove
  i. injection
  i. nerve
  i. nerve block
  i. notch
  i. region
  i. space
  i. space abscess
  i. suture
  i. vein
infrapatellar
  i. bursa
  i. fat body
  i. tendon rupture
infrapopliteal
  i. bypass
  i. transluminal angioplasty
  i. vessel
infrared
  i. coagulation
  i. photocoagulation
  i. spectroscopy
  i. therapy
  i. transillumination gastroscopy
infrarenal
  i. aorta
  i. aortic cross-clamping
  i. aortic reconstruction
  i. cava
  i. endograft placement
  i. template procedure
infrascapular
  i. artery
  i. region
infraspinatus
  i. bursa
  i. insertion erosion
infraspinous fossa
infrasplenic
infrasternal angle
infrastructure
  implant i.
infratemporal
  i. crest
  i. fossa
  i. fossa approach
  i. space

infratentorial
  i. arteriovenous malformation
  i. structure
  i. supracerebellar approach
  i. tumor
infrathoracic
infratrochlearis
infratrochlear nerve
infraumbilical
  i. incision
  i. omphalocele
  i. position
infraversion
infundibula (*pl. of* infundibulum)
infundibular wedge resection
infundibulectomy
  Brock i.
infundibuliform
  i. fascia
  i. sheath
infundibuloma
infundibuloovarian ligament
infundibulopelvic ligament
infundibulotomy
infundibulum, pl. **infundibula**
  caliceal i.
  ethmoidal i.
infused fluid
infusion
  analgesic i.
  i. cholangiography
  chronic subcutaneous i.
  computer-assisted controlled i.
    (CACI)
  drip i.
  drug i.
  epidural opioid i.
  i. graft
  hepatic arterial i. (HAI)
  intravariceal i.
  lipid i.
  mesenteric vasodilator i.
  nerve block i.
  phentolamine i.
  i. port
  portal i.
  propofol i.
  protracted venous i.
  i. rate
  steady-state i.
  target-controlled i. (TCI)
  triple-lumen i.
  vasodilator i.
infusional chemotherapy
Ingelman-Sundberg gracilis muscle
  procedure
ingested foreign body
Inglis-Cooper technique

Inglis-Ranawat-Straub
> I.-R.-S. elbow synovectomy
> I.-R.-S. technique

Inglis triaxial total elbow arthroplasty
Ingram bony bridge resection
Ingram-Canle-Beaty epiphysial-metaphysial osteotomy
Ingram-Withers-Speltz motor test
ingrowing toenail
ingrown nail
ingrowth
> fibrous i.
> i. fixation
> local i.

inguen
inguinal
> i. aponeurotic fold
> i. approach
> i. branch
> i. canal
> i. canal dissection
> i. crest
> i. field block
> i. fossa
> i. gland
> i. hernia
> i. herniorrhaphy
> i. incision
> i. ligament
> i. lymphadenectomy
> i. lymph node metastasis
> i. neuralgia
> i. perivascular block
> i. plexus
> i. region
> i. ring
> i. triangle
> i. trigone

inguinal-femoral node dissection
inguinocrural hernia
inguinodynia
> herniorrhaphy chronic i.
> mesh i.
> post herniorrhaphy i.

inguinofemoral hernia
inguinolabial hernia
inguinoperitoneal
inguinoproperitoneal hernia
inguinoscrotal hernia
inguinosuperficial hernia
inhalant anesthesia

inhalation
> i. aerosol
> i. agent
> i. analgesia
> i. anesthetic technique
> i. mask anesthesia
> i. method
> i. pneumonia
> i. therapy
> i. tuberculosis

inhalational anesthesia
inhaled
> i. anesthetic
> i. nitrous oxide (INO)

inherent risk
inherited
> i. cancer syndrome
> i. neuropathy

inhibition
> polymerase i.
> pyruvate dehydrogenase i.

inhibitor
> ACE i.
> COX-2 i.
> cytokine receptor i.
> direct thrombin i.
> phosphodiesterase III i.
> proton pump i. (PPI)
> selective serotonin reuptake i. (SSRI)

inhibitory
> i. nerve
> i. reflex
> i. role

inhibitory-excitatory mechanism
in-hospital mortality rate
inion
initial
> i. colostomy
> i. consonant position
> i. manifestation
> i. necrosectomy
> i. operation
> i. preparation
> i. primary pathogen
> i. resection
> i. screening procedure
> i. syphilitic lesion
> i. systemic chemotherapy

initialization
initiation
> tumor i.

NOTES

injected
injection
    air i.
    block i.
    blood patch i.
    bolus i.
    cervical nerve root i.
    ciliary i.
    circumcorneal i.
    collagen i.
    conjunctival i.
    continuous subcutaneous insulin i.
    contrast i.
    corticoid i.
    CT with hepatic arterial i.
    dermal i.
    dermal route of i.
    dye i.
    endoscopic India ink i.
    epidural steroid i. (ESI)
    ethanol i.
    extraarachnoid i.
    facet joint i.
    fluoroscopically guided
      corticosteroid i.
    fluoroscopically guided low-volume
      peritendinous corticosteroid i.
    heavy metal i.
    infraorbital i.
    i. injury
    intraarticular i.
    intraarticular facet i.
    intracavernosal i.
    intracavernous i.
    intracordal silicone i.
    intracytoplasmic sperm i. (ICSI)
    intradermal i.
    intralesional i.
    intramuscular i.
    intraosseous i.
    intrapulpal i.
    intratendinous i.
    intrathecal i.
    intratumoral i.
    intravariceal i.
    intravascular i.
    intravenous i.
    intraventricular i.
    intravitreal i.
    ipsilateral i.
    isotope i.
    local i.
    i. of local anesthetic
    lumbar facet i.
    lumbar nerve root i.
    i. mass
    mental block i.
    i. method
    i. molding

    morphine sulfate extended-release
      liposome i.
    nasopalatine i.
    nerve root sleeve i.
    paracervical i.
    paramagnetic contrast i.
    paravariceal i.
    parenchymal route of i.
    percutaneous alcohol i.
    percutaneous ethanol i. (PEI)
    peribulbar i.
    periocular i.
    peroneal tendon sheath i.
    retrobulbar i.
    retrogasserian glycerol i.
    root i.
    route of i.
    saline i.
    i. sclerotherapy
    selective i.
    sensitizing i.
    sham i.
    i. site
    steroid i.
    i. study
    subarachnoid i.
    subconjunctival i.
    subcutaneous i.
    tangential colonic submucosal i.
    i. technique
    test i.
    i. therapy
    trigger point i.
    ultrasonographically-guided i.
    Van Lint i.
    vocal cord i.
    i. volume
injection-molded method
injury
    acceleration i.
    acceleration/deceleration i.
    Ajmalin liver i.
    anal sphincter i.
    anterior abdominal i.
    arterial i.
    associated i.
    axial compression i.
    axillary vascular i.
    axonal i.
    bile duct i.
    blast gut i.
    blast lung i.
    blunt carotid i.
    blunt liver i.
    blunt torso i.
    bowel i.
    brachial plexus traction i.
    brain i.
    burn i.

Callahan extension of cervical i.
carotid i.
cerebral i.
cervical i.
closed head i.
closed soft tissue i.
combined i.'s
complement-induced lung i.
compression i.
concomitant spinal cord i.
crush i.
cutaneous burn i.
decompensation i.
diaphragm i.
diaphragmatic i.
duct i.
endothelial i.
epiphysial plate i.
explosion i.
extension i.
extension-type cervical spine i.
extensor tendon i.
extraabdominal i.
extravasation i.
extremity i.
first-degree radiation i.
flexion-extension i.
fourth-degree radiation i.
geriatric i.
head i.
hemorrhagic radiation i.
hepatic i.
hollow visceral i.
hollow viscus i.
hyperextension-hyperflexion i.
hyperfiltration i.
iatrogenic bowel i.
inadvertent venous i.
injection i.
innominate vascular i.
intestinal radiation i.
intraabdominal i.
intraoperative inadvertent venous i.
intrathoracic i.
I/R i.
irradiation i.
ischemia and reperfusion i.
ischemia-reperfusion i.
ischemic liver i.
isolated arterial i.
isolated liver i.
isolated venous i.

kneecapping i.
lateral compression i.
left-sided i.
levator i.
liver i.
major vascular i.
manipulation-induced PGID i.
medication-induced i.
microwave radiation i.
mild traumatic brain i. (MTBI)
minor splenic i.
missile i.
needlestick i.
nerve i.
neurologic i.
nonsevered i.
obstetrical traction i.
obturator nerve i.
occult diaphragmatic i.
open head i.
organ-specific pattern of i.
osteochondral i.
pediatric i.
penetrating liver i.
penetrating thoracoabdominal i.
percutaneous i. (PI)
perigenicular vascular i.
peripheral nerve i.
peroneal nerve i.
i. prevention
pronation i.
pronation-abduction i.
pronation-eversion i.
pronation-eversion-external
   rotation i.
proximal subclavian i.
radiation i.
recurrent nerve i.
reperfusion i.
retroclavicular i.
right-sided i.
second-degree radiation i.
severe traumatic brain i.
I. Severity Score (ISS)
soft tissue extremity i.
sphincter i.
spinal cord i.
splenic i.
stretch i.
subclavian i.
suction i.
supination i.

NOTES

injury *(continued)*
    supination-external rotation i.
    supination-inversion rotation i.
    supination-plantar flexion i.
    thermal i.
    third-degree radiation i.
    thoracic inlet vascular i.
    thoracoabdominal i.
    torso i.
    transfusion-related acute lung i.
      (TRALD)
    transfusion-related lung i. (TRLI)
    translation i.
    traumatic brain i. (TBI)
    trifurcation i.
    trocar i.
    trocar-related i.
    ureteral i.
    urinary tract i.
    valgus-external rotation i.
    vascular i.
    venous i.
    ventilator-induced lung i. (VILI)
    visceral i.
    viscus i.
    whiplash i.
injury-prevention strategy
inlay
    i. bone graft
    corneal i.
    direct method for making i.'s
    epithelial i.
    i. restoration
inlet
    i. allotransplantation
    i. patch mucosa
    i. port
    thoracic i.
in-line perfusion
innate immunity gene
inner
    i. bevel incision
    i. cell mass
    i. ear tack procedure
    i. limiting membrane
    i. table
innervation
    cutaneous i.
    i. of head and neck
    i. problem
    striated muscle i.
innominate
    i. artery
    i. artery compression syndrome
    i. artery reconstruction
    i. bone
    i. bone resection
    i. cardiac vein
    i. line

    i. osteotomy
    i. vascular injury
    i. vessel
innovative therapy
INO
    inhaled nitrous oxide
inoperable
    i. canal
    i. patient
inoscopy
inotrope
    i. resuscitation
    i. resuscitation technique
inotropic state
inotropism
inotropy
    negative i.
Inoue balloon mitral valvotomy
inpatient
    i. dialysis
    i. dialysis unit
input layer
inquiry
    cognitive-attitudinal factor i.
INR
    international normalized ratio
Insall
    I. anterior cruciate ligament
      reconstruction
    I. ligament reconstruction technique
    I. patella alta method
    I. patellar injury classification
    I. procedure
    I. procedure
Insall-Burstein-Freeman knee
  arthroplasty
inscription
    tendinous i.
insemination
    artificial intravaginal i.
    cervical i.
    cup i.
    direct intraperitoneal i.
    heterologous i.
    high intrauterine i.
    homologous artificial i.
    intrafollicular i.
    intratubal i.
    intrauterine i.
    Makler i.
    subzonal i.
    i. swim-up technique
    therapeutic i.
    washed intrauterine i.
insert graft
insertion
    anatomic i.
    anomalous i.
    anuloplasty band i.

axillary i.
biliary endoprosthesis i.
blind i.
buttonhole puncture technique for
  hemodialysis needle i.
catheter i.
caval i.
depth of i. (DOI)
endovascular graft i.
flatus tube i.
fluoroscopic i.
jejunal tube i.
J-tube i.
i. loss
marginal i.
needle i.
path of i.
PEG i.
percutaneous catheter i.
percutaneous endoscopic
  gastrostomy i.
percutaneous pin i.
Pierrot-Murphy advancement i.
i. point
rerouting i.
retrograde catheter i.
route of i.
screw i.
subclavian central venous
  catheter i.
i. technique
tendinous i.
tensor i.
transjugular i.
velamentous i.
wire i.
insertional excursion
inside-out technique
inside-to-outside technique
insolation
hepatic venous i.
inspiration
crowing i.
degree of i.
end i.
shallow i.
suspended i.
i. time
inspiratory
i. bulbospinal neuron
i. intercostal activity
i. occlusion pressure

i. positive airway pressure
i. pressure support
i. rib cage depression
i. time (Ti)
i. vapor concentration
i. warmer
inspiratory/expiratory
inspiratory-to-expiratory ratio
inspired
i. air
i. gas
i. ventilation (VI)
inspissate
inspissation
instability
atlantoaxial i.
catheter i.
cervical i.
congenital cervical i.
detrusor i.
dorsal intercalary segmental i.
extension i.
hemodynamic i.
membrane i.
1-plane i.
sagittal plane i.
spinal i.
installation procedure
install method
instillation
i. of anesthetic
contrast material i.
lavage i.
i. therapy
institute
Cardiopulmonary Research I.
Dana-Farber Cancer I.
National Cancer I. (NCI)
instrument
i. migration
i. recirculation
instrumental perforation
instrumentation failure
instrument-tract seeding
insufficiency
aortic valve i.
atrioventricular valve i.
chronic venous i. (CVI)
degenerative mitral valve i.
exocrine pancreatic i.
i. fracture
glottic i.

NOTES

insufficiency *(continued)*
    left ventricular i. (LVI)
    mesenteric i.
    mitral valve i.
    pulmonary valve i.
    renal i.
    respiratory i.
    transverse plane motion i.
    venous i.
insufficient airway maintenance
insufflate
insufflation
    air i.
    i. anesthesia
    i. anesthetic technique
    constant flow i.
    cranial i.
    endotracheal i.
    extraperitoneal carbon dioxide i.
    extraperitoneal CO_2 i.
    gas i.
    gastric i.
    helium i.
    intraperitoneal carbon dioxide i.
    intraperitoneal CO_2 i.
    perirenal i.
    peritoneal i.
    presacral i.
    i. pressure
    retroperitoneal gas i.
    Rubin tubal i.
    i. of stomach
    talc i.
    i. test set
    thoracoscopic talc i.
    tubal i.
insula, pl. **insulae**
    Haller i.
insular
    i. artery
    i. carcinoma
insulated
    i. cautery
    i. epidural needle
insulin
    i. coma
    i. coma therapy
    i. coma treatment
    i. preparation
    i. resistance
    i. secretion
    i. shock therapy
insulin-like growth factor I (IGF-1)
insulinoma
insult
    macrotraumatic i.
    microtraumatic i.
intact
    i. gastric serosa

    i. membrane
    i. parathyroid hormone (iPTH)
    i. parathyroid hormone assay
integration
    binaural i.
    body side i.
    competing messages i.
    complete i.
    fibrous i.
    large-scale i.
    medium-scale i.
    very large scale i.
integrity
    anatomic i.
    soft tissue i.
integument
integumentary barrier
intensification
    image i.
intensity
    Descriptor Differential Scale of
        Pain I.
    fluorescence i.
intensity-encoded receptor
intensity-weighted center of gravity
intensive care unit (ICU)
intent
    curative i.
    palliative i.
intention
    first i.
    second i.
    secondary i.
    third i.
intentional
    i. rebreathing
    i. replantation
    i. rotation
    i. saccade
    i. tooth reimplantation
interaction
    additive i.
    synergistic i.
interactive volume rendering
interalveolar space
interarticular
    i. fibrocartilage
    i. joint
interarytenoid notch
interatrial septum
interaural attenuation
interbody
    i. bone graft
    i. spinal fusion
intercalary
    i. allograft procedure
    i. graft
    i. resection
intercalated disc

intercapillary
intercapitales
intercapitular vein
intercarotic
intercarotid nerve
intercarpal articulation
intercartilaginous incision
intercavernosus septum
intercavernous venous sinus
intercellular
    i. fenestration
    i. space
intercentral
interceptive conditioning
intercervical disc herniation
interchangeability
interchondral
    i. articulation
    i. ligament
interclavicular
    i. ligament
    i. notch
interclinoid ligament
intercoccygeal
intercolonoscopy
intercolumnar
    i. fascia
    i. fiber
intercondylar
    i. eminence
    i. femoral fracture
    i. fossa
    i. humeral fracture
    i. line
    i. space
    i. tibial fracture
intercondyloid
    i. fossa
    i. notch
intercoronary anastomosis
intercostal
    i. anesthesia
    i. artery
    i. bundle
    i. flap
    i. fossa block
    i. membrane
    i. nerve
    i. nerve block
    i. nerve block anesthetic technique
    i. neuralgia
    i. space

    i. vein
    i. vessel
intercostalia
intercostohumeral nerve
intercricothyrotomy
intercristal space
intercrural fiber
intercuspal position
intercuspation
intercutaneomucous
interdeferential
interdental
    i. canal
    i. denudation
    i. excision
    i. ligation
    i. papilla
    i. resection
    i. space
    i. tissue
interdigestive
    i. motility disturbance
    i. period
interdigit
interdigital
interdigitating skin flap
interdigitation
interendognathic suture
interface
    bone-cement i.
    bone-implant i.
    cement i.
    cement-bone i.
    cup-cement i.
    electrode-skin i.
    graft-host i.
    implant-cement i.
    long-term bone-instrumentation i.
    pin-bone i.
    prosthesis i.
    prosthesis-cement i.
    soft tissue i.
interfacetal disease
interfacet wiring and fusion
interfacial canal
interfascial
    i. approach
    i. space
interfascicular
    i. epineurectomy
    i. epineurotomy
    i. fibrous tissue

NOTES

interfemoral
interference
    i. dissociation
    electromagnetic i. (EMI)
    i. fit fixation
    i. modification
    i. screw technique
interferential therapy
interforniceal approach
interfoveolar ligament
interfragmentary compression
interfrontal
interganglionic rami
interglobular space of Owen
intergluteal
intergonial
interhemispheric
    i. approach
    i. propagation time
    i. subdural hematoma
interilioabdominal amputation
interincisor
    i. distance
    i. gap
interinnominoabdominal amputation
interischiadic
interlamellar space
interlesional therapy
interlobar
interlobular
    i. artery
    i. artery of kidney
    i. ductule
interlocking suture technique
intermaxilla
intermaxillary
    i. fixation
    i. relation
    i. suture
intermediary nerve
intermediate
    i. amputation
    i. anterior wall
    i. bronchus
    i. bundle
    i. cuneiform bone
    i. digastric tendon
    i. ganglion
    i. hemorrhage
    i. laryngeal cavity
    i. line
    i. mesoderm
    i. omohyoid tendon
    i. phalangectomy
    i. restoration
    i. sacral crest
    i. temporal artery
intermediolateral

intermesenteric
    i. abscess
    i. arterial anastomosis
    i. plexus
intermetacarpal articulation
intermetameric
intermittent
    i. acute porphyria
    i. apnea technique
    i. bolus technique
    i. catheterization
    i. demand ventilation
    i. inflow occlusion
    i. mandatory ventilation (IMV)
    i. mechanical ventilation
    i. pneumatic calf compression
    i. positive pressure (IPP)
    i. positive pressure breathing
    (IPPB)
    i. positive pressure ventilation
    (IPPV)
    i. self-obturation
    i. sterilization
    i. subclavian vein obstruction
    i. vascular exclusion
intermodulation
intermuscular
    i. gluteal bursa
    i. groove
    i. hernia
    i. membrane
    i. septum
internal
    i. abdominal ring
    i. anal sphincter (IAS)
    i. auditory artery
    i. auditory canal
    i. auditory foramen
    i. auditory vein
    i. bevel incision
    i. branch
    i. canthus
    i. carotid artery (ICA)
    i. carotid venous plexus
    i. clot
    i. decompression
    i. drainage
    i. ethmoidectomy
    i. female genital organ
    i. fixation, closed reduction
    i. fixation fracture
    i. hemipelvectomy
    i. hemorrhage
    i. hemorrhoid
    i. hemorrhoidal complex
    i. hernia
    i. iliac artery
    i. inguinal ring
    i. jugular vein

i. jugular vein cannulation anesthetic technique
i. jugular vein catheterization anesthetic technique
i. jugular vein puncture anesthetic technique
i. lacrimal fistula
i. male genital organ
i. mammary artery (IMA)
i. mammary graft
i. mammary lymphoscintigraphy (IML)
i. mammary node
i. mammary node biopsy
i. mammary plexus
i. maxillary artery
i. maxillary plexus
i. maxillary vein
i. neurocranial foramen
i. neurolysis
i. oblique aponeurosis
i. oblique line
i. oblique osteomuscular flap
i. occipital crest
i. pudendal artery
i. pudendal vein
i. radiation therapy
i. rectal artery
i. rectal nerve
i. reflection
i. respiration
i. rotation
i. rotation deformity
i. rotation in extension
i. rotator
i. spermatic artery
i. spermatic fascia
i. sphincterotomy
i. spinal fixation
i. spiral sulcus
i. surface
i. thoracic artery
i. thoracic lymphatic plexus
i. thoracic vein
i. urethral orifice
i. urethral sphincter
i. urethrotomy
internal-external
i.-e. ilium
i.-e. rotation
internasal suture

international
I. Association for the Study of Pain (IASP)
I. Cancer of Cervix Classification
I. Classification of Diseases, Adapted for Use in the United States (ICDA)
I. Classification of Diseases-9 Version of Injury Severity Score (ICISS)
I. Federation of Gynecology and Obstetrics (FIGO)
I. Federation of Gynecology and Obstetrics classification
i. normalized ratio (INR)
I. Pelvic Pain Society (IPPS)
i. stage classification
interne
fixator i.
internervous plane
internist
internodal tract of Bachmann
internus
interocclusal rest space
interorbital
interosseal
interosseous
i. border
i. cartilage
i. crest
i. groove
i. margin
i. muscle
i. nerve
i. sacroiliac ligament
i. wire fixation
interosseus, pl. interossei
interpalpebral
interparietal
i. bone
i. hernia
i. suture
interpediculate
interpeduncular
i. cistern
i. fossa lesion
interpelviabdominal amputation
interperiosteal fracture
interphalangeal
i. amputation
i. articulation
i. collateral ligament

NOTES

interphalangeal *(continued)*
    distal i. (DIP)
    i. joint dislocation
interpleural
    i. administration
    i. analgesia
    i. anesthesia
    i. anesthetic technique
    i. application
    i. block
interpolated
    i. curve
    i. flap
interpolation
    i. flap
    i. technique
interposing
interposition
    jejunal i.
    i. membrane
    i. mesocaval shunt
    i. saphenous vein graft
    soft tissue i.
    tissue i.
interpositional
    i. elbow arthroplasty
    i. shoulder arthroplasty
interpretation
    cholangiographic i.
    false-positive i.
    image i.
    intraoperative i.
    mirror-image i.
    i. variability
interprismatic space
interproximal
    i. reduction
    i. space
interpubic disc
interpulmonary septum
interradicular
    i. alveoloplasty
    i. lesion
    i. septum
    i. space
interrater reliability
interrenal
interrogation
    deep Doppler velocity i.
    Doppler i.
    stereoscopic i.
interrupted
    i. aortic arch
    i. respiration
    i. suture technique
interruption
    sympathetic i.
interscalene
    i. approach

    i. blockade
    i. block anesthetic technique
    i. brachial plexus block
    i. triangle
interscapular amputation
interscapulum
intersection syndrome
intersegmental rotation
intersheath space
intersigmoid
    i. hernia
    i. recess
interspace
    implant substructure i.
interspecific graft
intersphincteric
    i. abscess
    i. anal fistula
    i. anorectal space
    i. proctectomy
interspinal
    i. line
    i. muscle
    i. plane
interspinous
    i. ligament
    i. segmental spinal instrumentation
      technique
    i. wiring
interstice, pl. **interstices**
    graft i.
interstimulus interval (ISI)
interstitial
    i. brachytherapy
    i. cystitis
    i. hernia
    i. implantation
    i. inflammation
    i. irradiation
    i. loculated hematoma
    i. neovascularization
    i. nephritis
    i. photodynamic therapy
    i. pressure
    i. pulmonary fibrosis (IPF)
    i. radiation therapy
    i. rejection
    i. space
    i. tissue
intertendinous bursa
intertransverse
    i. fusion
    i. ligament
    i. muscle
intertrigo with ulceration
intertrochanteric
    i. crest
    i. femoral fracture
    i. line

i. 4-part fracture
i. varus osteotomy
intertubercular
  i. eminence
  i. groove
  i. line
  i. plane
  i. sheath
  i. sulcus
interureteral
interureteric fold
intervaginal space
interval
  i. appendectomy
  disease-free i. (DFI)
  interstimulus i. (ISI)
  i. operation
  pacemaker escape i.
  rupture-delivery i.
interval-strength relation
intervascular
intervening connective tissue
intervention
  angiographic i.
  endovascular i.
  medical i.
  neurosurgical i.
  operative i.
  prophylactic angiographic i.
  surgical i.
interventional
  i. cardiac catheterization
  i. cardiologist
  i. neuroradiology
  i. option
  i. procedure
  i. radiologist
  i. radiology
  i. technique
  i. therapy
interventricular
  i. septal rupture
  i. septum
intervertebral
  i. cartilage
  i. disc blockade
  i. disc herniation
  i. foramen
  i. ganglion
  i. notch
  i. symphysis
  i. vein

interview
  structured pain i. (SPI)
intervolar plate ligament
intestina (*pl. of* intestinum)
intestinal
  i. allograft
  i. anastomosis
  i. anastomotic healing
  i. anastomotic leakage
  i. angina
  i. arterial arcade
  i. artery
  i. biopsy
  i. bypass procedure
  i. calculus
  i. colic
  i. conduit
  i. content
  i. endoscopy
  i. failure
  i. fistula
  i. fixation
  i. flora
  i. gland
  i. hemorrhage
  i. infection
  i. ischemic disorder
  i. loop
  i. malrotation
  i. obstruction
  i. perforation
  i. radiation injury
  i. resection
  i. rotation
  i. surgery
  i. tract
  i. transplantation
  i. trunk
  i. ulceration
  i. vein
  i. villous atrophy
  i. villus
  i. web
  i. wound healing
intestine
  absorptive i.
  large i.
  small i.
intestinum, pl. **intestina**
in-the-bag implantation
intima

NOTES

intimal
- i. flap
- i. hyperplasia
- i. thrombosis

intolerance
- hemodynamic i.

intonation contour

intortor

intoxication
- i. amaurosis
- citrate i.

intraabdominal
- i. abscess
- i. adhesion
- i. arterial hemorrhage
- i. bleeding
- i. catastrophe
- i. disease
- i. friction
- i. hypertension
- i. infection
- i. injury
- i. lesion
- i. mass
- i. organ
- i. pressure (IAP)
- i. sepsis
- i. spillage
- i. surgery
- i. tip

intraabdominally insufflated carbon dioxide

intraadenoidal

intraalveolar hemorrhage

intraamniotic infection

intraanal pressure

intraaortic balloon counterpulsation

intraarterial
- i. chemoembolization
- i. chemotherapy (IAC)
- i. counterpulsation
- i. therapy

intraarticular
- i. anesthetic technique
- i. cartilage
- i. facet injection
- i. hip fusion
- i. injection
- i. knee fusion
- i. loose body
- i. osteotomy
- i. procedure
- i. proximal tibial fracture
- i. reconstruction
- i. sternocostal ligament

intraaxial parenchymal brain neoplasm

intrabuccal

intrabulbar fossa

intracanalicular irradiation

intracapsular
- i. approach
- i. cataract extraction
- i. cataract extraction operation
- i. dissection
- i. fracture
- i. hemorrhage
- i. incision
- i. ligament
- i. metastasis
- i. osteotomy
- i. partial tonsillectomy
- i. temporomandibular joint arthroplasty

intracardiac
- i. mass
- i. pressure
- i. pressure curve

intracatheter

intracath technique

intracavernosal
- i. injection
- i. injection treatment

intracavernous
- i. injection
- i. injection therapy
- i. plexus

intracavitary
- i. anesthesia
- i. implantation
- i. pressure-electrogram dissociation
- i. pressure gradient
- i. radiation boost therapy

intracellular-like, calcium-bearing crystalloid solution

intracellular protein degradation

intracerebral
- i. arteriovenous malformation
- i. ganglioma
- i. hematoma
- i. hemorrhage
- i. leukostasis
- i. vascular malformation

intracerebroventricular

intracholedochal pressure

intracisternal

intraclass correlation coefficients

intracolic

intraconal lesion

intracordal silicone injection

intracorneal

intracoronal-extracoronal retention

intracoronary thrombolysis balloon valvuloplasty

intracorporeal
- i. anastomosis
- i. injection therapy
- i. knot
- i. knotting technique

i. laser lithotripsy
i. shockwave lithotripsy
i. suturing
intracostal
intracranial
  i. anatomy
  i. aneurysm
  i. arteriovenous fistula
  i. arteriovenous malformation
  i. bleeding
  i. cavity
  i. circulation
  i. dural vascular anomaly
  i. ganglion
  i. hematoma
  i. hemorrhage (ICH)
  i. hypotension
  i. mass
  i. mass lesion
  i. pathology
  i. pressure (ICP)
  i. pressure monitoring
  i. pressure value
  i. rhizotomy
  i. stimulation
  i. tumor
  i. vascular malformation
  i. venous system
intracranial-extracranial nerve graft
intracranial-intratemporal nerve graft
intracristal space
intractable
  i. epilepsy
  i. pain
intracutaneous segment
intracuticular stitch
intracystic hepatojejunostomy
intracytoplasmic sperm injection (ICSI)
intradermal
  i. anesthetic
  i. injection
  i. mattress suture technique
  i. tattooing technique
intradiploic pseudomeningocele
intradiscal
  i. electrothermal therapy (IDET)
  i. pressure
intraductal
  i. cancer
  i. carcinoma
  i. cholangioscopy
  i. component

i. hyperplasia
i. oncocytic papillary neoplasm
i. papillary mucinous neoplasm
  (IPMN)
i. papillary mucinous tumor
  (IPMT)
i. pressure
intradural
  i. abscess
  i. approach
  i. dissection
  i. dorsal spinal root rhizotomy
  i. epidermoidoma
  i. extramedullary lesion
  i. extramedullary mass
  i. tumor surgery
intraepidermal carcinoma
intraepiphysial osteotomy
intraepiploic hernia
intraepithelial
  i. excementosis
  i. nonkeratinizing carcinoma
intraesophageal
  i. peristaltic pressure
  i. variceal pressure
intrafaradization
intrafascial space
intrafollicular insemination
intragalvanization
intragastric
  i. anastomosis
  i. hydrolysis
  i. pressure
  i. prosthesis migration
  i. provocation under endoscopy
  i. resection
intraglandular fluid collection
intraglomerular pressure
intragraft expression
intrahepatic
  i. abscess
  i. anatomy
  i. arterioportal fistula
  i. A-V fistula
  i. bile duct
  i. biliary cystic dilation
  i. biliary tree
  i. control
  i. course
  i. ductal dilation
  i. hematoma
  i. hepatolithiasis

NOTES

intrahepatic *(continued)*
    i. hypertension
    i. lesion
    i. metastasis
    i. pathology
    i. portosystemic shunt
    i. spontaneous arterioportal fistula
    i. vascular division
intrahyoid
intrailiac hernia
intrajugular process
intralabyrinthine fistula
intralacrimal
    i. endoscopy
    i. surgery
intralesional
    i. excision
    i. injection
    i. therapy
intraligamentary anesthesia
intralobular
    i. connective tissue
    i. inflammation
intraluminal
    i. cyst
    i. esophageal pressure
    i. flow
    i. foreign body
    i. hemorrhage
    i. intubation
    i. pH-pressure relationship
    i. pouch
    i. seeding
    i. tonometry
    i. tumor
    i. urethral pressure
intramammary sentinel node
intramedullary
    i. anesthesia
    i. arteriovenous malformation
    i. bouquet fixation
    i. canal
    i. demyelination
    i. graft
    i. lesion
    i. nail extractor
    i. nailing
    i. rod fixation
    i. tractotomy
    i. tumor
    i. tumor biopsy
intramembranous
    i. formation
    i. space
intramucosal metastasis
intramural
    i. abscess
    i. air dissection
    i. artery

    i. blood perfusion
    i. colonic air
    i. esophageal rupture
    i. extramucosal lesion
    i. fistulous tract
    i. hematoma
    i. intestinal hemorrhage
    i. involvement
    i. pH
intramuscular (IM)
    i. abscess
    i. anesthetic
    i. injection
    i. preanesthetic medication
      anesthetic technique
    i. venous malformation
intramyocardial
    i. air
    i. pressure
    i. tumor
intranasal
    i. analgesic
    i. anesthesia
    i. approach
    i. ethmoidectomy
    i. hydromorphone hydrochloride
    i. nicotine
    i. polypectomy
    i. sinus surgery
intraneural pressure
in-transit
    i.-t. disease
    i.-t. metastasis
intraoccipital joint
intraocular
    i. administration
    i. cataract extraction
    i. fistula
    i. foreign body
    i. hemorrhage
    i. lens
    i. lens dislocation
    i. lens implantation
    i. pressure
intraoperative
    i. assessment
    i. bile sample
    i. biliary endoscopy
    i. biopsy
    i. bleeding
    i. blood loss
    i. bowel lavage
    i. bowel preparation
    i. cavernous nerve stimulation
    i. cholangiogram (IOC)
    i. clonidine administration
    i. colonic lavage
    i. complication

i. computer-assisted spinal orientation technique
i. confirmation
i. contamination
i. core body temperature
i. core hypothermia
i. CVP
i. death
i. dynamic cholangiography
i. enteroscopy
i. fluid management
i. fracture
i. frozen section
i. hemorrhage
i. imaging
i. imaging method
i. inadvertent venous injury
i. interpretation
i. iPTH assay
i. lymphatic mapping
i. monitor
i. morbidity
i. MRI
i. multiplane transesophageal echocardiogram
i. neurophysiologic monitoring (IOM)
i. normothermia
i. parathyroid hormone monitoring
i. penile erection
i. plateletpheresis
i. procedure
i. radiation
i. radiation therapy
i. rupture
i. stress relaxation
i. touch prep cytology
i. transcranial Doppler monitoring
i. ultrasonography (IOUS)
i. ultrasound (IOUS)
i. ultrasound finding
i. urine output
i. vascular accident
i. verification
intraoperatively donated autologous blood
intraoral
i. anesthesia
i. antrostomy
i. cone irradiation
i. flap
i. incision

i. pressure
i. trauma
intraorbital
i. anesthesia
i. foreign body
i. groove
i. surgery
intraosseous
i. abscess
i. anesthesia
i. bone lesion
i. fixation
i. injection
i. membrane
intrapancreatic portion
intraparavariceal procedure
intraparenchymal
i. digital dissection
i. hematoma
i. hemorrhage
intraparotid plexus
intrapartum
i. asphyxiation
i. hemorrhage
intrapatellar bursa
intrapelvic hernia
intrapericardial pressure
intraperitoneal
i. abscess
i. adhesion
i. air
i. anesthesia
i. anesthetic
i. blood transfusion
i. carbon dioxide insufflation
i. cavity
i. CO_2 insufflation
i. dissemination
i. drug administration
i. endometrial metastatic disease
i. fetal transfusion
i. hemorrhage
i. hyperthermic chemotherapy (IPHC)
i. hyperthermic perfusion
i. incision
i. method
i. mobilization
i. onlay mesh technique
i. perforation
i. position
i. pressure

NOTES

intraperitoneal *(continued)*
- i. procedure
- i. radiation therapy
- i. recurrence
- i. seeding
- i. spillage
- i. technique
- i. viscus
- i. viscus rupture
- i. volume

intraperitoneally
intrapharyngeal space
intrapial
intraplaque hemorrhage
intrapleural
- i. approach
- i. block
- i. catheter placement
- i. pressure
- i. rupture

intraportal vein
intraprostatic
intrapulmonary
- i. metastasis (IPM)
- i. shunt ratio

intrapulpal
- i. anesthesia
- i. injection
- i. pressure

intrapyretic amputation
intrarenal chemolysis
intrarrhachidian
intrascrotal
intrasellar
- i. extension
- i. lesion
- i. mass

intraseptal alveoloplasty
intrasheath tenotomy
intraspinal
- i. administration
- i. anesthesia
- i. therapy

intrasplenic
intrasynovial
intratendinous injection
intratentorial supracerebellar approach
intrathecal
- i. administration
- i. analgesic
- i. anesthesia
- i. anesthetic
- i. antinociception
- i. cannulation anesthetic technique
- i. injection
- i. morphine anesthetic technique
- i. neurolysis
- i. opioid

- i. opioid labor analgesia
- i. therapy

intrathoracic
- i. anastomosis
- i. bleeding
- i. disease
- i. esophagogastroscopy
- i. esophagogastrostomy
- i. esophagoplasty
- i. injury
- i. mass
- i. Nissen fundoplication
- i. position
- i. pressure
- i. stomach

intrathyroidal pathology
intrathyroid cartilage
intratracheal
- i. anesthesia
- i. ectopic thyroid
- i. ectopic thyroid tissue
- i. intubation

intratubal insemination
intratumoral
- i. calcification
- i. injection

intraurethral pressure
intrauterine
- i. amputation
- i. device (IUD)
- i. foreign body
- i. fracture
- i. growth retardation
- i. infection
- i. insemination
- i. intraperitoneal fetal transfusion
- i. pressure measurement
- i. respiration
- i. resuscitation

intravaginal
- i. electrical stimulation
- i. pouch
- i. space
- i. torsion

intravariceal
- i. infusion
- i. injection
- i. pressure
- i. sclerotherapy

intravasation
- venous i.

intravascular
- i. coagulation screen
- i. endothelial proliferative lesion
- i. fluid therapy
- i. foreign body
- i. foreign body retrieval
- i. injection
- i. lipolysis

i. mass
i. pressure
i. volume
i. volume expansion
intravelar veloplasty
intravenous (I.V.)
i. administration
i. alimentation
i. analgesic
i. anesthetic
i. antibiotic therapy
i. block
i. block anesthesia
i. blood
i. cannulation
i. cannulation anesthetic technique
i. contrast
i. digital subtraction imaging
i. drip
i. hydration
i. hydration therapy
i. hyperalimentation
i. hypnotic
i. injection
i. medication
i. oxygen-15 water bolus technique
i. ozone therapy
i. regional anesthesia (IVRA)
i. regional blockade
i. regional block with guanethidine
i. saline
i. sedation
i. sedation anesthesia
i. sheath
i. vasopressin
intraventricular
i. aberration
i. endoscopy
i. hemorrhage
i. injection
i. mass
i. therapy
intravesical
i. alum irrigation
i. anastomosis
i. chemotherapeutic treatment
i. chemotherapy
i. migration
i. pressure
i. ureterolysis
intravital microscopy
intravitreal injection

intrinsic
i. brainstem lesion
i. circuitry
i. compression
i. end-expiratory pressure
i. minus deformity
i. minus position
i. muscle
i. plus deformity
i. positive end-expiratory pressure (PEEPi)
i. restoration
i. sphincter
i. spinal cord catheter placement
introduction site
introflexion
introgastric
introitus
introjection
intromittent organ
introspective method
introvert
intrusive implantation
intubate
intubated ureterotomy
intubating laryngeal mask airway
intubation
altercursive i.
i. anesthetic technique
aqueductal i.
awake fiberoptic i.
blind nasotracheal i.
bronchoscope-guided i.
catheter-guided endoscopic i.
double-lumen i.
emergency tracheal i.
emergent i.
endobronchial i.
endotracheal i.
esophageal i.
esophagogastric i.
failed i.
i. failure
flexible lightwand-guided i.
heal i.
intraluminal i.
intratracheal i.
lighted stylet-guided oral i.
mainstem i.
nasal i.
nasogastric i.
nasotracheal i. (NTI)

NOTES

385

intubation (*continued*)
    O'Dwyer i.
    oral endotracheal i.
    oral lighted-stylet i.
    orotracheal i.
    prophylactic i.
    pyloric i.
    rapid sequence induction i.
    RSI orotracheal i.
    silicone i.
    terminal ileum i.
    total time to i. (TTI)
    tracheal i.
    translaryngeal tracheal i.
intumescence
intumescent
intumescentia
intussuscepted mass
intussuscepting
intussusception
    adult i.
    appendiceal i.
    cecal i.
    colocolic i.
    colonic i.
    enteric i.
    gastroenterostomy i.
    idiopathic adult i.
    idiopathic ileocecal i.
    ileocolic i.
    pediatric i.
    sigmoid-rectal i.
    stomal i.
inundation fever
invaded furcation
invaginate
invaginated membrane
invaginating
    i. anastomosis
    end-to-end i.
    i. suture technique
invagination
    basilar i.
    epithelial i.
    stomal i.
    stump i.
    i. technique
invasion
    advanced local i.
    blood vessel i. (BVI)
    cancer i.
    capsular i.
    chest wall i.
    extrathyroid i.
    local i.
    lymphatic i.
    lymphovascular i.
    lymph vessel i. (LVI)
    margin i.

    microscopic i.
    mucosal i.
    perineural i.
    serosa i.
    submucosal i.
    tumor i.
    vascular i.
    venous i.
    wall i.
invasive
    i. adenocarcinoma
    i. blood pressure (IBP)
    i. breast cancer
    i. breast carcinoma
    i. ductal cancer
    i. ductal carcinoma
    i. hemodynamic monitoring
    i. lobular carcinoma
    i. localization
    i. pressure measurement
    i. procedure
    i. recurrence
    i. technique
    i. therapy
    i. tumor
inventory
    Brief Pain I. (BPI)
    Multidimensional Pain I. (MPI)
    Neonatal Facial Pain I. (NFCS)
    Pain Appraisal I. (PAI)
    State-Trait Anxiety I. (STAI)
inverse bevel incision
inverse-ratio ventilation
inversion appendectomy
inversion-eversion rotation
inversion-ligation appendectomy
inversus
inverted
    i. bevel incision
    i. L-form osteotomy
    i. pelvis
    i. scarf osteotomy
    i. skin flap
inverted-U
    i.-U abdominal incision
    i.-U approach
    i.-U pouch
inverted-V peritoneotomy
inverted-Y
    i.-Y fracture
    i.-Y incision
inverting knot technique
invertor
investigation
    diagnostic i.
    direct histologic i.
    histologic i.
    preoperative i.
    soft x-ray i.

investing
  i. cartilage
  i. fascia
investment expansion
involuntary
  i. guarding
  i. sterilization
involution cyst
involved-field radiation
involvement
  bifurcation i.
  border i.
  celiac nodal i.
  diffuse breast i.
  extramedullary i.
  extraocular muscle i.
  intramural i.
  lymph node i.
  macroscopic i.
  margin resection i.
  mesocolic i.
  metastatic i.
  nervous system i.
  nodal i.
  node i.
  portal nodal i.
  pulmonary i.
  retinal i.
  segmental i.
  serosal i.
  trifurcation i.
inward-going rectification
inward rotation
IOC
  intraoperative cholangiogram
iodide-containing medication
iodine-131 whole-body scan
iodine treatment
iodized oil
IOM
  intraoperative neurophysiologic
    monitoring
ionization
  i. chamber pocket
  root canal i.
  specific i.
ionizing irradiation
iontophoresis
IOUS
  intraoperative ultrasonography
  intraoperative ultrasound

IPAA
  ileal pouch-anal anastomosis
IPC
  ischemic preconditioning
IPF
  idiopathic pulmonary fibrosis
  interstitial pulmonary fibrosis
IPHC
  intraperitoneal hyperthermic
    chemotherapy
IPM
  intrapulmonary metastasis
    macroscopic IPM
    microscopic IPM
IPMN
  intraductal papillary mucinous neoplasm
IPMT
  intraductal papillary mucinous tumor
IPP
  intermittent positive pressure
IPPB
  intermittent positive pressure breathing
IPPS
  International Pelvic Pain Society
    IPPS Pelvic Pain Assessment Form
IPPV
  intermittent positive pressure ventilation
IPSID
  immunoproliferative small intestine
    disease
ipsilateral
  i. acetabular fracture
  i. adrenalectomy
  i. femoral neck fracture
  i. femoral shaft fracture
  i. gland
  i. hemispheric symptom
  i. injection
  i. nerve root lesion
  i. pelvic fracture
  i. portal vein obstruction
  i. shoulder
  i. side
  i. thyroid lobectomy
  i. tibial fracture
iPTH
  intact parathyroid hormone
    iPTH assay
    iPTH level
I/R
  ischemia and reperfusion
    I/R injury

NOTES

IRA
>ileorectal anastomosis

IRDS
>infant respiratory distress syndrome

iridectomy
>argon laser i.
>basal i.
>Bethke i.
>buttonhole i.
>Castroviejo i.
>central i.
>Chandler i.
>complete i.
>Elschnig central i.
>laser i.
>i. operation
>optic i.
>optical i.
>patent i.
>peripheral i.
>preliminary i.
>preparatory i.
>pupil-to-root i.
>i. scar
>sector i.
>stenopeic i.
>superior sector i.
>therapeutic i.

iridencleisis
>Holth i.
>i. operation

irides (*pl. of* iris)
iridization
iridocapsulotomy
iridocele
iridocoloboma
iridocorneal
>i. angle
>i. endothelial syndrome
>i. epithelial syndrome

iridocorneosclerectomy
iridocyclectomy
iridocyclochoroidectomy
>Peyman i.

iridocystectomy
iridodialysis operation
iridodiastasis
iridogoniocyclectomy
iridoplasty
iridosclerotomy
iridotasis operation
iridotomy
>Abraham i.
>Castroviejo radial i.
>laser i.
>i. operation
>radial i.

iris, pl. **irides**
>i. diastasis

>i. ectasia
>i. incarceration
>i. neovascularization
>i. ring

iritoectomy
iritomy
iron-Hudson-Stähli line
iron line
iron-stocker line
irotomy
irradiated melanoma cell
irradiation
>abdominal i.
>abdominopelvic i.
>adjuvant i.
>breast i.
>cardiac i.
>i. cataract
>cataract i.
>cesium i.
>charged-particle i.
>childhood thyroid i.
>convergent beam i.
>cranial i.
>craniospinal i.
>i. damage
>external beam i.
>external orthovoltage i.
>extracorporeal i.
>i. failure
>fractionated external beam i.
>gamma i.
>half-body i.
>heavy-ion i.
>hemibody i.
>hyperfractionated total body i.
>i. injury
>interstitial i.
>intracanalicular i.
>intraoral cone i.
>ionizing i.
>linearly polarized near-infrared i.
>local i.
>low-dose i.
>mantle i.
>mediastinal i.
>Nd:YAG laser i.
>paraaortic node i.
>partial-breast i.
>pelvic i.
>postoperative i.
>prophylactic i.
>selective i.
>single-fraction total body i.
>surface i.
>therapeutic i.
>total axial node i.
>total body i.
>total lymphoid i.

total nodal i.
ultraviolet blood i.
UV i.
whole-abdomen i.
whole abdominopelvic i.
whole-body i.
whole-pelvis i.
irreducible
i. fracture
i. hernia
irregular bone
irregularly widened lumen
irresectability
irresectable
carcinoma stage i.
i. disease
i. finding
irrespirable
irresuscitable
irreversible
i. coma
i. shock
irrigating solution
irrigation
acetohydroxamic acid i.
antral i.
i. and aspiration
i. burn
caloric i.
canal i.
closed i.
continuous bladder i.
copious i.
endodontic i.
hemiacidrin i.
heparin i.
intravesical alum i.
on-table i.
oral i.
pulsed i.
pulse lavage i.
rectal pulsed i.
rectum i.
sinus i.
i. solution
whole-gut i.
wound i.
irrigation-suction
postoperative i.-s.
irritability
soft tissue i.
irritable lesion

irritant
i. patch-test reaction
i. patch-test response
irritation
i. callus
i. index
parastomal i.
peritoneal i.
irritative lesion
irruption
irruptive
Irvine operation
Irving tubal ligation
Irwin osteotomy
Isaacson classification (IC)
ischemia, ischaemia
acute limb i. (ALI)
chronic mesenteric i.
contralateral i.
exercise i.
exercise-induced silent myocardial i.
extremity i.
hepatic i.
left ventricular i. (LVI)
limb i.
lower limb i.
mesenteric i. (MI)
myocardial i.
nonocclusive mesenteric i. (NOMI)
normothermic i.
radiation-induced i.
i. and reperfusion (I/R)
i. and reperfusion injury
tourniquet i.
warm i.
ischemia-guided medical therapy
ischemia-reperfusion
i.-r. injury
i.-r. phenomenon
ischemic
i. aortic disease
i. cardiomyopathy
i. colitis
i. compression
i. encephalopathy
i. heart disease
i. hypoxia
i. infected ulceration
i. liver injury
i. mesenteric change
i. ocular inflammation
i. preconditioning (IPC)

NOTES

ischemic *(continued)*
    i. stroke
    i. ulcer
ischemic-tourniquet technique
ischia (*pl. of* ischium)
ischiadic
    i. plexus
    i. spine
ischiadicum
ischial
    i. bone
    i. bursa
    i. spine
    i. weightbearing ring
ischiatic hernia
ischioanal fossa
ischiobulbar
ischiocavernosus
ischiocavernous muscle
ischiocele
ischiococcygeal
ischiococcygeus
ischiofemoral
ischioperineal
ischiopubiotomy
    Farabeuf i.
ischiorectal
    i. abscess
    i. anorectal space
    i. fat pad
    i. fossa
    i. fossa plane
ischiovertebral
ischium, pl. **ischia**
ischuretic
I-shaped scalp flap
ISI
    interstimulus interval
island
    endometrial i.
    i. graft
    i. nail transfer
    i. pedicle scalp flap
    i. skin flap
    i. wound dressing
island-flap procedure
islet
    i. cell
    i. cell cancer
    i. cell engineering
    i. cell tumor
    i.'s of Langerhans
    pancreatic i.
isobaric spinal anesthesia
isobologram analysis
isobolographic analysis
isobolography
isocapnia
isocapnic hyperventilation

isodense subdural hematoma
isodose line
isoelectric
    i. line
    i. point
isoenzyme
    pancreas-specific amylase i.
isoflurane-induced vasoconstriction
isogeneic graft
isograft
isoinertial
isokinetic collection
isolated
    i. anuloplasty
    i. arterial injury
    i. dislocation
    i. fashion
    i. hepatic perfusion
    i. iliac artery aneurysm
    i. limb perfusion (ILP)
    i. liver injury
    i. metastatic tumor
    i. NCRLM
    i. procedure
    i. venous injury
isolation
    hepatic vascular i. (HVI)
    lung i.
    i. perfusion therapy
    i. technique
    total vascular i. (TVI)
isologous graft
isolysis
isometric
    i. cervical extension strength
    i. force dynamometry
    i. point
    i. technique
    i. tubular vacuolization
    i. venous tension
isoperistaltic anastomosis
isoplastic graft
isoproterenol
isoquinoline
isorhythmic dissociation
isosbestic point
isosulfan blue-dye mapping
isotope
    i. dilution-mass spectrometry
    i. injection
    i. localization
isotopic lymphoscintigraphy
isotransplantation
isotropic tissue
isovolemic hemodilution
isovolumetric
    i. relaxation
    i. relaxation time

isovolumic
>   i. relaxation
>   i. relaxation time

Israel method

ISS
>   Injury Severity Score

isthmectomy

isthmorrhaphy

isthmus

isthmusectomy

Italian
>   I. flap
>   I. method
>   I. operation
>   I. rhinoplasty

itchy soft palate

iterative reconstruction

Itis
>   bundle of I.

Ito
>   I. method
>   I. procedure

IUD
>   intrauterine device
>   IUD-related infection

I.V.
>   intravenous
>   I.V. contrast
>   I.V. fluid therapy
>   I.V. sedation

Ivalon
>   I. sponge-wrap operation
>   I. suture technique

IVC
>   inferior vena cava
>   inferior vena cavum
>   IVC ligation
>   IVC occlusion
>   IVC pressure
>   IVC reconstruction
>   retrohepatic IVC
>   suprahepatic IVC
>   thrombosis of IVC

IVCO
>   inferior vena cava balloon occlusion

IVCP
>   inferior vena cava pressure

IVCT
>   in vitro contracture test

Ivor
>   I. Lewis approach
>   I. Lewis esophagogastrectomy
>   I. Lewis 2-stage subtotal
>   esophagectomy

Ivor-Lewis resection

ivory membrane

IVRA
>   intravenous regional anesthesia

Ivy
>   I. loop wiring
>   I. method of bleeding time

NOTES

J

J loop technique
J point
J versus S versus W pelvic ileal
pouch
Jaboulay
J. amputation
J. gastroduodenostomy
J. pyloroplasty
Jaboulay-Doyen-Winkleman
J.-D.-W. operation
J.-D.-W. technique
jackknife position
Jackson
J. incision
J. membrane
J. and Parker classification
J. and Parker classification of
Hodgkin disease
Jackson-Babcock operation
Jacobaeus procedure
Jacob membrane
**Jacobs locking-hook spinal rod
technique**
Jacobson
J. cartilage
J. nerve
Jacoby
border tissue of J.
Jacod syndrome
Jacquart facial angle
Jacquemet recess
Jacques plexus
Jaeger-Hamby procedure
Jaesche-Arlt operation
Jaesche operation
Jaffe procedure
Jahss
J. maneuver
J. procedure
Jaime lacrimal operation
James
J. bundle
J. position
Jameson operation
jamming knot
Janecki-Nelson shoulder girdle resection
Janeway
J. gastrostomy
J. lesion
**Jannetta microvascular decompression
procedure**
Jansey
J. procedure
J. technique

Jansky classification
Japanese
J. approach
J. cancer classification
J. Classification for Gastric
Carcinoma (JCGC)
J. standard operation
Japanese-style
J.-s. gastrectomy
J.-s. lymphadenectomy
J.-s. operation
Japas
J. osteotomy
J. V-osteotomy
Jarjavay ligament
Jatene arterial switch procedure
jaundice
breast-milk j.
cholestatic j.
obstructive j.
preoperative j.
regurgitation j.
jaw
j. bone
Hapsburg j.
j. joint
j. relation
j. relation record
j. thrust maneuver
upper j.
Jaworski body
jaw-to-jaw
j.-t.-j. position
j.-t.-j. relation
JCGC
Japanese Classification for Gastric
Carcinoma
Jefferson fracture
Jeffery
J. radial fracture classification
J. technique
jejunal
j. artery
j. biopsy
j. fasting motor activity
j. free flap
j. interposition
j. interposition of Henle loop
j. lumen
j. manometry
j. motility
j. pouch
j. puncture
j. puncture area
j. Roux-en-Y limb

jejunal *(continued)*
    j. Roux-en-Y loop
    j. serosa
    j. submucosa
    j. tube insertion
jejunectomy
jejunization
jejunocolic fistula
jejunocolostomy
jejunoileal
    j. anastomosis
    j. bypass (JIB)
    j. bypass reversal method
    j. bypass reversal procedure
    j. bypass reversal technique
    j. bypass surgery
jejunoileostomy
    Roux-en-Y distal j.
jejunojejunal anastomosis
jejunojejunostomy
jejunoplasty
    Hoffman j.
jejunostomy
    afferent j.
    decompression j.
    j. elemental diet feeding
    endoscopic j.
    hepaticocutaneous j.
    laparoscopic j.
    loop j.
    needle catheter j. (NCJ)
    percutaneous endoscopic j. (PEJ)
    j. tract choledochoscopy
    j. tube feeding
    Witzel j.
jejunotomy
jejunum
    j. loop
    proximal j.
    upper j.
Jena method
Jendrassik-Grof method
Jendrassik maneuver
jennerization
Jensen
    J. classification
    J. operation
    J. transposition procedure
Jergesen incision
jerky respiration
Jerne technique
jet
    high-frequency j. (HFJ)
    j. lesion
    j. pilot position
    transtracheal j.
    j. ventilation
    j. ventilation anesthetic technique
Jeune syndrome

Jewett
    J. and Strong staging
    J. and Whitmore classification
JIB
    jejunoileal bypass
    JIB reversal
J-loop ileostomy
job capacity evaluation
Jobe-Glousman capsular shift procedure
Jobert
    J. de Lamballe fossa
    J. suture technique
Johner-Wruhs tibial fracture classification
Johnson
    J. chevron osteotomy
    J. esophagogastroscopy
    J. esophagogastrostomy
    J. operation
    J. pelvic fracture technique
    J. procedure
    J. pronator advancement
    J. root canal filling method
    J. staple technique
Johnson-Spiegl
    J.-S. hallux varus correction
    J.-S. procedure
Johnston
    J. buttonhole procedure
    J. method
    J. pursestring suture technique
joint
    anterior intraoccipital j.
    arthrodial j.
    j. aspiration
    atlantoaxial j.
    atlantooccipital j.
    axial rotation j.
    ball-and-socket j.
    biaxial j.
    bicondylar j.
    bilocular j.
    j. branch
    capitular j.
    j. capsule
    j. cavity
    coccygeal j.
    composite j.
    compound j.
    costochondral j.
    costotransverse j.
    costovertebral j.
    cotyloid j.
    cricothyroid j.
    j. deformity
    dentoalveolar j.
    j. depression fracture
    diarthrodial j.
    j. disarticulation

ellipsoid j.
ellipsoidal j.
enarthrodial j.
extraarticular subtalar j.
facet j.
fibrous j.
j. fusion
ginglymoid j.
glenohumeral j.
gliding j.
hinge j.
immovable j.
incudomalleolar j.
interarticular j.
intraoccipital j.
jaw j.
lateral atlantoaxial j.
j. line
j. line pain
lumbosacral j.
Luschka j.
mandibular j.
j. manipulation
manubriosternal j.
j. mobilization
j. mouse
movable j.
multiaxial j.
neurocentral j.
j. oil
peg-and-socket j.
petrooccipital j.
pivot j.
plane j.
polyaxial j.
posterior intraoccipital j.
j. protection training
j. reconstruction
j. replacement
rotary j.
rotation j.
sacrococcygeal j.
screw j.
SI j.
simple j.
socket j.
j. space
j. space narrowing
sphenooccipital j.
spheroid j.
spiral j.
sternal j.

sternoclavicular j.
sternocostal j.
suture j.
synarthrodial j.
synchondrodial j.
syndesmodial j.
synovial j.
talocrural j.
temporomandibular j.
thigh j.
trochoid j.
uncovertebral j.
uniaxial j.
unilocular j.
wedge-and-groove j.
xiphisternal j.
zygapophysial j.

Jonas modification of Norwood procedure
Jones
    J. first-toe repair
    J. fracture
    J. and Jones wedge technique
    J. position
    J. resection arthroplasty
    J. tube procedure
Jones-Barnes-Lloyd-Roberts classification
Jones-Brackett technique
Jones-Politano technique
Jonnesco fossa
Jonnson maneuver
Joplin bunionectomy
Jorgensen technique
Joseph rhinoplasty
J-pexy
    omental J-p.
J-pouch
    colonic J-p.
    ileal J-p.
J. R. Moore procedure
J-sella deformity
J-shaped
    J-s. ileal pouch
    J-s. ileal pouch-anal anastomosis
    J-s. skin incision
J-sign
J-tube insertion
J-type maneuver
Judd-Mayo overlap midline incisional hernioplasty
Judd pyloroplasty technique

NOTES

Judet
    J. graft
    J. quadricepsplasty
Judkins-Sones
    J.-S. technique
    J.-S. technique of cardiac
      catheterization
Judkins technique
juga (*pl. of* jugum)
jugal
    j. bone
    j. point
jugomaxillary point
jugular
    j. bulb anomaly
    j. bulb catheter placement
      assessment
    j. bulb oxyhemoglobin desaturation
    j. bulb venous oxygen saturation
    j. compression maneuver
    j. duct
    j. foramen
    j. foramen syndrome
    j. fossa
    j. ganglion
    j. lymphatic trunk
    j. nerve
    j. plexus
    j. process
    j. sinus
    j. technique
    j. tubercle
    j. vein
    j. vein dissection
    j. venous arch
    j. venous bulb
    j. venous oxygen saturation
      ($SjVO_2$)
    j. venous pressure
juguloomohyoid node
jugum, pl. **juga**
juice
    cancer j.
jumbo biopsy
jump
    j. flap
    j. graft
jumper-knee position
junction
    anorectal j.
    atypical j.
    cavohepatic j.
    choledochoduodenal j.
    choledochopancreatic ductal j.
    costochondral j.
    cystic duct-infundibulum j.

    duodenojejunal j.
    esophagogastric j.
    gastroesophageal j.
    hard-soft palate j.
    ileocecal j.
    manubriosternal j.
    mucocutaneous j.
    neuroeffector j.
    neuromuscular j.
    rectosigmoid j.
    sacrococcygeal j.
    sclerocorneal j.
    scotoma j.
    squamocolumnar j.
    sternoclavicular j.
    sternomanubrial j.
    ureteropelvic j. (UPJ)
    xiphisternal j.
junctional
    j. dilatation
    j. dilation
    j. ectopic tachycardia
    j. epithelium
junctura, pl. **juncturae**
Jung muscle
Junod procedure
Jurkat T-cell line
Juvara procedure
juvenile
    j. angiofibroma
    j. ankylosing spondylitis
    j. embryonal carcinoma
    j. hemangiofibroma
    j. nevoxanthoendothelioma
    j. pelvis
    j. polyp
    j. rheumatoid arthritis
juxta-anal colostomy
juxtaarticulation
juxta-auricular fossa
juxtacardiac pleural pressure
juxtacortical
    j. fracture
    j. osteogenic sarcoma
juxtacrine stimulation
juxtacubital reconstruction
juxtaepiphysial
juxtaglomerular
    j. body
    j. complex
    j. granulation index
juxtahepatic vein
juxtaposition
juxtarenal aneurysm
juxtarestiform body

k
k space
k space segmentation
K562 erythroid line
KACT
kaolin-activated clotting time
Kader gastrostomy
Kader-Senn
K.-S. gastrotomy technique
K.-S. operation
Kaes
line of K.
Kajava classification
kala-azar infection
Kalamchi classification
Kaliscinski ureteral procedure
Kalish osteotomy
Kalt suture technique
Kammerer-Battle incision
kangaroo
k. pouch
k. tendon suture technique
kaolin-activated clotting time (KACT)
Kapandji technique
Kapel elbow dislocation technique
Kaplan
K. oblique line
K. open reduction
K. osteotomy
K. technique
Kaplan-Meier method
Karakousis-Vezeridis
K.-V. procedure
K.-V. resection
Karapandzic flap
Karhunen-Loeve procedure
Karlsson procedure
Karnofsky
K. rating scale classification
K. scale
Karr method
Karydakis flap
Kasabach-Merritt syndrome
Kasai
K. operation
K. portoenterostomy
K. procedure
Kasai-type hepatoportoenterostomy
Kashin-Beck disease
Kashiwagi technique
Kasser-Kennedy method
Kasugai classification
Kates-Kessel-Kay technique
Kato thick smear technique
Katzin operation

Kaufer tendon technique
Kauffman-White classification
Kaufmann technique
Kausch-Whipple pancreatoduodenectomy
Kavanaugh-Brower-Mann fixation
Kawaii-Yamamoto procedure
Kawamura
K. dome osteotomy
K. pelvic osteotomy
Kazanjian operation
Keating-Hart method
Kebab graft
Keen
K. operation
K. point
Kehr
K. incision
K. technique
Keil tumor cell classification
Keith bundle
Keith-Wagener-Barker classification
Keith-Wagener classification
Kelami classification
Kelikian-Clayton-Loseff
K.-C.-L. surgical syndactyly
K.-C.-L. technique
Kelikian-McFarland procedure
Kelikian procedure
Kelikian-Riashi-Gleason
K.-R.-G. patellar tendon repair
K.-R.-G. technique
Kellam-Waddel classification
Keller
K. bunionectomy
K. procedure
K. resection arthroplasty
Keller-Madlener operation
Kelling-Madlener procedure
Kellogg-Speed
K.-S. fusion technique
K.-S. lumbar spinal fusion
Kelly
K. plication
K. plication procedure
K. suture technique
Kelly-Keck osteotomy
Kelly-Kennedy modification
Kelman operation
keloid
k. fibroblast
k. formation
keloplasty
kelotomy
Kelsey unloading exercise therapy
Kelvin body

K

Kempf-Grosse-Abalo Z-step osteotomy
Kendrick
  K. method
  K. method below-knee amputation
  K. procedure
  K. technique
Kendrick-Sharma-Hassler-Herndon
  technique
Kennedy
  K. area-length method
  K. classification
  K. ligament technique
  K. procedure
Kennedy-Pacey operation
Kent
  K. bundle
  K. bundle ablation
  bundle of Stanley K.
Kent-His bundle
keratectomy
  Castroviejo k.
  excimer laser photorefractive k.
  k. operation
  photorefractive k. (PRK)
  phototherapeutic k.
  superficial k.
keratinized tissue
keratin scale
keratitis-deafness cornification disorder
keratitis lesion
keratoacanthoma
keratoangioma
keratocele
keratocentesis operation
keratoconjunctivitis
keratocricoid
keratodermatocele
keratoepithelioplasty
keratoglossus
keratohyal
keratoleukoma
keratolysis
  pitted k.
keratoma
keratometry
  surgical k.
keratomileusis
  laser-assisted in situ k. (LASIK)
  laser in situ k. (LASIK)
  k. operation
keratomy
keratopathy
  band k.
  exposure k.
keratophakic keratoplasty
keratopharyngeus
keratoplasty
  allopathic k.

Arroyo k.
Arruga k.
autogenous k.
automated lamellar therapeutic k.
  (ALTK)
Durr nonpenetrating k.
Elschnig k.
epikeratophakic k.
Filatov k.
heterogeneous k.
homogenous k.
Imre k.
keratophakic k.
lamellar refractive k.
layered k.
Morax k.
nonpenetrating k.
k. operation
optic k.
optical k.
partial k.
Paufique k.
penetrating k.
perforating k.
photorefractive k.
punctate epithelial k.
refractive k.
Sourdille k.
superficial lamellar k.
tectonic k.
thermal k.
total k.
keratoscopy
keratostomy
keratotomy
  arcuate transverse k.
  astigmatic k.
  delimiting k.
  laser k.
  k. operation
  radial k. (RK)
  refractive k.
  Ruiz trapezoidal k.
  trapezoidal k.
Kerckring fold
kerectomy
kerion formation
Kerley A, B, C lines
Kernohan
  K. notch
  K. system of glioma classification
Kern technique
Kerr cesarean section
KESS constipation scoring system
  classification
Kessel-Bonney
  K.-B. extension osteotomy
  K.-B. procedure

Kessler
  K. repair
  K. suture technique
Kestenbaum procedure
ketoacidosis
  diabetic k. (DKA)
ketone body formation
ketoprofen analgesic therapy
Kety-Schmidt
  K.-S. inert gas saturation technique
  K.-S. method
Kevorkian punch biopsy
Key-Conwell pelvic fracture classification
Keyes punch biopsy
keyhole
  k. approach
  k. coronary bypass procedure
  k. deformity
  k. incision
  k. mastopexy
  k. method
  k. surgery
  k. tenodesis technique
keyhole-shaped craniectomy
key-in-lock maneuver
Key operation
Keystone
  K. graft
  K. mastopexy
  K. technique
kg/m^2
  kilogram per meter squared
KHC
  knot holding capacity
Khodadoust line
Kidde cannula technique
Kidner foot procedure
kidney
  abdominal k.
  k. abscess
  k. adenocarcinoma
  k. adenoma
  amyloid k.
  k. anomaly
  arciform vein of k.
  arteriosclerotic k.
  artificial k.
  Ask-Upmark k.
  atrophic k.
  k. biopsy
  cake k.

  k. carbuncle
  cicatricial k.
  k. colic
  contracted k.
  cortical arch of k.
  cystic k.
  donor k.
  ectopic k.
  floating k.
  Goldblatt k.
  granular k.
  interlobular artery of k.
  k. internal splint/stent (KISS)
  medullary sponge k.
  mortar k.
  movable k.
  pelvic k.
  k. position
  putty k.
  pyelonephritic k.
  rosette k.
  sclerotic k.
  sigmoid k.
  simultaneous pancreas and k. (SPK)
  thoracic k.
  k. transplantation
  tumor-bearing k.
  unicaliceal k.
  wandering k.
  waxy k.
kidney-sparing operation
Kiehn-Earle-DesPrez procedure
Kiel
  K. classification
  K. graft
  K. Pediatric Tumor Registry
Kienböck dislocation
Kiernan space
Kiesselbach area
Kikuchi-MacNap-Moreau approach
Kilfoyle humeral medial condylar fracture classification
Kilian line
killer
  flow artifact k. (FLAK)
Killian
  K. bundle
  K. frontal sinusotomy
  K. frontoethmoidectomy procedure
  K. incision
Killian-Jamieson area

K

NOTES

Killip
K. classification
K. classification of heart disease
Killip-Kimball heart failure classification
kilogram per meter squared (kg/m²)
kilovolt (kV)
Kimerle anomaly
Kimmelstiel-Wilson lesion
Kimura cartilage graft
Kinast indirect reduction
kinesthetic method
kinetic venous drainage
King
K. ASD umbrella closure
K. biopsy method
K. curve posterior correction (type IV)
K. intraarticular hip fusion
K. open reduction
K. operation
K. technique
King-Richards dislocation technique
King-Steelquist
K.-S. hindquarter amputation
K.-S. technique
kinking
catheter k.
Kinsey
K. atherectomy
K. rotation atherectomy extrusion angioplasty
Kinzie method
Kirby-Bauer disc diffusion method
Kirby operation
Kirchner cell
Kirk thigh amputation technique
Kirner deformity
Kirschner
K. pin fixation
K. suture technique
K. wire fixation
K. wire placement
Kirstein method
KISS
kidney internal splint/stent
kissing
k. balloon angioplasty
k. balloon technique
Kitano knot
Kitaoka-Leventen medial displacement metatarsal osteotomy
Kitzinger
K. method
K. method of childbirth
Kjeldahl method
Kjolbe technique
kleeblattschädel deformity

Klein
K. muscle
K. technique
Kleinert
K. modification
K. repair
Klippel-Feil
K.-F. anomaly
K.-F. deformity
K.-F. syndrome
Klippel-Trenaunay syndrome
Klippel-Trenaunay-Weber syndrome
Kluge method
Knapp
K. operation
K. procedure
Knapp-Wheeler-Reese operation
knee
k. anatomy
k. arthroplasty
descending artery of k.
k. dislocation
k. extension
k. extensor
flail k.
k. fracture
k. fusion
lateral k.
posterior k.
k. region
k. replacement
k. replacement surgery
k. rotation
kneecap
kneecapping injury
knee-chest position
knee-elbow position
kneeling position
kneeling-squatting position
knife-edged finishing line
knob
aortic k.
lateral deflection control k.
Knobby-Clark procedure
Knobloch modification
knock-knee deformity
Knoll
K. gland
K. refraction technique
Knoop hardness indenter point
knot
Aberdeen k.
Ahern k.
bow-tie k.
capstan k.
clinch k.
curved-needle surgeon's k.
enamel k.
externally releasable k.

extracorporeal jamming k.
false k.
fisherman's k.
friction k.
granny k.
half-hitch k.
1-handed k.
k. holding capacity (KHC)
ileosigmoid k.
intracorporeal k.
jamming k.
Kitano k.
laparoscopic extracorporeal k.
partial-throw surgeon's k.
primitive k.
Roeder loop k.
secure intracorporeal k.
self-tightening slip k.
surgeon's k.
syncytial k.
Tim k.
Topel k.
Tripier operation throw square k.
true k.
vital k.
wire k.
knotting
    catheter k.
Knott technique
Knowles pinning
knuckle of tube
Ko-Airan
    K.-A. bleeding control procedure
    K.-A. maneuver
Koch
    K. conduit
    K. continent ileostomy
    K. pouch
    K. pouch cutaneous urinary diversion
    K. pouch modified procedure
    K. reservoir ileostomy
    K. technique
Kocher
    K. anastomosis
    K. classification
    K. curved L approach
    K. fracture
    K. lateral J approach
    K. maneuver
    K. method
    K. point

    K. pylorectomy
    K. pyloromyotomy
    K. ureterosigmoidostomy procedure
Kocher-Gibson posterolateral approach
Kocher-Langenbeck
    K.-L. approach
    K.-L. exposure
Kocher-Lorenz fracture
Kocher-McFarland hip arthroplasty
Koenig graft
Koenig-Schaefer
    K.-S. incision
    K.-S. medial approach
Koerner flap
Koffler operation
Köhler
    K. illumination
    K. line
Kohlrausch muscle
Kolmogorov-Smirnov procedure
Kolobow membrane lung
Kondoleon operation
Kondoleon-Sistrunk elephantiasis procedure
Konno
    K. biopsy method
    K. operation
    K. procedure
    K. repair
Korean hand acupressure
koronion
koroscopy
Korotkoff test
Kotz-Salzer rotationplasty
Koutsogiannis
    K. calcaneal displacement osteotomy
    K. procedure
Koutsogiannis-Fowler-Anderson osteotomy
Kovalevsky canal
Krackow
    K. maneuver
    K. point
Kramer-Craig-Noel basilar femoral neck osteotomy
Kraske
    K. operation
    K. parasacral approach
    K. position
    K. procedure
    K. transsacral proctectomy

NOTES

Kraupa operation
Krause
- K. bone
- K. denervation
- K. ligament
- K. method
- K. muscle
- K. respiratory bundle
- transverse suture of K.

Krause-Wolfe graft
Krawkow-Cohn technique
Krawkow-Thomas-Jones technique
Krempen-Craig-Sotelo tibial nonunion technique
Krempen-Silver-Sotelo nonunion operation
Kreuscher bunionectomy
Krimsky method
Kristeller
- K. maneuver
- K. method

Kroner tubal ligation
Krönig technique
Krönlein
- K. hernia
- K. operation
- K. orbitotomy
- K. procedure

Krönlein-Berke operation
Kronner external fixation
Kropp
- K. cystourethroplasty
- K. operation
- K. procedure

Krukenberg
- K. corneal spindle
- K. hand reconstruction
- K. procedure

Kruskal-Wallis
- K.-W. nonparametric analysis
- K.-W. test

Kugel
- K. anastomosis
- K. approach
- K. hernia repair

Kugelberg reconstruction
Kuhnt
- K. eyelid operation
- K. tarsectomy

Kuhnt-Helmbold operation
Kuhnt-Junius repair
Kuhnt-Szymanowski procedure
Kuhnt-Thorpe operation
Kulchitsky cell carcinoma
Kumar
- K. application
- K. spica cast technique

Kumar-Cowell-Ramsey technique
Küntscher technique
Kussmaul
- K. coma
- K. respiration

Kussmaul-Kien respiration
Küstner
- K. incision
- K. uterine inversion correction

Kutler
- K. digital flap
- K. double lateral advancement flap
- K. finger amputation technique
- K. V-Y flap
- K. V-Y flap graft

Kuzmak
- K. gastric banding
- K. gastroplasty

kV
- kilovolt

KWB classification
K-wire placement
Kwitko operation
Kyle-Gustilo classification
Kyle-Gustilo-Premer classification
Kyle internal fixation
kyphectomy
- Sharrard-type k.

kyphosis
- k. correction
- k. creation
- postlaminectomy k.
- postradiation k.

kyphos resection
kyphotic
- k. angulation
- k. deformity
- k. deformity pathomechanics

λ (*var. of* lambda)
LA
    laparoscopic appendectomy
    lateral apical
    LA segment
Labat sciatic nerve block
Labbé
    L. gastrotomy technique
    L. triangle
    L. vein
labia (*pl. of* labium)
labial
    l. cavity
    l. fusion
    l. gland
    l. hernia
    l. line
    l. pad
    l. tubercle
    l. ulceration
    l. vein
    l. vestibule
labialization
labile blood pressure
labioglossolaryngeal
labioglossomandibular approach
labioglossopharyngeal
labioincisal line angle
labiolingual
    l. plane
    l. technique
labiomandibular
    l. approach
    l. glossotomy
labiomental
labionasal
labiopalatine
labioplasty
labioscrotal fold
labium, pl. **labia**
    l. majus
    ungual labia
labor
    l. augmentation induction
    l. pain
laboratory
    l. monitoring
    l. parameter
Laborde method
labored respiration
labral lesion
labrum
labyrinth
    bony l.
    ethmoidal l.

    Ludwig l.
    osseous l.
    renal l.
    Santorini l.
    vestibular l.
labyrinthectomy
labyrinthine
    l. artery
    l. fistula
    l. fistula test
    l. surgery
    l. vein
labyrinthotomy
labyrinthus
lacerable
lacerated foramen
laceration
    aortic l.
    birth canal l.
    bladder l.
    brain l.
    burst-type l.
    canalicular l.
    central stellate l.
    cervical l.
    chevron l.
    concurrent hepatic l.
    conjunctival l.
    corneal l.
    corneoscleral l.
    diaphragm l.
    diaphragmatic l.
    eyebrow l.
    flexor tendon l.
    hallucis longus l.
    inadvertent l.
    lid margin l.
    liver l.
    longitudinal l.
    lower pole l.
    parenchymal l.
    perineal l.
    peripheral l.
    rectal l.
    scalp l.
    splenic l.
    stellate l.
    tarsal l.
    tentorial l.
    through-and-through l.
    vaginal l.
    vascular l.
lace suture technique
Lachman maneuver
lacmoid staining solution

L

lacrimal, lachrymal
- l. angle duct anomaly
- l. apparatus
- l. artery
- l. bone
- l. canal
- l. canaliculus
- l. crest
- l. fascia
- l. fistula
- l. fold
- l. ganglion
- l. gland repair
- l. gland tumor
- l. irrigation test
- l. lake
- l. margin
- l. mass
- l. nerve
- l. notch
- l. papilla
- l. point
- l. punctum
- l. sac
- l. sac fossa
- l. surgery
- l. system
- l. vein

lacrimation
- excessive l.
- l. reflex

lacrimoconchal suture
lacrimomaxillary suture
lacrimotomy
Lacroix
- fibroosseous ring of L.
- osseous ring of L.

lactate
- blood l. (BL)
- l. clearance
- l. extraction
- l. level
- normalizing l.
- normal serum l.

lactation letdown response
lacteal
- l. fistula
- l. vessel

lactic
- l. acidosis
- l. acidosis and stroke-like syndrome

lactiferous
- l. duct
- l. gland
- l. sinus

lactoperoxidase radioiodination
lacuna, pl. **lacunae**
- Morgagni l.

- osteocytic l.
- urethral l.

lacunar
- l. abscess
- l. ligament

Ladd
- L. band
- L. operation
- L. procedure

Lafora body disease
lag
- dilation l.
- l. dilation
- l. screw fixation
- l. screw thread hole
- l. time

Lagleyze-Trantas operation
Lagrange operation
LAH
- laparoscopic-assisted hepatectomy

Lahey operation
Laimer area
Laird-McMahon anorectoplasty
laissez-faire lid operation
lake
- lacrimal l.
- lateral l.

Lallemand body
Lallemand-Trousseau body
Lallouette pyramid
LAMA
- laser-assisted microanastomosis

Lamaze
- L. method
- L. method of childbirth
- L. technique

lambda, λ
- l. suture line

lambdoid
- l. margin
- l. suture

Lambert canal
Lambl excrescence
Lamb-Marks-Bayne technique
Lambrinudi
- L. osteotomy
- L. technique

lamella, pl. **lamellae**
- corneal l.
- elastic l.

lamellar
- l. bone
- l. corneal transplant
- l. exfoliation
- l. refractive keratoplasty

lamellation
lamina, pl. **laminae**
- alar l.
- basal l.

basilar l.
cribrous l.
deep l.
external elastic l.
fusca l.
pterygoid l.
suprachoroid l.
thyroid l.
laminaplasty
expansive l.
Tsuji l.
laminar
l. cortex posterior aspect
l. flow hood
l. fracture
laminated
l. acellular mass
l. clot
lamination
laminectomy
cervical spine l.
decompression l.
decompressive l.
Gill l.
Girdlestone l.
multilevel l.
4-place l.
radial l.
laminoforaminotomy
laminoplasty
laminotomy and discectomy
Lancaster operation
Lancefield classification
lanceolate deformity
Lanchner operation
landmark
anatomic l.
anatomical l.
bony l.
cephalometric l.
developmental l.
pedicle l.
surface l.
thoracic spine l.
Winnie l.
Landolt
L. body
L. operation
Landzert fossa
Lane
L. band

L. operation
L. procedure
Langenbeck
L. operation
L. triangle
Langendorff
L. heart preparation
L. method
L. perfusion
Langenskiöld
L. bone graft
L. bony bridge resection
L. fusion
L. procedure
Langer
L. arch
L. line
Langerhans
islets of L.
Lange tendon lengthening and repair
Langevin updating procedure
Langhans line
Lannelongue ligament
lanugo
Lanz
L. incision
L. line
L. point
Lanza scale for drug-induced mucosal damage classification
LAO
left anterior oblique
left anterior occipital
LAO position
LAP
left atrial pressure
laparectomy
laparocele
laparocystidotomy
laparoenterotomy
laparogastroscopy
laparogastrostomy
laparogastrotomy
laparohepatotomy
laparohysterectomy
laparohystero-oophorectomy
laparohysteropexy
laparohysterosalpingo-oophorectomy
laparohysterotomy
laparoileotomy
laparomyomectomy
laparomyositis

L

NOTES

laparorrhaphy
laparosalpingectomy
laparosalpingo-oophorectomy
laparosalpingotomy
laparoscopic
l. adjustable silicone gastric banding
l. adrenalectomy
l. antegrade transcystic sphincterotomy
l. anterior adrenalectomy
l. anterior partial fundoplication
l. appendectomy (LA)
l. artery ligation
l. assistance
l. autopsy
l. bariatric surgery
l. bilioenteric anastomosis
l. bladder neck suture suspension procedure
l. bowel resection
l. Burch procedure
l. bypass procedure
l. cardiomyotomy
l. cecopexy
l. celiac plexus pain block
l. cholecystectomy (LC)
l. cholecystotomy
l. clip application
l. colectomy
l. colorectal cancer surgery
l. colposuspension technique
l. common bile duct exploration
l. common bile duct exploration choledochotomy
l. common bile duct exploration transcystic approach
l. cyst decortication
l. dismembered pyeloplasty
l. dissection and manipulation
l. distal pancreatectomy
l. Döderlein hysterectomy
l. donor nephrectomy (LDN)
l. Dorr antireflux surgery
l. duodenoileostomy ileoileostomy
l. esophageal myomectomy
l. esophagogastric fundoplasty
l. esophagogastroplasty with Nissen fundoplication
l. esophagomyotomy
l. esophagoplasty
l. evaluation
l. examination
l. extracorporeal knot
l. feeding tube replacement
l. fenestration
l. gallbladder removal
l. gas
l. gastric banding

l. gastric bypass
l. gastroenterostomy
l. gastroplasty
l. gastrostomy
l. guidance
l. Hassab operation
l. Heller myotomy
l. hepatectomy
l. hepatojejunostomy
l. hernioplasty
l. hysterosalpingectomy
l. intracorporeal ultrasonography (LICU)
l. intragastric resection
l. intraoperative ultrasonography (LIOUS)
l. IPOM repair
l. jejunostomy
l. laser cholecystectomy (LLC)
l. left hemicolectomy
l. live donor nephrectomy
l. liver biopsy
l. lymph node dissection method
l. lymph node dissection procedure
l. lymph node dissection technique
l. lymphocelectomy
l. lysis of adhesions
l. management
l. needle colposuspension
l. Nissen fundoplication (LNF)
l. Nissen fundoplication method
l. Nissen fundoplication procedure
l. Nissen fundoplication technique
l. Nissen fundoplication with esophageal lengthening
l. Nissen and Toupet fundoplication
l. orchiopexy
l. paraaortic lymph node sampling
l. paraaortic lymph node sampling method
l. paraaortic lymph node sampling procedure
l. paraaortic lymph node sampling technique
l. paraesophageal hernia repair (LPHR)
l. pelvic lymphadenectomy
l. pelvic lymph node dissection
l. photography
l. pneumodissection
l. port site metastasis
l. posterior hemifundoplication
l. proctectomy
l. PROST
l. prosthetic mesh repair
l. pyloromyotomy
l. radical hysterectomy
l. radical prostatectomy

l. repair of paraesophageal hernia (LRPH)
l. retropubic colposuspension
l. Roux-en-Y choledochojejunostomy
l. seromyotomy
l. sigmoidopexy
l. splenectomy
l. staging
l. stone extraction
l. stripping technique
l. surgical procedure
l. technology
l. total extraperitoneal herniorrhaphy
l. total gastrectomy
l. total occlusion (LTO)
l. total proctocolectomy
l. Toupet anti-reflux surgery
l. transcystic common bile duct exploration (LTCBDE)
l. transcystic duct exploration
l. transcystic lithotripsy (LTCL)
l. transcystic papillotomy
l. transcystic sphincter of Oddi manometry
l. transhiatal esophagectomy
l. transhiatal view
l. treatment
l. trocar wound
l. tubal banding procedure
l. ultrasonography (LUS)
l. ultrasound
l. ureteral reanastomosis
l. ureterolithotomy
l. uterine nerve ablation
l. uterolysis
l. vagotomy
l. varicocelectomy
l. varicocele repair
l. varix ligation
l. ventral hernia repair
l. vision

laparoscopically
l. assisted endorectal pull-through procedure
l. assisted surgery
l. assisted vaginal hysterectomy (LAVH)
l. guided cryoablation
l. guided transcystic exploration

laparoscopic-assisted
l.-a. aneurysmectomy
l.-a. aortic reconstructive surgery
l.-a. esophagectomy
l.-a. gastropexy
l.-a. hemicolectomy
l.-a. hepatectomy (LAH)
l.-a. living donor nephrectomy
l.-a. procedure
l.-a. small bowel resection
l.-a. subtotal gastrectomy
l.-a. vaginal hysterectomy
l.-a. vaginal hysteroscopy

laparoscopic-induced neuralgia
laparoscopist
laparoscopy
ambulatory gynecologic l.
bedside l.
closed l.
diagnostic l.
double-puncture l.
flexible l.
full diagnostic l.
gaseous l.
gasless l.
gynecologic l.
hand-assisted l.
laser l.
mandatory l.
needle l.
open l.
pelvic l.
revision l.
robot-assisted l.
second-look l.
single-port l.
single-puncture l.
staging l.
therapeutic l.

laparostomy technique
laparotomy
elective l.
emergency l.
exploratory l.
formal l.
l. incision
negative l.
open l.
routine l.
second-look l. (SLL)
staging l.
standard midline l.

laparotrachelotomy
laparotyphlotomy
laparouterotomy

L

NOTES

Lapides-Ball urethropexy
Lapidus
    L. bunionectomy
    L. hammertoe technique
lappet formation
lap seatbelt fracture
LAR
    low anterior resection
lardaceous liver
large
    l. canal
    l. cell carcinoma
    l. humeral head hemiarthroplasty
    l. intestine
    l. mask airway
    l. pelvis
    l. restoration
    l. vestibular aqueduct syndrome
large-core
    l.-c. needle aspiration biopsy
    l.-c. technique
large-particle biopsy
large-scale integration
Larmon
    L. forefoot arthroplasty
    L. forefoot procedure
LaRoque herniorrhaphy incision
Laroyenne operation
Larrey
    L. cleft
    L. hernia
Larsen syndrome
Larson
    L. ligament reconstruction
    L. technique
laryngeal
    l. anesthesia
    l. anomaly
    l. aperture
    l. bursa
    l. carcinoma
    l. cartilage fracture
    l. cavity
    l. cyst
    l. diaphragm
    l. edema
    l. electromyography
    l. framework surgery
    l. gland
    l. hemorrhage
    l. infection
    l. keel operation
    l. mask airway (LMA)
    l. mask insertion anesthetic
    technique
    l. muscle
    l. nerve
    l. nerve paralysis
    l. oscillation

    l. pharynx
    l. pouch
    l. prominence
    l. repair
    l. respiration
    l. sinus
    l. skeleton
    l. vein
    l. ventricle
    l. web
laryngectomy
    anterior partial l.
    frontolateral l.
    narrow-field l.
    near-total l.
    partial l.
    subtotal supraglottic l.
    supracricoid partial l.
    supraglottic l.
    total l.
    vertical partial l.
    wide-field total l.
larynges (*pl. of* larynx)
laryngocele
laryngology
laryngopharyngeal reflux
laryngopharyngectomy
    partial l.
    total l.
laryngopharyngeus
laryngopharynx
laryngoplasty
    sternothyroid muscle flap l.
laryngopyocele
laryngoscopy
    l. anesthetic technique
    direct l.
    fiber optic l.
    indirect l.
    laser l.
    mirror-image l.
    suspension l.
laryngospasm
    postextubation l.
laryngotomy
    inferior l.
laryngotracheal anesthesia (LTA)
laryngotracheoplasty (LTP)
larynx, pl. **larynges**
    external auditory l.
    folding l.
    polypoid hyperplasia of l.
    posterior l.
    superficial anterior l.
    superior l.
laser
    l. arthroscopy
    l. biliary lithotripsy
    l. bronchoscopy

l. cavity
l. cervical conization
l. coagulation
l. coagulation vaporization procedure (LCVP)
l. controlled area
l. Doppler flowmetry (LDF)
l. Doppler fluxmetry
l. hemorrhoidectomy
l. hemorrhoid excision
l. iridectomy
l. iridotomy
l. keratotomy
l. laparoscopic cholecystectomy (LLC)
l. laparoscopic vagotomy
l. laparoscopy
l. laryngoscopy
l. manipulation
l. method
l. partial nephrectomy
l. photoablation
l. photocoagulation
l. photovaporization
l. plume
l. recanalization
l. in situ keratomileusis (LASIK)
l. surgery
l. therapy
l. tissue weld
l. tissue welding
l. trabeculoplasty
l. uterosacral nerve ablation
l. uvulopalatoplasty
l. vaporization
l. welding technique

laser-assisted
l.-a. appendectomy
l.-a. balloon angioplasty
l.-a. microanastomosis (LAMA)
l.-a. in situ keratomileusis (LASIK)
l.-a. spinal endoscopy
l.-a. uvulopalatoplasty (LAUP)
laser-evoked potential
laser-filtering surgery
laser-induced
l.-i. fragmentation
l.-i. intracorporeal shockwave lithotripsy
lasering
lasertripsy

Lash
L. operation
L. procedure
LASIK
laser-assisted in situ keratomileusis
laser in situ keratomileusis
LAST
limited anterior small thoracotomy
LAST coronary bypass procedure
lata
fascia l.
Latarget
L. nerve
L. procedure
late
l. complication
l. graft dysfunction
l. graft failure
l. infection rate
l. transplant nephrectomy
l. wound failure
latency
postdrug l.
latent herpes simplex virus infection
late-onset
l.-o. disease
l.-o. hepatic failure (LOHF)
latera (*pl. of* latus)
lateral
l. aberration
l. adenoidectomy
l. apex
l. apical (LA)
l. aspiration
l. atlantoaxial joint
l. band mobilization
l. basal (LB)
l. bending technique
l. bicipital groove
l. calcaneal branch
l. canal
l. canal entrapment
l. canthotomy
l. canthus
l. cartilage flap
l. central palmar space
l. cerebral aperture
l. cervical node dissection
l. chest x-ray
l. closing wedge osteotomy
l. column
l. compartment reconstruction

L

NOTES

lateral *(continued)*
- l. compression
- l. compression injury
- l. condensation
- l. condylar humeral fracture
- l. condylar inclination
- l. condyle
- l. cord
- l. corticospinal tract
- l. crus
- l. decubitus position
- l. deflection control knob
- l. deltoid splitting approach
- l. edge
- l. excursion
- l. extensor expansion
- l. extensor release
- l. extracavitary approach
- l. fluoroscopy
- l. fusion
- l. Gatellier-Chastang approach
- l. geniculate body
- l. ginglymus
- l. glossoepiglottic fold
- l. ground (LG)
- l. ground bundle
- l. head
- l. illumination
- l. J approach
- l. jaw projection
- l. joint of ankle
- l. joint line
- l. joint space
- l. knee
- l. Kocher approach
- l. lake
- l. ligament
- l. lithotomy
- l. mass
- l. mass fracture
- l. meniscectomy
- l. muscle
- l. nail fold
- l. nasal branch
- l. orbit
- l. perforation
- l. pole
- l. portion
- l. process
- l. prone position
- l. rectus recession
- l. rectus resection
- l. rectus tendon
- l. recumbent position
- l. region
- l. retraction
- l. rhachotomy
- l. root
- l. sac
- l. sector
- l. sinus
- l. tarsal strip procedure
- l. thoracotomy
- l. utility incision
- l. ventricle
- l. wall
- l. window technique
- l. wound
- l. x-ray view

laterality

lateralization
- cortical l.

lateral-lateral pouch

lateral-sector pedicle

lateriflexion

lateroabdominal

lateroaortic
- l. lymph node dissection
- l. metastasis

laterodeviation

lateroflexion

lateropharyngeum

lateroposition

later postoperative period

late-stage disease

latex
- l. allergy
- l. closure

lathing procedure

latissimus
- l. dorsi island flap
- l. dorsi muscle flap
- l. dorsi musculocutaneous flap
- l. dorsi myocutaneous flap
- l. dorsi procedure
- l. dorsi tendon

latissimus-scapular muscle flap

latissimus-serratus muscle flap

lattice space

latus, pl. **latera**

Latzko
- L. cesarean section
- L. partial colpocleisis
- L. radical abdominal hysterectomy
- L. vesicovaginal fistula repair

laudable

Lauenstein procedure

Lauge-Hansen ankle fracture classification

Laugier
- L. fracture
- L. hernia

Laumonier ganglion

LAUP
- laser-assisted uvulopalatoplasty

Laurell
- L. method
- L. technique

Lauren gastric carcinoma classification
Lauth
    L. canal
    L. ligament
lavage
    abdominal l.
    bowel l.
    l. bowel preparation
    colonic l.
    continuous postoperative closed l.
    copious peritoneal l.
    diagnostic peritoneal l. (DPL)
    Exeter bone l.
    external biliary l.
    l. instillation
    intraoperative bowel l.
    intraoperative colonic l.
    on-table l.
    peritoneal l.
    pulsatile pressure l.
    saline l.
    l. solution
    l. and suction
    unilateral l.
LAVH
    laparoscopically assisted vaginal
    hysterectomy
law
    l. of association
    l. of denervation
    Hilton l.
    Le Chatelier l.
Lawson operation
layer
    aponeurotic l.
    barrier l.
    echographic l.
    echo-poor l.
    fascial l.
    hidden l.
    input l.
    meningeal l.
    mesothelial cell l.
    molecular external l.
    musculoaponeurotic l.
    nerve fiber bundle l.
    nuclear external l.
    orbital l.
    output l.
    parietal l.
    plexiform external l.

    posterior l.
    pretracheal l.
    prevertebral l.
    seromuscular l.
    serous l.
    superficial l.
    suprachoroid l.
    l. technique
    visceral l.
2-layer
    2-l. anastomosis
    2-l. enteroenterostomy
    2-l. latex closure
    2-l. open technique
layered
    l. closure
    l. keratoplasty
layer-to-layer gastroplasty
laying-open fistulotomy
Lazaro da Silva technique colostomy
Lazarus-Nelson technique
Lazepen-Gamidov anteromedial approach
lazy-C incision
lazy-H incision
lazy-S incision
lazy-Z incision
LB
    lateral basal
    LB segment
LC
    laparoscopic cholecystectomy
LCA
    left carotid artery
    left coronary artery
LCAT
    lecithin-cholesterol acyltransferase
L-curved incision
LCVP
    laser coagulation vaporization procedure
LCVP-aided
    LCVP-a. hepatectomy
    LCVP-a. hepatic resection
    LCVP-a. technique
LCVP-assisted
    LCVP-a. hepatectomy
    LCVP-a. major liver resection
LDF
    laser Doppler flowmetry
LDN
    laparoscopic donor nephrectomy
    LDN technique

L

NOTES

LDR
low dose rate
LDR intracavitary radiation therapy

Le
Le Chatelier law
Le Chatelier principle
Le Dentu suture
Le Dran suture technique
Le Fort classification
Le Fort fibular fracture
Le Fort I-III fracture
Le Fort mandibular fracture
Le Fort-Neugebauer operation
Le Fort operation
Le Fort osteotomy
Le Fort partial colpocleisis
Le Fort procedure
Le Fort suture technique
Le Fort-Wagstaffe fracture
Le Fort-Wehrbein-Duplay
hypospadias repair

Leach-Igou step-cut medial osteotomy
Leach-Schepsis-Paul augmentation
Leach technique
lead
l. colic
l. line

Leadbetter
L. cystourethroplasty
L. hip manipulation
L. maneuver
L. modification technique
L. procedure

Leadbetter-Politano
L.-P. procedure
L.-P. ureterovesicoplasty

lead-pipe
l.-p. appearance
l.-p. colon
l.-p. fracture

leaf
superior l.

leaflet
aortic valve l.
heart valve l.
mitral valve l.
posterior mitral valve l.
valve l.

Leahey operation
leak
anastomotic stump l.
bile l.
chylous l.
cystic duct stump l.
duodenal stump l.
glue patch l.
mask l.
pancreatic stump l.
periprosthetic l.

l. point pressure
postoperative anastomotic l.
Roux limb stump l.
stump l.
trocar gas l.

leakage
anastomotic l.
bile l.
biliary l.
cervical l.
chylous l.
corneal l.
intestinal anastomotic l.
local l.
l. rate
silicone implant l.
tube l.

lean
l. body mass
l. body weight

leapfrog position
leather-bottle stomach
Leboyer
L. method
L. technique

lecithin-cholesterol acyltransferase
(LCAT)
Lecompte maneuver
ledge
eccentric l.

LeDuc
L. anastomosis
L. technique

LeDuc-Camey
L.-C. ileocolostomy
L.-C. ileocystoplasty

Lee
L. anterosuperior iliac spine graft
L. bone graft
L. ganglion
L. procedure
L. reconstruction
L. technique

leech
mechanical l.

LEEP
loop electrocautery excision procedure
loop electrosurgical excision procedure
LEEP conization

leeway space
Lee-White
L.-W. clotting time
L.-W. clotting time method

Lefèvre gastrectomy technique
LeFort III facial advancement
left
l. anterior oblique (LAO)
l. anterior oblique position
l. anterior oblique projection

l. anterior occipital (LAO)
l. atrial isolation procedure
l. atrial pressure (LAP)
l. atrium-to-femoral artery
circulatory bypass
l. brachiocephalic vein
l. bundle branch block
l. carotid artery (LCA)
l. colectomy
l. coronary artery (LCA)
l. coronary valve
l. decubitus position
l. dominant coronary circulation
l. frontal craniotomy (LFC)
l. gutter
l. heart catheterization
l. hemicolectomy
l. hemidiaphragm
l. hepatectomy
l. hypochondriac region
l. inguinal hernia (LIH)
l. lateral decubitus position
l. lateral projection
l. lateral region
l. lower extremity (LLE)
l. lower quadrant (LLQ)
l. rotation
l. subclavian vein (LSV)
l. thorax
l. upper extremity (LUE)
l. upper quadrant (LUQ)
l. upper quadrant peritonectomy
l. ventricle
l. ventricular end-diastolic area
(LVEDa)
l. ventricular end-diastolic pressure
l. ventricular end-systolic area
(LVESa)
l. ventricular insufficiency (LVI)
l. ventricular ischemia (LVI)
l. ventricular outflow tract (LVOT)
l. ventricular pressure-volume
relationship (LVPVR)
l. ventricular puncture
l. ventricular systolic pressure
l. vertebral artery

left-sided
l.-s. colorectal obstruction
l.-s. injury
l.-s. nail
l.-s. thoracotomy

left-side-down position

left-to-right subtotal pancreatectomy
leg
bandy l.
Legat point
legged
1-l. stork test
Lehman technique
Leibolt technique
leiomyoblastoma
leiomyofibroma
leiomyoma enucleation
leiomyomectomy
leiomyosarcoma
recurrent l.
Leishman classification
Lejour mastopexy
Lejour-type breast reduction
Leksell technique
Lembert suture technique
Lempert
L. fenestration
L. incision
Lenart-Kullman technique
length
bowel l.
pedicle screw path l.
peripheral capillary filtration slit l.
restriction fragment l.
l. of stay (LOS)
length-breadth index
lengthening
distal catheter l.
extensor l.
laparoscopic Nissen fundoplication
with esophageal l.
surgical crown l.
tendon l.
length-height index
length-resting tension relation
length-tension relation
lengthwise slit
Lennert
L. classification
L. lesion
lens
l. aberration
C-loop intraocular l.
corneal l.
l. dislocation
l. equator
l. exchange
intraocular l.

L

NOTES

413

lens *(continued)*
 l. plane
 l. removal
 suture of l.
 l. suture technique
lensectomy
 Charles l.
 coal-mining l.
lentectomy
lenticular
 l. loop
 l. papilla
 l. process
 l. ring
lenticulostriate artery
lentiform bone
lentigo melanoma
Lepird procedure
L'Episcopo hip reconstruction
L'Episcopo-Zachary procedure
leprosy
 anesthetic l.
leptomeningeal
 l. anastomosis
 l. carcinoma
 l. metastasis
 l. space
leptomeninges
leptomyelolipoma
Leriche
 L. operation
 L. sympathectomy
Leri-Weill disease
LES
 lower esophageal sphincter
 LES pressure
Lesgaft
 L. hernia
 L. space
lesion
 accessible l.
 acetowhite l.
 acneform l.
 acute gastric mucosal l.
 acute traumatic l.
 admixture l.
 aggressive l.
 anal squamous intraepithelial l.
 angiocentric immunoproliferative l.
 angiocentric lymphoproliferative l.
 angiodysplastic l.
 angioinvasive l.
 angioproliferative l.
 angulated l.
 anterior labrum periosteum shoulder arthroscopic l.
 anular constricting l.
 aphthous-type l.
 apple-core l.

l. architecture
l. arrangement
articular cartilage l.
atherosclerotic carotid artery l.
atlantoaxial l.
axial l.
axillary skin l.
Baehr-Lohlein l.
Bankart shoulder l.
barrel-shaped l.
basal ganglionic l.
benign bone l.
benign lymphoepithelial l.
benign lymphoproliferative l.
benign vascular l.
Bennett l.
biceps interval l.
bifurcation l.
bilobed polypoid l.
bird's nest l.
blanchable red l.
blastic l.
bleeding l.
blue-gray l.
Blumenthal l.
bone marrow l.
bony l.
boomerang-shaped l.
Bracht-Wachter l.
braidlike l.
brainstem l.
branch l.
bridgelike l.
brown-black l.
bubbly bone l.
bullous skin l.
bull's eye macular l.
Bywaters l.
calcified l.
cancer l.
carpet l.
cavitary lung l.
cavitary small bowel l.
cemental l.
central l.
centrilobular l.
cerebral l.
cervical l.
chest l.
chiasmal l.
choroidal l.
circular cherry-red l.
cleavage l.
cochlear l.
coin l.
cold l.
colonic vascular l.
complete common peroneal nerve l.
concentric l.

congenital l.
conjunctival melanotic l.
constricting l.
cornea guttate l.
corneal punctate l.
cortical l.
Councilman l.
culprit l.
cutaneous l.
cylindromatous l.
cystic bone l.
cystic lymphoepithelial AIDS-
  related l.
demyelinating l.
dendritic l.
de novo l.
depigmented l.
depressed l.
dermal l.
desmoid l.
destructive bone l.
Dieulafoy l.
Dieulafoy-like l.
diffuse ulcerative l.
dilatable l.
disc l.
discoid skin l.
discrete l.
l. distribution
division I–IV l.
dorsal root entry zone l.
DREZ l.
ductal-dependent l.
Duret l.
dye sham intrarenal l.
dysarthric l.
dysplasia-associated l.
early cancer l.
ectatic vascular l.
eczematous l.
elementary l.
elevated l.
enhancing brain l.
entry zone l.
eosinophilic fibrohistiocytic l.
epididymis l.
epidural extramedullary l.
erysipelas-like skin l.
erythrodermatous l.
l. evolution
excavated l.

expansile unilocular well-demarcated
  bone l.
extracranial mass l.
extrahepatic l.
extramural l.
extratesticular l.
extremity l.
extrinsic l.
fibrocalcific l.
fibrohistiocytic l.
fibromusculoelastic l.
fibroosseous l.
fibrous bone l.
fibrous polypoid l.
firm l.
flat depressed l.
flat elevated l.
floor-of-mouth l.
florid duct l.
focal parenchymal brain l.
focal splenic l.
follicular l.
Forest I, II l.
gastrointestinal l.
genetic l.
genital papulosquamous l.
Ghon primary l.
giant cell l.
Gill l.
glomerular tip l.
gross l.
ground-glass l.
gunpowder l.
hamartomatous l.
hemorrhagic l.
hepatic mass l.
herpetoid l.
high-grade squamous
  intraepithelial l.
high-intensity l.
high neurological l.
Hill-Sachs shoulder l.
histologic l.
honeycomb l.
hot l.
hyperdense brain l.
hyperintense brain l.
hyperkeratotic l.
hyperpigmented l.
hypodense brain l.
hypoechoic l.
l. identification

L

NOTES

lesion *(continued)*

immunoproliferative l.
impaction l.
indiscriminate l.
infarctive l.
inflammatory l.
initial syphilitic l.
interpeduncular fossa l.
interradicular l.
intraabdominal l.
intraconal l.
intracranial mass l.
intradural extramedullary l.
intrahepatic l.
intramedullary l.
intramural extramucosal l.
intraosseous bone l.
intrasellar l.
intravascular endothelial
  proliferative l.
intrinsic brainstem l.
ipsilateral nerve root l.
irritable l.
irritative l.
Janeway l.
jet l.
keratitis l.
Kimmelstiel-Wilson l.
labral l.
Lennert l.
Libman-Sacks l.
lichenified l.
lipocytic l.
localized l.
Löhlein-Baehr l.
long l.
low-attenuation l.
lower motor neuron l.
low-grade squamous
  intraepithelial l.
lucent lung l.
lumbar spinal cord l.
lumbar spine l.
lumbosacral plexus l.
lumbosacral root l.
lymphoepithelial l.
lymphoproliferative l.
lytic bone l.
macrofollicular l.
macroscopic l.
macrovascular coronary l.
malignant pituitary l.
Mallory-Weiss l.
mammographic l.
l. margination
mass l.
medium l.
melanocytic conjunctival l.
melanotic l.

mesencephalic low-density l.
mesenchymal l.
mesenteric vascular l.
metastatic l.
minute polypoid l.
mixed fat-water density l.
mixed sclerotic and lytic bone l.
molecular l.
monotypic l.
Monteggia equivalent l.
Morel-Lavele l.
morphea-like l.
l. morphology
mucocutaneous l.
mucosal l.
mucous membrane l.
mulberry l.
multifocal enhancing l.
multilocular cystic l.
napkin-ring annular l.
neoplastic l.
neural l.
neurovascular l.
nickel-and-dime l.
nodular l.
nodule-in-nodule l.
nonbacterial thrombotic
  endocardial l.
nonblanchable, abnormally
  colored l.
nonerosive gastric mucosal l.
nonmeningiomatous malignant l.
nonneoplastic tumor-like l.
nonperforative l.
nucleus ambiguus l.
nummular l.
occult talar l.
ocular adnexal l.
oil drop l.
onion scale l.
orbital l.
organic l.
Osgood-Schlatter l.
osseous l.
osteoblastic l.
osteochondral l.
osteolytic bone l.
osteopathic l.
osteosclerotic l.
ostial l.
papillary l.
papulopustular l.
papulosquamous l.
papulovesicular l.
paraorbital l.
parasagittal l.
patch l.
pathologic l.
perforative l.

periodontal l.
peripheral nerve l.
perisellar vascular l.
periventricular hyperintense l.
periventricular white matter l.
Perthes l.
photon-deficient bone l.
pigmented l.
pigment epithelial l.
plaquelike l.
plexiform l.
polypoid l.
postfracture l.
potentially resectable l.
precancerous l.
prechiasmal optic nerve l.
precipitating l.
precursor l.
preexisting l.
premalignant l.
preoperative l.
presacral cystic l.
primary l.
proliferative l.
pruritic l.
pseudocancerous l.
pseudomedial longitudinal
  fasciculus l.
pulpoperiapical l.
punched-out l.
purpuric l.
pustular l.
pyodermatous skin l.
radial sclerosing l.
radiodense l.
radiofrequency l.
radiofrequency-generated thermal l.
radiolucent l.
radiopaque l.
reactive lymphoid l.
recurrent nerve l.
regurgitant l.
residual l.
restenosis l.
reticular l.
retroacetabular l.
retrochiasmal l.
retrogeniculate l.
reverse Hill-Sachs l.
right-sided l.
rim-enhancing l.
ring l.

ring-wall l.
rolled shoulder l.
rotationally induced shear-strain l.
rotator cuff l.
ruptured peliotic l.
saddle l.
satellite l.
scaling skin-colored l.
scirrhous l.
sclerosing l.
sclerotic bone l.
secondary l.
semipedunculated l.
sessile l.
shagreen l.
short-segment l.
SIL/ASCUS l.
Sinding-Larsen-Johansson l.
sinonasal l.
sinusoidal l.
l. size
skeletal l.
skin-colored l.
skip l.
SLAP l.
slope-shouldered l.
smooth skin-colored l.
soft tissue l.
space-occupying brain l.
special l.
spiculated l.
spinal l.
splenic l.
spontaneous l.
squamous intraepithelial l. (SIL)
square-shouldered l.
stellate border breast l.
Stener l.
stenotic l.
stereotactic l.
stress l.
structural l.
subtentorial l.
supranuclear l.
suprasellar low-density l.
supratentorial l.
suspicious l.
synchronous l.
systemic l.
tandem l.
target l.
thoracic l.

L

NOTES

lesion *(continued)*
  trabeculated bone l.
  transient l.
  traumatic l.
  trophic l.
  truncal l.
  tuberculous l.
  tubulovillar l.
  type B-1, -2 l.
  typical skin l.
  uncommitted metaphysial l.
  undifferentiated l.
  unifocal optic nerve l.
  unilocular cystic l.
  unresectable l.
  uremic gastrointestinal l.
  varicelliform l.
  vasculitic l.
  vegetative l.
  venular l.
  verrucous l.
  vesicobullous l.
  violaceous l.
  visceral l.
  vulvar pigmented l.
  vulvovaginal l.
  Waldeyer ring l.
  weeping l.
  well-circumscribed l.
  white l.
  white-spot l.
  wire-loop l.
  Woofry-Chandler classification of
    Osgood-Schlatter l.
  wraparound periapical l.
  Wrisberg l.
  yellow l.
lesioning
  stereotactic radiofrequency l.
Leslie-Ryan anterior axillary approach
LESR
  lower esophageal sphincter relaxation
lesser
  l. cul-de-sac
  l. curvature
  l. horn
  l. omentectomy
  l. omentum
  l. palatine artery
  l. pancreas
  l. pelvis
  l. peritoneal cavity
  l. peritoneal sac
  l. resection
  l. ring
  l. sac approach
  l. sac hernia
  l. sac technique
  l. sciatic notch

  l. supraclavicular fossa
  L. triangle
  l. trochanter
  l. trochanter fracture
  l. vestibular gland
Lesshaft triangle
Lester
  L. Martin modification
  L. Martin modification of Duhamel
    operation
Lester-Jones operation
lethal
  l. concentration
  l. osteogenesis imperfecta
Letournel-Judet
  L.-J. acetabular fracture
    classification
  L.-J. approach
letterbox technique
leukemia
leukemic infiltration
leukochloroma
leukocyte infiltration
leukocytic
  l. infiltration
  l. margination
leukocytoclastic vasculitis
leukocytoma
leukodepletion
leukoencephalopathy
  radiation-induced l.
leukolymphosarcoma
leukolysis
leukoma
  adherent l.
leukosarcoma
leukostasis
  intracerebral l.
leukotomy
  prefrontal l.
  transorbital l.
Leung thumb loss classification
Levaditi method
levator
  l. ani syndrome
  l. aponeurosis repair
  l. hernia
  l. injury
  l. palpebrae
  l. resection
  l. scapulae syndrome
  l. span
  l. swelling
levatorplasty
level
  anterior midpapillary l.
  antithrombin III plasma l.
  arterial lactate l.
  attenuation l.

bilirubin l.
CEA l.
Clark l.
collagenase l.
endothelin plasma l.
l. foundation
heparin cofactor II plasma l.
iPTH l.
lactate l.
motilin l.
multiple shunt l.'s
overall sound l.
pain tolerance l.
parathyroid hormone l.
pentane excretion l.
plasma l.
plasminogen plasma l.
postinjury l.
pretreatment l.
protein C, S plasma l.
PTH l.
saturation sound pressure l.
sensation l.
serum lidocaine l. (SLL)
serum total bilirubin l.
sound pressure l.
total bilirubin l.
uterine lysosome l.
level-dependent
blood oxygenation l.-d.
leverage
Levine
L. dislocation operation
L. gradation 1–6
Levine-Harvey classification
levitation
levodopa dopaminergic medication
levodopa-induced dyskinesia
levo-transposed position
Levret maneuver
Levy, Rowntree, and Marriott method
Lewis
L. and Benedict method
L. intercalary resection
L. operation
L. thoracotomy
Lewis-Chekofsky resection
Lewissohn method
Lewis-Tanner
L.-T. procedure
L.-T. subtotal esophagectomy and
reconstruction

Lewit stretch technique
Lewy body
Lexer operation
LFC
left frontal craniotomy
LFT
liver function test
LG
lateral ground
LG bundle
Liang and Pardee method
liberation
Libman-Sacks lesion
Lich
L. extravesical technique
L. procedure
lichenification
lichenified lesion
lichenoid graft-versus-host disease
Lich-Gregoir
L.-G. anastomosis
L.-G. kidney transplant surgery
L.-G. repair
L.-G. technique
L.-G. ureterolysis
Lichtblau osteotomy
Lichtenstein
L. hernial repair
L. herniorrhaphy
L. mesh repair
L. operation
L. tension-free hernioplasty
Lichtman technique
LICU
laparoscopic intracorporeal
ultrasonography
lid
l. closure reaction
l. margin laceration
upper l.
lid-loading technique
lidocaine
nebulized l.
lid-splitting procedure
Lieberkühn
L. crypt
L. gland
Liebolt radioulnar technique
lienal artery
lienculus
lienectomy
lienis

NOTES

lienopancreatic
lienophrenic ligament
lienorenal ligament
lienunculus
Lieutaud
    L. body
    L. triangle
    L. trigone
    L. uvula
life
    l. expectancy
    no signs of l.
    perceived quality of l. (PQOL)
    quality of l. (QOL)
    l. space
    l. table method
life-saving form of therapy
life-sustaining hepatic reserve
life-threatening
    l.-t. cancer
    l.-t. complication
    l.-t. illness
lift-and-cut
    l.-a.-c. biopsy
    l.-a.-c. method
lifting
    abdominal wall l.
    sternal l.
ligament
    accessory plantar l.
    accessory volar l.
    acromioclavicular l.
    alar l.
    anococcygeal l.
    anterior costotransverse l.
    anterior cruciate l. (ACL)
    anterior sternoclavicular l.
    anterior tibiotalar l.
    Arantius l.
    arcuate pubic l.
    atlantooccipital l.
    auricular l.
    Berry l.
    broad uterine l.
    Camper l.
    capsular l.
    cardinal l.
    caroticoclinoid l.
    caudal l.
    ceratocricoid l.
    cervical l.
    cholecystoduodenal l.
    chondroxiphoid l.
    ciliary l.
    Civinini l.
    Clado l.
    Cloquet l.
    collateral l.
    Colles l.

Cooper l.
coracoacromial l.
coracoclavicular l.
coracohumeral l.
costoclavicular l.
costocolic l.
costotransverse l.
costoxiphoid l.
cotyloid l.
Cowper l.
cricoarytenoid l.
cricothyroid l.
cricotracheal l.
cruciform l.
cystoduodenal l.
Denonvilliers l.
denticulate l.
digital retinacular l.
duodenorenal l.
epihyal l.
external l.
falciform l.
fallopian l.
Ferrein l.
fibulocalcaneal l.
fundiform l.
gastrocolic l.
gastrodiaphragmatic l.
gastrohepatic l.
gastrolienal l.
gastrophrenic l.
gastrosplenic l.
genitoinguinal l.
Gimbernat l.
l. graft
Gruber l.
Hensing l.
hepatocolic l.
hepatoduodenal l.
hepatoesophageal l.
hepatogastric l.
hepatorenal l.
Hesselbach l.
Holl l.
Hueck l.
hyalocapsular l.
hyoepiglottic l.
iliolumbar l.
inferior glenohumeral l.
inferior pubic l.
inferior transverse scapular l.
infundibuloovarian l.
infundibulopelvic l.
inguinal l.
interchondral l.
interclavicular l.
interclinoid l.
interfoveolar l.
interosseous sacroiliac l.

interphalangeal collateral l.
interspinous l.
intertransverse l.
intervolar plate l.
intraarticular sternocostal l.
intracapsular l.
Jarjavay l.
Krause l.
lacunar l.
Lannelongue l.
lateral l.
Lauth l.
lienophrenic l.
lienorenal l.
Lockwood l.
longitudinal l.
lumbocostal l.
Luschka l.
Mackenrodt l.
mallear l.
Mauchart l.
Meckel l.
nuchal l.
palpebral l.
pancreaticosplenic l.
pectineal l.
peridental l.
periodontal l.
Petit l.
petroclinoid l.
petrosphenoid l.
phrenicocolic l.
phrenicolienal l.
phrenicosplenic l.
phrenoesophageal l.
phrenogastric l.
phrenosplenic l.
prostatic l.
pterygomandibular l.
pterygospinal l.
pterygospinous l.
pubic arcuate l.
puboprostatic l.
pulmonary l.
radiate sternocostal l.
radiocapitate l.
radiotriquetral l.
radioulnar l.
l. reconstruction
reflected inguinal l.
reflex l.
rhomboid l.

right prostatic l.
right triangular l.
round uterine l.
l. rupture
sacrococcygeal l.
sacrodural l.
sacroiliac l.
sacrospinous l.
sacrotuberous l.
serous l.
sphenomandibular l.
spiral l.
splenocolic l.
splenorenal l.
stellate l.
sternoclavicular l.
sternopericardial l.
stylohyoid l.
stylomandibular l.
stylomaxillary l.
suprascapular l.
supraspinous l.
suspensory l.
sutural l.
synovial l.
tarsal l.
temporomandibular l.
Teutleben l.
Thompson l.
thyroepiglottic l.
thyrohyoid l.
Treitz l.
triangular l.
urachal l.
uterosacral l.
uterovesical l.
venous l.
ventral sacrococcygeal l.
ventricular l.
vertebropelvic l.
vesicoumbilical l.
vesicouterine l.
vestibular l.
vocal l.
Whitnall l.
yellow l.
Zaglas l.
Zinn l.

ligamenta (*pl. of* ligamentum)
ligamental anesthesia
ligamentopexy
ligamentoplasty

L

NOTES

ligamentous support tissue
ligamentum, pl. **ligamenta**
ligand
> tissue l.

ligated
> circumferentially l.
> doubly l.
> staple l.
> suture l.

ligate-divide-staple technique
ligation
> aneurysm clip l.
> artery l.
> band l.
> Barron l.
> bidirectional l.
> bile duct l.
> Blalock-Taussig shunt l.
> bleeding site l.
> cecal l.
> common bile duct l.
> coronary vein l.
> direct l.
> distal l.
> elastic band l.
> endoscopic band l.
> endoscopic esophagogastric
>   variceal l.
> esophageal band l.
> l. of hemorrhoid
> l. hemorrhoidectomy
> high l.
> hunterian l.
> hypogastric artery l.
> inferior vena cava l.
> interdental l.
> Irving tubal l.
> IVC l.
> Kroner tubal l.
> laparoscopic artery l.
> laparoscopic varix l.
> modified Irving-type tubal l.
> open retroperitoneal high l.
> parotid duct l.
> pedicle l.
> pole l.
> Pomeroy tubal l.
> postureteral l.
> rubber-band l.
> sigmoid sinus l.
> sling l.
> spermatic vein l.
> stump l.
> subfascial l.
> surgical l.
> suture l.
> l. suture technique
> teeth l.
> tracheal l.

> transesophageal varix l.
> transgastric l.
> tubal l.
> variceal band l.
> varicose vein stripping and l.
> varix l.
> vessel l.

ligature
light
> l. coagulation
> L. criteria
> l. exposure
> l. guide bundle
> l. microscopy
> l. projection
> l. wire torque

light-around-wire technique
lighted stylet-guided oral intubation
light-reflecting wedge
LIH
> left inguinal hernia

Lilienthal incision
Liliequist
> membrane of L.

Lillie allochrome method
limb
> afferent l.
> alimentary l.
> biliopancreatic l.
> l. deformity
> distal l.
> efferent l.
> l. ischemia
> l. ischemia pain
> jejunal Roux-en-Y l.
> l. length angulation
> pelvic l.
> phantom l.
> proximal l.
> l. reduction
> l. reduction abnormality
> l. reduction anomaly
> l. replantation
> Roux l.
> Roux-en-Y l.
> l. salvage
> l. salvage index
> thoracic l.
> vertebral, anal, cardiac, tracheal,
>   esophageal, renal, l. (VACTERL)
> 4-l. Z-plasty

limbal
> l. approach
> l. compression
> l. incision
> l. parallel orientation

limbal-based flap
limb-body wall complex

Limberg
  L. flap
  L. technique
limbi (*pl. of* limbus)
limbic center
limb-lengthening procedure
limb-salvage
  l.-s. procedure
  l.-s. surgery
limb-saving
  l.-s. method
  l.-s. procedure
  l.-s. technique
limb-sparing
  l.-s. operation
  l.-s. procedure
  l.-s. surgery
limbus, pl. **limbi**
  conjunctival l.
  corneal l.
  l. mass
  Vieussens l.
limited
  l. anterior small thoracotomy
    (LAST)
  l. examination
  l. fasciectomy
  l. gastrectomy
  l. hemorrhoidectomy
  l. hepatectomy
  l. obturator node dissection
  l. pancreatectomy
  l. resection
  l. thoracotomy
limit of flocculation
limiting
  l. membrane
  l. plate erosion
Limoge current
LINAC
  linear accelerator
LINAC-based radiosurgery
Lincoff operation
Lindell classification
Lindeman procedure
Lindesmith operation
Linde Walker Oxygen Program
Lindholm
  L. technique
  L. tendo calcaneus repair

Lindner
  L. operation
  L. sclerotomy
Lindsay operation
Lindseth osteotomy
line
  accretion l.
  AC-PC l.
  action l.
  air-fluid l.
  alveolar point-nasal point l.
  alveolar point-nasion l.
  alveolobasilar l.
  alveolonasal l.
  Amberg lateral sinus l.
  aneuploid cell l.
  l. angle
  angular l.
  anocutaneous l.
  anorectal l.
  anterior axillary l.
  anterior commissure-posterior
    commissure l.
  antitension l.
  arcuate l.
  Arlt l.
  arterial mean l.
  atopic l.
  axillary l.
  azygoesophageal l.
  basal l.
  base l.
  basinasal l.
  B cell l.
  Beau l.
  l. of Bekhterev
  BeWo choriocarcinoma cell l.
  bimastoid l.
  bisector l.
  bismuth l.
  black l.
  Blaschko l.
  blue l.
  Blumensaat l.
  Bolton-nasion l.
  Brödel bloodless l.
  Burton l.
  calcification l.
  calciotraumatic l.
  Camper l.
  canthomeatal l.
  Cantlie l.

L

NOTES

line *(continued)*

CaSki cell l.
cell l.
cement l.
cemental l.
cementing l.
cervical l.
Chaussier l.
Clapton l.
cleavage l.
clivus canal l.
colonic mucosal l.
Conradi l.
contour l.
corneal iron l.
coronoid l.
Correra l.
costoclavicular l.
costophrenic septal l.
Crampton l.
craze l.
cross-arch fulcrum l.
curved radiolucent l.
CVP l.
cyma l.
D l.
Daubenton l.
delay l.
Dennie l.
Dennie-Morgan l.
dentate l.
developmental l.
digastric l.
l. of direction
Donders l.
Douglas l.
Ebner l.
Egger l.
Ehrlich-Türck l.
emission l.
epiphysial l.
equipotential l.
established cell l.
external oblique l.
face l.
Farre white l.
fat l.
fat-density l.
feather-edged proximal finishing l.
Feiss l.
femoral head l.
Ferry l.
fingerprint l.
Fishgold l.
l. of fixation
Fleischner l.
l. focus principle
foramen magnum l.
fracture l.

Fränkel white l.
Frankfort horizontal light l.
Fraunhofer l.
fulcrum l.
Futcher l.
gallbladder-vena cava l.
Garrett orientation l.
gas density l.
gaussian l.
l. of Gennari
George l.
germ l.
gingival finishing l.
gluteal l.
Granger l.
gravitational l.
gravity l.
gray l.
growth arrest l.
Gubler l.
gum l.
Hampton l.
Harris growth arrest l.
Hawkins l.
Head l.
Helmholtz l.
hemostatic staple l.
high lip l.
high smile l.
Hilgenreiner horizontal Y l.
Hilgenreiner-Perkins l.
Hilton white l.
His l.
Holdaway l.
Holden l.
hot l.
Hudson l.
Hudson-Stähli l.
Hueter l.
human AML cell l.
humeral l.
Hunter l.
Hunter-Schreger l.
iliopectineal l.
incision l.
l. infection
infracostal l.
innominate l.
intercondylar l.
intermediate l.
internal oblique l.
interspinal l.
intertrochanteric l.
intertubercular l.
iron l.
iron-Hudson-Stähli l.
iron-stocker l.
isodose l.
isoelectric l.

joint l.
Jurkat T-cell l.
l. of Kaes
Kaplan oblique l.
Kerley A, B, C l.'s
K562 erythroid l.
Khodadoust l.
Kilian l.
knife-edged finishing l.
Köhler l.
labial l.
lambda suture l.
Langer l.
Langhans l.
Lanz l.
lateral joint l.
lead l.
Linton l.
lip l.
load l.
long l.
lorentzian l.
lower midclavicular l.
low lip l.
lumbar gravitational l.
lymphoblastoid cell l.
M l.
Mach l.
MacNab l.
mamillary l.
mammary l.
mare's tail l.
McGregor basal l.
McKee l.
McRae foramen magnum l.
median l.
Mees l.
mercurial l.
Meyer l.
Meyerding spondylolisthesis
  classification l.
midaxillary l.
midclavicular l.
midheel l.
midhumeral l.
midmalleolar l.
midpoint to meatal l.
midscapular l.
midsternal l.
Moloney l.
Monro l.
Monro-Richter l.

Morgan l.
Morris hepatoma cell l.
mucogingival l.
mucosal l.
Muehrcke l.
murine mesangial cell l.
myelomonocytic cell l.
mylohyoid l.
nasion-alveolar point l.
nasobasilar l.
nasolabial l.
Nélaton l.
neonatal l.
neuronal cell l.
nipple l.
nuchal l.
Obersteiner-Redlich l.
obturator l.
odontoid perpendicular l.
Ohngren l.
orbital l.
orbitomeatal l.
Owen l.
oxygen supply l.
palatooccipital l.
pararectal l.
paraspinal l.
parasternal l.
paravertebral l.
Pastia l.
pectinate l.
pectineal l.
percutaneous l.
peripheral arterial l.
Perkins vertical l.
physial l.
Pickerill imbrication l.
pigmentary demarcation l.
pleural l.
pleuroesophageal l.
plumb l.
Poirier l.
Poupart l.
preaxillary l.
principal l.
properitoneal fat l.
protrusive l.
psoas l.
pubic hair l.
pubococcygeal l.
pupillary l.
radiocapitellar l.

L

NOTES

line *(continued)*
  radiolucent crescent l.
  radio signal l.
  recessional l.
  rectal floor l.
  Reid base l.
  rejection l.
  resonance l.
  resting l.
  retentive fulcrum l.
  l. of Retzius
  reversal l.
  Rex-Cantli-Serege l.
  Richter-Monro l.
  right midinguinal l.
  rolandic l.
  Roser-Nélaton l.
  sacral arcuate l.
  sacral horizontal plane l.
  sagittal suture l.
  Salter incremental l.
  Sampoelesi l.
  scapular l.
  Schreger l.
  Schwalbe l.
  sclerotic l.
  scurvy l.
  semicircular l.
  semilunar l.
  septal l.
  Sergent white l.
  Shenton l.
  simian l.
  sinus l.
  Snellen l.
  soleal l.
  spectral l.
  Spieghel l.
  Spigelius l.
  spinolamellar l.
  spinolaminar l.
  spinous interlaminar l.
  spiral l.
  stabilizing fulcrum l.
  Stähli pigment l.
  sternal l.
  Stocker l.
  stromal l.
  subclavian l.
  subcostal l.
  supracondylar l.
  supracrestal l.
  survey l.
  suture l.
  Sydney l.
  sylvian l.
  T-cell l.
  teardrop l.
  temporal l.

  tender l.
  terminal l.
  l. test
  Thompson l.
  tibiofibular l.
  l. of Toldt
  tram l.
  trapezoid l.
  triradiate l.
  trough l.
  Turk l.
  Twining l.
  Tycos pressure infusion l.
  Ullmann l.
  V l.
  venous l.
  Vesling l.
  vibrating l.
  visual l.
  Voigt l.
  Von Ebner l.
  Wackenheim clivus canal l.
  water density l.
  Wegner l.
  white l.
  l. width
  Winberger l.
  Z l.
  Zahn l.
  zero l.
  Zöllner l.
  Z-shaped suture l.

linear
  l. accelerator (LINAC)
  l. accelerator-based radiosurgery
  l. calcification
  l. craniectomy
  l. incision
  l. osteotomy
  l. salpingostomy
  l. skull fracture
  l. thermal expansion
  l. ulceration

linearly polarized near-infrared irradiation

lined flap

Linell-Ljungberg classification

lingual
  l. approach
  l. artery
  l. bone
  l. branch
  l. cavity
  l. frenulum
  l. gland
  l. inclination
  l. mucosa
  l. nerve
  l. plexus

l. split-bone technique
l. tongue flap
l. tonsil hyperplasia (LTH)
l. vein
lingualplasty
lingula, pl. **lingulae**
lingular branch
linguofacial trunk
linguoincisal line angle
linguoocclusal line angle
lining
cavity l.
linnaean system of nomenclature
Linton
L. flap
L. incision
L. line
L. operation
L. procedure
LIOUS
laparoscopic intraoperative
ultrasonography
lip
acetabular l.
l. adhesion operation
anterior l.
cleft l.
l. line
l. switch flap
upper l.
lipectomy
abdominal l.
lipid
l. infusion
l. peroxidation
l. peroxidation product
lipiodol transarterial embolization treatment
lipoatrophy
postinfection l.
lipoblastoma
lipocele
lipocytic lesion
lipofibroadenoma
lipofibroma
lipogranuloma
lipoid theory of narcosis
lipoleiomyoma
lipolysis
heparin-induced l.
intravascular l.
lipoma

lipomalike tissue
lipomatous
l. infiltration
l. tissue
lipomeningocele
lipomyelocele
lipomyelocystocele
lipomyelomeningocele
lipomyxoma
liponecrosis
lipophilic opioid
lipoprotein
liposarcoma
high-grade primary extremity l.
liposomal preparation
liposome-encapsulated tetracaine
liposuction
submental l.
ultrasonic-assisted l. (UAL)
liposuctioning
Lipscomb
L. procedure
L. technique
Lipscomb-Anderson procedure
lip-splitting incision
liquefaction necrosis
liquid
l. extraction
l. scintillation spectrometer
liquor
Scarpa l.
Lisfranc
L. amputation
L. articulation
L. disarticulation
L. dislocation
L. fracture
L. fracture-dislocation
L. tubercle
Lison-Dunn method
Lissauer
L. bundle
L. tract
lissencephaly syndrome
lissosphincter
Lister
L. method
L. technique
L. tubercle
listerism
listhesis
Listing plane

L

NOTES

lithagogue
lithectomy
lithiasis
    biliary l.
    pancreatic l.
lithium
lithocystotomy
litholapaxy
    Bigelow l.
litholysis
    chemical l.
litholyte
litholytic
lithotomist
lithotomy
    bilateral l.
    dorsal l.
    high l.
    lateral l.
    marian l.
    median l.
    percutaneous cholangioscopic l.
    percutaneous transhepatic
      cholangioscopic l. (PTCSL)
    perineal l.
    l. position
    prerectal l.
    suprapubic l.
    vaginal l.
    vesical l.
lithotresis
    ultrasonic l.
lithotripsy
    biliary l.
    blind l.
    candela l.
    cystoscopic electrohydraulic l.
    electrohydraulic l. (EHL)
    electrohydraulic shockwave l.
      (ESWL)
    endoscopic-controlled l.
    endoscopic electrohydraulic l.
    endoscopic pulsed dye laser l.
    external shockwave l.
    extracorporeal piezoelectric
      shockwave l.
    extracorporeal shock wave l.
    intracorporeal laser l.
    intracorporeal shockwave l.
    laparoscopic transcystic l. (LTCL)
    laser biliary l.
    laser-induced intracorporeal
      shockwave l.
    mechanical l.
    piezoelectric l.
    pressure regulated
      electrohydraulic l.
    l. retreatment
    rotational contact l.

    shock wave l. (SWL)
    tunable dye laser l.
    ultrasonic l.
lithotripsy-induced hypertension
lithotriptic
lithotriptoscopy
lithotrity
lithuresis
litigation reaction
little
    L. area
    l. finger sign
Littler-Cooley technique
Littler technique
Littré
    L. gland
    L. hernia
Littré-Richter hernia
Litwak aortic bypass
Livaditis circular myotomy
live
    l. donor liver transplantation
      without blood products
    l. donor nephrectomy
liver
    l. abscess
    alcoholic l.
    l. allograft
    l. allotransplantation
    l. bed
    l. biopsy
    l. capsule
    cirrhotic l.
    l. cyst
    l. cyst infection
    l. damage
    l. disease
    l. distention
    echogenic l.
    l. failure
    l. flap
    floating l.
    frosted l.
    l. function
    l. function test (LFT)
    l. hanging maneuver
    hobnail l.
    icing l.
    l. injury
    l. laceration
    lardaceous l.
    l. lobe
    l. lobule
    l. mass
    l. metastasis
    native l.
    nutmeg l.
    obstructed l.
    l. operation

l. parenchyma
polycystic l.
l. regeneration
l. resection
split l.
stasis l.
steatotic l.
sugar-icing l.
l. tissue
l. tract
l. transplant
l. transplantation
triangular ligament of l.
l. tumor
l. volume
wandering l.
waxy l.
l. wire TC ablation

living
l. donor nephrectomy
l. donor partial hepatectomy
l. donor renal transplantation
l. relative donor
l. will

living-related
l.-r. donor (LRD)
l.-r. donor transplantation
l.-r. liver transplantation (LRLT)
l.-r. small bowel transplant

Livingstone therapy
Livingston peribulbar wedge
LLC
laparoscopic laser cholecystectomy
laser laparoscopic cholecystectomy

LLE
left lower extremity

Lloyd Davis modified lithotomy position
Lloyd-Roberts-Catteral-Salamon classification
Lloyd-Roberts fracture technique
LLQ
left lower quadrant

LMA
laryngeal mask airway

LMVD
lymphatic microvessel density

LNF
laparoscopic Nissen fundoplication

load
fecal l.
l. line

load-bearing graft

load-deflection
l.-d. curve
l.-d. rate

load-deformation curve
load-displacement
l.-d. curve
l.-d. plot

loading
fecal l.
l. fracture

lobar
l. bronchus
l. collapse
l. hemorrhage
l. nephronia
l. resection

lobate
lobatum
hepar l.

lobe
caudate l.
inferior parietal l.
liver l.
native caudate l.
paracentral l.
renal l.
l. resection
Riedel l.
right caudate l.
Spiegel l.
spigelian l.
Spigelius l.
superior parietal l.
thyroid l.

lobectomy
Falconer l.
hepatic l.
ipsilateral thyroid l.
pulmonary l.
sleeve l.
temporal l.
thyroid l.
total l.
unilateral l.

lobi (*pl. of* lobus)
lobose
lobotomy
frontal l.
prefrontal l.
radical prefrontal l.
transorbital l.

Lobstein ganglion

NOTES

L

lobster-claw deformity
lobular
    l. acinus
    l. carcinoma
    l. hyperplasia
lobulate
lobulated
    l. contour
    l. mass
lobule
    l. of epididymis
    hepatic l.
    liver l.
    posterior l.
    posterior-lateral l.
    renal cortical l.
    secondary pulmonary l.
lobulet
lobulus, pl. **lobuli**
lobus, pl. **lobi**
local
    l. abscess
    l. acidosis
    l. anesthesia
    l. anesthetic
    l. anesthetic reaction
    l. anesthetic sympathetic blockade
    l. bloodletting
    l. epineurotomy
    l. excision
    l. excitatory state
    l. exhaust ventilation
    l. hepatectomy
    l. hypoxia
    l. infection
    l. ingrowth
    l. injection
    l. invasion
    l. irradiation
    l. leakage
    l. lymphatic uptake
    l. muscle flap
    l. radical resection
    l. recurrence
    l. skin flap
    l. standby anesthesia technique
    l. surgery
    l. therapy
    l. tissue infiltration
    l. treatment
    l. tumor extension
    l. twitch response (LTR)
localization
    anatomic l.
    bleeding site l.
    l. of disease
    estrogen receptor l.
    eye tumor l.
    focus l.

    gamma probe l.
    hooked wire l.
    invasive l.
    isotope l.
    methylene blue dye l.
    needle l.
    pancreatic tumor l.
    pedicle l.
    percutaneous l.
    placental l.
    preoperative l.
    radioisotope l.
    sentinel node l.
    l. signal
    SLN l.
    stereotactic l.
    stereotaxic l.
    l. study
    l. technique
    l. test
    wire l.
localized
    l. abdominal sign
    l. abscess
    l. inflammation
    l. lesion
    l. leukocyte mobilization
    l. plaque formation
    l. prostate cancer
locally advanced disease
locating canal
location
    extraperitoneal l.
    nonaxillary l.
    tumor l.
lock
    Howland l.
locking suture technique
lock-stitch suture technique
Lockwood ligament
locoregional
    l. management
    l. recurrence
    l. recurrence-free survival (LRRFS)
    l. relapse
    l. treatment
loculation
    l. of fluid
    l. syndrome
Loeffler-Ballard incision
Loesche classification
Loewenthal
    L. bundle
    L. tract
Löffler suture technique
logadectomy
logical
    l. method
    l. operation

log relative exposure
logrolling maneuver
LOHF
late-onset hepatic failure
Löhlein-Baehr lesion
Löhlein operation
loin pain hematuria syndrome
lollipop mastopexy
Londermann operation
lone atrial fibrillation
long
l. axis
l. bone
l. bone fracture
l. cone technique
l. lesion
l. line
l. QT syndrome
l. thoracic artery
l. thoracic vein
l. tract sign
longer-segment obstruction
longissimus muscle
longitudinal
l. aberration
l. canal
2-chamber l. (2C-L)
l. choledochotomy
l. dissociation
l. enterotomy
l. fold
l. fracture
l. incision
l. laceration
l. ligament
l. ligament rupture
l. method
l. myotomy
l. nephrotomy of Boyce
l. oval pelvis
l. pancreaticojejunostomy
l. relaxation
l. scanning
l. section
l. side-to-side anastomosis
l. vertebral venous sinus
long-limb gastric artery bypass
Longmire
L. operation
L. valvotomy
Longmire-Gutgeman gastric
reconstruction

Longo hemorrhoidectomy
long-segment spinal fusion
long- and short-lever rotational
manipulation
long-term
l.-t. bone-instrumentation interface
l.-t. central venous access catheter
placement
l.-t. epidural catheterization
l.-t. followup
l.-t. morbidity
l.-t. outcome
l.-t. oxygen therapy
l.-t. paralysis
l.-t. survival
longus
l. capitis muscle
l. colli muscle
extensor carpi radialis l. (ECRL)
extensor digitorum l.
extensor hallucis l. (EHL)
extensor pollicis l.
loop
air-filled l.
Biebl l.
bowel l.
central chemoreflex l.
cerebral-sacral l.
cervical l.
l. choledochojejunostomy
colonic l.
contiguous l.
l. diathermy cervical conization
distended afferent l.
l. distribution
duodenal l.
efferent l.
l. electrocautery excision procedure
(LEEP)
l. electrosurgical excision procedure
(LEEP)
l. electrosurgical excision procedure
conization
l. esophagojejunostomy
expressor l.
l. fixation
l. forearm graft
foreign body l.
l. gastric bypass
l. gastric bypass method
l. gastric bypass procedure
l. gastric bypass technique

NOTES

L

431

loop *(continued)*
    l. gastrojejunostomy
    Henle l.
    Hyrtl l.
    ileal l.
    l. ileostomy
    l. ileostomy construction
    intestinal l.
    jejunal interposition of Henle l.
    jejunal Roux-en-Y l.
    l. jejunostomy
    jejunum l.
    2-l. J-shaped ileal pouch
    lenticular l.
    nephronic l.
    N-shaped sigmoid l.
    open l.
    ostomy l.
    l. ostomy bridge
    peduncular l.
    peripheral chemoreflex l.
    puborectalis l.
    Roux-en-Y l.
    l. stoma
    subclavian l.
    l. transverse colostomy
    vascular l.
    venous l.
3-loop
    3-l. ileal pouch
    3-l. technique
looped cautery
loop-end ileostomy
loop-on mucosa suture technique
loose
    l. fracture
    l. fragment
    l. intraarticular body
loosening
    screw l.
Loosett maneuver
lop-ear
Lopez-Enriquez operation
LOR
    loss of resistance
Lord
    L. dilation
    L. dilation of hemorrhoid
    L. hemorrhoidectomy
    L. operation
lordosis
    l. creation
    l. preservation
lorentzian line
Lorenz procedure
Loreta operation
lorry driver fracture
Lortat-Jacob approach

LOS
    length of stay
Losee
    L. modification
    L. modification of MacIntosh
        technique
    L. sling and reef technique
loss
    anticipated blood l.
    articular bone l.
    blood l.
    bone l.
    cutaneous heat l.
    dermal l.
    discrimination l.
    excessive blood l.
    excessive weight l.
    extreme hearing l.
    insertion l.
    intraoperative blood l.
    memory l.
    operative blood l.
    percutaneous anesthetic l.
    l. of resistance (LOR)
    surgical weight l.
    third space l.
    tissue l.
loss-of-resistance technique
loss-of-waist sign
lost wax pattern technique
Lotheissen
    L. hernia repair
    L. operation
Lothrop frontoethmoidectomy procedure
lotus position
Lougheed-White coccygectomy
Louis
    L. angle
    L. mastopexy
loupe magnification
Lovset maneuver
low
    l. anterior resection (LAR)
    l. central venous pressure
        anesthesia
    l. cervical approach
    l. cervical cesarean section
    l. dose rate (LDR)
    l. intermittent suction
    l. lip line
    l. lumbar spine fracture
    l. rectal cancer
    l. spinal anesthesia
    l. thoracic level epidural anesthesia
    l. transverse cesarean section
    l. transverse incision
low-attenuation
    l.-a. lesion
    l.-a. mass

low-collar incision
low-current
    l.-c. electrocautery
    l.-c. monopolar coagulation
low-density mass
low-dose
    l.-d. anesthetic
    l.-d. irradiation
    l.-d. radioiodine
LowDye
    L. strapping
    L. taping technique
Lowell reduction
Löwenberg canal
low-energy fracture
Löwenstein operation
lower
    l. body negative pressure
    l. cervical spine fusion
    l. cervical spine posterior
      stabilization
    l. cervical spine procedure
    l. esophageal sphincter (LES)
    l. esophageal sphincter pressure
    l. esophageal sphincter relaxation
      (LESR)
    l. extremity
    l. extremity bypass
    l. extremity edema
    l. extremity fracture
    l. extremity nerve block
    l. extremity noninvasive
    l. extremity occlusive disease
    l. extremity reconstruction
    l. extremity revascularization
    l. extremity surgery
    l. gastrointestinal hemorrhage
    l. gastrointestinal tract foreign body
    l. genital tract infection
    l. incisor angulation
    l. jaw bone
    l. lateral quadrant
    l. lid sling procedure
    l. limb ischemia
    l. medial quadrant
    l. midclavicular line
    l. motor neuron lesion
    l. nephron syndrome
    l. panendoscopy
    l. plexus compression
    l. pole laceration

    l. quadrant abdominal incisional
      hernia
    l. respiratory tract infection
    l. thyroid artery
    l. trapezius flap
    l. uterine segment (LUS)
    l. uterine segment incision
    l. uterine segment transverse
      (LUST)
    l. uterine segment transverse
      cesarean section
    l. uterine segment transverse C-
      section
Lowery method
lowest
    l. lumbar artery
    l. thyroid artery
low-field contrast-enhanced body MRA
low-flow
    l.-f. anesthetic technique
    l.-f. circuit
low-flux
    l.-f. cellulose-based membrane
    l.-f. cuprophane membrane
    l.-f. dialysis membrane
low-frequency jet ventilation
low-grade
    l.-g. dysplasia
    l.-g. glioma
    l.-g. MALT lymphoma
    l.-g. squamous intraepithelial lesion
    l.-g. suction unit
low-loop cutaneous ureterostomy
Lown
    L. classification
    L. technique
    L. and Woolf method
low-pressure tamponade
low-resistance fundoplication
low-risk papillary cancer
Lowry method
low-segment transverse incision
Lowsley
    L. lobar anatomy
    L. ribbon gut method
low-speed rotational angioplasty
LPHR
    laparoscopic paraesophageal hernia repair
LRD
    living-related donor
LRLT
    living-related liver transplantation

L

NOTES

LRPH
laparoscopic repair of paraesophageal
hernia
LRRFS
locoregional recurrence-free survival
LSG
lymphoscintigraphy
preoperative LSG
L-shaped capsular incision
LSV
left subclavian vein
LTA
laryngotracheal anesthesia
LTCBDE
laparoscopic transcystic common bile
duct exploration
LTCL
laparoscopic transcystic lithotripsy
LTH
lingual tonsil hyperplasia
LTO
laparoscopic total occlusion
LTP
laryngotracheoplasty
LTR
local twitch response
lubrication
skin l.
Lucas groove
lucent lung lesion
lückenschädel
Ludloff
L. bunionectomy
L. incision
L. medial approach
L. osteotomy
L. technique
Ludwig
L. angle
L. ganglion
L. labyrinth
L. plane
LUE
left upper extremity
Luke procedure
Lukes and Butler Hodgkin disease
classification
Lukes-Collins classification
lumbar
l. accessory movement technique
l. anesthetic technique
l. approach
l. artery
l. branch
l. canal
l. cistern
l. discectomy
l. disc herniation
l. epidural abscess

l. epidural anesthesia
l. epidural endoscopy
l. epidural steroid
l. extension
l. extension test
l. facet injection
l. flexure
l. ganglion
l. gravitational line
l. hemilaminectomy
l. hernia
l. interbody fusion
l. lordosis preservation
l. nephrectomy
l. nerve
l. nerve root injection
l. pedicle fixation
l. plexus
l. plexus block
l. port
l. puncture
l. region
l. rib
l. rotation
l. rotation test
l. segment
l. spinal cord lesion
l. spinal fusion
l. spine biopsy
l. spine burst fracture
l. spine fusion
l. spine kyphotic deformity
l. spine lesion
l. spine segmental fixation
l. spine stabilization
l. spine transpedicular fixation
l. spine vertebral osteosynthesis
l. spondylodiscitis
l. sympathectomy
l. sympathetic block
l. triangle
l. triangle of Petit
l. trunk
l. tumor
l. vein
l. vertebra
l. vertebral interbody fusion
l. vessel
lumbarization
lumbar-peritoneal shunting
lumbi (*pl. of* lumbus)
lumboabdominal
lumbocolostomy
lumbocolotomy
lumbocostal ligament
lumbocostoabdominal triangle
lumbodorsal fascia
lumboinguinal nerve
lumbo-ovarian

lumbosacral
- l. angle
- l. canal
- l. dislocation
- l. fusion
- l. joint
- l. junction fracture
- l. plexus
- l. plexus lesion
- l. root lesion
- l. trunk

lumbrical muscle flap

lumbus, pl. **lumbi**

lumen, pl. **lumina**
- bile duct l.
- gut l.
- irregularly widened l.
- jejunal l.

luminal
- l. content
- l. factor
- l. mass
- l. side

lumpectomy
- endoscopic aspiration l.
- l. mastectomy

lunate
- l. bone
- l. dislocation

lung
- l. biopsy
- breathing l.
- l. cancer
- l. carcinoma
- l. cavity
- l. disease
- essential brown induration of l.
- fixed l.
- human l.
- inflated l.
- l. isolation
- Kolobow membrane l.
- membrane artificial l.
- nonventilated l.
- oblique fissure of l.
- pump l.
- l. rejection
- respirator l.
- shock l.
- l. transplant
- l. transplantation
- trapped l.

- l. tumor
- 2-l. ventilation
- 1-l. ventilation anesthetic technique
- l. volume reduction (LVR)
- l. volume reduction surgery
- l. water
- wet l.

1-lung
- 1-l. anesthesia
- 1-l. ventilation (OLV)

lung-imaging fluorescent endoscopy

lung-to-head
- l.-t.-h. circumference
- l.-t.-h. circumference ratio

lunotriquetral
- l. dissociation
- l. fusion

lunula, pl. **lunulae**
- azure l.

lupus
- l. anticoagulant
- l. erythematosus preparation
- systemic l.

lupus-associated valve disease

LUQ
- left upper quadrant

Luque
- L. instrumentation concave technique
- L. instrumentation convex technique
- L. loop fixation
- L. rod fixation
- L. sublaminar wiring technique

Luque-Galveston fixation

Luria-Delbruck fluctuation test

LUS
- laparoscopic ultrasonography
- lower uterine segment
- LUS examination
- LUS scanning technique

Luschka
- L. cartilage
- duct of L.
- L. gland
- L. joint
- L. ligament
- L. and Magendie foramen
- L. sinus

lusitropism

LUST
- lower uterine segment transverse
- LUST C-section

NOTES

435

luster
 corneal l.
lustrous central yellow point
luteal
luteinization
luteinized thecoma
luteinoma
luteolysis
luteoma
 pregnancy l.
luteus
luxatio erecta shoulder dislocation
luxation
 habitual temporomandibular joint l.
 rotatory l.
 temporomandibular l.
Luys
 L. body
 L. body syndrome
LVEDa
 left ventricular end-diastolic area
LVESa
 left ventricular end-systolic area
LVI
 left ventricular insufficiency
 left ventricular ischemia
 lymph vessel invasion
LVOT
 left ventricular outflow tract
LVPVR
 left ventricular pressure-volume
  relationship
LVR
 lung volume reduction
 LVR procedure
Lyden-Lehman technique
Lyden technique
Lyme arthritis
lymph
 l. gland
 l. nodal station
 l. node basin
 l. node biopsy
 l. node dissection
 l. node involvement
 l. node metastasis
 l. node sampling
 l. node stage
 l. node status
 l. space
 tissue l.
 l. vessel
 l. vessel invasion (LVI)
lymphadenectomy
 axillary l.
 bilateral l.
 D2 l.
 elective l.
 endocavitary pelvic l. (ECPL)

 extended pelvic l.
 3-field l.
 inguinal l.
 Japanese-style l.
 laparoscopic pelvic l.
 mediastinal l.
 Meigs pelvic l.
 paraaortic l.
 pelvic l.
 prophylactic l.
 regional l.
 retroperitoneal l.
 selective l.
 sentinel l.
 thoracoabdominal retroperitoneal l.
lymphadenocele
lymphadenoma
lymphadenopathy
 axillary l.
 en bloc l.
 portal l.
lymphadenotomy
lymphangiectasis
lymphangiectomy
lymphangioendothelioma
lymphangiogenesis
lymphangiohemangioma
lymphangioleiomyomatosis
 pulmonary l.
lymphangioma
lymphangiomyomatosis
 end-stage l.
 pulmonary l.
lymphangioplasty
 Handley l.
lymphangiosarcoma
lymphangiotomy
Lymphapress compression therapy
lymphatic
 l. canal
 l. chain
 dermal l.'s
 l. dissection
 l. drainage
 l. drainage pattern
 l. duct
 l. edema
 l. invasion
 l. malformation
 l. mapping
 l. metastasis
 l. microvessel density (LMVD)
 parenchymal l.
 l. pathway
 l. permeation
 l. plexus
 l. spread
 l. tissue
 l. uptake

l. valvule
l. vessel
lymphaticostomy
lymphaticovenous
l. anastomosis
l. bypass
lymphatolysis
lymphedema
lymphoadenoma
lymphoblastoid cell line
lymphocelectomy
laparoscopic l.
pelvic l.
lymphocele drainage
lymphocyte
B, T phenotypic l.
cytotoxic T l.
l. cell
l. migration
phenotypic l.
lymphocytic infiltration
lymphocytoma
lymphodepletion
lymphoepithelial lesion
lymphoepithelioma
lymphogenous metastasis
lymphogranuloma
lymphoid
l. infiltration
l. ring
l. tissue
lymphoidectomy
lymphoma
Ann Arbor Hodgkin l. (stage I,
IE, II, IIE, IIIE, IIIS, IIISE, IV)
gastric MALT l.
gastric non-Hodgkin l.
high-grade MALT l.
low-grade MALT l.
MALT l.
mucosa-associated lymphoid
tissue l.
node l.
primary gastric l. (PGL)
primary gastric non-Hodgkin l.
(PGL)
l. relapse
l. system
lymphomatosa
struma l.

lymphomyeloma
lymphoplasty
lymphoproliferation
lymphoproliferative
l. disorder
l. lesion
lymphosarcoma
lymphoscintigraphy (LSG)
internal mammary l. (IML)
isotopic l.
preoperative l.
lymphovascular invasion
Lynch
L. frontoethmoidectomy procedure
L. incision
L. operation
L. syndrome
Lynn technique
Lyon-Horgan procedure
lyophilization of bone
lyophilized
l. bone graft
l. dural patch
l. extract
lysate
melanoma cell l.
lyse
Lysholm
L. Knee Scale
L. score
lysis
adhesion l.
l. of adhesions
direct muscle l.
endothelial l.
muscle l.
lysogenic
l. induction
l. strain
lysosomal
l. enzyme disorder
l. membrane
l. storage disease
l. swelling
lytic
l. blockade
l. bone lesion
l. cocktail

NOTES

L

MAb
monoclonal antibody
MABP
mean arterial blood pressure
MAC
minimal anesthetic concentration
minimum alveolar anesthetic
concentration
minimum alveolar concentration
monitored anesthesia care
MAC anesthesia
MAC infection
MAC ratio
1-MAC
1-minimum alveolar concentration
1-MAC halothane
MacAndrew Alcoholism Scale
MacAusland procedure
MacCallan classification
MacCarthy procedure
maceration
Macewen
M. classification
M. hernia operation
M. herniorrhaphy
M. triangle
Macewen-Shands osteotomy
MacFee incision
Machek-Blaskovics operation
Machek-Brunswick operation
Machek-Gifford operation
Machek ptosis operation
Mach line
MacIntosh
M. extraarticular tenodesis
M. over-the-top ACL reconstruction
M. over-the-top repair
M. technique
MACIS
metastasis, age, completeness of
resection, local invasion, tumor size
MACIS criteria
MACIS score
Mack-Brunswick operation
Mackenrodt
M. incision
M. ligament
Mackenzie point
MacNab
M. line
M. line for facet imbrication
M. operation
M. shoulder repair
MacNichol-Voutsinas classification
macroadenoma

macrocalcification
macrocirculation
macrocolon
macrocyst
multiple m.
macroelectrode
m. recording
m. recording technique
macrofollicular lesion
macroglossia
macro-Kjeldahl method
macronodular
macroorchidism
macropenis
macroperforation
macrophage
peritoneal m.
macrophagic migration
macrophallus
macroprolactinoma
macroprosopia
macroscopic
m. appearance
m. evidence
m. involvement
m. IPM
m. lesion
m. portal
m. sphincter
m. tumor removal
m. type
macrosigmoid
macrotraumatic insult
macrovascular coronary lesion
macula, pl. **maculae**
retinal m.
macular
m. ectopia
m. photocoagulation
macule
hypomelanotic m.
maculopapillary bundle
maculopathy
Madden
M. incisional herniorrhaphy
M. repair
M. repair of incisional hernia
M. technique
Maddox
M. rod test
M. wing test
Madelung deformity
Madigan prostatectomy
Madlener operation
maduromycetoma

M

Maffucci syndrome
Magendie space
Magenstrasse
    M. and Mill (M&M)
    M. and Mill procedure
Magerl
    M. posterior cervical screw fixation
    M. translaminar facet screw
      fixation technique
maggot
    surgical m.
Magilligan measuring technique
Magitot keratoplasty operation
magna, pl. **magnae**
magnet
    m. operation
    m. therapy
magnetic
    m. control suturing (MCS)
    m. extraction
    m. imaging guidance
    m. induction
    m. operation
    m. radiation exposure
    m. resonance (MR)
    m. resonance angiography (MRA)
    m. resonance
      cholangiopancreatography (MRCP)
    m. resonance imaging (MRI)
    m. resonance imaging
      cholangiography
    m. resonance imaging scan
    m. resonance spectroscopy
    m. source imaging (MSI)
    m. stimulation
magnetization precession angle
magnetoelectric stimulation
magnification
    electronic m.
    loupe m.
    relative spectacle m.
    spot m.
magnitude preparation-rapid acquisition
  gradient echo (MP-RAGE)
magnum
    foramen m.
magnus
Magnuson-Stack
    M.-S. operation
    M.-S. procedure
    M.-S. shoulder arthrotomy
Magnuson technique
MAGPI
    meatal advancement and glansplasty
    meatal advancement, glansplasty,
      penoscrotal junction meatotomy
    MAGPI hypospadias repair
    MAGPI operation

Ma-Griffith
    M.-G. technique
    M.-G. tendo calcaneus repair
Mahaim bundle
Mahan procedure
MAI
    Mycobacterium avium-intracellulare
    MAI infection
Maier sinus
maim
main
    m. bundle
    m. pancreatic duct (MPD)
mainstem intubation
maintainer cast space
maintenance
    m. dialysis
    m. fluid
    insufficient airway m.
Mainz
    M. pouch augmentation
    M. pouch cutaneous urinary
      diversion
    M. pouch operation
Maisonneuve fibular fracture
Maissiat band
Maitland technique
Majestro-Ruda-Frost tendon technique
Majewsky operation
major
    m. abdominal surgery
    m. amputation
    m. artery
    m. calix
    m. duodenal papilla
    m. fissure
    m. histocompatibility complex
      (MHC)
    m. liver resection (MLR)
    m. manifestation
    m. myocutaneous flap
    m. nonvascular abdominal surgery
    m. operation
    m. sinistral branch
    trochanter m.
    m. vascular injury
    m. vascular structure
majus
    labium m.
Makler insemination
malabsorptive procedure
Malacarne space
malacotomy
Maladie de Graeffe operation
malar
    m. fat pad
    m. fold
    m. foramen

m. fracture
m. node
Malawer excision technique
Malbec operation
Malbran operation
maldistribution
male
m. breast
m. castration
m. gonad
m. urethra
malformation
angiographically occult intracranial
vascular m. (AOIVM)
anorectal m.
Arnold-Chiari m.
arteriovenous m. (AVM)
atrioventricular m.
A-V m.
Bing-Siebenmann m.
bronchopulmonary foregut m.
capillary m.
cardiac valvular m.
cardiovascular m.
cavernous m.
central nervous system m.
cerebral arteriovenous m.
cerebral vascular m.
cerebrovascular m.
Chiari I–III m.
cloacal m.
clomiphene fetal m.
congenital brain m.
congenital cystic adenomatoid m.
(CCAM)
congenital heart m.
congenital vascular m.
craniofacial m.
cutaneous m.
cystic adenomatoid m. (CAM)
Dandy-Walker m.
DeMyer system of cerebral m.
Dieulafoy vascular m.
dural arteriovenous m.
dysraphic m.
Ebstein m.
extremity m.
faciotelencephalic m.
fetal cystic adenomatoid m.
flocculonodular arteriovenous m.
foregut m.
frontal arteriovenous m.

frontoparietal arteriovenous m.
galenic venous m.
gastric arteriovenous m.
glomus arteriovenous m.
infratentorial arteriovenous m.
intracerebral arteriovenous m.
intracerebral vascular m.
intracranial arteriovenous m.
intracranial vascular m.
intramedullary arteriovenous m.
intramuscular venous m.
lymphatic m.
mermaid m.
Michel m.
mixed venous-lymphatic m.
Mondini-Alexander m.
Mondini pulmonary
arteriovenous m.
neural axis vascular m.
neural crest m.
occipital m.
occult cerebrovascular m.
occult vascular m.
orbital arteriovenous m.
pulmonary arterial m.
pulmonary arteriovenous m.
radiculomeningeal spinal
vascular m.
retinal arteriovenous m.
Scheibe m.
sink-trap m.
spinal vascular m.
split-cord m.
supratentorial arteriovenous m.
telencephalic m.
teratogen-induced m.
thalamocaudate arteriovenous m.
Uhl m.
vascular m.
vein of Galen m.
venous m.
malfunction
cuff m.
pacemaker m.
Malgaigne
M. fossa
M. hernia
M. pelvic fracture
M. triangle
malignancy
abdominal m.
digestive tract m.

M

NOTES

malignancy *(continued)*
    gastric m.
    gastrointestinal m.
    gynecologic m.
    hepatic m.
    hereditary m.
    metastatic m.
    nonhereditary m.
    pancreatic m.
    primary m.
malignant
    m. adenoma
    m. angiomyolipoma
    m. carcinoid syndrome
    m. cell
    m. degeneration
    m. etiology
    m. external otitis syndrome
    m. fasciculation
    m. glioma
    m. hyperpyrexia
    m. hypertension (MH)
    m. hyperthermia (MH)
    m. pancreatic disease
    m. pituitary lesion
    m. process
    m. reading
    m. renal mass
    m. synovioma
    m. transformation
    m. tumor
    m. tumor classification
malignant-appearing microcalcification
malingering questionnaire
malinterdigitation
Mallampati
    M. oropharyngeal classification
    M. pharyngeal visibility
      classification
Mallard incision
mallear
    m. fold
    m. ligament
    m. process
    m. prominence
mallei (*pl. of* malleus)
malleoincudal
malleolar
    m. fracture
    m. osteotomy
malleolus, pl. **malleoli**
    medial m.
mallet
    m. finger deformity
    m. fracture
    m. toe deformity
malleus, pl. **mallei**
Mallory technique

Mallory-Weiss
    M.-W. lesion
    M.-W. mucosal rupture
    M.-W. procedure
    M.-W. syndrome
    M.-W. tear
malnutrition
malocclusion
Malone
    M. ACE procedure
    M. antegrade continence enema
      procedure
malpighian
    m. body
    m. pyramid
    m. stigma
malposition
    catheter m.
    extension m.
    strut m.
malpositioning
malpresentation
    fetal m.
malrelation
malrotation
    intestinal m.
    renal m.
MALT
    mucosa-associated lymphoid tissue
    MALT lymphoma
malunion
    humeral fracture m.
malunited
    m. calcaneus fracture
    m. forearm fracture
    m. radial fracture
mamillary
    m. body
    m. duct
    m. line
    m. process
    m. tubercle
mamillothalamic tract
mamma, pl. **mammae**
mammalian cell membrane
mammaplasty, mammoplasty
    Aries-Pitanguy m.
    augmentation m.
    bellybutton augmentation m.
    postreduction m.
    reconstructive m.
    reduction m.
    Wise pattern m.
mammary
    m. atrophy
    m. branch
    m. duct
    m. duct ectasia
    m. fistula

m. gland
m. line
m. node
m. node biopsy
m. plexus
m. region
m. tissue
mammectomy
mammilla, pl. **mammillae**
mammillaplasty
mammogram
abnormal m.
mammographer
mammographic
m. abnormality
m. appearance
m. evaluation
m. finding
m. lesion
m. malignant-appearing
microcalcification
m. presentation
mammography
digital m.
screening m.
mammoplasty (*var. of* mammaplasty)
Mammotest Plus breast aspiration
mammotomy
management
airway m.
m. of anesthesia
anesthetic m.
anesthetic and fluid m.
aneurysm m.
emergency airway m.
endoscopic m.
expectant m.
fluid m.
foreign body m.
intraoperative fluid m.
laparoscopic m.
locoregional m.
mechanical endoscopic m.
medical m.
nonoperative m.
nonsurgical m.
obstetrical m.
operative m.
optimal intensive medical m.
pain m.
perioperative m.
postoperative m.

renal m.
risk m.
selective nonoperative m.
m. strategy
surgical m.
ventilator m.
Manchester-Fothergill operation
Manchester operation
Mancini technique
mandatory
m. celiotomy
m. laparoscopy
Mandelbaum-Nartolozzi-Carney patellar
tendon repair
mandible
mandibula, pl. **mandibulae**
mandibular
m. articulation
m. body fracture
m. canal
m. cartilage
m. centric relation
m. condyle
m. condylectomy
m. condyle fracture
m. disc
m. dislocation
m. equilibration
m. excess
m. fixation
m. foramen
m. fossa
m. head
m. hinge position
m. incisor angle
m. joint
m. nerve
m. nerve block
m. node
m. notch
m. osteotomy advancement
m. plane
m. plane angle
m. ramus fracture
m. ramus osteotomy
m. reconstruction
m. rest position
m. space
m. surgery
m. swing operation
m. swing technique
m. symphysis

M

NOTES

mandibular *(continued)*
    m. symphysis fracture
    m. tongue
mandibulectomy
    segmental m.
mandibulofacial dysotosis syndrome
mandibulomaxillary fixation
mandibulopharyngeal
mandibulotomy
mandibulum
mandrel graft
maneuver
    Addison m.
    Adson m.
    Allen m.
    Allis m.
    alpha-loop m.
    Apley m.
    avoidance m.
    Barlow m.
    Bielschowsky m.
    Bigelow m.
    Bill m.
    Bracht m.
    Brandt-Andrews m.
    bunching m.
    BURP m.
    Buzzard m.
    Cairns m.
    Carlo Traverso m.
    circumduction m.
    closed manipulative m.
    cold pressor testing m.
    corkscrew m.
    costoclavicular m.
    Credé m.
    Dandy m.
    décollement m.
    DeLee m.
    Dix-Hallpike m.
    doll's eye m.
    doll's head m.
    Ejrup m.
    Epley m.
    Finkelstein m.
    flexion-extension m.
    forceps m.
    Fowler-Stephens m.
    Frenzel m.
    grunting m.
    Hallpike m.
    Halsted m.
    Hampton m.
    heel-to-ear m.
    Heimlich m.
    hemodynamic m.
    Hillis-Müller m.
    Hippocratic m.
    Hodge m.

Hoguet m.
Hubscher m.
Hueter m.
hyperventilation m.
Jahss m.
jaw thrust m.
Jendrassik m.
Jonnson m.
J-type m.
jugular compression m.
key-in-lock m.
Ko-Airan m.
Kocher m.
Krackow m.
Kristeller m.
Lachman m.
Leadbetter m.
Lecompte m.
Levret m.
liver hanging m.
logrolling m.
Loosett m.
Lovset m.
Massini m.
Mattox m.
Mauriceau m.
Mauriceau-Levret m.
Mauriceau-Smellie-Veit m.
McDonald m.
McKenzie extension m.
McMurray circumduction m.
McRoberts m.
Mendelsohn m.
meticulous m.
midforceps m.
modified Ritgen m.
Mueller m.
Müller m.
Müller-Hillis m.
Munro-Kerr m.
notch-and-roll m.
Nylen-Barany m.
oculocephalic m.
Ortolani m.
osteoclasis m.
Pajot m.
peroral m.
Phalen m.
Pinard m.
postural fixation back m.
Prague m.
Prentiss m.
Pringle m.
Proetz m.
pull m.
push m.
recruiting m.
recruitment m.
reexpansion m.

relative response attributable to
   the m.
reverse Bigelow m.
Ritgen m.
rotation-compression m.
Rubin m.
Saxtorph m.
scalene m.
Scanzoni m.
Scanzoni-Smellie m.
scarf m.
Schatz m.
Schreiber m.
Sellick m.
Semont m.
shoeshine m.
Slocum m.
Spurling m.
Steel m.
Stimson m.
straightening m.
surgical m.
Thorn m.
U-turn m.
Valsalva m.
Van Hoorn m.
wall push m.
Wigand m.
Woods screw m.
Wright m.
Zavanelli m.

mangled
   m. extremity severity score
   m. extremity syndrome

manifestation
   allergic m.
   articular m.
   cardiopulmonary m.
   central nervous system m.
   clinical m.
   cutaneous m.
   digestive m.
   hepatobiliary m.
   initial m.
   major m.
   minor m.
   mucocutaneous m.
   neurologic m.
   neuroophthalmic m.
   ocular m.
   oral m.
   otolaryngologic m.

presenting clinical m.
pulmonary m.
renal m.
vascular m.

manipulation
   bile duct m.
   catheter m.
   cervical m.
   contact m.
   cranial nerve m.
   digital m.
   direct m.
   fine m.
   gamete m.
   general thrust m.
   gross m.
   guide wire m.
   Hippocrates m.
   indirect m.
   joint m.
   laparoscopic dissection and m.
   laser m.
   Leadbetter hip m.
   long- and short-lever rotational m.
   myofascial m.
   noncontact m.
   opening wedge m.
   optimal external laryngeal m.
   pancreatic duct m.
   passive joint m.
   pharmacologic m.
   physical m.
   postureteroscopic m.
   shunt m.
   specific thrust m.
   spinal m.
   thrust m.

manipulation-induced PGID injury
manipulative therapy
Mankin
   M. resection
   M. technique

Manktelow transfer procedure
Mann-Bollman fistula
Mann-Coughlin-DuVries cheilectomy
Mann-Coughlin procedure
Mann-DuVries arthroplasty
Mann procedure
Mann-Whitney test
Mann-Williamson operation
manometer
   saline m.

M

NOTES

manometric
- m. data
- m. evaluation
- m. finding
- m. recording session
- m. study
- m. technique

manometry
- anal m.
- anorectal m.
- esophageal m.
- jejunal m.
- laparoscopic transcystic sphincter of Oddi m.
- stationary m.

Mansfield Valvuloplasty Registry
Manske-McCarroll opponensplasty
Manske-McCarroll-Swanson centralization
Manske technique
mantle irradiation
Mantoux method
manual
- m. extraction
- m. method
- m. pressure
- m. push-pull technique
- m. rotation
- m. ventilation

manubriosternal
- m. joint
- m. junction
- m. symphysis

manubrium, pl. **manubria**
MAP
- mean arterial pressure

maple leaf flap
maplike skull
mapping
- activation-sequence m.
- advanced cardiac m.
- atrial activation m.
- body surface Laplacian m.
- breast lymphatic m.
- catheter m.
- dermatomal m.
- dermatome m.
- endocardial m.
- intraoperative lymphatic m.
- isosulfan blue-dye m.
- lymphatic m.
- neural m.
- retrograde atrial activation m.
- SLN m.

Maquet
- M. dome osteotomy
- M. procedure

Maragiliano body
marantic clot

Marbach-Weil technique
marbleization
Marcacci muscle
March
- M. fracture
- M. technique

Marchand adrenal
Marchi tract
Marcille triangle
Marckwald operation
Marcove-Lewis-Huvos shoulder girdle resection
Marcus-Balourdas-Heiple ankle fusion technique
Marcus Gunn phenomenon
Marcy
- M. hernia repair
- M. operation

mare's tail line
Marfan syndrome
margin
- carious restoration m.
- cavity m.
- close m.
- costal m.
- dentate m.
- dissection m.
- falciform m.
- free gastric m.
- frontal m.
- gastric m.
- hepatic m.
- interosseous m.
- m. invasion
- lacrimal m.
- lambdoid m.
- mastoid m.
- mesovarian m.
- negative m.
- obtuse m.
- occipital m.
- parietal m.
- positive resection m.
- positive surgical m.
- psoas m.
- pupillary m.
- m. resection
- resection m.
- m. resection involvement
- squamous m.
- superior m.
- supraorbital m.
- surgical m.
- tumor-free m.

marginal
- m. artery
- m. excess
- m. excision
- m. incision

m. insertion
m. mandibular branch
m. myotomy
m. resection
m. ridge fracture
m. sinus rupture
m. sphincter
m. tentorial branch
m. tubercle
m. ulceration
margination
lesion m.
leukocytic m.
marginoplasty
margo, pl. **margines**
marian lithotomy
marijuana
medical m.
Marin Amat syndrome
Marion disease
Marion-Moschcowitz culdoplasty
mark
ecchymotic m.
port-wine m.
tape m.
marked
m. ascites
m. tenderness
marker
biologic m.
blood m.
genetic m.
histologic m.
immunohistochemical m.
prognostic m.
m. stitch
tumor m.
viral m.
Marks-Bayne technique for thumb duplication
Marlex
M. closure
M. hernial repair
M. plug technique
Marquardt angulation osteotomy
Marquez-Gomez
Marquez-Gomez conjunctival graft
Marquez-Gomez operation
Marriott method
marrow
m. ablation
allogenic bone m.

m. cavity
m. graft rejection
m. space
spinal m.
Marseille pancreatitis classification
Marshall
M. ligament repair technique
M. method
M. oblique vein
M. test
Marshall-Marchetti
M.-M. procedure
M.-M. test
Marshall-Marchetti-Krantz (MMK)
M.-M.-K. operation
M.-M.-K. procedure
M.-M.-K. urethropexy
Marshall-McIntosh technique
Marshall-Taylor vacuum extraction
marsupialization
renal cyst m.
Spence and Duckett m.
m. technique
transurethral m.
Martin
M. anoplasty
M. incision
M. modification
M. osteotomy
M. patellar wiring technique
M. reduction technique
Martin-Gruber anastomosis
Martius
M. bulbocavernosus fat flap
M. procedure
masculina
vagina m.
masculine
m. pelvis
m. uterus
masculinization
ovarian m.
masculinizing genitoplasty
masculinovoblastoma
mask
ecchymotic m.
m. leak
masking technique
Mason
M. approach
M. incision
M. operation

M

NOTES

Mason *(continued)*
    M. radial head fracture
      classification
    M. vertical banded gastroplasty
Mason-Likar limb lead modification
masquerade technique
MASS
    mitral valve prolapse, aortic anomalies,
      skeletal changes, skin changes
    MASS syndrome
mass
    abdominal wall m.
    abdominopelvic m.
    acellular m.
    adnexal m.
    adrenal cystic m.
    anterior mediastinal m.
    appendiceal m.
    apperceptive m.
    asymptomatic m.
    atomic m.
    benign m.
    body cell m.
    bone m.
    bony m.
    brain m.
    calcified renal m.
    carbon gelatin m.
    cardiac m.
    cardiophrenic angle m.
    cicatricial m.
    circumscribed m.
    colonic m.
    complex chest m.
    m. concentration
    congenital nasal m.
    congenital renal m.
    conglomerate m.
    cortical m.
    critical m.
    cul-de-sac m.
    cystic m.
    m. defect
    dense brain m.
    discrete m.
    dominant m.
    doughy m.
    dumbbell m.
    duodenal m.
    dysplasia-associated m.
    echodense m.
    erythrocyte m.
    esophageal m.
    exchangeable m.
    m. excision
    exophytic gut m.
    expansile abdominal m.
    extracardiac m.
    extramedullary m.

extramucosal m.
extrarenal m.
extrauterine pelvic m.
extravascular m.
extrinsic m.
fallopian tube m.
fat-free m.
filar m.
firm m.
flank m.
fluctuant m.
fungating m.
gastric m.
groin m.
hard m.
high-attenuation m.
hilar m.
hyaline m.
ill-defined m.
m. infection
infraauricular m.
injection m.
inner cell m.
intraabdominal m.
intracardiac m.
intracranial m.
intradural extramedullary m.
intrasellar m.
intrathoracic m.
intravascular m.
intraventricular m.
intussuscepted m.
lacrimal m.
laminated acellular m.
lateral m.
lean body m.
m. lesion
limbus m.
liver m.
lobulated m.
low-attenuation m.
low-density m.
luminal m.
malignant renal m.
mediastinal high-attenuation m.
m. memory
mesenteric m.
mixed density m.
molecular m.
mulberry-shaped m.
multiloculated renal m.
mushroom-shaped m.
mycelial m.
myocardial m.
neoplastic renal m.
noncalcified nodular m.
nonmobile m.
nonopaque intraluminal m.
ovarian m.

ovoid m.
oyster m.
palpable m.
parasellar m.
parovarian m.
pediatric m.
pelvic m.
periampullary m.
perirectal m.
perivascular m.
persistent ovarian m.
phlegmonous m.
plantar-hindfoot-midfoot bony m.
pleural m.
polypoid m.
posterior mediastinal m.
postmenopausal body m.
presacral m.
pulmonary m.
pulsatile m.
questionable m.
rectal m.
red blood cell m.
m. reflex
renal m.
retrobulbar m.
retrocardiac m.
retrosternal m.
rubbery m.
salivary m.
sclerotic cemental m.
scrotal m.
soft tissue m.
solitary pulmonary m.
m. spectrometer
m. spectrometry
stellate m.
submucosal m.
suprasellar m.
testicular m.
thymic m.
tooth m.
transformary m.
traumatic renal m.
tubular excretory m.
tumor m.
umbilical m.
uncinate process m.
unit of m.
uterine m.
vaginal m.
vascular renal m.

vertebral bone m.
well-defined m.
massage
cardiac m.
connective tissue m.
external cardiac m.
hand m.
nerve-point m.
prostatic m.
soft tissue m.
masse
reduction en m.
masseter
m. muscle
m. muscle flap
m. spasm
m. tendon
masseteric
m. artery
m. fascia
m. nerve
m. space
m. tuberosity
masseter-mandibular-pterygoid space
Massie sliding graft
Massini maneuver
massive
m. ascites
m. autotransfusion
m. bowel resection
m. bowel resection syndrome
m. hemorrhage
m. incisional hernioplasty
m. lower gastrointestinal bleeding
m. malignant infiltration
m. pulmonary hemorrhagic edema
Masson trichrome method
MAST
Michigan Abuse Screening Test
minimal access spine technology
MAST technique
mastadenoma
mastectomy
Auchincloss modified radical m.
axillary node dissection m.
bilateral subcutaneous m.
breast-sparing m.
m. closure
complete skin-sparing m.
extended radical m.
m. for gynecomastia
Halsted radical m.

M

NOTES

mastectomy *(continued)*
    m. incision
    lumpectomy m.
    McKissock m.
    McWhirter simple m.
    modified radical m.
    partial m.
    Patey modified radical m.
    preventive m.
    prophylactic m.
    quadrantectomy m.
    radical m.
    segmental m.
    simple m.
    skin sparing m.
    m. specimen
    2-stage technique m.
    standard m.
    subcutaneous m.
    total m.
    transverse m.
master
    m. gland
    m. IG bundle
mastication
    m. disorder
    m. muscle
masticator
    m. nerve
    m. space
    m. space infection
masticatory
    m. fat pad
    m. space
mastitis
    granulomatous m.
    periductal m.
mastoccipital
mastocytoma
mastoid
    m. antrum
    m. branch
    m. canaliculus
    m. cavity
    m. cell
    m. foramen
    m. fossa
    m. incision
    m. margin
    m. node
    m. notch
    m. obliteration operation
mastoidectomy
    modified radical m.
    radical m.
    simple m.
    tympanoplasty m.
mastopexy
    anchor m.

areolar m.
Benelli lollipop m.
breast-lift m.
circumareolar m.
concentric m.
crescent m.
double-skin m.
doughnut m.
endoscopic m.
full m.
keyhole m.
Keystone m.
Lejour m.
lollipop m.
Louis m.
modified m.
periareolar m.
pursestring m.
reduction m.
Regnault type B m.
short scar technique of m.
simple m.
vertical m.
Wise m.
mastoplasty
mastotomy
Mast-Spieghel-Pappas classification
Matas
    M. aneurysmectomy
    M. operation
Matchett-Brown hip arthroplasty
matching
    cross-modality m.
matchstick
    m. graft
    m. test
mater
    dura m.
    pia m.
material
    colloid m.
    contrast m.
    m. failure break point
    hydatid m.
    nonabsorbable m.
    obstructive hydatid m.
    osteosynthetic m.
maternal
    m. abdominal pressure
    m. anesthesia
    m. birthing position
    m. deprivation syndrome
    m. fracture
    m. hydration
    m. infection
    m. mercury exposure
    m. rejection
    m. tissue
    m. venous (MV)

maternal-placental-fetal drug transfer
Mathews olecranon fracture
  classification
Mathieu
  M. island onlay flap
  M. procedure
  M. technique
Mathieu-Horton-Devine flip-flap
matricectomy (*var. of* matrixectomy)
matrilineal
matrix, pl. **matrices**
  bilayered cellular m.
  bone m.
  m. calculus
  cartilage m.
  distal nail m.
  extracellular m.
  germinal m.
  glomerular extracellular m.
  m. metalloproteinase (MMP)
  nail m.
  proximal nail m.
  sterile m.
matrixectomy, matricectomy
  chemical m.
  partial m.
  phenol m.
  Steindler m.
  Winograd partial m.
  Zadik total m.
Matroc femoral head
Matsura preparation
Matta-Saucedo fixation
matted node
matter
  periaqueductal gray
    matter/periventricular gray m.
    (PAG/PVG)
  white m.
Matti-Russe
  M.-R. bone graft
  M.-R. technique
Mattox maneuver
mattress
  m. stitch
  m. suture otoplasty
maturation
  m. division
  m. index
  m. phase
mature teratoma
maturing the stoma

Mauchart ligament
Mauck procedure
Maudsley Mentation Test
Mauksch-Maumenee-Goldberg operation
Maumenee-Goldberg operation
Maunsell-Weir operation
Mau osteotomy
Mauriceau-Levret maneuver
Mauriceau maneuver
Mauriceau-Smellie-Veit maneuver
maxilla, pl. **maxillae**
maxillary
  m. antrum
  m. antrum closure
  m. canal
  m. excess
  m. expansion
  m. fracture
  m. hiatus
  m. nerve
  m. nerve block
  m. osteotomy
  m. restoration
  m. sinus carcinoma
  m. sinus cavity
  m. sinuscopy
  m. sinus mucocele
  m. surgery
  m. tubercle
maxillectomy
  Cocke m.
  partial m.
  subtotal m.
  total m.
maxillofacial
  m. anomaly
  m. fracture
  m. surgery
maxillomandibular
  m. fixation (MMF)
  m. relation
maxillotomy
  extended m.
maximal
  4-m. breath preoxygenation
    technique
  m. drug concentration
  m. expiratory flow rate
  m. expiratory flow volume
  m. rectal diameter
  m. ventilation rate
  m. voluntary ventilation

M

NOTES

Maximally Discriminative Facial Coding System
maximum
  m. breathing capacity (MBC)
  m. mouth opening
  m. occipital point
  m. permissible concentration
  m. stimulation test
  m. urethral closure pressure
  m. voluntary ventilation (MVV)
maximum-intensity projection
Maxwell body
Maydl
  M. hernia
  M. procedure
  M. ureterosigmoidostomy
Mayer transfer operation
Mayfield incision
May-Hegglin body
Maylard incision
Mayo
  M. approach
  M. carpal instability classification
  M. hysterectomy
  M. modified total elbow arthroplasty
  M. operation
  M. resection arthroplasty
  M. rheumatoid elbow classification
Mayo-Fueth inversion procedure
Mayo-Heuter bunionectomy
Mayo-Robson
  M.-R. incision
  M.-R. position
May-Thurner syndrome
Maze III procedure
Mazet
  M. disarticulation
  M. technique
mazolysis
mazopexy
MBC
  maximum breathing capacity
MCA
  middle cerebral artery
  MCA occlusion
McArthur incision
McBride
  M. bunionectomy
  M. procedure
McBurney
  M. appendectomy
  M. appendectomy incision
  M. operation
  M. point
McCall
  M. culdoplasty
  M. stitch
McCall-Schumann procedure

McCarroll-Baker procedure
McCauley technique
McConnell
  M. extensile approach
  M. median and ulnar nerve approach
  M. technique
McCormick-Blount procedure
McCraw gracilis myocutaneous flap
McDonald
  M. cerclage
  M. maneuver
  M. procedure
McElfresh-Dobyns-O'Brien technique
McElvenny-Caldwell procedure
McElvenny technique
McFarland bone graft
McFarland-Osborne
  M.-O. lateral approach
  M.-O. technique
McFarlane
  M. skin flap
  M. technique
McGavic operation
McGill Pain Questionnaire (MPQ)
McGlamry-Downey procedure
McGoon technique
McGregor basal line
McGuire operation
mCi
  millicurie
McIndoe
  M. operation
  M. procedure
  M. vaginal creation
McIndoe-Hayes
  M.-H. construction
  M.-H. procedure
McKay-Simons clubfoot operation
McKee line
McKeever
  M. and MacIntosh hemiarthroplasty
  M. medullary clavicle fixation
  M. open reduction
McKeever-Buck
  M.-B. elbow technique
  M.-B. fragment excision
McKenzie extension maneuver
McKissock mastectomy
McLaughlin
  M. acromioplasty
  M. approach
  M. operation
  M. procedure
McLaughlin-Hay technique
McLaughlin-Ryder incision
McLean
  M. operation
  M. technique

McMaster
> M. bone graft
> M. Quality of Life Scale
> M. technique

McMurray circumduction maneuver

MCN
> mucinous cystic neoplasm

McNeer classification

McRae foramen magnum line

McReynolds
> M. method
> M. open reduction technique
> M. operation

McRoberts maneuver

MCS
> magnetic control suturing

McShane-Leinberry-Fenlin acromioplasty

McSpadden method

McVay
> M. herniorrhaphy
> M. incision
> M. inguinal hernial repair
> M. method
> M. operation
> M. procedure
> M. technique

McVay-Cooper ligament repair

McWhirter simple mastectomy

McWhorter posterior shoulder approach

MD
> muscular dystrophy

MDCT
> multidetector computed tomography

MDMQ
> Menstrual Distress Management
> Questionnaire

mean
> m. airway resistance
> m. arterial blood pressure (MABP)
> m. arterial pressure (MAP)
> m. circulation time
> m. diastolic left ventricular
>   pressure
> m. foundation plane
> m. normalized systolic ejection rate
> m. pulmonary artery wedge
>   pressure
> m. shunt index
> m. systolic left ventricular pressure
> m. UV/MV ratio

Meares-Stamey technique

Mears-Rubash approach

measure
> nonpharmacologic m.
> preventive m.

measurement
> acoustic reflection m.
> alveolar diffusion m.
> ankle-brachial pressure m.
> continuous intramucosal PCO_2 m.
> 4-cuff technique segmental
>   pressure m.
> diurnal intraocular pressure m.
> endpoint m.
> esophageal m.
> facial excursion m.
> Fick cardiac output m.
> hematocrit m.
> intrauterine pressure m.
> invasive pressure m.
> muscle m.
> near-infrared m.
> negative inspiratory pressure m.
> oxygen saturation m.
> pH m.
> pressure m.
> pulse-echo distance m.
> serial hematocrit m.
> skin m.
> skin temperature gradient m.
> tissue pressure m.
> total exchangeable potassium m.
> transcutaneous oxygen pressure m.
> transstenotic pressure gradient m.
> tympanic membrane m.
> urethral pressure m.
> vasodilator-stimulated rCBF single
>   photon emission computed
>   tomographic m.
> voiding urethral pressure m.

meatal
> m. advancement and glansplasty
>   (MAGPI)
> m. advancement and glansplasty
>   incorporated
> m. advancement, glansplasty,
>   penoscrotal junction meatotomy
>   (MAGPI)
> m. cartilage

meatoplasty
> V-flap m.

meatorrhaphy

meatoscopy

M

NOTES

453

meatotomy
> meatal advancement, glansplasty,
> penoscrotal junction m. (MAGPI)
> ureteral m.

meatus, pl. **meatus**
> anterior nasal m.
> external auditory m.
> inferior m.
> middle m.
> superior m.
> ureteral m.

meaty appearance

MEC
> minimum effective concentration

mechanical
> m. anastomosis
> m. endoscopic management
> m. esophagojejunostomy
> m. extrahepatic obstruction
> m. leech
> m. lithotripsy
> m. occlusion
> m. perforation
> m. pulp exposure
> m. stimulation
> m. thrombectomy
> m. ureteral dilation
> m. variceal compression
> m. ventilation
> m. ventilation anesthetic technique
> m. ventilatory support

mechanism
> antireflux flap-valve m.
> association m.
> central extensor m.
> cholinergic m.
> clotting m.
> countercurrent m.
> digital extensor m.
> extensor hood m.
> extrinsic m.
> fascial shutter m.
> flap-valve m.
> hematogenous m.
> hemolytic m.
> immune m.
> inhibitory-excitatory m.
> noradrenergic m.
> obstructive m.
> renal m.
> screw-home m.
> surveillance m.
> urethral closure m.

mechanoactivation
mechanogram
mechanomyography
mechanoreflex
mèche

Meckel
> M. band
> M. cartilage
> M. cave
> M. cavity
> M. diverticulectomy
> M. diverticulum
> M. ganglion
> M. ligament
> M. scan
> M. space
> M. sphenopalatine ganglionectomy

meconium
> m. aspiration
> m. aspiration syndrome
> m. plug syndrome

media (*pl. of* medium)

medial
> m. aspect
> m. aspiration
> m. basal segment
> m. canthus
> m. capsular imbrication
> m. capsulorrhaphy
> m. clear space
> m. condyle
> m. crus
> m. cutaneous branch
> m. displacement osteotomy
> m. dissection
> m. extradural approach
> m. flap
> m. malleolar network
> m. malleolar subcutaneous bursa
> m. malleolus
> m. malleolus fixation
> m. malleolus resection
> m. mammary branch
> m. meniscectomy
> m. parapatellar capsular approach
> m. parapatellar incision
> m. process
> m. repair
> m. rotation
> m. rotation procedure
> m. rotator
> m. sector
> m. tibial stress syndrome (MTSS)

medialis obliquus imbrication

medialization
> silicone elastomer m.

medial-sector pedicle

median
> m. biopsy volume
> m. corpectomy
> m. detection threshold
> m. episiotomy
> m. glossoepiglottic fold
> m. groove

m. jaw relation
m. labiomandibular glossotomy
m. line
m. lithotomy
m. longitudinal raphe
m. mandibular point
m. nerve
m. nerve compression
m. section
m. sternotomy
m. sternotomy incision
m. strumectomy
m. thoracotomy

medianum

mediastinal
m. artery
m. branch
m. CTD
m. enlargement
m. esophagojejunostomy
m. hematoma
m. hemorrhage
m. high-attenuation mass
m. irradiation
m. lymphadenectomy
m. lymph node biopsy
m. lymph node dissection
m. pleura
m. shed blood (MSB)
m. space
m. tumor
m. vein
m. wedge

mediastinitis

mediastinoscopic examination

mediastinoscopy
Chamberlain m.
transthoracic m.
video m.

mediastinoscopy-assisted transhiatal esophagectomy

mediastinotomy

mediastinum
anterior m.
inferior m.
middle m.
posterior m.
superior m.
upper m.

mediate transfusion

mediator
proinflammatory m.

medical
m. care
m. care evaluation
m. chemoprevention
m. diathermy
m. dilation
m. illness
m. intervention
m. management
m. marijuana
m. oncologist
m. ophthalmoscopy
m. problem
m. record
m. systemic condition
m. therapy
m. treatment
m. treatment option
m. vagotomy

medication
aerosolized m.
antalgic m.
anticholinergic m.
antiepileptic m.
antiinflammatory m.
base m.
beta-blocker m.
m. bezoar
concomitant m.
dopaminergic m.
intravenous m.
iodide-containing m.
levodopa dopaminergic m.
nonsteroidal antiinflammatory m.
oral antibiotic m.
over-the-counter m.
parenteral m.
preanesthetic m.
pressor m.
prophylactic m.
psychopharmacologic m.
psychotropic m.
M. Quantification Scale
teratogenic m.
vasoactive m.

medication-induced
m.-i. injury
m.-i. obesity

medicinal preparation

medicine
alternative m.

M

NOTES

medicine *(continued)*
    American Board of Pain M.
      (ABPM)
    anesthesiology critical care m.
    complementary and alternative m.
    critical care m. (CCM)
    emergency m.
    evidence-based m. (EBM)
    fetal m.
    herbal m.
    nuclear m.
    vascular m.
medicochirurgical
medicolegal aspect
medioccipital
mediocolic sphincter
mediolateral episiotomy
medisect
Mediterranean exanthematous fever
medium, pl. **media**
    adhesive otitis media
    contrast m.
    culture m.
    m. lesion
    otitis media
medium-scale integration
medium-sized artery
medius
medulla, pl. **medullae**
    renal m.
    rostral ventrolateral m.
    suprarenal m.
medullar
medullary
    m. adenocarcinoma
    m. bone graft
    m. canal
    m. carcinoma
    m. cavity
    m. clavicle fixation
    m. nail fixation
    m. oxygenation
    m. pyramid
    m. pyramidotomy
    m. ray
    m. space
    m. spinal artery
    m. spinothalamic tractotomy
    m. sponge kidney
    m. substance
    m. tube
medullated
medullation
medullectomy
medullization
medulloblastoma
    desmoplastic m.
    melanotic m.
    m. metastasis

medulloepithelioma
medullomyoblastoma
medullostomy
    tarsal m.
medullovasculosa
medusa
    caput m.
    M. head
Meek operation
Mees line
mefenamic acid
megacalycosis
megacolon
megacystic syndrome
megacystis
megacystis-megaureter
    m.-m. association
    m.-m. syndrome
megacystis-microcolon-intestinal
    hypoperistalsis syndrome
megadolichovertebrobasilar anomaly
megaloureter
megalourethra
megarectum
megasigmoid
megaureter
Mehn-Quigley technique
Meibom gland
meibomian
    m. gland
    m. gland carcinoma
Meigs
    M. pelvic lymphadenectomy
    M. suture technique
Meigs-Okabayashi procedure
Meigs-Werthein hysterectomy
Meissner plexus
melanization
melanoacanthoma
melanoameloblastoma
melanoblastoma
melanocarcinoma
melanocytic conjunctival lesion
melanocytoma
melanoma
    acral lentiginous m. (ALM)
    anorectal m.
    axial m.
    m. cell lysate
    CTL immunity against m.
    cutaneous m.
    extremity m.
    familial atypical mole and m.
      (FAM-M)
    lentigo m.
    node-negative m.
    node-positive m.
    thick cutaneous m. (TCM)

m. transferrin
truncal m.
melanoma-associated
m.-a. antigen GD2
m.-a. antigen GD3
m.-a. antigen GM2
melanosarcoma
melanotic
m. carcinoma
m. lesion
m. medulloblastoma
m. oncocytic metaplasia
m. whitlow
MELAS
mitochondrial myopathy, encephalopathy,
lactic acidosis, and strokelike syndrome
myopathy, encephapathy, lactic acidosis,
stroke-like episodes
Meleney
M. gangrene
M. infection
Meller operation
mellitus
diabetes m.
melocervicoplasty
melolabial flap
Melone distal radius fracture
classification
melonoplasty
melon seed body
meloplasty
meloschisis
melting point
Meltzer method
membrana, pl. **membranae**
membrane
acute inflammatory m.
acute pyogenic m.
adamantine m.
alveolocapillary m.
alveolodental m.
amniotic m.
antibasement m.
antiglomerular basement m.
antitubular basement m.
antral m.
arachnoid m.
m. artificial lung
asymmetric unit m.
atlantooccipital m.
Barkan m.
basal cell m.

basement m.
basilar m.
basolateral m.
Bichat m.
bilaminar m.
Bowman m.
m. bridge
Bruch m.
brush-border m.
m. catheter technique
cell m.
cellulose-based m.
chorioallantoic m.
choroidal neovascular m.
cloacal m.
collodion m.
congenital pyloric m.
conjunctival m.
connective tissue m.
cricothyroid m.
cricotracheal m.
cricovocal m.
croupous m.
cuprophane m.
m. current
cuticular m.
cyclitic m.
cytoplasmic m.
Debove m.
decidual m.
Demours m.
dentinoenamel m.
Descemet m.
dialysis m.
dialyzer m.
diphtheritic m.
drum m.
dry mucous m.
Duddell m.
dysmenorrheal m.
egg m.
enamel m.
endothelial cell basement m.
epipapillary m.
epiretinal m.
epithelial basement m.
erythrocyte m.
exocelomic m.
m. expansion theory
false m.
fenestrated m.
fetal m.

NOTES

M

457

membrane *(continued)*

    fibroproliferative m.
    Fielding m.
    m. filtration method
    filtration-slit m.
    Fresnel m.
    germinal m.
    glassy m.
    gliotic m.
    Golgi m.
    Haller m.
    Henle elastic m.
    Henle fenestrated m.
    Heuser m.
    high-flux dialysis m.
    hourglass m.
    Hovius m.
    hyaline basement m.
    hyalitis anterior m.
    hyaloid posterior m.
    hymenal m.
    hyoglossal m.
    idiopathic preretinal m.
    inflammatory m.
    inner limiting m.
    m. instability
    intact m.
    intercostal m.
    intermuscular m.
    interposition m.
    intraosseous m.
    invaginated m.
    ivory m.
    Jackson m.
    Jacob m.
    m. of Liliequist
    limiting m.
    low-flux cellulose-based m.
    low-flux cuprophane m.
    low-flux dialysis m.
    lysosomal m.
    mammalian cell m.
    microvillous m.
    moist mucous m.
    mucous m.
    NaK-ATPase m.
    Nasmyth m.
    neovascular m.
    neuronal m.
    nictitating m.
    onion skin-like m.
    otolithic m.
    outer limiting m.
    m. oxygenator
    Payr m.
    m. peeling
    peridental m.
    perineal m.
    periodontal m.

    periorbital m.
    m. permeability
    phrenoesophageal m.
    pial-glial m.
    placental m.
    plasma m.
    polyacrylonitrile m.
    porous filter m.
    postsynaptic m.
    m. potential
    preretinal m.
    presynaptic m.
    prophylactic m.
    pseudoserous m.
    pulpodentinal m.
    pupillary m.
    purpurogenous m.
    pyogenic m.
    quadrangular m.
    Reichert m.
    Reissner m.
    reticular m.
    retrocorneal m.
    rolling m.
    rupture of m.'s (ROM)
    m. rupture
    Ruysch m.
    ruyschian m.
    salpingopalatine m.
    salpingopharyngeal m.
    sarcolemmal m.
    schneiderian respiratory m.
    secondary m.
    semiimpermeable m.
    semipermeable m.
    serous m.
    Shrapnell m.
    Slavianski m.
    small intestinal m.
    spiral m.
    statoconic m.
    stripping m.
    stylomandibular m.
    subepithelial m.
    subimplant m.
    submucous m.
    subretinal neovascular m.
    suprapleural m.
    surface m.
    synovial m.
    tarsal m.
    tectorial m.
    Tenon m.
    thickened synovial m.
    thin basement m.
    thyrohyoid m.
    Toldt m.
    Tourtual m.
    trabecular m.

m. trafficking
tubular basement m.
tympanic m.
undulating m.
unit m.
urea-impermeable m.
urogenital m.
urorectal m.
urothelial basement m.
vernix m.
vestibular m.
virginal m.
vitelline m.
vitreal m.
vitreous m.
Wachendorf m.
wrinkling m.
yolk m.
Zinn m.
membrane-coating granule
membranectomy
membranocartilaginous
membranoproliferative glomerulonephritis
membranotomy
transcardiac m.
membranous
m. acute inflammation
m. adhesion
m. obstruction
m. septum
m. urethra
Memorial Pain Assessment Card (MPAC)
memory
explicit m.
m. guidance saccade test
implicit m.
indirect m.
m. loss
mass m.
m. recall
scratch-pad m.
MEN
multiple endocrine neoplasia
MEN syndrome
MEN-2a, -2b syndrome
Mendelsohn maneuver
Mendelson syndrome
Menghini
M. biopsy technique
M. technique for percutaneous liver biopsy

Ménière
M. disease
M. syndrome
meningeal
m. branch
m. carcinoma
m. groove
m. hernia
m. layer
m. plexus
m. vein
meningeorrhaphy
meninges (*pl. of* meninx)
meningioma
meningioma-en-plaque
meningiomatosis
meningitic respiration
meningitis
meningocele
meningoencephalitis
meningoencephalocele
meningomyelocele
meningorrhagia
meningosis
meninguria
meninx, pl. **meninges**
meniscal
m. excision
m. repair
meniscectomy
arthroscopic m.
lateral m.
medial m.
partial m.
Patel medial m.
subtotal lateral m.
total m.
meniscoplasty
meniscus, pl. **menisci**
Dickhaut-DeLee classification of discoid m.
Watanabe classification of discoid m.
Mensor-Scheck
M.-S. hanging hip operation
M.-S. technique
menstrual
m. aspiration
m. cycle induction
M. Distress Management Questionnaire (MDMQ)

M

NOTES

menstrual *(continued)*
    m. extraction
    m. extraction abortion
menstruation
    reflux m.
mental
    m. artery
    m. block injection
    m. branch
    m. canal
    m. foramen
    m. nerve
    m. nerve block
    m. point
    m. process
    m. projection
    m. region
    m. spine
    m. status evaluation
    m. status examination
    m. symphysis
    m. tubercle
mentalis muscle
menti (*pl. of* mentum)
mentoanterior position
mentolabial
    m. furrow
    m. sulcus
mentoplasty
mentoposterior position
mentotransverse position
mentum, pl. **menti**
    m. anterior position
    m. posterior position
    m. transverse position
Menzies method
MEP
    motor-evoked potential
    myogenic motor-evoked potential
MER
    motor-evoked response
meralgia paresthetica
Mercator projection
Mercier bar
mercurial line
mercuroscopic expansion
mercury pressure
Merendino technique
meridian
    corneal m.
meridional aberration
Merkel
    M. cell cancer
    M. cell carcinoma
    M. fossa
    M. muscle
mermaid malformation
Méry gland
mesangial matrix expansion

mesangiolysis
mesangium
    extraglomerular m.
mesatipellic pelvis
mesencephalic
    m. cistern
    m. hemorrhage
    m. low-density lesion
    m. reticular formation
    m. tractotomy
mesencephalotomy
mesenchymal
    m. lesion
    m. tissue
mesenchymoma
mesenteric
    m. angiogram
    m. angiography
    m. arterial system
    m. arteriovenous fistula
    m. artery
    m. border
    m. bypass graft
    m. circulation
    m. cyst
    m. ganglion
    m. gland
    m. hematoma
    m. hernia
    m. insufficiency
    m. ischemia (MI)
    m. lymph node (MLN)
    m. mass
    m. nodal disease
    m. node
    m. plexus
    m. portion
    m. rupture
    m. tear
    m. vascular lesion
    m. vasodilator
    m. vasodilator infusion
    m. vein
    m. venoconstriction
mesentericoparietal
    m. fossa
    m. recess
mesentericoportal axis
mesenteriopexy
mesenteriorrhaphy
mesenteriplication
mesenteritis
mesentery
    m. abscess
    edematous m.
mesethmoid bone
mesh
    m. herniorrhaphy
    m. implantation

m. inguinodynia
m. plug hernioplasty
m. removal
m. repair
surgical m.
mesial
mesioangular position
mesiobuccal
m. canal
m. line angle
mesiobuccoocclusal point angle
mesiodistal
m. fracture
m. plane
mesiolabial
m. bilobed transposition flap
m. line angle
mesiolabioincisal point angle
mesiolingual line angle
mesiolinguoincisal point angle
mesiolinguo-occlusal point line angle
mesioocclusal line angle
mesioocclusodistal (MOD)
mesoappendix
mesoatrial shunt
mesocaval
m. anastomosis
m. H-graft
mesocecal
mesocecum
mesocolic
m. hernia
m. involvement
m. tenia
mesocolon
ascending m.
descending m.
sigmoid m.
transverse m.
mesocolopexy
mesocoloplication
mesoderm
extraembryonic m.
intermediate m.
mesoduodenal
mesoduodenum
mesoenteriolum
mesoepididymis
mesoesophageal dissection
mesohepatectomy
mesoileum
mesojejunum

mesolepidoma
mesolimbic-mesocortical tract
mesometrium
mesonephric
m. adenocarcinoma
m. duct
m. ridge
m. tubule
mesonephroma
mesonephros
mesoneuritis
mesopexy
mesophryon
mesorchium
mesorectal excision
mesorectum
residual m.
mesorrhaphy
mesosalpinx
mesosigmoid
mesosigmoidopexy
mesostenium
mesosternum
mesostructure
implant m.
mesotendineum
mesotendon
mesothelial
m. cell
m. cell layer
m. tissue
mesothelioma
benign m.
mesothelium
mesovarian margin
mesovarium
Messerklinger technique
metabolic
m. acidosis
m. change
m. coma
m. complication
m. disorder
m. evaluation
m. heat production
m. rate
m. response
metabolism
aerobic m.
pyruvate m.
metabolite

NOTES

M

461

metacarpal
    m. artery
    m. bone
    m. neck fracture
    m. osteotomy
metacarpophalangeal
    m. articulation
    m. joint arthroplasty
metacarpus, pl. **metacarpi**
metachronous emergence
metadiaphysis
metafacial angle
metal-ceramic restoration
metallic
    m. cranioplasty
    m. foreign body
    m. fragment
    m. restoration
    m. rod fixation
metalloproteinase
    matrix m. (MMP)
metalloscopy
metamorphosing respiration
metanephric
    m. cap
    m. duct
metaphysial
    m. abscess
    m. osteotomy
    m. tibial fracture
metaphysis, pl. **metaphyses**
    distal m.
    femoral m.
    fibular m.
    funnelization of m.
    rachitic m.
    tibial m.
metaplasia
    apocrine m.
    Barrett m.
    columnar m.
    melanotic oncocytic m.
    squamous m.
metaplastic epithelium
metastasectomy
    pulmonary m.
metastasis
    adnexal m.
    adrenal m.
    m., age, completeness of resection,
      local invasion, tumor size
      (MACIS)
    aortic node m.
    axillary node m.
    bilobar liver m.
    biochemical m.
    biopsy-proven m.
    blastic m.
    blood-borne m.

    bone m.
    bony m.
    brain m.
    breast m.
    calcareous m.
    calcified liver m.
    calcifying m.
    cardiac m.
    cavitating m.
    celiac lymph node m.
    cerebral m.
    cervical m.
    chiasmal m.
    choroidal m.
    clivus m.
    colonic m.
    colorectal m.
    contact m.
    contralateral axillary m.
    cutaneous m.
    cystic m.
    diffuse m.
    distal m.
    distant m.
    drop m.
    duodenal m.
    echopenic liver m.
    extracapsular m.
    extrahepatic m.
    extralymphatic m.
    extrathoracic m.
    fallopian tube m.
    floxuridine in hepatic m.
    gastric bed m.
    gastrointestinal m.
    hematogenic m.
    hematogenous m.
    hematopoietic m.
    hemorrhagic m.
    hepatic colorectal m.
    hernia m.
    implantation m.
    incisional m.
    inguinal lymph node m.
    intracapsular m.
    intrahepatic m.
    intramucosal m.
    in-transit m.
    intrapulmonary m. (IPM)
    laparoscopic port site m.
    lateroaortic m.
    leptomeningeal m.
    liver m.
    lymphatic m.
    lymph node m.
    lymphogenous m.
    medulloblastoma m.
    necrotic m.
    neoplasm m.

nodal m.
noncolorectal liver m. (NCRLM)
nonneuroendocrine m.
occult m.
ocular m.
omental m.
orbital m.
osseous m.
osteoblastic m.
ovarian cancer m.
paracardiac m.
parasellar m.
parenchymal brain m.
peritoneal m.
placental m.
port site m.
pulmonary m.
regional m.
resectable liver m.
retrobulbar orbital m.
satellite m.
serosal m.
serosal-peritoneal m.
skeletal m.
skip m.
soft tissue m.
sphenoid sinus m.
spinal m.
stomach cancer m.
synchronous hepatic m.
testicular m.
tumor, node, m. (TNM)
unique noncolorectal liver m.
unresectable m.
uterine sarcoma m.
uveal m.
vascular m.
Virchow m.
metastatic
m. abscess
m. adenocarcinoma
m. adenopathy
m. colorectal cancer
m. colorectal carcinoma
m. contamination
m. disease
m. implantation
m. involvement
m. lesion
m. malignancy
m. nodule
m. prostatic carcinoma

m. renal cell carcinoma
m. spread
m. tumor
m. tumor removal
metasternum
metasynchronous bacterial urinary tract infection
metatarsal
m. artery
m. bone
m. fracture
m. head
m. head resection
m. pad
m. Reverdin osteotomy
m. V-shaped osteotomy
metatarsi (*pl. of* metatarsus)
metatarsocuneiform articulation
metatarsophalangeal
m. articulation
m. joint disarticulation
m. joint dislocation
metatarsus, pl. **metatarsi**
metathesis
meter-kilogram-second (mks)
methacholine bronchoprovocation challenge
methamphetamine exposure
methanol freezing method
methemoglobin
methemoglobinemia
method
Abbott m.
Abell m.
Abell-Kendall m.
acid anhydride m.
acid guanidine thiocyanate-phenol-chloroform m.
acoupedic m.
acoustic m.
acridine orange m.
agar diffusion m.
Allain m.
analytic m.
Anderson-Keys m.
Anel m.
antegrade m.
anthrone m.
antibody linkage m.
Antyllus m.
area-length m.
aristotelian m.

M

NOTES

method *(continued)*
    artificial m.
    Arvidsson dimension-length m.
    Ashby differential agglutination m.
    Astrand 30-beat stopwatch m.
    atrial extrastimulus m.
    Attwood staining m.
    auditory m.
    Autenrieth and Funk m.
    avidin-biotin-peroxidase complex m.
    Ayoub-Shklar m.
    bacterial agar m.
    Baker Sudan black m.
    bandage m.
    Bangerter m.
    Barnett-Bourne acetic alcohol-silver nitrate m.
    barostat m.
    Barraquer m.
    barrier m.
    Barrnett-Seligman dihydroxydinaphthyl disulfide m.
    Barrnett-Seligman indoxyl esterase m.
    Barroso-Moguel and Costero silver m.
    Bass m.
    Bassini m.
    Batch least-squares m.
    Baumgartner m.
    Beaver direct smear m.
    Beck m.
    Belsey fundoplication m.
    Benedict-Talbot body surface area m.
    Bengston m.
    Bennett sulfhydryl m.
    Bennhold Congo red m.
    Bensley aniline-acid fuchsin-methyl green m.
    benzo sky blue m.
    Berg chelate removal m.
    Bielschowsky m.
    Bier m.
    bilateral inguinal hernia repair m.
    Billings m.
    Billroth I m.
    bimodal m.
    bisensory m.
    black periodic acid m.
    Bland-Altman m.
    Bleck m.
    Bobath m.
    Bodian m.
    Bohr isopleth m.
    Bonnaire m.
    Borchgrevink m.
    Borggreve m.
    Bradley m.

    Brasdor m.
    breast-conserving m.
    breathing m.
    Brecher-Cronkite m.
    brine flotation m.
    Brisbane m.
    Brown dietary m.
    Brown-Dodge m.
    Brown and Wickham pressure profile m.
    Bruhn m.
    Buck m.
    Budin-Chandler m.
    Buist m.
    bulkhead m.
    Burch bladder suspension m.
    Burgess m.
    Burow quantitative m.
    bypass m.
    Cajal gold-sublimate m.
    Cajal uranium silver m.
    Caldwell-Moloy m.
    Callahan root canal filling m.
    Camp-Gianturco m.
    Carpue m.
    catheter introduction m.
    Celermajer m.
    cellophane tape m.
    Chang aniline-acid fuchsin m.
    Charters m.
    Chayes m.
    chewing m.
    Chiffelle and Putt m.
    chloranilate m.
    chromate m.
    chrome alum hematoxylin-phloxine m.
    chromogenic m.
    chromolytic m.
    Ciaccio m.
    cinefluoroscopic m.
    Clark-Collip m.
    Clausen m.
    clean-catch collection m.
    closed circuit m.
    cobaltinitrite m.
    Cockroft m.
    Colcher-Sussman m.
    cold knife m.
    collagen staining m.
    Collis-Nissen fundoplication m.
    combined m.
    composite pelvic resection m.
    computer-assisted design-controlled alignment m.
    confrontation m.
    Con-Lish polishing m.
    consonant-injection m.
    constitutive heterochromatin m.

contact m.
contoured adduction trochanteric-
  controlled alignment m.
contraceptive m.
conventional m.
cooled-knife m.
Cope m.
copper sulfate m.
Corning m.
correlational m.
Craigie tube m.
Crawford m.
Credé m.
Cribier m.
Crippa lead tetraacetate m.
cross-consonant injection m.
cross-sectional m.
crown-contouring m.
CryoLife Single Step dilution m.
Cuignet m.
cup-and-cone m.
Cüppers m.
Cutler-Ederer m.
cyanogen bromide m.
cysteic acid m.
Dale-Laidlaw clotting time m.
Dane m.
Danielson m.
Defares rebreathing m.
definitive m.
depth caliper-meter stick m.
Devereux-Reichek m.
diazo staining m.
Dick m.
Dieffenbach m.
Dieterle m.
diffusion root canal filling m.
digitonin m.
3-dimensional FATS m.
direct m.
disc diffusion m.
disc sensitivity m.
Distress Risk Assessment M.
  (DRAM)
Dixon fat suppression m.
Döderlein m.
Dodge area-length m.
Doppler m.
Dor fundoplication m.
double antibody m.
double-stapled ileoanal reservoir m.
Douglas bag collection m.

Dow m.
downstream sampling m.
2-dye m.
dye dilution m.
dyed starch m.
dye scattering m.
dynamic traction m.
edge-detection m.
Eggleston m.
Eicken m.
ellipsoid m.
Elmslie-Trillat patellar
  realignment m.
encu m.
endorectal ileoanal pull-through m.
endoscopic mucosal resection m.
end-to-end reconstruction m.
ensu m.
enucleation m.
Epstein m.
estimated Fick m.
Eve m.
excisional biopsy m.
experimental m.
extension block splinting m.
extraanatomic bypass m.
extracorporeal m.
Fahraeus m.
Fallat-Buckholz m.
Ferguson scoliosis measuring m.
fiberoptic intubation m.
fibrinogen m.
fibrin plate m.
Fick oxygen extraction m.
field m.
filtration m.
Fite m.
fixed sediment m.
flat substrate m.
floppy Nissen fundoplication m.
flow convergence m.
fluorescence polarization m.
fluoroscopic m.
flush m.
Folin and Wu m.
Fones m.
Fontana-Masson staining m.
Foot reticulin m.
formal m.
formaldehyde-induced
  fluorescence m.
formalin-ether sedimentation m.

M

NOTES

method *(continued)*
    forward triangle m.
    freehand m.
    freeze-cleave m.
    freeze-etch m.
    freeze-fracture-etch m.
    French m.
    frozen section m.
    Galanti-Giusti colorimetric m.
    Gärtner m.
    gas clearance m.
    gaseous laparoscopy m.
    gasless laparoscopy m.
    gastric valve tightening m.
    Gerbert-Mellilo m.
    German m.
    glass-bead retention m.
    glucose oxidase m.
    glycerin m.
    Gohil-Cavolo m.
    gradient m.
    gradient-echo m.
    gradient-reversal fat suppression m.
    grammatic m.
    Granger m.
    Gräupner m.
    gravity m.
    Greenwald and Lewman m.
    Grimelius argyrophil m.
    Grocott-Gomori methenamine-
      silver m.
    guidance m.
    Hagedorn and Jansen m.
    half-time m.
    Hall m.
    Hamilton m.
    Hammerschlag m.
    hanging chain m.
    Hanley-McNeil m.
    Harrison m.
    Hatle m.
    Hawkins m.
    head-tilt m.
    Heinecke m.
    helium dilution m.
    hemi-double stapling m.
    heuristic m.
    hexokinase m.
    Hilton m.
    Hirschberg m.
    Hirschfeld m.
    histochemical m.
    Hoechst dye m.
    hold-relax m.
    hole preparation m.
    Holmes m.
    Holmgren m.
    Holzer m.
    Howard m.

Howe silver precipitation m.
H.P. Wright m.
Hugenholtz m.
hydrogen washout m.
Ilizarov m.
imaging m.
Imanaga m.
immersion m.
immobilization m.
immunodiagnostic m.
immunofluorescence m.
immunohistochemical m.
immunologic m.
immunometric sandwich m.
immunoperoxidase m.
impedance m.
1-inclinometer m.
2-inclinometer m.
Indian m.
indirect restorative m.
indocyanine green m.
indophenol m.
informal m.
inhalation m.
injection m.
injection-molded m.
Insall patella alta m.
install m.
intraoperative imaging m.
intraperitoneal m.
introspective m.
Israel m.
Italian m.
Ito m.
jejunoileal bypass reversal m.
Jena m.
Jendrassik-Grof m.
Johnson root canal filling m.
Johnston m.
Kaplan-Meier m.
Karr m.
Kasser-Kennedy m.
Keating-Hart m.
Kendrick m.
Kennedy area-length m.
Kety-Schmidt m.
keyhole m.
kinesthetic m.
King biopsy m.
Kinzie m.
Kirby-Bauer disc diffusion m.
Kirstein m.
Kitzinger m.
Kjeldahl m.
Kluge m.
Kocher m.
Konno biopsy m.
Krause m.
Krimsky m.

Kristeller m.
Laborde m.
Lamaze m.
Langendorff m.
laparoscopic lymph node
  dissection m.
laparoscopic Nissen
  fundoplication m.
laparoscopic paraaortic lymph node
  sampling m.
laser m.
Laurell m.
Leboyer m.
Lee-White clotting time m.
Levaditi m.
Levy, Rowntree, and Marriott m.
Lewis and Benedict m.
Lewissohn m.
Liang and Pardee m.
life table m.
lift-and-cut m.
Lillie allochrome m.
limb-saving m.
Lison-Dunn m.
Lister m.
logical m.
longitudinal m.
loop gastric bypass m.
Lowery m.
Lown and Woolf m.
Lowry m.
Lowsley ribbon gut m.
macro-Kjeldahl m.
Mantoux m.
manual m.
Marriott m.
Marshall m.
Masson trichrome m.
McReynolds m.
McSpadden m.
McVay m.
Meltzer m.
membrane filtration m.
Menzies m.
methanol freezing m.
Metzer-Boyce m.
Meyerding m.
microinjection m.
micro-Kjeldahl m.
2-microphone acoustic reflection m.
microsurgery m.

microwave-assisted streptavidin-biotin
  peroxidase m.
minimal access m.
modified band lid m.
Monte Carlo multiway sensitivity
  analysis m.
Moore m.
Morison m.
mother m.
Movat pentachrome m.
Mueller m.
Mueller-Walle m.
multiple cone root canal filling m.
multiple-port incision m.
Murphy m.
nail length gauge m.
Narula m.
natural m.
Needles split cast m.
needle thoracentesis m.
Neufeld dynamic m.
Nichols m.
Nikiforoff m.
Nissen fundoplication m.
Nissen-Rossetti fundoplication m.
Nitchie m.
noninvasive m.
nonresectional m.
non-rib-spreading thoracotomy
  incision m.
nonsurgical m.
numerical cipher m.
odd-even m.
Ogata m.
O'Hara 2-clamp m.
Okamoto m.
Oliver-Rosalki m.
Ollier m.
open circuit m.
optical density m.
oral-aural m.
Orsi-Grocco m.
Ouchterlony m.
oxygen step-up m.
Pachon m.
Palmer m.
Papanicolaou m.
Paris m.
Parker-Kerr closed m.
Parks m.
pause-squeeze m.
Pavlov m.

M

NOTES

467

method (*continued*)

Payr clamp m.
pedicle m.
Penaz volume-clamp m.
Penfield m.
Penn m.
percutaneous sampling m.
Pfeiffer-Comberg m.
Pfiffner and Myers m.
pharmacologic m.
phosphotungstic acid-magnesium
  chloride precipitation m.
Pichlmayer m.
pin-and-plaster m.
pinprick m.
Pizzolato peroxide-silver m.
plasma thrombin clot m.
plateau m.
plosive-injection m.
polarographic m.
Politzer m.
Pólya m.
4-port m.
prick-test m.
Pringle vascular control m.
prism m.
Prochownik m.
Puchtler alkaline Congo red m.
Puchtler Sirius red m.
Purmann m.
Puzo m.
pyramid m.
Quick m.
m. of Quinones
Rackley m.
Raff-Glantz derivative m.
rag-wheel m.
Ranawat-Dorr-Inglis m.
Ranawat triangle m.
Read rebreathing m.
reconstruction m.
Reddick-Saye m.
reduction m.
Rees-Ecker m.
reference m.
Rehfuss m.
Reichel-Pólya m.
relaxation m.
retrofilling m.
retrograde root canal filling m.
Reverdin m.
rhythm m.
Rideal-Walker m.
Risser m.
Riva-Rocci m.
Rochester m.
Rodeck m.
Russe-Gerhardt m.
Sahli m.

Salzman m.
Sandler-Dodge area-length m.
Sargenti m.
Satterthwaite m.
Scarpa m.
Schäfer m.
Schede m.
Schick m.
Schiller m.
Schober m.
Schüller m.
Schwartz m.
scientific m.
Scudder m.
sectional root canal filling m.
segmentation root canal filling m.
Seldinger m.
Sengstaken-Blakemore m.
shadowing m.
Shaffer-Hartmann m.
Shimazaki area-length m.
sigma m.
silver cone m.
silver point root canal filling m.
Silvester m.
simultaneous m.
single cone root canal filling m.
single-stick m.
sliding scale m.
Smellie m.
Smellie-Veit m.
sniff m.
Somogyi m.
special reference m.
sperm washing insemination m.
sphincter-saving m.
sphincter-sparing m.
split-cast m.
Stammer m.
standard radioenzymatic m.
Stanford biopsy m.
stapled reconstruction m.
static m.
Stegemann-Stalder m.
stereotactic core biopsy m.
Stillman m.
Stimson gravity m.
Stovall-Black m.
Strauss m.
Stroganoff m.
suction m.
surgical enucleation m.
swallow m.
Sweet m.
symptothermal m.
synthetic m.
systematic m.
Tajima m.
Tarkowski m.

tetanic stimulation m.
Thal fundoplication m.
Thane m.
Theden m.
thermally active m.
thermodilution m.
Thiersch m.
Thom flap laryngeal
  reconstruction m.
Thompson-Hatina m.
threshold shift m.
Thrombo-Wellcotest m.
Tilden m.
total fundoplication m.
Toupe m.
Towako m.
traditional m.
trapezoid m.
triangulation stapling m.
triphenyltetrazolium staining m.
trocar drainage m.
Tweed m.
twin m.
twirling m.
ultropaque m.
uncut Collis-Nissen
  fundoplication m.
unilateral inguinal hernia repair m.
Vecchietti m.
verbotonal m.
vertical condensation root canal
  filling m.
vertical-cut m.
Victor Gomel m.
visual m.
Vogel m.
volumetric m.
von Claus chronometric m.
von Kossa m.
V-slope m.
Wardill 4-flap m.
Wardill-Kilner advancement flap m.
Wardrop m.
Warthin-Starry staining m.
Waterston m.
Watson m.
Watson-Crick m.
Weiss logarithmic m.
Welcker m.
Westergren sedimentation rate m.
Wheeler m.
Willett-Stampfer m.

Wilson-White m.
Winston-Lutz m.
Wintrobe and Landsberg m.
Wintrobe sedimentation rate m.
Wolfe m.
Woolf m.
Wroblewski m.
xenon m.
x-line m.
zeta sedimentation ratio m.
zinc sulfate flotation m.
Z-track intramuscular injection m.
methylation
methylene blue dye localization
methyl-*tert*-butyl ether (MTBE)
meticulous
  m. hemostasis
  m. maneuver
metopic point
metopion
metopoplasty
metoposcopy
metrectomy
metric ophthalmoscopy
metrofibroma
metromalacoma
metroperitoneal fistula
metroplasty
  Strassman m.
metrotomy
Metzer-Boyce method
Meuli arthroplasty
Meyer
  M. cartilage
  M. incision
  M. line
  M. operation
Meyerding
  M. method
  M. spondylolisthesis classification
    line
Meyerding-Van Demark technique
Meyer-Overton
  M.-O. rule
  M.-O. theory of narcosis
Meyer-Schwickerath
  M.-S. light coagulation
  M.-S. operation
**Meyers-McKeever tibial fracture
  classification**
**Meyers quadratus muscle-pedicle bone
  graft**

M

NOTES

Meynert
  M. decussation
  M. retroflex bundle
Meyn reduction
mg
  milligram
MH
  malignant hypertension
  malignant hyperthermia
MHA-TP
  microhemagglutination *Treponema pallidum*
    MHA-TP test
MHC
  major histocompatibility complex
MI
  mesenteric ischemia
  myocardial infarction
    occlusive MI
Miami
  M. Modular Orthopaedic Spinal (MOSS)
  M. Modular Orthopaedic Spinal System
  M. pouch
micelle formation
Michaelson
  M. counter pressure
  M. operation
Michal
  M. I, II procedure
  M. II technique
Michel
  M. anomaly
  M. deformity
  M. malformation
Michele vertebral aspiration
Michigan Abuse Screening Test (MAST)
microadenoma
  pituitary m.
microadenomectomy
microaerosol
microamperage
  m. electrical nerve stimulation
  m. neural stimulation
microanastomosis
  laser-assisted m. (LAMA)
microaneurysm
microaspiration
microatheroma
microbic dissociation
microbiliary inflammation
microbubble
microcalcification
  diffuse m.
  malignant-appearing m.

  mammographic malignant-appearing m.
  suspicious m.
microcavitation
microchromoendoscopy
microcirculation
  native myocardial m.
  pulp m.
microcirculatory
  m. disturbance
  m. dysregulation
  m. failure
  m. flow
microcoil
  computed tomography-guided localization using platinum m.
microcolon
microcolpohysteroscopy
microcorneal
microcurrent therapy
microcystic disease
microdialysis
microdiffusion
microdiscectomy, microdiskectomy
  arthroscopic m.
  uniportal arthroscopic m.
microdissection
microelectrode
  m. recording
  m. recording technique
microembolization
microfilament bundle
microfistulous communication
microfollicle
microfollicular
microgastria
microgenia
microgenitalism
microglioma
micrograph
microhamartoma
microhemagglutination *Treponema pallidum* **(MHA-TP)**
microincineration
microincision
microinjection method
microinvasion
microinvasive
  m. carcinoma
  m. carcinoma classification
  m. technique
micro-Kjeldahl method
microlaparoscopic
  m. cholecystectomy
  m. Nissen fundoplication
microlaparoscopy
microlaryngoscopy
  Thornell m.
microlight guide spectrophotometry

micro liquid extraction
microlith
microlithiasis
microlumbar
    m. discectomy
    m. disc excision
micromanipulation
    gamete m.
    oocyte m.
    m. technique
micrometastasis, pl. **micrometastases**
    hematogenous m.
micrometastatic peritoneal disease
micromyelia
micron
microneurography
    sympathetic m.
microneurolysis
microneurorrhaphy
microneurovascular anastomosis
microoperative procedure
microorganism
    Gram-negative m.
    Gram-positive m.
micropapillary
    m. carcinoma
    m. subtype
micropenis
microperforation
microphone
    2-m. acoustic reflection method
microprolactinoma
microproliferation
micropuncture
microscopic
    m. absence
    m. diagnosis
    m. disease
    m. epididymal sperm aspiration
    m. invasion
    m. IPM
    m. multifocal medullary carcinoma
    m. resection
    m. sphincter
microscopically controlled surgery
microscopy
    binocular m.
    cryoelectron m.
    dark-field m.
    electron m.
    epifluorescent m.
    fluorescence m.

    fundus m.
    immersion m.
    immune electron m.
    immunofluorescence m.
    intravital m.
    light m.
    paraffin-section light m.
    polarization m.
    rotary shadowing electron m.
    scanning electron m.
    scanning force m.
    specular m.
    television m.
    transmission electron m.
microspectrofluorometry
microspectroscopy
microsphere
    radioactive m.
microstomia
microsurgery
    m. method
    m. procedure
    m. technique
    transanal endoscopic m. (TEM)
    videoendoscopic-assisted m.
microsurgical
    m. discectomy
    m. epididymal sperm aspiration
    m. epididymal sperm aspiration
     procedure
    m. free flap
    m. inguinal varicocelectomy
    m. reconstruction
    m. technique
    m. tubocornual anastomosis
microtia
microtrabecular hepatocellular carcinoma
microtransducer technique
microtraumatic insult
microtremor
    ocular m.
micro-tubulotomy technique
microvascular
    m. decompression (MVD)
    m. free flap
    m. free flap transfer
    m. surgical anastomosis
    m. technique
microvessel
microvillous membrane
microwave
    m. coagulation

M

NOTES

microwave *(continued)*
    m. fixation
    m. radiation injury
    m. therapy
    m. thermotherapy
microwave-assisted streptavidin-biotin peroxidase method
microwelding
micrurgical
micturition pain
midabdominal transverse incision
midaxillary
    m. line
    m. line incision
midazolam-induced excitatory reaction
midbody tumor
midbrain reticular formation
MIDCAB
    minimally invasive direct coronary artery bypass
midcarpal
    m. arthroscopy
    m. dislocation
    m. fusion
midcarpal fusion
midclavicular
    m. line
    m. port
midcoronal plane
middle
    m. cerebral artery (MCA)
    m. cerebral artery occlusion
    m. ear infection
    m. latency auditory evoked potential (MLAEP)
    m. latency auditory evoked response (MLAER)
    m. meatus
    m. mediastinum
    m. phalanx
midesophageal traction diverticulum
midexpiratory/midinspiratory flow ratio
midface
    m. degloving technique
    m. fracture
midfoot fracture
midforceps maneuver
midfrontal
    m. plane
    m. plane coronal section
midgastric transverse sphincter
midgut volvulus
midheel line
midhumeral line
midlateral approach
midline
    m. abdominal crease
    m. aponeurotic closure
    m. disc herniation

    m. exposure
    m. forehead flap
    m. incisional hernia
    m. incisional hernioplasty
    m. lower abdominal incision
    m. medial approach
    m. myelotomy
    m. oblique incision
    m. position
    m. spinal approach
    m. upper abdominal incision
midmalleolar line
midoccipital
midpalatal suture opening
midpalmar
    m. abscess
    m. space
midpapillary
    anterior m. (AM)
midpapillary-longitudinal (MP-L)
midpapillary-transverse (MP-T)
midpelvis
midpoint to meatal line
midriff
midsagittal
    m. plane
    m. section
midscapular line
midsection
midshaft fracture
midsigmoid sphincter
midsternal line
midsternum
midthalamic plane
Mielke bleeding time
MIGET
    multiple inert gas elimination technique
migraine
    abdominal m.
    m. abortive therapy
    basilar artery m.
    familial hemiplegic m.
    retinal m.
    vertiginous m.
migrating abscess
migration
    m. abnormality
    calculus m.
    cell m.
    cellular m.
    electrode m.
    embolus m.
    epithelial m.
    fibroblast m.
    gallstone m.
    graft m.
    implant m.
    instrument m.
    intragastric prosthesis m.

intravesical m.
lymphocyte m.
macrophagic m.
neural crest m.
neuronal m.
neutrophil m.
phagocyte m.
physiologic mesial m.
pigmentary m.
placental m.
rod m.
stage m.
tooth m.
trochanteric m.
tube m.
m. velocity
mika operation
Mikulicz
M. colostomy
M. incision
M. operation
M. pyloroplasty
M. sac
Milch
M. condylar fracture classification
M. cuff resection
M. cuff resection of ulna technique
M. elbow fracture classification
M. elbow technique
M. humeral fracture classification
mild traumatic brain injury (MTBI)
Miles
M. abdominoperineal resection
M. operation
Milford mallet finger technique
miliary
m. abscess
m. aneurysm
m. granulomatous inflammation
military
m. brace position
m. tuck position
milk
m. duct
m. gland
m. spot
milk-ejection reflex
milk-filled cyst
milkmaid elbow dislocation
milkman fracture
milky ascites

Mill
Magenstrasse and M. (M&M)
Millard
M. advancement rotation flap reconstruction
M. rotation-advancement lip repair
Millender arthroplasty
Millen-Read modification
Millen technique
mille pattes technique
Miller
M. flatfoot operation
M. procedure
Miller-Galante knee arthroplasty
Millesi
M. interfascicular graft
M. modified technique
M. nerve graft
millibar
millicurie (mCi)
Milligan-Morgan hemorrhoidectomy
milligram (mg)
milligram-hour
millimicrogram
milliosmole/kilogram
Miltner-Wan calcaneus resection
mimetic muscle
MIN
multiple intestinal neoplasia
mind-body therapy
mineral
m. oil aspiration
m. oil foreign body
mineralized tissue
Ming gastric carcinoma classification
miniature
m. end-plate potential
m. uterine cavity
minicholecystostomy
surgical-radiologic m.
minification
minikeratoplasty
Castroviejo m.
minilaparoscopic cholecystectomy
minilaparotomy
m. incision
m. technique
minimal
m. access general surgery
m. access method
m. access procedure

M

NOTES

minimal *(continued)*
- m. access spine technology (MAST)
- m. access technique
- m. air
- m. alveolar concentration
- m. anesthetic concentration (MAC)
- m. bactericidal concentration
- m. change disease
- m. change nephrotic syndrome
- m. incision pubovaginal suspension
- m. incision total hip retractor
- m. leak technique
- m. lesion nephrotic syndrome
- m. transurethral resection

minimally
- m. displaced fracture
- m. invasive approach
- m. invasive biopsy
- m. invasive direct coronary artery bypass (MIDCAB)
- m. invasive esophagectomy
- m. invasive mitral valve repair
- m. invasive nature
- m. invasive parathyroidectomy
- m. invasive procedure
- m. invasive robotic heart valve surgery
- m. invasive surgery (MIS)
- m. invasive surgical access
- m. invasive surgical technique
- m. invasive video-assisted parathyroidectomy (MIVAP)

minimum
- m. alveolar anesthetic concentration (MAC)
- m. alveolar concentration (MAC)
- 1-m. alveolar concentration (1-MAC)
- m. audible pressure
- m. bactericidal concentration
- m. detectable concentration
- m. effective analgesic concentration
- m. effective concentration (MEC)
- m. lethal concentration
- m. local analgesic concentration (MLAC)

ministernotomy

minithoracotomy

Minkoff-Jaffe-Menendez posterior approach

Minkoff-Nicholas procedure

Minnesota EKG classification

minor
- m. amputation
- m. calix
- m. duodenal papilla
- m. fissure
- m. manifestation

- m. operation
- m. splenic injury
- m. sublingual duct
- m. surgery
- trochanter m.

Minsky operation

minute
- alveolar ventilation per m.
- 1-m. endoscopy room test
- physiological dead space ventilation per m.
- m. polypoid lesion
- m. volume

Mirizzi syndrome

mirror-image
- m.-i. breast biopsy
- m.-i. interpretation
- m.-i. laryngoscopy
- m.-i. reflection

MIS
- minimally invasive surgery

misarticulation

misdirection phenomenon

mismatch
- prosthesis-patient m.
- ventilation/perfusion m.

misregistration
- chemical shift m.
- flow m.
- oblique flow m.

missed fracture

missile
- m. injury
- m. track abscess
- m. trajectory

missionary position

mistranslation

Mital elbow release technique

Mitchell osteotomy

miter technique

mitochondrial myopathy, encephalopathy, lactic acidosis, and strokelike syndrome (MELAS)

mitomycin transarterial embolization treatment

mitosis

mitotic activity

mitral
- m. balloon commissurotomy
- m. balloon valvotomy
- m. regurgitation murmur
- m. valve
- m. valve aneurysm
- m. valve anulus
- m. valve area
- m. valve closure index
- m. valve disorder
- m. valve gradient
- m. valve homograft graft

m. valve insufficiency
m. valve leaflet
m. valve prolapse, aortic anomalies, skeletal changes, skin changes (MASS)
m. valve prolapse syndrome
m. valve repair
m. valve replacement
m. valve-transverse (MV-T)
m. valve valvotomy
m. valvuloplasty

mitralization

Mitrofanoff
M. appendicovesicostomy
M. conduit
M. continent urinary diversion technique
M. principle
M. procedure
M. stoma

mittelschmerz

MIVAP
minimally invasive video-assisted parathyroidectomy

mixed
m. acid fermentation
m. chancre
m. connective tissue disease
m. connective tissue disorder
m. density mass
m. fat-water density lesion
m. fungal/bacterial infection
m. fungal organism
m. hemorrhoid
m. malignant glioma
m. nail infection
m. nerve
m. nodule
m. sclerotic and lytic bone lesion
m. tumor
m. venous-lymphatic malformation
m. venous oxygen content
m. venous oxygen saturation

mixture
anesthetic gas m.
epinephrine-anesthetic m.
racemic m.

Mize-Bucholz-Grogen approach

Mizuno-Hirohata-Kashiwagi technique

Mizuno technique

mks
meter-kilogram-second

MLAC
minimum local analgesic concentration

MLAEP
middle latency auditory evoked potential

MLAER
middle latency auditory evoked response

M line

MLN
mesenteric lymph node

MLR
major liver resection

M&M
Magenstrasse and Mill
M&M procedure

MMF
maxillomandibular fixation

MMK
Marshall-Marchetti-Krantz
MMK procedure

MMP
matrix metalloproteinase

Moberg
M. advancement flap
M. key-pinch procedure

Moberg-Gedda
M.-G. fracture
M.-G. open reduction

mobile
m. arc
m. sternum

mobility
abdominal wall m.
impaired m.
muscle tissue m.
rotation m.
translation m.

mobilization
circumferential m.
colonic m.
dorsal thyroid m.
esophageal m.
grade 1–5 m.
intraperitoneal m.
joint m.
lateral band m.
localized leukocyte m.
nonthrust m.
rectal m.
soft tissue m.
spinal joint m.
stapes m.
stem cell m.

M

NOTES

mobilization (*continued*)
m. test
thoracoscopic esophageal m.
m. with impulse

MOD
mesioocclusodistal
multiple organ dysfunction

modality
adjuvant diagnostic m.
diagnostic m.
imaging m.
implantable pain m.
nonexcisional m.
therapeutic m.
treatment m.

mode
Effler-Groves m.
tumor dormancy m.

model
corpectomy m.
Emory Pain Estimate M. (EPEM)
Gail m.
guidance-cooperation m.
implant m.
mutual participation m.
tumor kinetic m.
Zimmerman-Brittin exchange m.

modeling-derivation

moderate
m. hyperplasia
m. pain
m. resuscitative hypothermia

moderator band

modification
activator m.
Al-Ghorab m.
appliance m.
Astler-Coller m.
A-V nodal m.
Bateman m.
beak m.
Bloom-Raney m.
Bonfiglio m.
bracket m.
Bunnell m.
Burch m.
Burwell-Scott m. of Watson-Jones
incision
C-D screw m.
Clark-Southwick-Odgen m.
Counsellor-Flor m.
Deller m.
Duncan-Lovell m.
environment m.
fiber tip m.
Fielding m.
Furlow-Fisher m.
Gesell test with Knobloch m.
glutathione m.

Gunderson-Sosin m.
Harriluque sublaminar wiring m.
Hughes m.
interference m.
Kelly-Kennedy m.
Kleinert m.
Knobloch m.
Lester Martin m.
Losee m.
Martin m.
Mason-Likar limb lead m.
Millen-Read m.
Mullins m.
Muzsnai m.
Neer m.
Pereyra-Lebhertz m.
posttranslation m.
racemic m.
Raz m.
Rosch m.
Rossetti m.
Sade m.
Sammarco-DiRaimondo m.
Schoemaker m.
Seddon m.
Sequeira-Khanuja m.
Sever m.
Smith m.
Soper m.
Stamey m.
Stauffer m.
Strickland m.
thiol m.
Van Herick m.
Weinberg m.
Youngwhich m.

modified
m. band lid method
m. Bassini herniorrhaphy
m. Belsey fundoplication
m. Belsey fundoplication procedure
m. Belsey fundoplication technique
m. Blalock-Taussig shunt
m. brachial technique
m. Cantwell technique
m. Child technique
m. coracoid approach infraclavicular
brachial plexus block
m. dorsalis pedis myofascial flap
m. Essed-Schroeder corporoplasty
m. flap operation
m. Gibson incision
m. Hassan open technique
m. Heller esophagomyotomy
m. Hoke-Miller flatfoot procedure
m. Irving-type tubal ligation
m. Konno procedure
m. lithotomy position
m. mastopexy

m. McVay herniorrhaphy
m. method of Pugh
m. mold and surface replacement arthroplasty
m. Norfolk procedure
m. piggyback (MPB)
m. piggyback technique
m. Pomeroy technique
m. 2-portal endoscopic carpal tunnel release
m. radical hysterectomy
m. radical mastectomy
m. radical mastoidectomy
m. radical neck dissection
m. Raynaud phenomenon
m. Ritgen maneuver
m. Sacks-Vine push-pull technique
m. Seldinger procedure
m. Seldinger technique
m. Shouldice hernioplasty
m. Sugiura procedure
m. surgical approach
m. TAPP hernioplasty
The M. Somatic Pain Questionnaire
m. Toupe procedure
m. Toupe technique
m. tumescent technique
m. ultrafiltration
m. Van Lint anesthesia
m. V-Y advancement technique
m. Weber-Fergusson procedure
m. Whitehead hemorrhoidectomy
m. Wies procedure
m. Young urethroplasty
M. Zung Depression Scale

modiolus, pl. **modioli**

MODS
multiple organ dysfunction syndrome

modulation
amplitude m.
antigenic m.
autonomic m.
biochemical m.
brightness m.
frequency m.
immune m.
obstruction-induced m.
pain m.
m. potential
pressure amplitude m.
sex steroid m.
specific m.

module
dialysate preparation m.

Moebius anomaly

Moe scoliosis technique

MOF
multiorgan failure
multiple organ failure

Mogensen procedure

Mohrenheim
M. fossa
M. space

Mohr syndrome

Mohs
M. fresh tissue chemosurgery technique
M. micrographic surgery
M. microsurgery technique
M. microsurgical resection

moist
m. gangrene
m. mucous membrane

molar
anchor m.
m. teeth
m. tooth fracture
m. tube

mold acetabular arthroplasty

molding
compression m.
injection m.
tissue m.

molecular
m. biology
m. external layer
m. genetics
m. lesion
m. mass
m. sieve
m. technique

Molesworth-Campbell elbow approach

Molesworth osteotomy

Moll gland

Moloney
M. hernia repair
M. line

Molteno
M. drainage
M. episcleral explant

moment
activation m.
3-point bending m.

M

NOTES

477

Monakow
M. bundle
M. tract
Moncrieff operation
Mondini
M. anomaly
M. deformity
M. pulmonary arteriovenous
malformation
Mondini-Alexander malformation
Mondor disease
Monfort operation
monilial infection
monitor
intraoperative m.
monitored
m. anesthesia care (MAC)
m. anesthesia care anesthesia
m. anesthesia care anesthetic
technique
m. anesthesia control
monitoring
airway gas m.
ambulatory blood pressure m.
anesthetic m.
anticoagulant m.
anticoagulation m.
bispectral index m.
blood pressure m.
central venous pressure m.
close m.
depth of anesthesia m.
2-dimensional m.
ECoG m.
electrophysiologic m.
epicardial m.
esophageal pH m.
evoked external urethral sphincter
potential m.
external fetal m.
fetal heart rate m.
hemodynamic m.
hospital m.
intracranial pressure m.
intraoperative neurophysiologic m.
(IOM)
intraoperative parathyroid
hormone m.
intraoperative transcranial
Doppler m.
invasive hemodynamic m.
laboratory m.
neuromuscular blockade m.
outcome m.
posttetanic count m.
radiation m.
screw position perioperative m.
standard patient m.
m. technique

tissue pH m.
transcutaneous oxygen m.
vigilance m.
water vapor m.
monoamine reuptake-inhibitor
monobloc
monochromatic aberration
monoclonal
m. adenoma
m. antibody (MAb)
m. component
m. expansion
m. growth
monoclonality
monocular fixation
monodermoma
monodisperse
monofixation syndrome
monoinfection
monomalleolar ankle fracture
mononuclear cell infiltration
monoparesis
monopolar
m. coagulation
m. electrocautery
m. electrocoagulation
m. radiofrequency probe
monorchidic
monorchidism
monorecidive chancre
monospherical total shoulder
arthroplasty
monotherapy
oral m.
monotypic lesion
monoxide
carbon m. (CO)
dinitrogen m.
nitrogen m.
Monro
bursa of M.
M. foramen
M. line
Monro-Richter line
mons, pl. **montes**
m. plasty
m. pubis
Monte Carlo multiway sensitivity
analysis method
Monteggia
M. dislocation
M. equivalent lesion
M. forearm fracture
Montercaux fracture
montes (*pl. of* mons)
Montgomery
M. gland
M. tracheostomy
Monticelli-Spinelli distraction technique

mood state
Moore
> M. fracture
> M. method
> M. osteotomy-osteoclasis
> M. posterior approach
> M. technique
> M. tibial plateau fracture classification

Moran operation
Morax
> M. keratoplasty
> M. operation

morbidity
> cumulative operative m.
> m. excess
> febrile m.
> intraoperative m.
> long-term m.
> m. and mortality
> perioperative m.
> postoperative m.

morbidly obese patient
morcel
morcellation
> m. operation
> Robinson m.
> m. technique

morcellement
morcellized bone graft
Moreland-Marder-Anspach femoral stem removal
Morel-Fatio-Lalardie operation
Morel-Lavele lesion
Morgagni
> M. cartilage
> M. caruncle
> M. crypt
> M. foramen
> M. fossa
> M. fovea
> M. frenum
> M. hernia
> M. lacuna
> M. retinaculum
> M. sinus
> M. tubercle
> M. ventricle

Morgagni-Larrey type hernia
Morgan-Casscells meniscus suturing technique
Morganella morganii

morganii
> *Morganella m.*

Morgan line
moribund
Morison
> M. incision
> M. method
> M. pouch

morning glory optic disc anomaly
morphallactic regeneration
morpheaform basal cell carcinoma
morphea-like lesion
morphine
> m. narcotic analgesic therapy
> m. sulfate extended-release liposome injection

morphogenesis
> branching m.

morphological difference
morphologic classification
morphology
> endometrial m.
> Gram stain m.
> lesion m.

Morquio syndrome
Morrey-Bryan total elbow arthroplasty
Morris hepatoma cell line
Morrison
> M. neurovascular free flap
> M. pouch
> M. technique

Morse head
mortality
> cause-specific m.
> cumulative operative m.
> disease-associated m.
> hospital m.
> morbidity and m.
> operative m.
> perioperative m.
> postoperative m.
> m. rate

mortar kidney
mortification
Morton plane
mosaicplasty
> autologous osteochondral m.

Moschcowitz procedure
Mose technique
Mosher operation
Mosher-Toti operation

M

NOTES

MOSS
    Miami Modular Orthopaedic Spinal
Moss
    M. classification
    M. operation
Motais operation
moth-eaten
    m.-e. appearance
    m.-e. bone destruction
mother
    m. cyst
    m. method
moth patch
motilin
    m. effect
    m. level
motility
    contractile m.
    cyclic fasting m.
    m. disturbance
    ineffective esophageal m.
    jejunal m.
    postoperative m.
    upper jejunal m.
motion
    abdominal respiratory m.
    angulation m.
    m. barrier
    helical axis of m.
    osteokinematic m.
    pattern of m.
    range of m. (ROM)
    m. segment
    translation m.
motion-preserving procedure
motivating operation
motor
    m. activity
    m. anomaly
    m. change
    m. decussation
    m. disturbance
    m. examination
    m. fusion
    m. nerve
    m. oil peritoneal fluid
    m. paraplegia
    m. pattern
    m. perseveration
    m. point
    m. point block
    m. point block anesthetic technique
    m. recording
    m. response
motor-evoked
    m.-e. potential (MEP)
    m.-e. response (MER)
    m.-e. response to transcranial
      stimulation (tc-MER)

Mott body
mottled appearance
Mouchet fracture
Mould arthroplasty
mounted point stone
mouse
    joint m.
    peritoneal m.
mouth preparation
mouth-to-mouth
    m.-t.-m. respiration
    m.-t.-m. resuscitation
    m.-t.-m. ventilation
movable
    m. joint
    m. kidney
    m. spleen
    m. testis
Movat pentachrome method
movement
    anterosuperior external ilium m.
    border tissue m.
    bowel m.
    m. disorder
    dissociation m.
    external ilium m.
    extraneous m.
    extraocular m.
    fetal body m.
    head m.
    posteroinferior external m.
    primary rotation m.
    saccadic eye m.
    segmentation m.
    sound-stimulated fetal m.
    vocal cord m.
movement-related pain
moving time average (MTA)
Moynihan
    M. operation
    M. position
MPAC
    Memorial Pain Assessment Card
MPB
    modified piggyback
    MPB technique
MPD
    main pancreatic duct
MPGR
    multiple planar gradient-recalled
    MPGR technique
MPI
    Multidimensional Pain Inventory
MP-L
    midpapillary-longitudinal
    MP-L image
MPQ
    McGill Pain Questionnaire

MP-RAGE
magnitude preparation-rapid acquisition
gradient echo
MP-RAGE technique
MP-T
midpapillary-transverse
MP-T image
MPT
multidisciplinary pain treatment
MR
magnetic resonance
MR spectroscopy
MRA
magnetic resonance angiography
low-field contrast-enhanced body
MRA
MRCP
magnetic resonance
cholangiopancreatography
MRI
magnetic resonance imaging
MRI cholangiography
intraoperative MRI
MSB
mediastinal shed blood
MSI
magnetic source imaging
MSOF
multisystem organ failure
MTA
moving time average
MTBE
methyl-*tert*-butyl ether
MTBE therapy
MTBI
mild traumatic brain injury
MTSS
medial tibial stress syndrome
**Mubarak-Hargens decompression
technique**
mucilaginous gland
mucinous
m. adenocarcinoma
m. ascites
m. cystadenocarcinoma
m. cystic neoplasm (MCN)
muciparous gland
mucobuccal
m. fold
m. reflection
mucocele
appendix m.

breast m.
frontal sinus m.
frontoethmoidal m.
maxillary sinus m.
orbital m.
paranasal m.
retention m.
sinus m.
sphenoid m.
mucociliary
m. clearance
m. function
mucocutaneous
m. hemorrhoid
m. junction
m. lesion
m. lymph node syndrome
m. manifestation
m. muscle
m. pigmentation of Peutz-Jeghers
syndrome
mucoepidermal carcinoma
mucoepidermoid
m. carcinoma
m. tumor
mucogingival
m. line
m. surgery
mucoid ascites
mucoperichondrial flap
mucoperiosteal
m. periodontal flap
m. periodontal graft
m. sliding flap
mucopolysaccharidosis
mucopurulent exudate
mucopyocele
Mucor **infection**
mucormycosis
mucosa
bursa m.
colorectal m.
devitalize the tracheal m.
ectopic gastric m.
endocervical m.
gastric m.
gastroduodenal m.
inlet patch m.
lingual m.
multifocal ectopic gastric m.
oral m.
pharyngeal m.

M

NOTES

mucosa *(continued)*
    ulcerated m.
    upper respiratory tract m.
mucosa-associated
    m.-a. lymphoid tissue (MALT)
    m.-a. lymphoid tissue lymphoma
mucosal
    m. ablation
    m. abnormality
    m. advancement
    m. atrophy
    m. barrier
    m. biopsy
    m. bridge
    m. destruction
    m. esophageal ring
    m. hernia
    m. homeostasis
    m. inflammation
    m. invasion
    m. lesion
    m. line
    m. needle aspiration
    m. neuroma syndrome
    m. patch replacement
    m. periodontal flap
    m. periodontal graft
    m. proctectomy
    m. reconditioning
    m. relaxing incision technique
    m. remnant
    m. repair
    m. tunic
    m. ulceration
    m. vascular dilation
    m. web
    m. weight
mucosa-to-mucosa
    m.-t.-m. anastomosis
    m.-t.-m. Roux-en-Y
      hepaticojejunostomy
mucosectomy
    endoanal m.
    endoscopic m.
    rectal m.
    transabdominal m.
    transanal m.
mucositis
    radiation m.
mucous
    m. colic
    m. desiccation
    m. fistula
    m. gland
    m. membrane
    m. membrane graft
    m. membrane lesion
    m. membrane ulceration

    m. patch
    m. plug syndrome
    m. sheath
mucronate
mucus
    excess m.
mud bed
Muehrcke line
Mueller
    M. femoral supracondylar fracture
      classification
    M. hip arthroplasty
    M. intertochanteric varus osteotomy
    M. maneuver
    M. method
    M. operation
    M. patellar tendon graft
    M. technique
    M. tibial fracture classification
    M. transposition osteotomy
Mueller-type femoral head replacement
Mueller-Walle method
MUGA
    multiple gated acquisition
      MUGA exercise stress test
mulberry
    m. calculus
    m. lesion
mulberry-shaped mass
Mules
    M. graft
    M. operation
Mulholland sphincterotomy
Müller
    M. capsule
    M. duct
    M. duct body
    M. maneuver
Müller-Hillis maneuver
müllerian
    m. duct anomaly
    m. duct derivation syndrome
    m. duct fusion
    m. inhibiting substance
Mullins
    M. blade technique
    M. modification
multangular
    m. bone
    m. ridge fracture
multiaxial
    m. classification
    m. joint
multicentricity
multicentric study
multidetector computed tomography
    (MDCT)
Multidimensional Pain Inventory (MPI)

multidisciplinary
 m. approach
 m. pain treatment (MPT)
multidose vial
multifactorial
multifetal pregnancy reduction
multifetation
multifidus muscle
multifocal
 m. change
 m. ectopic gastric mucosa
 m. enhancing lesion
 m. extensive DCIS
 m. extensive disease
 m. inflammation
 m. tumor
 m. variety
multigated angiogram
multigland
 m. disease
 m. hyperplasia
multiglandular
 m. disease
 m. parathyroid hyperplasia
multi-infection
multilamellar body
multilevel
 m. atherosclerotic arterial occlusive
  disease
 m. fracture
 m. laminectomy
multilocular
 m. cyst
 m. cystic lesion
multiloculated renal mass
multimerization
multimodal
 m. adjuvant therapy
 m. analgesia
multimodality therapy
multinodular goiter
multiorgan
 m. failure (MOF)
 m. hernia
 m. system dysfunction
 m. system failure
multiparameter sensor
multiplanar image
multiple
 m. calcification
 m. cone root canal filling method
 m. core biopsy

 m. endocrine neoplasia (MEN)
 m. endocrine neoplasia type 2a
  (MEN-2a)
 m. endocrine neoplasia syndrome
  (type 2a, 2b)
 m. endocrinopathy
 m. exostoses
 m. fracture
 m. gated acquisition (MUGA)
 m. gland hyperplasia
 m. hamartoma syndrome
 m. hepatitis virus infection
 m. hydatid disease
 m. inert gas elimination technique
  (MIGET)
 m. inert gas exchange
 m. intestinal neoplasia (MIN)
 m. line scan imaging
 m. macrocyst
 m. mucosal neuroma syndrome
 m. myeloma staging
 m. organ dysfunction (MOD)
 m. organ dysfunction syndrome
  (MODS)
 m. organ failure (MOF)
 m. organ failure syndrome
 m. organ system failure
 m. planar gradient-recalled (MPGR)
 m. pterygium syndrome
 m. ray amputation
 m. sensitive point
 m. shunt levels
 m. site
 m. spin-echo imaging
 m. system atrophy
 m. system organ failure
 m. therapy
multiple-balloon valvuloplasty
multiple-echo imaging
multiple-mechanism inhaled anesthetic
multiple-plane imaging
multiple-point sacral fixation
multiple-port
 m.-p. incision
 m.-p. incision method
 m.-p. incision procedure
 m.-p. incision technique
multiple-punch resection
multiple-site inhaled anesthetic
multiple-stage approach
multipolar
 m. coagulation

M

NOTES

multipolar *(continued)*
    m. electrocautery
    m. electrocoagulation
multipotential stem cell
multiray fracture
multisegmental resection
multistaged carrier flap
**Multistage Maximal Effort exercise
  stress test**
multisystem
    m. disorder
    m. failure
    m. organ failure (MSOF)
multivessel PTCA
multiviscera
multivisceral graft
Muma Assessment Program
Mumford
    M. procedure
    M. resection
Mumford-Gurd arthroplasty
mummification
    m. necrosis
    pulp m.
Munro
    M. and Parker laparoscopic
      hysterectomy classification
    M. point
Munro-Kerr maneuver
mu receptor
murine
    m. graft
    m. mesangial cell line
murmur
    aortic regurgitation m.
    Austin Flint m.
    diamond ejection m.
    ejection m.
    endocardial m.
    exit block m.
    exocardial m.
    expiratory m.
    extracardiac m.
    mitral regurgitation m.
    reduplication m.
    systolic ejection m.
Murphy method
muscarinic
    m. agonist
    m. receptor
muscle
    abdominal external oblique m.
    abdominal internal oblique m.
    abductor hallucis m.
    abductor longus m.
    abductor magnus m.
    abductor pollicis brevis m.
    abductor pollicis longus m.
    Aeby m.

airway smooth m. (ASM)
Albinus m.
anconeus m.
antagonistic m.
anterior auricular m.
anterior cervical intertransverse m.
anterior rectus m.
anterior scalene m.
anterior serratus m.
anterior tibial m.
antigravity m.
antitragicus m.
appendicular m.
aryepiglottic m.
arytenoid m.
auricular m.
axial m.
Bell m.
2-bellied m.
belt m.
m. biopsy
bipennate m.
Bovero m.
brachial m.
brachioradial m.
branchiomeric m.
Braune m.
m. breakdown
broadest m.
bronchoesophageal m.
buccinator m.
bulbocavernosus m.
bulbospongiosus m.
m. cachexia
Casser perforated m.
ceratocricoid m.
cervical rotator m.
cheek m.
chin m.
chondroglossus m.
circular pharyngeal m.
coccygeal m.
coccygeus m.
Coiter m.
compressor naris m.
coracobrachial m.
coracobrachialis m.
corrugator cutis m.
corrugator supercilii m.
cowl m.
cremasteric m.
cricoarytenoid m.
cricopharyngeus m.
cricothyroid m.
cruciate m.
crus m.
cutaneomucous m.
cutaneous m.
dartos m.

deepithelialized rectus abdominis m. (DRAM)
deltoid m.
detrusor m.
digastric m.
dilator m.
m. dissection
m. distraction
dorsal sacrococcygeal m.
Duverney m.
m. dystonia
elevator m.
m. energy technique
epicranial m.
epicranius m.
erector spinae m.
extensor carpi radialis brevis m.
extensor carpi radialis longus m.
extensor carpi ulnaris m.
extensor digiti minimi m.
extensor digiti quinti m.
extensor digitorum brevis m.
extensor digitorum communis m.
extensor digitorum longus m.
extensor hallucis brevis m.
extensor hallucis longus m.
extensor indicis proprius m.
extensor pollicis brevis m.
extensor pollicis longus m.
extraocular m.
extrinsic m.
facial m.
femoral m.
fibularis brevis m.
fibularis longus m.
fibularis tertius m.
fixator m.
m. flap
flexor hallucis brevis m.
frontalis m.
Gavard m.
genioglossal m.
geniohyoid m.
glossopalatine m.
gluteus maximus m.
greater rhomboid m.
Guthrie m.
hamstring m.
m. hernia
Horner m.
Houston m.
hyoglossal m.

hyoid m.
hypothenar m.
iliac m.
iliococcygeal m.
iliocostal m.
iliohypogastric m.
iliopsoas m.
infrahyoid m.
interosseous m.
interspinal m.
intertransverse m.
intrinsic m.
ischiocavernous m.
Jung m.
Klein m.
Kohlrausch m.
Krause m.
laryngeal m.
lateral m.
longissimus m.
longus capitis m.
longus colli m.
m. lysis
Marcacci m.
masseter m.
mastication m.
m. measurement
mentalis m.
Merkel m.
mimetic m.
mucocutaneous m.
multifidus m.
muscular fascia
mylohyoid m.
nasal m.
oblique abdominal m.
oblique arytenoid m.
oblique auricular m.
occipitofrontal m.
occipitofrontalis m.
ocular m.
omohyoid m.
orbicular m.
orbital m.
orbitalis m.
palatoglossus m.
palatopharyngeal sphincter m.
palatopharyngeus m.
palpebral m.
pectoralis m.
pectorodorsal m.
pennate m.

NOTES

M

muscle *(continued)*

perineal m.
peroneal m.
peroneus brevis m.
peroneus longus m.
peroneus tertius m.
piriform m.
plantar interosseous m.
plantar quadrate m.
platysma m.
pleuroesophageal m.
popliteal m.
posterior cricoarytenoid m.
procerus m.
pronator quadratus m.
pronator teres m.
m. proteolysis
psoas major m.
psoas minor m.
pubococcygeal m.
puboprostatic m.
puborectal m.
pubovaginal m.
pubovesical m.
pupillae sphincter m.
pupillary m.
pyramidal auricular m.
quadrate m.
radial dilator m.
rectococcygeal m.
rectourethral m.
rectouterine m.
rectovesical m.
rectus abdominis m.
red m.
Reisseisen m.
m. relaxant
m. repositioning
m. resection
rhomboid major m.
rhomboid minor m.
ribbon m.
Riolan m.
risorius m.
rotator cuff m.
salpingopharyngeal m.
scalenus anterior m.
scalenus medius m.
scalenus minimus m.
scalenus posterior m.
scalp m.
scapular m.
Sebileau m.
second tibial m.
semimembranosus m.
semispinal m.
semispinalis capitis m.
semispinalis cervicis m.
semitendinosus m.

serratus anterior m.
serratus posterior inferior m.
serratus posterior superior m.
shunt m.
Sibson m.
skeletal m.
m. sliding operation
smooth m.
Soemmerring m.
sphincter m.
spinal m.
stapedius m.
sternal m.
sternochondroscapular m.
sternoclavicular m.
sternocleidomastoid m.
sternohyoid m.
sternomastoid m.
sternothyroid m.
strap m.
striated m.
styloauricular m.
styloglossus m.
stylohyoid m.
stylopharyngeal m.
subclavian m.
subcostal m.
suboccipital m.
subscapular m.
subscapularis m.
supinator m.
supraclavicular m.
suprahyoid m.
supraspinalis m.
supraspinatus m.
supraspinous m.
suspensory m.
synergistic m.
temporal m.
temporoparietal m.
tensor fascia lata m.
teres major m.
Theile m.
thenar m.
thoracic interspinal m.
thoracic intertransverse m.
thoracic longissimus m.
thoracic rotator m.
thyroarytenoid m.
thyroepiglottic m.
thyrohyoid m.
thyroid m.
tibial m.
m. tissue mobility
toe extensor m.
Toynbee m.
trachealis m.
tracheloclavicular m.
tragicus m.

transverse abdominal m.
transverse arytenoid m.
transverse rectus abdominis m.
  (TRAM)
transversospinal m.
transversus abdominis m.
Treitz m.
triangular m.
true m.
unipennate m.
unstriated m.
uvular m.
Valsalva m.
ventral sacrococcygeus m.
vestigial m.
visceral m.
vocal m.
vocalis m.
m. wasting
m. weakness
white m.
Wilson m.
wrinkler m.
zygomaticus major m.
zygomaticus minor m.
muscle-balancing procedure
muscle-periosteal flap
muscle-plasty
Speed V-Y m.-p.
muscle-sparing
m.-s. incision
m.-s. thoracotomy
muscle-splitting
m.-s. incision
m.-s. technique
muscle-tendon transplantation
muscular
m. anesthesia
m. artery
m. atrophy
m. change
m. coat
m. contraction
m. dystrophy (MD)
m. esophageal ring
m. fascia
m. pulley
m. substance
m. tissue
m. triangle
m. tunic

muscularis tunnel closure
musculature
musculi (*pl. of* musculus)
musculoaponeurotic layer
musculocutaneous
m. free flap
m. nerve
musculomembranous
musculophrenic
m. artery
m. vein
musculoplasty
Rambo m.
musculoskeletal
m. disorder
m. infection
m. system
m. tissue
m. tumor
musculospiral
m. groove
m. nerve
musculotendinous
m. cuff
m. flap
musculotubal canal
musculus, pl. **musculi**
mushroom
corneal m.
m. corneal graft
mushroom-shaped mass
mussitation
Mustard
M. intraatrial procedure
M. operation
Mustardé
M. operation
M. otoplasty
M. rotational cheek flap
mutation
m. analysis
breast cancer-related m.
m. carrier
m. carrier status
factor V Leiden m.
somatic m.
true m.
mutator gene
mutilation
mutual participation model
Muzsnai modification

M

NOTES

MV
maternal venous
MV blood
MVD
microvascular decompression
MV-T
mitral valve-transverse
MV-T image
MVV
maximum voluntary ventilation
mycelial mass
mycobacterial infection
Mycobacterium
M. avium complex infection
M. avium-intracellulare (MAI)
M. avium-intracellulare infection
Mycoplasma **infection**
mycotic
m. aneurysm
m. club nail
m. infection
m. pseudoaneurysm
myectomy
anorectal m.
m. operation
rectal m.
septal m.
myectopy
myelination
nerve fiber m.
optic pathway m.
myelinization
myelinolysis
central pontine m.
pontine m.
myelitis
myeloablation
myeloblastoma
myelocele
myelocystocele
myelocystomeningocele
myelocytoma
myelodiastasis
myelodysplasia
myeloid tissue
myelolipoma
myelolysis
myeloma
myelomalacia
myelomeningocele
m. operation
m. repair
myelomonocytic cell line
myelonic
myelopathic symptom
myelopathy
cervical spondylitic m.
radiation m.
spondylitic m.

myelophthisic
myelophthisis
myelopoiesis
extramedullary m.
myelorrhagia
myelorrhaphy
commissural m.
myelosarcoma
myeloschisis
myeloscopy
flexible fiberoptic m.
myelotomy
Bischof m.
commissural m.
midline m.
T m.
myenteric
m. plexus
m. reflex
myenteron
mylohyoid
m. artery
m. bridge
m. fossa
m. groove
m. line
m. muscle
m. nerve
m. ridge
mylohyoideus
mylopharyngeus
myoablative therapy
myoarchitectonic
myoblastoma
myocardial
m. contusion
m. cytochrome
m. hibernation
m. infarction (MI)
m. inflammation
m. ischemia
m. ischemic preconditioning
m. mass
m. perforation
m. protection
m. revascularization
m. rupture
m. tissue
myocardiorrhaphy
myocarditis
myocardium
postischemic stunned m.
m. retrograde
stunned m.
myocele
myocutaneous
m. flap
m. graft

myocytolysis
    coagulative m.
myocytoma
myodegeneration
myodermal flap
myodesis
myodiastasis
myoelastic-aerodynamic theory of phonation
myoepithelioma
myofascial
    m. dysfunction
    m. flap
    m. manipulation
    m. pain
    m. pain syndrome
    m. trigger point
myofibroblastoma
myofibroma
myofunctional therapy
myogenic
    m. headache
    m. motor-evoked potential (MEP)
myoglobin tubular obstruction
myoid cyst
myolipoma
myolysis
    cardiotoxic m.
myoma
myomatectomy
myomectomy
    abdominal m.
    laparoscopic esophageal m.
    vaginal m.
myomedulloblastoma
myometrial
myometrium
myomotomy
myonecrosis
    clostridial m.
myoneural blockade
myoneurectomy
myoneuroma
myoneurotization
myopathy, encephapathy, lactic acidosis, stroke-like episodes (MELAS)
myopectineal orifice
myopia
    space m.
myoplastic muscle stabilization

myoplasty
myorrhaphy
myorrhexis
myosalpinx
myosarcoma
myositis
myosteoma
myotenontoplasty
myotenotomy
myotomy
    circular m.
    cricoid m.
    cricopharyngeal m.
    diverticulectomy with m.
    esophageal m.
    extended m.
    Heller m.
    laparoscopic Heller m.
    Livaditis circular m.
    longitudinal m.
    marginal m.
    m. operation
    septal m.
    Z m.
myotomy-myectomy-septal resection
myotonia fluctuans
myotonic dystrophy
myotoxicity
myovascular sphincter
myovenous sphincter
myringitis
    chronic granular m.
myringoplasty
myringostapediopexy
myringotomy with aspiration
myxadenoma
myxedema
    m. ascites
    m. coma
myxochondrofibrosarcoma
myxochondroma
myxofibroma
myxofibrosarcoma
myxolipoma
myxoliposarcoma
myxoma sarcomatosum
myxomatosis
myxoneuroma
myxopapilloma
myxosarcoma

M

NOTES

N

newton

N2-Sargenti technique

nabothian cyst

Naclerio

V-sign of N.

NACS

Neurologic and Adaptive Capacity Score

nadir pressure

Naffziger operation

Nagamatsu incision

nail

anteroposterior n.
beak n.
n. bed
boat n.
brittle n.
cannulated n.
n. change
closed n.
clubbed n.
n. clubbing
condylocephalic n.
convex n.
digital n.
n. disorder
dystrophic n.
egg-shell n.
n. fold
n. fold capillaroscopy
n. fold removal
n. groove
half-and-half n.
hooked intramedullary n.
n. horn
ingrown n.
left-sided n.
n. length gauge method
n. matrix
mycotic club n.
nested n.
onychocryptosis n.
open-section n.
parrot-beak n.
pincer n.
n. pit
pitted n.
n. pitting
n. plate fixation
n. plate removal
racket n.
ram horn n.
reamed n.
reedy n.
n. root

shell n.
sliding n.
telescoping n.
thickened n.
titanium flexible humeral n.
n. wall
yellow n.

nailing

antegrade n.
femoral n.
intramedullary n.
reamed femoral n.
retrograde n.
tibiocalcaneal medullary n.
unreamed n.

nail-patella-elbow syndrome

nail-patella syndrome

nail-to-nail bed angle

naive recipient

NaK-ATPase membrane

Nakayama anastomosis

Nalebuff classification

**Nalebuff-Millender lateral band
mobilization technique**

naloxone

Nance leeway space

nanogram (ng)

napkin-ring

n.-r. annular lesion
n.-r. carcinoma
n.-r. compression
n.-r. defect

narcosis

adsorption theory of n.
colloid theory of n.
lipoid theory of n.
Meyer-Overton theory of n.
nitrogen n.
oxygen deprivation theory of n.
permeability theory of n.
surface tension theory of n.
thermodynamic theory of n.

narcotic

n. analgesic
n. reversal

narcotism

naris, pl. **nares**

narrowed pulse pressure

narrow-field laryngectomy

narrowing

disc space n.
eccentric n.
joint space n.

narrow internal ring

narrow-slit illumination

N

Narula method
nasal
n. airway
n. antrostomy
n. border
n. canal
n. cavity
n. cavity cancer
n. concha
n. crest
n. deformity
n. dissection
n. endoscopic surgery
n. endoscopy
n. foramen
n. fracture
n. granuloma gravidarum
n. height
n. hemorrhage
n. index
n. intubation
n. mucosal identification
n. mucosal ulceration
n. muscle
n. oxygen (NO)
n. pharynx
n. placode
n. port
n. provocation test
n. pyramid
n. reconstruction
n. respiration
n. septal perforation
n. septum
n. tip
n. tract
n. trumpet
n. vestibule
n. wall
NASCET
North American Symptomatic Carotid Endarterectomy Trial
NASH
nonalcoholic steatohepatitis
nasioiniac
nasion-alveolar point line
nasion soft tissue
Nasmyth membrane
nasobasilar line
nasobregmatic arc
nasociliary
n. ganglion
n. nerve
nasoendoscopy
nasofrontal
n. duct
n. vein
nasofrontalis
nasogastric (NG)

n. intubation
n. suction
n. tonometry
nasoileal
nasojejunal
nasojugal fold
nasolabial
n. groove
n. line
n. rotation flap
nasolacrimal
n. canal
n. sac
nasomandibular fixation
nasomaxillary suture
nasooccipital arc
nasooral
nasoorbital fracture
nasopalatine injection
nasopharyngeal
n. airway
n. biopsy
n. carcinoma (NPC)
n. groove
n. hematoma
n. hemorrhage
n. passage
n. suction
nasopharyngoscopy
nasopharynx
nasorostral
nasotracheal
n. intubation (NTI)
n. intubation anesthetic technique
n. suction
n. tube fixation using infant feeding tube
nasovesicular catheter technique
natal cleft
natatorium
nates (*pl. of* natis)
Nathan-Trung modification of Krukenberg hand reconstruction
national
N. Cancer Data Base (NCDB)
N. Cancer Institute (NCI)
N. Football Head and Neck Injury Registry
N. Marrow Donor Program
N. Pediatric Trauma Registry (NPTR)
N. Surgical Adjuvant Breast and Bowel Project (NSABP)
natis, pl. **nates**
native
n. caudate lobe
n. coronary anatomy
n. liver
n. myocardial microcirculation

n. portal vein
n. renal biopsy
natriuresis
pressure n.
natural method
nature
benign n.
dense n.
minimally invasive n.
n. root canal filling
secretomotor n.
navel
navicular
n. abdomen
n. bone
n. fracture
naviculocapitate
n. fracture
n. fracture syndrome
naviculocuneiform fusion
navigated
n. brain tumor surgery
n. neurosurgery
navigation
image-guided n.
surgical microscope n. (SMN)
n. system
navigational surgery
NCDB
National Cancer Data Base
NCI
National Cancer Institute
NCJ
needle catheter jejunostomy
NCPB
neurolytic celiac plexus block
NCRLM
noncolorectal liver metastasis
isolated NCRLM
unique NCRLM
NDSA
nondermatomal sensory abnormality
Nd:YAG
neodymium:yttrium-aluminum-garnet
Nd:YAG cyclophotocoagulation
Nd:YAG laser ablation
Nd:YAG laser irradiation
Nd:YAG laser therapy
Nealon technique
near
n. fixation
n. visual point

near-anatomic position
near-and-far suture technique
near-infrared (NIR)
n.-i. measurement
n.-i. spectrophotometry
n.-i. spectroscopy
near-point relative
near-total
n.-t. esophagectomy
n.-t. gastrectomy
n.-t. laryngectomy
n.-t. pancreatectomy
n.-t. thyroidectomy
NEB
New England Baptist
NEB hip arthroplasty
nebula, pl. **nebulae**
corneal n.
nebulization
nebulized lidocaine
nebulizer
spinning disc n.
ultrasonic n.
NEC
necrotizing enterocolitis
neck
anterolateral n.
aortic n.
deep anterior n.
N. Disability Index
n. dissection
n. exploration
n. extension position
n. flap
n. fracture
gallbladder n.
implant n.
implant superstructure n.
innervation of head and n.
pancreatic n.
residual n.
superficial n.
surgical n.
virgin n.
necrectomy
necrolysis
epidermal n.
toxic epidermal n.
necrolytic migratory erythema
necropsy
necroscopy

N

NOTES

necrosectomy
  initial n.
  operative n.
  reoperative n.
necrosis
  acute tubular n. (ATN)
  aminoglycoside tubular n.
  avascular n.
  bloodless zone of n.
  bony n.
  caseation n.
  centrilobular n.
  cerebral radiation n. (CRN)
  cheesy n.
  coagulation n.
  cumarin n.
  cystic medial n.
  diffuse n.
  electrocoagulation n.
  Erdheim cystic medial n.
  ethanol-induced tumor n.
  fat n.
  flap n.
  frank n.
  hepatic n.
  infected n.
  liquefaction n.
  mummification n.
  pancreatic n.
  periodontal membrane n.
  peripancreatic n.
  pressure n.
  radiation n.
  skin flap n.
  soft tissue n.
  splenic n.
  strangulation n.
  subcutaneous n.
  thermal n.
  tissue n.
  tumor n.
necrotic
  n. abscess
  n. flap
  n. focus
  n. hemorrhoid
  n. hyalinized tissue
  n. inflammation
  n. metastasis
  n. remain
  n. ulceration
necrotic/fibrotic tissue
necrotizing
  n. angiitis
  n. enterocolitis (NEC)
  n. granulomatous inflammation
  n. infection
  n. pancreatitis (NP)

necrotomy
  osteoplastic n.
needle
  n. ablation
  n. arthroscopy
  n. aspiration
  n. aspiration cytology
  n. catheter jejunostomy (NCJ)
  n. core biopsy
  n. holder
  n. insertion
  insulated epidural n.
  n. laparoscopy
  n. localization
  noninsulated n.
  n. prick
  n. reaction
  n. suspension procedure
  n. thoracentesis
  n. thoracentesis method
  n. thoracentesis procedure
  n. thoracentesis technique
  n. tracheoesophageal puncture
  n. tract
  n. tract implantation
  n. tract tumor seeding
2-needle
  2-n. technique
needle-free system
needle-knife
  n.-k. papillotomy
  n.-k. sphincterotomy
  n.-k. technique
needleless
  n. intravenous administration system
  n. suturing
needle-localized open biopsy (NLOB)
needlepoint electrocautery
needlescopic laparoscopic
  cholecystectomy
needlescopy
Needles split cast method
needlestick injury
needle-through-needle single interspace
  technique
needling
  dry n.
Neer
  N. acromioplasty
  N. capsular shift procedure
  N. femur fracture classification
  N. hemiarthroplasty
  N. modification
  N. open reduction
  N. posterior shoulder reconstruction
  N. shoulder fracture classification
  N. unconstrained shoulder
  arthroplasty

negative
- n. abdominal pressure
- n. appendectomy
- n. aspiration
- axillary node n.
- n. breast biopsy
- n. celiotomy
- n. control enzyme induction
- n. correlation
- n. cytology
- n. effect
- n. end-expiratory pressure
- false n.
- n. inotropy
- n. inspiratory breathing
- n. inspiratory pressure measurement
- n. laparotomy
- n. margin
- n. peritoneal cytology (NPC)
- n. predictive value (NPV)
- n. pressure
- n. pressure therapy
- n. pressure ventilation (NPV)
- true n.
- tumor receptor protein n.

negative-pressure
neglected rupture
neglectlike phenomena
Neher operation
Nehra-Mack operation
Neill-Mooser body
neisserial infection
Nélaton
- N. ankle dislocation
- N. fiber
- N. fold
- N. line
- N. sphincter

nematode infection
neoadjuvant
- n. therapy
- n. total androgen ablation

neobladder
neocartilage formation
neocystostomy
neodymium:YAG laser therapy
neodymium:yttrium-aluminum-garnet (Nd:YAG)
neoesophagus
neoformation
neoglottic reconstruction
neointima formation

neonatal
- n. anesthesia
- N. Facial Pain Inventory (NFCS)
- N. Infant Pain Scale (NIPS)
- n. infection
- n. intracranial hemorrhage
- n. intraventricular hemorrhage
- n. line
- n. pulmonary transplantation
- n. resuscitation
- n. ring
- n. severe hyperparathyroidism
- n. testicular torsion
- n. thymectomy

neonate
- n. examination
- surgical n.
- n. ventilation

neoplasia
- multiple endocrine n. (MEN)
- multiple endocrine n. type 2a
- multiple endocrine n. type 2b
- multiple intestinal n. (MIN)
- thyroid n.

neoplasm
- asymptomatic n.
- brain n.
- colonic n.
- follicular n.
- hepatic n.
- intraaxial parenchymal brain n.
- intraductal oncocytic papillary n.
- intraductal papillary mucinous n. (IPMN)
- n. metastasis
- mucinous cystic n. (MCN)
- parenchymal brain n.
- pediatric n.
- second malignant n. (SMN)
- vascular n.

neoplastic
- n. dissemination
- n. fracture
- n. lesion
- n. pathology
- n. port site implant
- n. renal mass
- n. tissue
- n. transformation

neorectal function
neosalpingostomy
- terminal n.

NOTES

N

neostigmine toxicity
neostomy
neoumbilicus
neovagina
    skin graft n.
neovascular
    n. bundle
    n. membrane
    n. network
neovascularization
    choroidal n.
    corneal n.
    disc n.
    disseminated asymptomatic
      unilateral n.
    interstitial n.
    iris n.
    pathologic n.
    preretinal n.
    retinal quadrant n.
    stromal n.
    subretinal n.
    vitreous n.
neovasculature
    tumor n.
nephradenoma
nephralgia
nephralgic
nephratonia
nephrectomy
    abdominal n.
    adjuvant n.
    anterior n.
    apical polar n.
    Balkan n.
    extracorporeal partial n.
    extraperitoneal laparoscopic n.
    hand-assisted laparoscopic live-
      donor n.
    laparoscopic-assisted living donor n.
    laparoscopic donor n. (LDN)
    laparoscopic live donor n.
    laser partial n.
    late transplant n.
    live donor n.
    living donor n.
    lumbar n.
    open partial n.
    paraperitoneal n.
    partial n.
    perifascial n.
    posterior n.
    radical n.
    retroperitoneoscopic n.
    transperitoneal laparoscopic n.
    transplant n.
    unilateral n.
nephredema
nephrelcosis

nephric
nephritic
    n. calculus
    n. colic
    n. syndrome
nephritis
    interstitial n.
nephritogenic
nephroblastoma
nephrocalcinosis
nephrocapsectomy
nephrocardiac
nephrocele
nephrogenetic
nephrogenic
    n. cord
    n. tissue
nephrogenous
nephrohydrosis
nephroid
nephrolith
nephrolithiasis
nephrolithotomy
    anatrophic n.
    percutaneous n.
    simultaneous bilateral
      percutaneous n.
nephrolithotripsy
    percutaneous n. (PCNL)
nephrology
nephrolysis
nephrolytic
nephroma
nephron
nephronia
    lobar n.
nephronic loop
nephron-sparing surgery
nephropathic
nephropathy
    end-stage reflux n.
nephropexy
nephrophthisis
nephroptosis
nephropyeloplasty
nephropyosis
nephrorrhaphy
nephros
nephrosclerosis
nephroscopic fulguration
nephroscopy
    anatrophic n.
    flexible n.
    percutaneous n.
nephrosis
nephrospasia
nephrostolithotomy
    caliceal n.
    percutaneous n. (PCNL)

nephrostomy
    circle wire n.
    n. drainage
    percutaneous n.
    n. puncture
nephrotic edema
nephrotomic cavity
nephrotomy
    anatrophic n.
nephrotoxic
nephrotoxicity
nephrotoxin
nephrotrophic
nephrotropic
nephrotuberculosis
nephroureterectomy
    bilateral n.
    radical n.
    transperitoneal laparoscopic n.
nephroureterocystectomy
nephroureteroscopy
nerve
    abdominopelvic splanchnic n.
    abducens n.
    accelerator n.
    accessory n.
    acoustic n.
    n. allografting
    alveolar n.
    n. anastomosis
    Andersch n.
    ansa cervicalis n.
    anterior auricular n.
    anterior cutaneous n.
    anterior ethmoidal n.
    anterior labial n.
    anterior scrotal n.
    anterior supraclavicular n.
    Arnold n.
    articular recurrent n.
    auditory tube n.
    augmentor n.
    auricular n.
    auriculotemporal n.
    autonomic n.
    axillary n.
    baroreceptor n.
    Bell respiratory n.
    n. biopsy
    n. block
    n. block anesthesia
    n. block infusion

    Bock n.
    brachial plexus n.
    buccal n.
    buccinator n.
    cardiac n.
    caroticotympanic n.
    cavernous n.
    centrifugal n.
    centripetal n.
    cervical splanchnic n.
    chorda tympani n.
    ciliary n.
    circumflex n.
    n. coaptation
    coccygeal n.
    cochlear n.
    common peroneal n.
    communicating n.
    n. compression anesthesia
    n. compression-degeneration syndrome
    n. conduction velocity examination
    corneal n.
    cranial n. (I–XII)
    n. cross section
    cutaneous cervical n.
    n. decompression
    deep peroneal n.
    deep petrosal n.
    deep temporal n.
    dental n.
    descending n.
    dorsal interosseous n.
    dorsal rami n.
    dorsal scapular n.
    eighth cranial n.
    eleventh cranial n.
    entrapped n.
    esodic n.
    ethmoidal n.
    n. excitability test
    excitor n.
    excitoreflex n.
    exodic n.
    external nasal n.
    external saphenous n.
    external spermatic n.
    extrinsic n.
    facial n.
    femoral n.
    n. fiber bundle
    n. fiber bundle layer

NOTES

nerve *(continued)*
    n. fiber myelination
    fifth cranial n.
    first cranial n.
    fold of laryngeal n.
    fourth cranial n.
    fourth lumbar n.
    furcal n.
    Galen n.
    gangliated n.
    genitocrural n.
    genitofemoral n.
    glossopharyngeal n.
    great auricular n.
    n. growth factor receptor
    gustatory n.
    hemorrhoidal n.
    Hering n.
    hypogastric n.
    iliohypogastric n.
    ilioinguinal n.
    n. implantation
    inferior alveolar n.
    inferior hemorrhoidal n.
    inferior palpebral n.
    inferior rectal n.
    inferior vesical n.
    infraorbital n.
    infratrochlear n.
    inhibitory n.
    n. injury
    intercarotid n.
    intercostal n.
    intercostohumeral n.
    intermediary n.
    internal rectal n.
    interosseous n.
    Jacobson n.
    jugular n.
    lacrimal n.
    laryngeal n.
    Latarget n.
    lingual n.
    lumbar n.
    lumboinguinal n.
    mandibular n.
    masseteric n.
    masticator n.
    maxillary n.
    median n.
    mental n.
    mixed n.
    motor n.
    musculocutaneous n.
    musculospiral n.
    mylohyoid n.
    nasociliary n.
    ninth cranial n.
    obturator n.

occipital n.
oculomotor n.
olfactory n.
olivocochlear n.
Oort n.
ophthalmic n.
optic n.
palatine n.
palpebral n.
n. paralysis
parasympathetic n.
pericardiophrenic n.
perineal n.
peripheral n.
peritonsillar n.
peroneal communicating n.
petrosal n.
phrenic n.
plantar digital n.
pneumogastric n.
popliteal communicating n.
presacral n.
pterygoid n.
pterygopalatine n.
pudendal n.
pudic n.
rectal n.
recurrent laryngeal n. (RLN)
recurrent meningeal n.
n. regeneration
right common iliac n.
n. root
n. root compression
n. rootlet ablation
n. root sleeve injection
sacral splanchnic n.
second cranial n.
secretory n.
sensory n.
seventh cranial n.
sinocarotid n.
sinuvertebral n.
sixth cranial n.
somatic n.
sphenopalatine n.
spinal accessory n.
splanchnic n.
statoacoustic n.
n. stimulator anesthetic technique
subclavian n.
subcostal n.
suboccipital n.
subscapular n.
supraclavicular n.
supraorbital n.
suprascapular n.
supratrochlear n.
sural n.
n. suture technique

sympathetic n.
temporal n.
temporomandibular n.
tenth cranial n.
tentorial n.
third cranial n.
third occipital n.
thoracic cardiac n.
thoracic spinal n.
thoracoabdominal n.
thoracodorsal n.
Tiedemann n.
n. tract
trifacial n.
trigeminal n.
trochlear n.
n. trunk
twelfth cranial n.
upper subscapular n.
vaginal n.
vagus n.
vascular n.
vasomotor n.
vesical n.
vestibular n.
vestibulocochlear n.
vidian n.
visceral n.
vomeronasal n.
Wrisberg n.
zygomatic n.
nerve-containing plate
nerve-point massage
nerve-preserving parotidectomy
nerve-sparing
n.-s. dissection
n.-s. radical retropubic
prostatectomy
nervi (*pl. of* nervus)
nervosa
foramina n.
nervous
n. damage
n. exhaustion
n. respiration
n. system
n. system involvement
nervus, pl. **nervi**
Nesbit
N. operation
N. plication
N. tuck procedure

nesidiectomy
nesidioblastoma
nest
Brunn n.
choristoma n.
nested nail
net
vascular n.
network
acromial arterial n.
articular vascular n.
calcaneal arterial n.
Cancer Genetics N.
cytokine n.
medial malleolar n.
neovascular n.
neural n.
patellar n.
peritarsal n.
plantar venous n.
Purkinje n.
trabecular n.
Neubauer artery
Neufeld dynamic method
Neugebauer-LeFort procedure
neural
n. arch
n. arch resection technique
n. axis vascular malformation
n. canal
n. crest malformation
n. crest migration
n. lesion
n. mapping
n. network
n. plasticity
n. spine
n. tissue
n. tube
n. tube defect
neuralgia
geniculate n.
inguinal n.
intercostal n.
laparoscopic-induced n.
petrosal n.
postherpetic n.
posttraumatic gustatory n.
secondary n.
Sluder n.
trigeminal n.
vidian n.

N

NOTES

neurapophysis
neurasthenia
    experimental n.
neuraxial
    n. medication trial
    n. neurolytic block
neurectasis
neurectomy
    cochleovestibular n.
    Cotte presacral n.
    Eggers n.
    genitofemoral n.
    iliohypogastric n.
    ilioinguinal n.
    obturator n.
    occipital n.
    opticociliary n.
    peripheral n.
    pharyngeal plexus n.
    Phelps n.
    presacral n.
    retrogasserian n.
    retrolabyrinthine-retrosigmoid
      vestibular n.
    retrolabyrinthine vestibular n.
    Sonnenberg n.
    transcochlear cochleovestibular n.
    transcochlear vestibular n.
    transtympanic n.
    tympanic n.
    ulnar motor n.
    vestibular n.
neurenteric canal
neurilemmosarcoma
neurilemoma, neurilemmoma
neurilemosarcoma
neurinoma
neuritic plaque
neuritis
    vibration n.
neuroablation
    cryogenic n.
neuroablative technique
neuroadenolysis
    pituitary n.
neuroanastomosis
neuroanatomy
neuroanesthesia
neuroastrocytoma
neuroaugmentation
neuroaxial opioid
neuroblastoma
neurocele
neurocentral
    n. joint
    n. suture
neurochronaxic theory of phonation
neurocirculation
neurocladism

neurocognitive change
neurocranium
neurocutaneous island flap
neurocytolysis
neurocytoma
neurodiagnostic evaluation
neuroectomy
neuroeffector junction
neuroelectric event
neuroendocrine
    n. cancer
    n. skin carcinoma
    n. tumor
neuroepithelioma
neuroepithelium
neurofibroma
    plexiform n.
neurofibromatosis
neurofibrosarcoma
neuroganglion
neurogastric
neurogenic
    n. bladder
    n. fracture
    n. hypertension
    n. incontinence
    n. PGID
    n. pulmonary edema (NPE)
neurogliomatosis
neurohypophysial
neurohypophysis
neuroimaging
neuroleptanalgesia
    n. anesthesia
    n. anesthetic technique
neuroleptanesthesia
neuroleptic
    n. agent
    n. malignant syndrome (NMS)
neurologic
    N. and Adaptive Capacity Score
      (NACS)
    n. complication
    n. deficit
    n. disease
    n. disorder
    n. examination
    n. function
    n. injury
    n. manifestation
    n. recovery
    n. surgery
    n. symptom
neurological
    n. evaluation
    n. surgery
neurology
    surgical n.

neurolysis
distal n.
internal n.
intrathecal n.
neurolytic
n. blockade
n. celiac plexus block (NCPB)
neuroma
acoustic n.
n. relocation surgery
neuroma-in-continuity
neuromatosis
neuromodulation
neuromotor dysfunction
neuromuscular
n. block
n. blockade (NMB)
n. blockade monitoring
n. blocking agent
n. electrical stimulation
n. facilitation
n. junction
n. pedicle graft
n. relaxant
n. system electric induction
n. transmission
neuron
inspiratory bulbospinal n.
nondopaminergic n.
neuronal
n. cell line
n. membrane
n. migration
n. nicotinic receptor activation
n. regeneration
neuronavigational system
neuronephric
neuronoma
neuroophthalmic manifestation
neuroophthalmologic examination
neuropathic
n. bladder
n. fracture
n. pain
n. ulcer
neuropathicum
papilloma n.
neuropathologist
neuropathology
neuropathophysiology
normalization of n.

neuropathy
inherited n.
optic n.
stretch-induced n.
traumatic optic n.
neurophysiologic examination
neuroplasticity
neuroplasty
epidural n.
neuropsychological deficit
neuroradiologic evaluation
neuroradiology
interventional n.
neurorrhaphy
epineurial n.
perineurial n.
neurosarcocleisis
neurosarcoma
neuroschwannoma
neurostimulating procedure
neurostimulation trial
neurosurgeon
pediatric n.
neurosurgery
functional stereotactic n.
image-guided interactive n.
navigated neurosurgery
stereotactic n.
neurosurgical
n. anesthesia
n. approach
n. intensive care unit (NICU)
n. intervention
n. procedure
neurosuture
neurotendinous
neurothekeoma
neurotic excoriation
neurotization
neurotize
neurotologic examination
neurotomy
opticociliary n.
retrogasserian n.
neurotoxicology
neurotransmitter system
neurotrauma
neurotripsy
neurotrosis
neuroureterectomy
neurourology
neurovaricosis

N

NOTES

neurovascular
n. anatomy
n. bundle
n. complication
n. compression syndrome
n. cross compression
n. free flap
n. island graft
n. island pedicle flap
n. lesion
n. sheath
neuroxanthoendothelioma
neutral
n. hip position
n. point
n. rotation
n. spine position
neutralization
n. plate fixation
serum n.
n. test
neutron
n. activation analysis
n. beam therapy
n. capture therapy
neutropenia-related bacterial infection
neutrophil
n. activation
n. migration
polymorphonuclear n. (PMN)
neutrophilic
n. infiltration
n. inflammation
nevi (*pl. of* nevus)
Neviaser
N. acromioclavicular technique
N. operation
Neviaser-Wilson-Gardner technique
nevocarcinoma
nevoid
n. anomaly
n. basal cell carcinoma syndrome
nevoxanthoendothelioma
juvenile n.
nevus, pl. **nevi**
bathing trunk n.
new
N. England Baptist (NEB)
N. York Heart Association heart
disease classification
newborn
n. anesthesia
n. examination
n. resuscitation
Newman
N. procedure
N. radial neck and head fracture
classification
newton (N)

newtonian
n. aberration
n. body
NFCS
Neonatal Facial Pain Inventory
NG
nasogastric
NG suction
ng
nanogram
NHBD
non-heart-beating donor
NIBP
noninvasive blood pressure
Nicholas
N. ligament technique
N. 5-in-1 reconstruction technique
Nichols
N. method
N. procedure
N. sacrospinous fixation
nick
skin n.
nickel-and-dime lesion
Nicks procedure
Nicola
N. incision
N. shoulder procedure
Nicoll
N. cancellous bone graft
N. cancellous insert graft
N. classification
N. fracture operation
N. fracture repair procedure
nicotine
intranasal n.
nicotinic
n. excitation
n. receptor
nictation, nictitation
nictitating membrane
NICU
neurosurgical intensive care unit
nidus, pl. **nidi**
cellular n.
Niebauer-King technique
Niebauer trapeziometacarpal arthroplasty
Niemeier
N. classification
N. gallbladder perforation
nightstick fracture
nigroid body
nigrostriatal tract
Nikaidoh-Bex technique
Nikiforoff method
nil disease
ninth cranial nerve
nipple
accessory n.

aortic n.
n. aspiration cytology
n. line
n. reconstruction
n. retraction
n. stimulation test
nipple-areolar reconstruction
nippled stoma
nipple-flat duct resection
NIPS
Neonatal Infant Pain Scale
NIR
near-infrared
Nirschl
N. operation
N. technique
Nissen
N. antireflux operation
N. 360-degree wrap fundoplication
N. fundoplasty
N. fundoplication method
N. fundoplication operation
N. fundoplication procedure
N. fundoplication technique
N. fundoplication wrap
N. repair
Nissen-Rossetti
N.-R. fundoplication
N.-R. fundoplication method
N.-R. fundoplication procedure
N.-R. fundoplication technique
Nitchie method
nitrate-induced venodilation
nitric
n. oxide bioavailability
n. oxide blocked sphincter
relaxation
n. oxide signaling
nitrogen
n. concentration
expiratory n.
n. monoxide
n. narcosis
n. partial pressure
nitrous
n. oxide (NO)
n. oxide-opioid-barbiturate anesthetic
technique
n. oxide-oxygen (N_2O-O_2)
n. oxide-oxygen-opioid anesthetic
technique (N_2O-O_2-opioid anesthetic
technique)

nitrovasodilator
Nizetic operation
NLOB
needle-localized open biopsy
NMB
neuromuscular blockade
NMR
nuclear magnetic resonance
NMR spectroscopy
NMS
neuroleptic malignant syndrome
NO
nasal oxygen
nitrous oxide
no
no infection-no rejection
no rejection
no signs of life
Noble
N. bowel plication
N. position
N. surgical plication of bowel
Noble-Mengert perineal repair
nocebo
nociception
nociceptive stimulation
nociceptor afferent peripheral terminal
nocturia
nocturnal
n. enuresis
n. painful tonic spasm (NPTS)
nodal
n. disease
n. extirpation
n. involvement
n. metastasis
n. plane
n. point
n. recurrence
n. tissue
n. yield
node
atrioventricular n.
n. biopsy
buccinator n.
Cloquet n.
companion lymph n.
coronary n.
cystic n.
diaphragmatic n.
n. dissection
foraminal n.

N

NOTES

node *(continued)*
    free n.
    gastroomental n.
    hot sentinel n.
    internal mammary n.
    intramammary sentinel n.
    n. involvement
    juguloomohyoid n.
    n. lymphoma
    n. lymphoma system
    malar n.
    mammary n.
    mandibular n.
    mastoid n.
    matted n.
    mesenteric n.
    mesenteric lymph n. (MLN)
    nonsentinel n.
    occipital n.
    paratracheal n.
    parietal n.
    parotid n.
    perigastric n.
    prelaryngeal n.
    pretracheal n.
    radiolabeled sentinel n.
    Ranvier n.
    regional n.
    retroauricular n.
    retroperitoneal n.
    retropharyngeal n.
    retropyloric n.
    Rosenmüller n.
    sentinel n.
    sentinel lymph n. (SLN)
    sinoatrial n.
    n. station
    subdigastric n.
    submandibular n.
    submental n.
    subpyloric n.
    suprapyloric n.
    Tawara n.
    tracheal n.
    tracheobronchial n.
    visceral n.
node-negative
    n.-n. disease
    n.-n. melanoma
node-positive
    n.-p. breast cancer
    n.-p. disease
    n.-p. melanoma
nodi (*pl. of* nodus)
nodose ganglion
nodoventricular tract
nodular
    n. chondrodermatitis

    n. hidradenoma
    n. lesion
nodulation
nodule
    cold n.
    hot n.
    hyperfunctioning n.
    metastatic n.
    mixed n.
    posterior n.
    subependymal brain n.
    thyroid n.
nodulectomy
nodule-in-nodule lesion
nodulus, pl. **noduli**
    n. cutaneus
nodus, pl. **nodi**
noise
    n. detection threshold
    n. exposure
no-leak technique
nomenclature
    Anglo-Saxon n.
    Couinaud n.
    linnaean system of n.
NOMI
    nonocclusive mesenteric ischemia
nomogram
    prognostic n.
    Radford n.
nonabsorbable material
nonadherent
nonalcoholic steatohepatitis (NASH)
nonanatomic
    n. renal bypass
    n. wedge resection
nonanesthetic gas
nonaneurysmal perimesencephalic subarachnoid hemorrhage
nonappendiceal carcinoid
nonarticular distal radial fracture
nonaxillary location
nonbacterial thrombotic endocardial lesion
nonbench surgery
nonbiologic liver support
nonblanchable, abnormally colored lesion
nonbullous emphysema
noncalcified nodular mass
noncancer death
noncardiac surgery
noncausal association
noncemented total hip arthroplasty
noncircumferential antireflux procedure
noncirrhotic metabolic liver disease
nonclassic nodal basin

noncolorectal
　　n. liver metastasis (NCRLM)
　　n. primary
noncontact manipulation
noncontiguous fracture
nondepolarizer
nondepolarizing
　　n. block
　　n. blockade
　　n. muscle relaxant
　　n. relaxant
nondermatomal sensory abnormality
　　(NDSA)
nondermatophyte fungal infection
nondiabetic
nondiagnostic FNA
nondismembered anastomosis
nondisplaced fracture
nondistended abdomen
nondominant gland
nondopaminergic neuron
nondysgerminoma
nonencapsulated
nonerosive gastric mucosal lesion
nonexcisional modality
nonfamilial
　　n. malignant endocrine tumor
　　n. multiglandular disease
　　n. untreated HPT
nonfatal
　　n. complication
　　n. stroke
nonfenestrated Fontan procedure
nonfunction
　　primary graft n.
nonfunctional malignant tumor
nonfunctioning islet cell tumor
non-heart-beating donor (NHBD)
nonhereditary malignancy
nonideal solution
nonimmunologic complication
noninfective extraabdominal complication
noninhalation
noninsulated needle
noninvasive
　　n. assessment
　　n. blood pressure (NIBP)
　　n. diagnosis
　　n. evaluation
　　n. infestation
　　n. localization study
　　lower extremity n.

　　n. method
　　n. positive-pressure ventilation
　　　(NPPV)
　　n. procedure
　　n. programmed stimulation
　　n. recurrence
　　n. technique
　　n. venous study
nonisometric graft
nonkeratinization
nonlaparoscopic
　　n. series
　　n. technique
nonmalignant
　　chronic n.
　　n. disease
nonmeningiomatous malignant lesion
nonmobile mass
nonmucosal hemorrhoidectomy
nonnecrotizing granulomatous
　　inflammation
nonneoplastic tumor-like lesion
nonneuroendocrine metastasis
nonocclusive
　　n. mesenteric ischemia (NOMI)
　　n. mesenteric ischemia syndrome
nonopaque intraluminal mass
nonoperative
　　n. approach
　　n. closure
　　n. diagnosis
　　n. management
　　n. reduction
　　n. staging
nonoperatively
nonophthalmologic surgical specialty
nonopportunistic infection
nonoptimal technique
nonorganic stridor
nonpalpable
　　n. invasive breast cancer
　　n. mammographic abnormality
nonparametric test
nonpathologic scar
nonpenetrating
　　n. keratoplasty
　　n. rupture
　　n. wound
nonperforative lesion
nonpharmacologic measure
nonphysial fracture
nonphysiologic position

N

NOTES

nonplicated appendicocystostomy
nonprosthetic closure
nonpulmonary route of elimination (NPE)
nonrebreathing anesthesia
nonresectional method
non-rib-spreading
    n.-r.-s. thoracotomy incision
    n.-r.-s. thoracotomy incision method
    n.-r.-s. thoracotomy incision procedure
    n.-r.-s. thoracotomy incision technique
nonrigid registration algorithm
nonrotation
nonrotational burst fracture
nonsecretory sigmoid cystoplasty
nonselective opioid receptor antagonist
nonseminomatous
    n. component
    n. testicular tumor
nonsentinel node
nonseptate cavity
nonsevered injury
nonshivering thermogenesis
nonspecific
    n. symptom
    n. therapy
nonstereospecific action
nonsteroidal
    n. antiinflammatory drug (NSAID)
    n. antiinflammatory medication
nonsurgical
    n. clinician
    n. management
    n. method
    n. therapy
    n. treatment
nonsurvivor
nonsympathetically mediated pain
nontherapeutic
nonthoracotomy
nonthrust mobilization
nontraumatic hernia
nontuberculous mycobacterial infection
nontumoral gastric wall
nonunion fracture
nonunited fracture
nonvascular abdominal surgery
nonventilated lung
nonviable tissue
nonvisualization
nonvital tissue
N_2O-O_2
    nitrous oxide-oxygen
N_2O-O_2-opioid anesthetic technique
noose
    Dormia n.
    n. suture technique

no-punch technique
noradrenergic mechanism
Norfolk
    N. procedure
    N. technique
norma, pl. normae
normal
    n. anatomic alignment
    n. anatomic position
    n. base deficit
    n. body temperature
    n. CI
    n. colon
    n. intravascular pressure
    n. ovariotomy
    n. planar MR anatomy
    n. saline
    n. saline solution
    n. serum lactate
    n. tissue
    n. transformation zone
normalization
    assay n.
    n. of neuropathophysiology
normalizing lactate
normal-pressure hydrocephalus
Norman Miller vaginopexy
normocalcemia
normocalcemic
normocapnia
normocephalic
normotensive
normothermia
    intraoperative n.
normothermic
    n. ischemia
    n. temperature
normoventilation
normovolemic hemodilution
North American Symptomatic Carotid Endarterectomy Trial (NASCET)
Northern blot technique
Norton operation
Norwood
    N. operation
    N. univentricular heart procedure
no-scalpel vasectomy
nose
    n. anesthesia
    artificial n.
    cleft n.
    external n.
nosocomial
    n. fire
    n. fungal infection
    n. gangrene
    n. pneumonia
nostril
notal

notancephalia
notch
    acetabular n.
    n. of acetabulum
    anacrotic n.
    angular n.
    auricular n.
    costal n.
    craniofacial n.
    ethmoidal n.
    frontal n.
    greater sciatic n.
    inferior thyroid n.
    inferior vertebral n.
    infraorbital n.
    interarytenoid n.
    interclavicular n.
    intercondyloid n.
    intervertebral n.
    Kernohan n.
    lacrimal n.
    lesser sciatic n.
    mandibular n.
    mastoid n.
    pancreatic n.
    parietal n.
    parotid n.
    preoccipital n.
    presternal n.
    pterygoid n.
    scapular n.
    sciatic n.
    sternal n.
    superior thyroid n.
    superior vertebral n.
    supraorbital n.
    suprascapular n.
    suprasternal n.
    tentorial n.
    thyroid n.
    tympanic n.
    umbilical n.
    vertebral n.
notch-and-roll maneuver
notching
    rib n.
notchplasty procedure
notencephalocele
notochord
no-touch technique
NovoSeven recombinant factor VIIa

noxious
    n. event
    n. stimulus
Noyes flexion rotation drawer test
NP
    necrotizing pancreatitis
NPC
    nasopharyngeal carcinoma
    negative peritoneal cytology
NPE
    neurogenic pulmonary edema
    nonpulmonary route of elimination
NPPV
    noninvasive positive-pressure ventilation
NPTR
    National Pediatric Trauma Registry
NPTS
    nocturnal painful tonic spasm
NPV
    negative predictive value
    negative pressure ventilation
NSABP
    National Surgical Adjuvant Breast and
      Bowel Project
NSAID
    nonsteroidal antiinflammatory drug
      NSAID analgesic
N-shaped sigmoid loop
NTI
    nasotracheal intubation
nub
    fibrotic n.
nucha
nuchal
    n. fascia
    n. ligament
    n. line
    n. plane
    n. region
Nuck canal
nuclear
    n. atypia
    n. external layer
    n. grade
    n. magnetic resonance (NMR)
    n. medicine
    n. tissue
nucleation time
nucleolysis
    percutaneous laser n.
nucleus, pl. **nuclei**
    n. ambiguus lesion

N

NOTES

nucleus *(continued)*
    Edinger-Westphal n.
    external cuneate n.
    extrapyramidal n.
    ossifying n.
    n. pulposus herniation
    n. rotator
Nuhn gland
nulliparity
null point
numbness
numerary renal anomaly
numerical cipher method
nummular lesion
nummulation
nurse
    n. anesthetist
    visiting n.
nutcracker
    n. esophagus
    n. fracture
nutmeg
    n. appearance
    n. liver
nutricius
nutrient
    n. absorption
    n. artery

    n. canal
    n. flap
    n. foramen
    hepatotrophic n.
    n. vessel
nutrition
    enteral n.
    parenteral n.
    tissue n.
    total parenteral n. (TPN)
nutritional
    n. assessment
    n. status
Nuttall operation
nycturia
Nyhus classification
Nylen-Barany maneuver
nympha
nymphal
nymphectomy
nymphocaruncularis
nymphocaruncular sulcus
nymphohymenal sulcus
nymphotomy
nystagmogram
nystagmoid-like oscillation
nystagmus
nyxis

O₂
    oxygen
OA
    open appendectomy
Oakley-Fulthorpe technique
oat cell carcinoma
OAV
    oculoauriculovertebral
    OAV syndrome
obcecation
O'Beirne sphincter
Ober
    O. incision
    O. tendon technique
Ober-Barr
    O.-B. procedure for brachioradialis
      transfer
    O.-B. transfer technique
Obersteiner-Redlich line
obese patient
obesity
    androgenic o.
    central o.
    clinically severe o. (CSO)
    o. hypoventilation syndrome (OHS)
    medication-induced o.
obex
object
    O. Classification Test
    fixation o.
    o. program
    o. space
objective
    O. Pain Scale
    surgical treatment o.
object-space focus
oblique
    o. abdominal muscle
    o. aberration
    o. arytenoid muscle
    o. auricular muscle
    o. base wedge osteotomy
    o. cord
    o. coronal plane
    o. displacement osteotomy
    external o.
    o. facial cleft
    o. fissure of lung
    o. flap
    o. flow misregistration
    o. fracture
    o. head
    o. hernia
    o. illumination
    left anterior o. (LAO)

    o. pericardial sinus
    o. projection
    right anterior o. (RAO)
    o. sagittal gradient-echo MR
      imaging
    o. section
obliterans
    arteriosclerosis o. (ASO)
    thromboangiitis o.
obliteration
    balloon-occluded retrograde
      transvenous o. (B-RTO)
    endoscopic extirpation cicatricial o.
    fibrous o.
    percutaneous transhepatic o.
    radiographic o.
    subdeltoid fat plane o.
    total ear o.
obliterative
    o. bronchiolitis
    o. inflammation
    o. scarring
oblongata
    rostral ventrolateral medulla o.
O'Brien
    O. akinesia technique
    O. anesthesia
    O. capsular shift procedure
    O. pelvic halo operation
obscuration
    transient visual o.
observation
    o. period
    o. ward
observer-dependent criteria
obstetric
    o. anesthesia
    o. pain
    o. position
obstetrical
    o. complication
    o. hysterectomy
    o. management
    o. operation
    o. traction injury
obstetrics
    International Federation of
      Gynecology and O. (FIGO)
obstipation
obstructed
    o. bowel
    o. liver
obstructing
    o. colorectal cancer
    o. pathology

O

obstruction
    acute intestinal o.
    adherence o.
    adhesive small bowel o.
    airway o.
    anorectal outlet o.
    ball-valve o.
    biliary tract o.
    bowel o.
    catheter o.
    closed loop intestinal o.
    clot-induced urinary tract o.
    colon o.
    colonic o.
    common duct o.
    complete o.
    complex left ventricular outflow
      tract o.
    ductal o.
    esophageal o.
    extrahepatic bile duct o.
    extrahepatic biliary o.
    extrahepatic binary o.
    extrahepatic portal vein o. (EHPO)
    extramural upper airway o.
    gastric outlet o. (GOO)
    hepatic venous outflow o.
    intermittent subclavian vein o.
    intestinal o.
    ipsilateral portal vein o.
    left-sided colorectal o.
    longer-segment o.
    mechanical extrahepatic o.
    membranous o.
    myoglobin tubular o.
    outflow tract o.
    partial mechanical o.
    portal vein o.
    postoperative airway o.
    shunt o.
    site of o.
    stop-valve airway o.
    superior venal caval o.
    upper airway o.
    ureteropelvic o.
    ureterovesical o.
    urinary tract o.
    vein o.
    ventricular inflow tract o.
    ventricular outflow tract o.
obstruction-induced modulation
obstructive
    o. apnea
    o. esophagogastric cancer
    o. hydatid material
    o. hydrocephalus
    o. jaundice
    o. lung disease (OLD)
    o. mechanism

    o. pulmonary dysfunction
    o. uropathy
obstruent
obtundation
Obtura injectable technique
obturation
    canal o.
    intermittent self-o.
    retrograde o.
    root canal filling technique o.
obturator
    o. artery
    o. avulsion fracture
    o. bypass
    o. canal
    o. crest
    o. fascia
    o. foramen
    o. groove
    o. hernia
    o. line
    o. lymphatic chain
    o. nerve
    o. nerve block
    o. nerve damage
    o. nerve injury
    o. neurectomy
    o. shelf cystourethropexy
    o. sign
    o. test
    o. tubercle
obtuse margin
obviate
OC
    operative cholangiography
occipital
    o. angle
    o. artery
    o. belly
    o. bone
    o. border
    o. branch
    o. cephalocele
    o. cerebral vein
    o. condyle
    o. condyle fracture
    o. condyle syndrome
    o. emissary vein
    o. fontanelle
    o. groove
    left anterior o. (LAO)
    o. malformation
    o. margin
    o. nerve
    o. neurectomy
    o. node
    o. plane
    o. plexus
    o. point

right anterior o. (RAO)
o. sinus
o. suture
o. triangle
occipitalization
occipitoanterior position
occipitoatlantal dislocation
occipitoatlantoaxial anomaly
occipitoatloid
occipitoaxial
occipitobregmatic
occipitocervical
o. approach
o. fixation
o. fusion
o. stabilization
occipitocollicular tract
occipitofacial
occipitofrontal muscle
occipitomastoid suture
occipitomental projection
occipitoparietal suture
occipitopontine tract
occipitoposterior position
occipitosphenoid suture
occipitotectal tract
occipitotemporal
occipitothalamic radiation
occipitotransverse position
occiput
occluded segment
occluding
o. centric relation record
o. relation
occlusal
o. cavity
o. correction
o. equilibration
o. plane
o. plane angle
o. position
o. pressure
o. projection
o. relation
o. therapy
occlusion
angioplasty-related vessel o.
aortic o.
arterial o.
artery o.
carotid artery o.
centric relation o.

clip o.
contralateral carotid artery o.
eccentric o.
endovascular balloon o.
graft o.
hemihepatic vascular o.
inferior vena cava balloon o.
(IVCO)
inflow o.
intermittent inflow o.
IVC o.
laparoscopic total o. (LTO)
MCA o.
mechanical o.
middle cerebral artery o.
2-plane o.
plastic stent o.
o. pressure
rapid o.
subclavian artery o.
temporary balloon o.
o. therapy
tourniquet o.
vascular o.
vein o.
venous o.
occlusive
o. carotid artery disease
o. coronary artery disease
o. ileus
o. MI
o. patch test
o. therapy
occult
o. bleeding
o. blood
o. cerebrovascular malformation
o. diaphragmatic injury
o. enterotomy
o. extrahepatic disease
o. fracture
o. hepatic disease
o. irresectable disease
o. metastasis
o. spinal dysraphism
o. systemic disease
o. talar lesion
o. vascular malformation
occupational
o. therapy
o. toxin exposure
Ochsenbein gingivectomy

O

NOTES

511

Ockerblad-Boari flap
O'Connor operation
O'Connor-Peter operation
OCR
 oculocardiac reflex
octanol/water coefficient
octogenarian
octreotide
ocular
 o. adnexa
 o. adnexal lesion
 o. barrier
 o. cul-de-sac
 o. inflammation
 o. manifestation
 o. metastasis
 o. microtremor
 o. microtremor during general anesthesia
 o. motility disorder
 o. muscle
 o. oscillation
 o. radiation therapy
 o. tumor
ocular-mucous membrane syndrome
oculi (*pl. of* oculus)
oculoauriculovertebral (OAV)
 o. dysplasia
oculobuccogenital syndrome
oculocardiac reflex (OCR)
oculocephalic
 o. maneuver
 o. vascular anomaly
oculofacial
oculogyration
oculomandibulofacial syndrome
oculomotor
 o. decussation
 o. foramen
 o. ganglion
 o. nerve
oculopharyngeal muscular dystrophy
oculoplastic
 o. surgeon
 o. surgery
oculovertebral syndrome
oculozygomatic
oculus, pl. oculi
odd-even method
Oddi sphincter
O'Donnell operation
O'Donoghue
 O. ACL reconstruction
 O. facetectomy
 O. procedure
odontectomy
odontoameloblastoma
odontoblastoma
odontocele

odontoclastoma
odontogenic infection
odontoid
 o. condyle fracture
 o. fracture internal fixation
 o. fracture stabilization
 o. neck fracture
 o. perpendicular line
 o. process osteosynthesis
 o. screw fixation
 o. screw placement
odontoidectomy
odontolysis
odontoplasty
odontoscopy
odontosteophyte
odontotomy
 prophylactic o.
odoriferous gland
ODQ
 Oswestry Disability Questionnaire
O'Dwyer intubation
OFD
 orofaciodigital
 OFD syndrome
off-center isoperistaltic technique
office
 Surgeon General's O. (SGO)
off-label use
off-pump coronary artery bypass (OPCAB)
off-set V-osteotomy
Ogata
 O. method
 O. technique
Ogden
 O. epiphysial fracture classification
 O. knee dislocation classification
Ogilvie
 O. operation
 O. syndrome
Ogston-Luc operation
Ogura operation
O'Hara 2-clamp method
Ohngren line
OHS
 obesity hypoventilation syndrome
 open heart surgery
OI
 oxygenation index
oil
 o. drop lesion
 o. gland
 iodized o.
 joint o.
oil-aspiration pneumonia
Okamoto method
Okamura technique

Okuda transhepatic obliteration of varix
OLD
    obstructive lung disease
old posterior cyst
olecranization
olecranon
    o. bursa
    o. fracture
    o. process
oleogranuloma
oleoma
olfactoria
olfactory
    o. anesthesia
    o. bulb
    o. bundle
    o. nerve
    o. tract
oligoanalgesia
oligoastrocytoma
    recurrent vermian o.
oligoclonal growth
oligodendroblastoma
oligodendroglioma
oligomerization
oligosegmental correction
oligospermia
oligozoospermatism
oliguresia
oliguria
olisthesis
olivary body
Oliver-Rosalki method
olivocerebellar tract
olivocochlear
    o. bundle
    o. nerve
olivospinal tract
Ollier
    O. arthrodesis approach
    O. incision
    O. lateral approach
    O. method
    O. technique
    O. thick split free graft
Ollier-Thiersch graft
Olshausen
    O. procedure
    O. suspension
OLT
    orthotopic liver transplant

    orthotopic liver transplantation
    OLT recipient
OLV
    1-lung ventilation
Olympus gastrostomy
Ombrédanne operation
omega-shaped incision
omenta (*pl. of* omentum)
omental
    o. appendage
    o. branch
    o. bursa
    o. cyst
    o. enterocleisis
    o. flap
    o. hammock
    o. hernia
    o. J-pexy
    o. metastasis
    o. nodal disease
    o. patch
    o. pedicle
    o. pedicle wrapping
    o. pouch
    o. recess
    o. reinforcement
    o. sac
    o. spread
    o. tenia
    o. tuber
omentectomy
    greater o.
    lesser o.
omentitis
omentofixation
omentopexy
omentoplasty
    pedicled o.
omentorrhaphy
omentosplenopexy
omentotomy
omentovolvulus
omentulum
omentum, pl. **omenta**
    colic o.
    gastrocolic o.
    gastrohepatic o.
    gastrosplenic o.
    greater o.
    lesser o.
    o. majus flap procedure
    pancreaticosplenic o.

O

NOTES

omentum *(continued)*
    permanent mesh o.
    splenogastric o.
omentumectomy
omentum-to-brain transposition
Omer-Capen
    O.-C. carpectomy
    O.-C. technique
omniplane scan
omocervical flap
omoclavicular
    o. fossa
    o. triangle
omohyoideus
omohyoid muscle
omothyroid
omotracheal triangle
omphalectomy
omphalic
omphalocele
    infraumbilical o.
omphalomesenteric
omphalos
omphalospinous
omphalotomy
omphalotripsy
omphalovesical
omphalus
oncho-osteodysplasia
oncocytoma
oncogene
    tumor suppressor o.
oncologic
    o. clearance
    o. consideration
oncologist
    medical o.
    radiation o.
    surgical o.
oncology
    GI o.
    surgical o.
    urologic o.
oncolysate
    polyvalent melanoma o.
    vaccinia melanoma o. (VMO)
oncoma
oncometric
oncoplastic surgery
oncotic pressure
oncotomy
Ondine curse
oneirogmus
oneiroscopy
ONF
    open Nissen fundoplication
onion
    o. peel appearance

    o. scale lesion
    o. skin-like membrane
onion-bulb
    o.-b. changes
    o.-b. changes on biopsy
onlay
    o. island flap
    o. island flap urethroplasty
    o. patch anastomosis
    o. technique
onlay-tube-onlay urethroplasty technique
on-line data
onset of blockade
on-table
    o.-t. irrigation
    o.-t. lavage
onychectomy
onychocryptosis nail
onychogryposis
onycholysis
onychoma
onychomycosis
onycho-osteodysplasia
onychoplasty
onychotomy
oocyte
    o. extrusion
    o. micromanipulation
oophorectomy
    prophylactic o.
oophorocystectomy
oophorohysterectomy
oophoroma
oophoropeliopexy
oophoropexy
oophoroplasty
oophororrhaphy
oophorosalpingectomy
oophorostomy
oophorotomy
Oort nerve
opacification
opacity
OPCAB
    off-pump coronary artery bypass
open
    o. adjustable silicone gastric
      banding
    o. adrenalectomy
    o. amputation
    o. anesthesia system
    o. antireflux surgery
    o. appendectomy (OA)
    o. application test
    o. bone graft epiphysiodesis
    o. brain biopsy
    o. cavity
    o. cholecystectomy
    o. circuit method

o. colectomy
o. common bile duct exploration
o. disc surgery
o. diverticulectomy
o. drainage
o. drop anesthesia
o. drop technique
o. endarterectomy
o. esophagectomy
o. esophagomyotomy
o. flap
o. flap technique
o. fundoplication
o. Hasson technique
o. head injury
o. heart surgery (OHS)
o. hemorrhoidectomy
o. hernia operation
o. herniorrhaphy
o. intraoperative ultrasonography
o. laparoscopic approach
o. laparoscopic technique
o. laparoscopy
o. laparotomy
o. liver biopsy
o. loop
o. lung biopsy
o. Nissen fundoplication (ONF)
o. Nissen operation
o. osteotomy
o. palm technique
o. partial nephrectomy
o. patch test
o. pinning
o. pneumothorax
o. pyelolithotomy
o. pyelotomy
o. reconstruction
o. reconstructive procedure
o. reduction
o. reduction and internal fixation
 (ORIF)
o. repair
o. retroperitoneal high ligation
o. skull fracture
o. sphincteroplasty
o. splenectomy
o. stereotactic craniotomy
o. surgical biopsy
o. surgical cordotomy
o. surgical therapy
o. surgical treatment

o. thoracotomy
o. venous channel
o. vertical banded gastroplasty
o. wedge
o. wound
open-book fracture
open-break fracture
open-end ostomy pouch
open-gloving technique
opening
 appendiceal o.
 o. flap
 ileocecal o.
 maximum mouth o.
 midpalatal suture o.
 o. pressure
 saphenous o.
 tendinous o.
 urethral o.
 vaginal o.
 o. wedge manipulation
open-section nail
open-sky
 o.-s. cryoextraction operation
 o.-s. technique
 o.-s. trephination
 o.-s. vitrectomy
operable
opera-glass deformity
operant
 o. conditioning
 o. procedure
operating
 o. room (OR)
 o. theater
 o. time
operation
 Abbe o.
 Abbe-Estlander o.
 Abbott-Lucas shoulder o.
 Abernethy o.
 ab externo filtering o.
 Adams hip o.
 Adler o.
 Agnew o.
 Agrikola o.
 Alexander o.
 Allen o.
 Allport o.
 Alvis o.
 Ammon o.
 Amsler o.

NOTES

operation *(continued)*

Amussat o.
Anagnostakis o.
anastomotic o.
Anel o.
Angelucci o.
Anson-McVay o.
antiperistaltic o.
antireflux o.
anular corneal graft o.
Appolito o.
Argyll-Robertson o.
Aries-Pitanguy o.
Arion o.
Arlt o.
Arlt-Jaesche o.
Armistead ulnar lengthening o.
Arrowhead o.
Arroyo o.
Arruga o.
Arruga-Berens o.
arterial switch o.
Ashford retracted nipple o.
atrial baffle o.
Auchincloss o.
Aylett o.
Babcock o.
Bacon-Babcock o.
Badal o.
Baker patellar advancement o.
Baker translocation o.
Baldy o.
Baldy-Webster o.
Ball o.
Ball-Hoffman o.
Band-Aid o.
Bangerter pterygium o.
Bankart o.
Bankart-Putti-Platt o.
bariatric o.
Barkan-Cordes linear cataract o.
Barkan double cyclodialysis o.
Barkan goniotomy o.
Barnard o.
Barraquer enzymatic zonulolysis o.
Barraquer keratomileusis o.
Barrie-Jones
  canaliculodacryorhinostomy o.
Barrio o.
Barr tendon transfer o.
Bassini o.
Bateman modification of Mayer
  transfer o.
Battle o.
Baudelocque o.
Bauer-Tondra-Trusler o.
Baynton o.
Beard o.
Beard-Cutler o.

Beck I, II o.
Beer o.
Belsey Mark IV antireflux o.
Benedict orbit o.
Berens pterygium transplant o.
Berens sclerectomy o.
Berens-Smith o.
Berger o.
Berke o.
Berke-Motais o.
Bernard o.
Bethke o.
Bielschowsky o.
biliary-enteric anastomosis o.
Billroth I, II o.
Bircher o.
Birch-Hirschfeld entropion o.
Blair o.
Blalock-Hanlon o.
Blalock-Taussig o.
Blasius lid flap o.
Blaskovics canthoplasty o.
Blaskovics dacryostomy o.
Blaskovics lid o.
Blatt o.
Bloch-Paul-Mikulicz o.
bloodless o.
Böhm o.
Bonaccolto-Flieringa vitreous o.
Bonnet enucleation o.
Bonzel o.
Bora o.
Bose o.
Bossalino blepharoplasty o.
Bowman o.
Boyd o.
Bozeman o.
Brailey o.
Brenner o.
Bricker o.
Bridge o.
bridge pedicle flap o.
Briggs strabismus o.
Bristow o.
Brock o.
Bromley foreign body o.
Bronson foreign body removal o.
Brophy o.
Brunschwig o.
Bryant o.
Budinger blepharoplasty o.
Burch eye evisceration o.
Burow flap o.
Butler fifth toe o.
buttonhole o.
Buzzi o.
bypass o.
Byron Smith ectropion o.
Cairns o.

Caldwell-Luc o.
Calhoun-Hagler lens extraction o.
Callahan o.
Camey I, II o.
Campodonico o.
capital o.
Carmody-Batson o.
Carrel o.
Carter o.
Casanellas lacrimal o.
Casey o.
Castroviejo o.
Castroviejo-Scheie cyclodiathermy o.
cataract extraction o.
Cattell o.
cautery o.
Cawthorne o.
Celsus-Hotz o.
Celsus spasmodic entropion o.
cerclage o.
cesarean o.
Chandler-Verhoeff o.
Chandler vitreous o.
Chaput o.
Chaput anal o.
Charles o.
Cheyne o.
Child o.
Cibis o.
cinching o.
Clagett o.
clean o.
clean-contaminated o.
Cleasby iridectomy o.
Cloward o.
cluster o.
Collin-Beard o.
Collis antireflux o.
colorectal o.
Comberg foreign body o.
commando o.
comparison o.
complete wrap Nissen o.
Conn o.
Conrad orbital blowout fracture o.
conventional o.
Cooper o.
corneal graft o.
Cotte o.
Cotting toenail o.
Counsellor-Davis artificial vagina o.
Crawford sling o.

crescent o.
Crespo o.
Crile-Matas o.
Critchett o.
Crock encircling o.
cryoextraction o.
cryotherapy o.
Csapody orbital repair o.
curative-intent o.
curative sphincter-saving o.
Cushing o.
Cusick o.
Cusick-Sarrail ptosis o.
Cutler o.
Cutler-Beard o.
cyclodiathermy o.
Czermak pterygium o.
Czerny o.
dacryoadenectomy o.
dacryocystectomy o.
dacryocystorhinotomy o.
dacryocystostomy o.
Dailey o.
Dalgleish o.
Dallas o.
Damus-Kaye-Stansel o.
Dana o.
Dandy o.
Danforth fetal o.
Daviel o.
day-case o.
debulking o.
de Grandmont o.
Deiter o.
Delorme rectal prolapse o.
Del Toro o.
Denker sinus o.
Derby o.
Desmarres o.
de Vincentiis o.
DeWecker o.
Diamond-Gould syndactyly o.
Dianoux o.
diathermy o.
Dickey o.
Dickey-Fox o.
Dickson-Wright o.
Dieffenbach o.
DKS o.
Döderlein roll-flap o.
Dohlman o.
D'ombrain o.

NOTES

operation *(continued)*

Donald-Fothergill o.
Doyle o.
Drummond-Morison o.
Duhamel colon o.
Duke-Elder o.
Dunnington o.
Dupuy-Dutemps o.
Durham flatfoot o.
Durr o.
Duverger-Velter o.
Dwyer clawfoot o.
Eagleton o.
Eaton-Malerich fracture-dislocation o.
Edlan-Mejchar o.
effector o.
Ekehorn o.
Elliot o.
Elschnig canthorrhaphy o.
Ely o.
emergency o.
emergent o.
Emmet o.
equilibrating o.
Escapini cataract o.
Esser inlay o.
Estes o.
Estlander o.
Eversbusch o.
eversion o.
evisceration o.
Ewing o.
exploratory o.
extraabdominal o.
extracapsular cataract extraction o.
Faden o.
Falk-Shukuris o.
Fanta cataract o.
Farmer o.
Fasanella o.
Fasanella-Servat ptosis o.
fenestrated Fontan o.
fenestration o.
Fergus o.
Filatov o.
Filatov-Marzinkowsky o.
filtering o.
Fink o.
Finney o.
Flajani o.
flap o.
floating forehead o.
Föerster o.
Foley o.
Fontan o.
Fothergill o.
Fothergill-Donald o.
Fothergill-Hunter o.

Fox o.
Franceschetti coreoplasty o.
Franceschetti corepraxy o.
Franceschetti deviation o.
Franceschetti keratoplasty o.
Franceschetti pupil deviation o.
Franke tabes o.
Frazier-Spiller o.
Fredet-Ramstedt o.
French supracondylar fracture o.
Freund o.
Fricke o.
Friede o.
Friedenwald o.
Friedenwald-Guyton o.
Frost-Lang o.
Fuchs canthorrhaphy o.
Fuchs iris bombe transfixation o.
Fukala o.
Furlow-Fisher modification of Virag 1 o.
Galeazzi patellar o.
Gallie o.
Gardner o.
Gauderer-Ponsky PEG o.
Gayet o.
Gifford delimiting keratotomy o.
Gigli o.
Gilles o.
Gilliam o.
Gilliam-Doleris o.
Gillies scar correction o.
Gil-Vernet o.
Giordano o.
Girard keratoprosthesis o.
Gittes o.
Glenn o.
Goldmann-Larson foreign body o.
Goldsmith o.
gold weight and wire spring o.
Gomez-Marquez lacrimal o.
Gonin cautery o.
goniotomy o.
Goodall-Power o.
Gradle keratoplasty o.
Graefe o.
Grant-Ward o.
Graves o.
Grimsdale o.
Grondahl-Finney o.
Gross o.
Grossmann o.
Gussenbauer o.
Gutzeit dacryostomy o.
Guyton ptosis o.
Halsted o.
Hampton o.
Handley o.
hanging hip o.

hanging toe o.
Harmon o.
Harms-Dannheim trabeculotomy o.
Hartmann o.
Hasner o.
Hassab o.
Haultain o.
Heaney o.
Heaton o.
Heine o.
Heineke o.
Heisrath o.
Heller o.
Heller-Belsey o.
Heller-Dor o.
Heller-Nissen o.
hemi-Fontan o.
Henry o.
Herbert o.
Hess eyelid o.
Hess ptosis o.
Hiff o.
Hill antireflux o.
Hinsberg o.
Hippel o.
Hirst o.
Hochenegg o.
Hofmeister o.
Hogan o.
Hoguet o.
Holth o.
Hopkins o.
Horay o.
Hotz-Anagnostakis o.
Hotz entropion o.
Huggins o.
Hughes o.
Hummelsheim o.
Hunt o.
Hunter o.
Hunt-Transley o.
Hutch ureteral reflux o.
I-beam hip o.
indentation o.
Indian o.
initial o.
interval o.
intracapsular cataract extraction o.
iridectomy o.
iridencleisis o.
iridodialysis o.
iridotasis o.

iridotomy o.
Irvine o.
Italian o.
Ivalon sponge-wrap o.
Jaboulay-Doyen-Winkleman o.
Jackson-Babcock o.
Jaesche o.
Jaesche-Arlt o.
Jaime lacrimal o.
Jameson o.
Japanese standard o.
Japanese-style o.
Jensen o.
Johnson o.
Kader-Senn o.
Kasai o.
Katzin o.
Kazanjian o.
Keen o.
Keller-Madlener o.
Kelman o.
Kennedy-Pacey o.
keratectomy o.
keratocentesis o.
keratomileusis o.
keratoplasty o.
keratotomy o.
Key o.
kidney-sparing o.
King o.
Kirby o.
Knapp o.
Knapp-Wheeler-Reese o.
Koffler o.
Kondoleon o.
Konno o.
Kraske o.
Kraupa o.
Krempen-Silver-Sotelo nonunion o.
Krönlein o.
Krönlein-Berke o.
Kropp o.
Kuhnt eyelid o.
Kuhnt-Helmbold o.
Kuhnt-Thorpe o.
Kwitko o.
Ladd o.
Lagleyze-Trantas o.
Lagrange o.
Lahey o.
laissez-faire lid o.
Lancaster o.

O

NOTES

operation *(continued)*
    Lanchner o.
    Landolt o.
    Lane o.
    Langenbeck o.
    laparoscopic Hassab o.
    Laroyenne o.
    laryngeal keel o.
    Lash o.
    Lawson o.
    Leahey o.
    Le Fort o.
    Le Fort-Neugebauer o.
    Leriche o.
    Lester-Jones o.
    Lester Martin modification of
      Duhamel o.
    Levine dislocation o.
    Lewis o.
    Lexer o.
    Lichtenstein o.
    limb-sparing o.
    Lincoff o.
    Lindesmith o.
    Lindner o.
    Lindsay o.
    Linton o.
    lip adhesion o.
    liver o.
    logical o.
    Löhlein o.
    Londermann o.
    Longmire o.
    Lopez-Enriquez o.
    Lord o.
    Loreta o.
    Lotheissen o.
    Löwenstein o.
    Lynch o.
    Macewen hernia o.
    Machek-Blaskovics o.
    Machek-Brunswick o.
    Machek-Gifford o.
    Machek ptosis o.
    Mack-Brunswick o.
    MacNab o.
    Madlener o.
    Magitot keratoplasty o.
    magnet o.
    magnetic o.
    Magnuson-Stack o.
    MAGPI o.
    Mainz pouch o.
    Majewsky o.
    major o.
    Maladie de Graeffe o.
    Malbec o.
    Malbran o.
    Manchester o.

    Manchester-Fothergill o.
    mandibular swing o.
    Mann-Williamson o.
    Marckwald o.
    Marcy o.
    Marquez-Gomez o.
    Marshall-Marchetti-Krantz o.
    Mason o.
    mastoid obliteration o.
    Matas o.
    Mauksch-Maumenee-Goldberg o.
    Maumenee-Goldberg o.
    Maunsell-Weir o.
    Mayer transfer o.
    Mayo o.
    McBurney o.
    McGavic o.
    McGuire o.
    McIndoe o.
    McKay-Simons clubfoot o.
    McLaughlin o.
    McLean o.
    McReynolds o.
    McVay o.
    Meek o.
    Meller o.
    Mensor-Scheck hanging hip o.
    Meyer o.
    Meyer-Schwickerath o.
    Michaelson o.
    mika o.
    Mikulicz o.
    Miles o.
    Miller flatfoot o.
    minor o.
    Minsky o.
    modified flap o.
    Moncrieff o.
    Monfort o.
    Moran o.
    Morax o.
    morcellation o.
    Morel-Fatio-Lalardie o.
    Mosher o.
    Mosher-Toti o.
    Moss o.
    Motais o.
    motivating o.
    Moynihan o.
    Mueller o.
    Mules o.
    muscle sliding o.
    Mustard o.
    Mustardé o.
    myectomy o.
    myelomeningocele o.
    myotomy o.
    Naffziger o.
    Neher o.

Nehra-Mack o.
Nesbit o.
Neviaser o.
Nicoll fracture o.
Nirschl o.
Nissen antireflux o.
Nissen fundoplication o.
Nizetic o.
Norton o.
Norwood o.
Nuttall o.
O'Brien pelvic halo o.
obstetrical o.
O'Connor o.
O'Connor-Peter o.
O'Donnell o.
Ogilvie o.
Ogston-Luc o.
Ogura o.
Ombrédanne o.
open hernia o.
open Nissen o.
open-sky cryoextraction o.
optical iridectomy o.
orbital implant o.
orthotopic hemi-Koch o.
outpatient thyroid o.
Owen o.
Pagenstecher o.
palliative o.
Palma o.
Palomo o.
Panas o.
pancreatic o.
parallel o.
parathyroid o.
Partsch o.
Patey o.
pattern cut corneal graft o.
Payne o.
pedicle flap o.
Peet o.
Pemberton o.
peripheral iridectomy o.
Peter o.
Physick o.
Pico o.
Pirogoff o.
plastic o.
plombage o.
pocket o.
Pollock o.

Pólya o.
Polyak o.
Pomeroy o.
Porro o.
portacaval shunt o.
Portmann interposition o.
Potts o.
Poulard o.
Power o.
Preziosi o.
probing lacrimonasal duct o.
protective antireflux o.
pubovaginal o.
Puestow-Gillesby o.
pull-through o.
pulsed-mode o.
Putenney o.
Putti-Platt o.
Quaglino o.
Ramstedt o.
Ransohoff o.
Rashkind o.
Rastan o.
Rastelli o.
Raverdino o.
Ray-Brunswick-Mack o.
Ray-McLean o.
Récamier o.
reconstructive o.
Redmond-Smith o.
Reese-Cleasby o.
Reese-Jones-Cooper o.
Reese ptosis o.
repeat o.
resectional phase of o.
resurfacing o.
Richet o.
Ripstein rectal prolapse o.
Rizzoli o.
Rosenburg o.
Rosengren o.
Roux-en-Y o.
Roux-Goldthwait dislocation o.
Roveda o.
Rovsing o.
Rowbotham o.
Rowinski o.
Rubbrecht o.
Ruedemann o.
Rycroft o.
sacrofixation o.
Saemisch o.

O

NOTES

521

operation *(continued)*

Saenger o.
Safar o.
Sanders o.
Sato o.
Savin o.
Sawyer o.
Sayoc o.
Scarpa o.
Schauta vaginal o.
Scheie o.
Schepens o.
Schimek o.
Schirmer o.
Schlatter o.
Schmalz o.
Schönbein o.
Schroeder o.
Schuchardt o.
scleral buckling o.
scleral fistulectomy o.
scleral shortening o.
scleroplasty o.
sclerotomy o.
Scott o.
scrotal pouch o.
Scudder o.
second-look o.
sector iridectomy o.
Selinger o.
semielective o.
Senn o.
Senning o.
sensor o.
serial o.
seton o.
sex change o.
Shaffer o.
Shirodkar o.
Shugrue o.
Sichi o.
Silva-Costa o.
Silver-Hildreth o.
single-stage o.
slant muscle o.
Smith-Boyce o.
Smith eyelid o.
Smith-Gibson o.
Smith-Indian o.
Smith-Kuhnt-Szymanowski o.
Smith-Robinson o.
Snellen ptosis o.
1-snip punctum o.
3-snip punctum o.
Soave o.
Soria o.
Soriano o.
Sorrin o.
Sourdille keratoplasty o.

Sourdille ptosis o.
Spaeth cystic bleb o.
Spaeth ptosis o.
Speas o.
Spencer-Watson Z-plasty o.
sphincter-saving o.
Spinelli o.
splitting lacrimal papilla o.
stage o.
staging o.
Stallard eyelid o.
Stallard flap o.
Stallard-Liegard o.
Stamey o.
State o.
step graft o.
stereotactic o.
Stock o.
Stocker o.
Stoffel o.
Stookey-Scarff o.
Straith eyelid o.
Strampelli-Valvo o.
Streatfield o.
Streatfield-Fox o.
Streatfield-Snellen o.
Stretta o.
Sturmdorf o.
Suarez-Villafranca o.
subcutaneous o.
Sugarbaker o.
Sugiura o.
Summerskill o.
suprapubic urethrovesical
  suspension o.
suspensory sling o.
switch o.
symmetry o.
synchrocyclotron o.
Szymanowski o.
Szymanowski-Kuhnt o.
tagliacotian o.
talc o.
Tanner o.
Tansini o.
Tansley o.
Tasia o.
Taussig o.
Taussig-Morton o.
Teale-Knapp o.
TeLinde o.
tenotomy o.
Terson o.
Tessier craniofacial o.
Thal fundic patch o.
Thiersch anal incontinence o.
Thiersch graft o.
Thomas o.
Thomson o.

thyroid o.
Tillett o.
tongue-in-groove o.
Torek o.
total excisional o.
Toti o.
Toti-Mosher o.
Townley-Paton o.
trabeculectomy o.
Trainor o.
transsphenoidal o.
Trantas o.
Trendelenburg o.
Treves o.
Tripier o.
Troutman o.
Truc o.
Tudor-Thomas o.
tumbling technique o.
Turnbull multiple ostomy o.
Turner o.
Ulloa o.
unattended laboratory o.
Urban o.
urologic o.
Uyemura o.
van Buren o.
Vecchietti o.
Verhoeff o.
Verhoeff-Chandler o.
Vermale o.
Verneuil o.
Verwey eyelid o.
Viers o.
Virag o.
Vogt o.
Von Ammon o.
von Blaskovics-Doyen o.
von Graefe o.
von Hippel o.
Waldhauer o.
Walter Reed o.
Waters o.
Waterston o.
Watson o.
Watzke o.
Waugh o.
Way o.
Webster o.
Weeker o.
Weeks o.
Weir o.

Weisinger o.
Wendell Hughes o.
Werb o.
Wertheim o.
Wertheim-Schauta o.
West o.
Weve o.
Wharton-Jones o.
Wheeler o.
Wheeler-Reese o.
Wheelhouse o.
Whipple o.
Whitehead o.
Whitnall sling o.
Wicherkiewicz eyelid o.
Wiener o.
Wies o.
Williams copulating pouch o.
Wilmer o.
Winiwarter o.
Wise o.
Witzel o.
Wolfe ptosis o.
Worst o.
Worth ptosis o.
Wright o.
Young o.
Young-Dees o.
Young-Dees-Leadbetter o.
Zickel subtrochanteric fracture o.
Ziegler o.
Zimmerman o.
Zylik o.

operational homeostasis
operative
  o. approach
  o. arthroscopy
  o. arthrotomy
  o. biliary bypass
  o. blood loss
  o. cholangiography (OC)
  o. choledochoscopy
  o. correction
  o. débridement
  o. diagnosis
  o. drainage
  o. excision
  o. exposure
  o. field
  o. finding
  o. intervention
  o. management

NOTES

O

operative *(continued)*
   o. mortality
   o. mortality rate
   o. necrosectomy
   o. perforation
   o. procedure
   o. reconstruction
   o. reexploration
   o. result
   o. site complication
   o. specimen
   o. stabilization
   o. stress
   o. technique
   o. therapy
   o. time
   o. treatment
operatively stabilized
operator exposure
operculectomy
operculum, pl. **opercula**
O'Phelan technique
ophryon
ophryospinal angle
ophthalmectomy
ophthalmic
   o. activating solution
   o. anesthesia
   o. artery
   o. cul-de-sac
   o. examination
   o. nerve
   o. vein
ophthalmocarcinoma
ophthalmocele
ophthalmologic anesthesia
ophthalmomyotomy
ophthalmopathy
ophthalmophlebotomy
ophthalmoplasty
ophthalmoplegia
ophthalmoscopy
   binocular indirect o.
   direct o.
   indirect o.
   medical o.
   metric o.
   slit-lamp o.
ophthalmospectroscopy
ophthalmostasis
ophthalmotomy
opiate
opioid
   o. agonist
   o. analgesia
   o. analgesic
   o. anesthesia
   o. anesthetic
   o. antinociceptive activity

   endogenous o.
   epidural o.
   esterase-metabolized o.
   intrathecal o.
   lipophilic o.
   neuroaxial o.
   o. prescreening
   o. receptor
   o. rotation
   single-shot intrathecal o.
   o. system
opioid-based technique
opioid-insensitive pain
opisthion
opisthionasial
opisthotonos, opisthotonus
   o. position
OPO
   organ procurement organization
opponensplasty
   abductor digiti minimi o.
   Bunnell o.
   Huber adductor digiti quinti o.
   Manske-McCarroll o.
opportunistic
   o. complication
   o. organism
   o. systemic fungal infection
opposition respiration
opposure
opsonization
optic
   o. canal
   o. chiasm compression
   o. cul-de-sac
   o. cup
   o. cup-to-disc ratio
   o. decussation
   o. disc
   o. evagination
   o. foramen
   o. ganglion
   o. iridectomy
   o. keratoplasty
   o. nerve
   o. nerve atrophy
   o. nerve head
   o. nerve tumor
   o. neuropathy
   o. papilla
   o. papilla cavity
   o. pathway myelination
   o. radiation
   o. sheath
   o. tract
   o. tract compression
   o. tract syndrome
   o. vesicle

optical
- o. aberration
- o. biopsy
- o. correction
- o. density method
- o. iridectomy
- o. iridectomy operation
- o. keratoplasty
- o. nodal point
- o. rotation
- o. system
- o. tracking

opticociliary
- o. neurectomy
- o. neurotomy

optimal
- o. external laryngeal manipulation
- o. intensive medical management
- O. Observation Score
- o. technique
- o. therapy

opting
- o. in
- o. out

option
- interventional o.
- medical treatment o.
- surgical treatment o.
- therapeutic o.
- treatment o.

optometrist

OR
- operating room
- OR technician

ora, pl. **orae**

orad

O'Rahilly limb deficiency classification

oral
- o. administration
- o. analgesic
- o. anesthetic
- o. anesthetic technique
- o. anomaly
- o. antibiotic medication
- o. anticoagulant
- o. anticoagulation
- o. antimotility agent
- o. aphthous ulcer
- o. cavity
- o. cavity abnormality
- o. cavity cytology
- o. cavity tumor

- o. cephalocele
- o. complication
- o. condyloma planus
- o. endotracheal intubation
- o. feeding
- o. fissure
- o. immediate-release oxymorphone
- o. infection
- o. irrigation
- o. lighted-stylet intubation
- o. manifestation
- o. and maxillofacial surgery
- o. monotherapy
- o. mucosa
- o. peripheral examination
- o. pharyngeal airway
- o. pharynx
- o. reconstruction
- o. region
- o. respiration
- o. tissue
- o. transmucosal fentanyl citrate
- o. ulceration

oral-aural method

oral-facial-digital

Orandi technique

orbicular
- o. muscle
- o. zone

orbit
- deep o.
- lateral o.
- superficial o.
- superior o.

orbita, pl. **orbitae**

orbital
- o. adipose tissue
- o. anesthesia
- o. angioma
- o. apex syndrome
- o. arteriovenous malformation
- o. blow-out fracture
- o. branch
- o. canal
- o. cavity
- o. decompression
- o. eminence
- o. exenteration
- o. exenteration gastroscopic access technique
- o. extension
- o. fascia

O

NOTES

orbital *(continued)*
- o. fat pad
- o. fissure
- o. floor fracture
- o. height
- o. hematoma
- o. hernia
- o. implant operation
- o. index
- o. layer
- o. lesion
- o. line
- o. metastasis
- o. mucocele
- o. muscle
- o. phlebogram
- o. plane
- o. pyramid
- o. region
- o. rim fracture
- o. rim reconstruction
- o. section
- o. septum
- o. surface
- o. surgery
- o. tumor
- o. vein
- o. wall
- o. wall fracture

orbitalis muscle
orbitofrontal artery
orbitomaxillectomy
orbitomeatal line
orbitonasal
- o. index
- o. tissue

orbitosphenoid
orbitotomy
- Berke-Krönlein o.
- Krönlein o.

orbitozygomatic
- o. mandibular osteotomy
- o. temporopolar approach

orchalgia
orchectomy
orchialgia
orchichorea
orchidectomy
- partial o.
- radical o.

orchidic
orchiditis
orchidoblastoma
orchidoptosis
orchidorraphy
orchiectomy
- prophylactic o.
- radical inguinal o.

orchiepididymitis

orchioblastoma
orchiocele
orchiodynia
orchioneuralgia
orchiopathy
orchiopexy
- Bevan o.
- Cabot-Nesbit o.
- eversion o.
- Fowler-Stephens o.
- laparoscopic o.
- Prentiss o.
- scrotal pouch o.
- staged o.
- 2-step o.
- Torek o.
- transseptal o.

orchioplasty
orchiorrhaphy
orchiotherapy
orchiotomy
orchis, pl. **orchises**
orchitic
orchitis
orchotomy
ordinal classification
orexigenic factor
organ
- o. ablation
- o. allograft
- o. compromise
- Corti o.
- o. donation
- o. donor
- o. dysfunction
- effector o.
- external female genital o.
- external male genital o.
- o. failure criteria
- floating o.
- genital o.
- o. harvest
- internal female genital o.
- internal male genital o.
- intraabdominal o.
- intromittent o.
- o. perfusion
- o. procurement organization (OPO)
- O. Procurement Program
- ptotic o.
- secondary retroperitoneal o.
- size-matched o.
- solid o.
- supernumerary o.
- o. system
- o. transplantation
- urinary o.
- wandering o.
- Weber o.

organa (*pl. of* organum)
organic
    o. articulation disorder
    o. lesion
    o. short bowel syndrome
organism
    aerobic Gram-negative o.
    Campylobacter-like o. (CLO)
    colonizing o.
    commensal o.
    enteric o.
    fungal o.
    Gram-negative aerobic o.
    gut-derived Gram-negative
     aerobic o.
    mixed fungal o.
    opportunistic o.
    pure fungal o.
organization
    organ procurement o. (OPO)
    World Health O. (WHO)
organized
    o. clot
    o. hematoma
organizing inflammation
organoaxial
    o. rotation
    o. volvulus
organology
organopexy
organoscopy
organ-specific
    o.-s. pattern
    o.-s. pattern of injury
organum, pl. **organa**
Oriental
    O. cholangiohepatitis
    O. V-Y flap
orientation
    angle of o.
    limbal parallel o.
    phalangeal articular o.
    temporal o.
    visual o.
ORIF
    open reduction and internal fixation
orifice
    anal o.
    appendiceal o.
    esophagogastric o.
    eustachian tube o.
    exocranial o.

    external urethral o.
    gastroduodenal o.
    golf-hole ureteral o.
    ileocecal o.
    internal urethral o.
    myopectineal o.
    pharyngeal o.
    pulmonary o.
    pyloric o.
    renal artery o.
    root canal o.
    vaginal o.
    vein o.
orificium, pl. **orificia**
origin
    aberrant bronchial o.
    biliodigestive o.
    ectal o.
    flexor-pronator o.
    pancreatic head o.
    pectoralis major muscle o.
    primary o.
    sternocleidomastoid muscle o.
    tumor o.
oris
Ormond disease
oroantral fistula
orocutaneous fistula
oroendotracheal
orofacial
    o. carcinoma
    o. fistula
orofaciodigital (OFD)
    o. syndrome
orogastric
    o. pathway
    o. suction
oromandibular
    o. defect
    o. reconstruction
oronasal fistula
oropharyngeal
    o. airway
    o. anesthesia
    o. approach
    o. carcinoma
    o. hemorrhage
    o. passage
    o. reconstruction
    o. wall
oropharynx
ororespiratory tract

O

NOTES

orostoma
orotracheal intubation
Orr
    O. incision
    O. rectal prolapse repair
Orr-Loygue transabdominal proctopexy
Orsi-Grocco method
orthodontia
    surgical o.
orthodontic
    o. procedure
    o. therapy
orthodontics
    surgical o.
orthodox procedure
Orthofix large-pin fixation
orthognathic surgery
orthogonal
    o. plane
    o. projection
orthokeratinization
orthopaedic, orthopedic
    o. anesthesia
    o. anomaly
    o. problem
    o. surgical procedure
    o. Trauma Association classification
    o. traumatologist
orthoptic transplantation
orthoradioscopy
orthoscopy
orthosis
    cervicothoracic o. (CTO)
    o. drop-lock ring
orthotopic
    o. appendicocystostomy
    o. bladder
    o. graft
    o. heart transplantation
    o. hemi-Koch operation
    o. liver transplant (OLT)
    o. liver transplantation (OLT)
    o. liver transplant recipient
    o. ureterocele
    o. urinary diversion
Orticochea
    O. procedure
    O. scalping technique
Ortner syndrome
Ortolani maneuver
os, pl. ossa
    o. calcis osteotomy
    external o.
Osborne-Cotterill
    O.-C. elbow technique
    O.-C. procedure
Osborne posterior approach
oscheal
oscheoplasty

oscillation
    grade I, II o.
    high-frequency o.
    laryngeal o.
    nystagmoid-like o.
    ocular o.
oscillatory ventilation
oscillometric calibration
oscillometry
Osgood
    O. modified technique
    O. rotational osteotomy
Osgood-Schlatter lesion
osmication
osmification
Osmond-Clarke technique
osmotic pressure
ossa (pl. of os)
osseointegration
osseoligamentous ring
osseous
    o. anomaly
    o. fixation
    o. flap
    o. labyrinth
    o. lesion
    o. metastasis
    o. ring of Lacroix
    o. surgery
    o. tissue
osseus
ossicle
ossicula (pl. of ossiculum)
ossicular
    o. chain reconstruction
    o. prosthesis
ossiculectomy
ossiculoplasty
    tympanoplasty o.
ossiculum, pl. ossicula
ossification
ossifying
    o. epiphysis
    o. fibroma
    o. inflammation
    o. nucleus
ostectomy
    buccal o.
    fibular o.
    partial o.
    periodontal o.
osteitis
    bone flap o.
osteoaneurysm
osteoarthritis disease
osteoarthropathy
osteoarticular
    o. allograft
    o. allograft transplantation

o. defect
o. graft
osteoblast
osteoblastic
o. bone regeneration
o. lesion
o. metastasis
osteoblastoma
osteobunionectomy
osteocachexia
osteocarcinoma
osteocartilaginous
o. graft
o. loose body
osteocementum
osteochondral
o. allograft
o. defect
o. fragment
o. graft
o. injury
o. lesion
o. loose body
o. prominence
o. ridge
osteochondritis
osteochondrodesmodysplasia
osteochondrodysplasia
osteochondrodystrophy
familial o.
osteochondrofibroma
osteochondrolysis
osteochondroma
osteochondromatosis
osteochondropathy
osteochondrophyte
osteochondrosarcoma
osteochondrosis
osteochrondral slice fracture
osteoclasia
osteoclasis
Blount technique for o.
o. maneuver
osteoclastic
osteoclastoma
osteoconduction
osteocranium
osteocutaneous flap
osteocystoma
osteocyte
osteocytic lacuna
osteocytoma

osteodentin
osteodentinoma
osteodermatopoikilosis
osteodermatous
osteodermia
osteodiastasis
osteodysplasty
osteodystrophia
osteodystrophy
osteoectasia
osteoectomy
osteoenchondroma
osteoepiphysis
osteofibrochondrosarcoma
osteofibroma
osteofibromatosis
osteofibrosis
osteogenesis
distraction o.
o. imperfecta
o. imperfecta congenita syndrome
osteogenetic fiber
osteogenic sarcoma
osteohalisteresis
osteohypertrophy
osteoid osteoma
osteoinduction
osteointegration phenomenon
osteokinematic motion
osteokinematics
osteolathyrism
osteolipochondroma
osteolipoma
osteologia
osteologist
osteology
osteolysis
osteolytic bone lesion
osteoma
extraspinal osteoid o.
osteoid o.
osteomalacia
osteomalacic pelvis
osteomatoid
osteomatosis
osteomere
osteomesopyknosis
osteometry
osteomized
osteomuscular flap
osteomusculocutaneous flap
osteomyelitic sinus

NOTES

O

osteomyelitis
osteomyelodysplasia
osteomyelofibrosis
osteomyelofibrotic syndrome
osteomyelosclerosis
osteomyocutaneous flap
osteon
osteonal
    o. bone union
    o. lamellar bone
osteoncus
osteonecrosis
osteonectin
osteoneogenesis
osteoneuralgia
osteopathia striata syndrome
osteopathic lesion
osteopathy
osteopedion
osteopenia
osteoperiosteal
    o. bone graft
    o. flap
osteoperiostitis
osteopetrosis
    cranial o.
osteopetrotic scar
osteophlebitis
osteophyma
osteophyte formation
osteophytosis
osteoplastic
    o. bone flap
    o. craniotomy
    o. flap
    o. flap approach
    o. frontal sinus procedure
    o. necrotomy
    o. reconstruction
osteoplasty
osteopoikilosis
osteopontin
osteoporosis pseudoglioma syndrome
osteoporotic
    o. bone
    o. fracture
    o. spine
osteopsathyrosis
osteopulmonary arthropathy
osteoradionecrosis
osteosarcoma
osteosarcomatosis
osteosclerotic lesion
osteosis
osteospongioma
osteosteatoma
osteosynovitis
Osteosynthesefragen
    Arbeitsgemeinschaft für O. (AO)

osteosynthesis
    anterior column o.
    cranial o.
    facial o.
    lumbar spine vertebral o.
    odontoid process o.
    plate-screw o.
    posterior column o.
    thoracic spine vertebral o.
    thoracolumbar spine vertebral o.
    vertebral o.
    wire o.
osteosynthetic material
osteotelangiectasia
osteothrombophlebitis
osteothrombosis
osteotomize
osteotomy
    Abbott-Gill o.
    abduction o.
    abductor o.
    abductory wedge o.
    adduction o.
    Agliette supracondylar o.
    Akin proximal phalangeal o.
    Amspacher-Messenbaugh closing
      wedge o.
    Amstutz-Wilson o.
    Anderson-Fowler calcaneal
      displacement o.
    angular o.
    angulation o.
    anterior calcaneal o.
    anterior innominate o.
    Austin o.
    Axer lateral opening wedge o.
    Axer varus derotational o.
    Bailey-Dubow o.
    Baker-Hill o.
    Balacescu closing wedge o.
    ball-and-socket trochanteric o.
    base-of-neck o.
    base wedge o.
    basilar o.
    Bellemore-Barrett closing wedge o.
    Berman-Gartland metatarsal o.
    Bernese periacetabular o.
    bifurcation o.
    biplane trochanteric o.
    blind o.
    block o.
    Blount displacement o.
    Brackett o.
    Brett-Campbell tibial o.
    calcaneal L o.
    Campbell o.
    Canale o.
    canal innominate o.
    Carstan reverse wedge o.

Cartam-Treander reverse wedge o.
cervical o.
C-form o.
Chambers o.
chevron o.
chevron-type transmalleolar o.
Chiari innominate o.
Chiari-Salter-Steel pelvic o.
closed intramedullary o.
closed wedge o.
closing abductory wedge o.
closing base wedge o.
Cole o.
compensatory basilar o.
controlled rotational o.
countersinking o.
Coventry distal femoral o.
Coventry vagal o.
craniofacial o.
Crego femoral o.
crescentic o.
crescentic calcaneal o.
C sliding o.
cuneiform o.
cup-and-ball o.
cylindrical o.
Dega pelvic o.
delayed femoral o.
derotational o.
dial pelvic o.
dial periacetabular o.
diaphysial o.
Dickinson-Coutts-Woodward-
  Handler o.
Dickson geometric o.
Dillwyn-Evans o.
Dimon-Hughston intertrochanteric o.
displacement o.
dome o.
dome-shaped o.
dorsal closing wedge o.
dorsal proximal metatarsal o.
dorsal V o.
dorsiflexory wedge o.
double o.
Dunn o.
Dunn-Hess trochanteric o.
Dwyer o.
Elizabethtown o.
Emmon o.
endoscopic vertical ramus o.
epiphysial-metaphysial o.

Eppright dial o.
Estersohn o.
ethmoidal o.
Evans anterior calcaneal o.
eversion o.
extension o.
failed femoral o.
femoral o.
Fernandez o.
flexion o.
French lateral closing wedge o.
frontonasomaxillary o.
frontoorbital o.
geometric supracondylar
  extension o.
Gerbert o.
Giannestras oblique metatarsal o.
Gibson-Piggott o.
glabellar exposure o.
Gleich o.
glenoid o.
Golden closing wedge o.
Grant-Small-Lehman supracondylar
  extension o.
Greenfield o.
Green-Reverdin o.
greenstick dorsal proximal
  metatarsal o.
Green-Watermann o.
Gudas scarf Z-plasty o.
Haber-Kraft o.
Haddad metatarsal o.
Herman-Gartland o.
high tibial o.
hinge o.
Hirayma o.
horizontal o.
iliac o.
Ingram-Canle-Beaty epiphysial-
  metaphysial o.
innominate o.
intertrochanteric varus o.
intraarticular o.
intracapsular o.
intraepiphysial o.
inverted L-form o.
inverted scarf o.
Irwin o.
Japas o.
Johnson chevron o.
Kalish o.
Kaplan o.

NOTES

osteotomy *(continued)*
    Kawamura dome o.
    Kawamura pelvic o.
    Kelly-Keck o.
    Kempf-Grosse-Abalo Z-step o.
    Kessel-Bonney extension o.
    Kitaoka-Leventen medial
      displacement metatarsal o.
    Koutsogiannis calcaneal
      displacement o.
    Koutsogiannis-Fowler-Anderson o.
    Kramer-Craig-Noel basilar femoral
      neck o.
    Lambrinudi o.
    lateral closing wedge o.
    Leach-Igou step-cut medial o.
    Le Fort o.
    Lichtblau o.
    Lindseth o.
    linear o.
    Ludloff o.
    Macewen-Shands o.
    malleolar o.
    mandibular ramus o.
    Maquet dome o.
    Marquardt angulation o.
    Martin o.
    Mau o.
    maxillary o.
    medial displacement o.
    metacarpal o.
    metaphysial o.
    metatarsal Reverdin o.
    metatarsal V-shaped o.
    Mitchell o.
    Molesworth o.
    Mueller intertochanteric varus o.
    Mueller transposition o.
    oblique base wedge o.
    oblique displacement o.
    open o.
    orbitozygomatic mandibular o.
    os calcis o.
    Osgood rotational o.
    Pauwels proximal o.
    Pauwels valgus o.
    pedicle subtraction o.
    peg-in-hole o.
    Peimer reduction o.
    pelvic o.
    Pemberton pericapsular o.
    perforation o.
    pericapsular o.
    phalangeal o.
    Platou o.
    posterior iliac o.
    posterior spinal wedge o.
    Pott eversion o.
    radial wedge o.

    Ranawat-DeFiore-Straub o.
    Rappaport o.
    reduction o.
    Reverdin o.
    Reverdin-Laird o.
    reverse Dillwyn-Evans calcaneal o.
    reverse wedge o.
    Root-Siegal varus derotational o.
    rotational o.
    sagittal-split mandibular o.
    Sakoff o.
    Salter innominate o.
    Salter pelvic o.
    Samilson crescentic calcaneal o.
    Sarmiento intertrochanteric o.
    scarf o.
    Schanz angulation o.
    Schanz femoral o.
    Schwartz dorsiflexory o.
    segmental alveolar o.
    Siffert intraepiphysial o.
    Siffert-Storen intraepiphysial o.
    Simmonds-Menelaus metatarsal o.
    Simmonds-Menelaus proximal
      phalangeal o.
    Simmons o.
    o. site
    sliding oblique o.
    Smith-Petersen o.
    Sofield o.
    Southwick biplane trochanteric o.
    spinal o.
    Sponsel oblique o.
    Stamm metatarsal o.
    Steel triple innominate o.
    step o.
    step-cut o.
    stepdown o.
    Stren intraepiphysial o.
    subcapital o.
    subcondylar oblique o.
    subtrochanteric o.
    Sugioka transtrochanteric
      rotational o.
    supracondylar varus o.
    supramalleolar varus derotation o.
    Sutherland-Greenfield o.
    tarsal wedge o.
    Tessier o.
    Thompson telescoping V o.
    through-and-through V-shaped
      horizontal o.
    tibial tuberosity o.
    transtrochanteric rotational o.
    trapezoidal o.
    Trethowan metatarsal o.
    triplane o.
    triple innominate o.
    trochanteric o.

tubercle o.
unplanned valgus o.
valgus wedge-prop o.
valgus Y-shaped prop o.
varus rotation shortening o.
vertical o.
V-shaped o.
Waterman o.
Weber humeral o.
Weber subcapital o.
wedge o.
wedge-shaped o.
Whitman o.
Wilson oblique displacement o.
Wiltse ankle o.
Wiltse varus supramalleolar o.
Yancey o.
Yu o.

osteotomy-bunionectomy
scarf o.-b.

osteotomy-osteoclasis
Moore o.-o.

osteotripsy
osteotrite
osteotympanic bone conduction
ostia (*pl. of* ostium)
ostial
o. lesion
o. sphincter

ostiomeatal
ostium, pl. **ostia**
abdominal o.
celiac o.
o. primum
o. secundum

ostomate
ostomy
o. loop
o. skin

Ostrum-Furst syndrome
Ostrup
O. harvesting technique
O. vascularized rib graft

Oswestry Disability Questionnaire (ODQ)
Osypka rotational angioplasty
otic
o. ganglion
o. periotic shunt procedure
o. vesicle

otitis
o. externa
o. media

otoconia
degenerating o.

otolaryngologic manifestation
otolaryngologist
otolaryngology
pediatric o.

otolith
otolithic membrane
otomandibular syndrome
otomicrosurgical transtemporal approach
otoplasty
mattress suture o.
Mustardé o.

otorhinolaryngology
otorrhea
clear o.

otosclerosis
otoscopy
pneumatic o.

Otto pelvis dislocation
ouabain
Ouchterlony
O. gel diffusion technique
O. method

Oudard procedure
out
opting o.

outcome
clinical o.
cosmetic o.
final o.
long-term o.
o. monitoring
perioperative o.
short-term o.
surgical o.

Outerbridge classification
outer limiting membrane
outermost
outflow
cerebrospinal fluid o.
o. control
craniosacral o.
thoracolumbar o.
o. tract
o. tract obstruction
venous o.

out-in-out technique
outlet strut fracture

O

NOTES

out-of-phase endometrial biopsy
outpatient
    o. anesthesia
    o. biopsy
    o. dialysis
    o. dialysis clinic
    o. endoscopy
    o. physical therapy
    o. surgical setting
    o. thyroidectomy
    o. thyroid operation
output
    cardiac o. (CO)
    chest tube o. (CTO)
    intraoperative urine o.
    o. layer
    pacemaker o.
    radiation o.
    saturation o.
    thermodilution cardiac o. (TDCO)
outside-to-outside arthroscopy technique
outward rotation
ova (*pl. of* ovum)
oval
    o. cup erysiphake
    o. window
ovale
    patent foramen o. (PFO)
oval-shaped crushing
ovarian
    o. ablation
    o. artery
    o. branch
    o. bursa
    o. cancer
    o. cancer metastasis
    o. carcinoma
    o. carcinoma debulking
    o. clear cell adenocarcinoma
    o. cortex
    o. cystectomy
    o. dermoid cyst
    o. fimbria
    o. follicle exhaustion
    o. hernia
    o. hyperstimulation syndrome
    o. incision
    o. masculinization
    o. mass
    o. overstimulation syndrome
    o. plexus
    o. stimulation
    o. surface
    o. thecoma
    o. tumor
    O. Tumor Registry
    o. vein
    o. vein syndrome
    o. wedge resection

ovariectomy
ovariocele
ovariohysterectomy
ovariosalpingectomy
ovariostomy
ovariotomy
    Beatson o.
    normal o.
ovary
    premenopausal o.
    right o.
overall sound level
over-and-over suture technique
overangulation
overbite
overcirculation
    pulmonary o.
overcompensation
overcorrected position
overcorrection
overdetermination
overdilation
overfilled canal
overflow incontinence
overgrafting
overgrowth
    bacterial o.
    cartilage o.
    fungal o.
overhang
overhanging restoration
Overhauser technique
Overholt procedure
overinflation
overinstrumentation
overlap
    o. midline incisional hernioplasty
    suture o.
overlapping
    o. incision
    o. suture technique
overlay restoration
overload
    circulatory o.
    compression o.
    pressure o.
overprojecting nasal tip
overrotation
oversedation
oversewing
    early o.
oversewn
overshoot
    calibration o.
    o. phenomenon
overstimulation
over-the-counter medication
over-the-top position
over-the-wire technique

Overton dowel graft
overventilation
overwhelming postsplenectomy infection
oviduct
oviductal
ovoid mass
ovotestis
ovular transmigration
ovulation
    estimated time of o. (ETO)
    o. induction
    o. rate
    o. stimulation
ovum, pl. **ova**
Owen
    interglobular space of O.
    O. line
    O. operation
owl's eye inclusion body
oxalate calculus
Oxford technique
oxidation
    o. of solution
    o. state
oxidation-reducing potential
oxide
    ethylene o. (ETO)
    inhaled nitrous o. (INO)
    nitrous o. (NO)
oxide-oxygen
    nitrous o.-o. (N_2O-O_2)
oximetry
    forehead reflectance o.
    pulse o.
    spinal o.
    transesophageal echocardiograph-guided left ventricular o.
    transesophageal echocardiograph-guided right ventricular o.
oxycarbonate
oxycardiorespirogram
oxycephalia
oxycephalic
oxycephaly
oxygen (O_2)
    o. administration
    o. in air
    o. analyzer
    o. concentration
    o. concentration in pulmonary capillary blood
    o. consumption

    o. debt
    o. deprivation theory of narcosis
    o. desaturation
    o. dissociation curve
    o. effect
    o. extraction rate
    flow-dependent o.
    hyperbaric o.
    nasal o. (NO)
    partial pressure of o. (PO_2)
    partial pressure of alveolar o. (PAO_2, PaO_2)
    partial pressure of arterial o. (PAO_2, PaO_2)
    o. poisoning
    rapid recompression-high pressure o.
    o. reduction product
    o. saturation
    o. saturation of hemoglobin of arterial blood
    o. saturation index
    o. saturation measurement
    o. step-up method
    supplementary o.
    o. supply line
    o. tension
    o. therapy
    o. toxicity
    transcutaneous partial pressure of o.
    o. under high pressure
    o. utilization
oxygenation
    apneic o.
    bubble o.
    cell o.
    disc o.
    extracorporeal membrane o. (ECMO)
    fetal scalp o.
    film o.
    hyperbaric o.
    o. index (OI)
    medullary o.
    pump o.
    rotating disc o.
    screen o.
    splanchnic o.
    tissue o.
    tumor o.

O

NOTES

oxygenator
    membrane o.
oxygen-carrying resuscitative fluid
oxygen-enriched atmosphere
oxygen-hemoglobin dissociation curve
oxygen-ratio monitoring controller
oxygen-related response

Oxyglobin
oxyhemoglobin dissociation curve
oxymorphone
    oral immediate-release o.
oyster mass
ozonization
ozonolysis

P2 prolongation
p53 tumor suppressor gene analysis
PA
    prophylactic antibiotic
    pulmonary artery
    pulmonary autograft
        PA filling pressure
        PA projection
        PA therapy
pacchionian granulation
pacemaker
    p. adaptive rate
    p. artifact
    p. burst pacing
    p. capture
    p. escape interval
    p. failure
    p. impedance
    p. lead fracture
    p. malfunction
    p. output
    p. pocket
    p. potential
    p. syndrome
    p. threshold
    p. undersensing
pacemaker-mediated tachycardia
Pacey technique
Pachon
    P. method
    P. test
pachydermatocele
pachymeningitis
pachyperitonitis
pachyvaginalitis
pacing
    external transcutaneous p.
    implantable cardioverter-
      defibrillator/atrial tachycardia p.
    pacemaker burst p.
    transesophageal atrial p. (TEAP)
    transesophageal echocardiography
      with p.
    transesophageal ventricular p.
      (TEVP)
packed red blood cells (PRBC)
Pack-Ehrlich deep iliac dissection
Pack technique
PaCO₂
    partial pressure of arterial carbon dioxide
Pacquin ureterolysis
PACU
    postanesthesia care unit
PAD
    percutaneous abscess drainage

pad
    abdominal fat p.
    adenoid p.
    adenoidal p.
    antimesenteric fat p.
    artificial fat p.
    axillary fat p.
    Bichat fat p.
    branch p.
    buccal fat p.
    bulbocavernosus fat p.
    buttocks p.
    digital p.
    epicardial fat p.
    esophagogastric fat p.
    fat p.
    heel fat p.
    herniated presacral fat p.
    Hoffa fat p.
    ileocecal fat p.
    ischiorectal fat p.
    labial p.
    malar fat p.
    masticatory fat p.
    metatarsal p.
    orbital fat p.
    patellar fat p.
    pericardial fat p.
    pubic p.
    retrodiscal p.
    retromolar p.
    retropatellar fat p.
PAF
    paroxysmal atrial fibrillation
    pulmonary arteriovenous fistula
Pagenstecher
    P. circle
    P. operation
    P. suture technique
Paget
    P. carcinoma
    P. extramammary disease
Paget-Eccleston stain
Paget-von Schrötter syndrome
PAG/PVG
    periaqueductal gray matter/periventricular
    gray matter
      PAG/PVG region
PAH
    pulmonary artery hypertension
PAI
    Pain Appraisal Inventory
pain
    p. anxiety symptoms scale
    P. Appraisal Inventory (PAI)

P

pain (*continued*)
    back p.
    p. behavior
    bone p.
    burn p.
    burning p.
    cancer p.
    P. Catastrophizing Scale (PCS)
    cementum p.
    central p.
    central poststroke p. (CPSP)
    chronic nonmalignant p.
    colicky p.
    colorectal distention p.
    P. Coping Questionnaire (PCQ)
    cyclic p.
    deafferentation p.
    p. deception
    dentin p.
    diffuse abdominal p.
    dysesthetic p.
    dystonic p.
    Edmonton Staging System for
      Cancer P.
    epigastric p.
    exacerbation of p.
    existential p.
    experimental p.
    p. expression
    expulsive p.
    exquisite p.
    facial p.
    herpes zoster p.
    IASP Classification of Chronic P.
    incisional p.
    p. induction
    inflammatory p.
    International Association for the
      Study of P. (IASP)
    intractable p.
    joint line p.
    labor p.
    limb ischemia p.
    p. management
    micturition p.
    moderate p.
    p. modulation
    movement-related p.
    myofascial p.
    neuropathic p.
    nonsympathetically mediated p.
    obstetric p.
    opioid-insensitive p.
    palliation of p.
    pancreatic cancer p.
    pediatric p.
    p. perception profile
    phantom foot p.
    phantom limb p.

    pillar p.
    postherniorrhaphy p.
    postoperative cesarean section p.
    poststroke p.
    postsurgical truncal p.
    postthoracotomy p.
    p. projection
    psychogenic p.
    referred trigger point p.
    P. Relief Scoring System
    scleratomal distribution of p.
    p. sensitivity range
    shortcut sciatic p.
    somatic p.
    spinal cord injury p.
    stump p.
    sympathetically maintained p.
      (SMP)
    p. syndrome
    temporomandibular p.
    thalamic p.
    p. threshold reduction
    p. tolerance level
    tourniquet p.
    tourniquet-induced p.
    tourniquet ischemic p.
    visceral p.

painful
    p. anesthesia
    p. point

painless rectal bleeding

Painter colic

paired
    p. electrical stimulation
    p. vasomotor response

Pais fracture

PAJB
    primary antecubital jump bypass

Pajot maneuver

PAK
    pancreas after kidney transplant
    pancreas after kidney transplantation

palatal
    p. approach
    p. expansion
    p. flap
    p. implant
    p. index
    p. lengthening procedure
    p. vein

palate
    Byzantine arch p.
    cleft p.
    hard p.
    itchy soft p.
    p. reconstruction
    soft p.

palatine
    p. bone

p. canal
p. flap
p. foramen
p. gland
p. nerve
p. suture
palatoethmoidal suture
palatoglossal fold
palatoglossus muscle
palatomaxillary
p. canal
p. index
p. suture
palatooccipital line
palatopharyngeal
p. closure
p. fold
p. ring
p. sphincter
p. sphincter muscle
palatopharyngeus muscle
palatopharyngoplasty
palatopharyngorrhaphy
palatoplasty
palatorrhaphy
palatosalpingeus
palatostaphylinus
palatovaginal
p. canal
p. groove
Paley classification
Palfyn
P. sinus
P. suture technique
palliation of pain
palliative
p. bypass
p. care
p. cerebrospinal shunt procedure
p. esophagostomy
p. exeresis
p. gastrostomy
p. hepatojejunostomy
p. intent
p. operation
p. resection
p. surgery
p. surgical procedure
p. technique
p. therapy
p. total gastrectomy
pallidectomy

pallidoamygdalotomy
pallidoansotomy
pallidotomy
posteroventral p.
stereotactic p.
unilateral p.
VPL p.
pallor
Palma operation
palmar
p. advancement flap
p. angulation
p. approach
p. branch
p. crease
p. cross-finger flap
p. incision
p. interosseous artery
p. synovectomy
palmate fold
Palmer
P. method
P. technique
P. transscaphoid perilunar
dislocation
Palmer-Dobyns-Linscheid ligament repair
Palmer-Widen shoulder technique
palmoscopy
palm space
Palomo
P. operation
P. procedure
P. technique
palpable
p. mass
p. rib diastasis
palpation
bimanual p.
p. testing
palpatory examination
palpebra, pl. **palpebrae**
levator palpebrae
palpebral
p. artery
p. branch
p. fascia
p. fissure
p. ligament
p. muscle
p. nerve
p. rim
palpebration

NOTES

P

palpebronasal fold
palpitation
    paroxysmal p.
    premonitory p.
palsy
    Bell p.
    temporary p.
    vocal cord p.
pampiniform
    p. body
    p. venous plexus
pampinocele
Panas operation
panclavicular dislocation
Pancoast
    P. suture technique
    P. tumor
pancolectomy
pancolonoscopy
pancreas
    aberrant p.
    accessory p.
    p. after kidney transplant (PAK)
    p. after kidney transplantation
      (PAK)
    anular p.
    artificial endocrine p.
    Aselli p.
    p. cancer
    distal p.
    ectopic p.
    endocrine p.
    exocrine p.
    lesser p.
    retroperitoneal p.
    small p.
    p. transplant (PTX)
    p. transplant alone (PTA)
    p. transplantation
    uncinate p.
    Willis p.
    Winslow p.
pancreas-kidney transplantation
pancreas-specific amylase isoenzyme
pancreatectomy
    Child radical p.
    complete laparoscopic distal p. (C-
      LDP)
    conventional distal p.
    distal p. (DP)
    distal laparoscopic p.
    donor p.
    en bloc distal p.
    laparoscopic distal p.
    left-to-right subtotal p.
    limited p.
    near-total p.
    partial p.
    proximal subtotal p.

    spleen-preserving distal p.
    subtotal distal p.
    total p.
    transduodenal p.
    Whipple p.
pancreatemphraxis
pancreatic
    p. abscess
    p. adenocarcinoma
    p. anastomosis
    p. artery
    p. autotransplantation
    p. bacterial infection
    p. biopsy
    p. body
    p. branch
    p. bypass
    p. calculus
    p. cancer pain
    p. capsule
    p. carcinoma
    p. colic
    p. complication
    p. cyst
    p. cystoduodenostomy
    p. disease
    p. duct
    p. duct dilatation
    p. duct manipulation
    p. duct pressure
    p. duct sphincterotomy
    p. endocrine tumor
    p. endoscopy
    p. enzyme
    p. enzyme secretion
    p. extract
    p. fascia
    p. fluid
    p. fluid collection
    p. fungal detection
    p. fungus
    p. head
    p. head cancer
    p. head origin
    p. imaging
    p. intraluminal radiation therapy
    p. islet
    p. lithiasis
    p. malignancy
    p. neck
    p. necrosis
    p. necrosis prognostic score
    p. notch
    p. operation
    p. parenchyma
    p. plexus
    p. pseudocyst
    p. pseudocystogastrostomy
    p. resection

p. sphincter
p. sphincteroplasty
p. stump
p. stump closure
p. stump leak
p. surgeon
p. surgery
p. tail
p. tail resection
p. tissue
p. transplantation
p. transplantation alone (PTA)
p. trauma
p. tumor localization
p. vein
pancreaticae
pancreatic-cutaneous fistula
pancreatici
pancreaticobiliary
p. endoscopy
p. tract
pancreaticoblastoma
pancreaticocystostomy
pancreaticoduodenal
p. allograft
p. arcade vessel
p. arterial arcade
p. artery
p. resection
p. transplantation
p. vein
pancreaticoduodenectomy
pylorus-preserving p.
pylorus-sparing p.
Whipple p.
pancreaticoduodenostomy
Child p.
Dennis-Varco p.
Waugh-Clagett p.
Whipple p.
pancreaticoenterostomy
pancreaticogastric anastomosis
pancreaticogastrointestinal anastomosis
pancreaticogastrostomy
p. anastomosis (PGA)
p. reconstruction
pancreaticojejunal anastomosis
pancreaticojejunostomy
p. anastomosis (PJA)
Cattell-Warren p.
caudal p.
distal p.

duct-to-mucosa p.
Duval p.
end-to-end intussuscepted p.
end-to-end inverting p.
Frey p.
longitudinal p.
Puestow p.
Roux-en-Y p.
pancreaticopleural fistula
pancreaticosplenectomy
pancreaticosplenic
p. ligament
p. omentum
pancreatic-preserving total gastrectomy
pancreatic-renal
simultaneous p.-r. (SPR)
pancreatitis
acute p. (AP)
biliary p.
centrilobular p.
chronic p.
clinical acute p.
diffuse hemorrhagic p.
p. dysfunction
gallstone p.
necrotizing p. (NP)
severe acute p. (SAP)
pancreatitis-related hemorrhage
pancreatobiliary canal
pancreatoblastoma
pancreatocholecystostomy
pancreatoduodenectomy
Billroth II p.
conventional p.
extended p.
Kausch-Whipple p.
partial p.
pylorus-preserving p. (PPPD)
radical p.
2-step p.
subtotal p.
Whipple p.
pancreatoduodenostomy
pancreatoenterostomy
pancreatogastrostomy
pancreatography
pancreatojejunostomy
retrocolic end-to-end p.
pancreatolith
pancreatolithectomy
pancreatolithiasis
pancreatolithotomy

NOTES

P

pancreatologist
pancreatolysis
pancreatolytic
pancreatomy
pancreatoscopy
    peroral p.
pancreatotomy
pancreectomy
pancreolith
pancreolithotomy
pancreoscopy
    infragastric p.
pandiculation
panel
    bleeding time coagulation p.
    clot retraction coagulation p.
    clotting time coagulation p.
    partial thromboplastin time
      coagulation p.
    plasma assay coagulation p.
    prediluted antibody p.
    prothrombin time coagulation p.
panendoscopy
    fiberoptic p.
    lower p.
    primary p.
    upper gastrointestinal p.
panhysterectomy
panmetatarsal head resection
panmucosal inflammatory cell
  infiltration
panni (*pl. of* pannus)
pannicular hernia
panniculectomy
panniculus, pl. panniculi
    abdominal p.
    p. retraction
pannus, pl. panni
    p. formation
panoramic surface projection
PANP
    pelvic autonomic nerve preservation
panphotocoagulation
panproctocolectomy
panretinal
    p. ablation
    p. argon laser photocoagulation
pantalar fusion
pantaloon
    p. hernia
    p. patch
pants-over-vest
    p.-o.-v. capsulorrhaphy
    p.-o.-v. hernial repair
    p.-o.-v. herniorrhaphy
    p.-o.-v. technique
Panum fusion area

PAO$_2$, PaO$_2$
    partial pressure of alveolar oxygen
    partial pressure of arterial oxygen
PAOD
    popliteal artery occlusive disease
PAOP
    pulmonary artery occlusion pressure
PAP
    positive airway pressure
    pulmonary artery pressure
Papanicolaou method
Papavasiliou olecranon fracture
  classification
paper point
papilla, pl. papillae
    bile p.
    circumvallate p.
    foliate p.
    inferior lacrimal p.
    interdental p.
    lacrimal p.
    lenticular p.
    major duodenal p.
    minor duodenal p.
    optic p.
    renal p.
    retrocuspid p.
    retromolar p.
    sublingual p.
    superior lacrimal p.
    urethral p.
    vallate p.
    Vater p.
papillary
    p. adenoma
    p. cancer
    p. cystadenocarcinoma
    p. duct
    p. ectasia
    p. foramen
    p. gastric carcinoma
    p. hidradenoma
    p. hyperplasia
    p. lesion
    p. muscle rupture
    p. muscle tip
    p. pedicle graft
    p. process
    p. projection
    p. reconstruction
    p. subtype
papillectomy
papillitis
papilloadenocystoma
papillocarcinoma
papillogram
papilloma
    choroid plexus p.
    p. neuropathicum

papillomacular nerve fiber bundle
papillomatosis
    diffuse p.
papillomavirus infection
Papillon-Léage and Psaume syndrome
papillotomy
    accessory p.
    endoscopic p.
    laparoscopic transcystic p.
    needle-knife p.
    precut p.
Papineau
    P. bone graft
    P. technique
Pap smear classification
papulopustular lesion
papulosis
papulosquamous lesion
papulovesicular lesion
papyracea
Paquin technique
paraaortic
    p. hematoma
    p. lymphadenectomy
    p. lymph node dissection
    p. node irradiation
    p. region
paraaortica
paraappendicitis
parabiosis
parabiotic flap
paracancerous tissue
paracanthoma
paracardiac metastasis
paracentesis
    abdominal p.
paracentetic
paracentral
    p. lobe
    p. nerve fiber bundle
paracervical
    p. block
    p. block anesthesia
    p. injection
paracervix
parachroma
parachute
    p. deformity
    p. jumper dislocation
paraclavicular thoracic outlet
  decompression
paracoagulation

paracolic
    p. gutter
    p. recess
paracollicular biopsy
paracolpium
paracystic pouch
paracystitis
paracystium
paradidymal
paradidymis
paradoxical
    p. embolism
    p. embolus
    p. extensor reflex
    p. incontinence
    p. reaction
    p. respiration
    p. technique
paraduodenal
    p. fossa
    p. hernia
    p. recess
paraesophageal
    p. diaphragmatic hernia
    p. hiatal hernia
paraesophagogastric devascularization
paraexstrophy skin flap
paraffin graft
paraffinoma
paraffin-section light microscopy
parafunctional habit
paraganglioma
paragenital tubule
paraglenoid groove
paraglottic
    p. area
    p. space
paragranuloma
parahepatic
parahiatal hernia
parahypophysis
paraileostomal hernia
parainfluenza virus infection
parainguinal incision
parajejunal fossa
parakeratinization
parakeratosis
paralaryngeal space
parallel
    p. operation
    p. robot
    p. technique

NOTES

P

paralleling
    p. cone position
    p. technique
parallelism
paralysis, pl. **paralyses**
    compression p.
    cord p.
    hernia p.
    laryngeal nerve p.
    long-term p.
    nerve p.
    permanent p.
    pharmacologic p.
    pharmacologically induced p.
    pressure p.
    recurrent nerve p.
    soft palate p.
    thoracic motor p.
    tourniquet p.
    unilateral laryngeal p.
    vocal cord p. (VCP)
paralytic
    p. ileus
    p. strabismus
paramagnetic
    p. contrast injection
    p. enhancement accentuation
    p. enhancement accentuation by
      chemical shift imaging
    p. shift relaxation
paramedial incision
paramedian
    p. approach
    p. incision
    p. pontine reticular formation
    p. sagittal plane
    p. sheath
paramedical personnel
paramesonephric duct
paramesonephricus
parameter
    canonical univariate p.
    clinical p.
    clotting p.
    conventional p.
    effect p.
    laboratory p.
    postprandial motor p.
parametrectomy
    radical p.
parametrial
parametric test
parametritis
    posterior p.
parametrium
paranalgesia
paranasal
    p. cell

    p. mucocele
    p. sinus
paraneoplastic ectopic ACTH production
paranephric
    p. abscess
    p. body
paranephros, pl. **paranephroi**
paranesthesia
paraneural infiltration
paraomphalic
paraoperative
paraoral tissue
paraorbital lesion
paraovarian
parapancreatic
paraparesis
parapatellar
    p. arthrotomy
    p. incision
paraperitoneal
    p. hernia
    p. nephrectomy
parapharyngeal
    p. space
    p. space abscess
paraphasia
    extended jargon p.
paraphimosis
paraphysis
parapineal
paraplegia
    complete motor p.
    p. in extension
    motor p.
    postoperative p.
parapneumonic empyema
paraproctium
paraprostatitis
parapubic hernia
pararectal
    p. fistula
    p. fossa
    p. line
    p. pouch
pararectus
    p. approach
    p. incision
pararenal space
parasaccular hernia
parasacral approach
parasagittal
    p. incision
    p. lesion
    p. plane
    p. section
parascapular
    p. flap
    p. incision

parasellar
p. mass
p. metastasis
p. syndrome
parasinoidal
parasitic
p. castration
p. cyst
p. flap
p. infection
paraspinal
p. approach
p. line
p. rod application
paraspinous aspect
parasternal
p. examination
p. line
parastomal
p. hernia
p. infection
p. irritation
parasympathectomy
sinoatrial nodal p.
parasympathetic
p. fiber
p. ganglion
p. nerve
p. projection
parasympathetic fiber
paraterminal body
parathyroid
p. adenoma
p. artery
p. autograft
p. biopsy
p. carcinoma
p. extract
p. gland
p. hormone (PTH)
p. hormone chemiluminescent assay
p. hormone level
p. hyperplasia
p. operation
p. remnant
superior p.
p. surgeon
p. surgery
p. tissue
p. tumor
p. tumor ablation

parathyroidectomy
endoscopic p.
incidental p.
minimally invasive p.
minimally invasive video-assisted p.
(MIVAP)
radioguided p.
reoperative p.
subtotal p.
total p.
unilateral p.
paratonsillar vein
paratracheal
p. node
p. tissue stripe
paratrachoma
paratrigeminal syndrome
paratrooper fracture
paraumbilical
p. hernia
p. incision
p. vein
paraurethral
p. duct
p. gland
parauterini
paravaccinia virus infection
paravaginal
p. defect repair
p. hysterectomy
p. incision
p. soft tissue
paravariceal
p. injection
p. sclerotherapy
paravertebral
p. anesthesia
p. ganglion
p. gutter
p. line
p. lumbar sympathetic block
p. somatic nerve blockade
paravesical
p. fossa
p. pouch
parecoxib sodium
parectasis
parencephalia
parencephalocele
parenchyma
breast p.
cirrhotic liver p.

NOTES

P

parenchyma *(continued)*
    damaged p.
    functional p.
    hepatic p.
    liver p.
    pancreatic p.
parenchymal
    p. brain metastasis
    p. brain neoplasm
    p. cell
    p. change
    p. destruction
    p. dissection
    p. hematoma
    p. laceration
    p. lymphatic
    p. route of injection
    p. sparing surgery
    p. tissue
    p. transection
parenchymatous intracerebral
  hemorrhage
parenteral
    p. administration
    p. analgesia
    p. analgesic
    p. anesthesia
    p. hyperalimentation
    p. medication
    p. nutrition
    p. nutritional support
    p. therapy
parent vessel
parepicele
parepididymis
Pare reduction
paresis
    elevation p.
    paresthesia pressure p.
paresthesia
    p. anesthetic technique
    p. pressure paresis
paresthetica
    meralgia p.
    postlaparoscopy meralgia p.
Paré suture technique
paries, pl. **parietes**
parietal
    p. angle
    p. artery
    p. bone
    p. border
    p. branch
    p. cell vagotomy
    p. defect
    p. eminence
    p. emissary vein
    p. fistula
    p. foramen

    p. hernia
    p. layer
    p. margin
    p. node
    p. notch
    p. pelvic fascia
    p. pericardiectomy
    p. pericardium
    p. peritoneum
    p. pleura
    p. region
    p. suture
    p. tuber
    p. wall
parietofrontal
parietography
parietomastoidea
parietomastoid suture
parietooccipital
    p. approach
    p. artery
parieto-occipitalis
parietopontine tract
parietosphenoid
parietosplanchnic
parietosquamosal
parietotemporal
parietovisceral
Paris
    P. classification
    P. method
park-bench position
Parker incision
Parker-Kerr
    P.-K. closed method
    P.-K. suture technique
Parkinson disease
parkinsonian tremor
Parks
    P. hemorrhoidectomy
    P. ileoanal anastomosis
    P. method
    P. method of anal fistulotomy
    P. partial sphincterotomy
    P. staged fistulotomy
Parks-Bielschowsky 3-step, head-tilt test
paroccipital process
parolivary
paromphalocele
Parona space
paronychial infection
parorchidium
parorchis
parosteal
parotic
parotid
    p. bed
    p. branch
    p. carcinoma

p. dissection
p. duct
p. duct ligation
p. fascia
p. gland
p. node
p. notch
p. plexus
p. recess
p. resection
p. sheath
p. space
p. vein
parotidectomy
facial nerve-preserving p.
nerve-preserving p.
radical p.
superficial p.
supraneural p.
total p.
parotideomasseteric fascia
parotidoauricularis
parovarian mass
parovariotomy
parovarium
paroxysmal
p. atrial fibrillation (PAF)
p. nocturnal hemoglobinuria
p. palpitation
Parrish-Mann hammertoe technique
Parrish procedure
parrot-beak nail
Parry-Jones vulvectomy
pars, pl. **partes**
p. flaccida
p. flaccida cholesteatoma
Parsonage-Turner syndrome
Parsonnet score
part
1-p. fracture
2-p. fracture
3-p. fracture
4-p. fracture
partes (*pl. of* pars)
partial
p. alveolectomy
p. atrioventricular canal
p. breech extraction
p. cardiopulmonary bypass
p. central hypophysectomy
p. colectomy
p. cricotracheal resection

p. cystectomy
p. discectomy
p. dislocation
p. duplication
p. encircling endocardial
    ventriculotomy
p. ethmoidectomy
p. facetectomy
p. fasciectomy
p. fibulectomy
p. gastrectomy (PG)
p. gastric resection
p. glossectomy
p. hemilaminectomy
p. hepatectomy
p. hepatic vascular exclusion
    (PHVE)
p. ileal bypass
p. inferior retrocolic end-to-side
    gastrojejunostomy
p. internal hemipelvectomy
p. keratoplasty
p. lamellar sclerouvectomy
p. laryngectomy
p. laryngopharyngectomy
p. lateral internal sphincterotomy
p. left ventriculectomy
p. liquid ventilation
p. mastectomy
p. matrixectomy
p. maxillectomy
p. mechanical obstruction
p. meniscectomy
p. mesh excision
p. nephrectomy
p. orchidectomy
p. ostectomy
p. pancreatectomy
p. pancreatoduodenectomy
p. patellectomy
p. pericystectomy
p. pressure
p. pressure of alveolar oxygen
    (PAO_2, PaO_2)
p. pressure of arterial carbon
    dioxide ($PaCO_2$)
p. pressure of arterial oxygen
    (PAO_2, PaO_2)
p. pressure of carbon dioxide
    (PCO_2)
p. pressure of CO_2 gas

NOTES

P

partial *(continued)*
    p. pressure of intramuscular carbon dioxide (PiCO$_2$)
    p. pressure of mesenteric venous carbon dioxide (PmvCO$_2$)
    p. pressure of oxygen (PO$_2$)
    p. pressure of water vapor
    p. proctectomy
    p. pulpectomy
    p. pulpotomy
    p. saturation
    p. saturation spin-echo
    p. superior retrocolic end-to-side gastrojejunostomy
    p. thromboplastin time coagulation panel
    p. wrist fusion
    p. zonal dissection
partial-breast irradiation
partial-thickness
    p.-t. burn
    p.-t. craniectomy
    p.-t. flap
partial-throw surgeon's knot
particle
    p. beam radiation therapy
    free-floating p.
particulate cancellous bone graft
Partipilo gastrostomy
partition
Partsch operation
parturient canal
parumbilical
paruresis
Parvin
    P. gravity technique
    P. reduction
PAS
    peripheral access system
    PAS Port
    PAS technique
passage
    nasopharyngeal p.
    oropharyngeal p.
    p. pressure
    transforaminal p.
    transperineurial p.
    wire p.
Passavant
    P. bar
    P. fold
    P. ridge
passé
    coma dé p.
passive
    p. clot
    p. gliding technique
    p. incontinence
    p. joint manipulation

    p. reciprocation
    p. tissue cooling
Pastia line
patch
    achromic p.
    p. amnesia
    aortic p.
    p. aortoplasty
    ash-leaf p.
    autologous pericardial p.
    blood p.
    butterfly p.
    cardiac p.
    p. clamp electrophysiology
    colic p.
    colonic p.
    cotton-wool p.
    eczematous p.
    electrodispersive skin p.
    epidural blood p. (EBP)
    p. esophagoplasty
    glue p.
    gray p.
    herald p.
    Hutchinson p.
    p. lesion
    lyophilized dural p.
    moth p.
    mucous p.
    omental p.
    pantaloon p.
    pericardial p.
    peritoneal p.
    Peyer p.
    pigskin p.
    prophylactic epidural blood p.
    prosthetic p.
    pruritic erythematous p.
    salmon p.
    sandwich p.
    sclerotic calvarial p.
    shagreen p.
    soldier p.
    p. stage
    p. technique
    2-p. technique
    p. testing
    p. test scarring
    vein p.
    venous sheath p.
    white p.
patch-graft angioplasty
patchplasty
patchy
    p. colonic ulceration
    p. infiltration
patefaction
patella, pl. **patellae**
    p. turndown approach

patellapexy
patellar
    p. fat pad
    p. intraarticular dislocation
    p. network
    p. retinaculum
    p. sleeve fracture
    p. tendon graft donor site
      (PTGDS)
    p. tendon repair
patellectomy
    partial p.
    total p.
    West-Soto-Hall p.
patelliform
patellofemoral articulation
Patel medial meniscectomy
patency
    biliary stent p.
    catheter p.
    graft p.
    shunt p.
    stent p.
    valve p.
patent
    p. ductus arteriosus (PDA)
    p. foramen ovale (PFO)
    p. iridectomy
    p. portal vein
Paterson
    P. procedure
    P. technique
Patey
    P. modified radical mastectomy
    P. operation
path
    p. of insertion
    p. of removal
pathogen
    fungal p.
    initial primary p.
    primary p.
pathogenesis
pathologic
    p. amputation
    p. barrier
    p. breast discharge
    p. cause
    p. characteristic
    p. diagnosis
    p. dislocation
    p. entity

    p. examination
    p. lesion
    p. neovascularization
    p. perforation
    p. retraction ring
    p. specimen
    p. sphincter
pathological
    p. anatomy
    p. fracture
pathology
    adrenal p.
    anatomic p.
    clinical p.
    colorectal p.
    p. examination
    experimental p.
    inciting p.
    intracranial p.
    intrahepatic p.
    intrathyroidal p.
    neoplastic p.
    obstructing p.
    p. scarring
    surgical p.
    synchronous p.
    thyroid p.
    venous p.
pathomechanics
    kyphotic deformity p.
    spinal fusion p.
pathophysiologic factor
pathophysiology
pathostimulation
pathway
    ascending p.
    beta-oxidation p.
    effector p.
    extrapyramidal p.
    extrinsic p.
    lymphatic p.
    orogastric p.
    proteolytic p.
    receptor-mediated endocytosis p.
    shunt p.
    somatosensory p.
    spinothalamic p.
    taste p.
    visual p.
PATI
    penetrating abdominal trauma index

NOTES

P

patient
    adult p.
    asymptomatic p.
    bariatric p.
    brain-dead p.
    diabetic p.
    dialysis-dependent p.
    disease-free p.
    endoscopically normal p.
    head-injured p.
    hemodialysis-dependent p.
    high-risk p.
    inoperable p.
    morbidly obese p.
    obese p.
    pediatric p.
    poor-risk p.
    p. population
    p. state analyzer
    p. state index (PSI)
    surgically treated p.
    symptomatic p.
    toxic-traumatized p.
    trauma p.
    tube-fed p.
    vascular access p.
patient-controlled
    p.-c. analgesia (PCA)
    p.-c. analgesia anesthetic technique
    p.-c. epidural analgesia (PCEA, PEA)
    p.-c. epidural with intravenous analgesia
    p.-c. intranasal analgesia (PCINA)
    p.-c. regional analgesia (PCRA)
patient-dependent factor
patrilineal
pattern
    abdominal wall venous p.
    airway p.
    p. arborization
    architectural p.
    p. of breathing
    butterfly p.
    chromatin p.
    p. cut corneal graft operation
    distribution p.
    p. of distribution
    p. of drainage
    drainage p.
    flow p.
    histologic p.
    lymphatic drainage p.
    p. of motion
    motor p.
    organ-specific p.
    p. recognition
    sinusoidal p.
    p. of staining
    upper jejunal motor p.
pattern-cut corneal graft
patulous
Pauchet procedure
paucity
Paufique
    P. keratoplasty
    P. synechiotomy
Pauli exclusion principle
Pauling theory
Paul-Mikulicz resection
Paulos ligament technique
Pauly point
pause-squeeze method
Pauwels
    P. femoral neck fracture classification
    P. fracture
    P. proximal osteotomy
    P. technique
    P. valgus osteotomy
    P. Y-osteotomy
PAV
    proportional assist ventilator
Pavlov method
Payne-DeWind jejunoileal bypass
Payne operation
Payr
    P. clamp method
    P. membrane
PBS
    phosphate buffered saline
    prune-belly syndrome
PCA
    patient-controlled analgesia
PCC
    percutaneous catheter cecostomy
    propagating clustered contraction
PCEA
    patient-controlled epidural analgesia
PCINA
    patient-controlled intranasal analgesia
PCIRV
    pressure control inverse ratio ventilation
    pressure-controlled inverse ratio ventilation
PCNA
    proliferating cell nuclear antigen
PCNL
    percutaneous nephrolithotripsy
    percutaneous nephrostolithotomy
PCO$_2$
    partial pressure of carbon dioxide
PCQ
    Pain Coping Questionnaire
PCRA
    patient-controlled regional analgesia

PCS
Pain Catastrophizing Scale
PCV
pressure control ventilation
PDA
patent ductus arteriosus
PDPH
postdural puncture headache
PDT
photodynamic therapy
PE
pulmonary embolism
submassive PE
PEA
patient-controlled epidural analgesia
pulseless electrical activity
Peabody-Mitchell bunionectomy
Peacock transposing technique
peak
p. exercise oxygen consumption
p. expiratory flow
p. expiratory flow rate (PEFR)
p. inspiratory ventilator pressure
p. pressure analysis
p. systolic aortic pressure
p. systolic gradient
p. systolic gradient pressure
p. transaortic valve gradient
Péan incision
pearl
cholesteatoma p.
perineal p.
PEBB
percutaneous excisional breast biopsy
Pecquet
P. cistern
P. duct
pecten
anal p.
p. band
pectinata
pectinate
p. body
p. line
p. zone
pectineal
p. fascia
p. hernia
p. ligament
p. line
pectiniform septum

pectoral
p. branch
p. fascia
p. groove
pectoralis
p. fascia
p. major muscle origin
p. major myocutaneous flap
p. muscle
p. myocutaneous esophagoplasty
p. myocutaneous flap
p. myofascial flap
pectoriloquy
whispered p.
pectorodorsal muscle
pectus
p. carinatum deformity
p. excavatum deformity
p. excavatum repair
p. index
PED
percutaneous external drainage
pedes (*pl. of* pes)
pediatric
p. airway
p. analgesic
p. anesthesia system
p. anesthetic
p. cardiovascular surgery
p. circle
p. colonoscopy
p. endoscopy
p. esophagogastroduodenoscopy
p. esophagoplasty
p. hepatojejunostomy
p. hernia
p. hypothermia
p. injury
p. intussusception
p. laparoscopic surgical procedure
p. mass
p. neoplasm
p. neurosurgeon
P. Oncology Group (POG)
p. ophthalmic surgery
p. otolaryngology
p. pain
p. patient
p. population
p. portal hypertension
p. radiotherapy anesthesia
p. surgeon

NOTES

P

pediatric *(continued)*
    p. trauma scale (PTS)
    p. urologist
    p. urology
    p. vaginoscopy
pedicellation
pedicle
    p. anatomy
    p. cannulation
    p. entrance point
    p. evaluation
    p. fat graft
    Filatov-Gillies tubed p.
    p. flap operation
    p. flap urethroplasty
    p. fracture
    glissonian p.
    p. groin flap
    hepatic p.
    p. landmark
    lateral-sector p.
    p. ligation
    p. localization
    medial-sector p.
    p. method
    omental p.
    portal p.
    posterior p.
    p. screw construct
    p. screw hardware prominence
    p. screw path length
    p. screw plating
    p. screw-rod fixation
    sectoral p.
    p. subtraction osteotomy
    vascular p.
    vasculobiliary p.
    p. wrapping
pedicled
    p. jejunal reconstruction
    p. myocutaneous flap
    p. omentoplasty
pedicolaminar fracture-dislocation
pedicular fixation
pediculation
pediculus, pl. **pediculi**
pediphalanx
pedis
    dorsalis p. (DP)
pedodontic endodontics
peduncle
peduncular loop
pedunculated loose body
pedunculation
pedunculotomy
peel
    fibrin p.
peeling
    membrane p.

PEEP
    positive end-expiratory pressure
PEEP/CPAP
    positive end-expiratory
      pressure/continuous positive airway
      pressure
PEEPi
    intrinsic positive end-expiratory pressure
Peet
    P. operation
    P. splanchnic resection
    P. Z-plasty
PEFR
    peak expiratory flow rate
PEG
    percutaneous endoscopic gastrostomy
      PEG insertion
peg
    p. bone graft
    p. flap
peg-and-socket
    p.-a.-s. articulation
    p.-a.-s. joint
    p.-a.-s. technique
peg-in-hole osteotomy
PEI
    percutaneous ethanol injection
Peimer reduction osteotomy
PEJ
    percutaneous endoscopic jejunostomy
pelidnoma
pelioma
peliosis hepatitis
Pell and Gregory classification
pellucidum
pelma
pelmatic
peltation
pelves (*pl. of* pelvis)
pelvic
    p. abscess
    p. adhesive disease
    p. appendix
    p. aspiration biopsy
    p. autonomic nerve preservation
      (PANP)
    p. autonomic plexus
    p. avulsion fracture
    p. axis
    p. brim
    p. canal
    p. cavity
    p. colonic surgery
    p. diaphragm
    p. direction
    p. examination
    p. exenteration
    p. fascia
    p. fixation

p. floor dysfunction
p. ganglion
p. girdle
p. hematocele
p. ileal reservoir construction
p. inclination
p. infection
p. inflammation
p. irradiation
p. kidney
p. laparoscopy
p. limb
p. lymphadenectomy
p. lymph node dissection (PLND)
p. lymphocelectomy
p. mass
p. node dissection
p. osteotomy
p. peritonectomy
p. plane
p. pouch
p. pouchoscopy
p. pouch procedure
p. promontory
p. relaxation
p. ring
p. ring fracture
p. rotation
p. sidewall
p. skeleton
p. stimulation
p. straddle fracture
pelvicaliceal
pelvifixation
pelvilithotomy
pelviolithotomy
pelvioplasty
pelvioscopy
pelviotomy
pelvirectal sphincter
pelvis, pl. **pelves**
android p.
anthropoid p.
assimilation p.
brachypellic p.
contracted p.
cordate p.
Deventer p.
dolichopellic p.
dwarf p.
extrarenal renal p.
false p.

flat p.
funnel-shaped p.
greater p.
gynecoid p.
heart-shaped p.
inclinatio p.
inverted p.
juvenile p.
large p.
lesser p.
longitudinal oval p.
masculine p.
mesatipellic p.
osteomalacic p.
platypellic p.
platypelloid p.
pseudoosteomalacic p.
renal p.
reniform p.
Robert p.
round p.
small p.
spider p.
transverse oval p.
true p.
ureteric p.
pelvisacral
pelviscopic
p. clip ligation technique
p. intrafascial hysterectomy
pelviscopy
pelvitomy
pelvivertebral angle
pelvoscopy
Pemberton
P. acetabuloplasty
P. operation
P. pericapsular osteotomy
PEMF
pulsed electromagnetic field
PEMF therapy
pemphigoid
pemphigus
penalization
Pena procedure
Penaz volume-clamp method
pencil-in-cup deformity
pendulous abdomen
pendulum
penectomy
penes (*pl. of* penis)
penetrance

NOTES

P

penetrating
  p. abdominal trauma index (PATI)
  p. corneal transplant
  p. fracture
  p. keratoplasty
  p. liver injury
  p. rupture
  p. thoracoabdominal injury
  p. trauma
  p. ulcer
  p. wound
penetration
  peritoneal p.
  serosal p.
  p. test
Penfield method
penial
penicillary
penicillate
penicillus
penile
  p. amputation
  p. block
  p. cancer
  p. carcinoma
  p. deformity
  p. erection
  p. extensibility
  p. incarceration
  p. injection testing
  p. injection therapy
  p. island flap
  p. raphe
  p. revascularization
  p. rupture
  p. urethra
  p. vein occlusion therapy
  p. venous ligation surgery
penile-brachial pressure index
penis, pl. penes
  bifid p.
  buried p.
  clubbed p.
  concealed p.
  deep p.
  dorsal p.
  glans p.
  webbed p.
penischisis
peniscopy
penitis
Pennal classification
pennate muscle
Penn method
penoplasty
penoscrotal transposition
penotomy
PENS
  percutaneous electrical nerve stimulation

pentadactyl
pentagonal block excision
pentane excretion level
pentoxifylline
  preincisional intravenous p.
penumbral region
Peptavlon stimulation test
peptic
  p. aspiration pneumonitis
  p. gland
  p. stricture
  p. ulcer
  p. ulcer disease
peptide
  atrial natriuretic p. (ANP)
  brain natriuretic p. (BNP)
  connective tissue activating p.
  endogenous opioid p.
  fusion p.
per
  p. anum
  p. contiguum
  p. continuum
peraxillary
perceived
  p. exertion
  p. quality of life (PQOL)
perceptual expansion
perched facet
percolation
Percoll technique
percussion
  hard p.
  p. therapy
percutaneous
  p. abscess drainage (PAD)
  p. access
  p. alcohol injection
  p. anesthetic loss
  p. anterior gastropexy
  p. appendectomy
  p. arterial cannulation
  p. aspirate
  p. aspiration thromboembolectomy
  p. balloon angioplasty
  p. balloon aortic valvuloplasty
  p. balloon aspiration
  p. balloon compression
  p. balloon dilation
  p. balloon mitral valvuloplasty
  p. balloon pericardiotomy
  p. balloon pulmonic valvuloplasty
  p. bone marrow infection
  p. catheter cecostomy (PCC)
  p. catheter drainage
  p. catheter insertion
  p. cholangioscopic lithotomy
  p. cholecystectomy
  p. cholecystolithotomy

p. cholecystostomy
p. compression device-tow
  deformity
p. cordotomy
p. coronary rotational atherectomy
p. corticotomy
p. CT-guided aspiration
p. dilational tracheostomy
p. electrical nerve stimulation
  (PENS)
p. embolization therapy
p. endofluoroscopy
p. endopyeloureterotomy
p. endoscopic gastrojejunostomy
p. endoscopic gastrostomy (PEG)
p. endoscopic gastrostomy insertion
p. endoscopic jejunostomy (PEJ)
p. endoscopic removal
p. endoscopy
p. endovascular treatment
p. enterostomy
p. epididymal sperm aspiration
p. ethanol ablation
p. ethanol injection (PEI)
p. ethanol injection therapy
p. excisional breast biopsy (PEBB)
p. external drainage (PED)
p. fetal cystoscopy
p. fetal tissue sampling
p. fine-needle aspiration
p. fine-needle aspiration biopsy
p. fine-needle pancreatic biopsy
p. fixation
p. FNA
p. gastroenterostomy
p. glycerol rhizolysis
p. injury (PI)
p. insertion technique
p. interventional technique
p. intraaortic balloon
  counterpulsation
p. laser nucleolysis
p. line
p. localization
p. low-stress angioplasty
p. lumbar discectomy
p. mechanical thrombectomy (PMT)
p. microwave coagulation therapy
p. mitral balloon commissurotomy
p. mitral balloon valvotomy
p. native renal biopsy
p. needle liver biopsy

p. needle puncture
p. nephrolithotomy
p. nephrolithotripsy (PCNL)
p. nephroscopy
p. nephrostolithotomy (PCNL)
p. nephrostomy
p. nephrostomy tube placement
p. neurolytic intercostal block
p. pancreas biopsy
p. patent ductus arteriosus closure
p. pin insertion
p. pinning
p. plantar fasciotomy
p. portocaval anastomosis
p. pressure ureteral perfusion test
p. radical cryosurgical ablation
p. radiofrequency catheter ablation
p. radiofrequency dorsal rhizotomy
p. radiofrequency gangliolysis
p. radiofrequency rhizolysis
p. reduction
p. renal puncture
p. retrogasserian glycerol
  chemoneurolysis
p. retrogasserian glycerol rhizolysis
p. rotational thrombectomy
p. sampling method
p. stimulation
p. stone removal
p. stricture dilatation (PSD)
p. tenotomy
p. transatrial mitral
  commissurotomy
p. transcatheter therapy
p. transhepatic approach
p. transhepatic balloon dilatation
  (PTBD)
p. transhepatic biliary drainage
  (PTBD)
p. transhepatic biliary procedure
p. transhepatic cardiac
  catheterization
p. transhepatic cholangiography
  (PTC)
p. transhepatic cholangioscopic
  lithotomy (PTCSL)
p. transhepatic cholangioscopy
p. transhepatic cholecystoscopy
p. transhepatic obliteration
p. transhepatic obliteration of
  esophageal varix
p. transhepatic placement

NOTES

P

percutaneous *(continued)*
    p. transluminal angioscopy
    p. transluminal balloon
      valvuloplasty
    p. transluminal coronary angioplasty
      (PTCA)
    p. transluminal coronary
      revascularization
    p. transluminal renal angioplasty
    p. transtracheal jet ventilation
      (PTJV, PTV)
    p. transtracheal ventilation
    p. transvenous mitral
      commissurotomy
    p. tumor ablation
    p. venoablation
Pereyra
    P. bladder neck suspension
    P. needle suspension
    P. procedure
Pereyra-Lebhertz modification
Pereyra-Raz cystourethropexy
perflation
perforans
perforated
    p. cancer
    p. cholecystitis
    p. peptic ulcer
    p. space
perforating
    p. abscess
    p. branch
    p. canal
    p. keratoplasty
    p. wound
perforation
    advanced tumor p.
    amebic p.
    appendiceal p.
    barogenic esophageal p.
    bladder p.
    bowel p.
    cardiac p.
    colon p.
    colonic p.
    corneal p.
    cortical p.
    diaphragm p.
    ductal system p.
    duodenal p.
    esophageal p.
    frank p.
    gallbladder p.
    gastric p.
    guide wire p.
    ileal p.
    inflammatory p.
    instrumental p.
    intestinal p.

    intraperitoneal p.
    lateral p.
    mechanical p.
    myocardial p.
    nasal septal p.
    Niemeier gallbladder p.
    operative p.
    p. osteotomy
    pathologic p.
    peritoneal p.
    p. peritonitis
    prepyloric p.
    retroduodenal p.
    retroperitoneal p.
    p. risk
    root p.
    sealing p.
    septal p.
    spontaneous p.
    spontaneous intestinal p. (SIP)
    strip p.
    sublabial p.
    tooth p.
    traumatic p.
    ureteral p.
    uterine p.
    vascular p.
    ventricular p.
perforative lesion
perforator
    superior gluteal artery p.
performance status
perfrigeration
perfusate
perfusion
    aortic p.
    blood p.
    cerebral p.
    continuous hyperthermic
      peritoneal p.
    continuous sanguineous p.
    distal aortic p.
    distal visceral p.
    extracorporeal liver p.
    ex vivo p.
    p. flow rate
    hepatic p.
    hyperthermic isolated limb p.
      (HILP)
    p. hypothermia technique
    hypothermic hepatic p.
    in-line p.
    in situ hypothermic p.
    intramural blood p.
    intraperitoneal hyperthermic p.
    isolated hepatic p.
    isolated limb p. (ILP)
    Langendorff p.
    p. measurement technique

organ p.
p. pressure
sanguineous p.
splanchnic p.
superficial renal cortical p. (SRCP)
p. system
systemic p.
p. therapy
tissue p.
visceral p.
perfusion/ventilation
periadvential tissue
periadventitial dissection
periampullary
p. cancer
p. carcinoma
p. mass
perianal
p. anorectal space
p. condyloma
p. fistula
p. fistula abscess
p. hematoma
p. incision
p. infection
perianesthetic thermoregulation
perianeurysmal hemorrhage
periangiocholitis
periaortic mediastinal hematoma
periaortitis
periapical
p. curettage
p. infection
p. pressure
p. surgery
p. tissue
p. tooth repair
periappendiceal abscess
periappendicitis
periappendicular
periaqueductal
p. gray area
p. gray matter stimulation
periaqueductal gray
matter/periventricular gray matter
(PAG/PVG)
periaqueductal-periventricular
p.-p. region
p.-p. stimulation
periareolar
p. incision
p. mastopexy

periarterial
p. plexus
p. sympathectomy
periarticular
p. fluid collection
p. fracture
p. tissue
periauricular
periaxial
periaxillary
peribronchial
peribronchiolar lymphocyte infiltration
peribuccal
peribulbar
p. anesthesia
p. anesthetic technique
p. block
p. injection
peribursal
pericallosal artery
pericanalicular connective tissue
pericapsular
p. fat infiltration
p. osteotomy
pericardectomy
pericardiacae
pericardiacophrenic
p. artery
p. vein
pericardial
p. biopsy
p. branch
p. decompression
p. fat pad
p. flap
p. fluid examination
p. hematoma
p. patch
p. pressure
p. puncture
p. reflection
p. reflex
p. reinforcement
p. sac
p. sinus
p. vein
p. window
pericardiectomy
parietal p.
thoracoscopic p.
visceral p.
pericardiocentesis

NOTES

P

pericardiophrenic nerve
pericardioplasty in pectus excavatum
   repair
pericardiorrhaphy
pericardioscopy
pericardiostomy
pericardiotomy, pericardotomy
      percutaneous balloon p.
      subxiphoid limited p.
      p. syndrome
pericarditis
      constrictive p.
pericardium
      parietal p.
      visceral p.
pericardotomy (*var. of* pericardiotomy)
pericecal
pericholecystic
      p. edema
      p. fluid collection
pericholecystitis
perichondral, perichondrial
      p. circulation
      p. ring
      p. sheath
perichondrium
perichoroidal space
pericolic membrane syndrome
pericolonitis
pericolostomy
      p. area
      p. hernia
pericorneal plexus
pericoronal flap
pericostal suture technique
pericranial temporalis flap
pericranium
pericystectomy
      partial p.
      total p.
pericystic
pericystitis
pericystium
peridectomy
peridental
      p. ligament
      p. membrane
      p. space
peridentinoblastic space
peridesmic
peridesmium
peridiaphragmatic hematoma
perididymis
perididymitis
periductal
      p. fibrosis
      p. mastitis
peridural anesthesia
perienteric

periependymal
periesophageal
      p. abscess
      p. blood vessel
      p. fat
      p. lymph node dissection
      p. structure
      p. tissue
perifascial nephrectomy
periganglionic
perigastric
      p. node
      p. node station
perigenicular vascular injury
perigraft hematoma
perihepatic
      p. abscess
      p. lymph nodal station
      p. space
perihepatitis
      gonococcal p.
perihernial
periimplant
      p. space
      p. tissue
periimplantation
perikaryon
perilaryngeal
perilenticular space
periligamentous
perilimbal
      p. incision
      p. suction
perilobular connective tissue
perilunar transscaphoid dislocation
perilunate
      p. carpal dislocation
      p. fracture-dislocation
perilymphatic
      p. cavity
      p. duct
      p. fistula
      p. fluid
      p. space
perilymph fistula
perimesencephalic cistern
perimeter
      p. corneal reflex test
      p. projection
perimetric
perimetrium
perimyelis
perimylolysis
perimysium
perinatal
      p. infection
      p. torsion
perinea (*pl. of* perineum)

perineal
    p. abscess
    p. analgesia
    p. anesthesia
    p. artery
    p. body
    p. defect
    p. flap
    p. flexure
    p. hernia
    p. impact trauma
    p. incision
    p. infection
    p. laceration
    p. lithotomy
    p. membrane
    p. muscle
    p. nerve
    p. nerve terminal motor latency
     test
    p. pearl
    p. polyp
    p. proctectomy
    p. prostatectomy
    p. raphe
    p. region
    p. repair
    p. scar
    p. section
    p. sinus
    p. sinus tract
    p. space
    p. urethrostomy
    p. urethrotomy
    p. urinary fistula
perineocele
perineoplasty
perineorrhaphy
    vaginal p.
perineoscrotal
perineostomy
perineosynthesis
perineotomy
perineovaginal fistula
perinephrial
perinephric
    p. abscess
    p. fluid collection
    p. hematoma
    p. space hemorrhage
    p. tissue
perinephritis

perinephrium
perineum, pl. **perinea**
perineural
    p. anesthesia
    p. infiltration
    p. invasion
    p. tissue
perineurial neurorrhaphy
perineurium
perinodal tissue
perinuclear
    p. cisterna
    p. space
periocular injection
period
    early postoperative p.
    immediate postoperative p.
    interdigestive p.
    later postoperative p.
    observation p.
    postoperative p.
    postprandial p.
    postresuscitation p.
    preoperative p.
    resuscitation p.
periodic respiration
periodontal
    p. disease
    p. flap
    p. inflammation
    p. lesion
    p. ligament
    p. ligament anesthesia
    p. membrane
    p. membrane necrosis
    p. ostectomy
    p. therapy
periodontium, pl. **periodontia**
periodontolysis
periomphalic
perioperative
    p. analgesia
    p. antibiotic
    p. antibiotic prophylaxis
    p. antibiotic therapy
    p. bacteremia
    p. complication
    p. corneal abrasion
    p. death
    p. management
    p. morbidity
    p. mortality

NOTES

P

perioperative *(continued)*
    p. outcome
    p. reduction
    p. risk factor
    p. shock
    p. standardized protocol
    p. stroke
    p. transfusion
perioptic subarachnoid space
periorbital
    p. infection
    p. membrane
periostea *(pl. of* periosteum)
periosteal
    p. elevation
    p. flap
    p. implantation
    p. new bone formation
    p. tissue
periosteoma
periosteophyte
periosteotomy
periosteous
periosteum, pl. **periostea**
    posterior p.
periostoma
periotic
    p. bone
    p. duct
    p. space
peripancreatic
    p. abdominal drainage
    p. fat plane
    p. infection
    p. necrosis
    p. tissue
peripartum endoscopy
peripenial
peripharyngeal space
peripheral
    p. access system (PAS)
    p. aneurysm
    p. antinociceptive action
    p. arterial aneurysmal disease
    p. arterial line
    p. balloon angioplasty
    p. bruit
    p. capillary filtration slit length
    p. cavity wall
    p. chemoreflex loop
    p. circulation
    p. examination
    p. extremity edema
    p. fusion
    p. hepatojejunostomy
    p. hyperalimentation
    p. hyperinsulinemia
    p. insulin resistance
    p. intravenous alimentation

    p. iridectomy
    p. iridectomy operation
    p. laceration
    p. laser angioplasty
    p. lymphoid tissue
    p. nerve
    p. nerve allografting
    p. nerve block
    p. nerve block anesthesia
    p. nerve block anesthetic technique
    p. nerve injury
    p. nerve lesion
    p. nerve regeneration
    p. neurectomy
    p. panretinal ablation
    p. pressure
    p. pulse
    p. thrombus
    p. vascular disease
    p. vascular surgery
    p. vein
    p. venous cannulation
periportal
    p. sinusoidal dilatation
    p. sinusoidal dilation
periproctic
periprostatic tissue
periprostatitis
periprosthetic
    p. fracture
    p. leak
peripylephlebitis
peripylic
peripyloric
perirectal
    p. abscess
    p. inflammation
    p. mass
    p. pelvic dissection
perirenal
    p. fascia
    p. hematoma
    p. insufflation
    p. space
perisalpinx
periscapular incision
periscleral space
perisellar vascular lesion
perisinusoidal space
perisplanchnic
perisplenic
perispondylic
peristalsis
    absent p.
peristaltic
peristasis
peristomal
    p. infection
    p. varix

peritarsal network
peritectomy
peritendineum
perithelioma
perithoracic
peritomist
peritomy
peritonea (*pl. of* peritoneum)
peritoneal
    p. access
    p. adenocarcinoma
    p. adhesion
    p. anatomy
    p. aspiration
    p. band
    p. biopsy
    p. cancer
    p. carcinomatosis
    p. cavity
    p. cavity abscess
    p. cavity fluid
    p. cytological assessment
    p. cytology
    p. cytology sample
    p. defect
    p. dialysis
    p. disease
    p. dissemination
    p. drainage
    p. encapsulation
    p. envelope
    p. equilibration test
    p. exchange volume
    p. fluid examination
    p. friction rub
    p. fungal infection
    p. hernia
    p. incision
    p. insufflation
    p. irritation
    p. lavage
    p. macrophage
    p. membrane permeability
    p. metastasis
    p. mouse
    p. patch
    p. penetration
    p. perforation
    p. pocket
    p. reconstruction
    p. recurrence
    p. reflection

    p. reinforcement
    p. sac
    p. seeding
    p. sepsis
    p. soilage
    p. space
    p. spill
    p. spread
    p. studding
    p. surface
    p. tap
    p. toilet
    p. transfusion
    p. tuberculosis
    p. vein
    ventricular p. (VP)
    p. villus
    p. violation
    p. washing
    p. washout
    p. window
peritonectomy
    left upper quadrant p.
    pelvic p.
    right upper quadrant p.
peritoneocentesis
peritoneoclysis
**peritoneopericardial diaphragmatic
  hernia**
peritoneopexy
peritoneoplasty
peritoneoscopy
peritoneotomy
    inverted-V p.
peritoneovenous shunt patency scan
peritoneum, pl. **peritonea**
    abdominal p.
    parietal p.
    visceral p.
peritonitis
    adhesive p.
    amebic p.
    aseptic p.
    barium p.
    chemical p.
    diffuse p.
    focal p.
    gastric perforation p.
    generalized p.
    perforation p.
    purulent p.

NOTES

P

peritonitis *(continued)*
  P. Severity Score (PSS)
  talc p.
peritonization
peritonize
peritonsillar
  p. nerve
  p. space
peritracheal
peritrochanteric fracture
peritubal syndrome
peritumoral site
perityphlic
periumbilical
  p. abscess
  p. hernia
  p. incision
  p. port
periureteral abscess
periureteric venous ring
periurethral abscess
periurethritis
periuterine
perivascular
  p. canal
  p. mass
  p. space
peri-vaterian therapeutic endoscopic procedure
periventricular
  p. hyperintense lesion
  p. white matter lesion
periventricular-intraventricular hemorrhage
perivertebral
perivesical
perivisceral
perivitelline space
Perkins vertical line
permanent
  p. anticoagulant therapy
  p. bipolar magnet placement
  p. end colostomy
  p. hypoparathyroidism
  p. loop ileostomy
  p. mesh omentum
  p. pacemaker placement
  p. paralysis
  p. pedicle flap
  p. proctectomy
  p. restoration
  p. section
  p. stoma
permeability
  capillary p.
  membrane p.
  peritoneal membrane p.
  sarcoplasmic reticulum p.
  p. theory of narcosis

permeation
  analgesia p.
  lymphatic p.
permissive hypercapnia (PHC)
permutation
perone
peroneal
  p. artery
  p. brevis tendon
  p. communicating nerve
  p. compartment syndrome
  p. dislocation
  p. groove
  p. island flap
  p. longus tendon
  p. muscle
  p. muscle atrophy
  p. nerve entrapment
  p. nerve injury
  p. phenomenon
  p. pulley
  p. retinaculum
  p. somatosensory evoked potential
  p. spastic flatfoot
  p. tendon sheath injection
  p. vein
peroneus
  p. brevis muscle
  p. longus muscle
  p. tertius muscle
peroral
  p. approach
  p. cholangiopancreatoscopy
  p. cholangioscopy
  p. endoscopy
  p. esophageal dilation
  p. intestinal biopsy
  p. maneuver
  p. pancreatoscopy
peroxidation
  lipid p.
perpendicular
  p. of ethmoid plate
  p. fashion
  p. plane
Perry
  P. extensile anterior approach
  P. technique
Perry-Nickel technique
Perry-O'Brien-Hodgson technique
Perry-Robinson cervical technique
perseveration
  infantile p.
  motor p.
persistent
  p. anovulation
  p. breast abnormality
  p. common atrioventricular canal
  p. fetal circulation

p. hypercalcemia
p. müllerian duct syndrome
p. occiput posterior position
p. ovarian mass
p. sciatic artery (PSA)
p. tolerant infection
personnel
paramedical p.
perspective
surgical p.
p. volume rendering (pVR)
perspiratory gland
Perthes
P. incision
P. lesion
P. procedure
P. test
perturbation
hemodynamic p.
pes, pl. **pedes**
p. planus deformity
PET
positron emission tomography
PETCO₂
extrapolated end-tidal carbon dioxide tension
petechia, pl. **petechiae**
petechial hemorrhage
Peter operation
Peters anomaly
PET-guided biopsy
Petit
P. aponeurosis
P. canal
P. hernia
P. herniotomy
P. ligament
lumbar triangle of P.
P. lumbar triangle
P. suture technique
petrobasilar suture
petroccipital
petroclinoid ligament
petromastoid
petrooccipital
p. fissure
p. joint
petropharyngeus
petrosa, pl. **petrosae**
petrosal
p. approach
p. artery

p. bone
p. branch
p. foramen
p. fossa
p. fossula
p. ganglion
p. nerve
p. neuralgia
p. vein
p. venous sinus
petrosectomy
total p.
petrositis
petrosomastoid
petrosphenoid ligament
petrospheno-occipital suture
petrosquamosal
petrosquamous
p. fissure
p. suture
p. venous sinus
petrostaphylinus
petrotympanic
p. fissure
p. suture
p. tissue
petrous
p. apex cell
p. pyramid
p. pyramid air cell exploration
p. pyramid exenteration
p. pyramid fracture
p. ridge
petrousitis
petrous-to-supraclinoid bypass
Peutz-Jeghers syndrome
Peyer
P. gland
P. patch
Peyman
P. full-thickness eye wall resection
P. iridocyclochoroidectomy
Peyronie disease
Peyrot thorax
Pfannenstiel
P. incision
P. transverse approach
Pfeiffer-Comberg method
Pfiffner and Myers method
PFO
patent foramen ovale

NOTES

PG
 partial gastrectomy
PGA
 pancreaticogastrostomy anastomosis
  PGA afferent
  PGA efferent
PGID
 postoperative gastrointestinal tract
  dysfunction
  analgesia-induced PGID
  anesthesia-induced PGID
  hypoperfusion-induced PGID
  inflammation-induced PGID
  neurogenic PGID
  surgery-induced PGID
PGL
 primary gastric lymphoma
 primary gastric non-Hodgkin lymphoma
pH
 hydrogen ion concentration
  pH electrode placement
  esophageal pH
  gastric mucosal pH
  intramural pH
  pH measurement
phaco-anaphylactic-endophthalmitis
phacocele
phacocystectomy
phacoemulsification
phacofragmentation
phacoglaucoma
phacolysis
phacoma, phakoma
 retinal p.
phacomatosis, phakomatosis
phacoscopy
phagocyte migration
phagolysis
phakoma (*var. of* phacoma)
phakomatosis (*var. of* phacomatosis)
phalangeal
 p. articular orientation
 p. diaphysial fracture
 p. dislocation
 p. fracture fixation
 p. malunion correction
 p. osteotomy
phalangectomy
 intermediate p.
phalangization
phalanx, pl. **phalanges**
 distal p.
 middle p.
 proximal p.
Phalen
 P. maneuver
 P. position
 P. sign
phallalgia

phallectomy
phallic
phalliform
phallitis
phallocampsis
phallocrypsis
phallodynia
phalloid
phalloncus
phalloplasty
phallotomy
Phaneuf-Graves repair
phantasmoscopia
phantasmoscopy
phantom
 p. aneurysm
 p. foot pain
 p. limb
 p. limb pain
pharaonic circumcision
pharmacodynamics
pharmacologic
 p. immunosuppression
 p. manipulation
 p. method
 p. paralysis
pharmacologically
 p. induced erection
 p. induced paralysis
pharyngeal
 p. airway
 p. anesthesia
 p. branch
 p. bursa
 p. canal
 p. cell
 p. exudate
 p. flap
 p. fornix
 p. gland
 p. gonococcal infection
 p. mucosa
 p. orifice
 p. plexus
 p. plexus neurectomy
 p. pouch
 p. pouch syndrome
 p. raphe
 p. recess
 p. region
 p. residue
 p. ridge
 p. space
 p. tissue
 p. tubercle
 p. vein
 p. wall carcinoma
pharyngealis
pharyngectomy

pharyngei
pharynges (*pl. of* pharynx)
pharyngobasilar fascia
pharyngocutaneous fistula
pharyngoepiglottic fold
pharyngoesophageal
    p. diverticulectomy
    p. reconstruction
pharyngoesophagogastroduodenoscopy
pharyngoesophagoplasty
pharyngoglossal
pharyngoglossus
pharyngolaryngeal
pharyngolaryngectomy
pharyngomaxillary space
pharyngometer
pharyngometry
    acoustic p.
pharyngonasal cavity
pharyngooral
pharyngopalatine
pharyngoplasty
    Hynes p.
    sphincter p.
    Wardill p.
pharyngoscleroma
pharyngoscopy
pharyngostoma
pharyngotomy
    transhyoid p.
pharyngotympanic groove
pharynx, pl. pharynges
    laryngeal p.
    nasal p.
    oral p.
    posterior p.
phase
    anhepatic p.
    eclipse p.
    ejection p.
    end-expiratory p.
    excitement p.
    exponential p.
    extradural p.
    granulation p.
    p. I, II block
    implantation p.
    maturation p.
    posthepatic resection p.
    prehepatic resection p.
    preinduction p.
    presensitization p.

    prolonged expiratory p.
    resectional p.
    reservoir p.
    1-p. subperiosteal implant technique
    transverse magnetization p.
    vector p.
phase-encoding direction
phase-sensitive gradient-echo MR imaging
phasic pressure wave
PHC
    permissive hypercapnia
PHCA
    profoundly hypothermic circulatory arrest
Pheasant elbow technique
Phelps
    P. neurectomy
    P. partial resection
    P. scapulectomy
Phemister
    P. acromioclavicular pin fixation
    P. incision
    P. medial approach
    P. onlay bone graft
    P. onlay bone graft technique
Phemister-Bonfiglio technique
phenol
    p. cauterization
    p. matrixectomy
phenolization
    angular p.
phenol-preserved extract
phenomenon, pl. phenomena
    all-or-nothing p.
    anoxic preconditioning p.
    Ascher glass-rod p.
    common cavity p.
    declamping p.
    doll's head p.
    entry p.
    extinction p.
    extravasation p.
    gelling p.
    glass-rod negative p.
    glass-rod positive p.
    Goldblatt p.
    hesitation p.
    identification p.
    ischemia-reperfusion p.
    Marcus Gunn p.
    misdirection p.
    modified Raynaud p.

NOTES

P

phenomenon *(continued)*
    neglectlike phenomena
    osteointegration p.
    overshoot p.
    peroneal p.
    preconditioning p.
    Raynaud p.
    referred trigger point p.
    relaxation p.
    specificity p.
    staircase p.
    steal p.
    temporary cavity p.
    tip-of-the-tongue p.
    truncation p.
    yo-yo weight fluctuation p.
phenotypic lymphocyte
phenozygous
phentolamine infusion
phenylethylbarbituric acid
pheochromoblastoma
pheochromocytoma
    adrenal p.
    p. crisis
philtrum, pl. **philtra**
phimosis, pl. **phimoses**
phimotic
phlebectomy
    greater saphenous p.
    transilluminated power p.
phlebitis
phlebogram
    orbital p.
phlebolite
phlebolith
phlebophlebostomy
phlebophthalmotomy
phleboplasty
phleborrhagia
phleborrhaphy
phleborrhexis
phlebostasis
phlebostrepsis
phlebotomy
    bloodless p.
    therapeutic p.
phlegmon
phlegmonous
    p. abscess
    p. gastritis
    p. mass
Phocas syndrome
phonation
    hypervalvular p.
    myoelastic-aerodynamic theory of p.
    neurochronaxic theory of p.
    reverse p.
    ventricular p.
    voice disorder of p.

phonomyography
phonophoresis
phonoscopy
phosphatase
    serum alkaline p.
phosphatase-antiphosphatase
    alkaline p.-a.
phosphate
    p. buffered saline (PBS)
    p. excretion index
    primary sodium p.
phosphodiesterase III inhibitor
phosphotungstic acid-magnesium chloride precipitation method
photic stimulation
photoablation
    laser p.
photoactivation
photoaged skin
photocoagulation
    argon laser p.
    infrared p.
    in situ p.
    laser p.
    macular p.
    panretinal argon laser p.
    retinal scatter p.
    scatter p.
    transendoscopic laser p.
    p. treatment
    xenon arc p.
photodisintegration
photodissociation
photodocumentation
photodynamic therapy (PDT)
photoepilation
photoexcitation
photography
    cross-polarization p.
    endoscopic p.
    laparoscopic p.
photoinactivation
photoirradiation
photolysis
    flash p.
photomicrograph
photomicroscopy
photon-deficient bone lesion
photoonycholysis
photopatch
photophore
photoplethysmographic waveform
photoplethysmography
photopolymerize
photopsia
photoradiation therapy
photorefractive
    p. keratectomy (PRK)
    p. keratoplasty

photoresection
photoscopy
photosensitive cell
phototherapeutic keratectomy
photothermal laser ablation
photothermolysis
   selective p.
photovaporization
   laser p.
phrenectomy
phrenemphraxis
phrenic
   p. ganglion
   p. nerve
   p. nerve block
   p. nerve block anesthetic technique
   p. pleura
   p. plexus
   p. stimulation
   p. vein
phrenicectomy
phreniclasia
phrenicoabdominal branch
phrenicocolic ligament
phrenicocostal sinus
phrenicoexeresis
phrenicogastric
phrenicoglottic
phrenicohepatic
phrenicolienal ligament
phrenicomediastinalis
phrenicomediastinal recess
phreniconeurectomy
phrenicopleural fascia
phrenicosplenic ligament
phrenicotomy
phrenicotripsy
phrenocolic
phrenocolopexy
phrenoesophageal
   p. ligament
   p. membrane
phrenogastric ligament
phrenohepatic
phrenosplenic ligament
phrictopathic
phrygian
   p. cap
   p. cap deformity
PHVE
   partial hepatic vascular exclusion

phyllodes
   cystosarcoma p.
   p.'s tumor
physial
   p. fracture
   p. line
physical
   p. barrier
   p. capacity evaluation
   p. examination
   p. finding
   p. manipulation
   p. problem
   p. restoration
   p. therapy
   p. therapy index
Physick operation
physiologic
   p. aspect
   p. barrier
   p. breast discharge
   p. change
   p. dose
   p. excavation
   p. mesial migration
   p. pattern release
   p. rest position
   p. retraction ring
   p. saline solution (PSS)
   p. salt solution
physiological
   p. dead space
   p. dead space ventilation per
     minute
   p. sphincter
physiology
   colorectal p.
   exercise p.
   flap p.
physiolysis
   central p.
physis
physocele
phytobezoar
PI
   percutaneous injury
pial-glial membrane
pia mater
piano-wire adhesion
PIC
   plasmin-inhibitor complex

NOTES

P

Pichlmayer
>P. method
>P. procedure
>P. technique

Pick bundle

Pickerill
>P. imbrication line
>imbrication line of P.

pickling solution

PiCO$_2$
>partial pressure of intramuscular carbon dioxide

Pico operation

Picot incision

picrotoxin

picture
>clinical p.
>p. frame vertebra

piece
>1-p. ostomy pouch

2-piece
>2-p. dental implant
>2-p. ostomy pouch

pie-crusting skin graft

Piedmont fracture

Pierre Robin anomalad

Pierrot-Murphy
>P.-M. advancement insertion
>P.-M. tendon technique

Piersol point

piezoelectric lithotripsy

pigeon-breast deformity

piggyback
>p. approach
>p. liver transplantation
>modified p. (MPB)

piggybacking

pigment
>p. cell transplantation
>p. epithelial lesion

pigmentary
>p. demarcation line
>p. migration

pigmented lesion

pigskin
>p. graft
>p. patch

pileus

pili (*pl. of* pilus)

pilimiction

pillar
>p. pain
>p. rib

pill-induced esophagitis

pillion fracture

pillow fracture

pill-rolling tremor

piloerection

pilojection

piloleiomyoma

pilomatrixoma

pilon ankle fracture

pilonidal
>p. abscess
>p. cyst
>p. cystectomy
>p. fistula

pilorum
>arrectores p.

pilot application

pilus, pl. **pili**
>arrector p.

pin
>cranial p.
>p. fixation
>p. retention
>p. site
>p. suture technique
>p. track
>p. tract infection

pin-and-plaster
>p.-a.-p. fixation
>p.-a.-p. method

Pinard maneuver

pin-bone interface

pincer nail

pinch
>p. biopsy
>p. restoration
>p. skin graft

pinch-grasp injection technique

pin-cushion distortion

pineal
>p. body
>p. eye
>p. gland
>p. recess
>p. region
>p. teratocarcinoma

pinealectomy

pinealoma

pineoblastoma

pineocytoma

ping-pong
>p.-p. ball deformity
>p.-p. fracture

piniform

pin-index safety system

pink frothy sputum

pinning
>closed p.
>hip p.
>in situ p.
>Knowles p.
>open p.
>percutaneous p.
>Sherk-Probst percutaneous p.

Sofield p.
Wagner closed p.

pinpoint
    p. electrocoagulation
    p. gastric mucosal defect
    p. gastric mucosal defect bleeding

pinprick
    p. analgesia
    p. method

pin-supported restoration
pinworm preparation
PIP
    positive inspiratory pressure
    prolactin inducible protein

pipe bone
Pipelle biopsy
Pipkin
    P. femoral fracture classification
    P. posterior hip dislocation
    classification
    P. subclassification of Epstein-
    Thomas classification

PIPP
    Premature Infant Pain Profile

Pirie bone
piriform
    p. fossa
    p. muscle
    p. recess
    p. sinus

piriformis syndrome
Pirogoff
    P. amputation
    P. angle
    P. operation
    P. triangle

pisiform
    p. bone
    p. fracture

pisotriquetral arthritis
pit
    p. of atlas for dens
    commissural lip p.
    costal p.
    p. and fissure cavity
    gastric p.
    granular p.
    herniation p.
    inferior articular p.
    inferior costal p.
    nail p.
    pterygoid p.

sublingual p.
superior costal p.
suprameatal p.

pitted
    p. keratolysis
    p. nail

pitting
    nail p.

pituicytoma
pituitary
    p. ablation
    p. adenoma
    p. body
    p. endocrine disorder
    p. fossa
    p. gland
    p. gland transplantation
    p. microadenoma
    p. neuroadenolysis
    p. stalk section
    p. tumor
    p. tumor cell

pituitectomy
pituitous
pivot
    p. joint
    p. point

Pizzolato peroxide-silver method
PJA
    pancreaticojejunostomy anastomosis
    PJA afferent
    PJA efferent

PKD
    polycystic kidney disease

place
    4-p. laminectomy

place of articulation
placebo therapy
placement
    aortic graft p.
    band p.
    biliary sphincterotomy and stent p.
    bone graft p.
    bur hole p.
    catheter tip p.
    clip p.
    dilator p.
    electrode p.
    endoscopic biliary stent p.
    endotracheal tube p.
    feeding tube p.
    filter p.

NOTES

P

placement *(continued)*
    fluoroscopic p.
    graft p.
    implant p.
    infrarenal endograft p.
    intrapleural catheter p.
    intrinsic spinal cord catheter p.
    Kirschner wire p.
    K-wire p.
    long-term central venous access
      catheter p.
    odontoid screw p.
    percutaneous nephrostomy tube p.
    percutaneous transhepatic p.
    permanent bipolar magnet p.
    permanent pacemaker p.
    pH electrode p.
    plate p.
    4-port diamond p.
    5-port fan p.
    posterolateral bone graft p.
    radiologic biliary stent p.
    rod p.
    sacral screw p.
    screw p.
    shunt p.
    stent p.
    suprarenal filter p.
    surgical p.
    temporary pacemaker p.
    T-tube p.
    tube p.
    ultrasound-guided caudal epidural
      needle p.
    ureteral stent p.
    variable screw p.
    ventriculoperitoneal shunt p.
    wire-guided p.
placenta, pl. **placentae**
    endotheliochorial p.
    endothelio-endothelial p.
    extrachorial p.
    premature separation of p.
placental
    p. barrier
    p. circulation
    p. extrusion
    p. fragment
    p. hemangioma syndrome
    p. hematoma
    p. hemorrhage
    p. implantation
    p. localization
    p. membrane
    p. metastasis
    p. migration
    p. respiration
    p. tissue
    p. tissue transplant

    p. transfer
    p. uptake
placentation bleeding
placentoma
Placido ring
placode
    nasal p.
pladaroma
plafond fracture
plagiocephaly
plain
    p. abdominal film
    p. abdominal radiography
plana (*pl. of* planum)
plane
    Aeby p.
    alveolar point-meatus p.
    anatomic p.
    auriculoinfraorbital p.
    axial p.
    axiobuccolingual p.
    axiolabiolingual p.
    axiomesiodistal p.
    base p.
    bite p.
    Broca visual p.
    buccolingual p.
    Camper p.
    cleavage p.
    coronal p.
    cove p.
    cusp p.
    datum p.
    Daubenton p.
    3-p. deformity
    diffuse p.
    p. of dissection
    equatorial p.
    equivalent refracting p.
    eye-ear p.
    facet p.
    facial p.
    fascial p.
    fat p.
    first parallel pelvic p.
    flexion-extension p.
    focal p.
    fourth parallel pelvic p.
    Frankfort horizontal p.
    French p.
    frontal p.
    guide p.
    guiding p.
    Hensen p.
    His p.
    Hodge p.
    horizontal p.
    internervous p.
    interspinal p.

intertubercular p.
ischiorectal fossa p.
p. joint
labiolingual p.
lens p.
Listing p.
Ludwig p.
mandibular p.
mean foundation p.
mesiodistal p.
midcoronal p.
midfrontal p.
midsagittal p.
midthalamic p.
Morton p.
nodal p.
nuchal p.
oblique coronal p.
occipital p.
occlusal p.
orbital p.
orthogonal p.
paramedian sagittal p.
parasagittal p.
pelvic p.
peripancreatic fat p.
perpendicular p.
preglenoid p.
primary movement p.
principal p.
sagittal p.
scan p.
second parallel pelvic p.
sensitive p.
short-axis p.
slant of occlusal p.
spectacle p.
spinous p.
sternal p.
sternoxiphoid p.
subcostal p.
subcutaneous p.
subpectoral p.
supracrestal p.
supracristal p.
suprasternal p.
symmetry p.
temporal p.
terminal p.
thalamic p.
third parallel pelvic p.

thoracic p.
tooth p.
transaxial scan p.
transection p.
transpyloric p.
transtubercular p.
transverse p.
umbilical p.
varus-valgus p.
vertical p.
visual p.
wide p.
1-plane
    1-p. deformity
    1-p. instability
    1-p. view
2-plane
    2-p. deformity
    2-p. fluoroscopy
    2-p. occlusion
planimetry
planithorax
planned
    p. awakening
    p. extracapsular cataract extraction
    p. reoperation
planning
    image-integrated surgery
      treatment p.
planta
plantar
    p. angulation
    p. approach
    p. aspect
    p. compartmental anatomy
    p. condylectomy
    p. digital nerve
    p. fasciotomy
    p. flexion-inversion deformity
    p. interosseous muscle
    p. longitudinal incision
    p. plate release
    p. pressure
    p. quadrate muscle
    p. space
    p. tendon sheath
    p. venous network
plantar-hindfoot-midfoot bony mass
plantaris tendon
planum, pl. **plana**
planuria

NOTES

P

planus
  condyloma p.
  oral condyloma p.
plaque
  atheromatous p.
  atherosclerotic p.
  augmentation p.
  carotid p.
  echogenic p.
  echolucent p.
  eczematoid pruritic p.
  p. formation
  p. fracture
  p. incision
  neuritic p.
  Randall p.
  p. rupture
  senile p.
  p. technique
plaquelike
  p. hamartoma
  p. lesion
plaquing
plasma
  p. assay coagulation panel
  p. atrial natriuretic protein
  p. cell portal infiltration
  p. clotting time
  p. colloid osmotic pressure
  p. endotoxin concentration
  p. exchange
  p. exchange therapy
  expanded p.
  extracellular p.
  fresh frozen p. (FFP)
  p. gastrin concentration
  p. half-life
  p. iron concentration
  p. level
  p. membrane
  p. norepinephrine concentration
  p. oncotic pressure
  p. renin concentration
  p. separation rate
  p. substitute
  target p.
  p. thrombin clot method
  p. urea concentration
  p. volume expansion
plasmacytoma
plasmapheresis
plasmin coagulation
plasmin-inhibitor complex (PIC)
plasminogen plasma level
plasmocytoma
plasmolysis
plaster cast application burn
plastic
  p. bowing fracture

  p. clot
  p. induration
  p. matrix technique
  p. operation
  p. reconstruction
  p. and reconstructive surgery
  p. repair
  p. section
  p. stent occlusion
  p. surgeon
  p. suture technique
plasticity
  connective tissue p.
  neural p.
plastron
plasty
  Coleman p.
  Durham p.
  endoventricular circular patch p.
  Foley Y-V p.
  mons p.
  posterior bladder flap p.
  rotation p.
  skin p.
  sliding p.
  V-Y p.
  Y-V p.
plate
  p. of Arantius
  cribriform p.
  dorsal p.
  ethmoidal p.
  p. fixation
  gallbladder p.
  hilar p.
  nerve-containing p.
  perpendicular of ethmoid p.
  p. placement
  pterygoid p.
  tarsal p.
  umbilical p.
  vessel-containing p.
  volar p.
plateau
  alveolar p.
  p. method
plate-guided
  p.-g. distraction device
  p.-g. distractor
platelet
  p. aggregation
  p. concentrate
  p. gene polymorphism
  p. nucleotide content
plateletpheresis
  intraoperative p.
plate-screw
  p.-s. fixation
  p.-s. osteosynthesis

platform
    dual-delivery p.
    p. posturography
plating
    compression p.
    pedicle screw p.
    posterior cervical lateral p.
Platou osteotomy
platybasia
platycephaly
platycrania
platyhieric
platymeric
platyopia
platyopic
platypellic pelvis
platypelloid pelvis
platyrrhine
platyrrhiny
platysma, pl. **platysmas, platysmata**
    p. muscle
    p. myocutaneous flap
platyspondylia
platystencephaly
Pleatman sac
pleoptics
    Bangerter method of p.
    Cüppers method of p.
plethysmography
    air p.
    forearm p.
    impedance p.
    venous-occlusion volume p.
    volume p.
pleura, pl. **pleurae**
    cervical p.
    costal p.
    diaphragmatic p.
    mediastinal p.
    parietal p.
    phrenic p.
    pulmonary p.
    visceral p.
pleuracentesis
pleuracotomy
pleurae (*pl. of* pleura)
pleural
    p. biopsy
    p. calculus
    p. cavity
    p. cupula
    p. effusion

    p. fluid
    p. fluid aspiration
    p. fluid collection
    p. fluid examination
    p. line
    p. mass
    p. patch reinforcement
    p. recess
    p. reflection
    p. sac
    p. sinus
    p. space
    p. stoma
    p. symphysis
    p. villus
    p. violation
pleurapophysis
pleurectomy
    thorascopic apical p.
pleurisy
pleurobiliary fistula
pleurocele
pleurocentesis
pleurocentrum
pleuroclysis
pleurodesis
    talc p.
pleuroesophageal
    p. fistula
    p. line
    p. muscle
pleuroesophageus
pleurolith
pleuroparietopexy
pleuropericardial
pleuropericarditis
pleuroperitoneal
    p. canal
    p. fold
    p. foramen
    p. hernia
    p. hiatus
    p. shunting
    p. space
pleuropneumonectomy
pleuropulmonary
pleuroscopy
pleurotomy
pleurovisceral
plexectomy
plexiform
    p. external layer

NOTES

P

plexiform *(continued)*
    p. lesion
    p. neurofibroma
plexopathy
    brachial p.
    idiopathic brachial p.
    postradiation p.
plexus, pl. **plexuses, plexus**
    abdominal aortic p.
    ascending pharyngeal p.
    Auerbach p.
    axillary p.
    basilar venous p.
    Batson p.
    brachial p.
    cardiac p.
    carotid venous p.
    cavernous p.
    celiac nervous p.
    cervical p.
    choroid p.
    coccygeal p.
    colic p.
    colonic mesenteric p.
    common carotid p.
    coronary p.
    Cruveilhier p.
    deep cardiac p.
    deferential p.
    enteric p.
    esophageal p.
    Exner p.
    external carotid p.
    external iliac p.
    external maxillary p.
    extrapancreatic nerve p.
    facial p.
    femoral p.
    gastroesophageal variceal p.
    Heller p.
    hemorrhoidal p.
    hepatic p.
    hypogastric p.
    hypoglossal canal venous p.
    iliac p.
    inferior hemorrhoidal p.
    inferior hypogastric p.
    inferior mesenteric p.
    inferior rectal p.
    inferior thyroid p.
    inferior vesical p.
    infraclavicular part of brachial p.
    inguinal p.
    intermesenteric p.
    internal carotid venous p.
    internal mammary p.
    internal maxillary p.
    internal thoracic lymphatic p.
    intracavernous p.

    intraparotid p.
    ischiadic p.
    Jacques p.
    jugular p.
    lingual p.
    lumbar p.
    lumbosacral p.
    lymphatic p.
    mammary p.
    Meissner p.
    meningeal p.
    mesenteric p.
    myenteric p.
    occipital p.
    ovarian p.
    pampiniform venous p.
    pancreatic p.
    parotid p.
    pelvic autonomic p.
    periarterial p.
    pericorneal p.
    pharyngeal p.
    phrenic p.
    popliteal p.
    posterior auricular p.
    posterior coronary p.
    prostaticovesical p.
    prostatic venous p.
    pterygoid p.
    pulmonary p.
    Quénu hemorrhoidal p.
    rectal venous p.
    Remak p.
    renal p.
    sacral venous p.
    Santorini p.
    Sappey p.
    sciatic p.
    solar p.
    spermatic p.
    splenic p.
    subclavian periarterial p.
    submucosal p.
    suboccipital venous p.
    superficial cardiac p.
    superficial temporal p.
    superior hemorrhoidal p.
    superior hypogastric p.
    superior mesenteric p.
    superior rectal p.
    superior thyroid p.
    suprarenal p.
    testicular p.
    thoracic aortic p.
    thyroid p.
    tympanic p.
    ureteric p.
    uterine venous p.
    uterovaginal p.

vaginal venous p.
vascular p.
venous p.
vertebral venous p.
vesical p.
vesicular venous p.
Walther p.
plica, pl. **plicae**
plicated appendicocystostomy
plicating suture technique
plication
bowel p.
buccinator p.
Child-Phillips bowel p.
disc p.
fundal p.
Graham p.
Kelly p.
Nesbit p.
Noble bowel p.
Rehne-Delorme p.
retractor p.
soft tissue p.
surgical p.
suture p.
tongue p.
transgastric p.
transmesenteric p.
plicectomy
plicotomy
PLIF
posterior lumbar interbody fusion
PLIF procedure
PLND
pelvic lymph node dissection
ploidy
tumor p.
plombage operation
plop
cardiac tumor p.
tumor p.
plosive-injection method
plot
load-displacement p.
pressure-flow p.
plug
p. flow
p. prosthetic mesh repair
plumb line
plume
laser p.
Plummer disease

plyometric exercise
PMN
polymorphonuclear neutrophil
PMT
percutaneous mechanical thrombectomy
PmvCO$_2$
partial pressure of mesenteric venous
carbon dioxide
pneumatic
p. bag esophageal dilation
p. balloon catheter dilation
p. bone
p. compression
p. dilatation
p. otoscopy
p. reduction
p. retinopexy
p. space
pneumatization
pneumatocele
pneumatorrhachis
pneumaturia
pneumectomy
pneumobulbar
pneumocardial
pneumocele
pneumocentesis
pneumocephalus
pneumococcal infection
pneumococcolysis
pneumoconiosis, pl. **pneumoconioses**
pneumoconstriction
pneumocystography
pneumocystosis
pneumodissection
laparoscopic p.
pneumogastric nerve
pneumography
impedance p.
retroperitoneal p.
pneumohydroperitoneum
pneumolysis
pneumonectomy
p. chest
sleeve p.
pneumonia
aspiration p.
congenital aspiration p.
endogenous lipid p.
extensive bilateral p.
Gram-negative p.
inhalation p.

NOTES

P

pneumonia *(continued)*
    nosocomial p.
    oil-aspiration p.
    postoperative p.
    ventilator-associated p.
pneumonic
pneumonitis
    acute radiation p.
    aspiration p.
    peptic aspiration p.
    radiation p.
pneumonocele
pneumonocentesis
pneumonopexy
pneumonoresection
pneumonorrhaphy
pneumonotomy
pneumoorbitography
pneumopericardium
    tension p.
    ventilator-induced p.
pneumoperitoneum
    ambulatory p.
    CO_2 p.
    hospital p.
    positive-pressure p.
    preoperative p.
    stent-induced p.
pneumopexy
pneumopleuroparietopexy
pneumopyelography
pneumoresection
pneumoretroperitoneum
    unilateral p.
pneumostatic dilation
pneumotachogram
pneumotachograph
pneumothorax, pl. **pneumothoraces**
    delayed p.
    extrapleural p.
    iatrogenic tension p.
    induced tension p.
    open p.
    posttraumatic persistent p. (PPP)
    pressure p.
    spontaneous p.
    tension p.
    ventilator-induced p.
pneumotomy
PNPB
    positive-negative pressure breathing
PO_2
    partial pressure of oxygen
POCD
    postoperative cognitive dysfunction
pocket
    circulating air p.
    elimination p.
    ionization chamber p.

    p. operation
    pacemaker p.
    peritoneal p.
    subpectoral p.
pocketed calculus
POD
    postoperative day
podalic extraction
PODVT
    postoperative deep venous thrombosis
POG
    Pediatric Oncology Group
pogonion
Pogrund lateral approach
point
    p. A
    abrasive p.
    p. of abscess
    absorbent p.
    Addison p.
    alveolar p.
    anchoring p.
    p. angle
    anterior focal p.
    APACHE-II p.
    apophysary p.
    apophysial p.
    p. of Arrhigi
    associated myofascial trigger p.
    auricular p.
    axial p.
    B p.
    p. B
    bleeding p.
    blur p.
    Boas p.
    Bolton p.
    bounce p.
    Boyd p.
    break p.
    Brinell hardness indenter p.
    Broadbent registration p.
    Cannon p.
    Capuron p.
    cardinal p.
    Castellani p.
    central bearing p.
    central yellow p.
    p. centric
    change p.
    Chauffard p.
    choroid p.
    Clado p.
    condenser p.
    conjugate p.
    contact area p.
    convenience p.
    convergence p.
    copular p.

corresponding p.
craniometric p.
Crowe pilot p.
cut p.
D p.
de Mussy p.
Desjardins p.
disparate p.
dorsal p.
E p.
electrodesiccated bleeding p.
end p.
entry p.
equivalence p.
Erb p.
ethmoid registration p.
exit p.
eye p.
far p.
faulty contact p.
F2 focal p.
fibromyalgia trigger p.
fixation p.
fixed p.
focal bleeding p.
focal image p.
freezing p.
fusing p.
gingival p.
glenoid p.
growing p.
Guéneau de Mussy p.
gutta-percha p.
Halle p.
Hartmann p.
hinge-axis p.
ice p.
identical p.
ignition p.
image p.
p. imaging
impaction p.
incident p.
incisal p.
incisor p.
p. of inflection
insertion p.
isoelectric p.
isometric p.
isosbestic p.
J p.
jugal p.

jugomaxillary p.
Keen p.
Knoop hardness indenter p.
Kocher p.
Krackow p.
lacrimal p.
Lanz p.
Legat p.
lustrous central yellow p.
Mackenzie p.
material failure break p.
p. of maximum impulse
maximum occipital p.
McBurney p.
median mandibular p.
melting p.
mental p.
metopic p.
motor p.
multiple sensitive p.
Munro p.
myofascial trigger p.
near visual p.
neutral p.
nodal p.
null p.
occipital p.
optical nodal p.
painful p.
paper p.
Pauly p.
pedicle entrance p.
Piersol p.
pivot p.
posterior focal p.
power p.
preauricular p.
pressure inversion p.
primary myofascial trigger p.
principal p.
purchase p.
Ramond p.
referred p.
respiratory inversion p.
restoration p.
retention p.
retrograde insertion p.
retromandibular p.
Robson p.
root canal p.
rotary mounted p.
sacral brim target p.

NOTES

P

point (*continued*)
    satellite myofascial trigger p.
    p. scanning
    secondary focal p.
    secondary myofascial trigger p.
    sensitive p.
    separation p.
    set p.
    p. source
    spinal p.
    Starlite p.
    stereo-identical p.
    Sudeck critical p.
    sulfur and silver p.
    supraauricular p.
    supraorbital p.
    sylvian p.
    tender p.
    thermal death p.
    trial p.
    trigger p.
    triple p.
    Trousseau p.
    Valleix p.
    virtual p.
    visual p.
    Weber p.
    white p.
    William Dixon Cratex p.
    wood p.
    yellow p.
    Z p.
    zygomaxillary p.
2-point
    2-p. discrimination test
    2-p. nerve block
3-point
    3-p. bending moment
    3-p. touch
4-point
    4-p. biopsy
    4-p. fixation
point-counting image
pointed condyloma
point-in-space stereotactic biopsy
Poirier
    P. gland
    P. line
    space of P.
Poiseuille space
poisoning
    oxygen p.
    radiation p.
Poland
    P. anomaly
    P. epiphysial fracture classification
    P. physical injury classification
polarimetry
    scanning laser p.

polariscopy
polarization microscopy
polarographic method
pole
    inferior p.
    lateral p.
    p. ligation
    superior p.
poli (*pl. of* polus)
poliomyelitis
Politano-Leadbetter
    P.-L. anastomosis
    P.-L. reimplantation
    P.-L. tunnel creation
    P.-L. ureterolysis
    P.-L. ureteroneocystostomy
Politzer method
pollakiuria
pollex, pl. **pollices, pollicis**
pollicization
    Buck-Gramcko p.
    index p.
    Riordan p.
pollination
Pollock operation
polus, pl. **poli**
Pólya
    P. anastomosis
    P. gastrectomy
    P. gastroenterostomy
    P. method
    P. operation
    P. procedure
    P. technique
polyacrylonitrile membrane
polyadenous
polyadenylation
polyagglutination
Polyak operation
polyaxial joint
polycentric rotation
polychondritis
    relapsing p.
polyclonal
    p. growth
    p. hyperplasia
polycystic
    p. kidney disease (PKD)
    p. liver
polydactylous
polydactyly
polydysplasia
polyembryoma
polyganglionic
polyglandular
polymer anesthetic
polymerase inhibition
polymicrobial infection

polymorphism
> platelet gene p.

polymorphonuclear neutrophil (PMN)
polymyalgia rheumatica
polyorchism
polyp
> adenomatous p.
> cellular p.
> colon p.
> colorectal p.
> cystic p.
> dental p.
> diffuse GI hamartoma p.
> endocervical p.
> endometrial p.
> hyperplastic p.
> juvenile p.
> perineal p.

polypapilloma
polypectomy
> colonoscopic p.
> duodenal endoscopic p.
> electrosurgical snare p.
> endoscopic sessile p.
> gastric p.
> incomplete p.
> intranasal p.

polypeptide growth factor
polypoid
> p. hyperplasia
> p. hyperplasia of larynx
> p. lesion
> p. mass
> p. superficial gastric carcinoma
> p. tissue

polypoid hyperplasia
polyposis
> carpetlike p.
> diffuse mucosal p.
> familial adenomatous p. (FAP)

polypropylene mesh herniorrhaphy
polyradiculoneuropathy
> chronic inflammatory
> demyelinating p. (CIDP)

polyradiculopathy
polysinusectomy
polyspermia
polysyndactyly
polytetrafluoroethylene graft
polythelia
polyuria

polyvalent
> p. melanoma oncolysate
> p. VMO

Pomeroy
> P. operation
> P. tubal ligation

Poncet perineal urethrostomy
pond fracture
Ponka
> P. herniorrhaphy
> P. technique for local anesthesia

pons, pl. **pontes**
Ponsky pull or guide wire insertion technique
Pontén fasciocutaneous flap
pontes (*pl. of* pons)
pontile
pontine
> p. artery
> p. cistern
> p. hemorrhage
> p. myelinolysis
> p. paramedian reticular formation
> p. spinothalamic tractotomy

PONV
> postoperative nausea and vomiting

pool
> abdominal p.
> p. therapy

poorly compliant bladder
poor-risk patient
popliteal
> p. artery
> p. artery entrapment
> p. artery occlusive disease (PAOD)
> p. artery trifurcation
> p. communicating nerve
> p. fascia
> p. fossa
> p. groove
> p. incision
> p. muscle
> p. plexus
> p. region
> p. space
> p. vein
> p. web syndrome

popliteus tendon
population
> adult p.
> patient p.

NOTES

P

population *(continued)*
 pediatric p.
 p. sample
population-based registry
porcelain
 p. cervical ditching technique
 p. condensation
 p. fracture
 p. gallbladder
 p. jacket restoration
porcelain-bonded restoration
porcelain-fused-to-metal restoration
pori (*pl. of* porus)
porocarcinoma
poroid hidradenoma
poroma
porotomy
porous
 p. filter membrane
 p. ingrowth fixation
 p. polyethylene implant
 p. tantalum implant
porphyria
 acute intermittent p.
 intermittent acute p.
Porro
 P. cesarean section
 P. operation
Porstmann technique
port
 chest p.
 p. displacement
 5-p. fan placement
 implantable infusion p.
 p. incision
 infusion p.
 inlet p.
 lumbar p.
 midclavicular p.
 nasal p.
 PAS P.
 periumbilical p.
 side p.
 p. site
 p. site hernia
 p. site metastasis
 subcostal p.
 subcutaneous implanted injection p.
 subxiphoid p.
 suprapubic p.
 umbilical p.
 velopharyngeal p.
 p. vitrectomy
4-port
 4-p. diamond placement
 4-p. method
 4-p. procedure
 4-p. technique
porta

portable C-arm image intensifier fluoroscopy
portacaval
 p. anastomosis
 p. H graft
 p. shunt
 p. shunt operation
port-access technique for coronary bypass surgery
portal
 arthroscopic entry p.
 aspiration p.
 p. bifurcation
 p. collateral
 p. decompression
 p. decompression surgery
 p. delta
 p. drainage
 p. eosinophilic inflammation
 p. fissure
 p. hypertension
 p. hypertensive bleeding
 p. inflow
 p. infusion
 p. lymphadenopathy
 p. lymph node basin
 macroscopic p.
 p. mesenteric shunting
 p. nodal involvement
 p. pedicle
 p. shunt index
 p. space
 p. steal
 6-p. synovectomy
 2-p. technique
 3-p. technique
 p. thrombosis
 p. tract
 p. tract inflammation
 p. triad
 p. triad clamping
 p. tumor thrombus
 p. vein
 p. vein approach
 p. vein catheterization
 p. vein obstruction
 p. vein reconstruction
 p. vein resection
 p. vein tumor thrombus (PVTT)
 p. venous pressure
 p. vessel
portal-collateral circulation
portal-hypophysial circulation
portal-systemic
 p.-s. anastomosis
 p.-s. collateral
 p.-s. collateral vein
 p.-s. encephalopathy (PSE)

p.-s. shunt
p.-s. shunt surgery
Porter fascia
Porter-Richardson-Vainio
    P.-R.-V. synovectomy
    P.-R.-V. technique
portio, pl. **portiones**
portion
    distal p.
    intrapancreatic p.
    lateral p.
    mesenteric p.
    proximal p.
    subcutaneous p.
portiplexus
Portmann interposition operation
portmanteau procedure
portobilioarterial
portoenterostomy
    Kasai p.
portography
    computed tomography arterial p.
     (CTAP)
    CT p.
    CT arterial p. (CTAP)
    indirect p.
portojejunostomy
    hepatic p.
portoportal anastomosis
portopulmonary venous anastomosis
portosystemic
    p. anastomosis
    p. collateral circulation
    p. shunt
    p. shunting
port-site wound recurrence
port-wine
    p.-w. hemangioma
    p.-w. mark
    p.-w. stain
porus, pl. **pori**
Posada fracture
position
    abdominal brace p.
    Adams p.
    airplane p.
    p. ametropia
    anatomic p.
    anatomical p.
    angular p.
    anomalous p.
    antecolic p.

anterior oblique p.
antiembolic p.
arch-and-slouch p.
arm p.
arm-extension p.
asynclitic p.
back-up p.
backward p.
barber chair p.
batrachian p.
bayonet fracture p.
beach chair p.
Bertel p.
birthing p.
bisecting angle cone p.
body p.
Bonner p.
Boyce p.
Bozeman p.
Brickner p.
brow p.
brow-anterior p.
brow-down p.
brow-posterior p.
brow-up p.
Buie p.
calcaneal stance p.
cardiac p.
cardinal p.
Casselberry p.
catheter p.
centric p.
cervical p.
chin p.
Concorde p.
condylar hinge p.
consonant p.
convergence p.
corrected sternal p.
cottonloader p.
curved flank p.
cuspid-molar p.
decubitus p.
deep extubation in tonsil p.
dissociated p.
distoangular p.
dorsal elevated p.
dorsal inertia p.
dorsal lithotomy p.
dorsal recumbent p.
dorsal rigid p.
dorsal supine p.

NOTES

P

position (*continued*)

dorsosacral p.
Duncan p.
eccentric jaw p.
Edebohls p.
electrical heart p.
Elliot p.
emprosthotonos p.
en face p.
English p.
equinus p.
exaggerated sniffing p.
extraabdominal p.
extrathoracic p.
face-down p.
face-to-pubes p.
Feist-Mankin p.
fetal head p.
Fick p.
figure-of-4 p.
final cone p.
final consonant p.
first cone p.
flank p.
flexed p.
forehead-nose p.
French p.
frogleg p.
frontoanterior p.
frontoposterior p.
frontotransverse p.
Fuchs p.
fusion-free p.
Gaynor-Hart p.
genucubital p.
genufacial p.
genupectoral p.
gingival p.
greater curve p.
head dependent p.
head-up tilt p.
heart p.
heterophoric p.
hinge p.
hook-lying p.
horizontal p.
hornpipe p.
infraumbilical p.
initial consonant p.
intercuspal p.
intraperitoneal p.
intrathoracic p.
intrinsic minus p.
jackknife p.
James p.
jaw-to-jaw p.
jet pilot p.
Jones p.
jumper-knee p.

kidney p.
knee-chest p.
knee-elbow p.
kneeling p.
kneeling-squatting p.
Kraske p.
LAO p.
lateral decubitus p.
lateral prone p.
lateral recumbent p.
leapfrog p.
left anterior oblique p.
left decubitus p.
left lateral decubitus p.
left-side-down p.
levo-transposed p.
lithotomy p.
Lloyd Davis modified lithotomy p.
lotus p.
mandibular hinge p.
mandibular rest p.
maternal birthing p.
Mayo-Robson p.
mentoanterior p.
mentoposterior p.
mentotransverse p.
mentum anterior p.
mentum posterior p.
mentum transverse p.
mesioangular p.
midline p.
military brace p.
military tuck p.
missionary p.
modified lithotomy p.
Moynihan p.
near-anatomic p.
neck extension p.
neutral hip p.
neutral spine p.
Noble p.
nonphysiologic p.
normal anatomic p.
obstetric p.
occipitoanterior p.
occipitoposterior p.
occipitotransverse p.
occlusal p.
opisthotonos p.
overcorrected p.
over-the-top p.
paralleling cone p.
park-bench p.
persistent occiput posterior p.
Phalen p.
physiologic rest p.
posterior border p.
postural resting p.
prayer p.

premuscular p.
primary p.
Proetz p.
prone split-leg p.
protrusive occlusal p.
proximal bow p.
pterygoid p.
pulmonary p.
quasistatic stressed p.
RAO p.
reclining p.
rectus p.
recumbent p.
rest p.
retrocolic p.
retromuscular p.
retruded p.
reverse Trendelenburg p.
Rhese p.
right acromiodorsoposterior p.
right anterior oblique p.
right-side-down p.
Robson p.
Rose p.
sacroanterior p.
sacroposterior p.
sacrotransverse p.
Samuel p.
scapuloanterior p.
scapuloposterior p.
Schüller p.
scissor-leg p.
Scultetus p.
sea lion p.
semi-Fowler p.
semilateral p.
semioblique p.
semiprone p.
semireclining p.
semirecumbent p.
semiupright p.
shock p.
shoe-and-stocking p.
Simon p.
Sims p.
sitting p.
ski p.
sniffing p.
p. in space
sphinx p.
spinal fusion p.

split-leg p.
static p.
steep Trendelenburg p.
sternal p.
subcostal p.
sulcus fixated p.
supine p.
terminal hinge p.
tooth p.
tooth-to-tooth p.
translational p.
Trendelenburg p.
tricuspid p.
tuck p.
upright p.
Valentine p.
vertex p.
vertical divergence p.
Walcher p.
Waters-Waldron p.
W-sitting p.
Zanelli p.

positional
p. release therapy
p. vertigo

positioner
hip p.

positioning
automated endoscopic system for optimal p. (AESOP)
surgical p.

positive
p. airway pressure (PAP)
p. control enzyme induction
p. correlation
p. cytology
p. end-expiratory pressure (PEEP)
p. end-expiratory pressure/continuous positive airway pressure (PEEP/CPAP)
p. expiratory pressure
extradomain A p.
false p.
p. inspiratory pressure (PIP)
p. peritoneal cytology (PPC)
p. predictive valve (PPV)
p. resection margin
p. surgical margin
true p.

positive-negative pressure breathing (PNPB)

NOTES

P

positive-pressure
 p.-p. pneumoperitoneum
 p.-p. ventilation (PPV)
positron
 p. emission tomography (PET)
 p. emission tomography-guided
  biopsy
 p. emission tomography scanning
post
 p. herniorrhaphy inguinodynia
 P. total shoulder arthroplasty
postactivation
 p. exhaustion
 p. facilitation
postadrenalectomy syndrome
postage stamp skin graft
postanal repair
postanesthesia care unit (PACU)
postanesthetic central nervous system
 dysfunction
postangioplasty
 p. intimal flap
 p. restenosis
postaugmentation
postauricular incision
postaxial
postballoon angioplasty restenosis
postbiopsy
 p. renal A-V fistula
 p. vascular complication
postbrachial
postbulbar ulceration
postburn
 p. bone marrow failure
 p. hypermetabolic response
postcardiotomy
 p. shock (PS)
 p. syndrome
postcatheterization
postcaval ureter
postcementation
postcentral
 p. gyrectomy
 p. sulcal artery
postcesarean anesthesia
postcholecystectomy
 p. flatulent dyspepsia
 p. syndrome
postclavicular
post-coiling
postcoital
 p. bleeding
 p. test
postcolonoscopy distention syndrome
postcommissurotomy syndrome
postcondensation
postcordial
postcore restoration
postcoronary angioplasty

postcostal
postcricoid web
postdiagnosis
postdischarge
postdrug latency
postductal coarctation
postdural puncture headache (PDPH)
postembolization syndrome
postendoscopy
posterior
 p. alveolar artery
 p. antebrachial region
 anterior and p. (A&P)
 p. anterior jugular vein
 p. arch
 p. arch fracture
 p. arm
 p. articular aorta
 p. aspect
 p. auricular artery
 p. auricular groove
 p. auricular plexus
 p. auricular vein
 p. basal branch
 p. basal segment
 p. belly
 p. bladder flap plasty
 p. border jaw relation
 p. border position
 p. brachial region
 p. capsular zonular barrier
 p. capsulorrhaphy
 p. capsulotomy
 p. cartilage graft
 p. cecal artery
 p. cerebral artery
 p. cervical fixation
 p. cervical fusion
 p. cervical lateral plating
 p. cervical space
 p. choroidal artery
 p. circulation aneurysm
 p. circumflex humeral artery
 p. clinoid process
 p. colporrhaphy
 p. column
 p. column cordotomy
 p. column fracture
 p. column osteosynthesis
 p. communicating artery
 p. condyloid foramen
 p. coronary plexus
 p. costotransversectomy approach
 p. cranial fossa
 p. cricoarytenoid muscle
 p. cyst
 p. diaphragmatic gastropexy
 p. element fracture
 p. explant

p. extraperitoneal approach
p. facial vein
p. flap
p. flap technique
p. flap vaginoplasty
p. focal point
p. fontanelle
p. fornix of vagina
p. fossa circulation
p. fossa decompression
p. fracture-dislocation
p. fundoplasty
p. glenoplasty
p. great vessel
p. hemicircular incision
p. hip dislocation
p. humeral circumflex artery
p. iliac osteotomy
p. inferior cerebellar artery
p. inferior iliac spine
p. innominate rotation
p. intercostal vein
p. intermuscular septum
p. interosseous artery
p. interosseous nerve compression
  syndrome
p. interosseous vein
p. intraoccipital joint
p. inverted-U approach
p. knee
p. knee region
p. labial artery
p. labial commissure
p. labial vein
p. laparoscopic approach
p. larynx
p. layer
p. limiting ring
p. lobule
p. longitudinal bundle
p. lower cervical spine surgery
p. lumbar approach
p. lumbar interbody fusion (PLIF)
p. lumbar spine and sacrum
  surgery
p. mediastinal artery
p. mediastinal esophagoplasty
p. mediastinal mass
p. mediastinum
p. meningeal artery
p. midline approach
p. mitral valve leaflet

p. neck region
p. nephrectomy
p. nodule
p. occipitocervical approach
p. oropharyngeal wall
p. pancreaticoduodenal artery
p. parametritis
p. parietal artery
p. parotid vein
p. pedicle
p. pelvic exenteration
p. periosteum
p. pharynx
p. Pólya procedure
p. primary division
p. proctotomy
p. radial approach
p. radicular artery
p. rectopexy
p. rectus sheath
p. rectus sheath wall
p. repair
p. rhizotomy
p. ring fracture
p. root
p. sclerotomy
p. screw fixation
p. scrotal vein
p. segmental fixation
p. shoulder approach
p. shoulder dislocation
p. side
p. spinal artery
p. spinal fusion
p. spinal wedge osteotomy
p. spinocerebellar tract
p. stomach
p. superior alveolar artery
p. superior iliac spine
superior labium anterior and p.
  (SLAP)
p. surface
p. synechia formation
p. temporal artery
p. thermal sclerostomy
p. thigh
p. tibialis tendon
p. tibial recurrent artery
p. tibiotalar
p. translation
p. transolecranon approach
p. transthoracic incision

NOTES

posterior *(continued)*
    p. truncal vagotomy
    p. ulnar recurrent artery
    p. upper cervical spine surgery
    p. urethra
    p. uveitis
    p. vaginal fornix
    p. vaginal hernia
    p. vaginal trunk
    p. vertical canal
    p. vitrectomy
    p. wall fracture
posterior-anterior pressure
posterior-interbody lumbar spinal fusion
posterioris
posterior-lateral
    p.-l. lobule
    p.-l. lumbar spinal fusion
posterior-superior oblique projection
posteroanterior projection
posteroinferior
    p. external
    p. external movement
posterolateral
    p. approach
    p. aspect
    p. bone graft placement
    p. bundle
    p. central artery
    p. costotransversectomy incision
    p. costotransversectomy technique
    p. herniation
    p. interbody fusion
    p. lumbosacral fusion
posteromedial
    p. approach
    p. central artery
    p. dislocation
posterosuperior segment
posteroventral pallidotomy
postesophageal
postevacuation
postexcision cavity
postextraction hemorrhage
postextubation
    p. croup
    p. laryngospasm
    p. stridor
postfixation radiography
postfracture lesion
postfundoplication syndrome
postganglionic
    p. parasympathetic fiber
    p. sympathetic fiber
postgastrectomy
    p. bleed
    p. cancer
    p. dysfunction

    p. hemorrhage
    p. syndrome
posthemorrhagic
posthepatic resection phase
postherniorrhaphy pain
postherpetic neuralgia
posthetomy
posthioplasty
posthitis
postholith
posthyoid
posthyperventilation apnea
posticus
postinfection lipoatrophy
postinflammatory hypopigmentation
postinjury
    p. immunologic defect
    p. level
postinsufflation
postintervention
postirradiation
    p. fracture
    p. study
    p. syndrome
postischemic
    p. administration
    p. stunned myocardium
postischial
postkeratoplasty
postlaminectomy
    p. kyphosis
    p. syndrome
postlaparoscopy meralgia paresthetica
postlumpectomy skin thickening
postlymphangiography abdomen
postmastectomy
postmastoid
postmedian
postmediastinal
postmediastinum
postmembrane
    p. pressure
    p. rupture
postmenopausal
    p. bleeding
    p. body mass
postmortem
    p. clot
    p. examination
    p. hypostasis
    p. suggillation
postnatal
    p. therapy
    p. torsion
postocular
postoperative
    p. abscess
    p. airway obstruction
    p. analgesia

p. analgesic
p. anastomotic leak
p. anesthesia
p. anisocoria
p. antibiotic
p. anticoagulation therapy
p. apnea
p. bleeding
p. cesarean section pain
p. choledochoscopy
p. cognitive dysfunction (POCD)
p. course
p. CT scan
p. day (POD)
p. death
p. deep venous thrombosis
   (PODVT)
p. diagnosis
p. dialysis
p. ductal dilation
p. dysphagia
p. ERCP
p. extubation
p. fatigue
p. followup evaluation
p. fracture
p. gastrointestinal tract dysfunction
   (PGID)
p. hemorrhage
p. hepatic failure
p. hernia
p. hour
p. hydrocele
p. hypocalcemia
p. ileus
p. immobilization
p. infection
p. irradiation
p. irrigation-suction
p. irrigation-suction drainage
p. liver failure
p. management
p. morbidity
p. mortality
p. motility
p. nausea and vomiting (PONV)
p. paraplegia
p. pelvic radiation
p. period
p. pleurobiliary fistula
p. pneumonia
p. recovery

p. regimen for oral early feeding
   (PROEF)
p. renal dysfunction
p. repair
p. respiratory complication
p. result
p. shivering
p. supplementation
p. survival
p. survival probability (PSP)
p. symptom
p. systemic chemotherapy
p. tetany
p. ventilation
postpartum
p. hemorrhage
p. infection
postpericardiotomy syndrome
postpharyngeal space
postphlebitic syndrome
postpneumonectomy tuberculous
   empyema
postpolypectomy
p. bleed
p. coagulation syndrome
p. hemorrhage
postprandial
p. AUC
p. distention
p. hour
p. motor activity
p. motor parameter
p. motor result
p. period
p. value
postprostatectomy incontinence
postpyloric sphincter
postradiation
p. change
p. fistula
p. kyphosis
p. plexopathy
p. therapy
postradical neck dissection
postreduction mammaplasty
postresection
p. defect
p. filling
p. filling technique
postresuscitation period
postreversal
postsacral

NOTES

postscapular
postsclerotherapy ulcer
postsensation
postshunt
postsphenoid bone
postsphincterotomy ERCP cannulation
postsplenectomy
    p. complication
    p. infection
    p. sepsis
postsplenic
poststenotic
    p. dilatation
    p. dilation
poststroke pain
post-subarachnoid hemorrhage
  hydrocephalus
postsulcal
postsurgical
    p. abdomen
    p. disturbance
    p. endoscopy
    p. motor anomaly
    p. motor change
    p. nervous damage
    p. truncal pain
postsynaptic membrane
posttecta
posttetanic
    p. count
    p. count monitoring
    p. facilitation
postthoracotomy
    p. change
    p. pain
posttranslation modification
posttransplant
    p. day
    p. immunosuppression therapy
    p. lymphoproliferative disease
    (PTLD)
    p. lymphoproliferative disorder
    (PTLD)
posttransverse
posttraumatic
    p. autotransplantation
    p. cervical dystonia
    p. chondrolysis
    p. gustatory neuralgia
    p. hemorrhage
    p. intradiploic pseudomeningocele
    p. pancreatic-cutaneous fistula
    p. persistent pneumothorax (PPP)
    p. renal failure
    p. seizure
    p. spinal deformity
    p. stress disorder (PTSD)
    p. subcapsular hepatic fluid
    collection

posttreatment hemorrhage
posttubal ligation syndrome
postural
    p. deformity
    p. drainage
    p. fixation back maneuver
    p. reduction
    p. resting position
    p. therapy
posture
    compensatory head p.
    forward head p.
    head p.
postureteral ligation
postureteroscopic manipulation
posturography
    platform p.
postuterine
postvagotomy
    p. dysphagia
    p. gastroparesis
    p. syndrome
postvalvar
postvasectomy
postvitrectomy fibrin
postzygomatic space
potassium space
potato tumor
potency
    anesthetic p.
    sphincteric p.
potential
    compound muscle action p.
    (CMAP)
    curative p.
    demarcation p.
    denervation p.
    electrode p.
    endogenous event-related p.
    excitatory junction p.
    excitatory postsynaptic p.
    extreme somatosensory evoked p.
    fasciculation p.
    fibrillation p.
    laser-evoked p.
    membrane p.
    middle latency auditory evoked p.
    (MLAEP)
    miniature end-plate p.
    modulation p.
    motor-evoked p. (MEP)
    myogenic motor-evoked p. (MEP)
    oxidation-reducing p.
    pacemaker p.
    peroneal somatosensory evoked p.
    reduction p.
    regeneration motor unit p.
    resting membrane p.

somatosensory evoked p. (SEP, SSEP)

standard electrode p.

standard reduction p.

potentially

    p. curative procedure

    p. lethal x-ray damage repair

    p. resectable lesion

potentiation

potentiometric titration

Pott

    P. aneurysm

    P. ankle fracture

    P. eversion osteotomy

    P. fracture

    P. gangrene

Potter

    P. classification

    P. facies

Potts

    P. anastomosis

    P. operation

    P. procedure

Potts-Smith anastomosis

pouch

    anal p.

    antibiotic bead p.

    arachnoid retrocerebellar p.

    bead p.

    p. biopsy

    bladder replacement urinary p.

    blind rectal p.

    blind upper esophageal p.

    Broca p.

    colonic p.

    coloplasty p.

    continent ileal p.

    continent urinary p.

    copulating p.

    deep perineal p.

    dermal p.

    p. development

    p. dilatation

    double-loop p.

    Douglas p.

    drainable ostomy p.

    endorectal ileal p.

    p. failure

    gastric p.

    Hartmann p.

    haustral p.

    heat-seal p.

hepatorenal p.

hernia p.

ileal neobladder urinary p.

p. ileitis

ileoanal p.

ileocecal p.

ileocolonic p.

inflamed synovial p.

intraluminal p.

intravaginal p.

inverted-U p.

jejunal p.

J-shaped ileal p.

J versus S versus W pelvic ileal p.

kangaroo p.

Koch p.

laryngeal p.

lateral-lateral p.

3-loop ileal p.

2-loop J-shaped ileal p.

Miami p.

Morison p.

Morrison p.

omental p.

open-end ostomy p.

paracystic p.

pararectal p.

paravesical p.

pelvic p.

pharyngeal p.

1-piece ostomy p.

2-piece ostomy p.

Prussak p.

p. reconstruction

rectal blind p.

rectouterine p.

rectovaginal p.

rectovaginouterine p.

rectovesical p.

renal p.

self-seal p.

sigmoid rectum p.

superficial perineal p.

suprapatellar p.

terminal ileal p.

triple loop p.

U p.

U-shaped jejunal p.

uterovesical p.

VBG p.

vertical banded gastroplasty p.

NOTES

P

pouch (*continued*)
    vesicouterine p.
    visceral p.
    W p.
    wallaby p.
    Willis p.
    Zenker p.
pouched ileostomy
pouchitis
pouchoscopy
    pelvic p.
Poulard operation
Poupart line
pour
    1-p. technique
    2-p. technique
powdered bone graft
power
    p. of attorney
    p. Doppler imaging
    P. operation
    p. point
    p. spectral analysis
Pozzi procedure
PPC
    positive peritoneal cytology
PPG
    pylorus-preserving gastrectomy
PPH
    primary pulmonary hypertension
PPI
    proton pump inhibitor
PPP
    posttraumatic persistent pneumothorax
PPPD
    pylorus-preserving
      pancreatoduodenectomy
PPS
    presurgical psychological screening
PPT
    pressure pain threshold
PPV
    positive predictive valve
    positive-pressure ventilation
PQOL
    perceived quality of life
practitioner
    alternative p.
Prague maneuver
Pratt
    P. open reduction
    P. technique
prayer position
PRBC
    packed red blood cells
preadaptation
preanal

preanesthetic
    p. medication
    p. skin-surface warming
preantiseptic
preaortic
preaseptic
preauricular
    p. cyst
    p. fistula
    p. fossa
    p. groove
    p. incision
    p. point
    p. sulcus
preauricularis
preaxial
preaxillary line
precancerous lesion
precapillary anastomosis
precatheterization
precaution
    full-stomach p.'s
    radiation p.'s
precentral
    p. cortical stimulation
    p. gyrectomy
    p. gyrus
    p. sulcal artery
prechiasmal
    p. compression
    p. optic nerve lesion
precipitate in solution
precipitating
    p. lesion
    p. noxious event
precise dissection
preclotted graft
precommissural bundle
preconditioning
    anesthetic p.
    ischemic p. (IPC)
    myocardial ischemic p.
    p. phenomenon
precordial wound
precordium, pl. **precordia**
precorneal
precostal
precuneal artery
precursor lesion
precut
    p. incision
    p. papillotomy
    p. sphincterotomy
predental space
**predialysis plasma phosphate
  concentration**
prediction
    breast cancer risk p.

Gail model of breast cancer
risk p.
predictive value
prediluted antibody panel
predisposing
p. condition
p. factor
predisposition
hereditary p.
predorsal bundle
preeclamptic liver disease
preemergence
preemptive
p. analgesia
p. anesthesia
preendoscopy
preepiglottic
p. soft tissue
p. space
preexcitation
p. syndrome
ventricular p.
preexisting lesion
prefabrication
prefrontal
p. leukotomy
p. lobotomy
preganglionic
p. cardiac sympathetic blockade
p. parasympathetic fiber
p. sympathectomy
p. sympathetic block
p. sympathetic denervation
p. sympathetic fiber
preglenoid plane
pregnancy
abdominal p.
p. complication
ectopic p.
p. luteoma
pregnancy-induced anesthesia
prehepatic resection phase
prehospital resuscitation
prehyoid gland
preincision
preincisional intravenous pentoxifylline
preincubation
preinduction phase
preinsufflation
preinterparietal bone
preintervention
preischemic administration

Preiser disease
prelabor membrane rupture
prelaryngeal node
prelimbic
preliminary iridectomy
preload
decreased p.
p. recruitable stroke work (PRSW)
p. reduction
premalignant
p. condition
p. lesion
premasseteric
p. space
p. space abscess
premature
p. airway closure
p. amnion rupture
p. ductus arteriosis closure
P. Infant Pain Profile (PIPP)
p. membrane rupture
p. separation
p. separation of placenta
premaxilla
premedicate
premedication
premembrane
p. pressure
p. rupture
premenopausal ovary
premicturition pressure
premolar teeth
premonitory palpitation
premorbid performance status
premuscular
p. mesh technique
p. position
p. prosthetic repair
prenatal
p. diethylstilbestrol exposure
p. dislocation
p. therapy
p. torsion
Prentiss
P. maneuver
P. orchiopexy
preoccipital notch
preoperative
p. analgesia
p. anesthetic
p. biopsy
p. chemoradiotherapy

NOTES

P

preoperative *(continued)*
    p. diagnosis
    p. dose
    p. ERCP
    p. evolution time
    p. factor
    p. fasting
    p. feature
    p. FNA specimen
    p. imaging
    p. induction chemotherapy
    p. investigation
    p. jaundice
    p. lesion
    p. liver function
    p. localization
    p. localization signal
    p. LSG
    p. lymphoscintigraphy
    p. percutaneous aspiration
    p. period
    p. pneumoperitoneum
    p. preparation
    p. retrograde cholangiogram
    p. scoring
    p. scoring system
    p. skin-surface warming
    p. staging
    p. staging evaluation
    p. study
    p. systemic chemotherapy
    p. therapy
    p. ultrasound
preoperatively donated autologous blood
preoxygenation
prepancreatic arch
prepapillary sphincter
preparation
    access p.
    bevel p.
    biomechanical p.
    bone-patellar tendon-bone p.
    bowel p.
    Brown dietary method for colon p.
    cavity p.
    chamfer p.
    colon p.
    corrosion p.
    crush p.
    p. and draping
    facet joint p.
    facial butt joint p.
    figure-of-8 p.
    fortified topical p.
    full shoulder p.
    galenic p.
    graft p.
    heart-lung p.
    impression p.

    incisal p.
    initial p.
    insulin p.
    intraoperative bowel p.
    Langendorff heart p.
    lavage bowel p.
    liposomal p.
    lupus erythematosus p.
    Matsura p.
    medicinal p.
    mouth p.
    pinworm p.
    preoperative p.
    renal proximal tubule p.
    rod contour p.
    shoulder with bevel p.
    skin p.
    slice p.
    slot p.
    slot-type p.
    Spälteholz p.
    step p.
    surgical p.
    unfiltered p.
    vertical versus horizontal p.
    wire contour p.
preparatory iridectomy
prepared
    p. cavity
    p. cavity impression
    p. large bowel
prepatellar
    p. bursa
    p. bursa inflammation
preperitoneal
    p. anesthesia
    p. approach
    p. fat
    p. space
    transabdominal p.
preplacental hemorrhage
prepontine
    p. cistern
    p. white epidermoidoma
prepped and draped
preprostate urethral sphincter
preprosthetic surgery
prepubic fascia
prepuce
preputial
    p. calculus
    p. continent vesicostomy
    p. gland
    p. sac
preputiotomy
prepyloric
    p. perforation
    p. sphincter
    p. vein

prepyramidal tract
prerecruitment
prerectal lithotomy
prerenal
preretinal
    p. hemorrhage
    p. membrane
    p. neovascularization
pre-rolandic artery
presacral
    p. anesthesia
    p. anomaly
    p. cystic lesion
    p. fascia
    p. insufflation
    p. mass
    p. nerve
    p. neurectomy
    p. rectopexy
    p. resection
    p. space
    p. sympathectomy
presaturation technique
presbyopia
presbyopic vision
prescreening
    opioid p.
presence
    arteriographic p.
presensitization phase
presentation
    acute p.
    chronic p.
    clinical p.
    p. of cord
    mammographic p.
presenting
    p. clinical manifestation
    p. symptom
preseptal space
preservation
    autonomic nerve p. (ANP)
    breast p.
    cadaver renal p.
    carotid p.
    extracorporeal renal p.
    extremity p.
    lordosis p.
    lumbar lordosis p.
    pelvic autonomic nerve p. (PANP)
    renal p.
    simple cold storage p.

    sphincter p.
    spleen p.
    p. technique
    p. time
    tissue p.
    visual p.
preservative solution
presigmoid-transtransversarium
  intradural approach
presphenoid bone
prespinal
presplenic fold
pressoreceptor
pressor medication
pressure
    abdominal p.
    acoustic p.
    airway p. (AP)
    p. alopecia
    alveolar carbon dioxide p.
    alveolar partial p.
    p. amaurosis
    p. amplitude modulation
    anal resting p.
    anal sphincter squeeze p.
    p. anesthesia
    aortic blood p.
    aortic dicrotic notch p.
    aortic pullback p.
    applanation p.
    p. area
    arterial blood p.
    arterial carbon dioxide p.
    arterial dicrotic notch p.
    arterial partial p.
    ascending aortic p.
    atmospheres of p.
    atrial filling p.
    p. atrophy
    average mean p.
    backward, upward, rightward p.
     (BURP)
    barometric p.
    basal anal canal p.
    basal anal sphincter p.
    bile duct p.
    bilevel positive airway p. (BiPAP)
    biliary tract p.
    BiPAP nasal continuous positive
     airway p.
    biting p.
    bladder p.

NOTES

P

pressure *(continued)*
    bleeding controlled with direct p.
    p. blister
    blood p.
    bone marrow p.
    capillary wedge p.
    carbon dioxide p.
    cardiovascular p.
    carotid artery stump p.
    central posterior-anterior p.
    central venous p. (CVP)
    cerebral perfusion p. (CPP)
    cerebrospinal fluid p. (CSFP)
    choledochal basal p.
    closing p.
    closure p.
    coaxial p.
    colloidal osmotic p.
    colloid osmotic p. (COP)
    compartmental p.
    compliance, rate, oxygenation, p.
      (CROP)
    p. condensation
    continuous distending airway p.
    continuous negative airway p.
    continuous positive airway p.
      (CPAP)
    p. control inverse ratio ventilation
      (PCIRV)
    p. control ventilation (PCV)
    p. conversion
    coronary perfusion p.
    coronary venous p.
    cricoid p.
    critical closing p.
    CSF p.
    detrusor p.
    diastolic blood p. (DBP)
    diastolic filling p.
    differential blood p.
    digital p.
    direct p.
    disc p.
    Donders p.
    downstream venous p.
    dynamic closure p.
    dynamic negative airway p.
      (DNAP)
    elastic recoil p.
    end-diastolic left ventricular p.
    end-expiratory intragastric p.
    end-systolic left ventricular p.
    p. epiphysis
    esophageal peristaltic p.
    esophageal sphincter p.
    expiratory positive airway p.
    external direct p.
    free hepatic venous p.
    p. gangrene

    gastric p.
    glomerular capillary p.
    p. gradient
    p. half-time technique
    high blood p.
    high-frequency positive p.
    high intraluminal p.
    hydrostatic p.
    hyperbaric p.
    increased p.
    p. increment rate
    inferior vena cava p. (IVCP)
    inspiratory occlusion p.
    inspiratory positive airway p.
    insufflation p.
    intermittent positive p. (IPP)
    interstitial p.
    intraabdominal p. (IAP)
    intraanal p.
    intracardiac p.
    intracholedochal p.
    intracranial p. (ICP)
    intradiscal p.
    intraductal p.
    intraesophageal peristaltic p.
    intraesophageal variceal p.
    intragastric p.
    intraglomerular p.
    intraluminal esophageal p.
    intraluminal urethral p.
    intramyocardial p.
    intraneural p.
    intraocular p.
    intraoral p.
    intrapericardial p.
    intraperitoneal p.
    intrapleural p.
    intrapulpal p.
    intrathoracic p.
    intraurethral p.
    intravariceal p.
    intravascular p.
    intravesical p.
    intrinsic end-expiratory p.
    intrinsic positive end-expiratory p.
      (PEEPi)
    invasive blood p. (IBP)
    p. inversion point
    IVC p.
    jugular venous p.
    juxtacardiac pleural p.
    labile blood p.
    leak point p.
    left atrial p. (LAP)
    left ventricular end-diastolic p.
    left ventricular systolic p.
    LES p.
    lower body negative p.
    lower esophageal sphincter p.

manual p.
maternal abdominal p.
maximum urethral closure p.
mean arterial p. (MAP)
mean arterial blood p. (MABP)
mean diastolic left ventricular p.
mean pulmonary artery wedge p.
mean systolic left ventricular p.
p. measurement
mercury p.
Michaelson counter p.
minimum audible p.
nadir p.
narrowed pulse p.
p. natriuresis
p. necrosis
negative p.
negative abdominal p.
negative end-expiratory p.
nitrogen partial p.
noninvasive blood p. (NIBP)
normal intravascular p.
occlusal p.
occlusion p.
oncotic p.
opening p.
osmotic p.
p. overload
oxygen under high p.
PA filling p.
p. pain threshold (PPT)
pancreatic duct p.
p. paralysis
partial p.
passage p.
peak inspiratory ventilator p.
peak systolic aortic p.
peak systolic gradient p.
perfusion p.
periapical p.
pericardial p.
peripheral p.
plantar p.
plasma colloid osmotic p.
plasma oncotic p.
p. pneumothorax
portal venous p.
positive airway p. (PAP)
positive end-expiratory p. (PEEP)
positive end-expiratory
 pressure/continuous positive p.
 (PEEP/CPAP)

positive expiratory p.
positive inspiratory p. (PIP)
posterior-anterior p.
postmembrane p.
premembrane p.
premicturition p.
proximal p.
pullback p.
pulmonary artery p. (PAP)
pulmonary artery occlusion p.
 (PAOP)
pulmonary artery occlusive
 wedge p.
pulmonary capillary wedge p.
pulmonary hypertension p.
pulmonary vascular p.
pulp p.
pulse p.
p. rate quotient
p. receptor
p. recovery
rectal resting p.
p. regulated electrohydraulic
 lithotripsy
p. relief valve
resting anal sphincter p.
p. reversal
right atrial p.
right ventricular end-diastolic p.
right ventricular systolic p.
p. ring
p. rise
screen filtration p.
selection p.
shock wave p.
sinusoidal capillary p.
p. sore
sphincter of Oddi p.
spinal cord perfusion p. (SCPP)
splanchnic capillary p.
squeeze p.
static closure p.
p. study
stump p.
subambient p.
subglottic p.
p. support ventilation (PSV)
systolic arterial p. (SAP)
systolic blood p. (SBP)
systolic left ventricular p.
p. technique filling
tentorial p.

NOTES

P

pressure *(continued)*
  time p.
  tissue p.
  p. tolerance
  tongue p.
  torr p.
  tourniquet p.
  transglomerular hydrostatic
    filtration p.
  transmembrane hydraulic p.
  p. transmission
  p. transmission ratio
  transmural p.
  transmyocardial perfusion p.
  ureteral p.
  urethral p.
  p. value
  vapor p.
  variable positive airway p.
  variceal p.
  vascular p.
  venous p.
  venous dialysis p. (VPd)
  ventilation peak p.
  ventricular diastolic p.
  ventricular filling p.
  p. wave
  p. waveform
  wedge p.
  wedged hepatic vein p. (WHVP)
  wedged hepatic venous p.
  p. welding
  white without p.
  zero end-expiratory p. (ZEEP)
  zero end-inspiratory p.
  z-point p.
pressure-controlled inverse ratio
  ventilation (PCIRV)
pressure-flow
  p.-f. electromyography study
  p.-f. plot
  p.-f. relation
  p.-f. relationship
pressure-natriuresis curve
pressure-point tension ring
pressure-regulated volume control
  ventilation
pressure-sensitive
  p.-s. area
  p.-s. tissue
pressure-supported ventilation (PSV)
pressure-tolerant tissue
pressure-volume
  p.-v. analysis
  p.-v. curve
  p.-v. index
  p.-v. relation
pressurized reservoir

prestenotic dilatation
presternal
  p. notch
  p. region
  p. space
presternum
presulcal
presumptive diagnosis
presurgical
  p. medical evaluation
  p. psychological screening (PPS)
  p. state
presynaptic
  p. membrane
  p. and postsynaptic nicotinic
    activation
presystolic pressure and volume
pretarsal space
pretecta
pretemporal space
prethyroid
pretracheal
  p. fascia
  p. layer
  p. node
  p. space
pretransplant evaluation
pretreatment
  p. evaluation
  p. level
pretympanic
prevention
  DVT p.
  extension for p.
  heterotopic ossification p.
  infection p.
  injury p.
  rod rotation p.
preventive
  p. intravesical therapy
  p. mastectomy
  p. measure
prevertebral
  p. fascia
  p. ganglion
  p. layer
  p. soft tissue
  p. space
  p. space abscess
prevesical fascia
prewarming
Preziosi operation
prezonular space
priapus
prick
  needle p.
  p. puncture test
prickle cell carcinoma

prick-test
    p.-t. concentration
    p.-t. method
Pridie incision
Pridie-Koutsogiannis procedure
primarily vascularized organ transplant
primarium
primary
    p. adenocarcinoma
    p. adhesion
    p. afferent depolarization
    p. amputation
    p. anesthetic
    p. antecubital jump bypass (PAJB)
    p. arteriovenous fistula
    p. bile duct carcinoma
    p. biliary cirrhosis
    p. cancer
    p. cesarean section
    p. closure
    colorectal p.
    p. diagnostic endoscopy
    p. endpoint
    p. end-to-end anastomosis
    p. fibrinolysis
    p. fungal infection
    p. gangrene
    p. gastric lymphoma (PGL)
    p. gastric lymphoma staging
    p. gastric non-Hodgkin lymphoma
    (PGL)
    p. graft nonfunction
    p. healing
    p. hemorrhage
    p. hepatic
    p. herpes simplex infection
    p. hyperparathyroidism
    p. indirect inguinal hernia
    p. inguinal herniorrhaphy
    p. intraosseous carcinoma
    p. lesion
    p. malignancy
    p. movement plane
    p. myofascial trigger point
    noncolorectal p.
    p. origin
    p. panendoscopy
    p. parathyroid hyperplastic tumor
    p. pathogen
    p. perineal hypospadias surgery
    p. position
    p. procedure

    p. proctocolectomy
    p. prophylaxis
    p. pulmonary hypertension (PPH)
    p. radiation
    p. rejection
    p. renal calculus
    p. repair
    p. resection
    p. rhabdomyosarcoma
    p. rotation movement
    p. sclerosing cholangitis
    p. shock
    p. sodium phosphate
    p. stenting
    p. surgeon
    p. suture technique
    p. tumor site
    p. union
    p. untreated HPT
    p. vascular incompetence
    p. yolk sac
primer
    Bowen cavity p.
    cavity p.
priming dose
primitive
    p. dislocation
    p. knot
    p. yolk sac
primordial cyst
primum
    ostium p.
primus
princeps, pl. **principes**
    p. cervicis artery
    p. pollicis artery
Princeteau tubercle
principal
    p. fiber bundle
    p. line
    p. plane
    p. point
    p. visual direction
principes (*pl. of* princeps)
principle
    anatomic fracture reduction p.
    axial compression p.
    clinical p.
    closure p.
    Fick p.
    Goodwin cup-patch p.
    image formation p.

NOTES

P

principle *(continued)*
    Le Chatelier p.
    line focus p.
    Mitrofanoff p.
    Pauli exclusion p.
    Venturi p.
Pringle
    P. maneuver
    P. vascular control
    P. vascular control method
    P. vascular control procedure
    P. vascular control technique
prior drug exposure
priority
    ICU care p.
prism
    p. adaptation test
    p. method
PRK
    photorefractive keratectomy
proactive hemostasis
probability
    bone cyst fracture p.
    postoperative survival p. (PSP)
proband
probe
    cryoablation p.
    monopolar radiofrequency p.
probing
    p. lacrimonasal duct operation
    robotic p.
probiotic bacteria
problem
    biliary p.
    clinical p.
    colon p.
    comorbid medical p.
    Coping with Health, Injuries,
      and P.'s (CHIP)
    cosmetic p.
    dermatologic p.
    functional p.
    gastrointestinal p.
    inflammatory p.
    innervation p.
    medical p.
    orthopaedic p.
    physical p.
    psychological p.
    rectal p.
    surgical p.
    wound p.
procallus formation
procedure
    Abbe-McIndoe p.
    Abbe-McIndoe-Williams p.
    Abbe-Wharton-McIndoe p.
    abdominal p.
    ablative p.

Adams p.
advancement p.
aesthetic p.
Akin p.
Akiyama p.
Aldridge sling p.
Al-Ghorab p.
Allison p.
anchovy p.
Anderson p.
Anderson-Fowler p.
anecdotal p.
antegrade continence enema p.
antenna p.
anterior Pólya p.
anterior stabilization p.
antiincontinence p.
antireflux p.
AO p.
arterial reconstructive p.
arterial switch p.
articulatory p.
Axer-Clark p.
Badgley combination p.
Baldy-Webster p.
balloon fenestration p.
Bandi p.
Bankart p.
Barsky p.
Bartlett p.
Bassini p.
Batista p.
Baxter-D'Astous p.
Bell-Tawse p.
Belsey fundoplication p.
Bentall p.
Berman-Gartland p.
Bernard lip reconstruction p.
B.H. Moore p.
Bickel-Moe p.
bilateral inguinal hernia repair p.
Bilhaut-Cloquet p.
Billroth I, II p.
Bing-Taussig heart p.
Björk method of Fontan p.
bladder chimney p.
Blair-Brown p.
Blalock-Hanlon p.
Blalock-Taussig p.
Blatt p.
Blatt-Ashworth p.
blocking p.
Boari bladder flap p.
bone block p.
bony p.
Bose p.
bowel refashioning p.
Boyce-Vest p.
Boyd-Bosworth p.

Boyd-McLeod p.
Boytchev p.
Brahms p.
Brantigan p.
Brantigan-Voshell p.
Braun p.
breast-conserving p.
Bricker p.
Bridle p.
Bristow-Helfet p.
Bristow-May p.
Brock p.
bronchial sleeve p.
Broström p.
Broström-Gould foot p.
Bryan p.
Bunnell-Williams p.
Burch bladder suspension p.
burn-out p.
Butler p.
bypass p.
Calandriello p.
Caldwell-Luc window p.
Camey p.
Campbell-Akbarnia p.
Campbell-Goldthwait p.
canalith repositioning p.
capsular shift p.
Carolinas Laparoscopic Advanced
  Surgery Program p.
carotid ablative p.
Castaneda p.
Castle p.
cataract p.
catheter-directed interventional p.
Cawthorne-Day p.
cecal imbrication p.
Cecil p.
Celestin p.
cervical spine stabilization p.
Chamberlain p.
Chambers p.
Charles p.
Chassar Moir-Sims p.
Chassar Moir sling p.
Cherry-Crandall p.
cherry-picking p.
Chester-Winter p.
Chrisman-Snook p.
Cibis liquid silicone p.
ciliary p.
circulatory arrest p.

CLASP p.
Clayton p.
Cleveland p.
Cloward p.
Cockett p.
Cohen antireflux p.
Cole intubation p.
Collis gastroplasty p.
Collis-Nissen esophageal
  lengthening p.
Collis-Nissen fundoplication p.
colon p.
coloplasty p.
commando p.
compartment p.
composite pelvic resection p.
concentration p.
Connolly p.
conventional p.
core drilling p.
coronary artery revascularization p.
coronary bypass p.
corporeal rotation p.
corridor p.
Cox Maze III p.
Cracchiolo p.
curative p.
curative-intent p.
Custodis nondraining p.
cyclodestructive p.
cyclops p.
Damian graft p.
Damus-Kaye-Stansel p.
Damus-Stansel-Kaye p.
Danus-Fontan p.
Darrach p.
dartos pouch p.
Das Gupta p.
Davis-Kitlowski p.
Davydov p.
DAWG p.
de-airing p.
debubbling p.
debulking p.
degloving p.
Delorme p.
dental prosthetic laboratory p.
Dewar posterior cervical fixation p.
diagnostic p.
Dickson-Diveley p.
DKS p.
Dohlman p.

NOTES

P

procedure *(continued)*
    domino p.
    Donald p.
    Donders p.
    Dor fundoplication p.
    Dorrance p.
    dorsal root entry zone p.
    dot-blot p.
    double-stapled ileoanal reservoir p.
    Douglas p.
    Downey-McGlamery p.
    DREZ p.
    Duckett p.
    Duhamel p.
    Dukes p.
    Duval p.
    Dwyer p.
    Ebbehoj p.
    Eden-Hybbinette p.
    Eden-Lange p.
    Edwards p.
    Effler-Groves mode of Allison p.
    elective surgical p.
    elimination p.
    Elmslie p.
    Elmslie-Trillat patellar p.
    emergency p.
    endolacrimal p.
    endorectal ileoanal pull-through p.
    endoscopic mucosal resection p.
    endoscopy p.
    end-to-end reconstruction p.
    enucleation p.
    esophageal sling p.
    Estes p.
    evacuation p.
    Evans p.
    Evans-Steptoe p.
    Everard Williams p.
    excisional biopsy p.
    EXIT p.
    ex situ-in vivo p.
    extended Ross p.
    extraanatomic bypass p.
    extraarticular p.
    extracorporeal p.
    ex utero intrapartum treatment p.
    Faden p.
    failed p.
    Fairbanks-Sever p.
    Fasanella-Servat p.
    fascial sling p.
    fiberoptic intubation p.
    Ficat p.
    filling p.
    filtering p.
    Fired-Hendel p.
    flip-flap p.
    floppy Nissen fundoplication p.

Fontan-Baudet p.
Fontan-Kreutzer p.
Fontan modification of Norwood p.
forage p.
Fowler-Stephens p.
Fox-Blazina p.
Frank p.
Fredet-Ramstedt p.
Fried-Green foot p.
Froimson p.
frontalis sling p.
Frost p.
Fulford p.
Furlow p.
Gallie p.
Gartland p.
gaseous laparoscopy p.
gasless laparoscopy p.
gastric bypass p. (GBP)
gastric emptying p. (GEP)
gastric partitioning p.
gastric pull-through p.
gastric pull-up p.
gastric valve tightening p.
Gelman p.
general laparoscopic surgical p.
Gilchrist p.
Gill p.
Gill-Jonas modification of
  Norwood p.
Gillquist p.
Gil-Vernet p.
Girard p.
Girdlestone hip p.
Girdlestone-Taylor p.
Gittes p.
Gittes-Loughlin p.
Glenn p.
Goebel p.
Goebel-Stoeckel-Frangenheim p.
Goldner-Hayes p.
Goldthwait-Hauser p.
Gould p.
Goulding p.
gracilis p.
Green p.
Gregoir-Lich p.
Gurd p.
Halban p.
hallux valgus p.
Hammon p.
hamular p.
Hancock p.
Hanley rectal bladder p.
Harada-Ito p.
Hark p.
Harmon p.
Hartmann p.
Hass p.

Haultain p.
Hauser patellar tendon p.
Hawkins p.
Hedley p.
Heifetz p.
hemi-Fontan p.
hemi-Koch p.
heparinization p.
Hepp-Couinaud biliary tract p.
hex p.
Heyman-Herndon clubfoot p.
Hibbs p.
Hill p.
Hinman p.
Hoffmann-Clayton p.
Hofmeister p.
Hohmann p.
Hoke p.
Hoke-Miller p.
Hood p.
Horton-Devine p.
Howorth p.
Howorth-Keillor p.
Hughston p.
Hughston-Hauser p.
Hui-Linscheid p.
Hummelsheim p.
Huntington p.
hypoglossal facial transfer p.
ileoanal pouch p.
ileoanal pull-through p.
iliac buttressing p.
4-incision p.
5-incision p.
infrarenal template p.
Ingelman-Sundberg gracilis
  muscle p.
initial screening p.
inner ear tack p.
Insall p.
in situ p.
installation p.
intercalary allograft p.
interventional p.
intestinal bypass p.
intraarticular p.
intraoperative p.
intraparavariceal p.
intraperitoneal p.
invasive p.
island-flap p.
isolated p.

Ito p.
Jacobaeus p.
Jaeger-Hamby p.
Jaffe p.
Jahss p.
Jannetta microvascular
  decompression p.
Jansey p.
Jatene arterial switch p.
jejunoileal bypass reversal p.
Jensen transposition p.
Jobe-Glousman capsular shift p.
Johnson p.
Johnson-Spiegl p.
Johnston buttonhole p.
Jonas modification of Norwood p.
Jones tube p.
J. R. Moore p.
Junod p.
Juvara p.
Kaliscinski ureteral p.
Karakousis-Vezeridis p.
Karhunen-Loeve p.
Karlsson p.
Kasai p.
Kawaii-Yamamoto p.
Kelikian p.
Kelikian-McFarland p.
Keller p.
Kelling-Madlener p.
Kelly plication p.
Kendrick p.
Kennedy p.
Kessel-Bonney p.
Kestenbaum p.
keyhole coronary bypass p.
Kidner foot p.
Kiehn-Earle-DesPrez p.
Killian frontoethmoidectomy p.
Knapp p.
Knobby-Clark p.
Ko-Airan bleeding control p.
Kocher ureterosigmoidostomy p.
Koch pouch modified p.
Kolmogorov-Smirnov p.
Kondoleon-Sistrunk elephantiasis p.
Konno p.
Koutsogiannis p.
Kraske p.
Krönlein p.
Kropp p.

NOTES

P

601

procedure *(continued)*

Krukenberg p.
Kuhnt-Szymanowski p.
Ladd p.
Lane p.
Langenskiöld p.
Langevin updating p.
laparoscopically assisted endorectal
  pull-through p.
laparoscopic-assisted p.
laparoscopic bladder neck suture
  suspension p.
laparoscopic Burch p.
laparoscopic bypass p.
laparoscopic lymph node
  dissection p.
laparoscopic Nissen
  fundoplication p.
laparoscopic paraaortic lymph node
  sampling p.
laparoscopic surgical p.
laparoscopic tubal banding p.
Larmon forefoot p.
laser coagulation vaporization p.
  (LCVP)
Lash p.
LAST coronary bypass p.
Latarget p.
lateral tarsal strip p.
lathing p.
latissimus dorsi p.
Lauenstein p.
Leadbetter p.
Leadbetter-Politano p.
Lee p.
Le Fort p.
left atrial isolation p.
Lepird p.
L'Episcopo-Zachary p.
Lewis-Tanner p.
Lich p.
lid-splitting p.
limb-lengthening p.
limb-salvage p.
limb-saving p.
limb-sparing p.
Lindeman p.
Linton p.
Lipscomb p.
Lipscomb-Anderson p.
loop electrocautery excision p.
  (LEEP)
loop electrosurgical excision p.
  (LEEP)
loop gastric bypass p.
Lorenz p.
Lothrop frontoethmoidectomy p.
lower cervical spine p.
lower lid sling p.

Luke p.
LVR p.
Lynch frontoethmoidectomy p.
Lyon-Horgan p.
MacAusland p.
MacCarthy p.
Magenstrasse and Mill p.
Magnuson-Stack p.
Mahan p.
malabsorptive p.
Mallory-Weiss p.
Malone ACE p.
Malone antegrade continence
  enema p.
Manktelow transfer p.
Mann p.
Mann-Coughlin p.
Maquet p.
Marshall-Marchetti p.
Marshall-Marchetti-Krantz p.
Martius p.
Mathieu p.
Mauck p.
Maydl p.
Mayo-Fueth inversion p.
Maze III p.
McBride p.
McCall-Schumann p.
McCarroll-Baker p.
McCormick-Blount p.
McDonald p.
McElvenny-Caldwell p.
McGlamry-Downey p.
McIndoe p.
McIndoe-Hayes p.
McLaughlin p.
McVay p.
medial rotation p.
Meigs-Okabayashi p.
Michal I, II p.
microoperative p.
microsurgery p.
microsurgical epididymal sperm
  aspiration p.
Miller p.
minimal access p.
minimally invasive p.
Minkoff-Nicholas p.
Mitrofanoff p.
M&M p.
MMK p.
Moberg key-pinch p.
modified Belsey fundoplication p.
modified Hoke-Miller flatfoot p.
modified Konno p.
modified Norfolk p.
modified Seldinger p.
modified Sugiura p.
modified Toupe p.

modified Weber-Fergusson p.
modified Wies p.
Mogensen p.
Moschcowitz p.
motion-preserving p.
multiple-port incision p.
Mumford p.
muscle-balancing p.
Mustard intraatrial p.
needle suspension p.
needle thoracentesis p.
Neer capsular shift p.
Nesbit tuck p.
Neugebauer-LeFort p.
neurostimulating p.
neurosurgical p.
Newman p.
Nichols p.
Nicks p.
Nicola shoulder p.
Nicoll fracture repair p.
Nissen fundoplication p.
Nissen-Rossetti fundoplication p.
noncircumferential antireflux p.
nonfenestrated Fontan p.
noninvasive p.
non-rib-spreading thoracotomy
   incision p.
Norfolk p.
Norwood univentricular heart p.
notchplasty p.
O'Brien capsular shift p.
O'Donoghue p.
Olshausen p.
omentum majus flap p.
open reconstructive p.
operant p.
operative p.
orthodontic p.
orthodox p.
orthopaedic surgical p.
Orticochea p.
Osborne-Cotterill p.
osteoplastic frontal sinus p.
otic periotic shunt p.
Oudard p.
Overholt p.
palatal lengthening p.
palliative cerebrospinal shunt p.
palliative surgical p.
Palomo p.
Parrish p.

Paterson p.
Pauchet p.
pediatric laparoscopic surgical p.
pelvic pouch p.
Pena p.
percutaneous transhepatic biliary p.
Pereyra p.
peri-vaterian therapeutic
   endoscopic p.
Perthes p.
Pichlmayer p.
PLIF p.
Pólya p.
4-port p.
portmanteau p.
posterior Pólya p.
potentially curative p.
Potts p.
Pozzi p.
Pridie-Koutsogiannis p.
primary p.
Pringle vascular control p.
psoas hitch p.
Puestow-Gillesby p.
pull-through p.
push-back p.
Putti-Platt shoulder p.
Quaegebeur p.
QUART p.
Quickert p.
Ramstedt p.
Ransley p.
Rastan-Konno p.
Rastelli p.
Raz p.
Raz-Leach p.
realignment p.
Récamier p.
reconstruction p.
reconstructive surgical p.
reefing p.
Rehbein p.
Reichel-Pólya p.
Reichenheim-King p.
repeat p.
restorative p.
resurfacing p.
retrogasserian p.
revascularization p.
reverse filling p.
reverse Mauck p.
reverse Putti-Platt p.

NOTES

P

procedure *(continued)*
    revision p.
    Richardson p.
    Richter and Albrich p.
    Ridlon p.
    Riedel frontoethmoidectomy p.
    Righini p.
    Ripstein p.
    Rockwood p.
    Rockwood-Matsen capsular shift p.
    Rose p.
    Ross p.
    Roux-en-Y p.
    Roux-Goldthwait p.
    Ruiz p.
    Ruiz-Mora p.
    Ryerson p.
    sacroiliac buttressing p.
    Sade modification of Norwood p.
    Salle p.
    salting-out p.
    salvage p.
    Samilson p.
    sartorial slide p.
    Sato p.
    Sauve-Kapandji p.
    Savin p.
    Sayoc p.
    Schauffler p.
    Schenk-Eichelter vena cava plastic
      filter p.
    Schoemaker p.
    Schonander p.
    Schrock p.
    scleral buckling p.
    Scopinaro p.
    screening p.
    Scudder p.
    Scuderi p.
    secondary p.
    segment-oriented p.
    Selakovich p.
    Seldinger p.
    semitendinosus p.
    Senning transposition p.
    septation p.
    Shauta-Aumreich p.
    Shea p.
    Shirodkar p.
    short lever specific contact p.
    Silfverskiöld p.
    Silver p.
    Simplate p.
    simultaneous pancreas and kidney
      transplant p.
    single-stage p.
    Sistrunk p.
    sling p.
    Smith-Robinson p.

Snow p.
Somerville p.
Sondergaard p.
Southwick slide p.
spatial localization p.
Spence p.
sphincter-saving p.
sphincter-sparing p.
spinal-locking p.
Spira p.
Spittler p.
SPLATT p.
split anterior tibial tendon p.
Stack shoulder p.
2-stage p.
3-stage p.
Staheli shelf p.
Stamey-Martius p.
Stamey modification of Pereyra p.
Stamm p.
standard gastric resection
  Whipple p.
standard stripping p.
standard surgical p.
Stanley Way p.
Stansel p.
stapled reconstruction p.
Steindler p.
2-step p.
stereotactic needle core biopsy p.
Stone p.
Stoppa p.
Strayer p.
Stretta p.
strip p.
Studer pouch p.
suburethral rectus fascial sling p.
Sugiura p.
supplementary sling p.
supramesocolic surgical p.
surgical enucleation p.
Swenson pull-through p.
switch p.
Syme p.
Tachdjian p.
takedown p.
tarsal strip p.
Taylor p.
terminal Syme p.
Thal fundoplication p.
thermal-assisted capsular shift p.
Thiersch p.
Thiersch-Duplay proximal tube p.
ThinPrep p.
Thomas p.
Thompson p.
Tikhoff-Linberg p.
p. time
TIPS p.

total fundoplication p.
Toti p.
touch-up p.
Toupe p.
Toupet p.
TRAM flap p.
transendoscopic p.
transhepatic antegrade biliary
 drainage p.
transvaginal Burch p.
transverse rectus abdominis muscle
 flap p.
Trillat p.
triple-wire p.
Tsai-Stillwell p.
tuck p.
tumbling p.
Turco p.
uncinate p.
uncut Collis-Nissen
 fundoplication p.
unilateral inguinal hernia repair p.
untethering p.
up-and-down staircases p.
UPLIFT p.
upper cervical spine p.
ureteral patch p.
urethral vesicle suspension p.
urologic laparoscopic surgical p.
vaginal needle suspension p.
vaginal wall sling p.
valvulotomy p.
Van de Kramer fecal fat p.
Van Ness p.
vascular p.
VATS p.
ventriculoperitoneal shunting p.
video-assisted thoracic surgical p.
Vineberg p.
Vulpius p.
Vulpius-Stoffel p.
V-Y p.
W p.
Waldhausen p.
Wardill-Kilner p.
Waterhouse transpubic p.
Waterston-Cooley p.
Watson-Cheyne-Burghard p.
Watson-Jones p.
Weaver-Dunn p.
Weber p.
Weber-Fergusson p.

Wheeler p.
Whipple p.
White slide p.
Whitman talectomy p.
Whitman-Thompson p.
Wies p.
Williams p.
Wilson p.
Winograd p.
Winter p.
Womack p.
Woodward p.
yoke transposition p.
York-Mason p.
Young p.
Young-Dees p.
Yount p.
Z p.
Zancolli-Lasso p.
Zancolli static lock p.
Zarins-Rowe p.
Zoellner-Clancy p.
Z-plasty p.

procephalic
procerus muscle
process
 accessory p.
 acromial p.
 alveolar p.
 anterior clinoid p.
 articular p.
 basilar p.
 benign p.
 calcaneal p.
 caudate p.
 ciliary p.
 Civinini p.
 clinoid p.
 cochleariform p.
 condylar p.
 condyloid p.
 conoid p.
 coracoid p.
 corniculate p.
 coronoid p.
 costal p.
 ensiform p.
 epileptogenic p.
 exocrinopathic p.
 falciform p.
 frontosphenoidal p.
 funicular p.

NOTES

process *(continued)*
    healing p.
    inferior articular p.
    intrajugular p.
    jugular p.
    lateral p.
    lenticular p.
    malignant p.
    mallear p.
    mamillary p.
    medial p.
    mental p.
    olecranon p.
    papillary p.
    paroccipital p.
    posterior clinoid p.
    pterygoid p.
    pterygospinous p.
    resuscitation p.
    space-occupying p.
    sphenoid p.
    spinous p.
    Stieda p.
    supracondylar p.
    supraepicondylar p.
    temporal p.
    thrombotic p.
    transverse p.
    trochlear p.
    vaginal p.
    vermiform p.
    vocal p.
    xiphoid p.
processus
procheilon
prochordal
Prochownik method
procidentia
procoagulant
procreate
procreation
    assisted medical p.
procreative
proctalgia fugax
proctectasia
proctectomy
    abdominoperineal p.
    intersphincteric p.
    Kraske transsacral p.
    laparoscopic p.
    mucosal p.
    partial p.
    perineal p.
    permanent p.
    proctomucosal p.
    radical p.
    restorative p.
    sphincter-preserving p.

    stapled ileal pouch-anal anastomosis
      without proctomucosal p.
    subtotal p.
    total p.
    transsacral p.
procteurynter
proctitis
    radiation p.
    radiation-induced p.
proctocele
proctoclysis
proctococcypexy
proctocolectomy
    abdominal p.
    laparoscopic total p.
    primary p.
    restorative p.
    secondary stage p.
    single-stage total p.
    subtotal p.
    total p.
    totally stapled restorative p.
proctocolitis
    radiation p.
proctocolonoscopy
proctocolpoplasty
proctocystocele
proctocystoplasty
proctocystotomy
proctodynia
proctoelytroplasty
proctography
proctologic
proctologist
proctology
proctomucosal proctectomy
proctoperineoplasty
proctoperineorrhaphy
proctopexy
    Orr-Loygue transabdominal p.
    transabdominal p.
proctoplasty
proctoptosia
proctorrhagia
proctorrhaphy
proctorrhea
proctoscopic examination
proctoscopy
    rigid p.
proctosigmoidectomy
proctosigmoidoscopy
    rigid p.
proctospasm
proctostasis
proctostat
proctostenosis
proctostomy
proctotomy
    posterior p.

proctotresia
proctovalvotomy
procumbent
procurement
    in situ split-liver p.
procurvation
product
    altered gene p.
    blood p.
    contact activation p.
    degradation p.
    fibrin degradation p.
    fibrinogen degradation p.
    fibrinogen-fibrin degradation p.
    lipid peroxidation p.
    live donor liver transplantation
      without blood p.'s
    oxygen reduction p.
    pyrolysis p.
    rate pressure p.
    tumor-cell p.
    vector p.
production
    biofilm p.
    collagen p.
    ectopic parathormone p.
    excessive heat p.
    metabolic heat p.
    paraneoplastic ectopic ACTH p.
productive inflammation
PROEF
    postoperative regimen for oral early
      feeding
Proetz
    P. displacement technique
    P. maneuver
    P. position
profile
    aortic valve velocity p.
    coagulation p.
    extraoral radiographic
      examination p.
    facial p.
    pain perception p.
    Premature Infant Pain P. (PIPP)
    projection p.
    resting urethral pressure p.
    sickness impact p.
    stress urethral pressure p.
    thrombogenic p.
    urethral closure pressure p.
    vector p.

profound hypothermia
profoundly hypothermic circulatory
  arrest (PHCA)
profunda
    p. brachii artery
    p. cervicalis artery
    colitis cystica p.
progenitalis
progestational
    p. protection
    p. therapy
prognosis, pl. prognoses
prognostic
    p. block
    p. determinant
    p. factor
    p. finding
    p. indicator
    p. information
    p. marker
    p. nomogram
    p. value
prognosticator
progonoma
prograde technique
program
    aquatic stabilization p.
    back-propagation neural network p.
    Cancer Surveillance P.
    Carolinas Laparoscopic Advanced
      Surgery P. (CLASP)
    conditioning p.
    diagnostic p.
    independent exercise p.
    Linde Walker Oxygen P.
    Muma Assessment P.
    National Marrow Donor P.
    object p.
    Organ Procurement P.
    Rothman Institute total hip p.
    safety p.
    SEER P.
    Solid Tumor Autologous Marrow
      Transplant P. (STAMP)
    source p.
    standard bone algorithm p.
    4-star exercise p.
    Starkey matrix p.
    stripping p.
    Surgical Education and Self-
      Assessment P. (SESAP)
    surveillance p.

NOTES

P

program *(continued)*
    survey p.
    walking p.
    Westcott Pyramid P.
    work hardening p.
programmed
    p. electrical stimulation
    p. therapy
progression
    tumor p.
progressive
    p. abdominal distention
    P. Ambulation Scale
    p. ascites
    p. bacterial synergistic gangrene
    p. compression
    p. dilation
    p. disease
    p. encephalopathy
    p. extraction
    p. liver failure
    p. parenchymal destruction
    p. respiratory failure
    p. spin saturation
proinflammatory mediator
project
    Breast Cancer Detection
      Demonstration P.
    National Surgical Adjuvant Breast
      and Bowel P. (NSABP)
projection
    afferent p.
    anterior oblique p.
    anteroposterior p.
    A&P p.
    apical lordotic p.
    ascending pathway of pain p.
    axial calcaneal p.
    axial sesamoid p.
    back p.
    base p.
    bony p.
    bregma-mentum p.
    bursal p.
    Caldwell p.
    convergence p.
    coronal oblique p.
    cross-sectional p.
    cross-table lateral p.
    Didiee p.
    divergent ray p.
    dorsoplantar p.
    enamel p.
    erroneous p.
    extradental p.
    false p.
    fan beam p.
    p. fiber
    p. fiber damage

    filtered-back p.
    Fischer p.
    frogleg lateral p.
    frontal p.
    Granger p.
    half-axial p.
    Harris-Beath p.
    Hermodsson tangential p.
    horizontal p.
    lateral jaw p.
    left anterior oblique p.
    left lateral p.
    light p.
    maximum-intensity p.
    mental p.
    Mercator p.
    oblique p.
    occipitomental p.
    occlusal p.
    orthogonal p.
    PA p.
    pain p.
    panoramic surface p.
    papillary p.
    parasympathetic p.
    perimeter p.
    posterior-superior oblique p.
    posteroanterior p.
    p. profile
    reverse topographic p.
    Rhese p.
    Rungstrom p.
    sagittal p.
    Schüller p.
    spider p.
    Stenvers p.
    stress dorsiflexion p.
    submental vertex p.
    submentovertical p.
    surface p.
    sympathetic p.
    tangential p.
    topographic p.
    Towne p.
    p. tract imaging
    transmandibular p.
    transorbital p.
    transverse p.
    visual p.
    Waters p.
projection-reconstruction
    p.-r. imaging
    p.-r. technique
projective technique
prolabial
prolabium
prolactin inducible protein (PIP)
prolapse
    Altemeier repair of rectal p.

anorectal mucosal p.
rectal p.
stomal p.
prolapsed
    p. hemorrhoid
    p. mitral valve syndrome
    p. stoma
proliferating cell nuclear antigen (PCNA)
proliferation
    p. area
    ductal p.
    fibroblast p.
    follicular p.
    p. zone
proliferative
    p. factor
    p. inflammation
    p. lesion
prolongation
    expiratory p.
    P2 p.
    pulse repetition time p.
prolonged
    p. expiratory phase
    p. postoperative ventilation
    p. prothrombin time
    p. rupture
prominence
    hypothenar p.
    laryngeal p.
    mallear p.
    osteochondral p.
    pedicle screw hardware p.
    styloid p.
    thenar p.
prominens
prominentia, pl. **prominentiae**
prominent indentation
promontory
    pelvic p.
    sacral p.
    p. stimulation test
promoter
    tumor p.
pronate
pronation
    p. control
    p. injury
pronation-abduction
    p.-a. fracture
    p.-a. injury

pronation-eversion
    p.-e. fracture
    p.-e. injury
pronation-eversion-external
    p.-e.-e. rotation
    p.-e.-e. rotation injury
pronation-supination
pronator
    p. quadratus muscle
    p. reflex
    p. teres muscle
    p. teres release
    p. teres syndrome
    p. teres tendon
prone
    p. extension test
    p. reduction
    p. split-leg position
pronephric duct
pronephros
pronglike excementosis
pronograde
pronuclear stage transfer (PROST)
prootic
prop
    rubber mouth p.
propagate
propagating clustered contraction (PCC)
propagation
    clot p.
propagative
proper
    p. hepatic artery
    p. palmar digital artery
    p. plantar digital artery
properitoneal
    p. fat
    p. fat line
    p. flank stripe
    p. inguinal hernia
    p. space
    transabdominal p. (TAPP)
property
    chemotactic p.
    vasodilatory p.
prophylactic
    p. angiographic intervention
    p. antibiotic (PA)
    p. antibiotic therapy
    p. anticoagulation
    p. antiemetic
    p. antifungal treatment

NOTES

P

prophylactic (*continued*)
    p. bone graft
    p. cholecystectomy
    p. colectomy
    p. epidural blood patch
    p. fasciotomy
    p. gastroenterostomy
    p. gastrojejunostomy
    p. intravenous antibiotic
    p. intubation
    p. irradiation
    p. lymphadenectomy
    p. mastectomy
    p. medication
    p. membrane
    p. odontotomy
    p. oophorectomy
    p. operative stabilization
    p. orchiectomy
    p. resection
    p. skeletal fixation
    p. surgery
    p. thyroidectomy
prophylaxis, pl. **prophylaxes**
    acustimulation antiemetic p.
    antibiotic p.
    antiemetic p.
    antifungal p.
    antithromboembolic p.
    aspiration p.
    CMV p.
    cytomegalovirus p.
    deep venous thrombosis p.
    DVT p.
    perioperative antibiotic p.
    primary p.
    stricture p.
propofol
    p. infusion
    p. rescue
proportional
    p. assist ventilation
    p. assist ventilator (PAV)
propria, pl. **propriae**
proprioceptive
    p. head-turning reflex
    p. neuromuscular facilitation
    p. neuromuscular facilitation
      approach
proptosis
prosection
prosector tubercle
prosopalgia
prospective study
prospermia
PROST
    pronuclear stage transfer
      laparoscopic PROST
prostacyclin

prostaglandin
    renal vasodilator p.
prostanoid
prostata
prostatalgia
prostate
    p. cancer
    contact laser ablation of p.
      (CLAP)
    female p.
    p. gland
    transurethral resection of p.
      (TURP)
    transurethral resection of p.
      (TURP)
    transurethral vaporization of p.
      (TUVP)
    visual laser ablation of p.
prostatectomy
    anatomical radical retropubic p.
    cavernous nerve-sparing p.
    laparoscopic radical p.
    Madigan p.
    nerve-sparing radical retropubic p.
    perineal p.
    radical perineal p.
    radical retropubic p.
    radical transcoccygeal p.
    salvage p.
    Stanford radical retropubic p.
    suprapubic p.
    total perineal p.
    transurethral ablative p.
    transurethral ultrasound-guided laser-
      induced p. (TULIP)
    visual laser-assisted p.
    Walsh radical retropubic p.
prostatic
    p. adenocarcinoma
    p. adenoma
    p. calculus
    p. carcinoma
    p. duct
    p. ductule
    p. fluid
    p. ligament
    p. massage
    p. sheath
    p. sinus
    p. urethra
    p. urethroplasty
    p. utricle
    p. venous plexus
prostaticovesicalis
prostaticovesical plexus
prostatism
prostatitis
prostatocystitis
prostatocystotomy

prostatodynia
prostatolith
prostatolithotomy
prostatomegaly
prostatomy
prostatorrhea
prostatoseminal vesiculectomy
prostatotomy
prostatovesiculectomy
prostatovesiculitis
prosthesis, pl. **prostheses**
    femoral p.
    p. interface
    ossicular p.
prosthesis-cement interface
prosthesis-patient mismatch
prosthetic
    p. arterial graft
    p. arthroplasty
    p. hemiarthroplasty
    p. incisional hernioplasty
    p. mesh repair
    p. patch
    p. restoration
    p. ring anuloplasty
    p. valve endocarditis (PVE)
prosthetist
prosthokeratoplasty
protamine correction
protection
    airway p.
    automated boundary p.
    barrier p.
    Baxter venous/arterial
      management p.
    cerebral p.
    digital artery p.
    endogenous p.
    gastroduodenal mucosal p.
    myocardial p.
    progestational p.
    radiation p.
    spinal cord p.
    p. test
    venous/arterial management p.
    (VAMP)
protective
    p. antireflux operation
    p. ventilatory strategy
protein
    p. C deficiency
    p. content

    p. C, S plasma level
    p. degradation
    heparin-binding p.
    plasma atrial natriuretic p.
    prolactin inducible p. (PIP)
    p. shock therapy
    p. truncation
    p. truncation test
    tumor necrosis factor-binding p.
    (TNF-bp)
proteinaceous aqueous exudation
proteinase
proteinuria
    steroid-resistant p.
proteolysis
    burn-induced muscle p.
    muscle p.
    sepsis-induced muscle p.
proteolytic pathway
prothrombin
    p. time
    p. time coagulation panel
prothrombogenic agent
protocol
    chemotherapy p.
    evaluation p.
    exsanguination p.
    flashback p.
    fractionation p.
    perioperative standardized p.
    reinjection p.
    resuscitation p.
    standardized p.
protoduodenum
proton
    p. beam therapy
    p. pump inhibition therapy
    p. pump inhibitor (PPI)
protopianoma
protoplasmolysis
protozoal infection
protracted venous infusion
protrude
protruded disc
protrusio
    p. deformity
    p. ring
protrusion
    corneal p.
protrusive
    p. excursion
    p. jaw relation

NOTES

protrusive *(continued)*
   p. line
   p. occlusal position
protuberance
protuberant abdomen
protuberantia
proud graft
Proust space
provesicalis
provisional
   p. fixation
   p. restoration
   p. stabilization
provocation test
provocative
   p. chelation test
   p. discography
   p. food thyroidectomy
Prowazek-Greeff body
proximad
proximal
   p. aorta
   p. bowel distention
   p. bowel tenderness
   p. bow position
   p. cavity
   p. centriole
   p. clot
   p. diverting stoma
   p. end
   p. endoleak
   p. esophagus
   p. femoral epiphysiolysis
   p. femoral fracture
   p. femoral resection
   p. gastrectomy
   p. gastric cancer
   p. gastric resection
   p. gastric vagotomy
   p. humeral fracture
   p. incision
   p. interphalangeal joint approach
   p. jejunum
   p. limb
   p. loop syndrome
   p. myofascial dysfunction
   p. nail matrix
   p. phalanx
   p. portion
   p. pressure
   p. radioulnar articulation,
   p. space
   p. subclavian injury
   p. subtotal pancreatectomy
   p. tendon rupture
   p. tibial metaphysial fracture
   p. tibiofibular joint dislocation
   p. tumor
   p. urethral sphincter

   p. vascular control
   p. vein
proximal-row carpectomy
proximal-to-distal ring
proximate space
proximity
   close p.
PRSW
   preload recruitable stroke work
prune-belly
   p.-b. abdomen
   p.-b. syndrome (PBS)
prune-juice
   p.-j. expectoration
   p.-j. peritoneal fluid
pruritic
   p. erythematous patch
   p. lesion
Prussak
   P. pouch
   P. space
PS
   postcardiotomy shock
PSA
   persistent sciatic artery
psammocarcinoma
psammoma body
psammomatoid ossifying fibroma
psammomatous
psammosarcoma
psauoscopy
PSD
   percutaneous stricture dilatation
PSE
   portal-systemic encephalopathy
   PSE index
pseudarthrosis repair
pseudesthesia
pseudoaddiction
pseudoagglutination
pseudoaneurysm
   p. formation
   mycotic p.
pseudoangiosarcoma
pseudoankylosis
pseudoarthritis
pseudoarthrosis repair
pseudoarticulation
pseudobiopsy technique
pseudo-blind loop syndrome
pseudoboutonnière deformity
pseudocalcification
pseudocancerous lesion
pseudocarcinoma
pseudocavitation
pseudocele
pseudocephalocele
pseudocholesteatoma
pseudochylous ascites

pseudoclaudication
pseudocoarctation of aorta
pseudocoloboma
pseudocoma
pseudocryptorchism
pseudocyst
    p. drainage
    pancreatic p.
pseudocystobiliary fistula
pseudocystogastrostomy
    pancreatic p.
pseudodefecation
pseudodislocation
pseudoepiphysis
pseudoepithelioma
pseudoexfoliation syndrome
pseudofacilitation
pseudoganglion
    Cloquet p.
pseudogestational sac
pseudoglioma
pseudohernia
pseudohydrocephaly
pseudoinfection
pseudolipoma
pseudolymphoma syndrome
pseudomasturbation
pseudomedial longitudinal fasciculus
  lesion
pseudomelanoma
pseudomembranous acute inflammation
pseudomeningocele
    intradiploic p.
    posttraumatic intradiploic p.
    traumatic p.
pseudomigration
Pseudomonas infection
pseudomucinous cystadenocarcinoma
pseudomyxoma
pseudoneurogenic bladder
pseudoneuroma
pseudoobstruction
    acute colonic p.
    colonic p.
pseudoomphalocele
pseudoosteomalacia
pseudoosteomalacic pelvis
pseudopod formation
pseudoprolactinoma
pseudoretinoblastoma
pseudosacculation
pseudosarcoma

pseudoserous membrane
pseudostoma
pseudostratified epithelium
pseudosubluxation
pseudotabes
    diabetic p.
pseudotrachoma
pseudotumor
    p. cerebrimeningeal biopsy pulmona
    p. formation
pseudotumor formation
pseudounipolar
pseudoureterocele
pseudoxanthoma elasticum syndrome
PSI
    patient state index
psoas
    p. fascia
    p. hitch procedure
    p. line
    p. major muscle
    p. margin
    p. minor muscle
    p. minor tendon
    p. sheath block
psoralens, ultraviolet A (PUVA)
psoriatic arthritis
PSP
    postoperative survival probability
PSS
    Peritonitis Severity Score
    physiologic saline solution
PSV
    pressure-supported ventilation
    pressure support ventilation
psychoactive
psychogenic
    p. colic
    p. pain
    p. symptom
psychologic
    p. consequence
    p. implication
psychological problem
psychological screening
psychomotor retardation
psychopharmacologic medication
psychorelaxation
psychosedation
    dental p.
psychosis
psychosurgery

NOTES

P

psychotropic medication
psychrophore
PTA
>pancreas transplant alone
>pancreatic transplantation alone

PTBD
>percutaneous transhepatic balloon
>dilatation
>percutaneous transhepatic biliary drainage

PTC
>percutaneous transhepatic
>cholangiography

PTCA
>percutaneous transluminal coronary
>angioplasty
>>multivessel PTCA

PTCSL
>percutaneous transhepatic
>cholangioscopic lithotomy

PTE
>pulmonary thromboendarterectomy

pterion
pterional
>p. approach
>p. craniotomy

pterygoid
>p. artery
>p. branch
>p. canal
>p. fissure
>p. fossa
>p. fovea
>p. hamulus
>p. lamina
>p. nerve
>p. notch
>p. pit
>p. plate
>p. plexus
>p. position
>p. process
>p. tubercle
>p. tuberosity

pterygomandibular
>p. ligament
>p. raphe
>p. space
>p. space abscess

pterygomaxillary
>p. fissure
>p. fossa
>p. space

pterygopalatine
>p. canal
>p. fossa
>p. fossa syndrome
>p. ganglion
>p. groove

>p. nerve
>p. space

pterygopharyngeal space
pterygospinal ligament
pterygospinous
>p. ligament
>p. process

PTGDS
>patellar tendon graft donor site

PTH
>parathyroid hormone
>>PTH chemiluminescent assay
>>PTH level

PTJV
>percutaneous transtracheal jet ventilation

PTLD
>posttransplant lymphoproliferative
>disease
>posttransplant lymphoproliferative
>disorder

ptosed
ptosis, pl. **ptoses**
ptotic organ
PTS
>pediatric trauma scale

PTSD
>posttraumatic stress disorder

PTV
>percutaneous transtracheal jet ventilation

PTX
>pancreas transplant

ptyalocele
pubes (*pl. of* pubis)
pubic
>p. angle
>p. arch
>p. arcuate ligament
>p. artery
>p. body
>p. bone
>p. branch
>p. crest
>p. diastasis
>p. fixation
>p. hair line
>p. pad
>p. region
>p. spine
>p. symphysis
>p. tubercle

pubiotomy
pubis, pl. **pubes**
>mons p.

pubocapsular
pubococcygeal
>p. line
>p. muscle

pubofemoral

puboprostatic
    p. ligament
    p. muscle
puboprostaticus
puborectalis loop
puborectal muscle
pubourethral triangle
pubovaginal
    p. muscle
    p. operation
pubovaginalis
pubovesical muscle
Puchtler
    P. alkaline Congo red method
    P. Sirius red method
Puddu tendon technique
pudendal
    p. anesthesia
    p. canal
    p. cleft
    p. hematocele
    p. hernia
    p. nerve
    p. sac
    p. slit
    p. vein
pudendum, pl. **pudenda**
pudic nerve
puerile respiration
puerperal
    p. hematoma
    p. infection
Puestow-Gillesby
    P.-G. operation
    P.-G. procedure
Puestow pancreaticojejunostomy
Pugh
    P. classification
    modified method of P.
Pugh-Child bleeding esophageal varices grading scale classification
Pulec and Freedman classification
pullback
    p. pressure
    p. pressure gradient
pulled-down colon
pull-enteroscopy
pulley
    muscular p.
    peroneal p.
    p. reconstruction
    p. suture technique

pull maneuver
pull-out wire suture technique
pull-through
    abdominal p.-t.
    Duhamel laparoscopic p.-t.
    endorectal ileal p.-t.
    endorectal ileoanal p.-t.
    ileoanal endorectal p.-t.
    p.-t. operation
    p.-t. procedure
    rapid p.-t. (RPT)
    sacroabdominoperineal p.-t.
    slow p.-t. (SPT)
    Soave endorectal p.-t.
    station p.-t. (SPT)
    p.-t. technique
pull-up
    gastric p.-u.
    total gastric p.-u.
pulmo, pl. **pulmones**
pulmoaortic canal
pulmona
    pseudotumor cerebrimeningeal biopsy p.
pulmonary
    p. acid aspiration syndrome
    p. angioma
    p. apoptosis
    p. arborization
    p. arterial malformation
    p. arterial web
    p. arteriovenous fistula (PAF)
    p. arteriovenous malformation
    p. artery (PA)
    p. artery catheter
    p. artery catheterization
    p. artery catheterization anesthetic technique
    p. artery hypertension (PAH)
    p. artery occlusion pressure (PAOP)
    p. artery occlusive wedge pressure
    p. artery pressure (PAP)
    p. artery wedge
    p. aspiration
    p. atresia
    p. autograft (PA)
    p. bacterial infection
    p. blastoma
    p. capillary blood
    p. capillary wedge pressure
    p. cavitation

NOTES

P

pulmonary *(continued)*
   p. cavity
   p. circulation
   p. circulation tear
   p. collateral
   p. compliance
   p. complication
   p. contusion
   p. dysfunction
   p. edema
   p. effect
   p. embolectomy
   p. embolism (PE)
   p. embolization
   p. epithelial cell
   p. fibrosis
   p. function
   p. fungal infection
   p. glomangiosis
   p. homograft
   p. hypertension pressure
   p. hypoplasia
   p. hypostasis
   p. intralobar sequestration
   p. involvement
   p. ligament
   p. lobectomy
   p. lymphangioleiomyomatosis
   p. lymphangiomyomatosis
   p. manifestation
   p. mass
   p. metastasectomy
   p. metastasis
   p. orifice
   p. outflow tract
   p. overcirculation
   p. parenchymal infection
   p. pleura
   p. plexus
   p. position
   p. resection
   p. sinus
   p. stenosis repair
   p. sulcus
   p. sulcus syndrome
   p. support
   p. suppuration
   p. sympathetic blockade
   p. thromboendarterectomy (PTE)
   p. tissue
   p. toilet
   p. transplantation
   p. trunk
   p. tuberous sclerosis
   p. tumor
   p. valve anomaly
   p. valve area
   p. valve disease
   p. valve gradient

   p. valve insufficiency
   p. valve replacement
   p. valve restenosis
   p. valve stenosis
   p. valvuloplasty
   p. vascular abnormality
   p. vascular pressure
   p. vascular resistance (PVR)
   p. vascular resistance index (PVRI)
   p. vein
   p. venous connection anomaly
   p. venous return
   p. venous return anomaly
   p. ventilation
   p. ventilation scan
pulmonary-gas exchange
pulmones (*pl. of* pulmo)
pulmonic valve stenosis
pulmonis
pulp, pl. **pulpa**
   p. amputation
   p. approach
   p. canal
   p. canal therapy
   p. cavity
   p. devitalization
   digital p.
   exposed p.
   p. extirpation
   p. flap
   p. microcirculation
   p. mummification
   p. pressure
   red p.
   splenic p.
   white p.
pulpal wall
pulpation
pulpectomy
   complete p.
   partial p.
pulpifaction
pulpiform
pulpify
pulpodentinal membrane
pulpoma
pulpoperiapical lesion
pulposus
pulpotomy
   complete p.
   formocresol p.
   partial p.
   total p.
pulsatile
   p. hematoma
   p. mass
   p. pressure lavage
pulsation

pulse
- abdominal p.
- p. dye laser therapy
- p. lavage irrigation
- p. oximetry
- peripheral p.
- p. pressure
- p. repetition time prolongation
- p. trisection
- p. value recording (PVR)
- p. width

pulsed
- p. electromagnetic field (PEMF)
- p. irrigation
- p. laser ablation

pulsed-mode operation
pulse-echo distance measurement
pulseless electrical activity (PEA)
pulsion
- p. diverticulum
- p. hernia

pultaceous
pulverization
Pulvertaft
- P. fishmouth incision
- P. weave technique

pump
- extracorporeal bypass p. (ECBP)
- p. lung
- p. oxygenation

punch
- p. biopsy
- p. graft
- p. resection

punched-out lesion
puncta (*pl. of* punctum)
punctate
- p. epithelial keratoplasty
- p. hemorrhage

punctation
punctoplasty
punctum, pl. **puncta**
- inferior lacrimal p.
- lacrimal p.
- renal p.
- scleral p.
- superior lacrimal p.

puncture
- antegrade p.
- anterior p.
- apical left ventricular p.
- Bernard p.

- bone marrow p.
- brain p.
- calix p.
- cecal ligation and p. (CLP)
- cisternal p.
- cystic p.
- dental p.
- diabetic p.
- diathermy p.
- direct cardiac p.
- direct cautery p.
- direct needle p.
- dural p.
- endoscopic fine-needle p.
- exploratory p.
- femoral p.
- p. incision
- jejunal p.
- left ventricular p.
- lumbar p.
- needle tracheoesophageal p.
- nephrostomy p.
- percutaneous needle p.
- percutaneous renal p.
- pericardial p.
- Quincke p.
- retrograde nephrostomy p.
- self-sealing scleral p.
- skin p.
- spinal p.
- splenic p.
- stereotactic p.
- sternal p.
- subdural p.
- suprapubic p.
- tracheoesophageal p.
- transseptal p.
- ultrasound-guided nephrostomy p.
- venous p.
- ventricular p.
- p. wound
- Ziegler p.

pupil
- p. dilation
- exit p.

pupilla, pl. **pupillae**
- pupillae sphincter muscle

pupillary
- p. dilatation
- p. line
- p. margin
- p. membrane

NOTES

P

pupillary *(continued)*
    p. membrane remnant
    p. muscle
    p. zone
pupillodilator fiber
pupilloscopy
pupil-to-root iridectomy
puppet technique
purchase point
pure
    p. cutting cautery
    p. fungal infection
    p. fungal organism
    p. insular carcinoma
    p. refractive surgery
    p. rotation
    p. translation
purgation
purging
    immunologic method of p.
    tumor cell p.
puriform aspect
Purkinje network
Purmann method
purpuric lesion
purpurogenous membrane
pursestring
    p. atriotomy
    p. mastopexy
    p. suture technique
purulence
purulent
    p. exudate
    p. exudation
    p. inflammation
    p. peritonitis
pus
    p. collection
    frank p.
push
    p. enteroscopy
    hemodynamic p.
    p. maneuver
    p. plus refraction technique
push-back
    p.-b. procedure
    p.-b. technique
push-pull T technique
push-type enteroscopy
pustular
    p. inflammation
    p. lesion
    p. patch-test reaction
pustulation
pustule
Putenney operation
Putti-Platt
    P.-P. arthroplasty

    P.-P. operation
    P.-P. shoulder procedure
Putti posterior approach
putty kidney
PUVA
    psoralens, ultraviolet A
    PUVA radiation
Puzo method
PVE
    prosthetic valve endocarditis
PVR
    pulmonary vascular resistance
    pulse value recording
pVR
    perspective volume rendering
PVRI
    pulmonary vascular resistance index
PVTT
    portal vein tumor thrombus
pyelectasis
pyelitic
pyelitis
pyelocaliceal
pyelocaliectasis
pyelocalyceal
pyelocalycotomy
pyelocystitis
pyeloileocutaneous
pyelolithotomy
    coagulum p.
    open p.
pyelolymphatic
pyelolysis
pyelonephritic kidney
pyelonephritis
    xanthogranulomatous p. (XCP)
pyelonephrosis
pyeloplasty
    Anderson-Hynes p.
    capsular flap p.
    Culp spiral flap p.
    disjoined p.
    dismembered p.
    Foley Y-plasty p.
    laparoscopic dismembered p.
    Scardino vertical flap p.
    Thompson capsule flap p.
pyeloplication
pyeloscopy
pyelostomy
pyelotomy
    extended p.
    open p.
pyeloureterectasis
pyeloureterography
pyeloureterostomy
pyelovenous backflow
pyelovesicostomy
pyencephalus

pyesis
pygal
pyknic
pyknotic body
pylemphraxis
pylephlebectasis
pylethrombosis
pylorectomy
    Kocher p.
pylori (*pl. of* pylorus)
pyloric
    p. antrum
    p. artery
    p. autotransplantation
    p. canal
    p. constriction
    p. dilation
    p. gland
    p. intubation
    p. orifice
    p. part of stomach
    p. ring
    p. sphincter
    p. vein
pyloricum
pyloricus
pyloristenosis
pylorodiosis
pylorogastrectomy
pyloromyotomy
    circumumbilical p.
    extramucosal p.
    Fredet-Ramstedt p.
    Kocher p.
    laparoscopic p.
    Ramstedt p.
    Ramstedt-Fredet p.
pyloroplasty
    double p.
    Finney p.
    Heineke-Mikulicz p.
    Jaboulay p.
    Mikulicz p.
    Ramstedt p.
    reconstructive p.
    transhiatal p.
    truncal vagotomy and p.
    vagotomy and p.
    Weinberg modification of p.
    Yu p.
pyloroptosis
pylorostenosis

pylorostomy
pylorotomy
pylorus, pl. pylori
pylorus-preserving
    p.-p. gastrectomy (PPG)
    p.-p. pancreaticoduodenectomy
    p.-p. pancreatoduodenectomy (PPPD)
    p.-p. surgery
pylorus-sparing pancreaticoduodenectomy
pyocele
pyocelia
pyocephalus
pyocolpocele
pyocystis
pyodermatous
    p. infection
    p. skin lesion
pyogen
pyogenesis
pyogenic
    p. arthritis
    p. hepatic abscess
    p. membrane
    p. spinal infection
pyomyoma
pyonephritis
pyonephrolithiasis
pyonephrosis
pyoperitoneum
pyoperitonitis
pyopneumothorax
pyopoiesis
pyopyelectasis
pyorrhea
pyosemia
pyosis
pyospermia
pyothorax
pyoureter ectopic ureterocele
pyramid
    Ferrein p.
    Lallouette p.
    malpighian p.
    medullary p.
    p. method
    nasal p.
    orbital p.
    petrous p.
    renal p.
pyramidal
    p. auricular muscle
    p. bone

NOTES

P

pyramidal *(continued)*
    p. decussation
    p. eminence
    p. epithelium
    p. fracture
    p. process of thyroid
    p. radiation
    p. tip
    p. tract
    p. tractotomy
pyramidale
pyramidalis
pyramidotomy
    medullary p.
    spinal p.

pyramis
pyretic therapy
pyriform
pyriformis
pyrogen
    endogenous p.
pyrolysis product
pyrosequencing
pyruvate
    p. dehydrogenase inhibition
    p. metabolism
pyuria

QOL
>quality of life

QST
>Quantitative Sensory Testing

Q-tip test

quadrangular
>q. cartilage
>q. membrane
>q. space
>q. therapy

quadrant
>circumareolar q.
>2-q. hemorrhoidectomy
>3-q. hemorrhoidectomy
>4-q. hemorrhoidectomy
>left lower q. (LLQ)
>left upper q. (LUQ)
>lower lateral q.
>lower medial q.
>right lower q. (RLQ)
>right upper q. (RUQ)
>q. sampling technique
>upper lateral q.
>upper medial q.

quadrantectomy
>q., axillary dissection, radiation
>therapy (QUART)
>q. mastectomy

quadrate
>q. femoral tubercle
>q. muscle

quadratus

quadriceps femoris tendon

quadricepsplasty
>Judet q.
>Thompson q.
>V-Y q.

quadrigeminal cistern

quadrilateral
>q. space
>q. space syndrome

quadripedal extensor reflex

quadripolar

quadruple
>q. amputation
>q. therapy

Quaegebeur procedure

Quaglino operation

quality
>q. of life (QOL)
>Q. of Well-Being Scale Self-
>Administered (QWB-SA)

quantification
>acoustic q.
>shunt q.

quantitative
>q. evaluation
>Q. Sensory Testing (QST)
>q. stool collection

quantity
>sound q.
>vector q.

QUART
>quadrantectomy, axillary dissection,
>radiation therapy
>QUART procedure
>QUART procedure for breast
>cancer

Quartey technique

quasistatic stressed position

Quatrefages angle

quenching
>thermal q.

Quénu
>Q. hemorrhoidal plexus
>Q. nail plate removal technique

**Quénu-Küss tarsometatarsal injury
classification**

questionable mass

questionnaire
>Acute Low Back Pain
>Screening Q. (ALBPSQ)
>Barriers Pain Q.
>Cognitive Errors Q.
>Coping Strategies Q. (CSQ)
>malingering q.
>McGill Pain Q. (MPQ)
>Menstrual Distress Management Q.
>(MDMQ)
>Oswestry Disability Q. (ODQ)
>Pain Coping Q. (PCQ)
>SF-McGill Pain Q.
>The Modified Somatic Pain Q.

quick
>q. angulation technique
>Q. method

Quickert
>Q. procedure
>Q. 3-suture technique

quilt suture technique

Quinby pelvic fracture classification

Quincke puncture

Quinones
>method of Q.

quinti
>extensor digiti q.

quotient
>pressure rate q.
>respiratory q.
>ventilation/perfusion q.

QWB-SA
  Quality of Well-Being Scale Self-
  Administered

QWB-SA form

R0, R1, R2 resection
racemate
racemic
    r. mixture
    r. modification
racemization
rachial
rachides (*pl. of* rachis)
rachidial
rachidian
rachiotomy
rachis, pl. **rachides, rachises**
rachitic metaphysis
rachitomy
racket nail
racket-shaped flap
Rackley method
racquet incision
racquet-shaped incision
radectomy
Radford nomogram
radiad
radial
    r. bursa
    r. club hand
    r. collateral artery
    r. dilator muscle
    r. forearm flap
    r. fracture reduction
    r. head
    r. head dislocation
    r. head fracture
    r. index artery
    r. iridotomy
    r. keratotomy (RK)
    r. laminectomy
    r. neck fracture
    r. recurrent artery
    r. scar
    r. sclerosing lesion
    r. skin incision
    r. styloid fracture
    r. suture track
    r. wedge osteotomy
    r. wrist extensor
radial-based flap
radiate sternocostal ligament
radiation
    r. angiopathy
    braking r.
    r. burn
    r. cataract
    characteristic r.
    r. chimera
    r. damage

diagnostic r.
r. enteritis
r. enteropathy
r. exposure
general r.
geniculocalcarine r.
Goldmann coherent r.
Gratiolet r.
r. hepatitis
r. hepatopathy
high dose r. (HDR)
homogenous r.
r. injury
intraoperative r.
involved-field r.
r. lung disease
r. monitoring
r. mucositis
r. myelopathy
r. necrosis
occipitothalamic r.
r. oncologist
optic r.
r. output
r. pneumonitis
r. poisoning
postoperative pelvic r.
r. precautions
primary r.
r. proctitis
r. proctocolitis
r. protection
PUVA r.
pyramidal r.
rectosigmoid r.
r. response
r. risk
single fraction r.
Sr-90 beta r.
superficial r.
r. survey
temporal lobe r.
r. therapy
r. treatment
Wernicke r.
whole abdominal r.
whole-body r.
radiation-induced
    r.-i. carcinoma
    r.-i. colitis
    r.-i. disease
    r.-i. ischemia
    r.-i. leukoencephalopathy
    r.-i. proctitis

R

radiation-induced (*continued*)
    r.-i. pulmonary toxicity
    r.-i. ulceration
radiatum
radical
    r. abdominal hysterectomy
    r. axillary dissection
    r. compartmental excision
    r. curative surgery
    r. cystectomy
    r. en bloc removal
    r. gastric resection
    r. glossectomy
    r. hemorrhoidectomy
    r. inguinal orchiectomy
    r. lymph node dissection
    r. mastectomy
    r. mastoidectomy
    r. mediastinal dissection
    r. neck dissection
    r. nephrectomy
    r. nephroureterectomy
    r. orchidectomy
    r. palmar fasciectomy
    r. pancreatoduodenectomy
    r. parametrectomy
    r. parotidectomy
    r. perineal prostatectomy
    r. prefrontal lobotomy
    r. proctectomy
    r. retropubic prostatectomy
    r. subtotal resection
    r. therapy
    r. total gastrectomy
    r. transcoccygeal prostatectomy
    r. vaginal hysterectomy
    r. vulvectomy
radices (*pl. of* radix)
radicle
radicotomy
radicular
    r. artery
    r. canal
radiculectomy
radiculomedullary fistula
radiculomeningeal spinal vascular
  malformation
radiculopathy
    thoracic r.
radiectomy
radii (*pl. of* radius)
radioactive
    r. concentration
    r. iodine uptake
    r. microsphere
    r. scan
    r. seed implantation
radioactivity
radiobicipital

radiocapitate ligament
radiocapitellar
    r. articulation
    r. line
radiocarpal
    r. arthroscopy
    r. articulation
    r. dislocation
radiocolloid
radiodense lesion
radiodigital
radiofluoroscopy
    televised r.
radiofrequency
    r. catheter ablation (RFCA)
    r. electrophrenic respiration
    r. lesion
    r. rhizotomy
    temperature-controlled r. (TCRF)
    r. thermal ablation (RFTA)
radiofrequency-generated thermal lesion
radiograph
    sequential r.'s
    serial r.'s
    specimen r.
radiographic
    r. evaluation
    r. examination
    r. image
    r. obliteration
    r. technique
    r. tooth repair
radiographic examination
radiography
    plain abdominal r.
    postfixation r.
radioguided
    r. parathyroidectomy
    r. technique
radiohumeral
radioimmunoglobulin therapy
radioimmunoguided surgery
radioimmunoscintimetry
radioiodination
    lactoperoxidase r.
radioiodine
    r. ablation
    r. ablation therapy
    low-dose r.
    r. treatment
radioisotope
    filtered r.
    r. localization
    unfiltered r.
    r. uptake
radiolabeled
    r. sentinel node
    r. serum albumin

radiolocalization
    gamma-probe r.
    SLN r.
radiologic
    r. biliary stent placement
    r. evaluation
    r. evidence
    r. study
    r. technique
radiological
    r. examination
    r. sphincter
radiologist
    interventional r.
    vascular r.
radiology
    interventional r.
radiolucent
    r. crescent line
    r. lesion
    r. operating room table extension
radiolunate fusion
radiolus
radiolysis
radiomuscular
radiomutation
radionecrosis
radionuclide
    r. scan
    r. technique
radiopalmar
radiopaque
    r. foreign body
    r. lesion
radiopharmaceutical therapy
radiopotentiation
radioprotector
radioscaphoid fusion
radiosensitization
radio signal line
radiosurgery
    LINAC-based r.
    linear accelerator-based r.
    stereotactic r.
radiotherapy
    adjuvant r.
    continuous hyperfractionated
      accelerated r. (CHART)
radiotriquetral ligament
radioulnar
    r. articulation

    r. dissociation
    r. ligament
radisectomy
radius, pl. **radii**
    r. of angulation
    scaphoid r.
radix, pl. **radices**
Radley-Liebig-Brown resection
radon seed implantation
Raeder syndrome
Raff-Glantz derivative method
rag-wheel method
Rai classification
Rainville technique
raise
    single heel r.
raising
    straight-leg r. (SLR)
rale
Ralston-Thompson pseudoarthrosis
  technique
Raman spectroscopy
Rambo musculoplasty
ram horn nail
rami (*pl. of* ramus)
ramicotomy
ramification
    apical r.
ramisection
Ramond point
Ramon flocculation
ramotomy
    superior pubic r.
Ramsay Hunt syndrome
Ramstedt
    R. operation
    R. procedure
    R. pyloromyotomy
    R. pyloroplasty
Ramstedt-Fredet pyloromyotomy
ramus, pl. **rami**
    cephalic arterial r.
Ranawat
    R. classification
    R. triangle method
Ranawat-DeFiore-Straub
    R.-D.-S. osteotomy
    R.-D.-S. technique
Ranawat-Dorr-Inglis method
Randall plaque
random
    r. bladder biopsy

R

NOTES

random *(continued)*
    r. cutaneous flap
    r. pattern flap
randomization
range
    r. of excursion
    r. of motion (ROM)
    pain sensitivity r.
Ransley-Cantwell repair
Ransley procedure
Ransohoff operation
Ranson
    R. acute pancreatitis classification
    R. pancreatitis criteria
    R. prognostic scoring index
Ranvier node
RAO
    right anterior oblique
    right anterior occipital
    RAO angulation
    RAO position
raphe
    anogenital r.
    median longitudinal r.
    penile r.
    perineal r.
    pharyngeal r.
    pterygomandibular r.
    scrotal r.
rapid
    r. acquisition radiofrequency-echo-
      steady state imaging
    r. bedside imaging
    r. intraoperative parathormone assay
    r. intraoperative parathormone
      immunoradiometric assay
    r. maxillary expansion
    r. occlusion
    r. pull-through (RPT)
    r. pull-through esophageal
      manometry technique
    r. recompression-high pressure
      oxygen
    r. scan fluoroscopy
    r. scan technique
    r. sequence induction intubation
    r. tumor lysis syndrome
    r. volume resuscitation
rapid-flush technique
rapid-sequence
    r.-s. induction (RSI)
    r.-s. induction of anesthesia
    r.-s. induction anesthetic technique
rapid-volume approach
Rapoport test
Rappaport
    R. classification
    R. osteotomy

RAPS
    recurrent abdominal pain syndrome
Rapunzel syndrome
rare system reaction
RAS
    robot-assisted surgery
rasceta
rash
    acneform r.
Rashkind
    R. balloon technique
    R. operation
raspberry-like density
Rastan-Konno procedure
Rastan operation
Rastelli
    R. classification
    R. classification of atrioventricular
      septal defect (type A–C)
    R. conduit
    R. graft
    R. operation
    R. procedure
    R. repair
rate
    anastomotic complication r.
    anastomotic stricture r.
    average flow r.
    beat-to-beat variation of fetal
      heart r.
    blood flow r.
    cerebral metabolic r. (CMR)
    circulation r.
    complication r.
    dipolë-dipolë relaxation r.
    disease recurrence r.
    disintegration r.
    early infection r.
    ejection r.
    expiratory flow r.
    fetal heart r.
    flotation r.
    r. of fluid filtration
    fusion nonunion r.
    gallbladder ejection r.
    glomerular filtration r. (GFR)
    heart r. (HR)
    high dose r. (HDR)
    implant survival r.
    infection r.
    infusion r.
    in-hospital mortality r.
    late infection r.
    leakage r.
    load-deflection r.
    low dose r. (LDR)
    maximal expiratory flow r.
    maximal ventilation r.

mean normalized systolic
   ejection r.
metabolic r.
mortality r.
operative mortality r.
ovulation r.
oxygen extraction r.
pacemaker adaptive r.
peak expiratory flow r. (PEFR)
perfusion flow r.
plasma separation r.
pressure increment r.
r. pressure product
recurrence r.
relapse r.
relaxation r.
resectability r.
Solomon-Bloembergen theory of
   dipole-dipole relaxation r.
stricture r.
stroke ejection r.
success r.
systolic ejection r.
transverse relaxation r.
T2 relaxation r.
vertebral osteosynthesis fusion r.
voiding flow r.

rated perceived exertion

Rathke

R. bundle
R. pouch cyst

rating of perceived exertion

ratio

adenoma-hyperplastic polyp r.
adenoma-nonadenoma r.
ankle-brachial blood pressure r.
body hematocrit-venous
   hematocrit r.
common mode rejection r.
cough-pressure transmission r.
cup-to-disc r.
dead space:tidal volume r.
external/internal rotation r.
fetal head:abdominal
   circumference r.
hand r.
head:body r.
head circumference:abdominal
   circumference r.
inspiratory-to-expiratory r.
international normalized r. (INR)
intrapulmonary shunt r.

lung-to-head circumference r.
MAC r.
mean UV/MV r.
midexpiratory/midinspiratory flow r.
optic cup-to-disc r.
pressure transmission r.
right-to-left shunt r.
sentinel node-to-background r.
   (SNBR)
shunt r.
stereoselectivity r.
tumor:cerebellum r.
UV/MV r.
ventilation/perfusion r.

rationalization

rat-tail deformity

Rauwolfia extract

rave

fracture en r.

Raverdino operation

raw hepatic surface

ray

r. amputation
medullary r.
r. resection

Ray-Brunswick-Mack operation

Ray-Clancy-Lemon technique

Rayhack technique

Ray-McLean operation

Raynaud

R. phenomenon
R. syndrome

Raz

R. bladder neck suspension
R. modification
R. needle suspension
R. procedure
R. 4-quadrant suspension
R. urethral suspension

Raz-Leach procedure

rCABG

reoperative coronary artery bypass graft

rCBF

regional cerebral blood flow

RDS

respiratory distress syndrome

reabsorb

reaction

anaphylactoid-type r.
anesthetic r.
compensation r.
cutaneous graft-versus-host r.

NOTES

R

reaction *(continued)*
    dextran r.
    eczematous r.
    elimination r.
    exergonic r.
    exitatory r.
    extrapyramidal r.
    foreign body r.
    r. formation
    general adaptation r.
    graft-versus-host disease r.
    homograft r.
    immediate asthmatic r. (IAR)
    implant r.
    inflammation r.
    irritant patch-test r.
    lid closure r.
    litigation r.
    local anesthetic r.
    midazolam-induced excitatory r.
    needle r.
    paradoxical r.
    pustular patch-test r.
    rare system r.
    reverse transcriptase-polymerase chain r. (RT-PCR)
    scar tissue r.
    whitegraft r.
reactivation tuberculosis
reactive
    r. arthritis
    r. dilation
    r. lymphoid lesion
reactivity
    airway r.
reading
    benign r.
    malignant r.
Read rebreathing method
real
    r. adaptive relaxation
    r. reconstruction
realignment procedure
reality
    virtual r.
real-time
    r.-t. colonoscopy
    r.-t. 3D biplanar transperineal prostate implantation
    r.-t. echo-planar image
    r.-t. endoscopic ultrasound-guided fine-needle aspiration
    r.-t. multiplanar image
    r.-t. sector scanning
reamed
    r. femoral nailing
    r. nail
reamputation
reanastomosed

reanastomosis
    laparoscopic ureteral r.
reanimation
    facial r.
reapproximation
reattachment
    Harris 4-wire trochanter r.
    4-wire trochanter r.
reattribution technique
reauditorization
rebound
    r. headache
    r. tenderness
rebreathing
    r. anesthesia
    intentional r.
    r. technique
Rebuck skin window technique
recalcification time
recall
    memory r.
Récamier
    R. operation
    R. procedure
recanalization
    balloon occlusive intravascular lysis enhanced r.
    excimer vascular r.
    laser r.
    TCD r.
    r. technique
    umbilical vein r.
    r. versus recannulization
recannulization
    recanalization versus r.
receiver saturation
recent dislocation
recently healed surgical incision
receptaculum
receptoma
receptor
    acetylcholine r.
    alpha-adrenergic r.
    alpha-2-adrenergic r.
    beta-adrenergic r.
    beta-2-adrenergic r.
    calcium-sensing r.
    dopamine r.
    endogenous opiate r.
    endometrial r.
    endothelin A, B r.
    high-affinity progestin r.
    high threshold r.
    intensity-encoded r.
    mu r.
    muscarinic r.
    nerve growth factor r.
    nicotinic r.
    opioid r.

pressure r.
silent r.
up-regulation of r.
receptor-mediated endocytosis pathway
recess
azygoesophageal r.
cecal r.
costodiaphragmatic r.
costomediastinal r.
duodenal r.
duodenojejunal r.
elliptical r.
epitympanic r.
frontal r.
hepatorenal r.
ileocecal r.
inferior duodenal r.
inferior ileocecal r.
inferior omental r.
intersigmoid r.
Jacquemet r.
mesentericoparietal r.
omental r.
paracolic r.
paraduodenal r.
parotid r.
pharyngeal r.
phrenicomediastinal r.
pineal r.
piriform r.
pleural r.
retrocecal r.
retroduodenal r.
Rosenmüller r.
sacciform r.
sphenoethmoidal r.
spherical r.
splenic r.
subhepatic r.
subphrenic r.
subpopliteal r.
superior duodenal r.
superior ileocecal r.
superior omental r.
suprabullar r.
suprapineal r.
supratonsillar r.
recession
clitoral r.
lateral rectus r.
recessional line
recession-resection

recessive
autosomal r.
recidivation
recipient
adult r.
r. hepatectomy
naive r.
OLT r.
orthotopic liver transplant r.
reciprocal relaxation
reciprocation
active r.
passive r.
recirculation
instrument r.
Recklinghausen disease type I
reclamping
reclination
reclining position
Reclus I syndrome
recoarctation of aorta
recognition
pattern r.
within-list r. (WLR)
recoil
elastic r.
recombinant
r. activated coagulation factor VII
r. DNA technique
r. factor VIIa
r. tissue-type plasminogen activator (RTPA, rtPA)
recommendation
FDA Anesthesia Apparatus Checkout R.'s
screening r.
reconciliation
reconditioning
mucosal r.
reconstruction
Abbe-McIndoe vaginal r.
ACL r.
alar r.
anal sphincter r.
analytic r.
Andrews iliotibial band r.
anterior capsulolabral r.
anterior cruciate ligament r. (ACLR)
aortic root r.
aortorenal r.
artery r.

NOTES

reconstruction *(continued)*

arthroscopic anterior cruciate ligament r. (AACLR)
Bankart r.
biliary r.
Billroth I, II r.
bladder outlet r.
breast r.
Brown knee joint r.
Cho anterior cruciate ligament r.
Chrisman-Snook r.
circumferential esophageal r.
Clancy cruciate ligament r.
columellar r.
constrained r.
coronal r.
corporeal r.
craniofacial r.
cruciate ligament r.
d'Aubigné femoral r.
d'Aubigné resection r.
3D computer r.
dermal pouch r.
Dibbell cleft lip-nasal r.
3-dimensional r.
distal vertebral artery r.
dural patch r.
Eaton-Littler ligament r.
Ellison lateral knee r.
endoscopic anterior cruciate ligament r.
endoscopic condylectomy and costochondral graft r.
end-to-end r.
epiglottic r.
Evans r.
exogenous r.
extraarticular r.
genital r.
Goldner r.
hand r.
Harmon hip r.
hemimandible r.
House r.
Hughston-Degenhardt r.
Hughston-Jacobson lateral compartment r.
immediate breast r.
index metacarpophalangeal joint r.
inferior vena cava r.
infrarenal aortic r.
innominate artery r.
Insall anterior cruciate ligament r.
in situ r.
intraarticular r.
iterative r.
IVC r.
joint r.
juxtacubital r.

Krukenberg hand r.
Kugelberg r.
Larson ligament r.
lateral compartment r.
Lee r.
L'Episcopo hip r.
Lewis-Tanner subtotal esophagectomy and r.
ligament r.
Longmire-Gutgeman gastric r.
lower extremity r.
MacIntosh over-the-top ACL r.
mandibular r.
r. method
microsurgical r.
Millard advancement rotation flap r.
nasal r.
Nathan-Trung modification of Krukenberg hand r.
Neer posterior shoulder r.
neoglottic r.
nipple r.
nipple-areolar r.
r. occlusal surface (RecOS)
O'Donoghue ACL r.
open r.
operative r.
oral r.
orbital rim r.
oromandibular r.
oropharyngeal r.
ossicular chain r.
osteoplastic r.
palate r.
pancreaticogastrostomy r.
papillary r.
pedicled jejunal r.
peritoneal r.
pharyngoesophageal r.
plastic r.
portal vein r.
pouch r.
r. procedure
pulley r.
real r.
renal artery r.
Rosenberg endoscopic anterior cruciate ligament r.
Roux-en-Y r.
Roux gastric r.
sagittal r.
secondary r.
septal r.
Sheen airway r.
socket r.
sphincter r.
S-pouch r.
staged r.

R

2-stage tendon graft r.
stapled r.
sternoclavicular joint r.
Swanson r.
synchronous bladder r.
Tanagho bladder neck r.
r. technique
tenoplastic r.
thumb r.
Torg knee r.
tracheal r.
tubular r.
tubularized bladder neck r.
urinary tract r.
vascular r.
Verdan osteoplastic thumb r.
vertebral artery r.
Watson-Jones r.
Whitman femoral neck r.
Wookey r.
Young-Dees bladder neck r.
Young-Dees-Leadbetter bladder
neck r.
Zancolli r.

reconstructive
r. mammaplasty
r. operation
r. preprosthetic surgery
r. pyloroplasty
r. surgical procedure
r. technique

record
anesthesia r.
anesthetic r.
automated anesthesia r.
centric occluding relation r.
eccentric interocclusal r.
eccentric maxillomandibular r.
jaw relation r.
medical r.
occluding centric relation r.
terminal jaw relation r.

recording
continuous on-line r.
duodenojejunal motor r.
fasting r.
macroelectrode r.
microelectrode r.
motor r.
pulse value r. (PVR)
segmental limb pressure r.
r. session

venous outflow r.
whole-cell patch clamp r.
RecOS
reconstruction occlusal surface
recovery
anesthetic immediate r.
fluid-attenuated inversion r.
(FLAIR)
neurologic r.
postoperative r.
pressure r.
r. and reorganization
r. room
r. room time
saturation r.
selective saturation r.
short tau inversion r. (STIR)
time to r.
r. time
recruiting maneuver
recruitment maneuver
recta (*pl. of* rectum)
rectal
r. alimentation
r. ampulla
r. anesthesia
r. anesthetic
r. anesthetic technique
r. blind pouch
r. cancer
r. carcinoma
r. column
r. diameter
r. dilation
r. distention
r. evacuation
r. examination
r. excision
r. fascia
r. fissure
r. fistula
r. flap
r. floor
r. floor line
r. fold
r. foreign body
r. hernia
r. laceration
r. mass
r. mobilization
r. mucosectomy
r. muscle cuff

NOTES

rectal *(continued)*
    r. myectomy
    r. nerve
    r. probe electroejaculation
    r. problem
    r. prolapse
    r. pulsed irrigation
    r. resting pressure
    r. shelf
    r. sinus
    r. stump
    r. suction biopsy
    r. surgery
    r. tip
    r. ulceration
    r. valvotomy
    r. venous plexus
rectalgia
rectalis
rectangular amputation
rectectomy
rectification
    anomalous r.
    inward-going r.
rectify
recto
    hernia in r.
rectoanal
    r. angulation
    r. inhibitory reflex
rectocele repair
rectoclysis
rectococcygeal muscle
rectococcygeus
rectococcypexy
rectolabial fistula
rectoperineal
rectoperineorrhaphy
rectopexy
    abdominal r.
    anterior r.
    Ekehorn r.
    posterior r.
    presacral r.
    Ripstein anterior sling r.
    Wells posterior r.
rectoplasty
rectorrhaphy
rectoscopic endometrial ablation
rectoscopy
rectosigmoid
    r. anastomosis
    r. carcinoma
    r. junction
    r. radiation
    r. sphincter
    r. stump
    r. vein
rectosigmoidoscopy

rectosphincteric reflex
rectostenosis
rectostomy
rectotomy
rectourethral
    r. fistula
    r. muscle
rectourinary fistula
rectouterine
    r. cul-de-sac
    r. fold
    r. muscle
    r. pouch
rectovaginal
    r. examination
    r. fistula
    r. pouch
    r. septum
    r. surgery
    r. surgical treatment
rectovaginouterine pouch
rectovesical
    r. fascia
    r. fistula
    r. fold
    r. muscle
    r. pouch
    r. septum
rectovestibular fistula
rectovulvar fistula
rectum, pl. **recta**
    aganglionic r.
    r. cancer
    colonoscopy per r.
    r. irrigation
rectus
    r. abdominis free flap
    r. abdominis muscle
    r. abdominis muscle flap
    r. abdominis musculocutaneous flap
    r. abdominis myocutaneous flap
    r. diastasis
    r. fascial wrap
    r. femoris flap
    r. femoris tendon
    r. muscle-splitting incision
    r. position
    r. sheath
    r. sheath hematoma
    r. sheath incision
    r. sheath wall
recumbent
    r. incision
    r. position
recurarization
recurrence
    distant r.
    goiter r.
    intraperitoneal r.

invasive r.
local r.
locoregional r.
nodal r.
noninvasive r.
peritoneal r.
port-site wound r.
r. rate
resectable extrahepatic r.
suprapubic midline r.
tumor r.
wound r.

recurrence-free survival
recurrent

r. abdominal pain syndrome
(RAPS)
r. arthralgia
r. ascites
r. aspiration
r. attack
r. corneal erosion
r. dysphagia
r. exophthalmos
r. hypercalcemia
r. incisional hernia
r. inflammation
r. interosseous artery
r. laryngeal nerve (RLN)
r. leiomyosarcoma
r. meningeal branch
r. meningeal nerve
r. nerve injury
r. nerve lesion
r. nerve lymphatic chain
r. nerve paralysis
r. patellar dislocation
r. pyogenic cholangiohepatitis
(RPC)
r. radial artery
r. thromboembolic complication
r. thromboembolic disease
r. thromboembolism
r. thrombophlebitis
r. thrombosis
r. tumor
r. ulnar artery
r. upper respiratory tract infection
r. vermian oligoastrocytoma

recurvation
recurvatum angulation deformity
red

r. blood cell mass

r. desaturation
r. ear syndrome
r. granulation
r. hepatization
r. induration
r. muscle
r. pulp

Reddick-Saye method
redébridement
red-eyed shunt syndrome
red-filter therapy
redilation
redintegration
redistribution hypothermia
Redman approach
Redmond-Smith operation
redo

r. CABG
r. fundoplication

redox indicator
redressement forcé
reduced liver transplant (RLT)
reduced-size

r.-s. graft
r.-s. transplant

reducible hernia
reduction

afterload r.
Agee force-couple splint r.
alar base r.
Allen r.
r. anuloplasty
Aries-Pitanguy breast r.
axillary endoscopic r.
Barsky macrodactyly r.
Becton open r.
r. before resection
Boitzy open r.
breast r.
calcaneal fracture r.
central cone technique r.
closed r.
cluster r.
concentric r.
Cooper r.
Cotton r.
Crosby r.
Cubbins open r.
delayed open r.
Dias-Giegerich open r.
r. division
Eaton closed r.

NOTES

reduction *(continued)*
Eaton-Malerich r.
embryo r.
r. en masse
Essex-Lopresti open r.
femoral neck fracture r.
fetal r.
Flynn femoral neck fracture r.
force-couple splint r.
Fowles open r.
fracture r.
fracture-dislocation r.
funic r.
Hankin r.
Hastings open r.
hip r.
Houghton-Akroyd open r.
incomplete r.
indirect r.
internal fixation, closed r.
interproximal r.
Kaplan open r.
Kinast indirect r.
King open r.
Lejour-type breast r.
limb r.
Lowell r.
lung volume r. (LVR)
r. mammaplasty
r. mastopexy
McKeever open r.
r. method
Meyn r.
Moberg-Gedda open r.
multifetal pregnancy r.
Neer open r.
nonoperative r.
open r.
r. osteotomy
pain threshold r.
Pare r.
Parvin r.
percutaneous r.
perioperative r.
pneumatic r.
postural r.
r. potential
Pratt open r.
preload r.
prone r.
radial fracture r.
r. ring
risk r.
short scar technique breast r.
shoulder r.
side posture r.
sigmoid loop r.
Speed-Boyd open r.
Speed open r.

spondylolisthesis r.
stable r.
stapled lung r.
sternoclavicular joint r.
stress r.
surgical r.
swan-neck deformity r.
r. syndactyly
r. technique
tongue base r.
trial r.
tuberosity r.
r. tuberosity
tumescent technique breast r.
r. ventriculoplasty
vertical pedicle technique breast r.
volvulus r.
Wayne County r.
Weber-Brunner-Freuler open r.
weight r.
wet technique with liposuction
    breast r.
reduction-stabilization
redundant
r. sac tissue
r. triangular-shaped skin
reduplication
r. cataract
r. murmur
redux
chancre r.
reedy nail
reefing
r. procedure
stomach r.
reendothelialization
reentry
bundle branch r.
reepithelialization
Rees-Ecker
R.-E. fluid
R.-E. method
Reese-Cleasby operation
Reese-Jones-Cooper operation
Reese ptosis operation
reexcision
reexpansion
r. maneuver
r. pulmonary edema (REPE)
reexploration
operative r.
reexplore
refashioning
reference method
referred
r. point
r. trigger point pain
r. trigger point phenomenon
refixation

reflectance
    endoscopic r.
reflected inguinal ligament
reflection
    angle of r.
    Campbell triceps r.
    corneal r.
    diaphragmatic r.
    diffuse r.
    guide wire r.
    hepatoduodenal r.
    hepatoduodenal-peritoneal r.
    internal r.
    mirror-image r.
    mucobuccal r.
    pericardial r.
    peritoneal r.
    pleural r.
    shiny cellophane r.
    specular r.
    total internal r.
reflectometry
    acoustic r.
reflex
    abdominal cardiac r.
    absent gag r.
    accommodation r.
    antebrachial r.
    Bezold-Jarisch r.
    body righting r.
    Breuer-Hering inflation r.
    cardiopressor r.
    celiac plexus r.
    copper-wire r.
    corneal light r.
    cremasteric r.
    crossed extension r.
    crossed extensor r.
    Cushing r.
    r. erection
    erector-spinal r.
    r. examination
    extensor thrust r.
    external oblique r.
    eyeball compression r.
    eye-closure r.
    eyelash r.
    eyelid-closure r.
    fixation r.
    flexion-extension r.
    fusion r.
    gastropancreatic vagovagal r.

    grasp r.
    Head paradoxical r.
    head-turning r.
    Hering-Breuer r.
    r. incontinence
    inflation r.
    inhibitory r.
    lacrimation r.
    r. ligament
    mass r.
    milk-ejection r.
    myenteric r.
    r. neurogenic bladder
    oculocardiac r. (OCR)
    paradoxical extensor r.
    pericardial r.
    pronator r.
    proprioceptive head-turning r.
    quadripedal extensor r.
    rectoanal inhibitory r.
    rectosphincteric r.
    renal r.
    silver-wire r.
    supination r.
    supinator longus r.
    r. sympathetic dystrophy (RSD)
    sympathoexcitation r.
    r. therapy
    vagovagal r.
    r. venoconstriction
    vertical suspension r.
    visceral traction r.
reflexive saccade
reflexogenic erection
reflux
    abdominal r.
    abdominojugular r.
    acid r.
    alkaline r.
    r. disease
    r. esophagitis
    gastric r.
    laryngopharyngeal r.
    r. menstruation
    saphenofemoral r.
    upright r.
    vesicoureteral r.
reformation
    fornix r.
    inferior fornix r.
reformulation
refractile body

NOTES

refractive
> r. keratoplasty
> r. keratotomy
> r. operative technique
> r. surgery

refractory
> r. ascites
> r. encephalopathy
> r. variceal hemorrhage

refrigeration anesthesia

regainer space

regenerate

regenerated esophageal epithelium

regeneration
> aberrant r.
> r. aberration
> atypical r.
> axonal r.
> carbon tetrachloride-induced liver r.
> compensatory r.
> epimorphic r.
> hepatic r.
> incomplete r.
> liver r.
> morphallactic r.
> r. motor unit potential
> nerve r.
> neuronal r.
> osteoblastic bone r.
> peripheral nerve r.
> squamous r.
> tibial bone defect r.
> tissue r.
> tubular r.

regimen
> adjuvant r.
> antifungal r.
> antiplatelet r.
> treatment r.

regio, pl. **regiones**

region
> abdominal r.
> anal r.
> ankle r.
> anterior antebrachial r.
> anterior brachial r.
> anterior knee r.
> argyrophilic nucleolar organizer r.
> axillary r.
> brachial r.
> brain r.
> calcaneal r.
> carpal r.
> choledochal r.
> epigastric r.
> femoral r.
> gastric pacemaker r.
> gluteal r.
> hilar r.

hypochondriac r.
hypogastric r.
ileocecal r.
iliac r.
inframammary r.
infraorbital r.
infrascapular r.
inguinal r.
knee r.
lateral r.
left hypochondriac r.
left lateral r.
lumbar r.
mammary r.
mental r.
nuchal r.
oral r.
orbital r.
PAG/PVG r.
paraaortic r.
parietal r.
penumbral r.
periaqueductal-periventricular r.
perineal r.
pharyngeal r.
pineal r.
popliteal r.
posterior antebrachial r.
posterior brachial r.
posterior knee r.
posterior neck r.
presternal r.
pubic r.
retroperitoneal r.
right hypochondriac r.
right iliac r.
right lateral r.
sacral r.
scapular r.
sternocleidomastoid r.
suboccipital r.
subphrenic r.
supraomental r.
suprapubic r.
sural r.
thoracoabdominal r.
umbilical r.
urogenital r.
vertebral r.
zygomatic r.

regional
> r. anesthetic
> r. anesthetic technique
> r. block
> r. cerebral blood flow (rCBF)
> r. flap
> r. hepatectomy
> r. hypoperfusion
> r. hypothermia

r. lymphadenectomy
r. lymph node basin
r. metastasis
r. node
r. saturation
r. ventilation
r. wall motion abnormality
regiones (*pl. of* regio)
registered nurse, first assist (RNFA)
registration
r. algorithm
image r.
robot-assisted r.
registry
Acoustic Neuroma R.
Autologous Bone and Marrow
Transplant R. (ABMTR)
Balloon Valvuloplasty R.
Brain Tumor R.
Kiel Pediatric Tumor R.
Mansfield Valvuloplasty R.
National Football Head and Neck
Injury R.
National Pediatric Trauma R.
(NPTR)
Ovarian Tumor R.
population-based r.
Renal Allograft Disease R.
St. Mark polyposis r.
tumor r.
United Kingdom Heart Valve R.
Regnault type B mastopexy
regression
clot r.
r. of thrombus
tumor r.
regressive-reconstructive approach
regular diet
regurgitant lesion
regurgitation
r. jaundice
r. test
rehabilitation stage
rehalation
Rehbein procedure
Rehfuss method
Rehne-Delorme plication
rehydrating solution
rehydration therapy
Reichel-Pólya
R.-P. method
R.-P. procedure

R.-P. stomach resection
R.-P. technique
Reichenheim-King procedure
Reichenheim technique
Reichert
R. cartilage
R. membrane
Reid base line
Reifenstein syndrome
Reilly body
reimplantation
aortorenal r.
Cohen cross-trigonal r.
end-to-side r.
intentional tooth r.
Politano-Leadbetter r.
ureteral r.
Reinert acetabular extensile approach
reinfection tuberculosis
reinforce
giant prosthetic r.
reinforcement
omental r.
pericardial r.
peritoneal r.
pleural patch r.
Stoppa giant prosthetic r.
reinjection protocol
Reinke
R. crystalloid
R. space
reinnervation
reinoculation
reinsemination
reintegrate
reintegration
reintubation
reinversion
reirrigation
Reisseisen muscle
Reissner membrane
Reis-Wertheim vaginal hysterectomy
Reiter
R. disease
R. syndrome
rejection
accelerated transplant r.
acute allograft r.
acute cellular r.
acute lung r.
acute vascular r.
allograft corneal r.

NOTES

rejection *(continued)*
r. cardiomyopathy transplant
cellular xenograft r.
chronic allograft r.
chronic transplant r.
delayed hyperacute transplant r.
ductopenic r.
fetal r.
fierce cellular r.
first-set graft r.
graft r.
homograft r.
hyperacute r.
interstitial r.
r. line
lung r.
marrow graft r.
maternal r.
no r.
no infection-no r.
primary r.
r. rejection
renal allograft r.
second-set graft r.
total graft area r.
transplant r.
vascular r.

rejuvenation

relapse
axillary r.
locoregional r.
lymphoma r.
r. rate

relapsing polychondritis

relation
acentric r.
acquired centric r.
acquired eccentric jaw r.
buccolingual r.
centric jaw r.
centric occluding r.
concentration-effect r.
convenience jaw r.
cusp-fossa r.
diastolic pressure-volume r.
Duane-Hunt r.
dynamic r.
eccentric jaw r.
end-systolic pressure-volume r.
end-systolic stress-dimension r.
equivalence r.
force-frequency r.
force-length r.
force-velocity r.
force-velocity-length r.
force-velocity-volume r.
Frank-Starling r.
intermaxillary r.
interval-strength r.

jaw r.
jaw-to-jaw r.
length-resting tension r.
length-tension r.
mandibular centric r.
maxillomandibular r.
median jaw r.
occluding r.
occlusal r.
posterior border jaw r.
pressure-flow r.
pressure-volume r.
protrusive jaw r.
resting length-tension r.
rest jaw r.
retruded jaw r.
ridge r.
static r.
tension-length r.
unstrained jaw r.
ventilation/perfusion r.
ventricular end-systolic pressure-volume r.
vertical r.
working bite r.

relationship
cause-effect r.
endoscope-body position r.
end-systolic pressure-length r. (ESPLR)
intraluminal pH-pressure r.
left ventricular pressure-volume r. (LVPVR)
pressure-flow r.
tissue-base r.
tumor cell-host bone r.
ventilation/perfusion r.

relative
r. curative resection
r. humidity
near-point r.
r. noncurative resection
r. response attributable to the maneuver
r. spectacle magnification

relaxant
depolarizing r.
muscle r.
neuromuscular r.
nondepolarizing r.
nondepolarizing muscle r.
r. reversal
smooth muscle r.

relaxation
adaptive r.
cardioesophageal r.
complete sphincter r.
diastolic r.
differential r.

dipolë-dipolë r.
dynamic r.
endothelial-dependent r.
endothelium-mediated r.
esophageal sphincter r.
incomplete r.
intraoperative stress r.
isovolumetric r.
isovolumic r.
longitudinal r.
lower esophageal sphincter r.
  (LESR)
r. method
nitric oxide blocked sphincter r.
paramagnetic shift r.
pelvic r.
r. phenomenon
r. rate
real adaptive r.
reciprocal r.
r. response
sinusoidal r.
smooth muscle r.
sphincter r.
stress r.
r. technique
r. time
r. time index
transverse r.
upper esophageal sphincter r.
uterine r.
ventricular r.

relaxing
r. incision
r. solution

release
de Quervain stenosing
  tenosynovitis r.
endoscopic carpal tunnel r. (ECTR)
endoscopic gastrocnemius r.
flexor-pronator origin r.
hilar r.
lateral extensor r.
modified 2-portal endoscopic carpal
  tunnel r.
physiologic pattern r.
plantar plate r.
pronator teres r.
soft tissue r.
suprahyoid laryngeal r.
sustained r. (SR)

reliability
interrater r.
relief
r. incision
r. space
symptomatic r.
relieving incision
remain
necrotic r.
Remak
R. ganglion
R. plexus
remargination
remedial
r. inguinal exploration
r. surgery
remifentanil
remission induction
remnant
cirrhotic liver r.
Cloquet canal r.
devascularized parathyroid r.
distal r.
esophageal r.
gastric r.
r. gland
r. liver volume
mucosal r.
parathyroid r.
pupillary membrane r.
remobilization
remodeling
extracellular matrix r.
tissue r.
r. of wound
remote
r. pedicle flap
r. tier
removable maintainer space
removal
Cameron femoral component r.
cast r.
cement r.
chordee r.
Collis-Dubrul femoral stem r.
colonoscopic r.
en bloc r.
endoscopic r.
excisional r.
extracorporeal CO_2 r. (ECOR)
femoral stem r.
forceps r.

NOTES

removal *(continued)*
    foreign body r.
    r. of foreign body
    gallbladder r.
    gastric coin r.
    gland r.
    Harris femoral component r.
    hump r.
    implant r.
    laparoscopic gallbladder r.
    lens r.
    macroscopic tumor r.
    mesh r.
    metastatic tumor r.
    Moreland-Marder-Anspach femoral
      stem r.
    nail fold r.
    nail plate r.
    path of r.
    percutaneous endoscopic r.
    percutaneous stone r.
    radical en bloc r.
    rib r.
    1-session r.
    small polyp r.
    stem r.
    stone r.
    through-the-scope balloon r.
    total surgical r.
    transsphenoidal r.
    tube r.
    tumor r.
    ureteral stoma r.
    Winograd nail plate r.

remyelination

remyelinization

renal
    r. abnormality
    r. adenocarcinoma
    r. adenoma
    r. allograft
    R. Allograft Disease Registry
    r. allograft rejection
    r. allograft rupture
    r. angiomyolipoma
    r. angioplasty
    r. anomaly
    r. arterial embolization
    r. artery
    r. artery occlusive disease
    r. artery orifice
    r. artery reconstruction
    r. artery response
    r. artery stenosis
    r. artery stenotic disease
    r. artery stenting
    r. artery thrombosis
    r. autotransplantation
    r. biopsy

r. branch
r. calculus
r. capsule
r. capsulotomy
r. cell carcinoma
r. colic
r. column
r. complication
r. compromise
r. cortex
r. cortical lobule
r. crush syndrome
r. cyst
r. cyst ablation
r. cyst decortication
r. cyst hemorrhage
r. cyst infection
r. cyst marsupialization
r. duplication
r. dysfunction
r. ectopia
r. failure
r. fascia
r. fistula
r. function
r. fungal infection
r. ganglion
r. hematoma
r. hyperfiltration
r. hypertension
r. impression
r. infarction
r. infusion therapy
r. injury repair
r. insufficiency
r. labyrinth
r. lobe
r. malrotation
r. management
r. manifestation
r. mass
r. mechanism
r. medulla
r. papilla
r. pelvis
r. pelvis carcinoma
r. plexus
r. pouch
r. preservation
r. proximal tubule preparation
r. punctum
r. pyramid
r. reflex
r. replacement therapy
r. revascularization
r. scintography
r. segment
r. sinus
r. sonography

r. stone
r. surface
r. thromboendarterectomy
r. transplantation
r. tubular acidosis
r. tumor
r. vascular disease
r. vasodilator prostaglandin
r. vein
r. vein renin concentration
vertebral, anus, tracheoesophageal, radial, and r. (VATER)
r. vessel

renal-sparing surgery
renal-splanchnic steal
renaturation
rendering
interactive volume r.
perspective volume r. (pVR)
renewal
tissue r.
renicapsule
renicardiac
reniculus, pl. **reniculi**
reniform pelvis
reninoma
reniportal
renocutaneous
renogastric fistula
renointestinal
renomegaly
renopathy
renoprival
renopulmonary
renorrhaphy
renovascular hypertension (RVH)
rent
dural r.
Rentrop classification
renunculus
reoperation
planned r.
reoperative
r. bariatric surgery
r. blepharoplasty
r. carotid surgery
r. coronary artery bypass graft (rCABG)
r. esthetic surgery
r. necrosectomy
r. parathyroidectomy

r. pelvic surgery
r. ureteroneocystostomy
reorganization
recovery and r.
reoxygenation
repair
Abraham-Pankovich tendo calcaneus r.
ACL r.
acromioclavicular joint r.
all-inside r.
Allison gastroesophageal reflux r.
Allison hiatal hernia r.
anal sphincter r.
anatomic r.
aneurysm r.
Anson-McVay hernia r.
anterior and posterior r.
aortic valve r.
A&P r.
Arlt epicanthus r.
Arlt eyelid r.
Atasoy-type r.
Bankart shoulder r.
Bassini inguinal hernia r.
Bassini-Stetten hernia r.
Belsey Mark IV r.
Belt-Fuqua hypospadias r.
bilateral inguinal hernia r.
bilayer patch hernia r.
Black r.
Blair epicanthus r.
blepharochalasis r.
blepharoptosis r.
Boari ureteral flap r.
Boerema hernia r.
bone graft r.
Bosworth tendo calcaneus r.
Boyd-Anderson biceps tendon r.
brachial plexus r.
Brom r.
Bunnell tendon r.
Cantwell-Ransley epispadias r.
Caspari r.
cemental r.
coarctation r.
Collis r.
columellar r.
complex syndactyly r.
cross-trigonal r.
crural r.
cystocele r.

NOTES

repair *(continued)*

Danus-Stanzel r.
DeBakey-Creech aneurysm r.
delayed primary r.
density-dependent r.
Devine hypospadias r.
diaphragmatic crural r.
dog-ear r.
dural r.
DuVries hammertoe r.
dynamic r.
early thoracoscopic r.
Ecker-Lotke-Glazer patellar
  tendon r.
Effler hiatal hernia r.
elective hernia r.
endoluminal r.
endoscopic mitral valve r.
endovascular r.
end-to-end tendon r.
end-to-side r.
epineural r.
episiotomy r.
epispadias r.
extensor tendon r.
exteriorized uterine r.
extracorporeal r.
extraperitoneal endoscopic hernia r.
fascicular r.
fibrous r.
first-stage r.
flexor tendon r.
Fontan r.
fracture r.
Froimson-Oh r.
functional r.
Gardner meningocele r.
glenohumeral dislocation r.
group fascicular r.
Halsted-Bassini hernia r.
Harrington-Allison r.
Harrington hernia r.
Hatafuku fundus onlay patch
  esophageal r.
hernia r.
Hill hiatus hernia r.
Hill median arcuate r.
histologic tooth r.
Hoguet pantaloon hernia r.
hypoplastic left heart r.
in situ uterine r.
in utero r.
Jones first-toe r.
Kelikian-Riashi-Gleason patellar
  tendon r.
Kessler r.
Kleinert r.
Konno r.
Kugel hernia r.
Kuhnt-Junius r.

lacrimal gland r.
Lange tendon lengthening and r.
laparoscopic IPOM r.
laparoscopic paraesophageal
  hernia r. (LPHR)
laparoscopic prosthetic mesh r.
laparoscopic varicocele r.
laparoscopic ventral hernia r.
laryngeal r.
Latzko vesicovaginal fistula r.
Le Fort-Wehrbein-Duplay
  hypospadias r.
levator aponeurosis r.
Lich-Gregoir r.
Lichtenstein hernial r.
Lichtenstein mesh r.
Lindholm tendo calcaneus r.
Lotheissen hernia r.
MacIntosh over-the-top r.
MacNab shoulder r.
Madden r.
MAGPI hypospadias r.
Ma-Griffith tendo calcaneus r.
Mandelbaum-Nartolozzi-Carney
  patellar tendon r.
Marcy hernia r.
Marlex hernial r.
McVay-Cooper ligament r.
McVay inguinal hernial r.
medial r.
meniscal r.
mesh r.
Millard rotation-advancement lip r.
minimally invasive mitral valve r.
mitral valve r.
Moloney hernia r.
myelomeningocele r.
Nissen r.
Noble-Mengert perineal r.
open r.
Orr rectal prolapse r.
Palmer-Dobyns-Linscheid ligament r.
pants-over-vest hernial r.
paravaginal defect r.
patellar tendon r.
pectus excavatum r.
periapical tooth r.
pericardioplasty in pectus
  excavatum r.
perineal r.
Phaneuf-Graves r.
plastic r.
plug prosthetic mesh r.
postanal r.
posterior r.
postoperative r.
potentially lethal x-ray damage r.
premuscular prosthetic r.
primary r.

prosthetic mesh r.
pseudarthrosis r.
pseudoarthrosis r.
pulmonary stenosis r.
radiographic tooth r.
Ransley-Cantwell r.
Rastelli r.
rectocele r.
renal injury r.
reverse sigma penoscrotal
 transposition r.
rod fracture r.
Rodney Smith biliary stricture r.
rotator cuff r.
Scuderi r.
secondary r.
Senning r.
Sever-L'Episcopo r.
shoulder r.
Shouldice-Bassini hernia r.
simple syndactyly r.
slipped Nissen r.
Speed sternoclavicular r.
sphincter r.
2-stage r.
staged abdominal r. (STAR)
1-stage hypospadias r.
Staples r.
Staples-Black-Broström ligament r.
Stoppa hernia r.
Stoppa-type laparoscopic r.
Strickland tendon r.
sublethal x-ray damage r.
surgical r.
suture r.
Talesnick scapholunate r.
tendon r.
Tennison-Randall lip r.
tension-free mesh r.
tension-free prosthetic mesh r.
TEP r.
Teuffer tendo calcaneus r.
Thal esophageal stricture r.
Theirsch-Duplay r.
thoracic aortic aneurysm r.
thoracoabdominal aortic aneurysm r.
thoracoscopic r.
tight Nissen r.
tissue r.
total extraperitoneal r.
tracheal r.
transabdominal preperitoneal r.

triad knee r.
trichiasis r.
tricuspid valve r.
triple ligamentous r.
Turco-Spinella tendo calcaneus r.
ultrasound-guided compression r.
 (UGCR)
unilateral inguinal hernia r.
vaginal-psoas suspension r.
vaginal wall r.
vascular laceration r.
Veirs canaliculus r.
vesicovaginal r.
vest-over-pants hernia r.
videoscopic r.
volar plate r.
Watson-Jones fracture r.
Wheeler halving r.
Y mesh hernia r.
York-Mason r.
Young type epispadias r.
Zancolli clawhand deformity r.

repairable parietal defect
reparative cardiac surgery
REPE
 reexpansion pulmonary edema
repeat
 r. balloon mitral valvotomy
 r. cesarean section
 r. operation
 r. procedure
 r. revascularization
repeated
 r. exposure
 r. respiratory infection
 r. tissue expansion
reperfusion
 r. injury
 ischemia and r. (I/R)
reperfusion-induced hemorrhage
reperitonealization
repetitive
 r. cluster
 r. nerve stimulation
rephasing
 echo r.
 even-echo r.
replacement
 anatomic porous r. (APR)
 aortic root r.
 aortic valve r.
 Cosgrove mitral valve r.

NOTES

replacement *(continued)*
    fluid r.
    heart valve r.
    hip r.
    homograft aortic valve r.
    joint r.
    knee r.
    laparoscopic feeding tube r.
    mitral valve r.
    mucosal patch r.
    Mueller-type femoral head r.
    pulmonary valve r.
    supraannular mitral valve r.
    tile plate facet r.
    total hip r.
    total joint r.
    total knee r.
    tube r.
    valve r.
    valve-sparing aortic root r.
replant
replantation
    intentional r.
    limb r.
repolarization
reposit
reposition
repositioning
    muscle r.
repreparation
reproductive
    r. tract
    r. tract abnormality
requirement
    anticoagulation monitoring r.
re-resected
re-resecting
re-resection
rerouting insertion
rerupture
rescue
    r. analgesia
    r. angioplasty
    r. antiemetic
    failure to r.
    propofol r.
    r. surgery
    r. technique
    r. therapy
resect
resectability
    r. rate
    surgical r.
    tumor r.
resectable
    r. carcinoma
    r. extrahepatic recurrence
    r. hepatic disease
    r. liver metastasis

    r. periampullary cancer
    r. tumor
resection
    abdominal-perineal r.
    abdominoperineal r. (APR)
    abdominosacral r.
    absolute curative r.
    absolute noncurative r.
    activation map-guided surgical r.
    anterior r.
    r. arthrodesis
    r. arthroplasty
    atrial septal r.
    Badgley iliac wing r.
    bar r.
    bilateral r.
    bilobar r.
    bleb r.
    bone r.
    bony bridge r.
    bowel r.
    breast r.
    bronchial sleeve r.
    calcaneonavicular bar r.
    Carrell r.
    caudal lamina r.
    cesarean r.
    classical subtotal r.
    Clayton procedure with
      panmetatarsal head r.
    cold-cup r.
    coloanal r.
    colon r.
    colonic r.
    colorectal cancer r.
    colosigmoid r.
    combined gastrointestinal r.
    combined organ r.
    complete r.
    composite pelvic r.
    condyle r.
    conservative r.
    craniofacial en bloc r.
    CRC r.
    cricotracheal r.
    cryo-assisted r.
    cuff r.
    curative r.
    D2 r.
    Darrach r.
    definitive r.
    r. dermodesis
    diathermic r.
    Dillwyn-Evans r.
    elective sigmoid r.
    electrocautery r.
    en bloc vein r.
    endocardial r.
    endometrial r.

R

endoscopic mucosal r. (EMR)
endoscopic snare r.
end-to-end ileoanal anastomosis
  without mucosal r.
epidermoid r.
epiphysial bar r.
esophageal r.
esophagogastric r.
ex situ-in situ liver r.
extended r.
extraarticular r.
ex vivo r.
femoral r.
formal hepatic r.
gastric leiomyoma r.
gastrointestinal r.
Girdlestone r.
Guller r.
gum r.
Gurd r.
Hartmann r.
Henry r.
hepatic r.
Hoffmann panmetatarsal head r.
hyoid bone r.
ileal r.
ileocolic r.
ileocolonic r.
iliac crest r.
iliac wing r.
incomplete tumor r.
infundibular wedge r.
Ingram bony bridge r.
initial r.
innominate bone r.
intercalary r.
interdental r.
intestinal r.
intragastric r.
Ivor-Lewis r.
Janecki-Nelson shoulder girdle r.
Karakousis-Vezeridis r.
kyphos r.
Langenskiöld bony bridge r.
laparoscopic-assisted small bowel r.
laparoscopic bowel r.
laparoscopic intragastric r.
lateral rectus r.
LCVP-aided hepatic r.
LCVP-assisted major liver r.
lesser r.
levator r.

Lewis-Chekofsky r.
Lewis intercalary r.
limited r.
liver r.
lobar r.
lobe r.
local radical r.
low anterior r. (LAR)
major liver r. (MLR)
Mankin r.
Marcove-Lewis-Huvos shoulder
  girdle r.
margin r.
r. margin
marginal r.
massive bowel r.
medial malleolus r.
metatarsal head r.
microscopic r.
Milch cuff r.
Miles abdominoperineal r.
Miltner-Wan calcaneus r.
minimal transurethral r.
Mohs microsurgical r.
mucosal r.
multiple-punch r.
multisegmental r.
Mumford r.
muscle r.
myotomy-myectomy-septal r.
nipple-flat duct r.
nonanatomic wedge r.
ovarian wedge r.
palliative r.
pancreatic r.
pancreaticoduodenal r.
pancreatic tail r.
panmetatarsal head r.
parotid r.
partial cricotracheal r.
partial gastric r.
Paul-Mikulicz r.
Peet splanchnic r.
Peyman full-thickness eye wall r.
Phelps partial r.
portal vein r.
presacral r.
primary r.
prophylactic r.
proximal femoral r.
proximal gastric r.
pulmonary r.

NOTES

resection *(continued)*
  punch r.
  radical gastric r.
  radical subtotal r.
  Radley-Liebig-Brown r.
  ray r.
  reduction before r.
  Reichel-Pólya stomach r.
  relative curative r.
  relative noncurative r.
  rim r.
  Rockwood r.
  root end r.
  R0, R1, R2 r.
  scleral r.
  sectoral r.
  sectorial r.
  segmental colonic r.
  segmental lung r.
  segmental pulmonary r.
  segment-oriented hepatic r.
  segment-oriented liver r.
  septal r.
  shoulder girdle r.
  sleeve r.
  sphincter-sparing r.
  spleen-preserving pancreatic r.
  standard gastric r.
  Stener-Gunterberg r.
  stomach r.
  strip r.
  subcomplete r.
  submucous r.
  subperiosteal r.
  subtotal gastric r.
  surgical r.
  synchronous r.
  terminal ileal r.
  Thompson r.
  thyroid r.
  Tikhoff-Linberg shoulder girdle r.
  Torek r.
  Torpin cul-de-sac r.
  tracheal r.
  transanal endoscopic
    microsurgical r.
  transcervical r.
  transoral odontoid r.
  transsphenoidal microsurgical r.
  transsphenoidal pituitary r.
  transthoracic vertebral body r.
  transurethral r.
  transverse r.
  tumor r.
  ultralow anterior r.
  unilateral r.
  VATS wedge r.
  vertebral r.
  Weaver-Dunn r.

  wedge r.
  Whipple r.
resectional
  r. phase
  r. phase of operation
  r. technique
resection-arthrodesis
  Enneking r.-a.
resection-realignment
resective
  r. colostomy
  r. surgery
resectoscopy
resedation
reserve
  hepatic function r.
  life-sustaining hepatic r.
reservoir
  r. host
  r. of infection
  r. mucosal absorption
  r. phase
  pressurized r.
residual
  r. abscess
  r. body
  r. cleft
  r. cyst
  r. cystic cavity
  r. DCIS
  r. disease
  r. ductal tissue
  r. focus
  r. fragment
  r. lesion
  r. mesorectum
  r. neck
  r. neuromuscular blockade
residue
  pharyngeal r.
resin
  r. condensation
  r. restoration
resistance
  activated protein C r.
  alkylation r.
  aortic valve r.
  cerebrovascular r. (CVR)
  drug r.
  extreme drug r. (EDR)
  increased systemic vascular r.
  insulin r.
  loss of r. (LOR)
  mean airway r.
  peripheral insulin r.
  pulmonary vascular r. (PVR)
  respiratory system r.
  systemic vascular r.
  tissue r.

resolution
    spontaneous r.
resolvent
resonance
    r. line
    magnetic r. (MR)
    nuclear magnetic r. (NMR)
resonant abdomen
resorption
respirable aerosol
respiration
    abdominal r.
    absent r.
    accelerated r.
    aerobic r.
    agonal r.
    amphoric r.
    anaerobic r.
    apneustic r.
    artificial r.
    assisted r.
    asthmoid r.
    Austin Flint r.
    Biot r.
    Bouchut r.
    bronchial r.
    bronchocavernous r.
    bronchovesicular r.
    cavernous r.
    central r.
    cerebral r.
    Cheyne-Stokes r.
    cogwheel r.
    collateral r.
    controlled diaphragmatic r.
    Corrigan r.
    cortical r.
    costal r.
    cyclic r.
    decreased r.
    diaphragmatic r.
    diaphragmatic-abdominal r.
    diffusion r.
    direct r.
    divided r.
    electrophrenic r.
    external r.
    forced r.
    granular r.
    grunting r.
    harsh r.
    internal r.

    interrupted r.
    intrauterine r.
    jerky r.
    Kussmaul r.
    Kussmaul-Kien r.
    labored r.
    laryngeal r.
    meningitic r.
    metamorphosing r.
    mouth-to-mouth r.
    nasal r.
    nervous r.
    opposition r.
    oral r.
    paradoxical r.
    periodic r.
    placental r.
    puerile r.
    radiofrequency electrophrenic r.
    rude r.
    Seitz metamorphosing r.
    shallow r.
    sighing r.
    slow r.
    sonorous r.
    stertorous r.
    stridulous r.
    supplementary r.
    suppressed r.
    temperature, pulse, r. (TPR)
    thoracic r.
    tissue r.
    transitional r.
    tubular r.
    ventilator-assisted r.
    vesiculocavernous r.
    vicarious r.
    wavy r.
respirator
    r. brain
    r. lung
respiratory
    r. ataxia
    r. bronchiole
    r. bundle
    r. care
    r. complication
    r. compromise
    r. depression
    r. distress syndrome (RDS)
    r. exchange
    r. excursion

R

NOTES

respiratory *(continued)*
- r. failure
- r. frequency
- r. insufficiency
- r. inversion point
- r. kinetic therapy
- r. minute volume
- r. quotient
- r. syncytial virus conduit
- r. syncytial virus infection
- r. system resistance
- r. tract
- r. tract fluid
- r. tract infection

respiratory-esophageal fistula

response
- anabolic r.
- auditory middle lateral r. (AMLR)
- baroreflex r.
- biobehavioral r.
- brainstem evoked r.
- callus r.
- canal resonance r.
- carbon dioxide r.
- central carbon dioxide ventilatory r.
- clinical r.
- Cushing pressure r.
- deconditioned exercise r.
- detector r.
- foreign body r.
- hemodynamic r.
- hepatic arterial buffer r.
- hypercapnic ventilatory r.
- hypercontractile external sphincter r.
- hypermetabolic r.
- hypnotic r.
- hypoxic ventilatory r.
- immune r.
- implantation r.
- inflammatory r.
- irritant patch-test r.
- lactation letdown r.
- local twitch r. (LTR)
- metabolic r.
- middle latency auditory evoked r. (MLAER)
- motor r.
- motor-evoked r. (MER)
- oxygen-related r.
- paired vasomotor r.
- postburn hypermetabolic r.
- radiation r.
- relaxation r.
- renal artery r.
- senior-level trauma-team r.
- sensitization r.
- skin potential r.
- snout r.
- steady-state auditory evoked r. (SSAER)
- steady-state ventilatory r.
- stress r.
- sympathoadrenal r.
- sympathoexcitatory r.
- transient auditory evoked r. (TAER)
- transient hyperemic r.
- twitch r.
- ventilatory r.
- white line r.

responsiveness
- airway r.
- baroreflex r.

rest
- r. jaw relation
- r. position
- thyroid r.
- thyrothymic thyroid r.

restenosis
- aortic valve r.
- r. lesion
- postangioplasty r.
- postballoon angioplasty r.
- pulmonary valve r.

restiform body

resting
- r. anal sphincter pressure
- r. energy expenditure
- r. length-tension relation
- r. line
- r. membrane potential
- r. urethral pressure profile

restoration
- acid-etched r.
- adhesive resin-bonded cast r.
- alloy r.
- amalgam r.
- Berens-Smith cul-de-sac r.
- bonded cast r.
- buccal r.
- ceramic r.
- ceramometal r.
- combination r.
- composite resin r.
- compound r.
- contour r.
- r. contour
- crown r.
- cul-de-sac r.
- cusp r.
- dental r.
- direct acrylic r.
- direct composite resin r.
- direct gold r.
- distal extension r.
- esthetic r.
- facial r.

R

facilitating r.
faulty r.
foreskin r.
full cast r.
implant r.
inlay r.
intermediate r.
intrinsic r.
large r.
maxillary r.
metal-ceramic r.
metallic r.
overhanging r.
overlay r.
permanent r.
physical r.
pinch r.
pin-supported r.
r. point
porcelain-bonded r.
porcelain-fused-to-metal r.
porcelain jacket r.
postcore r.
prosthetic r.
provisional r.
resin r.
root canal r.
silicate r.
silver amalgam r.
temporary r.
voice r.
restorative
r. colectomy
r. fixation
r. procedure
r. proctectomy
r. proctocolectomy
r. proctocolectomy technique
restriction
r. endonuclease analysis
extension r.
r. fragment length
soft tissue r.
result
angiographic r.
cosmetic r.
cytologic r.
false-negative r.
false-positive r.
histologic r.
indocyanine green clearance r.
operative r.

postoperative r.
postprandial motor r.
short-term r.
Surveillance, Epidemiology and
End R. (SEER)
true-negative r.
true-positive r.
resurfacing
facial laser r.
r. operation
r. procedure
resurgence
resuscitate
resuscitated by volume
resuscitation
blood substitute r.
cardiac r.
cardiopulmonary r. (CPR)
delayed r.
emergency department r.
r. endpoint
fluid r.
heart-lung r.
hypertonic-hyperoncotic fluid r.
hypotensive r.
inotrope r.
intrauterine r.
mouth-to-mouth r.
neonatal r.
newborn r.
r. period
prehospital r.
r. process
r. protocol
rapid volume r.
supranormal r.
supraphysiologic r.
resuscitation-induced pulmonary apoptosis
resuscitative
r. endpoint
r. fluid
r. thoracotomy
retained
r. foreign body
r. papilla technique
r. placental fragment
retainer closure
retard
expiratory r.
retardation
developmental r.

NOTES

retardation *(continued)*
    fetal growth r.
    growth r.
    healing r.
    intrauterine growth r.
    psychomotor r.
retching
rete, pl. **retia**
    r. cord
    Haller r.
retention
    r. cyst
    extracoronal r.
    intracoronal-extracoronal r.
    r. mucocele
    pin r.
    r. point
    surgical r.
    r. suture bridge
    r. suture technique
    throat pack r.
    urinary r.
    viscera r.
retentive fulcrum line
Rethi incision
retia (*pl. of* rete)
retial
reticula (*pl. of* reticulum)
reticular
    r. formation
    r. lesion
    r. membrane
    r. vein
reticulate pigmented anomaly
reticulation
reticuloendothelioma
reticulogranuloma
reticulohistiocytoma
reticulospinal tract
reticulotomy
reticulum, pl. **reticula**
    Ebner r.
    endoplasmic r.
    extraconal fat r.
retina
retinaculum, pl. **retinacula**
    antebrachial flexor r.
    caudal r.
    extensor r.
    Morgagni r.
    patellar r.
    peroneal r.
    superior peroneal r.
retinal
    r. arteriovenous malformation
    r. circulation
    r. examination
    r. excavation
    r. exudate

    r. flap
    r. fold
    r. hemorrhage
    r. imbrication
    r. involvement
    r. macula
    r. migraine
    r. phacoma
    r. pigment epithelial cell
    r. quadrant neovascularization
    r. scatter photocoagulation
    r. surgeon
    r. surgery
    r. treatment
retinectomy
retinitis
retinoblastoma
retinoblastoma-mental retardation syndrome
retinochoroidectomy
retinocytoma
retinoic acid
retinopathy
    diabetic r.
    r. hemorrhage
retinopexy
    pneumatic r.
retinophotoscopy
retinoscopy
    Copeland r.
    cylinder r.
    fogging r.
    streak r.
retinotomy
retothelioma
retract
retracted stoma
retractile testis
retraction
    r. of clot
    downward r.
    lateral r.
    nipple r.
    panniculus r.
    scar r.
    soft palate r.
    r. space
    stomal r.
    wound r.
retractor
    acetabular r.
    fan-type r.
    minimal incision total hip r.
    r. plication
    sciatic nerve r.
retraining
    computerized diaphragmatic
      breathing r. (CDBR)

retransplantation
    cardiac r.
retreat
    stabilization on r.
retreatment
    lithotripsy r.
retrenchment
retrieval
    foreign body r.
    intravascular foreign body r.
    transvaginal oocyte r. (TVOR)
    transvaginal ultrasonically guided
      oocyte r.
retroacetabular lesion
retroadductor space
retroarytenoidal edema
retroauricular
    r. free flap
    r. incision
    r. node
retrobulbar
    r. anesthesia
    r. anesthetic technique
    r. hemorrhage
    r. injection
    r. mass
    r. nerve block
    r. orbital metastasis
    r. space
retrocalcaneal bursa
retrocardiac
    r. mass
    r. space
retrocaval ureter
retrocecal
    r. abscess
    r. hernia
    r. recess
retrocervical
retrochiasmal
    r. lesion
    r. optic tract
retroclavicular injury
retroclination
retroclival structure
retroclusion
retrocolic
    r. end-to-end pancreatojejunostomy
    r. end-to-side choledochojejunostomy
    r. end-to-side gastrojejunostomy
    r. hernia
    r. position

retrocorneal membrane
retrocrural
    r. approach
    r. celiac plexus block
    r. space
retrocuspid papilla
retrodeviation
retrodiscal, retrodiskal
    r. pad
    r. temporomandibular joint pad
      inflammation
retrodisplacement
retroduodenal
    r. artery
    r. fossa
    r. perforation
    r. recess
retroesophageal
    r. artery
    r. space
retrofilling method
retroflected
retroflection
retroflexed
retroflexion
    endoscopic r.
retrogasserian
    r. glycerol injection
    r. neurectomy
    r. neurotomy
    r. procedure
retrogastric
    r. dissection
    r. space
retrogeniculate lesion
retrograde
    r. atrial activation mapping
    r. balloon rupture
    r. cannulation
    r. catheter insertion
    r. catheterization
    r. cholangiogram
    r. cholecystectomy
    r. collateral endoleak
    r. direction
    r. duodenogastroscopy
    r. endoscopic approach
    r. femoral approach
    r. hernia
    r. incarceration
    r. insertion point
    r. intrarenal surgery

R

NOTES

retrograde *(continued)*
    myocardium r.
    r. nailing
    r. nephrostomy puncture
    r. obturation
    r. root canal filling method
    r. sphincterotomy
    r. tracheal intubation anesthetic
      technique
    r. transurethral prostatic
      urethroplasty
    r. vascularization of superior
      mesenteric artery
retrohepatic
    r. inferior vena cava
    r. IVC
    r. vein
retrohyoid bursa
retroiliac ureter
retroillumination
retroinguinal space
retrojection
retrojector
retrolabyrinthine
    r. presigmoid approach
    r. vestibular neurectomy
**retrolabyrinthine-retrosigmoid vestibular
neurectomy**
retrolental space
retrolingual
retrolisthesis positional dyskinesia
retromammary space
retromandibular
    r. fossa
    r. point
    r. vein
retromastoid suboccipital craniectomy
retromolar
    r. fossa
    r. pad
    r. papilla
    r. triangle
retromuscular
    r. position
    r. prosthetic technique
    r. space
retromylohyoid space
retroocular space
retropancreatic lymph node basin
retropatellar fat pad
retroperitoneal
    r. adenopathy
    r. approach
    r. bleeding
    r. cavity
    r. cutaneous ureterostomy
    r. decompression
    r. fistula
    r. gas insufflation

    r. hematoma
    r. hemorrhage
    r. hernia
    r. infection
    r. lymphadenectomy
    r. lymph node dissection (RPLND)
    r. node
    r. pancreas
    r. pelvic lymph node dissection
      (RPLND)
    r. perforation
    r. pneumography
    r. primary rhabdomyosarcoma
    r. region
    r. soft tissue
    r. space
    r. structure
    r. viscus
retroperitoneal-iliopsoas abscess
retroperitoneoscopic nephrectomy
retroperitoneoscopy
retroperitoneum
retroperitonitis
retropharyngeal
    r. approach
    r. hematoma
    r. hemorrhage
    r. node
    r. soft tissue
    r. space
retropharynx
retroplacental hematoma
retroposed
retroposition
retropubic
    r. colpourethrocystopexy
    r. hernia
    r. Lapides-Ball bladder neck
      suspension
    r. space
    r. urethrolysis
    r. urethropexy
    r. urethroscopy
    r. vesiculoprostatectomy
retropulsed bone excision
retropulsion
retropyloric node
retrorectal abscess
retrosacral fascia
retrosellar structure
retrosigmoid approach
retrospection
retrospective analysis
retrosphenoidal syndrome
retrosternal
    r. air space
    r. approach
    r. dislocation
    r. gland

r. hernia
r. mass
r. route
retrotracheal space
retrouterine
retroversioflexion
retroversion
retroverted
retrovesical space
retrovirus infection
retrovisceral
r. fascia
r. space
retrozygomatic space
retruded
r. jaw relation
r. position
retrusive excursion
return
pulmonary venous r.
total anomalous pulmonary
venous r.
venous r.
Retzius
R. cavity
line of R.
R. space
reunient
reuptake-inhibitor
monoamine r.-i.
revaccination
revascularization
arrested-heart r.
arterial r.
brain r.
cerebral r.
coronary r.
heart laser r.
hybrid myocardial r.
lower extremity r.
myocardial r.
penile r.
percutaneous transluminal
coronary r.
r. procedure
renal r.
repeat r.
transmyocardial carbon dioxide
laser r.
transmyocardial laser r. (TMLR,
TMR)
revascularized tissue

reverberation
echo r.
r. room
Reverdin
R. bunionectomy
R. epidermal free graft
R. method
R. osteotomy
Reverdin-Laird
R.-L. bunionectomy
R.-L. osteotomy
Reverdin-McBride bunionectomy
reversal
ileostomy r.
r. jejunoileal bypass surgery
JIB r.
r. line
narcotic r.
r. pedicle flap
pressure r.
relaxant r.
sex r.
unfractionated heparin r.
vasectomy r.
reverse
r. augmentation
r. Barton fracture
r. bevel incision
r. Bigelow maneuver
r. Colles fracture
r. cross-finger flap
r. Dillwyn-Evans calcaneal
osteotomy
r. Eck fistula
r. filling procedure
r. forearm island flap
r. gastric tube esophagoplasty
r. Hill-Sachs lesion
r. Mauck procedure
r. Monteggia fracture
r. phonation
r. Putti-Platt procedure
r. sigma penoscrotal transposition
repair
r. steal effect
r. topographic projection
r. transcriptase-polymerase chain
reaction (RT-PCR)
r. Trendelenburg position
r. wedge osteotomy
r. wedge technique

R

NOTES

reversed
r. left saphenous vein bypass graft
r. reimplanted appendicocystostomy
reverse-Y incision
reversible
r. decortication
r. shock
revision
r. hip arthroplasty
r. laparoscopy
r. procedure
shunt r.
revivification
revulsion
rewarming
Rex-Cantli-Serege line
RFCA
radiofrequency catheter ablation
RFTA
radiofrequency thermal ablation
rhabdomyolysis
acute recurrent r.
exertional r.
familial paroxysmal r.
hypoxia-induced r.
idiopathic paroxysmal r.
rhabdomyoma
cardiac r.
clinically silent r.
rhabdomyosarcoma
abdominal wall r.
advanced retroperitoneal r.
alveolar r.
primary r.
retroperitoneal primary r.
vaginal r.
rhabdosarcoma
rhabdosphincter
rhachotomy
Capener lateral r.
decompression r.
lateral r.
rhegma
rhegmatogenous
rheologic therapy
rheolytic catheter thrombectomy
Rhese
R. position
R. projection
rheumatica
polymyalgia r.
rheumatoid arthritis
rheumatoid-related ulceration
rhexis
hemorrhage per r.
rhinitis
rhinocanthectomy
rhinocerebral infection
rhinocheiloplasty

rhinocleisis
rhinodymia
rhinokyphectomy
rhinology
rhinometry
acoustic r.
rhinopharyngeal
rhinopharynx
rhinoplasty
English r.
esthetic r.
Indian r.
Italian r.
Joseph r.
rhinoscleroma
rhinoscopy
rhinoseptal approach
rhinotomy
rhizolysis
chemical r.
percutaneous glycerol r.
percutaneous radiofrequency r.
percutaneous retrogasserian
glycerol r.
Rhizopus **infection**
rhizotomy
anterior r.
bilateral ventral r.
cranial nerve r.
Dana posterior r.
dorsal r.
facet r.
Frazier-Spiller r.
glycerol r.
intracranial r.
intradural dorsal spinal root r.
percutaneous radiofrequency
dorsal r.
posterior r.
radiofrequency r.
selective posterior r. (SPR)
selective sacral r.
thermal r.
trigeminal r.
rhombic
rhomboatloideus
rhombocele
rhomboid
r. ligament
r. major muscle
r. minor muscle
r. transposition flap
rhomboidal sinus
rhonchus, pl. **rhonchi**
expiratory rhonchi
rhoton suction
rhythm
ectopic r.
fibrillation r.

R

r. method
sinus r. (SR)
rhythmic
r. initiation technique
r. stabilization
rhytide
rhytidectomy
rhytidoplasty
rib
bicipital r.
bifid r.
cervical r.
costochondral r.
r. diastasis
double-exposed r.
false r.
floating r.
r. fracture
lumbar r.
r. notching
pillar r.
r. removal
slipping r.
r. tip syndrome
true r.
vertebral r.
vertebrochondral r.
vertebrosternal r.
ribbon
r. arch technique
r. muscle
rib-cage volume
Ribes ganglion
rice body
Richard fringe
Richardson
R. procedure
R. suture technique
Riche-Cannieu anastomosis
Richet operation
Richter
R. and Albrich procedure
R. hernia
R. suture technique
Richter-Monro line
rickets
celiac r.
Ricketts-Abrams technique
rickettsial infection
Rideal-Walker method
Rideau technique

ridge
bicipital r.
epidermal r.
r. extension
external oblique r.
mesonephric r.
mylohyoid r.
osteochondral r.
Passavant r.
petrous r.
pharyngeal r.
r. relation
sphenoidal r.
supraorbital r.
temporal r.
trapezoid r.
urogenital r.
Ridley sinus
Ridlon procedure
Riedel
R. frontoethmoidectomy procedure
R. lobe
Rieger syndrome
Rieux hernia
Righini procedure
right
r. acromiodorsoposterior position
r. anterior oblique (RAO)
r. anterior oblique angulation
r. anterior oblique position
r. anterior occipital (RAO)
r. anterior pararenal space
r. atrial pressure
r. branch
r. bundle branch block
r. caudate lobe
r. colic artery
r. common iliac nerve
r. coronary valve
r. crural area
deviation to the r.
r. femoral artery
r. fibrous trigone
r. heart catheterization
r. hemidiaphragm
r. hypochondriac region
r. iliac region
r. inguinal hernia (RIH)
r. lateral region
r. lobe hepatectomy
r. lower extremity (RLE)
r. lower quadrant (RLQ)

NOTES

right (*continued*)
    r. lymphatic duct
    r. main bronchus
    r. middle suprarenal artery
    r. midinguinal line
    r. obturator artery
    r. ovary
    r. prostatic ligament
    r. replaced hepatic artery
    r. rotation
    r. sagittal fissure
    r. septal valve
    r. sigmoid sinus
    r. subclavian artery
    r. subclavian vessel
    r. temporoparietal craniotomy
    r. testicular artery
    r. thorax
    r. triangular ligament
    r. umbilical fold
    r. upper extremity (RUE)
    r. upper quadrant (RUQ)
    r. upper quadrant peritonectomy
    r. ventricle
    r. ventricle-pulmonary artery
    conduit surgery
    r. ventricular end-diastolic pressure
    r. ventricular outflow tract (RVOT)
    r. ventricular outflow tract
    tachycardia
    R. Ventricular Stroke Work Index
    (RVSWI)
    r. ventricular systolic pressure
right-angled end-to-side anastomosis
right-angle technique
right-sided
    r.-s. injury
    r.-s. lesion
    r.-s. submandibular transverse
    incision
    r.-s. thoracotomy
right-side-down position
right-to-left shunt ratio
rigid
    r. body
    r. bronchoscopy
    r. cervical immobilization
    r. endofluoroscopy
    r. endoscopic surgery
    r. graft
    r. internal fixation
    r. plate fixation
    r. proctoscopy
    r. proctosigmoidoscopy
    r. ureteroscopy
rigidity
    abdominal r.
    boardlike r.
    spinal fixation r.

rigors
    frank r.
RIH
    right inguinal hernia
Riley-Day syndrome
Riley-Smith syndrome
rim
    r. incision
    palpebral r.
    r. resection
    surgical occlusion r.
rima, pl. **rimae**
rim-enhancing lesion
ring
    abdominal r.
    abscess r.
    r. abscess
    acetabular reinforcement r.
    amnion r.
    anorectal r.
    anterior limiting r.
    aortic r.
    r. apophysis
    arterial r.
    atrial r.
    atrioventricular r.
    B r.
    r. block
    r. block digital anesthetic
    cardiac lymphatic r.
    cataract mask r.
    choroidal r.
    ciliary r.
    Coats white r.
    collagenous trabecular r.
    common annular r.
    common tendinous r.
    congenital r.
    conjunctival r.
    constriction r.
    contractile r.
    coronary r.
    corrin r.
    cricoid r.
    crural r.
    deep inguinal r.
    distal esophageal r.
    double r.
    doughnut r.
    drop-lock r.
    dural r.
    enhancing r.
    epiphysial r.
    r. epiphysis
    esophageal A, B r.
    esophageal contractile r.
    esophageal contraction r.
    esophageal mucosal r.
    esophageal muscular r.

external inguinal r.
extracapsular arterial r.
femoral r.
fibrous r.
r. finger
r. fracture
glaucomatous r.
glial r.
gold r.
greater r.
head r.
hymenal r.
ilioinguinal r.
iliopsoas r.
inguinal r.
internal abdominal r.
internal inguinal r.
iris r.
ischial weightbearing r.
lenticular r.
r. lesion
lesser r.
lymphoid r.
mucosal esophageal r.
muscular esophageal r.
narrow internal r.
neonatal r.
orthosis drop-lock r.
osseoligamentous r.
palatopharyngeal r.
pathologic retraction r.
pelvic r.
perichondral r.
periureteric venous r.
physiologic retraction r.
Placido r.
posterior limiting r.
pressure r.
pressure-point tension r.
protrusio r.
proximal-to-distal r.
pyloric r.
reduction r.
rust r.
Schatzki esophageal r.
Schwalbe anterior border r.
scotoma r.
Soemmerring r.
r. structure
subcutaneous r.
symblepharon r.

tentorial r.
tracheal r.
trigonal r.
T-shaped constriction r.
tympanic r.
r. ulcer
umbilical r.
vascular r.
Vieussens r.
Waldeyer r.
white r.
wide internal inguinal r.
ring-disrupting fracture
Ringer arthroscopy
ring-form congenital cataract
ring-shaped cataract
ring-wall lesion
ringworm
Rinkel serial endpoint titration
Riolan
　　R. anastomosis
　　R. arc
　　R. arcade
　　R. bone
　　R. muscle
Riordan
　　R. pollicization
　　R. tendon transfer technique
Ripstein
　　R. anterior sling rectopexy
　　R. procedure
　　R. rectal prolapse operation
Risdon approach
rise
　　pressure r.
Riseborough-Radin intercondylar fracture classification
risk
　　anesthetic r.
　　bleeding r.
　　breast cancer r.
　　r. factor
　　Goldman classification operative r.
　　inherent r.
　　r. management
　　r. management of anesthesia
　　perforation r.
　　radiation r.
　　r. reduction
　　surgical r.
risorius muscle

NOTES

Risser
- R. method
- R. technique

Ritgen maneuver

Ritter-Oleson technique

Riva-Rocci method

Rives splenectomy

Rivinus
- R. canal
- R. duct
- R. gland

Rizzoli operation

RK
- radial keratotomy

RLE
- right lower extremity

RLN
- recurrent laryngeal nerve

RLQ
- right lower quadrant

RLT
- reduced liver transplant

RNFA
- registered nurse, first assist

Roaf syndrome

Robert pelvis

Roberts
- R. approach
- R. syndrome
- R. technique

robertsonian fusion

Robertson incision

Robinson
- R. anterior cervical discectomy
- R. cervical spine fusion
- R. morcellation

Robinson-Southwick fusion technique

robot
- parallel r.

robot-assisted
- r.-a. laparoscopy
- r.-a. registration
- r.-a. surgery (RAS)

robotic
- r. approach
- r. probing
- r. surgery

robotic-assisted laparoscopic bariatric surgery

robotic-enhanced Dresden technique

Robson
- R. point
- R. position

Rochester method

Rockwood
- R. acromioclavicular injury classification
- R. clavicular fracture classification
- R. posterior capsulorrhaphy

- R. procedure
- R. resection

Rockwood-Green technique

Rockwood-Matsen capsular shift procedure

rod
- r. cell
- r. contour preparation
- r. fiber
- r. fracture repair
- r. granule
- r. migration
- r. placement
- r. rotation prevention
- r. sleeve fixation
- r. spherule

Rodeck method

rodless end-loop stoma

Rodman incision

Rodney Smith biliary stricture repair

Roeder loop knot

roentgenographic evaluation

Rogers cervical fusion technique

Röhrer index

Rokitansky hernia

rolandic
- r. artery
- r. line
- r. vein

Rolando
- R. fissure
- R. fracture
- R. vein

role
- r. fixation
- inhibitory r.

roll
- iliac r.
- scleral r.
- r. stitch

rolled shoulder lesion

rollerball
- r. endometrial ablation
- r. technique

Rollet incision

rolling
- r. hiatal hernia
- r. membrane

roll-tube technique

ROM
- range of motion
- rupture of membranes

rongeured

Rood technique

roof fracture

roof-patch graft

room
- emergency r. (ER)
- operating r. (OR)

recovery r.
reverberation r.
surgical dressing r.
trauma r.
Roos approach
root
accessory nerve r.
r. amputation
anatomical r.
r. anomaly
ansa cervicalis r.
anterior r.
bifurcation of r.
r. canal
r. canal access
r. canal débridement
r. canal disinfection
r. canal electrosterilization
r. canal filling
r. canal filling technique obturation
r. canal ionization
r. canal orifice
r. canal point
r. canal restoration
r. canal shaping
r. canal sterilization
r. canal therapy
r. canal treatment
ciliary ganglion r.
r. compression
dorsal r.
dural nerve r.
r. end resection
facial r.
facial nerve r.
r. formation
r. fracture
r. furcation
r. fusion
glossopharyngeal nerve r.
r. infiltration
r. injection
lateral r.
nail r.
nerve r.
r. perforation
posterior r.
spinal r.
trigeminal nerve r.
vagus nerve r.
ventral r.
Root-Siegal varus derotational osteotomy

rope flap
Rorabeck fasciotomy
Rosalki technique
Rosch modification
Rose
R. position
R. procedure
rosebud stoma
Rosenberg endoscopic anterior cruciate ligament reconstruction
Rosenburg operation
Rosengren operation
Rosen incision
Rosenmüller
R. body
R. fossa
R. gland
R. node
R. recess
valve of R.
Rosenthal
basal vein of R.
R. fiber
R. nail injury classification
R. vein
Roser-Nélaton line
rosette kidney
Ross
R. body
R. procedure
R. technique
Rossetti
R. modification
R. modification of Nissen fundoplication
Ross-Jones test
rostra (*pl. of* rostrum)
rostrad
rostral
r. cingulotomy
r. transtentorial herniation
r. ventrolateral medulla
r. ventrolateral medulla oblongata
rostralis
rostrate
rostriform
rostrocaudal extent signal abnormality
rostrum, pl. **rostra**
rotary
r. joint
r. mounted point

R

NOTES

rotary *(continued)*
    r. shadowing electron microscopy
    r. subluxation

rotated
    externally r.

rotating
    r. aspiration thromboembolectomy
    r. disc oxygenation
    r. frame imaging
    r. frame zeugmatography

rotation
    abduction-external r.
    anisotropic r.
    anterior innominate r.
    axial r.
    axis of r.
    Borggreve limb r.
    caudal-cranial r.
    cervical general r.
    clockwise r.
    counterclockwise r.
    r. drawer test
    external r.
    external/internal r.
    eye r.
    r. flap
    flexion in abduction and
      external r.
    flexion in adduction and internal r.
    foot r.
    forceps r.
    r. fracture
    gantry r.
    hip r.
    horizontal external r.
    intentional r.
    internal r.
    internal-external r.
    intersegmental r.
    intestinal r.
    inversion-eversion r.
    inward r.
    r. joint
    knee r.
    left r.
    lumbar r.
    manual r.
    medial r.
    r. mobility
    neutral r.
    opioid r.
    optical r.
    organoaxial r.
    outward r.
    pelvic r.
    r. plasty
    polycentric r.
    posterior innominate r.
    pronation-eversion-external r.
    pure r.
    r. recurvatum test
    right r.
    sagittal r.
    shoulder r.
    specific r.
    spine r.
    sternal r.
    supination-external r.
    supination-external r. IV (SER-IV)
    synchronous scapuloclavicular r.
    r. testing
    r. therapy
    timed intermittent r.
    twin bracket tooth r.
    vertebral r.
    visceral r.
    wheel r.

rotational
    r. ablation
    r. angioplasty
    r. burst fracture
    r. contact lithotripsy
    r. coronary atherectomy
    r. correction
    r. deformity
    r. dislocation
    r. flap
    r. osteotomy
    r. thrombectomy

rotationally induced shear-strain lesion
rotation-compression maneuver
rotationplasty
    Kotz-Salzer r.
    Van Ness r.
    Winkelmann r.

rotator
    r. cuff
    r. cuff advancer
    r. cuff arthropathy
    r. cuff lesion
    r. cuff muscle
    r. cuff repair
    r. cuff tear
    r. cuff tear arthroplasty
    external r.
    r. flap
    internal r.
    medial r.
    nucleus r.

rotatory
    r. fixation
    r. luxation

rotavirus infection
Rothman Institute total hip program
Rotterdam Symptom Checklist
rotunda
Rouget bulb
rough tissue handling

rouleaux formation
round
   r. back deformity
   r. body
   r. foramen
   r. hemorrhage
   r. pelvis
   r. shoulder deformity
   r. spermatid
   r. uterine ligament
rounded contour
round-robin classification
route
   r. of administration
   endoscopic r.
   external r.
   r. of injection
   r. of insertion
   retrosternal r.
   subcutaneous r.
   transthoracic r.
routine
   r. bilateral neck exploration
   r. laparotomy
   r. unilateral exploration
Roux
   R. gastric reconstruction
   R. gastroenterostomy
   R. limb
   R. limb stump
   R. limb stump dehiscence
   R. limb stump leak
   R. stasis syndrome
Roux-duToit staple capsulorrhaphy
Roux-en-Y
   R.-e.-Y. biliary bypass
   R.-e.-Y. biliary bypass with
     antrectomy
   R.-e.-Y. choledochojejunostomy
   R.-e.-Y. cystojejunostomy
   R.-e.-Y. distal jejunoileostomy
   R.-e.-Y. esophagojejunostomy
   R.-e.-Y. gastric bypass (RYGB)
   R.-e.-Y. gastroenterostomy
   R.-e.-Y. gastrojejunostomy
   R.-e.-Y. hepaticojejunal anastomosis
   R.-e.-Y. hepaticojejunostomy
   R.-e.-Y. hepatojejunostomy
   R.-e.-Y. jejunal loop incision
   R.-e.-Y. limb
   R.-e.-Y. limb enteroscopy
   R.-e.-Y. loop

   R.-e.-Y. operation
   R.-e.-Y. pancreaticojejunostomy
   R.-e.-Y. procedure
   R.-e.-Y. procedure with vagotomy
   R.-e.-Y. reconstruction
Roux-Goldthwait
   R.-G. dislocation operation
   R.-G. procedure
Roveda operation
Rovsing operation
Rowbotham
   R. operation
   R. orbital decompression
Rowe
   R. calcaneal fracture classification
   R. posterior shoulder approach
Rowe-Lowell
   R.-L. hip dislocation classification
   R.-L. system for fracture-dislocation
     classification
Rowe-Zarins shoulder immobilization
Rowinski
   R. dacryostomy
   R. operation
Royle posterior approach
Royle-Thompson transfer technique
RPC
   recurrent pyogenic cholangiohepatitis
RPLND
   retroperitoneal lymph node dissection
   retroperitoneal pelvic lymph node
     dissection
RPT
   rapid pull-through
   RPT technique
RSD
   reflex sympathetic dystrophy
RSI
   rapid-sequence induction
   RSI orotracheal intubation
RTPA, rtPA
   recombinant tissue-type plasminogen
     activator
RT-PCR
   reverse transcriptase-polymerase chain
     reaction
rub
   peritoneal friction r.
   textured fabric r.
rubber
   r. mouth prop
   r. tissue

R

NOTES

rubber-band
  r.-b. extraction
  r.-b. hemorrhoidectomy
  r.-b. ligation
  r.-b. ligation of hemorrhoid
rubbery
  r. mass
  r. texture
rubbing
  desensitization with towel r.
Rubbrecht
  R. extirpation
  R. operation
Rubens breast flap
Rubin
  R. maneuver
  R. tubal insufflation
rubrobulbar tract
rubroreticular tract
rubrospinal
  r. decussation
  r. tract
Rucker body
Ruddy incision
rude respiration
RUE
  right upper extremity
Ruedemann operation
Ruedi-Allgower classification
ruffed canal
ruga, pl. **rugae**
rugal column
rugine
rugose
rugosity
rugous
Ruiz
  R. procedure
  R. trapezoidal keratotomy
Ruiz-Mora
  R.-M. correction
  R.-M. procedure
rule
  Fletcher r. of irradiation tolerance
  Meyer-Overton r.
  Simpson r.
Rungstrom projection
running
  r. continuous suture technique
  r. vascular technique
  r. vascular technique without
    tension
runoff
Runyon classification
rupture
  Achilles tendon r.
  acute hepatic r.
  adductor longus muscle r.
  amnion r.

aneurysmal r.
anterior talofibular ligament r.
aortic r.
balloon r.
cardiac r.
chamber r.
chordae tendineae r.
chordal r.
choroidal r.
collateral ligament r.
complete r.
contained r.
crescentic r.
diaphragmatic r.
distal biceps brachii tendon r.
ERCP-induced splenic r.
esophageal r.
flexor tendon r.
Frank intrabiliary r.
free r.
gastric r.
hemidiaphragm r.
hepatic r.
hernia r.
hydatid cyst intrahepatic r.
incidental r.
inflammatory r.
infrapatellar tendon r.
interventricular septal r.
intramural esophageal r.
intraoperative r.
intraperitoneal viscus r.
intrapleural r.
ligament r.
longitudinal ligament r.
Mallory-Weiss mucosal r.
marginal sinus r.
membrane r.
r. of membranes (ROM)
mesenteric r.
myocardial r.
neglected r.
nonpenetrating r.
papillary muscle r.
penetrating r.
penile r.
plaque r.
postmembrane r.
prelabor membrane r.
premature amnion r.
premature membrane r.
premembrane r.
prolonged r.
proximal tendon r.
renal allograft r.
retrograde balloon r.
scar r.
scleral r.
splenic r.

spontaneous r.
stress r.
tendon r.
testicular r.
total perineal r.
transverse ligament r.
traumatic aortic r.
traumatic choroidal r.
tubal r.
ulnar collateral ligament r.
umbilical hernia r.
urinary bladder r.
uterine r.
valve r.
ventricular septal r.

ruptured
    r. abdominal aortic aneurysm
    r. disc
    r. disc excision
    r. episiotomy
    r. peliotic lesion
rupture-delivery interval
RUQ
    right upper quadrant
Russe
    R. classification
    R. technique
Russe-Gerhardt method
Russell
    R. fibular head autograft

hooked bundle of R.
R. percutaneous endoscopic
    gastrostomy
R. technique
uncinate bundle of R.
Russell-Taylor classification
rust ring
Rüter classification
Rutkow-Robbins-Gilbert classification
Rutledge extended hysterectomy
    classification
ruyschian membrane
Ruysch membrane
RVH
    renovascular hypertension
RVOT
    right ventricular outflow tract
RVSWI
    Right Ventricular Stroke Work Index
Rycroft operation
Rye Hodgkin disease classification
Ryerson
    R. bone graft
    R. procedure
    R. technique
RYGB
    Roux-en-Y gastric bypass

NOTES

R

σ (*var. of* sigma)
SA
    septal apical
    spinal anesthesia
    splenic artery
      SA segment
S-A
    sinoatrial
SAA
    splenic artery aneurysm
SAAST
    Self-Administered Alcoholism Screening
      Test
saber-cut
    s.-c. approach
    s.-c. incision
saber-sheath trachea
sabre-shin deformity
sac
    abdominal s.
    air s.
    allantoic s.
    alveolar s.
    amniotic s.
    aneurysmal s.
    aortic s.
    bursal s.
    caudal s.
    chorionic s.
    common dural s.
    conjunctival s.
    cupular blind s.
    dental s.
    double decidual s.
    embryonic s.
    empty gestational s.
    enamel s.
    endolymphatic s.
    enterocele s.
    s. extirpation
    fluid-filled s.
    s. formation
    gestational s.
    giant prosthetic reinforcement of
      visceral s. (GPRVS)
    greater peritoneal s.
    heart s.
    hernia s.
    hydrocele s.
    indirect hernial s.
    lacrimal s.
    lateral s.
    lesser peritoneal s.
    Mikulicz s.
    nasolacrimal s.

    omental s.
    pericardial s.
    peritoneal s.
    Pleatman s.
    pleural s.
    preputial s.
    primary yolk s.
    primitive yolk s.
    pseudogestational s.
    pudendal s.
    secondary yolk s.
    serous s.
    Stoppa giant prosthetic
      reinforcement of visceral s.
    tear s.
    thecal s.
    tooth s.
    vestibular blind s.
    vitelline s.
    wide-mouth s.
    yolk s.
saccade
    intentional s.
    reflexive s.
    volitional s.
saccadic
    s. eccentric target
    s. eye movement
saccate
sacci (*pl. of* saccus)
sacciform recess
saccular
    s. aneurysm
    s. collection
    s. spot
sacculated
sacculation
saccule
sacculotomy
sacculus, pl. **sacculi**
saccus, pl. **sacci**
saclike cavity
sacra (*pl. of* sacrum)
sacrad
sacral
    s. ala
    s. anesthesia
    s. arcuate line
    s. bar technique
    s. bone tumor
    s. brim target point
    s. canal
    s. crest
    s. foramen
    s. fracture

S

sacral *(continued)*
    s. ganglion
    s. hiatus
    s. horizontal plane line
    s. horn
    s. index
    s. pedicle screw fixation
    s. promontory
    s. region
    s. screw placement
    s. spine fixation
    s. spine fusion
    s. spine stabilization
    s. splanchnic nerve
    s. triangle
    s. venous plexus
    s. vertebra
sacral-foraminal approach
sacralization
sacrectomy
sacred bone
sacroabdominoperineal pull-through
sacroanterior position
sacrococcygeal
    s. cyst
    s. disc
    s. joint
    s. junction
    s. ligament
    s. tumor
sacrococcygeus
sacrocolpopexy
    abdominal s.
sacrodural ligament
sacrofixation operation
sacrogenital fold
sacroiliac (SI)
    s. approach
    s. articulation
    s. buttressing procedure
    s. disarticulation
    s. dislocation
    s. extension fixation
    s. flexion fixation
    s. fracture
    s. ligament
sacrolisthesis
sacrolumbar
sacropelvic
sacroperineal approach
sacropexy
    abdominal s.
sacroposterior position
sacrosciatic
sacrospinal
sacrospinous
    s. ligament
    s. ligament suspension
    s. ligament vaginal fixation

sacrotomy
sacrotransverse position
sacrotuberous ligament
sacrouterine fold
sacrovaginal fold
sacrovertebral
sacrovesical fold
sacrum, pl. **sacra**
    assimilation s.
    s. fracture
    s. fusion screw fixation
saddle
    s. block
    s. block anesthesia
    s. connector base
    s. lesion
    Turkish s.
saddle-nose deformity
Sade
    S. modification
    S. modification of Norwood
      procedure
Saeed technique
Saemisch
    S. operation
    S. section
Saenger
    S. operation
    S. suture technique
Safar operation
safety program
Sage-Clark
    S.-C. cheilectomy
    S.-C. technique
SAGES
    Society of American Gastrointestinal
    Endoscopic Surgeons
Sage-Salvatore acromioclavicular joint injury classification
sagittal
    s. deformity
    s. fissure
    s. plane
    s. plane imaging
    s. plane instability
    s. projection
    s. reconstruction
    s. rotation
    s. section
    s. slice fracture
    s. spin-echo image
    s. suture line
    s. venous sinus
sagittal-split mandibular osteotomy
sag test
Saha
    S. shoulder muscle classification
    S. transfer technique
Sahli method

Sakati-Nyhan syndrome
Sakellarides calcaneal fracture
   classification
Sakellarides-DeWeese technique
Sakoff osteotomy
saline
   hypertonic lactated s.
   ice-cold s.
   s. injection
   s. injection therapy
   intravenous s.
   s. lavage
   s. manometer
   normal s.
   phosphate buffered s. (PBS)
   s. solution
   s. technique
saline-epinephrine
Salinem infection
saliva
salivary
   s. duct
   s. duct carcinoma
   s. EGF
   s. epithelium
   s. fistula
   s. gland
   s. gland carcinoma
   s. gland infection
   s. gland tumor
   s. mass
salivation
Salle procedure
salmon
   s. backcut incision
   s. patch
salmon-patch
   s.-p. hemorrhage
   s.-p. hue
salmon-pink epithelium
salpingectomy
salpinges (*pl. of* salpinx)
salpingian
salpingioma
salpingitis
salpingocele
salpingolysis
salpingoneostomy
salpingo-oophorectomy
   abdominal s.-o.
   bilateral s.-o. (BSO)

total abdominal hysterectomy and
   bilateral s.-o. (TAHBSO)
unilateral s.-o.
salpingo-oophorocele
salpingo-ovariectomy
salpingo-ovariolysis
salpingopalatine
   s. fold
   s. membrane
salpingopexy
salpingopharyngeal
   s. fascia
   s. fold
   s. membrane
   s. muscle
salpingoplasty
salpingorrhaphy
salpingoscopy
salpingostomatomy
salpingostomy
   linear s.
salpingotomy
   abdominal s.
salpinx, pl. **salpinges**
Salter
   S. epiphysial fracture classification
   S. incremental line
   S. innominate osteotomy
   S. I-VI fracture
   S. pelvic osteotomy
   S. technique
Salter-Harris
   S.-H. epiphysial fracture
      classification
   S.-H. fracture
salting-out procedure
saltwater solution
salvage
   s. balloon angioplasty
   s. cystectomy
   s. cytology
   limb s.
   s. procedure
   s. prostatectomy
   s. surgery
   s. therapy
Salzman method
SAMBA
   simultaneous areolar mastopexy and
   breast augmentation
same-day discharge

NOTES

Samilson
- S. crescentic calcaneal osteotomy
- S. procedure

Sammarco-DiRaimondo
- S.-D. modification
- S.-D. modification of Elmslie technique

sample
- bile s.
- biopsy s.
- cytology s.
- FNA s.
- intraoperative bile s.
- peritoneal cytology s.
- population s.
- wire-guided biopsy s.

sampling
- endocervical s.
- endometrial s.
- fetal tissue s.
- incremental blood s.
- laparoscopic paraaortic lymph node s.
- lymph node s.
- percutaneous fetal tissue s.
- selective venous s.
- tissue s.
- venous s.

Sampoelesi line
Sampson cyst
Samuel position
sand
- s. body
- urinary s.

Sanders
- S. incision
- S. operation
- S. technique

Sandler-Dodge area-length method
Sandström body
sandwich
- s. patch
- s. staghorn calculus therapy

sandwiched iliac bone graft
Sanger incision
sanguification
sanguineous
- s. exudate
- s. infiltration
- s. inflammation
- s. perfusion

sanitation
sanitization
Santiani-Stone classification
Santorini
- S. canal
- S. cartilage
- S. duct
- S. fissure

- S. labyrinth
- S. major caruncle
- S. minor caruncle
- S. plexus
- S. vein

SaO$_2$
- arterial oxygen saturation

SAP
- severe acute pancreatitis
- systolic arterial pressure

saphena
saphenectomy
saphenofemoral
- s. incompetence
- s. reflux

saphenous
- s. branch
- s. flap
- s. hiatus
- s. ICA bypass
- s. opening
- s. vein
- s. vein bypass
- s. vein bypass graft
- s. vein patch graft

Sappey
- S. fiber
- S. plexus

saprophyte
SAPS
- simplified acute physiology score

sarcocele
sarcoid
sarcoidosis
sarcolemmal membrane
sarcology
sarcoma
- Abernethy s.
- embryonal s.
- juxtacortical osteogenic s.
- osteogenic s.
- soft tissue s. (STS)
- spindle cell s.
- undifferentiated embryonal s.

sarcomatosis
sarcomatosum
- glioma s.
- myxoma s.

sarcoplasmic reticulum permeability
sarcotripsy
Sargenti method
Sarmiento
- S. intertrochanteric osteotomy
- S. trochanteric fracture technique

sartorial slide procedure
Sassouni classification
satellite
- s. abscess
- s. lesion

s. metastasis
s. myofascial trigger point
satellitosis
Sato
S. operation
S. procedure
Satterthwaite method
saturated solution
saturation
s. analysis
arterial oxygen s. (SaO_2)
arterial oxyhemoglobin s. (SpO_2)
color s.
s. current
s. index
jugular bulb venous oxygen s.
jugular venous oxygen s. ($SjVO_2$)
mixed venous oxygen s.
s. output
oxygen s.
partial s.
progressive spin s.
receiver s.
s. recovery
regional s.
secondary s.
selective s.
s. sound pressure level
step-up in oxygen s.
s. time
s. transfer
venous s.
saturnine colic
saucerization
saucerized biopsy
sausage-shaped appearance
Sauve-Kapandji procedure
Savage perineal body
Savary-Mille grading scale classification
Savin
S. operation
S. procedure
Sawyer operation
Saxtorph maneuver
Sayoc
S. operation
S. procedure
SB
septal basal
SB segment
SBP
systolic blood pressure

SC
subtotal colectomy
supracondylar
SC suspension
Scaglietti
S. closed reduction technique
S. procedure scale
scala, pl. **scalae**
scalar classification
scale
Abbreviated Injury S. (AIS)
addiction acknowledgment s.
addiction potential s.
alcohol dependence s.
Borg treadmill exertion s.
Bromage s.
Charrière s.
children's coma s.
Cleveland Clinic weighted s.
clinical grading s. (CGS)
Colored Visual Analogue S.
  (CVAS)
coma s.
dissociation, analgesia, immobility,
  and tension s.
ECoG performance status s.
Edinburgh 2 Coma S.
French s.
Glasgow Coma S. (GCS)
Glasgow Outcome S.
Hospital Anxiety and Depression S.
Karnofsky s.
keratin s.
Lysholm Knee S.
MacAndrew Alcoholism S.
McMaster Quality of Life S.
Medication Quantification S.
Modified Zung Depression S.
Neonatal Infant Pain S. (NIPS)
Objective Pain S.
pain anxiety symptoms s.
Pain Catastrophizing s.
pediatric trauma s. (PTS)
Progressive Ambulation S.
Scaglietti procedure s.
Sessing pressure ulcer
  assessment s.
Shea pressure ulcer assessment s.
sound pressure level s.
Symptom Distress S.
verbal descriptor s.
verbal-rank s.

NOTES

scale *(continued)*
    visual analog s. (VAS)
    Volpicelli functional ambulation s.
    Zung Depression S.
scalene
    s. fascia
    s. fat pad biopsy
    s. hiatus
    s. lymph node biopsy
    s. maneuver
    s. node biopsy (SNB)
    s. tubercle
scalenectomy
scalenotomy
    Adson-Coffey s.
scalenus
    s. anterior muscle
    s. anticus syndrome
    s. medius muscle
    s. minimus muscle
    s. posterior muscle
scaling skin-colored lesion
scalloped closure
scalp
    s. closure
    s. incision
    s. infection
    s. laceration
    s. muscle
    s. sickle flap
    subcutaneous s.
scalpel cricothyrotomy
scalping
    s. flap
    s. flap of Converse
scan
    biplane s.
    computed tomography s.
    contrast-enhanced CT s.
    cross-vector A s.
    CT s.
    EMI s.
    high-dose s.
    iodine-131 whole-body s.
    magnetic resonance imaging s.
    Meckel s.
    omniplane s.
    peritoneovenous shunt patency s.
    s. plane
    postoperative CT s.
    pulmonary ventilation s.
    radioactive s.
    radionuclide s.
    scintillation s.
    sector s.
    serial transverse s.
    sestamibi nuclear s.
    stimulation s.
    time position s.

    transesophageal echocardiography s.
    transverse s.
    ventilation lung s.
    ventilation/perfusion lung s.
scan-directed biopsy
Scanlon early neonatal neurobehavioral score
scanning
    body s.
    contrast-enhanced CT s.
    CT s.
    s. electron microscopy
    external s.
    fluorodeoxyglucose-positron emission
      tomography s.
    s. force microscopy
    functional activation PET s.
    s. laser Doppler flowmetry
    s. laser polarimetry
    longitudinal s.
    point s.
    positron emission tomography s.
    real-time sector s.
    scintillation s.
    sector s.
    sestamibi s.
    s. technique
    thallium-technetium s.
    total body s.
    transverse s.
    whole-body s.
Scanzoni maneuver
Scanzoni-Smellie maneuver
scaphocapitate fusion
scaphocephaly
scaphohydrocephalus
scaphoid
    s. abdomen
    s. bone
    s. fossa
    s. fracture
    s. radius
scapholunate
    s. dislocation
    s. dissociation
scaphotrapezial trapezoid arthritis
scaphotrapeziotrapezoidal fusion
scapi *(pl. of* scapus)
scapula, pl. **scapulae**
scapular
    s. approximation test
    s. elevation
    s. flap
    s. line
    s. muscle
    s. notch
    s. peroneal atrophy
    s. region

scapulectomy
    Das Gupta s.
    Phelps s.
scapuloanterior position
scapuloclavicular articulation
scapulohumeral
scapuloperoneal syndrome
scapulopexy
scapuloposterior position
scapulothoracic
    s. disarticulation
    s. dissociation
    s. fusion
scapulothoracic disarticulation
scapus, pl. **scapi**
scar
    s. carcinoma
    s. dehiscence
    episiotomy s.
    facetted corneal s.
    s. formation
    gray-white corneal s.
    hypertrophic s. (HS)
    incisional s.
    iridectomy s.
    nonpathologic s.
    osteopetrotic s.
    perineal s.
    radial s.
    s. retraction
    s. rupture
    sternotomy s.
    thoracotomy s.
    s. tissue
    s. tissue reaction
Scardino
    S. flap
    S. vertical flap pyeloplasty
scarf
    s. maneuver
    s. osteotomy
    s. osteotomy-bunionectomy
    s. Z-osteotomy
    s. Z-osteotomy-bunionectomy
    s. Z-plasty
scarification test
scarify
scarless endoscopic thyroidectomy
Scarpa
    S. fascia
    S. ganglion
    S. hiatus

    S. liquor
    S. method
    S. operation
    S. sheath
    S. triangle
scarred skin
scarring
    corneal s.
    corneal s.
    duodenal s.
    gastrostomy s.
    hypertrophic s.
    obliterative s.
    patch test s.
    pathology s.
scatoma
scatoscopy
scatter
    s. correction
    s. photocoagulation
scavenger
    superoxide s.
scavenging system
Schaberg-Harper-Allen technique
Schacher ganglion
Schäfer method
Schanz
    S. angulation osteotomy
    S. femoral osteotomy
Schatzker tibial plateau fracture
    classification
Schatzki esophageal ring
Schatz maneuver
Schauffler procedure
Schaumann body
Schauta vaginal operation
Schauwecker patellar wiring technique
Schede
    S. clot
    S. method
    S. thoracoplasty
schedule
    Edmonton Symptom Assessment S.
    Support Team Assessment S.
    (STAS)
Scheibe malformation
Scheie
    S. classification
    S. operation
    S. syndrome
    S. technique
    S. thermal sclerostomy

S

NOTES

671

schema
  body s.
schematic
scheme
  chemotherapeutic s.
Schenk-Eichelter vena cava plastic filter procedure
Schepens
  S. operation
  S. technique
Schepsis-Leach technique
Scher nail biopsy
Schick method
Schiller-Duvall body
Schiller method
Schimek operation
schindylesis
Schiotz tonometry
Schirmer operation
schistocystis
schistorrhachis
schistosomal
  s. bladder carcinoma
  s. cystitis
schistosomiasis
  ectopic cutaneous s.
schistothorax
Schlatter
  S. gastrectomy technique
  S. operation
Schlein elbow arthroplasty
Schlemm canal
Schmalz operation
Schmidel anastomosis
Schneider fixation
schneiderian
  s. carcinoma
  s. respiratory membrane
Schnute wedge resection technique
Schober
  S. method
  S. technique
Schobinger incision
Schoemaker
  S. anastomosis
  S. gastroenterostomy
  S. modification
  S. procedure
Schonander
  S. procedure
  S. technique
Schönbein operation
Schoonmaker-King single-catheter technique
Schreger line
Schreiber maneuver
Schrock procedure
Schroeder operation

Schuchardt
  S. operation
  S. relaxing incision
Schuknecht classification
Schüller
  S. duct
  S. method
  S. position
  S. projection
Schütz
  S. bundle
  tract of S.
Schwalbe
  S. anterior border ring
  S. line
  S. space
Schwann cell
schwannoma
Schwartz
  S. dorsiflexory osteotomy
  S. method
  S. tractotomy
sciatic
  s. hernia
  s. nerve block
  s. nerve palsy hematoma
  s. nerve retractor
  s. notch
  s. plexus
  s. spine
sciatic-femoral nerve block
scientific method
scimitar syndrome
scintigraphy
  hepatic s.
  sestamibi s.
  somatostatin receptor s. (SRS)
scintillation
  s. scan
  s. scanning
  s. vial
scintography
  renal s.
scirrhous lesion
scissor-leg position
scissors dissection
scissors-excision hemorrhoidectomy
scissura
sclera, pl. **sclerae**
scleral
  s. buckle
  s. buckling operation
  s. buckling procedure
  s. canal
  s. ectasia
  s. exoplant
  s. fistula
  s. fistulectomy operation
  s. flap

s. hemorrhage
s. punctum
s. resection
s. roll
s. rupture
s. search coil technique
s. shortening operation
s. sulcus
scleratomal distribution of pain
sclerectoiridectomy
sclerectomy
Holth s.
thermal s.
scleriritomy
scleroatrophic cholecystitis
sclerocorneal
s. junction
s. sulcus
scleroderma
sclerodermoid graft-versus-host disease
sclerokeratectomy
scleroma
scleroplasty operation
sclerosant
sclerosing
s. adenosis
s. inflammation
s. lesion
s. osteomyelitis of Garré
s. solution
s. therapy
sclerosis, pl. scleroses
pulmonary tuberous s.
tuberous s.
sclerostomy
posterior thermal s.
Scheie thermal s.
sclerotherapy
s. complication
emergent endoscopic s.
endoscopic injection s. (EIS)
endoscopic retrograde s.
endoscopic variceal s.
esophageal variceal s.
s. failure
fiberoptic injection s.
injection s.
intravariceal s.
paravariceal s.
variceal s.
sclerotic
s. bone lesion

s. calvarial patch
s. cemental mass
s. kidney
s. line
s. stomach
scleroticectomy
scleroticotomy
sclerotomy
anterior s.
foreign body s.
Lindner s.
s. operation
posterior s.
s. with drainage
s. with exploration
sclerouvectomy
partial lamellar s.
scolicidal fluid
scoliosis
s. correction
s. surgery
scoliotic
s. curve fixation
s. deformity
Scopinaro
S. pancreaticobiliary bypass
S. procedure
score
Abbreviated Injury S. (AIS)
airway s.
Aldrete s.
alertness/sedation s.
American Society of
Anesthesiology s.
APACHE-II s.
Apgar s.
BI-RADS s.
cosmetic s.
cumulative s.
cumulative pain s. (CPS)
defecation s.
discrimination s.
Dripps-American Surgical
Association s.
echo s.
evacuation s.
GIQLI s.
Glasgow Coma S.'s
Glasgow Outcome S. (GOS)
Gleason s.
Injury Severity S. (ISS)

NOTES

score (*continued*)
International Classification of Diseases-9 Version of Injury Severity S. (ICISS)
Lysholm s.
MACIS s.
mangled extremity severity s.
Neurologic and Adaptive Capacity S. (NACS)
Optimal Observation S.
pancreatic necrosis prognostic s.
Parsonnet s.
Peritonitis Severity S. (PSS)
Scanlon early neonatal neurobehavioral s.
simplified acute physiology s. (SAPS)
Steward Recovery S.
symptom s.
Trauma Score and Injury Severity S. (TRISS)
visual analog pain s. (VAPS)
Yale Optimal Observation S.

scoring
s. incision
preoperative s.
s. system

scotoma
s. junction
s. ring

scotomata

scotomization

scotoscopy

Scott
S. glenoplasty technique
S. jejunoileal bypass
S. operation
S. posterior glenoplasty

scotty
s. dog fracture
s. dog graft
s. dog sign

SCPP
spinal cord perfusion pressure

scratch-pad memory

scratch-type incision

screen
coagulation s.
s. filtration pressure
intravascular coagulation s.
s. oxygenation
throat s.

screening
colonoscopy s.
endocrine s.
s. mammography
presurgical psychological s. (PPS)
s. procedure
psychological s.

s. recommendation
s. test

screw
s. angulation
s. epiphysiodesis
s. fixation
headless bone s.
s. implantation
s. insertion
s. insertion technique
s. joint
s. loosening
s. placement
s. position perioperative monitoring
s. stabilization
s. stripout

screw-and-plate fixation

screw-and-wire fixation

screw-home mechanism

screw-in

screw-plate approach

screw-type abutment

scrota (*pl. of* scrotum)

scrotal
s. artery
s. hematocele
s. hernia
s. mass
s. pouch operation
s. pouch orchiopexy
s. raphe
s. septum
s. skin
s. skin ulcer
s. swelling
s. vein

scrotectomy
total s.

scrotiform

scrotitis

scrotocele

scrotoplasty

scrotoscopy

scrotum, pl. **scrota**

SCS
spinal cord stenosis
spinal cord stimulation

Scudder
S. method
S. operation
S. procedure
S. technique

Scuderi
S. procedure
S. repair
S. technique

Scultetus position

scurvy line

scyphiform

scyphoid
SEA
 spinal epidural abscess
seal
 cavity s.
sealed envelope technique
sealer extrusion
sealing perforation
sea lion position
Sealy-Laragh technique
seamless graft
seatbelt fracture
seat belt sign
Seattle classification
sebaceous
 s. adenocarcinoma
 s. cyst
 s. gland
sebaceum, pl. **sebacea**
 adenoma s.
Sebileau
 S. hollow
 S. muscle
seborrhea
second
 s. cranial nerve
 s. cuneiform bone
 forced expiratory volume in 1 s.
 (FEV$_1$)
 s. gas effect
 s. intention
 s. lumbar artery
 s. malignant neoplasm (SMN)
 s. pain wind-up
 s. parallel pelvic plane
 s. tibial muscle
secondary
 s. adhesion
 s. amputation
 s. anesthetic
 s. arrest
 s. arrest of dilatation
 s. articulation
 s. closure
 s. diagnostic biopsy
 s. expansion
 s. fixation
 s. focal point
 s. fracture
 s. fungal infection
 s. gangrene
 s. hemorrhage

 s. hernia
 s. HPT
 s. hyperalgesia
 s. intention
 s. lesion
 s. membrane
 s. myofascial trigger point
 s. neuralgia
 s. procedure
 s. ptosis correction
 s. pulmonary lobule
 s. reconstruction
 s. renal calculus
 s. repair
 s. retroperitoneal organ
 s. saturation
 s. stage proctocolectomy
 s. surgery
 s. suture technique
 s. union
 s. yolk sac
second-degree
 s.-d. burn
 s.-d. hemorrhoid
 s.-d. radiation injury
second-echo image
second-generation
second-grade fusion
second-line
 s.-l. chemotherapy
 s.-l. drug
second-look
 s.-l. laparoscopy
 s.-l. laparotomy (SLL)
 s.-l. operation
 s.-l. surgery
second-set graft rejection
secretin stimulation
secretion
 biliary s.
 cholecystokinin s.
 gastrin s.
 insulin s.
 pancreatic enzyme s.
 tracheal s.
secretomotor nature
secretory
 s. adenocarcinoma
 s. duct
 s. nerve
sectile
sectio, pl. **sectiones**

S

NOTES

section
  abdominal s.
  attached cranial s.
  axial s.
  bar s.
  cesarean s. (C-section)
  classical cesarean s.
  coronal s.
  cranial s.
  cross s.
  cryostat s.
  s. cutting
  detached cranial s.
  diagonal s.
  distal shave s.
  extraperitoneal cesarean s.
  s. freeze substitution technique
  frontal s.
  frozen s. (FS)
  Giemsa-stained s.
  horizontal s.
  intraoperative frozen s.
  Kerr cesarean s.
  Latzko cesarean s.
  longitudinal s.
  low cervical cesarean s.
  lower uterine segment transverse
    cesarean s.
  low transverse cesarean s.
  median s.
  midfrontal plane coronal s.
  midsagittal s.
  nerve cross s.
  oblique s.
  orbital s.
  parasagittal s.
  perineal s.
  permanent s.
  pituitary stalk s.
  plastic s.
  Porro cesarean s.
  primary cesarean s.
  repeat cesarean s.
  Saemisch s.
  sagittal s.
  tangential s.
  thin s.
  transperitoneal cesarean s.
  transverse s.
  vaginal birth after cesarean s.
    (VBAC)
  vertical s.
  vestibular nerve s.
sectional
  s. root canal filling method
  s. technique
sectiones (*pl. of* sectio)
sectioning
  surgical s.

sector
  s. cut
  end-viewing s.
  s. iridectomy
  s. iridectomy operation
  lateral s.
  medial s.
  s. scan
  s. scanning
sectoral
  s. pedicle
  s. resection
sectorial
  s. branch
  s. resection
secundarium
secundum
  ostium s.
secure intracorporeal knot
sedation
  adjunctive s.
  chemical s.
  conscious s.
  ICU s.
  intravenous s.
  I.V. s.
sedation-induced hypoventilation
sedative
  s. effect
  s. therapy
Seddon
  S. classification
  S. dorsal spine costotransversectomy
  S. modification
  S. nerve graft
  S. technique
sedimentation
  s. equilibrium
  s. index
seeding
  instrument-tract s.
  intraluminal s.
  intraperitoneal s.
  needle tract tumor s.
  peritoneal s.
  surgical s.
  tumor s.
SEER
  Surveillance, Epidemiology and End
  Results
  SEER Program
SEF
  spectral edge frequency
segment
  AA s.
  AB s.
  AM s.
  anterior basal s.
  anterior inferior s.

anterior superior s.
apical s.
apicoposterior s.
bronchopulmonary s.
cardiac s.
cervical s.
colorectal s.
demucosalized augmentation with
  gastric s. (DAWG)
extramedullary s.
gastric s.
hepatic s.
IA s.
IB s.
inferior lingular s.
intracutaneous s.
LA s.
LB s.
lower uterine s. (LUS)
lumbar s.
medial basal s.
motion s.
occluded s.
posterior basal s.
posterosuperior s.
renal s.
SA s.
SB s.
subapical s.
subsuperior s.
superior lingular s.
venous s.
segmenta (*pl. of* segmentum)
segmental
  s. alveolar osteotomy
  s. blocking technique
  s. bronchus
  s. colonic resection
  s. compression construct
  s. dilatation
  s. duct
  s. epidural anesthesia
  s. explant
  s. fixation
  s. fracture
  s. gastrectomy
  s. hepatectomy
  s. involvement
  s. limb pressure recording
  s. lung resection
  s. mandibulectomy
  s. mastectomy

s. neural blockade
s. peridural spinal anesthesia
s. pressure index
s. pulmonary resection
s. sphincter
s. surgery
s. tendon graft
s. vessel
s. wall motion deformity (SWMA)
segmentalis
segmentation
  s. anomaly
  k space s.
  s. movement
  s. root canal filling method
  s. sphere
  volume s.
segmentectomy
segmented flap
segment-oriented
  s.-o. hepatic resection
  s.-o. liver resection
  s.-o. procedure
  s.-o. technique
segmentum, pl. **segmenta**
Segond fracture
segregation
Seidelin body
Seiler cartilage
Seinsheimer femoral fracture
  classification
Seitz metamorphosing respiration
seizure
  posttraumatic s.
Selakovich procedure
Seldinger
  S. cystic duct catheterization
  S. method
  S. percutaneous technique
  S. procedure
  S. retrograde wire/intubation
    technique
selection pressure
selective
  s. anesthesia
  s. angiography
  s. arterial embolization
  s. arterial stimulation
  s. bowel decontamination
  s. bronchial catheterization
    anesthetic technique
  s. catheterization

NOTES

selective *(continued)*
- s. ductal cannulation
- s. excitation projection reconstruction imaging
- s. inguinal node dissection
- s. injection
- s. intracoronary thrombolysis
- s. irradiation
- s. lectin-triggered apoptosis
- s. lymphadenectomy
- s. nonoperative management
- s. obturator nerve block
- s. photothermolysis
- s. portal decompression
- s. posterior rhizotomy (SPR)
- s. proximal vagotomy
- s. sacral rhizotomy
- s. saturation
- s. saturation recovery
- s. serotonin reuptake inhibitor (SSRI)
- s. shunting
- s. thoracic spine fusion
- s. vascular clamping (SVC)
- s. venous sampling

selenoid body
self-administered
- S.-A. Alcoholism Screening Test (SAAST)
- Quality of Well-Being Scale S.-A. (QWB-SA)

self-breast examination
self-catheterization
- clean intermittent s.-c.

self-expandable
self-expanding
self-help
self-infection
self-mutilation
self-obturation
- intermittent s.-o.

self-reduction
self-sealing scleral puncture
self-seal pouch
self-tightening slip knot
Selinger operation
sella
- empty s.
- s. structure

sellar tumor
Sell-Frank-Johnson extensor shift technique
Sellheim incision
Sellick maneuver
Selye
- adaptation syndrome of S.

semantic conditioning

Semb
- S. apicolysis
- S. nephrectomy technique

semenuria
semicanal
semicanalis
semicartilaginous
semicircular
- s. canal
- s. duct
- s. line

semicircularis
semiclosed
- s. anesthesia
- s. circle

semicoma
semiconductor
- extrinsic s.

semiconstrained total elbow arthroplasty
semielective
- s. operation
- s. status

semiflexed incision
semi-Fowler position
semiimpermeable membrane
semilateral position
semilinear canonical correlation
semilunar
- s. bone
- s. cartilage
- s. fibrocartilage
- s. flap
- s. ganglion
- s. hiatus
- s. incision
- s. line
- s. valvular septum

semilunate cut
semimembranosus
- s. muscle
- s. tendon

semimembranous
seminal
- s. colliculus
- s. duct
- s. fluid
- s. gland
- s. granule
- s. hillock
- s. tract
- s. tract washout
- s. vesicle
- s. vesicle aspiration

semination
seminiferous
seminoma
seminomatous
seminuria
semioblique position

semiopen
- s. anesthesia
- s. hemorrhoidectomy
- s. sliding tenotomy

semipedunculated lesion
semipermeable membrane
semipronation
semiprone position
semireclining position
semirecumbent position
semispinalis
- s. capitis muscle
- s. cervicis
- s. cervicis muscle

semispinal muscle
semisulcus
semisupination
semisupine
semitendinosus
- s. muscle
- s. procedure
- s. technique
- s. tendon

semitendinous
semiupright position
Semm Z technique
Semont maneuver
Sengstaken-Blakemore method
senile
- s. ectasia
- s. plaque

senior-level trauma-team response
Senning
- S. operation
- S. repair
- S. transposition procedure

Senn operation
sensate
sensation
- s. level
- s. time

sense of defecation
sensitive
- s. plane
- s. plane projection reconstruction imaging
- s. point
- s. visceral postsurgical disturbance

sensitivity
sensitization
- central s.
- s. response

sensitizing injection
sensor
- calcium s.
- multiparameter s.
- s. operation

sensoria (*pl. of* sensorium)
sensorimotor stimulation approach
sensorineural acuity level technique
sensorium, pl. **sensoria, sensoriums**
sensory
- s. block
- s. blockade
- s. examination
- s. extinction
- s. fusion
- s. nerve
- s. nerve fiber bundle
- s. stimulation
- s. tract

sentence classification
sentinel
- s. blood clot
- s. lymphadenectomy
- s. lymph node (SLN)
- s. lymph node biopsy
- s. lymph node detection (SLND)
- s. node
- s. node biopsy (SNB)
- s. node excision
- s. node localization
- s. node staging
- s. node-to-background ratio (SNBR)
- s. spinous process fracture

SEP
- somatosensory evoked potential

separation
- cotton-wool s.
- s. point
- premature s.

sepsis, pl. **sepses**
- anorectal s.
- catheter s.
- Gram-negative s.
- Gram-positive s.
- intraabdominal s.
- peritoneal s.
- postsplenectomy s.
- severe human s.
- systemic s.

sepsis-induced
- s.-i. disseminated intravascular coagulation

NOTES

sepsis-induced *(continued)*
    s.-i. metabolic change
    s.-i. muscle breakdown
    s.-i. muscle proteolysis
septa (*pl. of* septum)
septal
    s. apical (SA)
    s. basal (SB)
    s. defect
    s. hematoma
    s. line
    s. myectomy
    s. myotomy
    s. perforation
    s. reconstruction
    s. resection
    s. space
septate
septation procedure
septectomy
    atrial s.
    balloon s.
    Blalock-Hanlon᾽ atrial s.
    Edwards s.
    transampullary s.
septic
    s. arthritis
    s. complication
    s. focus
    s. shock (SS)
septicemia
septodermoplasty
septomarginal tract
septoplasty
    frontal sinus s.
septorhinoplasty
    esthetic s.
septostomy
    atrial balloon s.
    balloon atrial s.
    blade atrial s.
septulum, pl. **septula**
septum, pl. **septa**
    anorectal s.
    anterior intermuscular s.
    Bigelow s.
    bridgelike s.
    cartilaginous s.
    Cloquet s.
    colorectal s.
    comblike s.
    crural s.
    deviated s.
    endovenous s.
    femoral s.
    interatrial s.
    intercavernosus s.
    intermuscular s.
    interpulmonary s.

    interradicular s.
    interventricular s.
    membranous s.
    nasal s.
    orbital s.
    pectiniform s.
    posterior intermuscular s.
    rectovaginal s.
    rectovesical s.
    scrotal s.
    semilunar valvular s.
    urogenital s.
    urorectal s.
    valvular s.
    ventricular s.
Sequeira-Khanuja modification
sequela, pl. **sequelae**
sequence
    caudal dysplasia s.
    fast spin-echo s.
    FLAIR s.
    turbo spin-echo s.
sequential
    s. administration
    s. line imaging
    s. plane imaging
    s. point imaging
    s. radiographs
sequestration
    s. bronchopneumonia
    pulmonary intralobar s.
sequestrectomy
sequestrotomy
sera (*pl. of* serum)
Serafini hernia
Sergent white line
serial
    s. blood gas
    s. dilation
    s. extraction
    s. hematocrit measurement
    s. imaging
    s. operation
    s. percutaneous liver biopsy
    s. radiographic evaluation
    s. radiographs
    s. sonography
    s. transverse scan
series
    diagnostic small bowel s.
    nonlaparoscopic s.
    upper gastrointestinal s.
serioscopy
seriscission
SER-IV
    supination-external rotation IV
        SER-IV fracture
serofibrinous inflammation
serofibrous

serologic
    s. adhesion
    s. examination
serological test
seroma cavity
seromembranous
seromucosa
seromucous gland
seromuscular
    s. coat
    s. colocystoplasty
    s. enterocystoplasty
    s. layer
    s. stitch
    s. suture technique
seromyectomy
    duodenal s.
seromyotomy
    anterior s.
    laparoscopic s.
seroprotection
serosa
    cecal s.
    gastric s.
    intact gastric s.
    s. invasion
    jejunal s.
serosal
    s. breach
    s. fluid
    s. involvement
    s. metastasis
    s. penetration
    s. tear
serosal-peritoneal metastasis
serosanguineous
seroserous suture technique
serotonergic
    s. system
    s. tract
serous
    s. acute inflammation
    s. adenocarcinoma
    s. cystadenocarcinoma
    s. exudate
    s. gland
    s. layer
    s. ligament
    s. membrane
    s. sac
serovaccination

serpentine
    s. aneurysm
    s. incision
serpent infection
serpiginous ulceration
serration
serratus
    s. anterior muscle
    s. anterior muscle flap
    s. posterior inferior muscle
    s. posterior superior muscle
Serres angle
Sertoli-cell-only syndrome
serum, pl. **sera**
    s. alanine amino transaminase
    s. alkaline phosphatase
    s. ALT
    s. bactericidal concentration
    s. bilirubin
    s. bilirubin concentration
    s. calcium concentration
    s. carcinoembryonic antigen
    s. CEA
    s. EGF
    fetal bovine s. (FBS)
    s. lidocaine level (SLL)
    s. lithium concentration
    s. neutralization
    s. total bilirubin level
service
    trauma s.
sesamoid
    s. bone
    s. cartilage
sesamoidectomy
    fibular s.
SESAP
    Surgical Education and Self-Assessment
    Program
sessile
    s. adenoma
    s. lesion
Sessing pressure ulcer assessment scale
session
    manometric recording s.
    recording s.
    1-s. removal
sestamibi
    s. nuclear scan
    s. scanning
    s. scintigraphy

S

NOTES

SET
   signal extraction technology
set
   insufflation test s.
   s. point
seton
   s. operation
   s. wound
setpoint
setting
   s. expansion
   outpatient surgical s.
setup
   ambulatory s.
seventh cranial nerve
Sever
   S. modification
   S. modification of Fairbanks
     technique
severe
   s. acute pancreatitis (SAP)
   s. deforming osteogenesis
     imperfecta
   s. human sepsis
   s. traumatic brain injury
Severin classification
Sever-L'Episcopo
   S.-L. repair
   S.-L. repair of shoulder
Sewall technique
sewing machine technique
sex
   s. change operation
   s. reversal
   s. steroid modulation
sextant technique
sexual
   s. aberration
   s. evaluation
   s. gland
sexualization
S-flap incision
SF-McGill Pain Questionnaire
SGO
   Surgeon General's Office
SGPA
   supragenicular popliteal artery
shadowing
   acoustic s.
   s. method
Shaffer-Hartmann method
Shaffer operation
Shaffer-Weiss classification
shaft
   femoral s.
   s. fracture
shagreen
   s. lesion
   s. patch

Shaher-Puddu classification
shallow
   s. inspiration
   s. respiration
sham
   s. injection
   s. surgery
Shambaugh incision
shank bone
shaping
   root canal s.
sharing
   United Network for Organ S.
     (UNOS)
sharp
   s. angle
   s. and blunt dissection
   s. dilaceration
   s. dissection technique
Sharpey fiber
Sharrard transfer technique
Sharrard-type kyphectomy
Shauta-Aumreich procedure
shave
   s. biopsy
   s. excision technique
Shea
   S. pressure ulcer assessment scale
   S. procedure
shear fracture
sheath
   anterior s.
   anterior rectus s.
   axillary s.
   carotid s.
   common flexor s.
   crural s.
   femoral s.
   fenestrated s.
   fibrous tendon s.
   flexor s.
   glissonian s.
   infundibuliform s.
   intertubercular s.
   intravenous s.
   mucous s.
   neurovascular s.
   optic s.
   paramedian s.
   parotid s.
   perichondral s.
   plantar tendon s.
   posterior rectus s.
   prostatic s.
   rectus s.
   Scarpa s.
   synovial tendon s.
   vascular s.
   Waldeyer s.

sheathed artery
shedding
    endometrial s.
Sheehan
    S. and Dodge technique
    S. syndrome
Sheen
    S. airway reconstruction
    S. tip graft
sheet mesh excision
shelf
    s. acetabuloplasty
    Blumer s.
    rectal s.
    vocal s.
shell
    s. nail
    total hip arthroplasty with internal
      eccentric s.'s (THARIES)
Shelton femoral fracture classification
shelving
    s. edge
    s. incision
Shenton line
shepherd
    s.'s crook deformity
    S. fracture
Sherk-Probst
    S.-P. percutaneous pinning
    S.-P. technique
shift
    fluid s.
Shigella **infection**
Shimazaki area-length method
shin bone
shiny cellophane reflection
ship
    Fabricius s.
Shirodkar
    S. cervical cerclage
    S. operation
    S. procedure
    S. suture technique
shish kebab technique
shivering
    postoperative s.
shock
    allergic s.
    anesthetic s.
    cardiogenic s.
    declamping s.
    deferred s.

    defibrillation s.
    defibrillatory s.
    early unequivocal s.
    endotoxic s.
    endotoxin s.
    heat s.
    hemorrhagic s.
    hyperdynamic s.
    hypovolemic s.
    irreversible s.
    s. lung
    perioperative s.
    s. position
    postcardiotomy s. (PS)
    primary s.
    reversible s.
    septic s. (SS)
    s. wave lithotripsy (SWL)
    s. wave pressure
shoe-and-stocking position
shoelace
    s. fasciotomy closure
    s. stitch
shoeshine maneuver
Shone anomaly
short
    s. bone
    s. bowel syndrome
    s. central artery
    s. duration, unilateral, neuralgic,
      conjunctival injection and tearing
      (SUNCT)
    s. esophagus type hiatal hernia
    s. gastric artery
    s. gastric vein
    s. gastric vessel
    s. head
    s. hepatic vein
    s. incubation hepatitis
    s. inversion recovery imaging
    s. lever accessory movement
      technique
    s. lever specific contact procedure
    s. limb Roux-en-Y
      gastroenterostomy
    s. oblique fracture
    s. saphenous vein
    s. scar technique breast reduction
    s. scar technique of mastopexy
    s. tau inversion recovery (STIR)
    s. wave diathermy
short-axis plane

S

NOTES

short-cone technique
shortcut sciatic pain
shortening
    chordal s.
    esophageal s.
short-pulse repetition time/echo time image
short-segment
    s.-s. disease
    s.-s. lesion
    s.-s. spinal fusion
short-term
    s.-t. convalescence
    s.-t. immunosuppression
    s.-t. outcome
    s.-t. result
    s.-t. total continence
shotgun wound
shoulder
    s. amputation
    s. arthroplasty
    s. blade
    s. deformity
    s. disarticulation
    s. dislocation
    s. dislocation bone bank
    s. flap
    s. girdle
    s. girdle resection
    ipsilateral s.
    S. Pain and Disability Index
    s. reduction
    s. repair
    s. rotation
    Sever-L'Episcopo repair of s.
    s. strap incision
    s. with bevel preparation
Shouldice
    S. hernioplasty
    S. herniorrhaphy
Shouldice-Bassini hernia repair
Shrapnell membrane
shrinkage
    thermal-assisted capsular s.
    tumor s.
Shugrue operation
shunt
    atriocaval s.
    bidirectional Glenn s.
    Blalock-Taussig s.
    s. blockage
    cavoatrial s.
    central systemic-to-pulmonary s.
    s. cyanosis
    distal splenorenal s. (DSRS)
    end-to-side portocaval s.
    end-to-side splenorenal s.
    Glenn s.
    s. index

    s. infection
    interposition mesocaval s.
    intrahepatic portosystemic s.
    s. manipulation
    mesoatrial s.
    modified Blalock-Taussig s.
    s. muscle
    s. obstruction
    s. patency
    s. pathway
    s. placement
    portacaval s.
    portal-systemic s.
    portosystemic s.
    s. quantification
    s. ratio
    s. revision
    side-to-side portacaval s. (SSPCS)
    s. surgery
    s. tap
    transjugular intrahepatic portosystemic s. (TIPS)
shunting
    airway s.
    distal splenoadrenal s.
    lumbar-peritoneal s.
    pleuroperitoneal s.
    portal mesenteric s.
    portosystemic s.
    selective s.
    splenoadrenal s.
    surgical portosystemic s.
    ventricular peritoneal s.
    ventriculoperitoneal s.
SHVC
    suprahepatic inferior vena cava
SI
    sacroiliac
    SI joint
SIADH
    syndrome of inappropriate antidiuretic hormone
sialadenitis
sialoadenectomy
sialoadenotomy
sialocarcinoma
sialocele
sialolithotomy
Sibson
    S. fascia
    S. groove
    S. muscle
Sichi operation
sick
    s. building syndrome
    s. sinus syndrome
sickle flap
sickle-shaped canal
sickness impact profile

side
    antimesenteric s.
    contralateral s.
    depressed s.
    ipsilateral s.
    luminal s.
    s. port
    posterior s.
    s. posture reduction
side-bending barrier
side-entry access
side-lying iliac compression test
sideration
sideswipe elbow fracture
side-to-side
    s.-t.-s. anastomosis
    s.-t.-s. gastroenterostomy
    s.-t.-s. hepatojejunostomy
    s.-t.-s. portacaval shunt (SSPCS)
sidewall
    pelvic s.
    s. structure
SIDS
    sudden infant death syndrome
sieve
    s. bone
    s. graft
    molecular s.
Siffert intraepiphysial osteotomy
Siffert-Storen intraepiphysial osteotomy
sighing respiration
sigma, σ
    s. method
sigmoid
    s. artery
    s. colon
    s. colon carcinoma
    s. cutaneous fistula
    s. cystoplasty
    s. end colostomy
    s. enterocystoplasty
    s. flexure
    s. fold
    s. fossa
    s. kidney
    s. loop reduction
    s. loop rod colostomy
    s. mesocolon
    s. rectum pouch
    s. sinus ligation
    s. sulcus

    s. venous sinus
    s. volvulus (SV)
sigmoidectomy
sigmoidocystoplasty
sigmoidopexy
    band s.
    endoscopic s.
    laparoscopic s.
sigmoidoproctostomy
sigmoidorectostomy
sigmoidoscopy
    fiberoptic s.
    flexible s.
sigmoidostomy
sigmoidotomy
sigmoidovesical fistula
sigmoid-rectal intussusception
sign
    Aaron s.
    absent bow tie s.
    accordion s.
    alien hand s.
    Allis s.
    Apley s.
    Aufrecht s.
    Babinski s.
    banana s.
    Battle s.
    bite s.
    blue dot s.
    Blumberg s.
    Boas s.
    bone bruise s.
    bow-tie s.
    brim s.
    Brudzinski s.
    Chadwick s.
    chain-of-lakes s.
    chandelier s.
    coiled spring s.
    Cole s.
    comb s.
    cortical ring s.
    cotton-wool s.
    Courvoisier s.
    crowded carpal s.
    Cullen s.
    dagger s.
    Dalrymple s.
    Dance s.
    David Letterman s.
    double bubble s.

S

NOTES

sign (*continued*)
 double-density s.
 double halo s.
 drawer s.
 echo s.
 extrapyramidal s.
 fabere s.
 fat pad s.
 Homans s.
 impingement s.
 little finger s.
 localized abdominal s.
 long tract s.
 loss-of-waist s.
 s. mechanism for ventilator
  breathing
 obturator s.
 Phalen s.
 scotty dog s.
 seat belt s.
 stacked coin s.
 target s.
 Thomas s.
 Tinel s.
signal
 abnormal preoperative
  localization s.
 s. attenuation
 Doppler s.
 electromagnetic s.
 s. extraction technology (SET)
 s. hemorrhage
 localization s.
 preoperative localization s.
signaling
 downstream s.
 nitric oxide s.
signature
 surgical s.
signet-ring
 s.-r. adenocarcinoma
 s.-r. appearance
 s.-r. cell carcinoma
significance
 atypical squamous cell of
  undetermined s. (ASCUS)
 squamous intraepithelial
  lesion/atypical squamous cell of
  undetermined s. (SIL/ASCUS)
SIH
 stress-induced hyperthermia
SIL
 squamous intraepithelial lesion
SIL/ASCUS
 squamous intraepithelial lesion/atypical
  squamous cell of undetermined
  significance
  SIL/ASCUS lesion

Silastic
 S. collar-reinforced stoma
 S. lunate arthroplasty
 S. ring vertical-banded gastric
  bypass (SRVGB)
Silber technique
silence
 electrocerebral s. (ECS)
silent
 s. aspiration
 s. autonephrectomy
 s. gallstone
 s. receptor
Silfverskiöld
 S. lengthening technique
 S. procedure
silhouette sign of Felson
silicate restoration
silicone
 s. elastomer medialization
 s. elastomer ring vertical
  gastroplasty
 s. implant arthroplasty
 s. implant leakage
 s. intubation
 s. rubber arthroplasty
 s. wrist arthroplasty
**Sillence type II-IV osteogenesis
 imperfecta**
Silva-Costa operation
silver
 s. amalgam restoration
 S. bunionectomy
 s. cone method
 s. dollar technique
 Gomori methenamine s. (GMS)
 s. point root canal filling method
 S. procedure
silver-fork deformity
Silver-Hildreth operation
silver-wire
 s.-w. arteriole
 s.-w. reflex
Silvester method
simian line
Simmonds-Menelaus
 S.-M. metatarsal osteotomy
 S.-M. proximal phalangeal
  osteotomy
Simmons
 S. cervical spine fusion
 S. osteotomy
Simon
 S. expansion arch
 S. incision
 S. position
 S. suture technique
Simonart band
Simonton technique

Simplate procedure
simple
    s. bypass
    s. cold storage preservation
    s. diversion
    s. external drainage
    s. hepatojejunostomy
    s. joint
    s. mastectomy
    s. mastoidectomy
    s. mastopexy
    s. periodontal flap
    s. shoulder test (SST)
    s. skull fracture
    s. sound source
    s. suture technique
    s. syndactyly repair
    s. transfusion
    s. vulvectomy
simplification
simplified acute physiology score
  (SAPS)
Simpson
    S. atherectomy
    S. rule
Sims
    S. position
    S. suture technique
simulation
    surgical s.
simultaneous
    s. areolar mastopexy and breast
      augmentation (SAMBA)
    s. bilateral percutaneous
      nephrolithotomy
    s. compression-ventilation CPR
    s. kidney-pancreas transplantation
    s. method
    s. pancreas and kidney (SPK)
    s. pancreas-kidney transplantation
    s. pancreas and kidney transplant
      procedure
    s. pancreatic-renal (SPR)
    s. segmental hepatectomy
SIMV
    spontaneous intermittent mandatory
      ventilation
    synchronized intermittent mandatory
      ventilation
    synchronized intermittent mechanical
      ventilation
sincipital

sinciput
S incision
Sinding-Larsen-Johansson lesion
sinew
Singer-Blom endoscopic
  tracheoesophageal puncture technique
Singh
    S. osteoporosis classification
    S. osteoporosis index
single
    s. adenoma
    s. biopsy
    s. cone root canal filling method
    s. denture construction
    s. fraction radiation
    s. fracture
    s. GSW
    s. heel raise
    s. hydatid disease
    s. injection ultrasound-assisted
      femoral nerve block
    s. lung ventilation
    s. midline extraperitoneal incision
    s. pedicle TRAM flap
    s. proximal portal technique
    s. site
    s. space technique
    s. strand conformation
      polymorphism analysis
single-armed suture technique
single-balloon
    s.-b. valvotomy
    s.-b. valvuloplasty
single-breath
    s.-b. diffusing capacity
    s.-b. induction
    s.-b. induction of anesthesia
single-echo diffusion imaging
single-fraction total body irradiation
single-incision fasciotomy
single-layer continuous closure
single-level spinal fusion
single-lung transplant
single-mechanism inhaled anesthetic
single-photon emission computed
  tomography
single-photon emission computer-aided
  tomography
single-port
    s.-p. laparoscopy
    s.-p. technique
single-pour technique

S

NOTES

single-puncture laparoscopy
single-shot
    s.-s. caudal block
    s.-s. imaging technique
    s.-s. intrathecal opioid
    s.-s. spinal
    s.-s. spinal anesthesia
    s.-s. subarachnoid block
single-site inhaled anesthetic
single-slice gradient-echo image
single-stage
    s.-s. operation
    s.-s. procedure
    s.-s. tissue transfer
    s.-s. total proctocolectomy
single-step esophagoplasty
single-stick method
Singleton incision
Singleton-Merten syndrome
single-trocar access thoracoscopy
sinister
sinistra
sinistrogyration
sinistrorotation
sinistrorse
sinistrotorsion
sinistrum
sink-trap malformation
sinoaortic denervation
sinoatrial (S-A)
    s. exit block
    s. nodal branch
    s. nodal function
    s. nodal parasympathectomy
    s. node
sinocarotid nerve
sinonasal
    s. carcinoma
    s. cavity
    s. disease
    s. lesion
    s. tumor
sinoscopy
sinus
    air s.
    anal s.
    basilar venous s.
    branchial s.
    carotid s.
    cavernous venous s.
    s. cavity
    cerebral s.
    cervical s.
    circular venous s.
    s. closure
    coronary s.
    costomediastinal s.
    cranial venous s.
    dural venous s.

endodermal s.
s. endoscopy
Englisch s.
s. exit block
frontal s.
Guérin s.
Huguier s.
inferior longitudinal s.
inferior petrosal s.
inferior sagittal s.
intercavernous venous s.
s. irrigation
jugular s.
lactiferous s.
laryngeal s.
lateral s.
s. line
longitudinal vertebral venous s.
Luschka s.
Maier s.
Morgagni s.
s. mucocele
oblique pericardial s.
occipital s.
osteomyelitic s.
Palfyn s.
paranasal s.
pericardial s.
perineal s.
petrosal venous s.
petrosquamous venous s.
s. petrosus superior
phrenicocostal s.
piriform s.
pleural s.
prostatic s.
pulmonary s.
rectal s.
renal s.
rhomboidal s.
s. rhythm (SR)
Ridley s.
right sigmoid s.
sagittal venous s.
sigmoid venous s.
sphenoidal s.
sphenoparietal venous s.
splenic s.
straight s.
s. surgery
s. tarsi syndrome
tentorial s.
s. tract
transverse pericardial s.
transverse venous s.
tympani s.
urogenital s.
s. venosus
venous s.

sinuscopy
> maxillary s.

sinusitis
> allergic fungal s.
> chronic s.
> fungal s.

sinusoid
> hepatic s.

sinusoidal
> s. capillary pressure
> s. congestion
> s. endothelium
> s. endothelium cornucopia
> s. lesion
> s. pattern
> s. relaxation

sinusotomy
> Killian frontal s.

sinuvertebral nerve

SIP
> spontaneous intestinal perforation

siphon
> carotid s.

siphonage

SIRS
> systemic inflammatory response
> syndrome

SIS
> small intestinal submucosa

Sistrunk procedure

site
> alternative introduction s.
> anatomic s.
> anatomical s.
> arterial bleeding s.
> arterial entry s.
> biopsy s.
> bleeding s.
> carcinoma of uncertain primary s.
> catheter s.
> coaptation s.
> contralateral s.
> endoscopic biopsy s.
> entry s.
> excisional biopsy s.
> exit s.
> extraabdominal s.
> extraction s.
> extrahepatic tumor s.
> extranodal s.
> extrapulmonary s.
> fracture s.

> graft s.
> implantation s.
> injection s.
> introduction s.
> multiple s.
> s. of obstruction
> osteotomy s.
> patellar tendon graft donor s.
> (PTGDS)
> peritumoral s.
> pin s.
> port s.
> primary tumor s.
> single s.
> stoma s.
> suprapubic extraction s.
> tumor s.
> wound s.

site-specific surgery

sitting
> 1-s. endodontics

sitting position

situ
> carcinoma in s. (CIS)
> ductal carcinoma in s. (DCIS)
> ex s.
> fusion in s.
> in s.
> tumor in s.

situation
> anatomical s.

situs

Siurala classification

sixth
> s. cranial nerve
> s. venereal disease

size
> aerodynamic s.
> age, distant metastases, extent of
> local s. (AMES)
> breast s.
> clot s.
> crosslink plate s.
> gland s.
> heterogeneous gland s.
> in-between s.
> lesion s.
> metastasis, age, completeness of
> resection, local invasion, tumor s.
> (MACIS)
> true s.
> tumor s.

S

NOTES

size-matched organ
Sjöqvist intramedullary tractotomy
SjVO$_2$
>   jugular venous oxygen saturation
skeletal
>   s. abnormality
>   s. biopsy
>   s. correction
>   s. deformity
>   s. fixation
>   s. lesion
>   s. metastasis
>   s. muscle
>   s. muscle atrophy
>   s. muscle hypotonia
>   s. tissue
skeletal-extraskeletal angiomatosis
skeletal fixation
skeletology
skeleton
>   appendicular s.
>   axial s.
>   cardiac fibrous s.
>   fibrous s.
>   laryngeal s.
>   pelvic s.
>   spine s.
skeletonization
Skene
>   external genitalia, Bartholin,
>   urethral, and S. (EG/BUS)
>   S. gland
skewer technique
skew flap
skier fracture
Skillern fracture
skin
>   alligator s.
>   s. approximation
>   atrophic s.
>   s. biopsy
>   s. closure
>   combination s.
>   s. conductance
>   s. crease
>   s. crease incision
>   s. deficit wound
>   s. expansion technique
>   s. flap
>   s. flap necrosis
>   s. folding
>   s. graft
>   s. graft neovagina
>   s. groove
>   hidden nail s.
>   s. infection
>   s. knife incision
>   s. lubrication
>   s. lubrication therapy

>   s. measurement
>   s. nick
>   ostomy s.
>   photoaged s.
>   s. plasty
>   s. potential response
>   s. preparation
>   s. puncture
>   s. puncture test
>   redundant triangular-shaped s.
>   scarred s.
>   scrotal s.
>   s. sparing mastectomy
>   s. surfacing technique
>   surplus s.
>   s. temperature
>   s. temperature gradient measurement
>   thin glossy s.
>   triangular-shaped s.
>   s. ulcer
>   s. window technique
skin-colored lesion
skin-epidural distance
skinfold thickness
skinned muscle fiber
Skinner classification
skinning
>   s. colpectomy
>   s. vulvectomy
skinny-needle biopsy
skin-to-tumor distance
skip
>   s. area
>   s. graft
>   s. lesion
>   s. metastasis
ski position
skived incision
Skoog
>   S. fasciotomy
>   S. technique
skull
>   s. base approach
>   s. base tumor
>   s. block
>   cloverleaf s.
>   s. deformity
>   s. fracture
>   maplike s.
>   steeple s.
skullcap
slack
>   tissue s.
slant
>   s. muscle operation
>   s. of occlusal plane
SLAP
>   superior labium anterior and posterior
>   SLAP lesion

slaved programmed electrical stimulation
Slavianski membrane
sleep
    s. apnea-hypoventilation syndrome
    s. dissociation
    twilight s.
sleeve
    s. fracture
    s. gastrectomy
    s. graft
    s. lobectomy
    s. pneumonectomy
    s. resection
    s. technique
    2-s. technique
slice
    s. fracture
    s. preparation
sliding
    s. abdominal hernia
    s. esophageal hiatal hernia
    s. flap
    s. inlay bone graft
    s. nail
    s. oblique osteotomy
    s. plasty
    s. scale method
    s. tenotomy
sling
    s. and blanket technique
    s. immobilization
    s. ligation
    s. procedure
    s. and reef technique
    s. suture technique
sling-ring complex
sling/wrapping technique
slippage
    stomach s.
slipped
    s. capital femoral epiphysis
    s. hernia
    s. Nissen fundoplication
    s. Nissen repair
    s. rib cartilage syndrome
    s. vertebral apophysis
slipping
    s. rib
    s. rib syndrome
slit
    s. catheter technique

    Cheatle s.
    s. hemorrhage
    s. illumination
    lengthwise s.
    pudendal s.
    s. valve
    s. ventricle syndrome
    vulvar s.
slit-lamp ophthalmoscopy
slitlike defect
SLL
    second-look laparotomy
    serum lidocaine level
SLN
    sentinel lymph node
    SLN biopsy
    SLN localization
    SLN mapping
    SLN radiolocalization
SLND
    sentinel lymph node detection
Sloan incision
Sloan-Kettering thyroid cancer staging
Slocum
    S. amputation technique
    S. fusion technique
    S. maneuver
slope-shouldered lesion
slot
    s. fracture
    s. preparation
slot-blot
    s.-b. hybridization analysis
    s.-b. technique
slotted acetabular augmentation
slot-type preparation
slow
    s. exchange soft tissue
    s. maxillary expansion
    s. pull-through (SPT)
    s. respiration
slow-pathway ablation
SLR
    straight-leg raising
    SLR with external rotation test
Sluder
    S. guillotine tonsillectomy
    S. neuralgia
sludge
    biliary s.
sludging of circulation

S

NOTES

slush
ice s.
SMA
superior mesenteric artery
Smead-Jones closure
smear
buccal s.
smegma
smegmalith
Smellie method
Smellie-Veit method
smile
endogenous s.
exogenous s.
smiley-face knotting technique
smiling incision
Smith
S. dislocation
S. eyelid operation
S. flexor pollicis longus abductorplasty
S. fracture
S. Indian technique
S. modification
S. physical capacity evaluation
S. trabeculectomy
Smith-Boyce operation
Smith-Gibson operation
Smith-Indian operation
Smith-Kuhnt-Szymanowski operation
Smith-Lemli-Opitz syndrome
Smith-Petersen
S.-P. approach
S.-P. cup arthroplasty
S.-P. hemiarthroplasty
S.-P. osteotomy
S.-P. sacroiliac joint fusion
S.-P. synovectomy
S.-P. technique
Smith-Petersen-Cave-Van Gorder anterolateral approach
Smith-Robinson
S.-R. anterior cervical discectomy
S.-R. anterior fusion
S.-R. cervical disc approach
S.-R. cervical fusion
S.-R. interbody fusion
S.-R. operation
S.-R. procedure
S.-R. technique
Smithwick sympathectomy
SMN
second malignant neoplasm
surgical microscope navigation
smoldering appendix
smooth
s. muscle
s. muscle relaxant
s. muscle relaxation
s. muscular sphincter
s. skin-colored lesion
s. surface cavity
s. wrap
smooth-brain syndrome
SMP
sympathetically maintained pain
SNA
sympathetic nerve activity
snap-frozen biopsy
snapping iliopsoas tendon
snapshot GRASS technique
snare
s. cautery
s. electrocoagulation
s. excision biopsy
s. loop biopsy
s. technique
SNB
scalene node biopsy
sentinel node biopsy
SNBR
sentinel node-to-background ratio
Snellen
S. line
S. ptosis operation
S. suture technique
sniffing position
sniff method
snip
1-s. punctum operation
3-s. punctum operation
snout response
Snow procedure
snuffbox
anatomical s.
Snyder classification
soaking solution
soak therapy
Soave
S. endorectal pull-through
S. operation
social
s. consequence
s. interaction therapy
society
S. of American Gastrointestinal Endoscopic Surgeons (SAGES)
International Pelvic Pain s. (IPPS)
socket
hard s.
s. joint
s. reconstruction
suspension-type s.
sodium
parecoxib s.
Soemmerring
S. muscle

S. ring
S. ring cataract
Sofield
S. femoral deficiency technique
S. osteotomy
S. pinning
soft
s. abdomen
s. callus stage
s. cataract
s. chancre
s. corn
s. event
s. exudate
s. palate
s. palate cancer
s. palate cleft
s. palate paralysis
s. palate retraction
s. pigment stone
s. sore
s. stool
s. tissue
s. tissue abnormality
s. tissue abscess
s. tissue curettage
s. tissue damage
s. tissue dissection
s. tissue envelope
s. tissue extremity injury
s. tissue flap
s. tissue healing
s. tissue hinge
s. tissue integrity
s. tissue interface
s. tissue interposition
s. tissue irritability
s. tissue lesion
s. tissue mass
s. tissue massage
s. tissue metastasis
s. tissue mobilization
s. tissue necrosis
s. tissue plication
s. tissue release
s. tissue restriction
s. tissue sarcoma (STS)
s. tissue stranding
s. tissue stretching
s. tissue structure
s. tissue swelling
s. tissue thickness

s. tissue undercut
s. tissue window
s. tissue xerography
s. tubercle
s. wall
s. x-ray examination
s. x-ray investigation
soilage
peritoneal s.
soiling
colostomy s.
fecal s.
solar
s. ganglion
s. plexus
Solcia classification
soldier patch
soleal line
sole laser therapy
solid
s. hidradenoma
s. hyperplasia
s. organ
s. phase extraction
s. subtype
s. tumor
S. Tumor Autologous Marrow Transplant Program (STAMP)
s. visceral hematoma
solitaire
cholesterol s.
solitary
s. bundle
s. foramen
s. gland
s. pulmonary arteriovenous fistula
s. pulmonary mass
s. rectal ulcer
s. rectal ulcer syndrome
s. tract
Solomon-Bloembergen theory of dipole-dipole relaxation rate
solubility
solubilization
soluble gas technique
solute
total body s.
solution
activating s.
aqueous s.
azeotropic s.
cardioplegic s.

NOTES

solution *(continued)*
    cleaning s.
    cold soak s.
    colloid s.
    colonic lavage s.
    s. of contiguity
    s. of continuity
    crystalloid cardioplegic s.
    disclosing s.
    disinfecting s.
    electrolyte flush s.
    electrolytic s.
    extracellular-like, calcium-free s.
    extravasation irrigation s.
    eye irrigating s.
    hardening s.
    hydrolysis of s.
    hypotonic s.
    ideal s.
    intracellular-like, calcium-bearing
      crystalloid s.
    irrigating s.
    irrigation s.
    lacmoid staining s.
    lavage s.
    nonideal s.
    normal saline s.
    ophthalmic activating s.
    oxidation of s.
    physiologic saline s. (PSS)
    physiologic salt s.
    pickling s.
    precipitate in s.
    preservative s.
    rehydrating s.
    relaxing s.
    saline s.
    saltwater s.
    saturated s.
    sclerosing s.
    soaking s.
    solvent s.
    standard s.
    sterility of s.
    surgical marking s.
    volumetric s.
    wetting s.
    whole-gut lavage activating s.
solvation
solvent
    s. extraction
    s. solution
solvolysis
soma
somatectomy
    subtotal s.
somatic
    s. gene-transfer approach
    s. hypoalgesia

    s. mutation
    s. nerve
    s. pain
    s. therapy
somaticosplanchnic
somaticovisceral
somatization disorder
somatoprosthetics
somatosensory
    s. evoked potential (SEP, SSEP)
    s. pathway
somatostatin
    s. analogue
    s. receptor scintigraphy (SRS)
somatostatinoma syndrome
somatotropinoma
somatovisceral
Somerville
    S. anterior approach
    S. procedure
    S. technique
somite formation
somnolence
Somogyi method
Sondergaard procedure
Sondermann canal
Sones technique
sonication technique
sonic thrombolysis
sonification
Sonnenberg
    S. classification
    S. neurectomy
sonographic evidence
sonography
    focused abdominal s.
    renal s.
    serial s.
sonography-guided aspiration
sonoguided biopsy
sonohysterography
sonolucent tissue
sonomicrometry
sonomicroscopy
sonorous respiration
Soper modification
Sorbie calcaneal fracture classification
sore
    fungating s.
    hard s.
    pressure s.
    soft s.
    venereal s.
Soren ankle fusion
soreness
    delayed onset muscle s. (DOMS)
Soriano operation
Soria operation
Sorondo-Ferré hindquarter amputation

Sorrin operation
sorter
    fluorescence-activated cell s.
      (FACS)
Soto-Hall bone graft
sound
    absent bowel s.'s
    s. analysis
    bowel s.'s
    hypoactive bowel s.'s
    s. pressure level
    s. pressure level scale
    s. quantity
sound-stimulated fetal movement
source
    discrete bleeding s.
    endoscopic light s.
    point s.
    s. program
    simple sound s.
Sourdille
    S. keratoplasty
    S. keratoplasty operation
    S. ptosis operation
Southern blot technique
Southwick
    S. biplane trochanteric osteotomy
    S. slide procedure
Southwick-Robinson anterior cervical
  approach
space
    abdominal s.
    acromioclavicular s.
    air s.
    alveolar dead s.
    anatomic dead s.
    anorectal s.
    antecubital s.
    anterior clear s.
    apical s.
    arachnoid s.
    axillary s.
    Berger s.
    Bogros s.
    Böttcher s.
    Bowman s.
    buccal s.
    buccinator s.
    buccopharyngeal s.
    Burns s.
    capsular s.
    carotid s.

    central palmar s.
    cervical s.
    Chassaignac s.
    circumlental s.
    Colles s.
    coracoclavicular s.
    costoclavicular s.
    Cotunnius s.
    cranial epidural s.
    craniospinal s.
    danger s.
    dead s.
    deep perineal s.
    deep postanal anorectal s.
    denture s.
    digastric s.
    disc s.
    Disse s.
    s. of Donders
    echo-free s.
    edentulous s.
    embrasure s.
    endolymphatic s.
    epidural s.
    episcleral s.
    extracellular s.
    extraction s.
    extradural s.
    extraperitoneal s.
    extrapleural s.
    extravascular s.
    fascial s.
    fat cell s.
    first web s.
    fixed maintainer s.
    Fontana s.
    s. of Fontana
    freeway s.
    geniohyoid s.
    gingival s.
    H s.
    Henke s.
    His perivascular s.
    Holzknecht s.
    incisural s.
    increased lateral joint s.
    infraglottic s.
    inframesocolic s.
    infraorbital s.
    infratemporal s.
    interalveolar s.
    intercellular s.

S

NOTES

space *(continued)*

intercondylar s.
intercostal s.
intercristal s.
interdental s.
interfascial s.
interlamellar s.
interocclusal rest s.
interprismatic s.
interproximal s.
interradicular s.
intersheath s.
intersphincteric anorectal s.
interstitial s.
intervaginal s.
intracristal s.
intrafascial s.
intramembranous s.
intrapharyngeal s.
intravaginal s.
ischiorectal anorectal s.
joint s.
k s.
Kiernan s.
lateral central palmar s.
lateral joint s.
lattice s.
leeway s.
leptomeningeal s.
Lesgaft s.
life s.
lymph s.
Magendie s.
maintainer cast s.
Malacarne s.
mandibular s.
marrow s.
masseteric s.
masseter-mandibular-pterygoid s.
masticator s.
masticatory s.
Meckel s.
medial clear s.
mediastinal s.
medullary s.
midpalmar s.
Mohrenheim s.
s. myopia
Nance leeway s.
object s.
palm s.
paraglottic s.
paralaryngeal s.
parapharyngeal s.
pararenal s.
Parona s.
parotid s.
perforated s.
perianal anorectal s.

perichoroidal s.
peridental s.
peridentinoblastic s.
perihepatic s.
periimplant s.
perilenticular s.
perilymphatic s.
perineal s.
perinuclear s.
perioptic subarachnoid s.
periotic s.
peripharyngeal s.
perirenal s.
periscleral s.
perisinusoidal s.
peritoneal s.
peritonsillar s.
perivascular s.
perivitelline s.
pharyngeal s.
pharyngomaxillary s.
physiological dead s.
plantar s.
pleural s.
pleuroperitoneal s.
pneumatic s.
s. of Poirier
Poiseuille s.
popliteal s.
portal s.
position in s.
posterior cervical s.
postpharyngeal s.
postzygomatic s.
potassium s.
predental s.
preepiglottic s.
premasseteric s.
preperitoneal s.
presacral s.
preseptal s.
presternal s.
pretarsal s.
pretemporal s.
pretracheal s.
prevertebral s.
prezonular s.
properitoneal s.
Proust s.
proximal s.
proximate s.
Prussak s.
pterygomandibular s.
pterygomaxillary s.
pterygopalatine s.
pterygopharyngeal s.
quadrangular s.
quadrilateral s.
regainer s.

Reinke s.
relief s.
removable maintainer s.
retraction s.
retroadductor s.
retrobulbar s.
retrocardiac s.
retrocrural s.
retroesophageal s.
retrogastric s.
retroinguinal s.
retrolental s.
retromammary s.
retromuscular s.
retromylohyoid s.
retroocular s.
retroperitoneal s.
retropharyngeal s.
retropubic s.
retrosternal air s.
retrotracheal s.
retrovesical s.
retrovisceral s.
retrozygomatic s.
Retzius s.
s. of Retzius abscess
right anterior pararenal s.
Schwalbe s.
septal s.
sphenomaxillary s.
sphenopalatine s.
subacromial s.
subaponeurotic s.
subarachnoid s.
subchorial s.
subcoracoid s.
subdiaphragmatic s.
subdural s.
subgingival s.
subhepatic s.
sublingual s.
submandibular s.
submasseteric s.
submaxillary s.
submental s.
submucosal s.
subperitoneal s.
subphrenic s.
subpulmonic pleural s.
subretinal s.
subumbilical s.
superficial perineal s.

superior joint s.
supracolic s.
suprahepatic s.
suprahyoid s.
supralevator anorectal s.
supraomental s.
suprasternal s.
supratentorial s.
Tarin s.
temporal s.
Tenon s.
thenar s.
tibiofibular clear s.
tissue s.
Traube semilunar s.
Trautmann triangular s.
triangular s.
vascular s.
vertebral epidural s.
vesicocervical s.
Virchow-Robin s.
visceral s.
Waldeyer s.
web s.
Westberg s.
widened retrogastric s.
yolk s.
Zang s.
zonular s.
zygomaticotemporal s.

space-occupying
s.-o. brain lesion
s.-o. disease
s.-o. process

spacing
excessive s.

Spaeth
S. cystic bleb operation
S. ptosis operation

spall

Spälteholz preparation

span
levator s.

sparganoma

sparing therapy

Sparks
S. mandrel graft
S. mandrel technique

spasm
diffuse esophageal s. (DES)
esophageal s.
masseter s.

S

NOTES

spasm (*continued*)
    nocturnal painful tonic s. (NPTS)
    tonic s.
spasmodic colic
spasmolysis
spastic
    s. colon
    s. thumb-in-palm deformity
spatial
    s. localization procedure
    S. Orientation Memory Test
spatium, pl. **spatia**
spatulate
spatulated
spatulation
    s. condensation
    graft s.
    ureteral s.
Spaulding classification
Speas operation
special
    s. lesion
    s. reference method
specialized intralobular connective tissue
specialty
    nonophthalmologic surgical s.
    surgical s.
species
    fungal s.
specific
    s. ionization
    s. modulation
    s. rotation
    s. survival
    s. thrust manipulation
specificity phenomenon
specimen
    biopsy s.
    catheter s.
    colorectal s.
    cytologic s.
    cytology s.
    excised s.
    gastrectomy s.
    mastectomy s.
    operative s.
    pathologic s.
    preoperative FNA s.
    s. radiograph
    s. volume
speckled appearance
spectacle
    s. correction
    s. plane
spectacular shrinking deficit syndrome
spectometry
    time-of-flight mass s.
spectral
    s. edge

    s. edge frequency (SEF)
    s. edge frequency capnography
    s. entropy
    s. line
spectrometer
    liquid scintillation s.
    mass s.
spectrometry
    gas chromatography-mass s.
    gas isotope ratio mass s.
    isotope dilution-mass s.
    mass s.
spectrophotometry
    endoscopic reflectance s.
    fluorescence s.
    microlight guide s.
    near-infrared s.
spectroscopic
spectroscopy
    clinical s.
    image-selected in vivo s.
    infrared s.
    in vivo optical s.
    magnetic resonance s.
    MR s.
    near-infrared s.
    NMR s.
    Raman s.
specular
    s. microscopy
    s. reflection
speculum examination
speech
    s. correction
    s. detection threshold
Speed
    S. arthroplasty
    S. open reduction
    S. osteotomy graft
    S. radial head fracture classification
    S. sternoclavicular repair
    S. V-Y muscle-plasty
Speed-Boyd
    S.-B. open reduction
    S.-B. radial-ulnar technique
Spemann induction
Spence
    S. and Duckett marsupialization
    S. procedure
Spencer plication of vena cava
Spencer-Watson
    S.-W. Z-plasty
    S.-W. Z-plasty operation
sperm
    s. aspiration
    epididymal s.
    s. immobilization test

s. microaspiration retrieval
technique
s. washing insemination method
spermagglutination
spermatic
s. cord
s. duct
s. fistula
s. plexus
s. vein
s. vein ligation
spermatid
round s.
spermatocele
spermatocelectomy
spermatocyst
spermatogram
spermatolysis
spermatorrhea
spermaturia
spermiduct
spermolith
spermolysis
Spetzler anterior transoral approach
Spetzler-Martin classification
sphacelation
sphenethmoid
sphenion
sphenobasilar
sphenoccipital
sphenocephaly
sphenoethmoid
sphenoethmoidal recess
sphenoethmoidectomy
sphenofrontal suture
sphenoid
s. bone
s. emissary foramen
s. emissary vein
s. mucocele
s. process
s. sinus metastasis
sphenoidal
s. angle
s. concha
s. fissure
s. herniation
s. ridge
s. sinus
s. spine
s. turbinated bone
sphenoidectomy

sphenoidostomy
sphenoidotomy
sphenomalar
sphenomandibular ligament
sphenomaxillary
s. fissure
s. fossa
s. space
s. suture
sphenooccipital
s. joint
s. suture
sphenoorbital suture
sphenopalantine ganglion blockade
sphenopalatine
s. artery
s. canal
s. foramen
s. ganglion
s. ganglionectomy
s. nerve
s. space
sphenoparietal
s. suture
s. venous sinus
sphenopetrosa
sphenopetrosal fissure
sphenorbital
sphenosalpingostaphylinus
sphenosquamosal
sphenosquamous suture
sphenotemporal
sphenotic foramen
sphenoturbinal
sphenovomerine suture
sphenozygomatic suture
sphere
segmentation s.
spherica
spherical
s. lens aberration
s. recess
spheroid
s. articulation
s. joint
spherule
rod s.
sphincter
anatomical s.
anorectal s.
antral s.
anular s.

S

NOTES

sphincter *(continued)*
  artificial s.
  basal s.
  bicanalicular s.
  Boyden s.
  canalicular s.
  choledochal s.
  colic s.
  deep anal s.
  duodenal s.
  duodenojejunal s.
  esophageal s.
  external rectal s.
  external urethral s.
  extrinsic s.
  functional s.
  Glisson s.
  hepatopancreatic s.
  hypertensive lower esophageal s.
    (HLES)
  Hyrtl s.
  ileal s.
  ileocecocolic s.
  iliopelvic s.
  incompetent s.
  s. injury
  internal anal s. (IAS)
  internal urethral s.
  intrinsic s.
  lower esophageal s. (LES)
  macroscopic s.
  marginal s.
  mediocolic s.
  microscopic s.
  midgastric transverse s.
  midsigmoid s.
  s. muscle
  myovascular s.
  myovenous s.
  Nélaton s.
  O'Beirne s.
  Oddi s.
  s. of Oddi dysfunction
  s. of Oddi pressure
  ostial s.
  palatopharyngeal s.
  pancreatic s.
  pathologic s.
  pelvirectal s.
  s. pharyngoplasty
  physiological s.
  postpyloric s.
  prepapillary s.
  preprostate urethral s.
  prepyloric s.
  s. preservation
  proximal urethral s.
  pyloric s.
  radiological s.

  s. reconstruction
  rectosigmoid s.
  s. relaxation
  s. repair
  segmental s.
  smooth muscular s.
  s. sphincter
  striated muscular s.
  unicanalicular s.
  urethral s.
  Varolius s.
  velopharyngeal s.

sphincteral
sphincteralgia
sphincterectomy
  endoscopic s.
sphincterial
sphincteric
  s. construction
  s. continence
  s. potency
sphincterismus
sphincteroid tract
sphincterolysis
sphincteroplasty
  open s.
  pancreatic s.
  transduodenal s.
sphincteroscopy
sphincterotomy
  antegrade transcystic s.
  biliary s.
  Doublet s.
  endoscopic s. (ES)
  endoscopic pancreatic duct s.
  Erlangen pull-type s.
  external s.
  Geenen s.
  internal s.
  laparoscopic antegrade transcystic s.
  Mulholland s.
  needle-knife s.
  pancreatic duct s.
  Parks partial s.
  partial lateral internal s.
  precut s.
  retrograde s.
  transduodenal s.
  transendoscopic s.
  transurethral s.
  urethral s.
  zipper s.
sphincter-preserving proctectomy
sphincter-saving
  s.-s. method
  s.-s. operation
  s.-s. procedure
  s.-s. surgery
  s.-s. technique

sphincter-sparing
  s.-s. method
  s.-s. procedure
  s.-s. resection
  s.-s. technique
sphinx position
sphygmopalpation
sphygmoscopy
SPI
  structured pain interview
spica cast immobilization
spiculated lesion
spider
  s. angioma
  s. pelvis
  s. projection
spider-web clot
Spiegel lobe
Spieghel line
spigelian
  s. hernia
  s. lobe
  s. vein
Spigelius
  S. hernia
  S. line
  S. lobe
spike burst on electromyogram of colon
spill
  peritoneal s.
spillage
  intraabdominal s.
  intraperitoneal s.
  tumor s.
Spiller-Frazier technique
spina, pl. **spinae**
  s. bifida
spinal
  s. accessory nerve
  s. accessory nerve-facial nerve
    anastomosis
  afferent s.
  s. analgesia
  s. analgesic
  s. anesthesia (SA)
  s. anesthetic
  s. anesthetic technique
  s. angioma
  s. artery
  s. block
  s. canal
  s. column

  s. column stabilization
  s. compression fracture
  s. cord
  s. cord circulation
  s. cord compression
  s. cord concussion
  s. cord injury
  s. cord injury pain
  s. cord perfusion pressure (SCPP)
  s. cord protection
  s. cord shock syndrome
  s. cord stenosis (SCS)
  s. cord stimulation (SCS)
  s. cord tumor
  s. coronal plane deformity
  s. decompression
  s. deformity-instability
  s. delivery
  s. dermal sinus tract
  s. dural arteriovenous fistula
  s. epidural abscess (SEA)
  failed s.
  s. fixation
  s. fixation rigidity
  s. fluid drainage
  s. fusion
  s. fusion pathomechanics
  s. fusion position
  s. fusion technique
  s. ganglion
  s. gate
  s. headache
  s. hematoma
  s. infection
  s. infection biopsy
  s. inflammation
  s. injury operative stabilization
  s. instability
  s. joint mobilization
  s. lesion
  s. manipulation
  s. marrow
  s. metastasis
  Miami Modular Orthopaedic s.
  s. mobilization technique
  s. muscle
  s. osteotomy
  s. osteotomy stabilization
  s. oximetry
  s. point
  s. puncture
  s. pyramidotomy

S

NOTES

spinal *(continued)*
    s. root
    single-shot s.
    s. surgery
    s. tractotomy
    s. trauma
    s. vascular malformation
    s. vein
spinal/epidural
    combined s./e. (CSE)
spinal-locking procedure
spinally administered
spinaloscopy
spinate
spindle
    s. cell carcinoma
    s. cell sarcoma
    s. cell thymoma
    Krukenberg corneal s.
spindle-shaped incision
spine
    alar s.
    angular s.
    anterior inferior iliac s.
    anterior superior iliac s.
    bamboo s.
    Chance fracture thoracolumbar s.
    s. deformity
    dorsal s.
    s. fracture
    hemal s.
    iliac s.
    inferior iliac s.
    ischiadic s.
    ischial s.
    mental s.
    neural s.
    osteoporotic s.
    posterior inferior iliac s.
    posterior superior iliac s.
    pubic s.
    s. rotation
    sciatic s.
    s. skeleton
    sphenoidal s.
    thoracic s.
spin-echo
    s.-e. image
    s.-e. magnetic resonance imaging
    partial saturation s.-e.
Spinelli operation
spinning disc nebulizer
spinning-top deformity
spinocerebellar tract
spinogalvanization
spinoglenoid
spinolamellar line
spinolaminar line
spinomuscular

spinoneural
spinoolivary tract
spinotectal tract
spinothalamic
    s. cordotomy
    s. pathway
    s. tract (STT)
    s. tractotomy
spinous
    s. aspect
    s. interlaminar line
    s. plane
    s. process
    s. process fracture
spiradenoma
spiral
    s. CT technique
    s. dissection
    s. fold
    s. foraminous tract
    s. ganglion
    s. groove
    s. incision
    s. joint
    s. ligament
    s. line
    s. membrane
    s. oblique fracture
    s. suture technique
    s. vein graft
Spira procedure
spirochetal infection
spirochete infection
spirochetolysis
spirogram
    forced expiratory s.
spiroscopy
Spittler procedure
Spitzka marginal tract
Spivack gastrotomy technique
SPK
    simultaneous pancreas and kidney
    SPK transplant
    SPK transplantation
splanchnapophysial
splanchnapophysis
splanchnectopia
splanchnemphraxis
splanchnic
    s. anesthesia
    s. A-V fistula
    s. capillary pressure
    s. circulation
    s. congestion
    s. ganglion
    s. hypoperfusion
    s. nerve
    s. oxygenation
    s. oxygen consumption

s. perfusion
s. venous stasis
s. vessel
s. wall
splanchnicectomy
chemical s.
splanchnicotomy
splanchnocele
splanchnocranium
splanchnodiastasis
splanchnolith
splanchnologia
splanchnology
splanchnomicria
splanchnoptosis
splanchnoscopy
splanchnoskeletal
splanchnoskeleton
splanchnosomatic
splanchnotomy
splanchnotribe
S-plasty
SPLATT
split anterior tibial tendon
SPLATT procedure
splayed carina
splayfoot deformity
spleen
accessory s.
adult wandering s.
ectopic s.
enlarged s.
floating s.
movable s.
s. preservation
s. tip
wandering s.
spleen-preserving
s.-p. distal pancreatectomy
s.-p. pancreatic resection
splenectomy
abdominal s.
Henry s.
incidental s.
laparoscopic s.
open s.
Rives s.
subcapsular s.
splenectopia
splenetic
splenia (*pl. of* splenium)
splenial

splenic
s. artery (SA)
s. artery aneurysm (SAA)
s. A-V fistula
s. branch
s. conservation
s. cord
s. cord of Billroth
s. cyst
s. flexure
s. flexure carcinoma
s. flexure colonoscopy
s. fossa
s. hilum
s. injury
s. laceration
s. lesion
s. necrosis
s. plexus
s. pulp
s. puncture
s. recess
s. rupture
s. sequestration syndrome
s. sinus
s. tissue
s. vein
s. vein deformity
s. vein stump
spleniform
spleniserrate
splenium, pl. **splenia**
splenius
splenoadrenal
s. anastomosis
s. shunting
splenobronchial fistula
splenocele
splenocleisis
splenocolic ligament
splenogastric omentum
splenogonadal fusion
splenoid
splenolymphatic
splenoma
splenomegaly
congenital s.
splenonephric
splenopancreatic
splenopexy
splenophrenic
splenoptosis

S

NOTES

splenorenal
    s. angle
    s. ligament
    s. venous anastomosis
splenorenale
splenorrhagia
splenorrhaphy
splenosis
splenotomy
splenule
splenulus, pl. **splenulus**
splenunculus, pl. **splenunculi**
splintered fracture
splinter hemorrhage
splinting
    s. of abdomen
    closed reduction/chemical s.
    extracoronal s.
    Strong dorsal extension block s.
splint/stent
    kidney internal s./s. (KISS)
split
    s. anterior tibial tendon (SPLATT)
    s. anterior tibial tendon procedure
    s. anterior tibial tendon transfer
    s. cuff nipple technique
    s. fixation
    s. fracture
    s. ileostomy
    s. incision
    s. liver
    s. renal function test
    upper sternal s.
split-and-roll technique
split-bone technique
split-cast method
split-cord malformation
split-course technique
split-hand deformity
split-heel
    s.-h. approach
    s.-h. fracture
    s.-h. incision
split-leg position
split-liver
    s.-l. transplant
    s.-l. transplantation
split-lung ventilation
split-nail deformity
split-patellar approach
split-thickness
    s.-t. periodontal flap
    s.-t. skin graft
splitting
    s. fracture
    s. lacrimal papilla operation
SpO$_2$
    arterial oxyhemoglobin saturation
spoiled gradient-echo imaging

spoke-wheel appearance
spondylectomy
spondylitic
    s. deformity
    s. myelopathy
spondylitis
    ankylosing s.
    juvenile ankylosing s.
spondylodesis
spondylodiscitis
    lumbar s.
spondylolisthesis reduction
spondylolysis
spondylophyte
spondylothoracic
spondylotomy
spondylous
sponge
    s. biopsy
    s. dissection
    s. explant
spongioblastoma
spongioplasty
spongiositis
spongy
    s. body
    s. urethra
Sponsel oblique osteotomy
spontaneous
    s. adenocarcinoma
    s. aliquorrhea
    s. amputation
    s. ascites filtration
    s. breathing
    s. breech extraction
    s. coronary artery dissection
    s. dialytic ultrafiltration
    s. fracture
    s. hyperemic dislocation
    s. intermittent mandatory ventilation (SIMV)
    s. intestinal perforation (SIP)
    s. lateral ventricle hernia
    s. lesion
    s. perforation
    s. pneumothorax
    s. renal hemorrhage
    s. resolution
    s. rupture
    s. ventilation
    s. ventilation anesthetic technique
    s. ventrolateral hernia
sporadic
    s. CRC
    s. islet cell tumor
    s. multigland disease
    s. multigland hyperplasia
    s. multiple gland parathyroid hyperplasia

s. pituitary adenoma
s. primary HPT
s. primary hyperparathyroidism
s. renal cell carcinoma

spot
ash-leaf s.
cold s.
s. compression
corneal s.
hottest s.
s. magnification
milk s.
saccular s.
utricular s.

S-pouch reconstruction
spout
ileostomy s.

SPR
selective posterior rhizotomy
simultaneous pancreatic-renal

Sprague arthroscopic technique
sprain fracture
spray-wipe-spray disinfection
spread
extrathyroid s.
lymphatic s.
metastatic s.
omental s.
peritoneal s.

spreader graft
spreading
s. fistulation
s. hypoperfusion

Sprengel
S. anomaly
S. deformity

spring fixation
sprinter fracture
sprouting
ephaptic s.
sympathetic s.

sprue
collagenous s.

SPT
slow pull-through
station pull-through
SPT technique

spur formation
spurious hyponatremia
Spurling maneuver
spurring
sputum, pl. **sputa**

s. induction
pink frothy s.

SQ
subcutaneous

squama, pl. **squamae**
frontal s.
temporal s.

squamatization
squamocolumnar junction
squamofrontal
squamomastoid suture
squamooccipital
squamoparietal
squamopetrosal
squamosal suture
squamosomastoidea
squamotemporal
squamotympanic fissure
squamous
s. border
s. cell carcinoma
s. epithelium
s. hyperplasia
s. intraepithelial lesion (SIL)
s. intraepithelial lesion/atypical
squamous cell of undetermined
significance (SIL/ASCUS)
s. margin
s. metaplasia
s. regeneration
s. suture

squamozygomatic
squared
kilogram per meter s. (kg/m^2)

3-square flap
square-shouldered lesion
squeak
bronchopleural leak s.

squeeze pressure
SR
sinus rhythm
sustained release

Sr-90 beta radiation
SRCP
superficial renal cortical perfusion

SRS
somatostatin receptor scintigraphy

SRVGB
Silastic ring vertical-banded gastric
bypass

SS
septic shock

NOTES

Ssabanejew-Frank gastrostomy
SSAER
    steady-state auditory evoked response
SSEP
    somatosensory evoked potential
S-shaped
    S-s. body
    S-s. deformity
    S-s. ileal pouch-anal anastomosis
    S-s. incision
SSI
    surgical site infection
    anterior-posterior fusion with SSI
SSPCS
    side-to-side portacaval shunt
    direct SSPCS
    emergency SSPCS
SSRI
    selective serotonin reuptake inhibitor
    SSRI discontinuation syndrome
SST
    simple shoulder test
ST
    systolic time
    ST segment elevation
stab
    s. avulsion technique
    s. wound
    s. wound incision
stability
    cardiovascular s.
    detrusor s.
    hemodynamic s.
stabilization
    anterior internal s.
    anterior short-segment s.
    s. approach
    atlantoaxial s.
    atlantooccipital s.
    cervical spine s.
    cervicothoracic junction s.
    chest wall s.
    coronoradicular s.
    definitive s.
    distal radioulnar joint s.
    dynamic lumbar s.
    flexion compression spine injury s.
    fracture s.
    Gruca s.
    iliac crest bone graft s.
    lower cervical spine posterior s.
    lumbar spine s.
    myoplastic muscle s.
    occipitocervical s.
    odontoid fracture s.
    s. on retreat
    operative s.
    prophylactic operative s.
    provisional s.

    rhythmic s.
    sacral spine s.
    screw s.
    spinal column s.
    spinal injury operative s.
    spinal osteotomy s.
    subluxation s.
    thoracolumbar spine s.
    s. training
    TSRH crosslink s.
    wire s.
stabilized
    operatively s.
stabilizing fulcrum line
stable
    s. burst fracture
    s. cavitation
    hemodynamically s.
    s. reduction
stacked coin sign
stacking
    breath s.
Stack shoulder procedure
Stafne idiopathic bone cavity
stage
    s. B, C carcinoma
    disease s.
    Dukes s.
    hard callus s.
    s. II_E tumor
    implant s.
    lymph node s.
    s. migration
    s. operation
    patch s.
    3-s. procedure
    rehabilitation s.
    soft callus s.
    symptom experience s.
    tumor s.
stage
1-stage
    1-s. amputation
    1-s. hypospadias repair
    1-s. left colectomy
2-stage
    2-s. hip fusion
    2-s. procedure
    2-s. repair
    2-s. Syme amputation
    2-s. technique mastectomy
    2-s. tendon grafting technique
    2-s. tendon graft reconstruction
staged
    s. abdominal repair (STAR)
    s. bilateral stereotactic thalamotomy
    s. orchiopexy
    s. reconstruction

s. repair of extensive aortic
aneurysm
s. tympanoplasty
staghorn calculus
staging
Ann Arbor classification of
Hodgkin disease s.
Astwood-Coller s.
Boden-Gibb tumor s.
s. celiotomy
s. evaluation
FAB s.
FIGO classification s.
Jewett and Strong s.
laparoscopic s.
s. laparoscopy
s. laparotomy
multiple myeloma s.
nonoperative s.
s. operation
preoperative s.
primary gastric lymphoma s.
sentinel node s.
Sloan-Kettering thyroid cancer s.
surgical s.
surgical-pathologic s.
TNM system for tumor s.
tumor s.
stagnant
s. anoxia
s. hypoxemia
s. hypoxia
s. loop syndrome
stagnation
Staheli
S. shelf procedure
S. technique
Stähli pigment line
STAI
State-Trait Anxiety Inventory
stain
endocardial s.
immunohistochemical s.
Paget-Eccleston s.
port-wine s.
staining
anal canal s.
argyrophilic nucleolar organizer
region s.
blue s.
corneal blood s.
extrinsic environmental s.

GMS s.
Gomori methenamine silver s.
immunohistochemical s.
pattern of s.
staircase phenomenon
stairstep fracture
stalk
body s.
Stallard
S. eyelid operation
S. flap operation
Stallard-Liegard operation
staltic
STA-MCA
superficial temporal artery-to-middle
cerebral artery
STA-MCA anastomosis
Stamey
S. modification
S. modification of Pereyra
procedure
S. needle suspension
S. operation
S. urethropexy
Stamey-Martius procedure
Stamm
S. gastroplasty
S. gastrostomy
S. metatarsal osteotomy
S. procedure
S. procedure for intraarticular hip
fusion
Stammer method
Stamm-Kader gastrotomy technique
STAMP
Solid Tumor Autologous Marrow
Transplant Program
STAMP therapy
standard
s. biopsy technique
s. bone algorithm program
s. clavicular incision
s. D1 gastrectomy
s. electrode potential
s. fashion
s. formalin fixation
s. gastric resection
s. gastric resection Whipple
procedure
s. Kocher incision
s. mastectomy
s. midline laparotomy

NOTES

standard *(continued)*
   s. neck exploration
   s. open approach
   s. organ failure criteria
   s. patient monitoring
   s. radioenzymatic method
   s. reduction potential
   s. retroperitoneal flank incision
   s. right hemicolectomy
   s. solution
   s. stripping procedure
   s. surgical procedure
   s. technique
   s. thoracotomy
standardization
standardized
   s. curative radical total gastrectomy
   s. hepatectomy
   s. protocol
   s. uptake value (SUV)
stand-off weapon
Stanford
   S. aortic dissection (type A, B)
   S. biopsy method
   S. radical retropubic prostatectomy
Stanford-type aortic dissection
Stanisavljevic technique
Stanley Way procedure
Stanmore shoulder arthroplasty
Stansel procedure
stapedectomy
   House s.
stapedius
   s. muscle
   s. tendon
stapedotomy
   small fenestra s.
stapes mobilization
staphylectomy
staphylococcal
   s. infection
   s. scalded skin syndrome
Staphylococcus epidermidis
staphylopharyngorrhaphy
staphyloplasty
staphylorrhaphy
staphylotomy
staple
   s. capsulorraphy bone bank
   s. capsulorrhaphy
   s. fixation
   s. ligated
   s. line dehiscence
stapled
   s. blind end
   s. coloanal anastomosis
   s. esophagojejunostomy
   s. hemorrhoidectomy
   s. ileal pouch-anal anastomosis

   s. ileal pouch-anal anastomosis
     without proctomucosal proctectomy
   s. ileoanal anastomosis
   s. lung reduction
   s. reconstruction
   s. reconstruction method
   s. reconstruction procedure
   s. reconstruction technique
   s. stricturoplasty
Staples
   S. repair
   S. technique
Staples-Black-Broström ligament repair
stapling
   s. diverticulotomy
   gastric s.
   surgical s.
   s. technique
STAR
   staged abdominal repair
   STAR technique
star
   s. construction test
   4-s. exercise program
   s. formation
starch
   hydroxyethyl s.
Stark
   S. classification
   S. graft
Starkey matrix program
Stark-Moore-Ashworth-Boyes technique
Starlite point
startle technique
Starzl technique
STAS
   Support Team Assessment Schedule
stasis
   s. edema
   s. gallbladder
   s. liver
   splanchnic venous s.
   s. syndrome
   s. ulceration
   venous s.
state
   central excitatory s.
   chronic hyperparathyroid s.
   dysphoric mood s.
   S. end-to-end anastomosis
   exhaustion s.
   hypercoagulable s.
   inotropic s.
   International Classification of
     Diseases, Adapted for Use in the
     United s.'s (ICDA)
   local excitatory s.
   mood s.
   S. operation

oxidation s.
presurgical s.
thrombin-mediated consumptive s.
State-Trait Anxiety Inventory (STAI)
static
s. closure pressure
s. compliance
s. compliance of the total respiratory system
s. compression
s. dilation technique
s. evaluation
s. fixation
s. gangrene
s. image
s. method
s. position
s. relation
s. storage allocation
station
lymph nodal s.
node s.
perigastric node s.
perihepatic lymph nodal s.
s. pull-through (SPT)
s. pull-through esophageal manometry technique
s. test
stationary manometry
statoacoustic nerve
statoconia
statoconic membrane
status
acid-base s.
ASA physical s.
cancer s.
carrier s.
s. cribriform
s. epilepticus
s. evaluation
hepatic intracellular energy s.
hydration s.
lymph node s.
mutation carrier s.
nutritional s.
performance s.
premorbid performance s.
semielective s.
Stauffer
S. modification
S. syndrome
staurion

staving
barrel s.
stay
hospital s.
length of s. (LOS)
s. suture technique
steady-state
s.-s. auditory evoked response (SSAER)
s.-s. gradient-echo imaging
s.-s. infusion
s.-s. ventilatory response
steal
circulatory s.
iliac s.
s. phenomenon
portal s.
renal-splanchnic s.
subclavian s.
steam autoclave sterilization
steamy appearance
steatocystoma
steatohepatitis
nonalcoholic s. (NASH)
steatoma
steatotic liver
steel
S. correction
S. maneuver
S. rule of thirds
S. triple innominate osteotomy
steep
s. head-down tilt
s. Trendelenburg position
steeple skull
steerable cystoscopy
Steffee
S. instrumentation technique
S. thumb arthroplasty
Stegemann-Stalder method
stegnosis
Steichen neurovascular free flap
Steinberg infiltration block
Steinbrocker classification
Steindler
S. flexorplasty
S. matrixectomy
S. procedure
Steinert disease
Steinmann pin fixation
stellate
s. border breast lesion

S

NOTES

709

stellate *(continued)*
   s. configuration
   s. ganglion
   s. ganglion block
   s. ganglion blockade
   s. ganglion block anesthesia
   s. ganglion block anesthetic
     technique
   s. incision
   s. laceration
   s. ligament
   s. mass
   s. skull fracture
stellectomy
stem
   s. bronchus
   s. cell
   s. cell gene therapy
   s. cell mobilization
   s. removal
stem-loop structure
Stener-Gunterberg resection
Stener lesion
stenion
stenobregmatic
stenocephalia
stenocephalous
stenocephaly
stenocrotaphy
stenopeic iridectomy
stenosal
stenosed
stenosis, pl. **stenoses**
   arterial s.
   artery s.
   atherosclerotic renal artery s.
   calcific aortic s.
   carotid artery atherosclerotic s.
   cervical s.
   choledochoduodenal junctional s.
   congenital pyloric s.
   discrete s.
   esophageal s.
   granulation s.
   idiopathic hypertrophic subaortic s.
   ileostomy s.
   pulmonary valve s.
   pulmonic valve s.
   renal artery s.
   spinal cord s. (SCS)
   subglottic tracheal s.
   subvalvular aortic s.
   supravalvular aortic s.
   tracheal s.
   vessel s.
stenothorax
stenotic
   s. cricoid

   s. disease
   s. esophagogastric anastomosis
   s. lesion
   s. stoma
Stensen
   S. canal
   S. duct
stent
   s. apposition
   s. construction
   s. deployment
   s. evaluation
   s. expansion
   s. graft
   s. implantation
   s. incrustation
   s. patency
   s. placement
stented
   s. bovine pericardial xenograft
   s. porcine xenograft
stent-induced
   s.-i. intimal hyperplasia
   s.-i. pneumoperitoneum
stenting
   accessory duct s.
   antral s.
   biliary s.
   carotid s.
   carotid angioplasty with s.
   endoluminal s.
   endoscopic ampullary s.
   endoscopic pancreatic s.
   endoscopic papillotomy and s.
   endoscopic retrograde biliary s.
   endovascular s.
   primary s.
   renal artery s.
   s. technique
   transhepatic s.
   tumor s.
stentless composite graft
stent-mounted
stent-through-wire mesh technique
Stenvers projection
step
   corneal graft s.
   diagnostic s.
   s. graft operation
   s. osteotomy
   s. preparation
   therapeutic s.
2-step
   2-s. orchiopexy
   2-s. pancreatoduodenectomy
   2-s. procedure
   2-s. technique
step-by-step technique

step-cut
  s.-c. osteotomy
  s.-c. transection
stepdown
  s. osteotomy
  s. therapy
stephanial
stephanion
stepladder incision technique
step-up in oxygen saturation
stercolith
stercoral
  s. abscess
  s. fecaloma
  s. fistula
  s. ulceration
stercoroma
stereoauscultation
stereochemistry
stereocolpogram
stereoencephalotomy
stereography
  3-dimensional s.
StereoGuide stereotactic needle core biopsy
stereo-identical point
stereomagnification
stereoscopic interrogation
stereoscopy
stereoselective
stereoselectivity ratio
stereospecific action
stereotactic
  s. aspiration
  s. aspiration biopsy
  s. automated technique
  s. brain biopsy
  s. catheter drainage
  s. cordotomy
  s. core biopsy method
  s. core biopsy technique
  s. core breast biopsy
  s. craniotomy
  s. guidance
  s. lesion
  s. localization
  s. needle core biopsy
  s. needle core biopsy procedure
  s. neurosurgery
  s. operation
  s. pallidotomy
  s. percutaneous needle biopsy

  s. puncture
  s. radiation therapy
  s. radiofrequency lesioning
  s. radiosurgery
  s. surgery
  s. surgical ablation
  s. trigeminal tractotomy
  s. Vim thalamotomy
  s. VL thalamotomy
stereotactic-assisted radiation therapy
stereotactic-focused radiation therapy
stereotactic-guided biopsy
stereotaxic
  s. localization
  s. surgery
  s. technique
stereotaxis
  volumetric s.
stereotaxy
  frame-based s.
  frameless s.
sterile
  s. abscess
  s. field barrier
  s. granuloma
  s. matrix
  s. technique
  s. vaginal examination
sterility of solution
sterilization
  chemical vapor s.
  cold gas s.
  defined s.
  discontinuous s.
  dry heat oven s.
  ethylene oxide s.
  ETO s.
  fractional s.
  gas s.
  glutaraldehyde s.
  intermittent s.
  involuntary s.
  root canal s.
  steam autoclave s.
  tubal s.
  unsaturated chemical vapor s.
  voluntary s.
sterilized
  cold gas s.
steri-stripped incision
sterna (*pl. of* sternum)
sternad

NOTES

sternal
- s. angle
- s. artery
- s. branch
- s. cartilage
- s. development
- s. fragment
- s. joint
- s. lifting
- s. line
- s. muscle
- s. notch
- s. part of diaphragm
- s. plane
- s. position
- s. puncture
- s. rotation

sternal-occipital-mandibular immobilization
sternal-splitting incision
Sternberger antibody sandwich technique
sternochondroscapularis
sternochondroscapular muscle
sternoclavicular
- s. angle
- s. disc
- s. joint
- s. joint dislocation
- s. joint reconstruction
- s. joint reduction
- s. junction
- s. ligament
- s. muscle

sternocleidal
sternocleidomastoid
- s. artery
- s. hemorrhage
- s. muscle
- s. muscle origin
- s. region
- s. vein

sternocostal
- s. articulation
- s. head
- s. joint
- s. triangle

sternodynia
sternofascialis
sternoglossal
sternohyoideus
sternohyoid muscle
sternoid
sternomanubrial junction
sternomastoid
- s. artery
- s. muscle

sternopericardial ligament

sternoschisis
sternothyroid
- s. muscle
- s. muscle flap laryngoplasty

sternothyroideus
sternotomy
- complete s.
- concomitant median s.
- s. incision
- median s.
- s. scar

sternotracheal
sternotrypesis
sternovertebral
sternoxiphoid plane
sternum, pl. **sterna**
- s. cartilage
- mobile s.

sternum-splitting approach
steroid
- s. concentration
- endogenous s.
- s. hormone
- s. injection
- lumbar epidural s.

steroid-dependent asthmatic
steroid-resistant proteinuria
stertorous respiration
stethalgia
stetharteritis
stethoscopy
Steward Recovery Score
Stewart
- S. distal clavicular excision
- S. incision
- S. styloidectomy
- S. test

Stewart-Hamilton cardiac output technique
Stewart-Treves syndrome
Stickler syndrome
stick-tie suture technique
Stieda
- S. fracture
- S. process

Stiegmann-Goff technique
stiff abdomen
stiffness
- fusion s.

stiff-person syndrome
stigma, pl. **stigmata**
- malpighian s.
- stigmata of recent hemorrhage

stigmatization
stigmatoscopy
Stiles-Bunnell transfer technique
Stilling
- canal of S.

Stillman
>   S. method
>   S. technique

still radiography technique

stilus

Stimson
>   S. anterior shoulder reduction
>   technique
>   S. gravity method
>   gravity method of S.
>   S. maneuver

stimulated gracilis neosphincter technique

stimulating effect

stimulation
>   anal electrical s.
>   anocutaneous s.
>   antidromic s.
>   brain s.
>   calibrated electrical s.
>   cervical carcinoma s.
>   cortical s.
>   direct brain s.
>   direct electrical nerve s.
>   direct neural s.
>   dorsal column s. (DCS)
>   dorsal cord s.
>   double-burst s.
>   double simultaneous s.
>   electric s.
>   electrical nerve s.
>   electrical surface s.
>   electro-acupoint s.
>   electrogalvanic s.
>   electronic bone s.
>   electrophysiological s.
>   external-coil electrical s.
>   follicle maturation s.
>   functional electrical s.
>   functional neuromuscular s.
>   galvanic s.
>   Ganzfeld s.
>   gastric electrical s.
>   gingival s.
>   high-voltage pulsed galvanic s.
>   hilum s.
>   implantable gastric s. (IGS)
>   intracranial s.
>   intraoperative cavernous nerve s.
>   intravaginal electrical s.
>   juxtacrine s.
>   magnetic s.

magnetoelectric s.
mechanical s.
microamperage electrical nerve s.
microamperage neural s.
motor-evoked response to
>   transcranial s. (tc-MER)
neuromuscular electrical s.
nociceptive s.
noninvasive programmed s.
ovarian s.
ovulation s.
paired electrical s.
pelvic s.
percutaneous s.
percutaneous electrical nerve s.
>   (PENS)
periaqueductal gray matter s.
periaqueductal-periventricular s.
photic s.
phrenic s.
precentral cortical s.
programmed electrical s.
repetitive nerve s.
s. scan
secretin s.
selective arterial s.
sensory s.
slaved programmed electrical s.
spinal cord s. (SCS)
subthreshold s.
supramaximal tetanic s.
tactile s.
s. test
tetanic s.
thermal s.
s. threshold
train-of-four s.
transcranial s. (TCS)
transcranial electrical s.
transcutaneous acupoint electrical s.
>   (TAES)
transcutaneous cranial electrical s.
>   (TCES)
transcutaneous electric s. (TES)
transcutaneous electrical nerve s.
transcutaneous electrode nerve s.
transesophageal atrial s.
transurethral electrical bladder s.
ultrarapid subthreshold s.
vagal nerve s.
vaginal electrical s.
ventricular-programmed s.

S

NOTES

stimulation *(continued)*
    vibroacoustic s.
    visual s.
stimulator
    cochlear s.
stimulus, pl. **stimuli**
    double extra s.
    external s.
    flicker-fusion s.
    noxious s.
    train-of-four s.
    transcutaneous tetanic s.
stippled epiphysis
stippling
    geographic s.
STIR
    short tau inversion recovery
    STIR technique
stitch
    s. abscess
    Allgöwer s.
    baseball s.
    bow-tie s.
    Bunnell s.
    Connell s.
    cuticular s.
    extramucosal s.
    figure-of-8 s.
    Fothergill s.
    Frost s.
    funnel s.
    intracuticular s.
    marker s.
    mattress s.
    McCall s.
    roll s.
    seromuscular s.
    shoelace s.
    tagging s.
    tilt s.
    tracheal safety s.
    triple-throw square knot s.
St. Mark polyposis registry
Stocker
    S. line
    S. operation
Stockholm technique for radium therapy
stocking anesthesia
stocking-glove
    s.-g. anesthesia
    s.-g. pain distribution
stocking-seam incision
Stock operation
Stoffel operation
Stoll dilution egg count technique
stoma, pl. **stomata**
    abdominal s.
    anastomotic s.

Benchekroun s.
bowel s.
s. button
catheterizable s.
s. closure
colonoscopy per s.
concealed umbilical s.
diverting s.
dusky s.
end s.
end-loop s.
gastroenterostomy s.
gastrointestinal s.
s. hernia
ileostomy s.
loop s.
maturing the s.
Mitrofanoff s.
nippled s.
permanent s.
pleural s.
prolapsed s.
proximal diverting s.
retracted s.
rodless end-loop s.
rosebud s.
Silastic collar-reinforced s.
s. site
stenotic s.
s. therapist
tracheostomy s.
ureteral s.
ureteric s.
Wang pleural s.
stomach
    aberrant umbilical s.
    s. acid
    s. adenocarcinoma
    bilocular s.
    s. cancer metastasis
    s. cardiomyotomy
    s. deformity
    Dieulafoy vascular malformation of s.
    drain-trap s.
    dumping s.
    hourglass s.
    insufflation of s.
    intrathoracic s.
    leather-bottle s.
    posterior s.
    pyloric part of s.
    s. reefing
    s. resection
    sclerotic s.
    s. slippage
    thoracic s.
    totally intrathoracic s.
    trifid s.

upside-down s.
wallet s.
watermelon s.
water-trap s.
stomachal
stomachic
stomal
s. colonoscopy
s. complication
s. intussusception
s. invagination
s. prolapse
s. retraction
s. ulceration
stomata (*pl. of* stoma)
stomatal
stomatic
stomatomy
stomatonoma
stomatoplastic
stomatoplasty
stomatoscopy
diagnostic fiberoptic s.
fiberoptic s.
stomatotomy
stomocephalus
stomodeum
stone
biliary tract s.
bladder s.
cholesterol s.
common bile duct s. (CBDS)
duct s.
endoscopic extraction pancreatic
duct s.
s. extraction
extraction bile duct s.
extraction pancreatic s.
extrahepatic s.
s. fragmentation
s. granuloma formation
mounted point s.
S. procedure
s. removal
renal s.
soft pigment s.
s. surgery
vein s.
stony-hard eye
Stookey-Scarff operation
stool
abdominal s.

s. evacuation
guaiac-negative s.
guaiac-positive s.
hard s.
heme-negative s.
heme-positive s.
s. impaction
soft s.
Stoppa
S. giant prosthetic reinforcemant
S. giant prosthetic reinforcement of
visceral sac
S. GPRVS
S. hernia repair
S. procedure
Stoppa-type laparoscopic repair
stop-valve airway obstruction
storage allocation
storm
thyroid s.
Stovall-Black method
stove-in chest
strabismus
paralytic s.
s. surgery
strabotomy
straddle fracture
straight
s. canal
s. catheter test
s. graft
s. incision
s. seminiferous tubule
s. sinus
straightening maneuver
straight-in ventriculostomy
straight-leg raising (SLR)
strain
compression s.
lysogenic s.
strain/counterstrain technique
straining
excessive s.
Straith eyelid operation
Strampelli-Valvo operation
stranding
fascial s.
soft tissue s.
strangulated
s. hemorrhoid
s. incisional hernia
s. paraesophageal hernia

NOTES

S

strangulation necrosis
strangury
strap muscle
strapping
 LowDye s.
Strassman
 S. metroplasty
 S. technique
 transverse fundal incision of S.
strata (*pl. of* stratum)
strategy
 imaging s.
 injury-prevention s.
 management s.
 protective ventilatory s.
 surgical s.
 treatment s.
stratification
stratified
 s. clot
 s. epithelium
stratiform fibrocartilage
stratum, pl. **strata**
Straub technique
Strauss method
strawberry angioma
straw-colored ascites
Strayer
 S. procedure
 S. tendon technique
streak retinoscopy
stream
 fecal s.
Streatfield-Fox operation
Streatfield operation
Streatfield-Snellen operation
strength
 bone-screw interface s.
 cervical extension s.
 extensor hallucis longus s.
 extrinsic muscle s.
 graft s.
 isometric cervical extension s.
 wound-breaking s.
strength-duration curve
Stren intraepiphysial osteotomy
streptococcal infection
Streptococcus **infection**
stress
 cold restraint s.
 s. dorsiflexion projection
 s. fracture
 s. lesion
 operative s.
 s. reduction
 s. relaxation
 s. response
 s. rupture
 surgical s.

 s. ulceration
 s. ulcer hemorrhage
 s. urethral pressure profile
 s. urinary incontinence
stress-induced
 s.-i. gastric ulceration
 s.-i. hyperthermia (SIH)
stress-redistribution-reinjection thallium-201 imaging
stretch
 anal s.
 s. injury
stretch-and-spray technique
stretcher
stretch-induced neuropathy
stretching
 soft tissue s.
Stretta
 S. operation
 S. procedure
stria, pl. **striae**
 corneal s.
 striae of Zahn
striate
 s. artery
 s. body
striated
 s. duct
 s. muscle
 s. muscle innervation
 s. muscular sphincter
striation
 tabby-cat s.
 tigroid s.
Strickland
 S. modification
 S. technique
 S. tendon repair
stricture
 anastomotic s.
 benign s.
 bile duct s.
 biliary s.
 bismuth type IV s.
 Caroli type I distal bile duct s.
 cicatricial s.
 clip-induced bile duct s.
 distal bile duct s.
 esophageal s.
 s. formation
 peptic s.
 s. prophylaxis
 s. rate
stricturoplasty
 Finney s.
 Heineke-Mikulicz s.
 stapled s.
 s. technique
 Thal s.

stricturoplasty
Finney s.
Heineke-Mikulicz s.
stapled s.
s. technique
Thal s.
stricturotomy
endoscopic s.
stridor
nonorganic s.
postextubation s.
stridulous respiration
string
s. cell carcinoma
s. test
string-of-beads appearance
strip
autogenous s.
s. biopsy
s. biopsy resection technique
circumferential s.
s. craniectomy
s. perforation
s. procedure
s. resection
stripe
paratracheal tissue s.
properitoneal flank s.
stripout
screw s.
stripping
s. membrane
s. program
stroboscope
Stroganoff method
stroke
acute ischemic s.
s. ejection rate
exploratory s.
hemorrhagic s.
ischemic s.
mitochondrial myopathy,
encephalopathy, lactacidosis, s.
(MELAS)
nonfatal s.
perioperative s.
s. volume (SV)
stroma
stromal
s. line
s. neovascularization
stromatolysis
stromatosis
Strombeck nipple transposition
Strong dorsal extension block splinting

strongyloma
strophocephaly
Stroud pectinated area
structural
s. abnormality
s. anomaly
s. lesion
structure
abdominal s.
anatomic s.
bony s.
cord s.
cystic s.
echodense s.
endosellar s.
extraarticular s.
graft s.
helix-loop-helix s.
implant s.
infratentorial s.
major vascular s.
periesophageal s.
retroclival s.
retroperitoneal s.
retrosellar s.
ring s.
sella s.
sidewall s.
soft tissue s.
stem-loop s.
underlying s.
vascular s.
structured pain interview (SPI)
struma lymphomatosa
strumectomy
median s.
strumiform
strut
s. allograft
s. fracture
s. fusion technique
s. graft
s. malposition
s. plate fixation
struvite
s. calculus
s. crystal formation
STS
soft tissue sarcoma
STT
spinothalamic tract
studding
peritoneal s.
Studebaker technique
Student-Newman-Keuls test

S

NOTES

Studer
    S. pouch procedure
    S. reservoir urinary diversion
study
    acoustic stimulation s.
    altitude simulation s.
    angiographic s.
    Asymptomatic Carotid
      Atherosclerosis S. (ACAS)
    barium swallow s.
    bead chain s.
    bulb-tip retrograde s.
    contrast s.
    coronary artery surgery s. (CASS)
    cytologic s.
    diagnostic s.
    Doppler s.
    electromyographic s.
    electrophysiology s.
    epidemiologic s.
    exercise s.
    histologic s.
    imaging s.
    injection s.
    localization s.
    manometric s.
    multicentric s.
    noninvasive localization s.
    noninvasive venous s.
    postirradiation s.
    preoperative s.
    pressure s.
    pressure-flow electromyography s.
    prospective s.
    radiologic s.
    tissue s.
    T-tube s.
    venographic s.
    venous s.
    Veterans Administration
      Cooperative s.
    volumetric s.
Stulberg classification
stump
    anastomotic s.
    cervical s.
    s. dehiscence
    distal s.
    duodenal s.
    s. embolization syndrome
    Hartmann s.
    s. invagination
    s. leak
    s. ligation
    s. pain
    pancreatic s.
    s. pressure
    rectal s.
    rectosigmoid s.

    Roux limb s.
    splenic vein s.
stunned myocardium
Sturmdorf
    S. operation
    S. suture technique
stuttering
    exteriorized s.
    urinary s.
stye
styliform
styloauricularis
styloauricular muscle
styloglossus muscle
stylohyal
stylohyoid
    s. branch
    s. ligament
    s. muscle
    s. process syndrome
styloid
    s. cornu
    s. prominence
    s. syndrome
styloidectomy
    Stewart s.
stylomandibular
    s. ligament
    s. membrane
stylomastoid
    s. artery
    s. foramen
    s. vein
stylomaxillary ligament
stylopharyngeal muscle
stylopharyngeus
stylostaphyline
stylosteophyte
styptic collodion
Suarez-Villafranca operation
Suave-Kapandji arthroplasty
subabdominal
subabdominoperitoneal
subacromial
    s. bursa
    s. space
subacute inflammation
subambient pressure
subanal
subanesthetic concentration
subapical segment
subaponeurotic space
subarachnoid
    s. anesthesia
    s. block
    s. cavity
    s. cistern
    s. hemorrhage

s. injection
s. space
subarcuata
subarcuate fossa
subareolar tenderness
subastragalar dislocation
subaural
subauricular
subaxial
subaxillary
subcapital
s. fracture
s. osteotomy
subcapsular
s. hemorrhage
s. renal hematoma
s. splenectomy
subcartilaginous
subcaudate tractotomy
subcecal fossa
subchondral
subchorial
s. hemorrhage
s. space
subchorionic
s. hematoma
s. hemorrhage
subchoroidal approach
subciliary incision
subclassification
subclavian
s. arteriovenous fistula
s. artery
s. artery aneurysm
s. artery occlusion
s. central venous catheter insertion
s. duct
s. groove
s. injury
s. line
s. loop
s. lymphatic trunk
s. muscle
s. nerve
s. periarterial plexus
s. perivascular block
s. steal
s. steal syndrome
s. sulcus
s. triangle
s. vein
s. vein catheterization

s. vein patch angioplasty
s. vessel exposure
subclavian-subclavian bypass
subclavicular approach
subclinical infection
subcoma therapy
subcomplete resection
subcondylar
s. deformity
s. oblique osteotomy
subconjunctival
s. hemorrhage
s. injection
subcoracoid
s. bursa
s. shoulder dislocation
s. space
subcorneal blister
subcortical hemorrhage
subcostal
s. artery
s. flank incision
s. groove
s. line
s. muscle
s. nerve
s. plane
s. port
s. position
s. transperitoneal incision
s. vein
subcostosternal
subcranial
subcruralis
subcrureus
subcutaneous (SQ)
s. acromial bursa
s. anastomosis
s. calcaneal bursa
s. cyst
s. dose
s. emphysema
s. fascia
s. fasciotomy
s. flap
s. fungal infection
s. hematoma
s. implantation
s. implanted injection port
s. infrapatellar bursa
s. injection
s. mastectomy

NOTES

subcutaneous *(continued)*
- s. necrosis
- s. necrotizing infection
- s. olecranon bursa
- s. operation
- s. plane
- s. portion
- s. ring
- s. route
- s. scalp
- s. tibialis posterior tenotomy
- s. tissue
- s. transfusion

subcuticular suture technique
subcutis
subdeltoid
- s. bursa
- s. fat plane obliteration

subdiaphragmatic
- s. abscess
- s. space

subdigastric node
subdorsal
subduce
subdural
- s. abscess
- s. block
- s. cavity
- s. cleft
- s. effusion
- s. electrode array
- s. grid implantation
- s. hematoma
- s. hematorrhachis
- s. hemorrhage
- s. hygroma
- s. puncture
- s. space

subendocardial
subependymal
- s. brain calcification
- s. brain nodule
- s. extension
- s. giant cell astrocytoma
- s. hemorrhage

subependymoma
subepithelial
- s. hemorrhage
- s. membrane

subepithelium
subfalcial herniation
subfascial
- s. hematoma
- s. ligation
- s. prepatellar bursa

subfrontal approach
subfrontal-transbasal approach
subgaleal
- s. abscess

- s. emphysema
- s. hematoma
- s. hemorrhage

subgingival space
subglenoid shoulder dislocation
subglottic
- s. cavity
- s. edema
- s. pressure
- s. tracheal stenosis

subgluteal hematoma
subgrundation
subhepatic
- s. abscess
- s. recess
- s. space

subhuman primate donor
subhyaloid hemorrhage
subhyoid bursa
subiliac
subilium
subimplant membrane
subinfection
subinguinal
- s. fossa
- s. incision
- s. microsurgical varicocelectomy
- s. triangle

subintimal hemorrhage
subjacent tissue
subject
- human s.
- supine human s.

subjugal
sublabial
- s. incision
- s. midline rhinoseptal approach
- s. perforation

sublaminar
- s. fixation
- s. wiring

sublation
sublesional ulceration
sublethal x-ray damage repair
subligamentous dissection
sublimation
sublimis
sublingual
- s. artery
- s. bursa
- s. caruncula
- s. crescent
- s. cyst
- s. duct
- s. fold
- s. fossa
- s. ganglion
- s. gland
- s. hematoma

s. papilla
s. pit
s. space
s. space abscess
s. vein
sublumbar
subluxation
rotary s.
s. stabilization
submammary incision
submandibular
s. duct
s. fossa
s. ganglion
s. node
s. space
s. space abscess
s. triangle
submandibulectomy
submasseteric
s. space
s. space abscess
submassive PE
submaxillary
s. duct
s. fossa
s. ganglion
s. space
s. triangle
submembranous placental hematoma
submental
s. artery
s. fistula
s. hematoma
s. liposuction
s. node
s. space
s. space abscess
s. triangle
s. vein
s. vertex projection
submentovertical projection
submucosa
jejunal s.
small intestinal s. (SIS)
submucosal
s. dissection
s. gastric hemorrhage
s. invasion
s. mass
s. plexus
s. space

s. urethral augmentation
s. vascular dilation
submucous
s. membrane
s. resection
submuscular implantation
subnarcotic
subnasal
subneural
suboccipital
s. decompression
s. muscle
s. nerve
s. region
s. triangle
s. venous plexus
suboccipital-subtemporal approach
suboccipital-transmeatal approach
suboptimal
s. examination
s. surgery
subparalyzing dose
subparietal
subpatellar
subpectoral
s. implantation
s. implantation technique
s. plane
s. pocket
subpelviperitoneal
subpericardial
subperichondrial excision
subperiosteal
s. abscess
s. dissection
s. exposure
s. fracture
s. hematoma
s. hemorrhage
s. implant abutment
s. implant 1-phase technique
s. infection
s. resection
subperiosteally
subperitoneal
s. fascia
s. space
subperitoneoabdominal
subperitoneopelvic
subpetrosal
subpharyngeal

NOTES

subphrenic
- s. abscess
- s. fluid
- s. recess
- s. region
- s. space

subpleural

subplexal

subpopliteal recess

subpopulation

subpreputial

subpubic
- s. angle
- s. hernia

subpubicus

subpulmonary

subpulmonic pleural space

subpylorici

subpyloric node

subretinal
- s. damage
- s. hemorrhage
- s. neovascularization
- s. neovascular membrane
- s. space
- s. surgery

subsarcolemma cisterna

subsartorial canal

subscale
- catastrophizing s.
- cognitive anxiety s.
- fear s.
- helplessness s.

subscapular
- s. artery
- s. branch
- s. bursa
- s. fossa
- s. muscle
- s. nerve
- s. vein

subscapularis
- s. muscle
- s. tendon

subsector

subsegmental hepatectomy

subsegmentectomy
- hepatic s.

subselective embolization

subserosa

subserous

subspinous

substance
- cement s.
- compact s.
- s. concentration
- corneal s.
- cortical s.
- exogenous s.

- exophthalmos-producing s.
- extracellular ground s.
- glandular s.
- medullary s.
- müllerian inhibiting s.
- muscular s.
- tumor polysaccharide s.
- vasoactive s.

substantia

substernal
- s. angle
- s. gland

substernomastoid

substitute
- blood s.
- bone graft s.
- hypooncotic plasma s.

substitutional cardiac surgery

substitution transfusion

substructure

subsuperior segment

subtalar
- s. articulation
- s. dislocation

subtemporal
- s. craniotomy
- s. decompression
- s. dissection

subtemporal-intradural approach

subtendinous
- s. iliac bursa
- s. prepatellar bursa

subtentorial lesion

subthreshold stimulation

subtotal
- s. colectomy (SC)
- s. distal pancreatectomy
- s. esophagectomy
- s. esophagoplasty
- s. gastrectomy
- s. gastric exclusion
- s. gastric resection
- s. glossectomy
- s. hepatectomy
- s. lateral meniscectomy
- s. maxillectomy
- s. pancreatoduodenectomy
- s. parathyroidectomy
- s. proctectomy
- s. proctocolectomy
- s. somatectomy
- s. supraglottic laryngectomy
- s. thyroidectomy

subtraction
- image s.
- s. technique

subtrochanteric
- s. femoral fracture

S

s. incision
s. osteotomy
subtrochlear
subtype
comedo s.
cribriform s.
micropapillary s.
papillary s.
solid s.
tumor s.
subumbilical
s. incision
s. infection
s. space
subungual hematoma
suburethral rectus fascial sling
procedure
subvaginal
subvalvular aortic stenosis
subvertebral
subvitrinal
subvolution
subvoxel accuracy
subxiphoid
s. limited pericardiotomy
s. port
subzonal insemination
subzygomatic
succenturiate
successive approximation
success rate
sucking chest wound
Sucquet
S. anastomosis
S. canal
Sucquet-Hoyer
S.-H. anastomosis
S.-H. canal
sucrose test
suction
airway s.
s. aspiration
s. biopsy
bulb s.
s. coagulator
continuous NG s.
s. curettage
diastolic s.
s. dissection
s. drainage
Frazier s.
Gomco s.

s. injury
lavage and s.
low intermittent s.
s. method
nasogastric s.
nasopharyngeal s.
nasotracheal s.
NG s.
orogastric s.
perilimbal s.
rhoton s.
s. suspension
suctioning
endotracheal s.
suction-irrigation technique
Suda papilla classification (type I–III)
sudation
sudden infant death syndrome (SIDS)
Sudeck critical point
sudomotor
s. axon reflex testing
s. evaluation
sudoriferous
s. duct
s. gland
Sugarbaker operation
sugar-icing liver
suggillation
postmortem s.
Sugioka transtrochanteric rotational
osteotomy
Sugiura
S. esophageal variceal transection
S. operation
S. procedure
suite
endoscopy s.
sulcal artery
sulcate
sulci (*pl. of* sulcus)
sulciform
sulcomarginal tract
sulcus, pl. **sulci**
ampullary s.
atrioventricular s.
calcaneal s.
carotid s.
cerebral s.
chiasmatic s.
cingulate s.
coronary s.
deltopectoral s.

NOTES

sulcus *(continued)*
    s. fixated position
    s. fixation
    implant gingival s.
    inferior petrosal s.
    internal spiral s.
    intertubercular s.
    mentolabial s.
    nymphocaruncular s.
    nymphohymenal s.
    preauricular s.
    pulmonary s.
    scleral s.
    sclerocorneal s.
    sigmoid s.
    subclavian s.
    superior petrosal s.
    supraacetabular s.
    talar s.
    terminalis s.
sulfacytine
sulfation
sulfonation
sulfur and silver point
Summerskill operation
sump syndrome
sun
    s. and chemical combination
      damage
    s. exposure
SUNCT
    short duration, unilateral, neuralgic,
    conjunctival injection and tearing
    SUNCT syndrome
Sunderland nerve injury classification
Sunna circumcision
Supartz joint fluid therapy
superacromial
superanal
superciliary arch
superduct
superexcitation
superfecundation
superfetation
superficial
    s. angioma
    s. anterior larynx
    s. anterior wall
    s. brachial artery
    s. branch
    s. burn
    s. cardiac plexus
    s. cervical artery
    s. circumflex iliac artery
    s. epigastric artery
    s. excision
    s. external pudendal artery
    s. forearm
    s. head

s. implantation
s. inguinal fascia
s. keratectomy
s. lamellar keratoplasty
s. layer
s. lymphatic vessel
s. neck
s. orbit
s. palmar arch
s. palmar artery
s. parotidectomy
s. perineal artery
s. perineal pouch
s. perineal space
s. radiation
s. renal cortical perfusion (SRCP)
s. subumbilical infection
s. suture technique
s. temporal artery
s. temporal artery/middle cerebral
    artery (STA-MCA)
s. temporal artery-to-MCA bypass
s. temporalis artery
s. temporal plexus
s. thrombophlebitis
s. type
s. volar artery
s. wound
superficialis
superficialization
supergenual
superimpregnation
superinfection
    fungal s.
superior
    s. aberrant ductule
    s. alveolar artery
    s. angle
    s. arcuate bundle
    s. boundary
    s. carotid triangle
    s. cerebellar artery
    s. cervical cardiac branch
    s. cervical ganglion
    s. cervical ganglionectomy
    s. costal facet
    s. costal pit
    s. dislocation
    s. duodenal fold
    s. duodenal fossa
    s. duodenal recess
    s. edge
    s. epigastric artery
    s. face
    s. fascia
    s. flap
    s. flexure
    s. gluteal artery
    s. gluteal artery perforator

s. gluteal neurovascular bundle
s. hemorrhoidal artery
s. hemorrhoidal plexus
s. horn
s. hypogastric plexus
s. hypophysial artery
s. ileocecal recess
s. intercostal artery
s. internal parietal artery
s. joint space
s. labial artery
s. labial branch
s. labium anterior and posterior (SLAP)
s. lacrimal duct
s. lacrimal papilla
s. lacrimal punctum
s. laryngeal cavity
s. laryngeal nerve external branch
s. larynx
s. lateral genicular artery
s. leaf
s. lingular segment
s. margin
s. meatus
s. medial genicular artery
s. mediastinum
s. mesenteric arterial system
s. mesenteric artery (SMA)
s. mesenteric ganglion
s. mesenteric plexus
s. mesenterorenal bypass technique
s. oblique tendon
s. omental recess
s. orbit
s. orbital fissure
s. orbital fissure syndrome
s. pancreaticoduodenal artery
s. parathyroid
s. parietal lobe
s. pelvic aperture
s. peroneal retinaculum
s. petrosal sulcus
s. phrenic artery
s. pole
s. pubic ramotomy
s. rectal artery
s. rectal fold
s. rectal plexus
s. sector iridectomy
sinus petrosus s.
s. suprarenal artery

s. tarsus
s. thoracic aperture
s. thoracic artery
s. thyroid artery
s. thyroid notch
s. thyroid plexus
s. thyroid tubercle
s. tibial articulation
s. ulnar collateral artery
s. vena cava (SVC)
s. vena cava syndrome
s. venal caval obstruction
s. vertebral notch
s. vesical artery
superior-intradural approach
superlactation
supernate
supernumerary
s. breast
s. gland
s. organ
superobese
superolateral
superovulation induction
superoxide-mediated endothelial cell dysfunction
superoxide scavenger
superpetrosal
superpigmentation
superselective
s. microcoil embolization
s. vagotomy
supersensitivity
superstructure
super-wet technique
supinate
supination
s. deformity
s. injury
s. reflex
supination-adduction fracture
supination-eversion
s.-e. fracture
supination-external
s.-e. rotation
s.-e. rotation injury
s.-e. rotation IV (SER-IV)
s.-e. rotation IV fracture
supination-inversion rotation injury
supination-plantar flexion injury
supinator
s. crest

S

NOTES

supinator *(continued)*
    s. longus reflex
    s. muscle
supine
    s. human subject
    s. hypotensive syndrome
    s. position
    s. sciatic block
supine-oblique approach
supple bowel
supplementary
    s. analgesia
    s. canal
    s. oxygen
    s. respiration
    s. sling procedure
supplementation
    calcitriol s.
    calcium carbonate s.
    postoperative s.
    temporary postoperative s.
    vitamin D s.
supply
    arterial s.
    blood s.
    compensatory blood s.
    tumor blood s.
support
    advanced trauma life s. (ATLS)
    biologic liver s.
    blood pressure s.
    excessive lip s.
    external s.
    extracorporeal life s. (ECLS)
    inspiratory pressure s.
    mechanical ventilatory s.
    nonbiologic liver s.
    parenteral nutritional s.
    pulmonary s.
    s. suture technique
    systemic pressure s.
    S. Team Assessment Schedule
      (STAS)
    ventilator s.
    ventilatory s.
    volume-assured pressure s.
supporting tissue
suppository
suppressed respiration
suppression
    twitch s.
suppressor
    tumor s.
suppurant
suppurate
suppuration
    alveodental s.
    pulmonary s.

suppurativa
    hidradenitis s.
suppurative
    s. acute inflammation
    s. cholecystitis
    s. chronic inflammation
    s. exudate
    s. granulomatous inflammation
    s. infection
supraacetabular
    s. groove
    s. sulcus
supraacetabularis
supraacromial
supraanal
supraannular mitral valve replacement
supraarytenoid cartilage
supraauricular point
supraaxillary
suprabuccal
suprabullar recess
supracerebellar approach
supracervical
    s. hysterectomy
    s. incision
suprachoroid
    s. lamina
    s. layer
suprachoroidal hemorrhage
suprachoroidea
supraciliary canal
supraclavicular
    s. approach
    s. brachial block
    s. brachial block anesthesia
    s. compression
    s. examination
    s. fracture
    s. lymph node biopsy
    s. muscle
    s. nerve
    s. triangle
supraclinoid aneurysm
supracolic space
supracondylar (SC)
    s. amputation
    s. humeral fracture
    s. line
    s. process
    s. suspension
    s. varus osteotomy
    s. Y-shaped fracture
supracondyloid
supracostal
supracotyloid
supracrestal
    s. line
    s. plane
supracricoid partial laryngectomy

supracristal plane
supradiaphragmatic
supraduodenal
  s. approach
  s. artery
supraepicondylar process
supraesophageal
  s. reflux changes
  s. reflux disease
supragenicular popliteal artery (SGPA)
supraglenoid tubercle
supraglottic
  s. edema
  s. laryngectomy
supraglottoplasty
suprahepatic
  s. cuff
  s. inferior vena cava (SHVC)
  s. IVC
  s. space
  s. vena cava
suprahyoid
  s. branch
  s. gland
  s. laryngeal release
  s. muscle
  s. neck dissection
  s. space
  s. triangle
suprainguinal
suprainterparietal bone
supraintestinal
supralevator
  s. anorectal space
  s. pelvic exenteration
  s. perirectal abscess
supralumbar
supramalleolar
  s. flap
  s. varus derotation osteotomy
supramammary
supramandibular
supramastoid fossa
supramaxillary
supramaximal tetanic stimulation
suprameatal
  s. pit
  s. triangle
supramental
supramesocolic surgical procedure
supranasal
Suprane

supraneural parotidectomy
supranormal
  s. CI
  s. hemodynamic therapy
  s. resuscitation
  s. value
supranuclear lesion
supraomental
  s. region
  s. space
supraomohyoid neck dissection
supraoptic
  s. anastomosis
  s. canal
supraopticohypophysial tract
supraorbital
  s. arch
  s. artery
  s. canal
  s. foramen
  s. margin
  s. nerve
  s. notch
  s. pericranial flap
  s. point
  s. ridge
  s. vein
supraorbital-pterional approach
supraorbitomeatal
suprapapillary Roux-en-Y
  duodenojejunostomy
suprapatellar
  s. bursa
  s. pouch
suprapelvic
supraperiosteal flap
supraphysiologic
  s. fluid
  s. fluid technique
  s. resuscitation
suprapineal recess
suprapleural membrane
supraprostatectomy
suprapubic
  s. cystotomy
  s. extraction site
  s. hernia
  s. lithotomy
  s. midline recurrence
  s. needle aspiration
  s. Pfannenstiel incision
  s. port

S

NOTES

suprapubic *(continued)*
- s. prostatectomy
- s. puncture
- s. region
- s. urethrovesical suspension operation

suprapyloric node

suprarenal
- s. body
- s. capsule
- s. cortex
- s. filter placement
- s. gland
- s. impression
- s. medulla
- s. plexus
- s. vein

suprarenalectomy

suprascapular
- s. artery
- s. ligament
- s. nerve
- s. nerve compression
- s. notch
- s. vein

suprasellar
- s. low-density lesion
- s. mass
- s. subarachnoid cistern

suprasphincteric fistula

supraspinale

supraspinalis muscle

supraspinatus muscle

supraspinous
- s. fossa
- s. ligament
- s. muscle

suprasternal
- s. bone
- s. examination
- s. notch
- s. plane
- s. space

suprasymphysary

supratemporal

supratentorial
- s. approach
- s. arteriovenous malformation
- s. craniotomy
- s. lesion
- s. space
- s. tumor

suprathoracic

Suprathreshold Adaptation Test

supratonsillar
- s. fossa
- s. recess

supratragic tubercle

supratrochlear
- s. artery
- s. nerve
- s. vein

supraumbilical incision

supravaginal

supravalvar

supravalvular aortic stenosis

supraventricular
- s. arrhythmia
- s. crest
- s. dysrhythmia

supraventricularis

supraversion

supravesical fossa

supreme
- s. intercostal artery
- s. intercostal vein

sural
- s. artery
- s. nerve
- s. nerve biopsy
- s. region

surface
- acromial articular s.
- articular s.
- auricular s.
- s. biopsy
- buccal s.
- s. cooling technique
- costal s.
- cut s.
- denture foundation s.
- diaphragmatic s.
- s. disinfection
- dorsal s.
- s. electrode
- endosteal s.
- s. epithelium
- extensor s.
- external s.
- foundation s.
- glenoid s.
- hepatic s.
- implant-bearing s.
- inferior s.
- internal s.
- s. irradiation
- s. landmark
- s. membrane
- orbital s.
- ovarian s.
- peritoneal s.
- posterior s.
- s. projection
- raw hepatic s.
- reconstruction occlusal s. (RecOS)
- renal s.
- s. replacement hip arthroplasty

temporal s.
s. tension theory of narcosis
tissue ingrowth s.
surface-projection rendering image
surfactant
hydrolysis of s.
surfer's ear
surgeon
American College of S.'s (ACS)
American Society for Colon and
Rectal S.'s (ASCRS)
colorectal s.
endocrine s.
Fellow of American College
of S.'s (FACS)
general s.
S. General's Office (SGO)
gynecologic s.
s.'s knot
oculoplastic s.
pancreatic s.
parathyroid s.
pediatric s.
plastic s.
primary s.
retinal s.
Society of American
Gastrointestinal Endoscopic S.'s
thoracic s.
thyroid s.
trauma s.
vascular s.
surgeon-dependent technique failure
surgery
ablative cardiac s.
adjustable suture strabismus s.
adult cardiovascular s.
adult scoliosis s.
AESOP-assisted laparoscopic s.
ambulatory s.
American Board of S. (ABS)
anorectal s.
anterior cervical spine s.
anterior cervicothoracic junction s.
anterior lower cervical spine s.
antiglaucoma s.
antireflux s.
aortic reconstructive s.
apically repositioned flap in
mucogingival s.
arterial reconstructive s.
arthroscopic laser s.

aseptic s.
asymmetric s.
bariatric s.
bat ear s.
beating-heart bypass s.
bench s.
breast-conserving s.
bypass s.
cardiac s.
cardiothoracic s.
cardiovascular s.
carotid s.
cataract s.
cervical decompression s.
cervical disc s.
cervicothoracic junction s.
ciliodestructive s.
clean-contaminated s.
closed s.
colon and rectal s.
colorectal s.
combination s.
s. complication
computer-assisted s. (CAS)
computer-assisted stereotactic s.
concomitant antireflux s.
conservation s.
conservative s.
conventional s.
corneal s.
cosmetic s.
craniofacial reconstructive s.
cranio-orbital s.
curative-intent s.
cytoreductive s.
debulking s.
decompressive s.
definitive s.
dental s.
dentofacial s.
dialysis access s.
dirty s.
double jaw s.
DREZ s.
ECA-PCA bypass s.
elective s.
elective cosmetic s. (ECS)
emergency s.
emergent s.
endocrine s.
endodontic s.
endoscopic cardiac s.

S

NOTES

surgery *(continued)*

endoscopic sinus s.
endoscopic video-assisted s.
endovascular s.
epilepsy s.
esthetic s.
excisional cardiac s.
exploratory s.
ex situ bench s.
extracorporeal s.
extracranial-intracranial bypass s.
eyelid s.
eye muscle s.
failed s.
featural s.
femorodistal reconstructive s.
fetal s.
filtration s.
first ray s.
fistulizing s.
flexible endoscopic s.
frameless stereotactic s.
functional endoscopic sinus s.
  (FESS)
gastric bypass s.
gastric reduction s.
gastrointestinal s.
general thoracic s.
glaucoma s.
hand-assisted laparoscopic s.
  (HALS)
hepatic resectional s.
hepatobiliary s.
hip replacement s.
hypotensive s.
hysteroscopic s.
ileal pouch s.
image-guided s. (IGS)
inadequate s.
intestinal s.
intraabdominal s.
intradural tumor s.
intralacrimal s.
intranasal sinus s.
intraorbital s.
jejunoileal bypass s.
keyhole s.
knee replacement s.
labyrinthine s.
lacrimal s.
laparoscopically assisted s.
laparoscopic-assisted aortic
  reconstructive s.
laparoscopic bariatric s.
laparoscopic colorectal cancer s.
laparoscopic Dorr antireflux s.
laparoscopic Toupet anti-reflux s.
laryngeal framework s.
laser s.

laser-filtering s.
Lich-Gregoir kidney transplant s.
limb-salvage s.
limb-sparing s.
local s.
lower extremity s.
lung volume reduction s.
major abdominal s.
major nonvascular abdominal s.
mandibular s.
maxillary s.
maxillofacial s.
microscopically controlled s.
minimal access general s.
minimally invasive s. (MIS)
minimally invasive robotic heart
  valve s.
minor s.
Mohs micrographic s.
mucogingival s.
nasal endoscopic s.
navigated brain tumor s.
navigational s.
nephron-sparing s.
neurologic s.
neurological s.
neuroma relocation s.
nonbench s.
noncardiac s.
nonvascular abdominal s.
oculoplastic s.
oncoplastic s.
open antireflux s.
open disc s.
open heart s. (OHS)
oral and maxillofacial s.
orbital s.
orthognathic s.
osseous s.
palliative s.
pancreatic s.
parathyroid s.
parenchymal sparing s.
pediatric cardiovascular s.
pediatric ophthalmic s.
pelvic colonic s.
penile venous ligation s.
periapical s.
peripheral vascular s.
plastic and reconstructive s.
port-access technique for coronary
  bypass s.
portal decompression s.
portal-systemic shunt s.
posterior lower cervical spine s.
posterior lumbar spine and
  sacrum s.
posterior upper cervical spine s.
preprosthetic s.

primary perineal hypospadias s.
prophylactic s.
pure refractive s.
pylorus-preserving s.
radical curative s.
radioimmunoguided s.
reconstructive preprosthetic s.
rectal s.
rectovaginal s.
refractive s.
remedial s.
renal-sparing s.
reoperative bariatric s.
reoperative carotid s.
reoperative esthetic s.
reoperative pelvic s.
reparative cardiac s.
rescue s.
resective s.
retinal s.
retrograde intrarenal s.
reversal jejunoileal bypass s.
right ventricle-pulmonary artery
  conduit s.
rigid endoscopic s.
robot-assisted s. (RAS)
robotic s.
robotic-assisted laparoscopic
  bariatric s.
salvage s.
scoliosis s.
secondary s.
second-look s.
segmental s.
sham s.
shunt s.
sinus s.
site-specific s.
sphincter-saving s.
spinal s.
stereotactic s.
stereotaxic s.
stone s.
strabismus s.
suboptimal s.
subretinal s.
substitutional cardiac s.
symmetric s.
targeted s.
telepresence s.
telerobotic-assisted laparoscopic s.
thoracic s.

thyroglossal cyst s.
total hip replacement s.
total knee replacement s.
transperitoneal hand-assisted
  laparoscopic s.
transsexual s.
transsphenoidal s.
transsphincteric s.
trauma s.
tubal reconstruction s.
tumor s.
upper gastrointestinal tract s.
urologic s.
vaginal s.
valvular heart s.
vascular abdominal s.
video-assisted thoracoscopic s.
  (VATS)
video-assisted thorascopic s.
  (VATS)
videoscopic hernia s.
vitreoretinal s.
vitreous s.
volume reduction s. (VRS)
weight reduction s.

surgery-induced PGID
surgical
　s. abdomen
　s. access
　s. adjunct
　s. admitting unit
　s. airway
　s. anatomy
　s. anesthesia
　s. approach
　s. autoimmunization
　s. bone impression
　s. change
　s. cholecystectomy
　s. cholecystostomy
　s. clinician
　s. correction
　s. crown lengthening
　s. cystgastrostomy
　s. débridement
　s. debulking
　s. defect
　s. diagnosis
　s. diathermy
　s. drape combustion
　s. dressing room

NOTES

surgical *(continued)*
S. Education and Self-Assessment Program (SESAP)
s. emergency
s. emphysema
s. endarterectomy
s. endodontics
s. enucleation
s. enucleation method
s. enucleation procedure
s. enucleation technique
s. eruption
s. erysipelas
s. estrogen ablation
s. excision
s. excision biopsy
s. extirpation
s. failure
s. field
s. flap
s. incision
s. indication
s. infection
s. intervention
s. keratometry
s. ligation
s. maggot
s. maggot therapy
s. management
s. maneuver
s. margin
s. marking solution
s. mesh
s. microscope navigation (SMN)
s. neck
s. neck fracture
s. neonate
s. neurangiographic technique
s. neurology
s. occlusion rim
s. oncologist
s. oncology
s. orthodontia
s. orthodontics
s. outcome
s. pancreatic disease
s. pathology
s. perspective
s. placement
s. plication
s. portal decompression
s. portosystemic shunting
s. positioning
s. preparation
s. problem
s. pulp exposure
s. reduction
s. repair
s. resectability

s. resection
s. retention
s. risk
s. sectioning
s. seeding
s. signature
s. simulation
s. site infection (SSI)
s. specialty
s. staging
s. stapling
s. strategy
s. stress
s. suture technique
s. thrombectomy
s. trauma
s. treatment
s. treatment objective
s. treatment option
s. tuberculosis
s. vagotomy
s. weight loss
s. wound
surgically
s. corrected hypertension
s. treated patient
surgical-pathologic staging
surgical-radiologic minicholecystostomy
surplus skin
surrenal
surveillance
endoscopic s.
s. endoscopy
S., Epidemiology and End Result (SEER)
graft s.
s. mechanism
s. program
s. technique
survey
s. line
s. program
radiation s.
survival
breast cancer-specific s. (BCSS)
s. curve
disease-free s. (DFS)
distant recurrence-free s. (DRFS)
graft s.
locoregional recurrence-free s. (LRRFS)
long-term s.
postoperative s.
recurrence-free s.
specific s.
TRISS probability of s.
Susac syndrome
susceptibility gene

suspended
    s. animation
    s. inspiration
suspended-pedicle approach
suspension
    Aldridge-Studdefort urethral s.
    Alexander-Adams uterine s.
    Baldy-Webster uterine s.
    bladder neck s.
    Burch bladder s.
    Burch iliopectineal ligament
      urethrovesical s.
    Coffey s.
    corporeal sacrospinous s.
    corset s.
    cuff s.
    endoscopic bladder neck s.
    extraperitoneal laparoscopic bladder
      neck s.
    fingertrap s.
    flexible hinge s.
    Gilliam-Doleris uterine s.
    Gittes-Loughlin bladder neck s.
    s. laryngoscopy
    minimal incision pubovaginal s.
    Olshausen s.
    Pereyra bladder neck s.
    Pereyra needle s.
    Raz bladder neck s.
    Raz needle s.
    Raz 4-quadrant s.
    Raz urethral s.
    retropubic Lapides-Ball bladder
      neck s.
    sacrospinous ligament s.
    SC s.
    Stamey needle s.
    suction s.
    supracondylar s.
    urethral s.
    uterine s.
suspension-type socket
suspensory
    s. ligament
    s. muscle
    s. sling operation
suspicion
    clinical s.
suspicious
    s. abnormality
    s. finding
    s. FNA

    s. lesion
    s. microcalcification
sustained
    s. pressure technique
    s. release (SR)
sustentacular tissue
sustentaculum tali
Sutherland-Greenfield osteotomy
Sutherland-Rowe incision
sutura, pl. **suturae**
sutural
    s. bone
    s. diastasis
    s. ligament
suture
    absorbable surgical s.
    s. anastomosis
    s. anchor technique
    apical s.
    basilar s.
    bregmatomastoid s.
    s. bridge
    cervical s.
    s. closure
    s. closure technique
    coronal s.
    cranial s.
    dentate s.
    ethmoidolacrimal s.
    ethmoidomaxillary s.
    s. failure
    false s.
    s. fatigue
    s. fixation
    frontal s.
    frontoethmoidal s.
    frontomaxillary s.
    frontonasal s.
    frontoparietal s.
    frontosphenoid s.
    frontozygomatic s.
    infraorbital s.
    interendognathic s.
    intermaxillary s.
    internasal s.
    interparietal s.
    s. joint
    lacrimoconchal s.
    lacrimomaxillary s.
    lambdoid s.
    Le Dentu s.
    s. of lens

S

NOTES

suture *(continued)*
s. ligated
s. ligation
s. line
s. line cancer
s. line dehiscence
nasomaxillary s.
neurocentral s.
occipital s.
occipitomastoid s.
occipitoparietal s.
occipitosphenoid s.
s. overlap
palatine s.
palatoethmoidal s.
palatomaxillary s.
parietal s.
parietomastoid s.
petrobasilar s.
petrospheno-occipital s.
petrosquamous s.
petrotympanic s.
s. plication
s. repair
sphenofrontal s.
sphenomaxillary s.
sphenooccipital s.
sphenoorbital s.
sphenoparietal s.
sphenosquamous s.
sphenovomerine s.
sphenozygomatic s.
squamomastoid s.
squamosal s.
squamous s.
temporal s.
transosseous s.
tympanomastoid s.
tympanosquamosal s.
zygomaticofrontal s.
zygomaticomaxillary s.
zygomaticotemporal s.
suturectomy
sutured
doubly s.
sutureless
s. bowel anastomosis
s. colostomy closure
s. laparoscopic extraperitoneal
inguinal herniorrhaphy
suturing
Bard endoscopic s.
conventional s.
direct s.
intracorporeal s.
magnetic control s. (MCS)
needleless s.
SUV
standardized uptake value

suxamethonium
SV
sigmoid volvulus
stroke volume
SVC
selective vascular clamping
superior vena cava
swage
swallow
barium s.
s. method
swamp carcinoma
Swan incision
swan-neck
s.-n. deformity reduction
s.-n. finger deformity
Swanson
S. classification
S. Convex condylar arthroplasty
S. radial head implant arthroplasty
S. reconstruction
S. silicone wrist arthroplasty
S. technique
sweat
s. duct
s. gland adenocarcinoma
s. gland adenoma
Swedish approach
Sweet method
swelling
external s.
genital s.
levator s.
lysosomal s.
scrotal s.
soft tissue s.
Swenson pull-through procedure
Swiss roll embedding technique
switch
biliopancreatic diversion with
duodenal s.
compression s.
s. operation
s. procedure
switched B-gradient technique
swivel dislocation
SWL
shock wave lithotripsy
SWMA
segmental wall motion deformity
sword-fighting
sycoma
sycosiform fungous infection
Sydney
S. line
S. system gastritis classification
sylvian
s. approach
s. aqueduct

s. cistern
s. dissection
s. fissure
s. fistula
s. hematoma
s. line
s. point
s. vein
Sylvius
    valve of S.
symblepharon ring
Syme
    S. ankle disarticulation amputation
    S. external urethrotomy
    S. procedure
Symington anococcygeal body
symmetric
    s. surgery
    s. thumb duplication
    s. vertebral fusion
symmetry
    s. operation
    s. plane
sympathectomy
    cervical perivascular s.
    cervicothoracic s.
    chemical s.
    endoscopic s.
    Leriche s.
    lumbar s.
    periarterial s.
    preganglionic s.
    presacral s.
    Smithwick s.
    transdermal s.
    upper dorsal s.
    visceral s.
sympathetic
    s. blockade
    s. blockade anesthetic technique
    s. branch
    s. denervation
    s. denitrogenation
    s. fiber
    s. ganglion block anesthetic
      technique
    s. interruption
    s. microneurography
    s. nerve
    s. nerve activity (SNA)
    s. nerve block
    s. projection

s. sprouting
s. trunk
sympathetically maintained pain (SMP)
sympathetoblastoma
sympathic
sympathicectomy
sympathicoblastoma
sympathicogonioma
sympathicotripsy
sympathicus
sympathoadrenal response
sympathoblastoma
sympathoexcitation reflex
sympathoexcitatory response
sympathogonioma
sympatholysis
sympatholytic agent
sympathomimetic agent
symperitoneal
symphyseotomy
symphyses (*pl. of* symphysis)
symphysialis
symphysic
symphysion
symphysiotomy
symphysis, pl. **symphyses**
    cardiac s.
    intervertebral s.
    mandibular s.
    manubriosternal s.
    mental s.
    pleural s.
    pubic s.
symptom
    acute s.
    chronic reflux s.
    S. Distress Scale
    s. experience stage
    s. formation
    ipsilateral hemispheric s.
    s. magnification syndrome
    myelopathic s.
    neurologic s.
    nonspecific s.
    postoperative s.
    presenting s.
    psychogenic s.
    s. score
    transient neurologic s. (TNS)
    unremitting s.
symptomatic
    s. infection

S

NOTES

symptomatic (*continued*)
   s. patient
   s. primary HPT
   s. relief
   s. traumatic dissection
symptomatology
symptothermal method
synadelphus
synanastomosis
synandrogenic
synapse, pl. **synapses**
   excitatory s.
synaptosome
synarthrodia
synarthrodial joint
synarthrosis, pl. **synarthroses**
syncephalus
synchondrodial joint
synchondroseotomy
synchondrosis, pl. **synchondroses**
   s. xiphosternalis
synchondrotomy
synchrocyclotron operation
synchronization
synchronized
   s. fibrillation
   s. intermittent mandatory ventilation
   (SIMV)
   s. intermittent mechanical
   ventilation (SIMV)
synchronous
   s. bladder reconstruction
   s. emergence
   s. hepatic metastasis
   s. intermittent mandatory ventilation
   s. lesion
   s. pathology
   s. resection
   s. scapuloclavicular rotation
   s. tumor
   s. urinary tract infection
syncope
syncytial knot
syndactylia
syndactylization
syndactylous
syndactyly
   Diamond-Gould reduction s.
   Kelikian-Clayton-Loseff surgical s.
   reduction s.
syndectomy
syndesmectomy
syndesmectopia
syndesmodial joint
syndesmopexy
syndesmophyte
   bridging s.
syndesmoplasty
syndesmorrhaphy

syndesmotic
syndesmotomy
syndrome
   abdominal compartment s.
   abdominal cutaneous nerve
    entrapment s.
   abdominal muscle deficiency s.
   acrofacial s.
   acute coronary s.
   acute disconnection s.
   acute respiratory distress s.
   (ARDS)
   acute tumor lysis s. (ATLS)
   adhesive s.
   adrenal feminization s.
   adult respiratory distress s. (ARDS)
   afferent loop s.
   aglossia-adactylia s.
   Alport s.
   amniotic infection s.
   angio-osteohypertrophy s.
   ankyloglossia superior s.
   anomalous innominate artery
    compression s.
   anterior cavernous sinus s.
   anterior chest wall s.
   anterior spinal artery s.
   Apert s.
   Arnold-Chiari s.
   Ascher s.
   Bannayan-Riley-Ruvalcaba s.
   Behçet s.
   bent-nail s.
   bile plug s.
   biliary sump s.
   billowing mitral valve s.
   black patch s.
   blind loop s.
   blind pouch s.
   Bloodgood s.
   blue toe s.
   body cast s.
   Boerhaave s.
   Bogorad s.
   bowel bypass s.
   brittle nail s.
   Budd-Chiari s.
   Burnett s.
   burning feet s.
   calcaneal spur s.
   callosal disconnection s.
   camptomelic s.
   cancer susceptibility s.
   capillary leak s.
   capsular exfoliation s.
   Caroli s.
   carpal tunnel s.
   cauda equina s.
   cavernous sinus s.

celiac artery compression s. (CCS)
celiac axis compression s.
celiac band s.
central anticholinergic s.
central cord s.
central heel pad s.
cerebellomedullary malformation s.
cerebellopontine angle s.
cervical acceleration-deceleration s.
cervical compression s.
cervical fusion s.
Cheatle s.
Chiari II s.
chronic hyperventilation s.
chronic intestinal
  pseudoobstruction s.
classic multiple organ failure s.
clinical s.
clivus s.
cloverleaf skull s.
cluster tic s.
coarctation s.
Cogan s.
common peroneal nerve s.
compartment compression s.
compensatory antiinflammatory
  response s. (CARS)
complex regional pain s. (I, II)
  (CRPS)
compression s.
congenital central hypoventilation s.
congenital long QT s.
congenital ring s.
Cooper s.
cord traction s.
coronary s.
Costen s.
Cronkhite-Canada s.
Crouzon s.
crush s.
cubital tunnel s.
cutaneomucouveal s.
Dandy-Walker s.
D chromosome ring s.
deafferentation pain s.
Dejerine-Roussy s.
delayed pulmonary toxicity s.
de Quervain s.
dialysis disequilibrium s.
dialysis encephalopathy s.
disconnection s.
DISH s.

dumping s.
dural shunt s.
Eagle s.
Eagle-Barrett s.
ectopic ACTH s.
embryonic fixation s.
entrapment s.
euthyroid sick s.
excited skin s.
exertional anterior compartment s.
exertional deep posterior
  compartment s.
exfoliation s.
exploding head s.
extraarticular pain s.
extrapyramidal s.
facet joint s.
failed back surgery s.
familial aortic ectasia s.
familial atypical multiple mole
  melanoma s.
familial cardiac myxoma s.
familial cholestasis s.
familial polyposis s.
FAM-M s.
female urethral s.
feminization s.
fetal aspiration s.
fibrocystic breast s.
fibrofascial compartment s.
first arch s.
flapping valve s.
floppy valve s.
Fraley s.
Franceschetti s.
Fraser s.
Frey s.
functional prepubertal castration s.
G s.
gastrojejunal loop obstruction s.
glomangiomatous osseous
  malformation s.
glucagonoma s.
Gorlin-Chaudhry-Moss s.
Hadju-Cheney acroosteolysis s.
Hallermann-Streiff s.
Hallermann-Streiff-François s.
Hanhart s.
head-bobbing doll s.
hemangioma-thrombocytopenia s.
hemispheric disconnection s.
hemolytic uremic s.

S

NOTES

syndrome *(continued)*
    hepatorenal s.
    hereditary cancer s.
    hereditary flat adenoma s.
    Hinman s.
    HNPCC s.
    Horner s.
    hungry bone s.
    Hutchison s.
    hyaline membrane s.
    hymenal s.
    hyoid s.
    hypersensitive xiphoid s.
    hyperventilation s.
    hypoplastic left heart s.
    hypothenar hammer s.
    immotile cilia s.
    impaired regeneration s.
    s. of inappropriate antidiuretic
      hormone (SIADH)
    infantile choriocarcinoma s.
    infant respiratory distress s. (IRDS)
    inherited cancer s.
    innominate artery compression s.
    intersection s.
    iridocorneal endothelial s.
    iridocorneal epithelial s.
    Jacod s.
    Jeune s.
    jugular foramen s.
    Kasabach-Merritt s.
    Klippel-Feil s.
    Klippel-Trenaunay s.
    Klippel-Trenaunay-Weber s.
    lactic acidosis and stroke-like s.
    large vestibular aqueduct s.
    Larsen s.
    levator ani s.
    levator scapulae s.
    lissencephaly s.
    loculation s.
    loin pain hematuria s.
    long QT s.
    lower nephron s.
    Luys body s.
    Lynch s.
    Maffucci s.
    malignant carcinoid s.
    malignant external otitis s.
    Mallory-Weiss s.
    mandibulofacial dysotosis s.
    mangled extremity s.
    Marfan s.
    Marin Amat s.
    MASS s.
    massive bowel resection s.
    maternal deprivation s.
    May-Thurner s.
    meconium aspiration s.

    meconium plug s.
    medial tibial stress s. (MTSS)
    megacystic s.
    megacystis-megaureter s.
    megacystis-microcolon-intestinal
      hypoperistalsis s.
    MEN s.
    MEN-2a, -2b s.
    Mendelson s.
    Ménière s.
    minimal change nephrotic s.
    minimal lesion nephrotic s.
    Mirizzi s.
    mitochondrial myopathy,
      encephalopathy, lactic acidosis,
      and strokelike s. (MELAS)
    mitral valve prolapse s.
    Mohr s.
    monofixation s.
    Morquio s.
    mucocutaneous lymph node s.
    mucocutaneous pigmentation of
      Peutz-Jeghers s.
    mucosal neuroma s.
    mucous plug s.
    müllerian duct derivation s.
    multiple endocrine neoplasia s.
      (type 2a, 2b)
    multiple hamartoma s.
    multiple mucosal neuroma s.
    multiple organ dysfunction s.
      (MODS)
    multiple organ failure s.
    multiple pterygium s.
    myofascial pain s.
    nail-patella s.
    nail-patella-elbow s.
    naviculocapitate fracture s.
    nephritic s.
    nerve compression-degeneration s.
    neuroleptic malignant s. (NMS)
    neurovascular compression s.
    nevoid basal cell carcinoma s.
    nonocclusive mesenteric ischemia s.
    OAV s.
    obesity hypoventilation s. (OHS)
    occipital condyle s.
    ocular-mucous membrane s.
    oculobuccogenital s.
    oculomandibulofacial s.
    oculovertebral s.
    OFD s.
    Ogilvie s.
    optic tract s.
    orbital apex s.
    organic short bowel s.
    orofaciodigital s.
    Ortner s.
    osteogenesis imperfecta congenita s.

osteomyelofibrotic s.
osteopathia striata s.
osteoporosis pseudoglioma s.
Ostrum-Furst s.
otomandibular s.
ovarian hyperstimulation s.
ovarian overstimulation s.
ovarian vein s.
pacemaker s.
Paget-von Schrötter s.
pain s.
Papillon-Léage and Psaume s.
parasellar s.
paratrigeminal s.
Parsonage-Turner s.
pericardiotomy s.
pericolic membrane s.
peritubal s.
peroneal compartment s.
persistent müllerian duct s.
Peutz-Jeghers s.
pharyngeal pouch s.
Phocas s.
piriformis s.
placental hemangioma s.
popliteal web s.
postadrenalectomy s.
postcardiotomy s.
postcholecystectomy s.
postcolonoscopy distention s.
postcommissurotomy s.
postembolization s.
posterior interosseous nerve
  compression s.
postfundoplication s.
postgastrectomy s.
postirradiation s.
postlaminectomy s.
postpericardiotomy s.
postphlebitic s.
postpolypectomy coagulation s.
posttubal ligation s.
postvagotomy s.
preexcitation s.
prolapsed mitral valve s.
pronator teres s.
proximal loop s.
prune-belly s. (PBS)
pseudo-blind loop s.
pseudoexfoliation s.
pseudolymphoma s.
pseudoxanthoma elasticum s.

pterygopalatine fossa s.
pulmonary acid aspiration s.
pulmonary sulcus s.
quadrilateral space s.
Raeder s.
Ramsay Hunt s.
rapid tumor lysis s.
Rapunzel s.
Raynaud s.
Reclus I s.
recurrent abdominal pain s. (RAPS)
red ear s.
red-eyed shunt s.
Reifenstein s.
Reiter s.
renal crush s.
respiratory distress s. (RDS)
retinoblastoma-mental retardation s.
retrosphenoidal s.
rib tip s.
Rieger s.
Riley-Day s.
Riley-Smith s.
Roaf s.
Roberts s.
Roux stasis s.
Sakati-Nyhan s.
scalenus anticus s.
scapuloperoneal s.
Scheie s.
scimitar s.
Sertoli-cell-only s.
Sheehan s.
short bowel s.
sick building s.
sick sinus s.
Singleton-Merten s.
sinus tarsi s.
sleep apnea-hypoventilation s.
slipped rib cartilage s.
slipping rib s.
slit ventricle s.
Smith-Lemli-Opitz s.
smooth-brain s.
solitary rectal ulcer s.
somatostatinoma s.
spectacular shrinking deficit s.
spinal cord shock s.
splenic sequestration s.
SSRI discontinuation s.
stagnant loop s.
staphylococcal scalded skin s.

S

NOTES

syndrome *(continued)*
  stasis s.
  Stauffer s.
  Stewart-Treves s.
  Stickler s.
  stiff-person s.
  stump embolization s.
  stylohyoid process s.
  styloid s.
  subclavian steal s.
  sudden infant death s. (SIDS)
  sump s.
  SUNCT s.
  superior orbital fissure s.
  superior vena cava s.
  supine hypotensive s.
  Susac s.
  symptom magnification s.
  systemic inflammatory response s.
  (SIRS)
  Takayasu s.
  talar compression s.
  tarsal tunnel s.
  terminal reservoir s.
  Terson s.
  testicular feminization s.
  tethered cord s.
  third and fourth pharyngeal
  pouch s.
  thoracic compression s.
  thoracic endometriosis s.
  thoracic outlet s. (TOS)
  Thorn s.
  Tillaux-Phocas s.
  Tolosa-Hunt s.
  tooth-and-nail s.
  Tourette s.
  transient bone marrow edema s.
  transient compartment s.
  translocation Down s.
  transplant lung s.
  transurethral resection s.
  Treacher Collins s.
  trisomy 8 s.
  trisomy C, D s.
  Trotter s.
  tumor lysis s.
  Turcot s.
  Turner s.
  twin-twin transfusion s. (TTTS)
  ulnocarpal abutment s.
  Unverricht-Lundborg s.
  urethral s.
  Usher s.
  uterine hernia s.
  uveoencephalitic s.
  valgus extension overload s.
  vanished testis s.
  vanishing lung s.

  vascular ring s.
  VATER association s.
  velocardiofacial s.
  venous leak s.
  Vernet s.
  vertebral subluxation s.
  vibration s.
  vibrator hand s.
  Villaret s.
  visual deprivation s.
  vitreoretinal traction s.
  Vogt-Koyanagi-Harada s.
  vulvar vestibulitis s.
  Wartenberg s.
  wasting s.
  Weyers-Thier s.
  white clot s.
  white dot s.
  Winchester s.
  yellow nail s.
  Yentl s.

synechia, pl. **synechiae**
  s. formation
synechiotomy
  Paufique s.
synechotomy
synectenterotomy
synencephalocele
synergism
synergistic
  s. effect
  s. interaction
  s. muscle
synergy
  drug s.
syngeneic
  s. graft
  s. tissue
  s. transplantation
syngenesioplastic transplantation
syngenesioplasty
syngenesiotransplantation
syngnathia
syngraft
synonychia
synorchidism
synoscheos
synostectomy
synosteology
synostosis
synotia
synovectomy
  Albright s.
  arthroscopic s.
  carpal s.
  dorsal s.
  Inglis-Ranawat-Straub elbow s.
  palmar s.
  6-portal s.

Porter-Richardson-Vainio s.
Smith-Petersen s.
volar s.
Wilkinson s.
synovia (*pl. of* synovium)
synovial
s. biopsy
s. bursa
s. cavity
s. fistula
s. fluid
s. fluid examination
s. fold
s. frenula
s. frenum
s. fringe
s. gland
s. hernia
s. herniation
s. joint
s. ligament
s. membrane
s. tendon sheath
s. tissue
s. villus
synovialis
synovioma
benign giant cell s.
malignant s.
synoviparous
synovitis
synovium, pl. **synovia**
synpolydactyly
synthesis, pl. **syntheses**
collagen s.
first-strand cDNA s.
synthetic
s. augmentation
s. method
syphilid
syphilis
syphilitic fever
syphiloma of Fournier
syringadenoma
syringeal
syringectomy
syringes (*pl. of* syrinx)
syringoadenoma
syringocarcinoma
syringocele
syringocisternostomy
syringocystadenoma

syringocystoma
syringohydromyelic cavity
syringoma
syringomeningocele
syringomyelia
syringomyelic
s. dissociation
s. hemorrhage
syringomyelocele
syringomyelus
syringotome
syringotomy
syrinx, pl. **syringes**
syssarcosic
syssarcosis
syssarcotic
system
anesthetic s.
APACHE-II s.
arterial s.
autologous melanoma s.
behavioral inhibition s. (BIS)
biliary s.
bioartificial liver support s.
Breast Imaging Reporting and
Data S. (BI-RADS)
cartilaginous part of skeletal s.
celiac arterial s.
central nervous s.
circle s.
Clinical Classification S. (CCS)
closed anesthesia s.
closed-loop s.
coronary sinus perfusion s.
digestive s.
duct s.
ductal s.
electromagnetic s.
endogenous opioid s.
enteric nervous s.
extracellular matrix s.
Facial Action Coding S.
Fatal Accident Reporting S.
force feedback s.
intracranial venous s.
lacrimal s.
lymphoma s.
Maximally Discriminative Facial
Coding S.
mesenteric arterial s.
Miami Modular Orthopaedic
Spinal S.

S

NOTES

741

system *(continued)*
  musculoskeletal s.
  navigation s.
  needle-free s.
  needleless intravenous
    administration s.
  nervous s.
  neuronavigational s.
  neurotransmitter s.
  node lymphoma s.
  open anesthesia s.
  opioid s.
  optical s.
  organ s.
  Pain Relief Scoring S.
  pediatric anesthesia s.
  perfusion s.
  peripheral access s. (PAS)
  pin-index safety s.
  preoperative scoring s.
  scavenging s.
  scoring s.
  serotonergic s.
  static compliance of the total
    respiratory s.
  superior mesenteric arterial s.
  Texas Scottish Rite Hospital hook-
    rod s.
  therapeutic intervention scoring s.
    (TISS)
  TNM staging s.
  trauma s.
  United States Renal Data S.
  Universal Spine S. (USS)
  vascular s.
  vein s.
  venous s.
  vertical vein s.
systematic
  s. method
  s. sextant biopsy

systematization
systemic
  s. absorption
  s. adjuvant therapy
  s. antibiotic
  s. anticoagulation
  s. antifungal therapy
  s. arteriovenous fistula
  s. chemotherapy
  s. condition
  s. disease
  s. dissection
  s. drainage
  s. endotoxemia
  s. examination
  s. fungal infection
  s. hypoperfusion
  s. hypotension
  s. immunotherapy
  s. inflammatory response syndrome
    (SIRS)
  s. lesion
  s. lupus
  s. oxygen extraction
  s. perfusion
  s. pressure support
  s. radioimmunoglobulin therapy
  s. sepsis
  s. vascular resistance
  s. venodilation
  s. venous circulation
systolic
  s. arterial pressure (SAP)
  s. blood pressure (SBP)
  s. ejection murmur
  s. ejection rate
  s. left ventricular pressure
  s. pressure time index
  s. time (ST)
Szymanowski-Kuhnt operation
Szymanowski operation

T

    T cell
    T condylar fracture
    T fracture
    T incision
    T lesion
    T myelotomy
    T sign

T1

    first twitch height

T1-weighted spin-echo image
T2 relaxation rate
T2-weighted spin-echo image
TAA

    thoracoabdominal aortic aneurysm

tabby-cat striation
tabetic dissociation
tablature
table

    inner t.
    vitreous t. '

tabulation
TAC

    total abdominal colectomy

TACC

    thoracic aortic cross-clamping

Tachdjian

    T. classification
    T. procedure

tachistoscopy
tachycardia

    atrial ectopic t.
    atrioventricular reentry t.
    automatic ectopic t.
    bundle branch reentrant t.
    ectopic atrial t.
    endless-loop t.
    exercise-induced ventricular t.
    junctional ectopic t.
    pacemaker-mediated t.
    right ventricular outflow tract t.
    torsade de pointes ventricular t.
    (TdPVT)

tachyphylaxis
tacrolimus-based immunosuppression
tactic

    thyroidectomy t.
    thyroid surgical t.

Tactilaze angioplasty
tactile

    t. anesthesia
    t. stimulation

TAER

    transient auditory evoked response

TAES

    transcutaneous acupoint electrical
    stimulation

tagging stitch
tagliacotian operation
TAH

    total abdominal hysterectomy

TAHBSO

    total abdominal hysterectomy and
    bilateral salpingo-oophorectomy

tail

    artery of pancreatic t.
    axillary t.
    t. bone
    pancreatic t.
    t. tumor
    t. vertebra

tailbone
tailor bunionectomy
Tait flap
Tajima

    T. method
    T. suture technique

Takayasu

    T. arteritis
    T. disease
    T. syndrome

takedown

    t. abdominal approach
    bilateral ureterostomy t.
    colostomy t.
    t. procedure

talar

    t. avulsion fracture
    t. canal
    t. compression syndrome
    t. dislocation
    t. neck fracture
    t. osteochondral fracture
    t. sulcus

talc

    t. insufflation
    t. operation
    t. peritonitis
    t. pleurodesis

talectomy

    Trumble t.

Talesnick scapholunate repair
tali

    sustentaculum t.

talipes

    t. cavus deformity
    t. equinovarus

talocalcaneal

    t. angle

T

talocalcaneal *(continued)*
    t. articulation
    t. fusion
talocalcaneonavicular articulation
talocrural joint
talonavicular
    t. bone
    t. fusion
taloscaphoid
talotibial
talus, pl. **tali**
tamp
    bone t.
tamponade
    balloon tube t.
    low-pressure t.
    t. needle tract
    tract t.
tamponage
tamponing
tamsulosin
Tanagho
    T. bladder flap urethroplasty
    T. bladder neck reconstruction
tandem
    t. clipping technique
    t. colonoscopy
    t. construction
    t. lesion
tangential
    t. biopsy
    t. colonic submucosal injection
    t. débridement
    t. excision
    t. incision
    t. projection
    t. section
    t. tract
    t. wound
tangent screen examination
Tanner operation
Tansini operation
Tansley operation
tantalum cranioplasty
tap
    abdominal t.
    peritoneal t.
    shunt t.
tape mark
tapered tip
taper point
tapetum
tapinocephalic
tapinocephaly
TAPP
    transabdominal properitoneal
tapping
    glabellar t.

target
    fixation t.
    t. gland
    t. lesion
    t. plasma
    t. plasma concentration (TPC)
    saccadic eccentric t.
    t. sign
target-controlled infusion (TCI)
targeted
    t. brain biopsy
    t. lobar deflation
    t. surgery
targeting
    tumor t.
Tarin space
Tarkowski method
tarsal
    t. amputation
    t. bone fracture
    t. canal
    t. dislocation
    t. fold
    t. gland
    t. joint infection
    t. laceration
    t. ligament
    t. medullostomy
    t. membrane
    t. plate
    t. strip procedure
    t. tunnel syndrome
    t. wedge osteotomy
tarsectomy
    Blaskovics t.
    Kuhnt t.
tarsen
tarsi (*pl. of* tarsus)
tarsocheiloplasty
tarsoconjunctival flap
tarsometatarsal
    t. amputation
    t. articulation
    t. dislocation
    t. fracture-dislocation
    t. truncated-wedge arthrodesis
tarsophalangeal
tarsoplasty
tarsorrhaphy
    bilateral temporary t.
tarsotomy
    transverse t.
tarsus, pl. **tarsi**
    inferior t.
    superior t.
tartrate
Tasia operation
taste pathway

tattooing
　　colonic t.
Taussig-Bing anomaly
Taussig-Morton
　　T.-M. node dissection
　　T.-M. operation
Taussig operation
Tawara node
Taylor
　　T. approach
　　T. procedure
　　T. suture technique
Taylor-Daniel-Weiland technique
**Taylor-Townsend-Corlett iliac crest bone
　graft**
TBF
　　tracheal blood flow
TBI
　　traumatic brain injury
TBSA
　　total body surface area
TBW
　　total body weight
TC
　　total colectomy
TCD
　　transcranial Doppler
　　TCD recanalization
T-cell
　　T-c. depleted bone marrow
　　　transplantation
　　T-c. line
TCES
　　transcutaneous cranial electrical
　　　stimulation
TCI
　　target-controlled infusion
TCM
　　thick cutaneous melanoma
Tc-99m
　　technetium-99m
tc-MER
　　motor-evoked response to transcranial
　　　stimulation
TCNB
　　Tru-Cut needle biopsy
T-configuration
TCRF
　　temperature-controlled radiofrequency
TCS
　　transcranial stimulation

TD
　　thermodilution
TDCO
　　thermodilution cardiac output
TdPVT
　　torsade de pointes ventricular tachycardia
TE
　　tracheoesophageal
　　TE fistula
TEA
　　thromboendarterectomy
teacup fracture
Teale-Knapp operation
team
　　2-t. dissection
　　trauma t.
TEAP
　　transesophageal atrial pacing
　　TEAP threshold
tear
　　bucket-handle t.
　　esophageal t.
　　flap meniscal t.
　　inadvertent serosal t.
　　Mallory-Weiss t.
　　mesenteric t.
　　pulmonary circulation t.
　　rotator cuff t.
　　t. sac
　　serosal t.
teardrop
　　t. fracture
　　t. line
tearing
　　excessive t.
　　short duration, unilateral, neuralgic,
　　　conjunctival injection and t.
　　　(SUNCT)
technetium-99m (Tc-99m)
technic
technical
　　t. consideration
　　t. factor
　　t. failure
technician
　　OR t.
technique
　　abdominal pressure t.
　　abduction traction t.
　　ablative t.
　　Ace-Colles frame t.
　　acid etch bonding t.

NOTES

T

technique *(continued)*

adduction traction t.
afterloading t.
agglutination t.
airbrasive t.
air-gap t.
airway occlusion t.
Albert suture t.
Alexander t.
Allison suture t.
alternating suture t.
American laryngectomy t.
Amplatz t.
Amspacher-Messenbaugh t.
Anderson-Hutchins t.
Andrews t.
anesthetic t.
angiographic road-mapping t.
angle bisection t.
angle suture t.
antegrade double balloon-double
 wire t.
antegrade/retrograde cardioplegia t.
anterior quadriceps
 musculocutaneous flap t.
anterior sandwich patch t.
anterograde transseptal t.
antireflux ureteral implantation t.
AO t.
APOLT t.
Appolito suture t.
apposition suture t.
approximation suture t.
Araki-Sako t.
arcuate suture t.
Argyll-Robertson suture t.
Arlt suture t.
Armaly-Drance t.
Armistead t.
Aronson-Prager t.
arrested-heart revascularization t.
arterial cannulation anesthetic t.
arthrographic capsular distention
 and rupture t.
ascending t.
aseptic t.
ASIF screw fixation t.
Asnis t.
assay t.
assisted reproductive t.
Atasoy V-Y t.
Atkinson t.
atraumatic suture t.
atrial-well t.
autosuture t.
Avila t.
avulsion t.
Axenfeld suture t.
axillary block anesthetic t.

axillary perivascular t.
Ayre spatula-Zelsmyr cytobrush t.
Babcock suture t.
back-and-forth suture t.
Badgley t.
bag-of-bones t.
Bailey-Badgley t.
Bailey-Dubow t.
Baker t.
Balacescu-Golden t.
balanced anesthetic t.
balloon catheter t.
balloon-catheter and basket-
 retrieval t.
balloon tamponade t.
Banks-Laufman t.
Barcat t.
bare scleral t.
Barkan t.
Barraquer suture t.
barrier t.
Barron hemorrhoidal banding t.
Barsky t.
baseball suture t.
basic t.
basilar suture t.
basket extraction t.
basket fragmentation t.
basketing t.
Bass t.
Bassini t.
bastard suture t.
Batch-Spittler-McFaddin t.
Bauer-Tondra-Trusler t.
Baumgard-Schwartz tennis elbow t.
Beall-Webel-Bailey t.
Beckenbaugh t.
Becker t.
Béclard suture t.
Becton t.
Begg light wire differential
 force t.
behavioral t.
Bell-Tawse open reduction t.
Belsey fundoplication t.
Belt t.
bench surgical t.
Bentall composite graft t.
Bentall inclusion t.
Bertrandi suture t.
Beverly-Douglas lip-tongue
 adhesion t.
bilateral inguinal hernia repair t.
Billroth I, II t.
bioprogressive t.
biopsy t.
biparietal suture t.
Bircher-Weber t.
bisecting angle t.

bisecting-the-angle t.
bitewing t.
Black t.
Black-Broström staple t.
Blackburn t.
bladder neck preserving t.
Blair t.
Blair-Byars hypospadias t.
blanket suture t.
Bleck recession t.
Blenderm patch t.
blind nasal intubation anesthetic t.
blind nasotracheal intubation
  anesthetic t.
blind-spot projection t.
Bloom-Raney modification of
  Smith-Robinson t.
Blount tracing t.
Blundell-Jones t.
Bohlman cervical fusion t.
Bohlman triple-wire t.
bolster suture t.
bolus intravenous anesthetic t.
bone t.
Bonfiglio-Bardenstein t.
Bonfiglio modification of
  Phemister t.
Bonola t.
boost t.
bootstrap 2-vessel t.
Bora t.
Borggreve-Hall t.
bougienage t.
Bowers t.
Bowles t.
Box t.
Boyd-Anderson t.
Boyden chamber t.
Boyd-McLeod tennis elbow t.
Boyes brachioradialis transfer t.
Bozeman suture t.
Braasch bulb t.
brachial plexus block anesthetic t.
Brackett-Osgood-Putti-Abbott t.
Brackin t.
Brady-Jewett t.
Brand tendon transfer t.
breast-conserving t.
breast reduction t.
Brecher-Cronkite t.
Brecher new methylene blue t.
bregmatomastoid suture t.

Brenner gastrojejunostomy t.
bridle suture t.
Brockenbrough t.
Brockhurst t.
bronchoscopy anesthetic t.
Brooks t.
Brooks-Jenkins atlantoaxial fusion t.
Brooks-Seddon transfer t.
Broström injection t.
Brown t.
Brown-Beard t.
Brown-Brenn t.
Brown-Wickham t.
Bruhat t.
Bruser t.
Bryan-Morrey t.
Buck-Gramcko t.
Bugg-Boyd t.
bulk pack t.
bunching suture t.
Buncke t.
Bunnell atraumatic t.
Bunnell suture t.
Bunnell tendon transfer t.
Burch bladder suspension t.
Burgess t.
buried mass far-and-near suture t.
Burkhalter modification of Stiles-
  Bunnell t.
Burkhalter transfer t.
Burrows t.
buttonhole suture t.
button suture t.
Buxton bolus suture t.
bypass t.
cable wire suture t.
Caldwell-Coleman flatfoot t.
Callahan fusion t.
Camino catheter t.
Camitz t.
Campbell t.
Canale t.
canal wall-up t.
Capello t.
Cape Town t.
capitonnage suture t.
capping t.
capsule flap t.
capsule forceps t.
cardiovascular imaging t.
Carey Ranvier t.
Carnesale t.

T

NOTES

technique *(continued)*

carotid preservation t.
Carrell fibular substitution t.
Carrel suture t.
catheterization t.
catheter-securing t.
caudal epidural anesthetic t.
cavernosal alpha blockade t.
Cave-Rowe shoulder dislocation t.
celiac plexus block anesthetic t.
cell separation t.
cement t.
cementless t.
central anesthetic t.
central slip sparing t.
central venous cannulation
  anesthetic t.
cephalotrigonal t.
cervical plexus block anesthetic t.
cervical screw insertion t.
cervical spondylotic myelopathy
  fusion t.
chain suture t.
channel shoulder pin t.
Charters t.
Chaves-Rapp muscle transfer t.
Cherney suture t.
chevron t.
chew-in t.
Chiari t.
Childress ankle fixation t.
chloramine T t.
cholangiographic t.
Cho tendon t.
Chow t.
Chrisman-Snook ankle t.
Cierny-Mader t.
Cincinnati t.
circular suture t.
circulatory arrest anesthetic t.
circumcision suture t.
clamp-and-sew t.
clamshell t.
Clancy ligament t.
Clark transfer t.
classic DSRS t.
Clayton-Fowler t.
clearance t.
Cleveland-Bosworth-Thompson t.
clip t.
closed circuit anesthetic t.
closed gloving t.
closed tubule fixation t.
Cloward t.
Coakley suture t.
coaptation suture t.
cobalt-60 moving strip t.
cobbler's suture t.
Cobb scoliosis measuring t.

Codivilla tendon lengthening t.
Coffey t.
Coffey-Witzel jejunostomy t.
Cofield t.
Cohen cross-trigonal t.
cold saline-induced paresthesia t.
Cole t.
Coleman flatfoot t.
Collis broken femoral stem t.
Collis-Nissen fundoplication t.
Coltart fracture t.
combination of isotonics t.
combined spinal/epidural t.
combined spinal/epidural
  anesthetic t.
compensation t.
composite addition t.
composite pelvic resection t.
compound suture t.
compression t.
computer-assisted continuous
  infusion anesthetic t.
computer-controlled drug
  administration anesthetic t.
computer-controlled infusion
  anesthetic t.
Connell suture t.
Connolly t.
continuous gum t.
continuous infusion anesthetic t.
continuous pull-through t.
continuous spinal anesthetic t.
continuous suture t.
continuous wave t.
contoured anterior spinal plate t.
contraceptive t.
contract-relax t.
controlled release anesthetic t.
controlled water-added t.
conventional t.
Conyers t.
Coomassie brilliant blue t.
Coonse-Adams t.
Cope t.
Copeland t.
coracoclavicular t.
Corbin t.
coronary flow reserve t.
costotransversectomy t.
cough CPR t.
Counsellor-Flor modification of
  McIndoe t.
Cozen-Brockway t.
crash t.
Crawford graft inclusion t.
Crawford-Marxen-Osterfeld t.
Creech t.
Crego tendon transfer t.
cricoid pressure anesthetic t.

cross-facial t.
Crown suture t.
cruciform suture t.
crushing t.
Crutchfield reduction t.
cryosurgical t.
Cubbins shoulder dislocation t.
Culcher-Sussman t.
culturing t.
cup-patch t.
Curtis t.
Curtis-Fisher knee t.
Cushing suture t.
cushioning suture t.
cutaneous suture t.
cutdown t.
cuticular suture t.
Czerny-Lembert suture t.
Czerny suture t.
Darrach-McLaughlin shoulder t.
Davey-Rorabeck-Fowler
  decompression t.
Davis drainage t.
decompression t.
decortication t.
DEFT t.
Deisting prostatic dilation t.
delayed primary suture t.
deliberate hypotension anesthetic t.
demand-adapted administration
  anesthetic t.
Denis Browne urethroplasty t.
Dennis t.
de novo needle-knife t.
DePalma modified patellar t.
depth pulse t.
dermal suture t.
descending t.
destructive interference t.
Devonshire t.
Dewar-Barrington clavicular
  dislocation t.
Dewar-Harris shoulder t.
Dewar posterior cervical fusion t.
Deyerle femoral fracture t.
diagnostic t.
Dias-Giegerich fracture t.
Dickinson calcaneal bursitis t.
Dickson transplant t.
Dieffenbach-Duplay hypospadias t.
differential force t.

differential spinal block
  anesthetic t.
digital subtraction t.
dilator-and-sheath t.
dilution-filtration t.
Dimon-Hughston t.
Diprivan t.
direct/indirect t.
direct insertion t.
distraction t.
Dixon t.
Dolenc t.
Doll trochanteric reattachment t.
Doppler auto-correlation t.
Dor fundoplication t.
dot-blot t.
Dotter t.
Dotter-Judkins t.
double-armed suture t.
double-balloon t.
double-button suture t.
double-dummy t.
double-folded cup-patch t.
double-freeze t.
double-looped semitendinosus t.
double-rod t.
double-sealant t.
double-staple t.
double-stapled ileoanal reservoir t.
double stapling t. (DST)
double-stick t.
double-tube t.
double-wire t.
Douglas bag t.
dowel t.
doweling spondylolisthesis t.
Drake tandem clipping t.
DREZ modification of Eriksson t.
drilling t.
driven equilibrium Fourier
  transform t.
Drummond spinous wiring t.
Drummond wire t.
dry field t.
dual impression t.
duct-to-mucosa t.
Dufourmentel t.
dunking t.
Dunn t.
Dunn-Brittain foot stabilization t.
Duplay I, II t.
Dupuytren suture t.

NOTES

technique *(continued)*

DuVries deltoid ligament reconstruction t.
Dyban t.
dye dilution t.
dynamic bolus tracking t.
Eastwood t.
Eaton-Littler t.
Eaton-Malerich fracture-dislocation t.
Eberle contracture release t.
ECG signal-averaging t.
Ecker-Lotke-Glazer tendon reconstruction t.
edge-to-edge suture t.
Eftekhar broken femoral stem t.
Eggers tendon transfer t.
Eisenberger t.
Eklund t.
elephant trunk t.
elliptical excision t.
Ellis-Jones peroneal tendon t.
Ellison t.
Ellis skin traction t.
Emmet suture t.
en bloc, no-touch t.
Ender femoral fracture t.
endobronchial intubation anesthetic t.
endodontic t.
endofluoroscopic t.
endorectal ileoanal pull-through t.
endoscope-assisted t.
endoscopic-assisted t.
endoscopic-assisted microsurgical t.
endoscopic mucosal resection t.
endovascular stenting t.
end-to-end reconstruction t.
end-to-side vasoepididymostomy t.
entangling t.
enucleation t.
epiaortic imaging t.
epidural blood patch anesthetic t.
epineural suture t.
epithelialization t.
Erickson-Leider-Brown t.
Eriksson brachial block t.
Eriksson ligament t.
erysiphake t.
esophageal banding t.
Essex-Lopresti axial fixation t.
Essex-Lopresti calcaneal fracture t.
Evans ankle reconstruction t.
eversion t.
everting interrupted suture t.
evoked potential t.
exchange t.
excisional biopsy t.
excision-curettage t.
ex situ-in situ t.

extraanatomical renal revascularization t.
extraanatomic bypass t.
extraarticular t.
extracorporeal t.
extraction balloon t.
extradural anesthetic t.
extravesical ureteral reimplantation t.
extremity mobilization t.
extubation anesthetic t.
ex vivo t.
facet excision t.
Fahey t.
Fahey-O'Brien t.
Fairbanks t.
Falk vesicovaginal fistula t.
far-and-near suture t.
Farmer t.
fast exposure t.
fat-suppression t.
feeder-frond t.
femoral 3-in-1 t.
Ferkel torticollis t.
ferning t.
fiberoptic bronchoscopy anesthetic t.
fiberoptic endoscopy anesthetic t.
fiberoptic tracheal intubation anesthetic t.
Fick t.
Ficoll-Hypaque t.
Fielding modification of Gallie t.
figure-of-8 suture t.
filling first t.
finger fracture t.
Finochietto-Billroth I gastrectomy t.
first-line screening t.
first-pass t.
first rib resection via subclavicular approach t.
Fish cuneiform osteotomy t.
fixation t.
fixation suture t.
FLAK t.
flap t.
Flatt t.
flicker-fusion frequency t.
Flick-Gould t.
flip-flap t.
floppy Nissen fundoplication t.
flow detection t.
flow interruption t.
flow mapping t.
fluid loading anesthetic t.
fluorescent antibody staining t. (FAST)
fluoroscopic pushing t.
flush-and-bathe t.
flushing t.

Flynn t.
Fones t.
Forbes modification of Phemister
 graft t.
Ford triangulation t.
fore-and-aft suture t.
Forest-Hastings t.
forward triangle t.
Fourier-acquired steady-state t.
 (FAST)
Fowles dislocation t.
Frank permanent gastrotomy t.
Fraunfelder no-touch t.
Freebody-Bendall-Taylor fusion t.
freehand suturing t.
free ligature suture t.
free-root insertion t.
French fracture t.
Fried-Hendel tendon t.
Froimson t.
frontalis sling t.
Frost suture t.
functional t.
furrier's suture t.
fusion t.
Gaenslen split-heel t.
Gallie atlantoaxial fusion t.
Gallie wiring t.
Galveston t.
Gambee suture t.
Ganley t.
Garceau tendon t.
gaseous laparoscopy t.
gasless laparoscopy t.
gastric valve tightening t.
gated t.
Gaur balloon distention t.
Gély suture t.
general anesthetic t.
George Lewis t.
Giannestras modification of
 Lapidus t.
Gibson suture t.
gift wrap suture t.
Gilbert-Tamai-Weiland t.
Gillies-Millard cocked-hat t.
Gill-Manning-White
 spondylolisthesis t.
Gill sliding graft t.
Gil-Vernet t.
Gittes t.
Glen Anderson t.

gliding-hole-first t.
gloved-fist t.
Glover suture t.
Glynn-Neibauer t.
Goebel-Frangenheim-Stoeckel t.
Goldberg t.
Goldmann kinetic t.
Goldmann static t.
Goldner-Clippinger t.
gold plate t.
gold seed implantation t.
Goldstein spinal fusion t.
Gomco t.
Goodwin t.
Goodwin-Hohenfellner t.
Goodwin-Scott t.
Gordon-Broström t.
Gordon joint injection t.
Gordon-Taylor t.
Gould suture t.
grabbing t.
gracilis flap t.
grasping t.
Graves t.
gravimetric t.
Green-Banks t.
Greulich-Pyle t.
Grice-Green t.
Grimelius t.
Gritti-Stokes knee amputation t.
groove suture t.
Grosse-Kempf tibial t.
Groves-Goldner t.
Gruber suture t.
Grüntzig t.
Guhl t.
guide wire exchange t.
guide wire and mini-snare t.
Gussenbauer suture t.
Guttmann t.
Guyon ankle amputation t.
guy suture t.
Guyton-Friedenwald suture t.
Hackethal stacked nailing t.
Håkanson t.
half-mouth t.
Hall t.
Halsted suture t.
Hamas t.
Hamou t.
Hardinge t.
harelip suture t.

T

NOTES

751

technique *(continued)*

Hark t.
Harmon transfer t.
Harriluque t.
Harris suture t.
Hartel t.
Hartmann reconstruction t.
Hassan method t.
Hassan open t.
Hassmann-Brunn-Neer elbow t.
Hauri t.
Hauser patellar realignment t.
Hawkins inside-out nephrostomy t.
Hawkins single-stick t.
head turn t.
Heaney t.
helical suture t.
hemostat t.
hemostatic suture t.
Hendler unitunnel t.
Henning inside-to-outside t.
Henry acromioclavicular t.
hepatic vascular isolation t.
Hermodsson internal rotation t.
Hey-Groves fascia lata t.
Hey-Groves-Kirk t.
Hey-Groves ligament
  reconstruction t.
Heyman-Herndon-Strong t.
high-amplitude sucking t.
high-heat casting t.
high-kV t.
high-tension suturing t.
Hill-Nahai-Vasconez-Mathes t.
Hitchcock tendon t.
Hodgson t.
Hofmeister t.
Hohl-Moore t.
Hoke-Kite t.
hold-relax t.
hole-in-1 t.
Hood t.
Hoppenfeld-Deboer t.
Hori t.
horizontal mattress suture t.
hot biopsy t.
Hotchkiss-McManus PAS t.
hot-dog t.
Houghton-Akroyd fracture t.
House t.
Howard t.
Hughes modification of Burch t.
Hughston-Jacobson t.
Hungerford t.
Hunt-Early t.
Huntington tibial t.
hybridization-subtraction t.
hybridoma t.
hydroflow t.

hydrogen inhalation t.
hygroscopic t.
hypogastric plexus block
  anesthetic t.
hypothermia anesthetic t.
Ilizarov limb-lengthening t.
image-related screening t.
imaging t.
imbricated suture t.
immediate extension t.
immersion t.
immunohistochemical t.
implanted suture t.
impression t.
indicator dilution t.
indirect t.
indocyanine green indicator
  dilution t.
induced hypotension anesthetic t.
induction anesthetic t.
infiltration anesthetic t.
Inglis-Cooper t.
Inglis-Ranawat-Straub t.
inhalation anesthetic t.
injection t.
inotrope resuscitation t.
Insall ligament reconstruction t.
insemination swim-up t.
insertion t.
inside-out t.
inside-to-outside t.
insufflation anesthetic t.
intercostal nerve block anesthetic t.
interference screw t.
interlocking suture t.
intermittent apnea t.
intermittent bolus t.
internal jugular vein cannulation
  anesthetic t.
internal jugular vein catheterization
  anesthetic t.
internal jugular vein puncture
  anesthetic t.
interpleural anesthetic t.
interpolation t.
interrupted suture t.
interscalene block anesthetic t.
interspinous segmental spinal
  instrumentation t.
interventional t.
intraarticular anesthetic t.
intracath t.
intracorporeal knotting t.
intradermal mattress suture t.
intradermal tattooing t.
intramuscular preanesthetic
  medication anesthetic t.
intraoperative computer-assisted
  spinal orientation t.

intraperitoneal t.
intraperitoneal onlay mesh t.
intrathecal cannulation anesthetic t.
intrathecal morphine anesthetic t.
intravenous cannulation anesthetic t.
intravenous oxygen-15 water
  bolus t.
intubation anesthetic t.
invaginating suture t.
invagination t.
invasive t.
inverting knot t.
ischemic-tourniquet t.
isolation t.
isometric t.
Ivalon suture t.
Jaboulay-Doyen-Winkleman t.
Jacobs locking-hook spinal rod t.
Jansey t.
Jeffery t.
jejunoileal bypass reversal t.
Jerne t.
jet ventilation anesthetic t.
J loop t.
Jobert suture t.
Johnson pelvic fracture t.
Johnson staple t.
Johnston pursestring suture t.
Jones-Brackett t.
Jones and Jones wedge t.
Jones-Politano t.
Jorgensen t.
Judd pyloroplasty t.
Judkins t.
Judkins-Sones t.
jugular t.
Kader-Senn gastrotomy t.
Kalt suture t.
kangaroo tendon suture t.
Kapandji t.
Kapel elbow dislocation t.
Kaplan t.
Kashiwagi t.
Kates-Kessel-Kay t.
Kato thick smear t.
Kaufer tendon t.
Kaufmann t.
Kehr t.
Kelikian-Clayton-Loseff t.
Kelikian-Riashi-Gleason t.
Kellogg-Speed fusion t.
Kelly suture t.

Kendrick t.
Kendrick-Sharma-Hassler-Herndon t.
Kennedy ligament t.
Kern t.
Kessler suture t.
Kety-Schmidt inert gas saturation t.
keyhole tenodesis t.
Keystone t.
Kidde cannula t.
King t.
King-Richards dislocation t.
King-Steelquist t.
Kirk thigh amputation t.
Kirschner suture t.
kissing balloon t.
Kjolbe t.
Klein t.
Knoll refraction t.
Knott t.
Koch t.
Krawkow-Cohn t.
Krawkow-Thomas-Jones t.
Krempen-Craig-Sotelo tibial
  nonunion t.
Krönig t.
Kumar-Cowell-Ramsey t.
Kumar spica cast t.
Küntscher t.
Kutler finger amputation t.
Labbé gastrotomy t.
labiolingual t.
lace suture t.
Lamaze t.
Lamb-Marks-Bayne t.
Lambrinudi t.
laparoscopic colposuspension t.
laparoscopic lymph node
  dissection t.
laparoscopic Nissen
  fundoplication t.
laparoscopic paraaortic lymph node
  sampling t.
laparoscopic stripping t.
laparostomy t.
Lapidus hammertoe t.
large-core t.
Larson t.
laryngeal mask insertion
  anesthetic t.
laryngoscopy anesthetic t.
laser welding t.
lateral bending t.

T

NOTES

technique *(continued)*

lateral window t.
Laurell t.
layer t.
2-layer open t.
Lazarus-Nelson t.
LCVP-aided t.
LDN t.
Leach t.
Leadbetter modification t.
Leboyer t.
Le Dran suture t.
LeDuc t.
Lee t.
Lefèvre gastrectomy t.
Le Fort suture t.
Lehman t.
Leibolt t.
Leksell t.
Lembert suture t.
Lenart-Kullman t.
lens suture t.
lesser sac t.
letterbox t.
Lewit stretch t.
Lich extravesical t.
Lich-Gregoir t.
Lichtman t.
lid-loading t.
Liebolt radioulnar t.
ligate-divide-staple t.
ligation suture t.
light-around-wire t.
Limberg t.
limb-saving t.
Lindholm t.
lingual split-bone t.
Lipscomb t.
Lister t.
Littler t.
Littler-Cooley t.
Lloyd-Roberts fracture t.
localization t.
local standby anesthesia t.
locking suture t.
lock-stitch suture t.
Löffler suture t.
long cone t.
3-loop t.
loop gastric bypass t.
loop-on mucosa suture t.
Losee modification of MacIntosh t.
Losee sling and reef t.
loss-of-resistance t.
lost wax pattern t.
LowDye taping t.
low-flow anesthetic t.
Lown t.
Ludloff t.

lumbar accessory movement t.
lumbar anesthetic t.
1-lung ventilation anesthetic t.
Luque instrumentation concave t.
Luque instrumentation convex t.
Luque sublaminar wiring t.
LUS scanning t.
Lyden t.
Lyden-Lehman t.
Lynn t.
MacIntosh t.
macroelectrode recording t.
Madden t.
Magerl translaminar facet screw
    fixation t.
Magilligan measuring t.
Magnuson t.
Ma-Griffith t.
Maitland t.
Majestro-Ruda-Frost tendon t.
Malawer excision t.
Mallory t.
Mancini t.
mandibular swing t.
Mankin t.
manometric t.
Manske t.
manual push-pull t.
Marbach-Weil t.
March t.
Marcus-Balourdas-Heiple ankle
    fusion t.
Marlex plug t.
Marshall ligament repair t.
Marshall-McIntosh t.
marsupialization t.
Martin patellar wiring t.
Martin reduction t.
masking t.
masquerade t.
MAST t.
Mathieu t.
Matti-Russe t.
4-maximal breath preoxygenation t.
Mazet t.
McCauley t.
McConnell t.
McElfresh-Dobyns-O'Brien t.
McElvenny t.
McFarland-Osborne t.
McFarlane t.
McGoon t.
McKeever-Buck elbow t.
McLaughlin-Hay t.
McLean t.
McMaster t.
McReynolds open reduction t.
McVay t.
Meares-Stamey t.

mechanical ventilation anesthetic t.
Mehn-Quigley t.
Meigs suture t.
membrane catheter t.
Menghini biopsy t.
Mensor-Scheck t.
Merendino t.
Messerklinger t.
Meyerding-Van Demark t.
Michal II t.
microelectrode recording t.
microinvasive t.
micromanipulation t.
microsurgery t.
microsurgical t.
microtransducer t.
micro-tubulotomy t.
microvascular t.
midface degloving t.
Milch cuff resection of ulna t.
Milch elbow t.
Milford mallet finger t.
Millen t.
mille pattes t.
Millesi modified t.
minilaparotomy t.
minimal access t.
minimal leak t.
minimally invasive surgical t.
Mital elbow release t.
miter t.
Mitrofanoff continent urinary
  diversion t.
Mizuno t.
Mizuno-Hirohata-Kashiwagi t.
modified Belsey fundoplication t.
modified brachial t.
modified Cantwell t.
modified Child t.
modified Hassan open t.
modified piggyback t.
modified Pomeroy t.
modified Sacks-Vine push-pull t.
modified Seldinger t.
modified Toupe t.
modified tumescent t.
modified V-Y advancement t.
Moe scoliosis t.
Mohs fresh tissue chemosurgery t.
Mohs microsurgery t.
molecular t.

monitored anesthesia care
  anesthetic t.
monitoring t.
Monticelli-Spinelli distraction t.
Moore t.
morcellation t.
Morgan-Casscells meniscus
  suturing t.
Morrison t.
Mose t.
motor point block anesthetic t.
MPB t.
MPGR t.
MP-RAGE t.
Mubarak-Hargens decompression t.
mucosal relaxing incision t.
Mueller t.
Mullins blade t.
multiple inert gas elimination t.
  (MIGET)
multiple-port incision t.
muscle energy t.
muscle-splitting t.
Nalebuff-Millender lateral band
  mobilization t.
nasotracheal intubation anesthetic t.
nasovesicular catheter t.
Nealon t.
near-and-far suture t.
2-needle t.
needle-knife t.
needle thoracentesis t.
needle-through-needle single
  interspace t.
nerve stimulator anesthetic t.
nerve suture t.
neural arch resection t.
neuroablative t.
neuroleptanalgesia anesthetic t.
Neviaser acromioclavicular t.
Neviaser-Wilson-Gardner t.
Nicholas ligament t.
Nicholas 5-in-1 reconstruction t.
Niebauer-King t.
Nikaidoh-Bex t.
Nirschl t.
Nissen fundoplication t.
Nissen-Rossetti fundoplication t.
nitrous oxide-opioid-barbiturate
  anesthetic t.

NOTES

technique (*continued*)

nitrous oxide-oxygen-opioid
anesthetic t. (N$_2$O-O$_2$-opioid
anesthetic technique)
no-leak t.
noninvasive t.
nonlaparoscopic t.
nonoptimal t.
non-rib-spreading thoracotomy
incision t.
N$_2$O-O$_2$-opioid anesthetic t.
nitrous oxide-oxygen-opioid
anesthetic technique
noose suture t.
no-punch t.
Norfolk t.
Northern blot t.
no-touch t.
N2-Sargenti t.
Oakley-Fulthorpe t.
Ober-Barr transfer t.
Ober tendon t.
O'Brien akinesia t.
Obtura injectable t.
off-center isoperistaltic t.
Ogata t.
Okamura t.
Ollier t.
Omer-Capen t.
onlay t.
onlay-tube-onlay urethroplasty t.
open drop t.
open flap t.
open-gloving t.
open Hasson t.
open laparoscopic t.
open palm t.
open-sky t.
operative t.
O'Phelan t.
opioid-based t.
optimal t.
oral anesthetic t.
Orandi t.
orbital exenteration gastroscopic
access t.
Orticochea scalping t.
Osborne-Cotterill elbow t.
Osgood modified t.
Osmond-Clarke t.
Ostrup harvesting t.
Ouchterlony gel diffusion t.
out-in-out t.
outside-to-outside arthroscopy t.
over-and-over suture t.
Overhauser t.
overlapping suture t.
over-the-wire t.
Oxford t.

Pacey t.
Pack t.
Pagenstecher suture t.
Palfyn suture t.
palliative t.
Palmer t.
Palmer-Widen shoulder t.
Palomo t.
Pancoast suture t.
pants-over-vest t.
Papineau t.
Paquin t.
paradoxical t.
parallel t.
paralleling t.
paresthesia anesthetic t.
Paré suture t.
Parker-Kerr suture t.
Parrish-Mann hammertoe t.
Parvin gravity t.
PAS t.
passive gliding t.
patch t.
2-patch t.
Paterson t.
patient-controlled analgesia
anesthetic t.
Paulos ligament t.
Pauwels t.
Peacock transposing t.
peg-and-socket t.
pelviscopic clip ligation t.
Percoll t.
percutaneous insertion t.
percutaneous interventional t.
perfusion hypothermia t.
perfusion measurement t.
peribulbar anesthetic t.
pericostal suture t.
peripheral nerve block anesthetic t.
Perry t.
Perry-Nickel t.
Perry-O'Brien-Hodgson t.
Perry-Robinson cervical t.
Petit suture t.
1-phase subperiosteal implant t.
Pheasant elbow t.
Phemister-Bonfiglio t.
Phemister onlay bone graft t.
phrenic nerve block anesthetic t.
Pichlmayer t.
Pierrot-Murphy tendon t.
pinch-grasp injection t.
pin suture t.
plaque t.
plastic matrix t.
plastic suture t.
plicating suture t.
Pólya t.

Ponsky pull or guide wire insertion t.
porcelain cervical ditching t.
Porstmann t.
4-port t.
2-portal t.
3-portal t.
Porter-Richardson-Vainio t.
posterior flap t.
posterolateral costotransversectomy t.
postresection filling t.
1-pour t.
2-pour t.
Pratt t.
premuscular mesh t.
presaturation t.
preservation t.
pressure half-time t.
primary suture t.
Pringle vascular control t.
Proetz displacement t.
prograde t.
projection-reconstruction t.
projective t.
pseudobiopsy t.
Puddu tendon t.
pulley suture t.
pull-out wire suture t.
pull-through t.
pulmonary artery catheterization anesthetic t.
Pulvertaft weave t.
puppet t.
pursestring suture t.
push-back t.
push plus refraction t.
push-pull T t.
quadrant sampling t.
Quartey t.
Quénu nail plate removal t.
quick angulation t.
Quickert 3-suture t.
quilt suture t.
radiographic t.
radioguided t.
radiologic t.
radionuclide t.
Rainville t.
Ralston-Thompson pseudoarthrosis t.
Ranawat-DeFiore-Straub t.
rapid-flush t.

rapid pull-through esophageal manometry t.
rapid scan t.
rapid-sequence induction anesthetic t.
Rashkind balloon t.
Ray-Clancy-Lemon t.
Rayhack t.
reattribution t.
rebreathing t.
Rebuck skin window t.
recanalization t.
recombinant DNA t.
reconstruction t.
reconstructive t.
rectal anesthetic t.
reduction t.
refractive operative t.
regional anesthetic t.
Reichel-Pólya t.
Reichenheim t.
relaxation t.
rescue t.
resectional t.
restorative proctocolectomy t.
retained papilla t.
retention suture t.
retrobulbar anesthetic t.
retrograde tracheal intubation anesthetic t.
retromuscular prosthetic t.
reverse wedge t.
rhythmic initiation t.
ribbon arch t.
Richardson suture t.
Richter suture t.
Ricketts-Abrams t.
Rideau t.
right-angle t.
Riordan tendon transfer t.
Risser t.
Ritter-Oleson t.
Roberts t.
Robinson-Southwick fusion t.
robotic-enhanced Dresden t.
Rockwood-Green t.
Rogers cervical fusion t.
rollerball t.
roll-tube t.
Rood t.
Rosalki t.
Ross t.

T

NOTES

technique *(continued)*
Royle-Thompson transfer t.
RPT t.
running continuous suture t.
running vascular t.
Russe t.
Russell t.
Ryerson t.
sacral bar t.
Saeed t.
Saenger suture t.
Sage-Clark t.
Saha transfer t.
Sakellarides-DeWeese t.
saline t.
Salter t.
Sammarco-DiRaimondo modification
  of Elmslie t.
Sanders t.
Sarmiento trochanteric fracture t.
Scaglietti closed reduction t.
scanning t.
Schaberg-Harper-Allen t.
Schauwecker patellar wiring t.
Scheie t.
Schepens t.
Schepsis-Leach t.
Schlatter gastrectomy t.
Schnute wedge resection t.
Schober t.
Schonander t.
Schoonmaker-King single-catheter t.
scleral search coil t.
Scott glenoplasty t.
screw insertion t.
Scudder t.
Scuderi t.
sealed envelope t.
Sealy-Laragh t.
secondary suture t.
sectional t.
section freeze substitution t.
Seddon t.
segmental blocking t.
segment-oriented t.
Seldinger percutaneous t.
Seldinger retrograde
  wire/intubation t.
selective bronchial catheterization
  anesthetic t.
Sell-Frank-Johnson extensor shift t.
Semb nephrectomy t.
semitendinosus t.
Semm Z t.
sensorineural acuity level t.
seromuscular suture t.
seroserous suture t.
Sever modification of Fairbanks t.
Sewall t.

sewing machine t.
sextant t.
sharp dissection t.
Sharrard transfer t.
shave excision t.
Sheehan and Dodge t.
Sherk-Probst t.
Shirodkar suture t.
shish kebab t.
short-cone t.
short lever accessory movement t.
Silber t.
Silfverskiöld lengthening t.
silver dollar t.
Simon suture t.
Simonton t.
simple suture t.
Sims suture t.
Singer-Blom endoscopic
  tracheoesophageal puncture t.
single-armed suture t.
single-port t.
single-pour t.
single proximal portal t.
single-shot imaging t.
single space t.
skewer t.
skin expansion t.
skin surfacing t.
skin window t.
Skoog t.
sleeve t.
2-sleeve t.
sling and blanket t.
sling and reef t.
sling suture t.
sling/wrapping t.
slit catheter t.
Slocum amputation t.
Slocum fusion t.
slot-blot t.
smiley-face knotting t.
Smith Indian t.
Smith-Petersen t.
Smith-Robinson t.
snapshot GRASS t.
snare t.
Snellen suture t.
Sofield femoral deficiency t.
soluble gas t.
Somerville t.
Sones t.
sonication t.
Southern blot t.
Sparks mandrel t.
Speed-Boyd radial-ulnar t.
sperm microaspiration retrieval t.
sphincter-saving t.
sphincter-sparing t.

Spiller-Frazier t.
spinal anesthetic t.
spinal fusion t.
spinal mobilization t.
spiral CT t.
spiral suture t.
Spivack gastrotomy t.
split-and-roll t.
split-bone t.
split-course t.
split cuff nipple t.
spontaneous ventilation anesthetic t.
Sprague arthroscopic t.
SPT t.
stab avulsion t.
2-stage tendon grafting t.
Staheli t.
Stamm-Kader gastrotomy t.
standard t.
standard biopsy t.
Stanisavljevic t.
stapled reconstruction t.
Staples t.
stapling t.
STAR t.
Stark-Moore-Ashworth-Boyes t.
startle t.
Starzl t.
static dilation t.
station pull-through esophageal
 manometry t.
stay suture t.
Steffee instrumentation t.
stellate ganglion block anesthetic t.
stenting t.
stent-through-wire mesh t.
2-step t.
step-by-step t.
stepladder incision t.
stereotactic automated t.
stereotactic core biopsy t.
stereotaxic t.
sterile t.
Sternberger antibody sandwich t.
Stewart-Hamilton cardiac output t.
stick-tie suture t.
Stiegmann-Goff t.
Stiles-Bunnell transfer t.
Stillman t.
still radiography t.
Stimson anterior shoulder
 reduction t.

stimulated gracilis neosphincter t.
STIR t.
Stoll dilution egg count t.
strain/counterstrain t.
Strassman t.
Straub t.
Strayer tendon t.
stretch-and-spray t.
Strickland t.
stricturoplasty t.
strip biopsy resection t.
strut fusion t.
Studebaker t.
Sturmdorf suture t.
subcuticular suture t.
subpectoral implantation t.
subperiosteal implant 1-phase t.
subtraction t.
suction-irrigation t.
superficial suture t.
superior mesenterorenal bypass t.
super-wet t.
support suture t.
supraphysiologic fluid t.
surface cooling t.
surgical enucleation t.
surgical neurangiographic t.
surgical suture t.
surveillance t.
sustained pressure t.
suture anchor t.
suture closure t.
Swanson t.
Swiss roll embedding t.
switched B-gradient t.
sympathetic blockade anesthetic t.
sympathetic ganglion block
 anesthetic t.
Tajima suture t.
tandem clipping t.
Taylor-Daniel-Weiland t.
Taylor suture t.
telescoping suture t.
tendon suture t.
tension band wiring t.
tension suture t.
Terzis t.
test dose anesthetic t.
Teuffer t.
Thal fundoplication t.
thermal expansion t.
thermocatalytic t.

NOTES

technique *(continued)*

thermodilution t.
Thiersch suture t.
thiopental-sufentanil-desflurane-nitrous oxide anesthetic t.
Thomas t.
Thomas-Thompson-Straub transfer t.
Thompson t.
Thompson-Henry t.
Thompson-Loomer t.
thoracic epidural anesthetic t.
thoracolumbar spondylosis surgical t.
threaded-hole-first t.
through-and-through suture t.
thyroidectomy t.
thyroid surgical t.
tissue-sparing t.
titration t.
Todd-Evans stepladder tracheal dilatation t.
Tohen tendon t.
Tom Jones suture t.
Tompkins median bivalving t.
tongue-and-groove suture t.
topical anesthetic t.
Torg t.
Torgerson-Leach modified t.
total etch t.
total fundoplication t.
total intravenous anesthetic t.
Toupe t.
tracheal extubation anesthetic t.
tracheal intubation anesthetic t.
tracheal suction anesthetic t.
traction suture t.
transanal stapling t.
transarterial anesthetic t.
transcranial electrical stimulation anesthetic t.
transdermal anesthetic t.
transfixing suture t.
transiliac bar t.
translaryngeal guided intubation anesthetic t.
transmucosal drug administration anesthetic t.
transoral t.
transtracheal jet ventilation anesthetic t.
trapezius stimulation anesthetic t.
Traverso-Longmire t.
Trethowan-Stamm-Simmonds-Menelaus-Haddad t.
triangulation t.
triple-wire t.
trocar t.
trocar-cannula t.
Trusler aortic valve t.

tubal ligation band t.
tube exchange t.
tube-shift t.
tube-within-tube t.
Tuffier morcellement t.
Tullos t.
tumbling t.
tumescent liposuction t.
Turco clubfoot release t.
turn-and-suction biopsy t.
Turnbull t.
twisted suture t.
twist-off t.
Uchida t.
ultrasonographic t.
ultrasound anesthetic t.
uncut Collis-Nissen fundoplication t.
underlay fascia t.
unilateral inguinal hernia repair t.
uninterrupted suture t.
unitunnel t.
unlocking spiral t.
upgated t.
Ussing chamber t.
Van Lint modified t.
vascular isolation t.
Vastamäki t.
Veleanu-Rosianu-Ionescu t.
velocity catheter t.
venous access t.
ventral bending t.
Verdan t.
Verhoeff suture t.
vertical-cut t.
vertical mattress suture t.
Vidal-Ardrey fracture t.
video-assisted t.
videofluoroscopic t.
video transurethral resection t.
Vim-Silverman t.
volumetric t.
Volz-Turner reattachment t.
Von Haberer-Finney gastrectomy t.
Vulpius-Compere tendon t.
V-Y advancement t.
Wadsworth t.
Wagner open reduction t.
Wagoner cervical t.
Waldhausen subclavian flap t.
Wallace t.
Wanger reduction t.
Warner-Farber ankle fixation t.
Warwick and Ashken t.
wash t.
washed field t.
water-suppression t.
Watkins fusion t.
Watson t.
Watson-Cheyne t.

wax-matrix t.
wax pattern thermal expansion t.
Weaver-Dunn acromioclavicular t.
Weber-Brunner-Freuler-Boitzy t.
Weber-Vasey traction-absorption
  wiring t.
Weckesser t.
Weinstein-Ponseti t.
Welch t.
Wertheim-Bohlman t.
West-Soto-Hall patellar t.
whiplash t.
whipstitch suture t.
Whitesides t.
Whitesides-Kelly cervical t.
whole blood lysis t.
Wick catheter t.
Wickham t.
Williams-Haddad t.
Willi glass crown t.
Wilson t.
Wilson-Jacobs tibial fracture
  fixation t.
Wilson-McKeever shoulder t.
window t.
Windson-Insall-Vince grafting t.
Winograd t.
Winter spondylolisthesis t.
wire removal t.
Wirth-Jager tendon t.
Wölfler suture t.
Woodward t.
^{133}Xe intravenous injection t.
xenon-washout t.
Young t.
Young-Dees t.
Y-suture t.
Zancolli rerouting t.
Zarins-Rowe ligament t.
Zavala t.
Zazepen-Gamidov t.
Zeier transfer t.
Zielke t.
Z-suture t.
Zuker and Manktelow t.
technocausis
technologist
  certified surgical t. (CST)
technology
  assisted reproduction t.
  controlled release silver t.
  endoluminal t.

endoscopic t.
endovascular t.
fluorescent optode t.
laparoscopic t.
minimal access spine t. (MAST)
signal extraction t. (SET)
tectobulbar tract
tectocephalic
tectocephaly
tectology
tectonic
  t. epikeratoplasty
  t. keratoplasty
tectopontine tract
tectorial membrane
tectospinal
  t. decussation
  t. tract
TEE
  transesophageal echocardiography
teeth
  canine t.
  central incisor t.
  extruded t.
  t. ligation
  molar t.
  premolar t.
TEF
  tracheoesophageal fistula
Teflon granuloma
teflurane
TEG
  thromboelastograph hemostasis analyzer
  thromboelastography
tegmentotomy
tela, pl. **telae**
telangiectasia
telangiectatic angioma
telangioma
telecobalt therapy
telelectrocardiogram
telemedicine
telencephalic malformation
telencephalization
telepresence surgery
telerobotic-assisted laparoscopic surgery
telescoping
  t. nail
  t. suture technique
telesurgery
televised radiofluoroscopy
television microscopy

NOTES

TeLinde operation
telomerase
TEM
    transanal endoscopic microsurgery
temperature
    ambient t.
    axilla t.
    basal body t.
    bladder t.
    body t.
    brain t.
    core body t.
    esophagus t.
    t. exchange apparatus
    flash-point t.
    t. gradient
    heat production t.
    hyperthermic t.
    intraoperative core body t.
    normal body t.
    normothermic t.
    t., pulse, respiration (TPR)
    skin t.
    t. threshold
temperature-compensated vaporizer
temperature-controlled
    t.-c. radiofrequency (TCRF)
    t.-c. radiofrequency tissue ablation
templating
    digital t.
tempora (*pl. of* tempus)
temporal
    t. aponeurosis
    t. apophysis
    t. arteritis
    t. artery
    t. artery biopsy
    t. bone
    t. bone fracture
    t. bone tumor
    t. branch
    t. canal
    t. fascia
    t. flap
    t. fossa
    t. incision
    t. line
    t. lobectomy
    t. lobe radiation
    t. muscle
    t. nerve
    t. orientation
    t. plane
    t. process
    t. ridge
    t. space
    t. space infection
    t. squama
    t. surface

    t. suture
    t. vein
    t. wedge
temporal-cerebral arterial anastomosis
temporalis
    t. fascia flap
    t. fascial flap
    t. muscle flap
    t. tendon
temporary
    t. balloon occlusion
    t. cavity phenomenon
    t. diverting colostomy
    t. end colostomy
    t. fecal diversion
    t. loop ileostomy
    t. nerve blockade
    t. pacemaker placement
    t. palsy
    t. postoperative supplementation
    t. restoration
temporization
temporoauricular
temporofrontal tract
temporohyoid
temporomalar
temporomandibular
    t. articular disc
    t. joint
    t. joint articulation
    t. joint dislocation
    t. ligament
    t. luxation
    t. nerve
    t. pain
temporomandibularis
temporomaxillary vein
temporooccipital
temporoparietal
    t. fascial flap
    t. muscle
temporopontine tract
temporosphenoid
tempus, pl. **tempora**
tenacious adhesion
tendency
    thrombotic t.
tender
    t. line
    t. point
tenderness
    abdominal t.
    diffuse abdominal t.
    marked t.
    proximal bowel t.
    rebound t.
    subareolar t.
tendineae
tendines (*pl. of* tendo)

tendinis
   vagina fibrosa t.
tendinitis
tendinomyoplastic amputation
tendinoplasty
tendinosuture
tendinous
   t. arch
   t. cord
   t. inscription
   t. insertion
   t. opening
tendinum
tendo, pl. **tendines**
   t. Achillis
tendolysis
tendon
   abductor pollicis longus t.
   Achilles t.
   adductor magnus t.
   anterior tibialis t.
   attenuation of t.
   biceps t.
   calcaneal t.
   calcanean t.
   central t.
   t. centralization
   central perineum t.
   common annular t.
   common extensor t.
   conjoined t.
   conjoint t.
   cricoesophageal t.
   digital extensor t.
   elbow extensor t.
   erector spinae t.
   t. excursion
   extensor carpi radialis brevis t.
   extensor carpi radialis longus t.
   extensor carpi ulnaris t.
   extensor digiti minimi t.
   extensor digiti quinti t.
   extensor digitorum t.
   extensor digitorum brevis t.
   extensor digitorum communis t.
   extensor digitorum longus t.
   extensor hallucis longus t.
   extensor indicis proprius t.
   extensor pollicis brevis t.
   extensor pollicis longus t.
   extensor quinti t.
   fibularis longus t.

   fibularis tertius t.
   t. flap
   flexor carpi radialis t.
   flexor digitorum longus t.
   flexor digitorum profundus t.
   flexor digitorum superficialis t.
   flexor hallucis brevis t.
   flexor hallucis longus t.
   flexor pollicis longus t.
   gracilis t.
   t. graft
   hamstring t.
   heel t.
   iliopsoas t.
   intermediate digastric t.
   intermediate omohyoid t.
   t. interposition arthroplasty
   lateral rectus t.
   latissimus dorsi t.
   t. lengthening
   masseter t.
   peroneal brevis t.
   peroneal longus t.
   plantaris t.
   popliteus t.
   posterior tibialis t.
   pronator teres t.
   psoas minor t.
   quadriceps femoris t.
   rectus femoris t.
   t. repair
   t. rupture
   semimembranosus t.
   semitendinosus t.
   snapping iliopsoas t.
   split anterior tibial t. (SPLATT)
   stapedius t.
   subscapularis t.
   superior oblique t.
   t. suture technique
   temporalis t.
   thumb extensor t.
   toe extensor t.
   t. transplantation
   trefoil t.
   triceps t.
   vastus medialis t.
   wrist extensor t.
   t. of Zinn
tendoplasty
tendotomy (*var. of* tenotomy)
tendovaginal

NOTES

763

tenectomy
tenesmus
tenia, pl. **teniae**
  free t.
  mesocolic t.
  omental t.
tenial
teniamyotomy
Tennison-Randall lip repair
tenodesis
  calcaneal t.
  extensor t.
  MacIntosh extraarticular t.
  Watson-Jones t.
tenolysis
tenomyoplasty
tenomyotomy
Tenon
  T. capsule
  T. membrane
  T. space
tenonectomy
tenontology
tenontomyoplasty
tenontomyotomy
tenontoplastic
tenontoplasty
tenontotomy
tenophyte
tenoplastic reconstruction
tenoplasty
tenorrhaphy
tenosuture
tenosynovectomy
  dorsal t.
  flexor t.
tenosynovitis
  de Quervain t.
tenotomy, tendotomy
  adductor t.
  Arroyo t.
  Arruga t.
  Braun shoulder t.
  curb t.
  extensor t.
  free t.
  graduated t.
  intrasheath t.
  t. operation
  percutaneous t.
  semiopen sliding t.
  sliding t.
  subcutaneous tibialis posterior t.
  transverse t.
  Veleanu-Rosianu-Ionescu adductor t.
  Z marginal t.
  Z-plasty t.
tensile

tension
  t. by applanation
  t. band fixation
  t. band wiring technique
  t. endothorax
  exhaled oxygen t.
  extrapolated end-tidal carbon
    dioxide t. (PETCO$_2$)
  t. fracture
  isometric venous t.
  oxygen t.
  t. pneumopericardium
  t. pneumothorax
  running vascular technique
    without t.
  t. suture technique
  tissue oxygen t.
  twitch t.
tension-free
  t.-f. anastomosis
  t.-f. hernioplasty
  t.-f. hiatoplasty
  t.-f. mesh implantation
  t.-f. mesh repair
  t.-f. prosthetic mesh repair
tension-length relation
tensor
  t. fascia femoris flap
  t. fascia lata muscle
  t. fascia lata muscle flap
  t. insertion
  t. tympani canal
tenth cranial nerve
tentorial
  t. herniation
  t. laceration
  t. nerve
  t. notch
  t. pressure
  t. ring
  t. sinus
tentorium, pl. **tentoria**
Tenzel rotational cheek flap
TEP
  totally extraperitoneal
    TEP repair
teratoblastoma
teratocarcinoma
  pineal t.
teratogenic medication
teratogen-induced malformation
teratologic dislocation
teratoma
  epignathus t.
  mature t.
teratomatous
teratoneuroma
teratospermia
terebration

teres major muscle
tergal
tergum
terminad
terminal
   t. bronchiole
   t. cisterna
   t. colostomy
   t. crest
   t. duct carcinoma
   t. head
   t. hinge position
   t. ileal pouch
   t. ileal resection
   t. ileostomy
   t. ileum
   t. ileum intubation
   t. infection
   t. jaw relation record
   t. line
   t. neosalpingostomy
   nociceptor afferent peripheral t.
   t. plane
   t. reservoir syndrome
   t. Syme procedure
   t. ventriculostomy
   t. web
terminalis sulcus
terminalization
termini (*pl. of* terminus)
terminolateral
terminoterminal anastomosis
terminus, pl. termini
territory
   hepatic t.
Terson
   T. operation
   T. syndrome
tertiary
   t. amputation
   t. care
   t. healing
   t. trauma center
Terzis technique
TES
   transcutaneous electric stimulation
Tessier
   T. classification
   T. craniofacial operation
   T. osteotomy
test
   abduction external rotation t.

acetowhite t.
acoustic stimulation t.
Adson t.
air t.
alcohol used disorders
   identification t.
Allen t.
anorectal function t.
Apley compression t.
articulation t.
artificial erection t.
Astrand 6-minute submaximal cycle
   ergometer t.
axial compression t.
balloon expulsion t.
baroreceptor t.
Behçet skin puncture t.
bentonite flocculation t.
Bielschowsky-Parks head-tilt, 3-
   step t.
Bielschowsky 3-step, head-tilt t.
bladder neck elevation t.
Bonney t.
brachial plexus tension t. (BPTT)
breast stimulation contraction t.
breath excretion t.
Brodie-Trendelenburg tourniquet t.
bronchial inhalation challenge t.
bronchoprovocation t.
caffeine and halothane
   contracture t. (CHCT)
Campylobacter-like organism t.
   (CLOtest)
carpal compression t.
Casoni t.
cavity t.
chlormerodrin accumulation t.
closed patch t.
CO_2 inhalation t.
cold pressor t. (CPT)
compression t.
concentration performance t.
confrontation visual field t.
corneal staining t.
Cortrosyn stimulation t.
Crampton t.
deep articulation t.
diagnostic articulation t.
differential ureteral catheterization t.
Digit Symbol Substitution T.
direct immunofluorescence t.
disc space saline acceptance t.

T

NOTES

test (*continued*)

t. dose anesthetic technique
double Maddox rod t.
DR-70 tumor marker t.
Dunnett t.
Dupuy-Dutemps
  dacryocystorhinostomy dye t.
Durkan carpal compression t.
dye exclusion t.
dye reduction spot t.
elevated arm stress t. (EAST)
ergonovine provocation t.
excitability t.
external rotation-abduction stress t.
external rotation-recurvatum t.
extrastimulus t.
extrinsic entrapment t.
fast-flush t.
Feagin shoulder dislocation t.
femoral nerve traction t.
fetal acoustic stimulation t.
Finger Oscillation T.
fistula t.
flexion-rotation-drawer knee
  instability t.
fluctuation t.
fluorescein instillation t.
fluorescein string t.
foramen compression t.
foraminal compression t.
forced duction t. (FDT)
forced generation t.
forearm ischemic exercise t.
forearm supination t.
forward traction t.
Friberg microsurgical
  agglutination t.
gastric accommodation t.
germ tube t.
Gruber t.
hair bulb incubation t.
head compression t.
head distraction t.
head-down tilt t.
head-dropping t.
head-tilt t.
head-up tilt t.
head-up tilt-table t.
hepaplastin t.
high-altitude simulation t.
Hollander t.
1-hour office pad t.
Howard t.
Hughston external rotation
  recurvatum t.
human ovum fertilization t.
hyperventilation t.
iliac compression t.
immunodiffusion t.

immunofluorescence t.
implantation t.
in vitro contracture t. (IVCT)
indirect hemagglutination t.
indocyanine green retention t.
Ingram-Withers-Speltz motor t.
t. injection
Korotkoff t.
Kruskal-Wallis t.
labyrinthine fistula t.
lacrimal irrigation t.
1-legged stork t.
line t.
liver function t. (LFT)
localization t.
lumbar extension t.
lumbar rotation t.
Luria-Delbruck fluctuation t.
Maddox rod t.
Maddox wing t.
Mann-Whitney t.
Marshall t.
Marshall-Marchetti t.
matchstick t.
Maudsley Mentation T.
maximum stimulation t.
memory guidance saccade t.
MHA-TP t.
Michigan Abuse Screening T.
  (MAST)
1-minute endoscopy room t.
mobilization t.
MUGA exercise stress t.
Multistage Maximal Effort exercise
  stress t.
nasal provocation t.
nerve excitability t.
neutralization t.
nipple stimulation t.
nonparametric t.
Noyes flexion rotation drawer t.
Object Classification T.
obturator t.
occlusive patch t.
open application t.
open patch t.
Pachon t.
parametric t.
Parks-Bielschowsky 3-step, head-
  tilt t.
penetration t.
Peptavlon stimulation t.
percutaneous pressure ureteral
  perfusion t.
perimeter corneal reflex t.
perineal nerve terminal motor
  latency t.
peritoneal equilibration t.
Perthes t.

2-point discrimination t.
postcoital t.
prick puncture t.
prism adaptation t.
promontory stimulation t.
prone extension t.
protection t.
protein truncation t.
provocation t.
provocative chelation t.
Q-tip t.
Rapoport t.
regurgitation t.
Ross-Jones t.
rotation drawer t.
rotation recurvatum t.
sag t.
scapular approximation t.
scarification t.
screening t.
Self-Administered Alcoholism
  Screening T. (SAAST)
serological t.
side-lying iliac compression t.
simple shoulder t. (SST)
skin puncture t.
SLR with external rotation t.
Spatial Orientation Memory T.
sperm immobilization t.
split renal function t.
star construction t.
station t.
Stewart t.
stimulation t.
straight catheter t.
string t.
Student-Newman-Keuls t.
sucrose t.
Suprathreshold Adaptation T.
Thompson t.
thymol tumidity t.
tilt t.
tissue compression t.
tourniquet t.
traction t.
transillumination t.
Trieger t.
trunk incurvation t.
Tsui t.
tube dilution t.
tube precipitin t.
tumor skin t.

twitch height t.
University of Pennsylvania Smell
  Identification T.
upper lip bite t.
vaginal cornification t.
vaginal mucification t.
Valpar whole body range of
  motion t.
vertical compression t.
vibration threshold t.
Visual-Motor Integration T.
Von Frey t.
walking ventilation t.
washout t.
Whitaker pressure-perfusion t.
Wilcoxon signed-rank t.
wire-loop t.

testalgia
testectomy
testes (*pl. of* testis)
testicle
testicular
  t. adrenal-like tissue
  t. appendage
  t. artery
  t. biopsy
  t. carcinoma
  t. cord
  t. duct
  t. ectopia
  t. feminization syndrome
  t. mass
  t. metastasis
  t. plexus
  t. rupture
  t. torsion
  t. tumor
  t. vein
testiculus
testing
  compression t.
  confrontation t.
  Doppler ultrasound segmental blood
    pressure t.
  fecal occult blood t. (FOBT)
  genetic t.
  palpation t.
  patch t.
  penile injection t.
  Quantitative Sensory T. (QST)
  rotation t.
  sudomotor axon reflex t.

NOTES

testing *(continued)*
    tilt-table t.
    wake-up t.
testis, pl. **testes**
    t. cord
    cryptorchid t.
    t. fracture
    impalpable t.
    movable t.
    retractile t.
    torsion t.
    undescended t.
testitis
testoid
tetanic
    t. fade
    t. stimulation
    t. stimulation method
tetanization
tetanus
    cephalic t.
    extensor t.
    head t.
    traumatic t.
tetany
    duration t.
    hyperventilation t.
    postoperative t.
tethered cord syndrome
tetracaine
    hyperbaric t.
    liposome-encapsulated t.
tetragonus
tetralogy of Fallot
Teuffer
    T. technique
    T. tendo calcaneus repair
Teutleben ligament
TEVP
    transesophageal ventricular pacing
Texas
    T. Scottish Rite Hospital (TSRH)
    T. Scottish Rite Hospital hook-rod
      system
texture
    echo t.
    firm t.
    rubbery t.
textured fabric rub
T-fastener gastropexy
TFCC
    triangular fibrocartilage complex
TG
    total gastrectomy
TGF
    transforming growth factor
Thal
    T. esophageal stricture repair
    T. esophagogastroscopy

    T. esophagogastrostomy
    T. fundic patch operation
    T. fundoplasty
    T. fundoplication
    T. fundoplication method
    T. fundoplication procedure
    T. fundoplication technique
    T. stricturoplasty
thalamectomy
thalamencephalic
thalamencephalon
thalamic
    t. circulation
    t. pain
    t. plane
thalamic-subthalamic hemorrhage
thalamocaudate arteriovenous
    malformation
thalamostriate vein
thalamotomy
    gamma t.
    staged bilateral stereotactic t.
    stereotactic Vim t.
    stereotactic VL t.
    Vim t.
thallium-technetium scanning
Thal-Nissen fundoplasty
thanatopsy
Thane method
THARIES
    total hip arthroplasty with internal
    eccentric shells
THE
    transhiatal esophagectomy
theater
    operating t.
    twin operating t.
thebesian
    t. circulation
    t. vein
theca, pl. **thecae**
thecal
    t. sac
    t. sac compression
theca-lutein cyst
thecoma
    luteinized t.
    ovarian t.
Theden method
Theile muscle
Theirsch-Duplay repair
thele
theleplasty
thenad
thenal
thenar
    t. eminence
    t. flap
    t. muscle

t. prominence
t. space
thenen
theory
gate-control t.
membrane expansion t.
Pauling t.
thoracic pump t.
therapeutic
t. alternative
t. anesthesia
t. angiogenesis
t. approach
t. arsenal
t. colonoscopy
t. dissection
t. effect
t. efficacy
t. endpoint
t. insemination
t. intervention scoring system (TISS)
t. iridectomy
t. irradiation
t. laparoscopy
t. lymph node dissection (TLND)
t. modality
t. nerve block
t. option
t. phlebotomy
t. step
t. upper endoscopy
therapist
stoma t.
therapy
ablation t.
ablative laser t.
ActiPatch t.
active appliance t.
active assistive motion t.
adjunct t.
adjunctive suppressive medical t.
adjuvant chemoradiation t.
adjuvant drug t.
aerosol t.
alternate-day t.
alternative t.
amplitude-summation interferential current t.
anaclitic t.
angina-guided t.
antiarrhythmic t.

antibiotic t.
anticoagulant t.
anticoagulation t.
antiemetic t.
antifungal t.
antihormonal t.
antilymphoid t.
antireflux t.
antithrombotic t.
apotreptic t.
argon laser t.
around-the-clock oral maintenance bronchodilator t.
augmentation t.
balloon photodynamic t.
belly bath t.
biomagnetic t.
bite plane t.
boron neutron-capture t.
Bragg peak proton-beam t.
breast conservation t. (BCT)
breast-conserving t.
breast-preservation t.
brisement t.
bronchoscopic photodynamic t.
buprenorphine narcotic analgesic t.
Cancell t.
cerebral protective t.
chest physical t.
chronic opioid analgesic t. (COAT)
Clinitron air-fluidized t.
coagulative laser t.
cobalt t.
cognitive-behavioral t.
combined chemoradiation t.
compartmental radioimmunoglobulin t.
complementary t.
concomitant t.
conditioning t.
conformal radiation t.
conservative t.
contact dissolution t.
continuous renal replacement t.
convulsive t.
3-cornered t.
corrective t.
Crozat t.
deep chest t.
definitive local t.
device t.
diagnostic surgical t.

T

NOTES

therapy *(continued)*
diathermic t.
dilation t.
3-dimensional conformal radiation t.
diuretic t.
dressing t.
dual t.
electrical stimulation t.
electric aversion t.
electric differential t.
electroconvulsive t.
electrotherapeutic sleep t.
endocavitary radiation t.
endoluminal t.
endoscopic hemostatic t.
endoscopic injection t.
endoscopic laser t.
endoscopic pancreatic t.
endoscopic photodynamic t.
endourological t.
endovascular t.
enterostomal t.
eradication t.
erythropoietin t.
esophageal photodynamic t.
ethanol injection t.
expansion and activator t.
extended field irradiation t.
external beam radiation t.
external vacuum t.
external x-ray t.
ex vivo gene t.
factor replacement t.
fast neutron radiation t.
fetal drug t.
focused radiation t.
fractionated radiation t.
frappage t.
frequency-difference interferential
  current t.
functional orthodontic t.
gene replacement t.
gene-transfer t.
grenz ray t.
HDR intracavitary radiation t.
hemofiltration t.
hepatic arterial t.
herbal t.
high-dose radioiodine t.
high-voltage t.
hydration t.
hyperbaric oxygen t. (HBO)
hyperthermia t.
ImmTher t.
immunocompetent tissue t.
implosive t.
incremental t.
indirect pulpal t.
Indoklon t.

infrared t.
inhalation t.
injection t.
innovative t.
instillation t.
insulin coma t.
insulin shock t.
interferential t.
interlesional t.
internal radiation t.
interstitial photodynamic t.
interstitial radiation t.
interventional t.
intraarterial t.
intracavernous injection t.
intracavitary radiation boost t.
intracorporeal injection t.
intradiscal electrothermal t. (IDET)
intralesional t.
intraoperative radiation t.
intraperitoneal radiation t.
intraspinal t.
intrathecal t.
intravascular fluid t.
intravenous antibiotic t.
intravenous hydration t.
intravenous ozone t.
intraventricular t.
invasive t.
ischemia-guided medical t.
isolation perfusion t.
I.V. fluid t.
Kelsey unloading exercise t.
ketoprofen analgesic t.
laser t.
LDR intracavitary radiation t.
life-saving form of t.
Livingstone t.
local t.
long-term oxygen t.
Lymphapress compression t.
magnet t.
manipulative t.
medical t.
microcurrent t.
microwave t.
migraine abortive t.
mind-body t.
morphine narcotic analgesic t.
MTBE t.
multimodal adjuvant t.
multimodality t.
multiple t.
myoablative t.
myofunctional t.
Nd:YAG laser t.
negative pressure t.
neoadjuvant t.
neodymium:YAG laser t.

neutron beam t.
neutron capture t.
nonspecific t.
nonsurgical t.
occlusal t.
occlusion t.
occlusive t.
occupational t.
ocular radiation t.
open surgical t.
operative t.
optimal t.
orthodontic t.
outpatient physical t.
oxygen t.
PA t.
palliative t.
pancreatic intraluminal radiation t.
parenteral t.
particle beam radiation t.
PEMF t.
penile injection t.
penile vein occlusion t.
percussion t.
percutaneous embolization t.
percutaneous ethanol injection t.
percutaneous microwave
  coagulation t.
percutaneous transcatheter t.
perfusion t.
periodontal t.
perioperative antibiotic t.
permanent anticoagulant t.
photodynamic t. (PDT)
photoradiation t.
physical t.
placebo t.
plasma exchange t.
pool t.
positional release t.
postnatal t.
postoperative anticoagulation t.
postradiation t.
posttransplant immunosuppression t.
postural t.
prenatal t.
preoperative t.
preventive intravesical t.
progestational t.
programmed t.
prophylactic antibiotic t.
protein shock t.

proton beam t.
proton pump inhibition t.
pulp canal t.
pulse dye laser t.
pyretic t.
quadrangular t.
quadrantectomy, axillary dissection,
  radiation t. (QUART)
quadruple t.
radiation t.
radical t.
radioimmunoglobulin t.
radioiodine ablation t.
radiopharmaceutical t.
red-filter t.
reflex t.
rehydration t.
renal infusion t.
renal replacement t.
rescue t.
respiratory kinetic t.
rheologic t.
root canal t.
rotation t.
saline injection t.
salvage t.
sandwich staghorn calculus t.
sclerosing t.
sedative t.
skin lubrication t.
soak t.
social interaction t.
sole laser t.
somatic t.
sparing t.
STAMP t.
stem cell gene t.
stepdown t.
stereotactic-assisted radiation t.
stereotactic-focused radiation t.
stereotactic radiation t.
Stockholm technique for radium t.
subcoma t.
Supartz joint fluid t.
supranormal hemodynamic t.
surgical maggot t.
systemic adjuvant t.
systemic antifungal t.
systemic radioimmunoglobulin t.
telecobalt t.
thermal t.
thrombolytic t.

T

NOTES

therapy *(continued)*
- timed-sequential t.
- tocolytic t.
- tongue thrust t.
- total push t.
- transcatheter arterial embolization t.
- transfusion t.
- transgenic t.
- transurethral collagen injection t.
- transvenous t.
- triadic t.
- trial of conservative t.
- trimodality t.
- triple intrathecal t.
- tumor t.
- ultrasonic t.
- ultrasound t.
- ultrasound-guided shockwave t.
- unfractionated heparin t.
- vocal fold fixation t.
- voice t.
- volume t.
- whole-brain radiation t.
- wide-field radiation t.
- wide-range radiation t.
- xenogenic cell t.
- x-ray t.

therencephalous

thermal
- t. ablation
- t. anesthesia
- t. balance
- t. coefficient expansion
- t. death point
- t. disinfection
- t. expansion technique
- t. injury
- t. keratoplasty
- t. necrosis
- t. quenching
- t. rhizotomy
- t. sclerectomy
- t. stimulation
- t. therapy

thermal-assisted
- t.-a. capsular shift procedure
- t.-a. capsular shrinkage

thermally active method

thermal/perfusion balloon angioplasty

thermic anesthesia

thermocatalytic technique

thermocauterectomy

thermocautery

thermochemotherapy

thermocoagulation

thermodilution (TD)
- bolus t. (BTD)
- t. cardiac output (TDCO)

- t. method
- t. technique

thermodynamic theory of narcosis

thermogenesis
- nonshivering t.

thermogram

thermographic examination

thermography

thermokeratoplasty

thermolysis

thermometry
- tympanic t.

thermopenetration

thermoregulation
- perianesthetic t.

thermoregulatory vasoconstriction

thermorhizotomy

thermosclerectomy

thermosclerostomy

thermosclerotomy

thermotherapy
- microwave t.
- transurethral microwave t. (TUMT)

thick cutaneous melanoma (TCM)

thickened
- t. nail
- t. synovial membrane

thickening
- endocardial t.
- heel pad t.
- postlumpectomy skin t.

thickness
- Breslow t.
- endometrial t.
- end-systolic wall t. (ESWT)
- skinfold t.
- soft tissue t.

Thiersch
- T. anal incontinence operation
- T. graft operation
- T. medium split free graft
- T. method
- T. procedure
- T. suture technique
- T. thin split free graft

Thiersch-Duplay
- T.-D. proximal tube procedure
- T.-D. tube graft
- T.-D. urethral construction
- T.-D. urethroplasty

thigh
- t. bone
- t. graft arteriovenous fistula
- t. joint
- posterior t.

thimble valvotomy

thin
- t. basement membrane
- t. basement membrane disease

t. glossy skin
t. section
thin-needle biopsy
thinning
corneal t.
ThinPrep procedure
thin-section axial image
thiol
t. augmentation
t. modification
thiopental-sufentanil-desflurane-nitrous oxide anesthetic technique
third
t. cranial nerve
t. and fourth pharyngeal pouch syndrome
t. intention
t. occipital nerve
t. parallel pelvic plane
t. space fluid accumulation
t. space loss
Steel rule of t.'s
t. trochanter
t. ventriculostomy
third-degree
t.-d. burn
t.-d. hemorrhoid
t.-d. radiation injury
third-grade fusion
Thiry fistula
Thiry-Vella fistula
Thoma ampulla
Thomas
T. classification
T. extrapolated bar graft
T. operation
T. procedure
T. sign
T. technique
Thomas-Thompson-Straub transfer technique
Thomas-Warren incision
Thom flap laryngeal reconstruction method
Thompson
T. anterolateral approach
T. anteromedial approach
T. capsule flap pyeloplasty
T. excision
T. ligament
T. line
T. posterior radial approach

T. procedure
T. quadricepsplasty
T. resection
T. technique
T. telescoping V osteotomy
T. test
Thompson-Epstein femoral fracture classification
Thompson-Hatina method
Thompson-Henry technique
Thompson-Loomer technique
Thomson operation
thoracentesis
needle t.
thoraces (*pl. of* thorax)
thoracic
t. anesthesia
t. aneurysm
t. aorta
t. aortic aneurysm repair
t. aortic cross-clamping (TACC)
t. aortic disease
t. aortic dissection
t. aortic plexus
t. approach
t. axis
t. bioimpedance
t. cage
t. cardiac branch
t. cardiac nerve
t. cavity
t. compression syndrome
t. discectomy
t. disc herniation
t. duct
t. duct fistula
t. endometriosis syndrome
t. epidural analgesia
t. epidural anesthetic technique
t. epidural catheterization
t. esophagogastrostomy
t. esophagus
t. facet fusion
t. ganglion
t. girdle
t. great vessel
t. index
t. inlet
t. inlet soft tissue
t. inlet vascular injury
t. interspinal muscle
t. intertransverse muscle

NOTES

thoracic *(continued)*
- t. kidney
- t. lesion
- t. limb
- t. longissimus muscle
- t. motor paralysis
- t. outlet compression
- t. outlet decompression
- t. outlet syndrome (TOS)
- t. plane
- t. pump theory
- t. radiculopathy
- t. respiration
- t. rotator muscle
- t. short esophagomyotomy
- t. spinal fusion
- t. spinal nerve
- t. spine
- t. spine biopsy
- t. spine fracture
- t. spine kyphotic deformity
- t. spine landmark
- t. spine scoliotic deformity
- t. spine vertebral osteosynthesis
- t. stomach
- t. surgeon
- t. surgery
- t. vein
- t. vertebra
- t. vertebral body
- t. wall

thoracicoabdominal
thoracicoacromial
thoracicohumeral
thoracis
thoracoabdominal
- t. aneurysm
- t. aortic aneurysm (TAA)
- t. aortic aneurysm repair
- t. esophagectomy
- t. esophagogastrectomy
- t. extrapleural approach
- t. gunshot wound
- t. incision
- t. injury
- t. intrapleural approach
- t. nerve
- t. region
- t. retroperitoneal lymphadenectomy
- t. trauma

thoracoacromial
- t. artery
- t. flap
- t. trunk
- t. vein

thoracoacromialis
thoracoceloschisis
thoracocentesis
thoracocyllosis

thoracocyrtosis
thoracodorsal
- t. artery
- t. nerve

thoracoepigastric
- t. flap
- t. vein

thoracofemoral bypass
thoracograph
thoracolaparotomy
thoracolumbar
- t. aponeurosis
- t. burst fracture
- t. fascia
- t. junction surgical exposure
- t. outflow
- t. retroperitoneal approach
- t. spine anterior exposure
- t. spine fracture
- t. spine fracture-dislocation
- t. spine stabilization
- t. spine vertebral osteosynthesis
- t. spondylosis surgical technique
- t. transdiaphragmatic approach

thoracolysis
thoracomelus
thoracopagus twins
thoracophrenolaparotomy
thoracoplasty
- conventional t.
- costoversion t.
- Delorme t.
- Schede t.
- Wilms t.

thoracopneumoplasty
thoracoschisis
thoracoscopic
- t. approach
- t. discectomy
- t. esophageal mobilization
- t. esophagomyotomy
- t. pericardiectomy
- t. repair
- t. talc insufflation

thoracoscopic-assisted esophagectomy
thoracoscopy
- single-trocar access t.
- video t.

thoracostenosis
thoracosternotomy
thoracostomy
- closed chest t.
- tube t.

thoracotomy
- anterior t.
- anterolateral t.
- t. approach
- axillary t.
- bilateral anterior t.

book t.
clamshell t.
emergency department t. (EDT)
emergency room t.
ER t.
esophagectomy with t.
t. incision
lateral t.
left-sided t.
Lewis t.
limited t.
limited anterior small t. (LAST)
median t.
muscle-sparing t.
open t.
resuscitative t.
right-sided t.
t. scar
standard t.
trapdoor t.
thorascopic
t. apical pleurectomy
t. drainage
thorax, pl. **thoraces**
left t.
Peyrot t.
right t.
Thorel bundle
thorn
T. maneuver
T. syndrome
Thornell microlaryngoscopy
threaded-hole-first technique
Three
T. Color Concept
T. Color Concept of wound
classification
threshold
apneic t.
atrial defibrillation t.
current perception t. (CPT)
defibrillation t.
detection t.
displacement t.
double-point t.
experimental t.
fibrillation t.
flicker-fusion t.
median detection t.
noise detection t.
pacemaker t.
pressure pain t. (PPT)

t. shift method
speech detection t.
stimulation t.
TEAP t.
temperature t.
ventilation t.
throat
t. anesthesia
t. pack retention
t. screen
thrombase
thrombasthenia
thrombectomy
chemical t.
early t.
mechanical t.
percutaneous mechanical t. (PMT)
percutaneous rotational t.
rheolytic catheter t.
rotational t.
surgical t.
thrombi (*pl. of* thrombus)
thrombin
human t.
thrombin-mediated consumptive state
thromboangiitis obliterans
thromboasthenia
thrombocythemia
thrombocytopenia
heparin-induced t. (HIT)
immune-mediated unfractionated
heparin-induced t.
unfractionated heparin-induced t.
thromboelastogram
thromboelastograph hemostasis analyzer
(TEG)
thromboelastography (TEG)
thromboembolectomy
percutaneous aspiration t.
rotating aspiration t.
thromboembolic
t. complication
t. disease
t. event
t. fistula
t. risk factor
thromboembolism
recurrent t.
venous t.
thromboendarterectomy (TEA)
pulmonary t. (PTE)
renal t.

T

NOTES

thrombogenesis
thrombogenic
    t. disorder
    t. foreign body
    t. profile
thrombolysis
    catheter-directed t.
    coronary t.
    T. in Myocardial Infarction (TIMI)
    T. in Myocardial Infarction
      classification
    selective intracoronary t.
    sonic t.
    urokinase t.
thrombolytic
    t. agent
    t. therapy
thrombopathy
thrombophlebitis
    recurrent t.
    superficial t.
thromboplastin
    tissue t.
thromboprophylaxis
thrombosed
    t. graft
    t. internal and external hemorrhoid
thrombosin
thrombosis, pl. **thromboses**
    acute mesenteric venous t.
    arterial t.
    chronic t.
    deep vein t.
    deep venous t. (DVT)
    diffuse microvascular t.
    early graft t.
    effort t.
    graft t.
    intimal t.
    t. of IVC
    portal t.
    postoperative deep venous t.
      (PODVT)
    recurrent t.
    renal artery t.
    vascular access t.
    venous effort t.
    widespread portal system t.
thrombostasis
thrombotic
    t. complication
    t. disease
    t. episode
    t. gangrene
    t. process
    t. tendency
Thrombo-Wellcotest method
thrombus, pl. **thrombi**
    deep venous t.

    t. extension
    peripheral t.
    portal tumor t.
    portal vein tumor t. (PVTT)
    regression of t.
    tumor t.
    vein tumor t.
through-and-through
    t.-a.-t. fracture
    t.-a.-t. laceration
    t.-a.-t. suture technique
    t.-a.-t. V-shaped horizontal
      osteotomy
through-knee amputation
through-the-scope
    t.-t.-s. balloon dilation
    t.-t.-s. balloon removal
thrower fracture
thrust manipulation
thumb
    t. deformity
    t. duplication
    t. extensor tendon
    t. metacarpophalangeal joint
      approach
    t. reconstruction
    t. web
thumb-in-palm deformity
thumbprinting
thymectomy
    cervical t.
    complete t.
    neonatal t.
    transcervical t.
    video-assisted thoracoscopic t.
thymi (*pl. of* thymus)
thymic
    t. artery
    t. branch
    t. carcinoma
    t. cyst
    t. duct
    t. mass
    t. vein
thymicolymphatic
thymocyte NA$^+$/H$^+$ exchanger
thymol
    t. flocculation
    t. tumidity test
thymolipoma
thymoma
    spindle cell t.
thymus, pl. **thymi**
    t. gland
    t. gland excision
    xenotransplantation t.
thymusectomy
thyroarytenoid muscle
thyrocele

thyrocervical
    t. artery
    t. trunk
thyrochondrotomy
thyroepiglottic
    t. ligament
    t. muscle
thyroglobulin
thyroglossal
    t. cyst surgery
    t. duct
    t. duct cyst
    t. fistula
thyrohyal
thyrohyoid
    t. ligament
    t. membrane
    t. muscle
thyroid
    t. adenoma
    t. axis
    t. body
    t. cancer
    t. carcinoma
    t. cartilage
    t. cystadenoma
    t. eminence
    t. endocrine disorder
    t. gland
    goitrous t.
    t. hormone serum concentration
    t. hyperplasia
    intratracheal ectopic t.
    t. lamina
    t. lobe
    t. lobectomy
    t. muscle
    t. needle biopsy
    t. neoplasia
    t. nodule
    t. nodule ablation
    t. notch
    t. operation
    t. pathology
    t. plexus
    pyramidal process of t.
    t. resection
    t. rest
    t. storm
    t. surgeon
    t. surgical tactic
    t. surgical technique

    t. tissue
    t. tumor
    t. vein
thyroidal hernia
thyroidectomize
thyroidectomy
    breast approach t.
    complete t.
    completion t.
    gasless endoscopic t.
    near-total t.
    outpatient t.
    prophylactic t.
    provocative food t.
    scarless endoscopic t.
    subtotal t.
    t. tactic
    t. technique
    total t.
    videoendoscopic t.
thyroiditis
    acute suppurative t.
thyrointoxication
thyrolaryngeal
thyrolingual duct
thyromental distance
thyropalatine
thyroparathyroidectomy
thyropharyngeal
thyroplasty
thyroptosis
thyrothymic thyroid rest
thyrotomy
thyrotoxic coma
Ti
    inspiratory time
TIA
    transient ischemic attack
tibia, pl. **tibiae**
tibiad
tibial
    t. acceleration
    t. augmentation block
    t. bending fracture
    t. bone defect regeneration
    t. condyle fracture
    t. crest
    t. diaphysial fracture
    t. distractor
    t. epiphysis
    t. fracture fixation
    t. intertendinous bursa

T

NOTES

tibial (*continued*)
    t. metaphysis
    t. muscle
    t. open fracture
    t. plafond fracture
    t. plateau fracture
    t. plateau fracture-dislocation
    t. shaft fracture
    t. triplane fracture
    t. tuberosity fracture
    t. tuberosity osteotomy
tibialis posterior dislocation
tibiocalcaneal
    t. arthrodesis
    t. medullary nailing
tibiofascialis
tibiofemoral articulation
tibiofibular
    t. articulation
    t. clear space
    t. diastasis
    t. fusion
    t. joint dislocation
    t. line
tibionavicular
tibioperoneal
    t. trunk angioplasty
    t. vessel angioplasty
tibioscaphoid
tibiotalar
    t. fusion
    posterior t.
tibiotalocalcaneal
    t. arthrodesis
    t. fusion
tic
    t. douloureux
    dystonic t.
tidal
    t. drainage
    t. volume
Tiedemann nerve
tier
    remote t.
ties-over-stent
tightening
    gastric valve t.
tight Nissen repair
tight-to-shaft (TTS)
tigroid
    t. appearance
    t. striation
tigrolysis
Tikhoff-Linberg
    T.-L. procedure
    T.-L. shoulder girdle resection
Tilden method

tile
    t. classification
    t. plate facet replacement
Tillaux
    extraocular muscles of T.
Tillaux-Chaput fracture
Tillaux-Kleiger fracture
Tillaux-Phocas syndrome
Tillett operation
tilt
    base-ring t.
    filter t.
    head-down t.
    head-up t.
    steep head-down t.
    t. stitch
    t. test
    Trendelenburg t.
tilt-table testing
time
    acceleration t.
    activated clotting t. (ACT)
    activated coagulation t.
    anesthesia t.
    anesthetic t.
    association t.
    average extubation t.
    bleeding t.
    blood-brain equilibration t.
    carotid ejection t.
    celite-activated clotting t. (CACT)
    cerebral circulation t.
    circulation t.
    cold ischemia t.
    concentration times t.
    correlation t.
    deceleration t. (DCT)
    decimal reduction t.
    2D transit t.
    Duke bleeding t.
    duration t.
    ejection t.
    electrode response t.
    evolution t.
    execution t.
    explosive doubling t.
    followup t.
    forced expiratory t.
    helium equilibration t.
    heparin neutralized thrombin t. (HnTT)
    hepatic ischemic t.
    high-dose thrombin t. (HiTT)
    inspiration t.
    inspiratory t. (Ti)
    interhemispheric propagation t.
    isovolumetric relaxation t.
    isovolumic relaxation t.
    Ivy method of bleeding t.

kaolin-activated clotting t. (KACT)
lag t.
Lee-White clotting t.
t. of maximum concentration
mean circulation t.
Mielke bleeding t.
nucleation t.
operating t.
operative t.
plasma clotting t.
t. position scan
preoperative evolution t.
preservation t.
t. pressure
procedure t.
prolonged prothrombin t.
prothrombin t.
recalcification t.
recovery t.
t. to recovery
recovery room t.
relaxation t.
saturation t.
sensation t.
systolic t. (ST)
total respiratory t.
total tourniquet t.
tourniquet t.
tumor doubling t.
ventilator t.
ventricular activation t.
voice termination t.
warm ischemic t.

time-concentration curve
time-cycled ventilation
timed
t. forced expiratory volume
t. intermittent rotation
timed-sequential therapy
time-of-flight
t.-o.-f. echoplanar imaging
t.-o.-f. mass spectometry
TIMI
Thrombolysis in Myocardial Infarction
TIMI classification
Tim knot
Tinel sign
tip
t. angle
intraabdominal t.
nasal t.
overprojecting nasal t.

papillary muscle t.
pyramidal t.
rectal t.
spleen t.
tip-of-the-tongue phenomenon
TIPS
transjugular intrahepatic portosystemic
shunt
TIPS procedure
TISS
therapeutic intervention scoring system
tissue
abdominal adipose t.
aberrant t.
t. ablation
acellular pannus t.
acinar t.
adipose connective t.
ampullary granulation t.
anechoic t.
aneurysm t.
aneurysmal t.
angiomatous neoplastic t.
anisotropic t.
aortic aneurysm t.
t. approximation
t. architecture
areolar connective t.
atrioventricular conduction t.
attenuating t.
t. bank
t. blocking
border t.
breast biopsy t.
bronchial-associated lymphoid t.
brown adipose t.
bursa-equivalent t.
bursal t.
cancellous t.
capsular support t.
cartilaginous t.
caseated t.
cementoid t.
cervical soft t.
chromaffin t.
cicatricial t.
t. coagulation
collagenous t.
t. compression
t. compression test
t. conductivity
t. confirmation

T

NOTES

tissue *(continued)*

conjunctiva-associated lymphoid t.
connective t.
corneal t.
coronal pulp t.
crushed t.
cryostat t.
cutaneous t.
denuded connective t.
t. detritus
devitalized t.
diffuse lymphatic t.
t. dissection
donor t.
t. Doppler imaging
dorsal t.
earlobe adipose t.
echogenic t.
ectopic endometrial t.
elastic t.
enveloping scar t.
episcleral t.
t. expansion
extraarticular t.
extracapsular t.
extraperitoneal t.
exuberant granulation t.
fatty prostatic t.
fetal lymphoid t.
fibroadipose t.
fibroblastic t.
fibroelastic t.
fibrofatty breast t.
fibrotic t.
fibrous connective t.
fibrous scar t.
t. fluke
functional renal t.
t. fusion
Gamgee t.
ganglial t.
gastrointestinal-associated
  lymphoid t. (GALT)
gingival t.
glandular t.
granulation t.
granulomatous t.
gut-associated lymphoid t. (GALT)
hard and soft t.
healthy t.
hemangiomatous t.
hematopoietic t.
hilar structure scar t.
His-Purkinje t.
histiocytic t.
t. homogeneity
hyperplastic t.
hypertrophic granulation t.
hypocellular fibrous t.

t. hypoxia
t. imprint
t. ingrowth surface
interdental t.
interfascicular fibrous t.
t. interposition
interstitial t.
intervening connective t.
intralobular connective t.
intratracheal ectopic thyroid t.
isotropic t.
keratinized t.
ligamentous support t.
t. ligand
lipomalike t.
lipomatous t.
liver t.
t. loss
t. lymph
lymphatic t.
lymphoid t.
mammary t.
maternal t.
mesenchymal t.
mesothelial t.
mineralized t.
t. molding
mucosa-associated lymphoid t.
  (MALT)
muscular t.
musculoskeletal t.
myeloid t.
myocardial t.
nasion soft t.
t. necrosis
necrotic/fibrotic t.
necrotic hyalinized t.
neoplastic t.
nephrogenic t.
neural t.
nodal t.
nonviable t.
nonvital t.
normal t.
nuclear t.
t. nutrition
oral t.
orbital adipose t.
orbitonasal t.
osseous t.
t. oxygenation
t. oxygen tension
pancreatic t.
paracancerous t.
paraoral t.
parathyroid t.
paravaginal soft t.
parenchymal t.
t. perfusion

periadvential t.
periapical t.
periarticular t.
pericanalicular connective t.
periesophageal t.
periimplant t.
perilobular connective t.
perinephric t.
perineural t.
perinodal t.
periosteal t.
peripancreatic t.
peripheral lymphoid t.
periprostatic t.
petrotympanic t.
pharyngeal t.
t. pH monitoring
placental t.
polypoid t.
preepiglottic soft t.
t. preservation
t. pressure
t. pressure measurement
pressure-sensitive t.
pressure-tolerant t.
prevertebral soft t.
pulmonary t.
redundant sac t.
t. regeneration
t. remodeling
t. renewal
t. repair
residual ductal t.
t. resistance
t. respiration
retroperitoneal soft t.
retropharyngeal soft t.
revascularized t.
rubber t.
t. sampling
scar t.
skeletal t.
t. slack
slow exchange soft t.
soft t.
sonolucent t.
t. space
specialized intralobular connective t.
splenic t.
t. study
subcutaneous t.
subjacent t.

supporting t.
sustentacular t.
syngeneic t.
synovial t.
testicular adrenal-like t.
t. texture abnormality
thoracic inlet soft t.
t. thromboplastin
thyroid t.
t. tolerance
t. tolerance dose
t. transfer
t. transplant
t. transplantation
t. trauma
t. trimming
trophoblastic t.
tuberculosis granulation t.
t. typing
vascular t.
viable t.
viscoelastic t.
vital t.
t. water content
t. welding
xenogeneic t.
tissue-base relationship
tissue-bearing area
tissue-borne
tissue-equivalent
tissue-sparing technique
tissue-supported base
tissue-tissue-supported base
titanium
    t. flexible humeral nail
    t. vocal fold medialization implant
titratable
titration
    coulometric t.
    Dean and Webb t.
    potentiometric t.
    Rinkel serial endpoint t.
    t. technique
titubation
    head t.
TIVA
    total intravenous anesthesia
TKA
    total knee arthroscopy
TLND
    therapeutic lymph node dissection

T

NOTES

T-lymphocyte
> cytolytic T-l. (CTL)
> cytotoxic T-l. (CTL)

TME
> total mesorectal excision

TMLR
> transmyocardial laser revascularization

TMR
> transmyocardial laser revascularization

TNF
> tumor necrosis factor

TNF-alpha
> tumor necrosis factor-alpha

TNF-bp
> tumor necrosis factor-binding protein

TNM
> tumor, node, metastasis
>> TNM carcinoma classification
>> TNM staging system
>> TNM system for tumor staging

TNS
> transient neurologic symptom

to-and-fro anesthesia

tocolysis

tocolytic therapy

Todd-Evans stepladder tracheal dilatation technique

toddler fracture

toe
> Butler procedure to correct overlapping t.'s
> catheter t.
> t. extensor
> t. extensor muscle
> t. extensor tendon
> great t.

toe-block anesthesia

toenail
> embedded t.
> ingrowing t.

toe-phalanx transplantation

TOF
> train-of-four

Tohen tendon technique

toilet
> cavity t.
> peritoneal t.
> pulmonary t.

tolazoline

Toldt
> T. fascia
> line of T.
> T. membrane

tolerance
> anesthetic t.
> histologic t.
> pressure t.
> tissue t.

Tolosa-Hunt syndrome

tomentum

Tom Jones suture technique

tomography
> automated computerized axial t.
> computed t. (CT)
> contrast-enhanced computed t.
> expiratory computed t.
> fluorodeoxyglucose-positron emission t.
> multidetector computed t. (MDCT)
> positron emission t. (PET)
> single-photon emission computed t.
> single-photon emission computer-aided t.
> ultrafast CT electron beam t.
> ultrafast spiral computed t.

Tompkins median bivalving technique

tongue
> t. base reduction
> t. bone
> t. fasciculation
> t. flap
> t. fracture
> mandibular t.
> t. plication
> t. pressure
> t. thrust classification
> t. thrust therapy

tongue-and-groove suture technique

tongue-in-groove operation

tongue-jaw-neck dissection

tongue-splitting transmandibular approach

tonic spasm

tonometer
> indentation t.

tonometry
> applanation t.
> gastric t.
> indentation t.
> intraluminal t.
> nasogastric t.
> Schiotz t.

tonsil
> Gerlach t.

tonsilla, pl. **tonsillae**

tonsillar
> t. branch
> t. crypt
> t. fold
> t. hernia
> t. herniation

tonsillectomy
> t. and adenoidectomy
> contact diode laser t.
> intracapsular partial t.
> Sluder guillotine t.

tonsilloadenoidectomy

tooth
>   anatomical t.
>   t. extraction
>   t. fracture
>   t. hemisection
>   t. immobilization
>   t. mass
>   t. migration
>   t. perforation
>   t. plane
>   t. position
>   t. sac
>   t. transplantation

tooth-and-nail syndrome
tooth-to-tooth position
topectomy
Topel knot
tophus, pl. **tophi**
topical
>   t. anesthetic
>   t. anesthetic technique
>   t. antibacterial agent
>   t. antibiotic
>   t. cooling
>   t. hemostatic agent
>   t. iodine application
>   t. oropharyngeal anesthesia

Topinard facial angle
topistic
topographic projection
top-up
>   epidural t.-u.

Torek
>   T. operation
>   T. orchiopexy
>   T. resection

Torg
>   T. classification
>   T. knee reconstruction
>   T. technique

Torgerson-Leach modified technique
tori (*pl. of* torus)
toric ablation
Torkildsen ventriculocisternostomy
Tornwaldt cyst
Torode-Zieg classification
Toronto pelvic fracture classification
Torpin cul-de-sac resection
torque
>   light wire t.
>   translation of t.

>   t. tube catheter
>   unwanted screw t.

torrential hemorrhage
torr pressure
torsade de pointes ventricular tachycardia (TdPVT)
torsion
>   angle of femoral t.
>   bilateral t.
>   biliary tract t.
>   extravaginal testicular t.
>   intravaginal t.
>   neonatal testicular t.
>   perinatal t.
>   postnatal t.
>   prenatal t.
>   testicular t.
>   t. testis
>   unilateral testicular t.

torsional fracture
torso
>   t. crease
>   t. injury

torsoclusion
tortipelvis
tortuous intercostal artery
toruloma
Torulopsis infection
torus, pl. **tori**
>   t. fracture

TOS
>   thoracic outlet syndrome

total
>   t. abdominal colectomy (TAC)
>   t. abdominal evisceration
>   t. abdominal hysterectomy (TAH)
>   t. abdominal hysterectomy and bilateral salpingo-oophorectomy (TAHBSO)
>   t. ankle arthroplasty
>   t. anomalous pulmonary venous return
>   t. articular replacement arthroplasty
>   t. articular resurfacing arthroplasty
>   t. axial node irradiation
>   t. bilateral vagotomy
>   t. bilirubin level
>   t. biopsy
>   t. body fat
>   t. body hypothermia
>   t. body irradiation
>   t. body scanning

NOTES

total *(continued)*
- t. body solute
- t. body surface area (TBSA)
- t. body water
- t. body weight (TBW)
- t. breech extraction
- t. colectomy (TC)
- t. colonic aganglionosis
- t. colonoscopy
- t. continence
- t. cystectomy
- t. dehiscence
- t. ear obliteration
- t. elbow arthroplasty
- t. endoscopic esophagectomy
- t. erythrocyte volume
- t. etch technique
- t. ethmoidectomy
- t. exchangeable potassium measurement
- t. excisional operation
- t. extraperitoneal repair
- t. fundoplication
- t. fundoplication method
- t. fundoplication procedure
- t. fundoplication technique
- t. gastrectomy (TG)
- t. gastric pull-up
- t. gastric wrap
- t. glossectomy
- t. graft area
- t. graft area rejection
- t. hip arthroplasty
- t. hip arthroplasty with internal eccentric shells (THARIES)
- t. hip replacement
- t. hip replacement surgery
- t. hypophysectomy
- t. internal reflection
- t. intravenous anesthesia (TIVA)
- t. intravenous anesthetic technique
- t. joint replacement
- t. keratoplasty
- t. knee arthroplasty
- t. knee arthroscopy (TKA)
- t. knee replacement
- t. knee replacement surgery
- t. laparoscopic esophagectomy
- t. laryngectomy
- t. laryngopharyngectomy
- t. L-chain concentration
- t. left hepatectomy
- t. lobectomy
- t. lymphoid irradiation
- t. mastectomy
- t. maxillectomy
- t. meniscectomy
- t. mesorectal excision (TME)
- t. nodal irradiation

- t. pancreatectomy
- t. parathyroidectomy
- t. parenteral alimentation
- t. parenteral nutrition (TPN)
- t. parotidectomy
- t. patellectomy
- t. patellofemoral joint arthroplasty
- t. pelvic exenteration
- t. pericystectomy
- t. perineal prostatectomy
- t. perineal rupture
- t. petrosectomy
- t. proctectomy
- t. proctocolectomy
- t. prostatoseminal vesiculectomy
- t. protein concentration
- t. pulpotomy
- t. push therapy
- t. respiratory time
- t. retrocolic end-to-side gastrojejunostomy
- t. scrotectomy
- t. shoulder arthroplasty
- t. space analysis
- t. spinal anesthesia
- t. surgical removal
- t. thoracic esophagectomy
- t. thyroidectomy
- t. time to intubation (TTI)
- t. tourniquet time
- t. transfusion
- t. vascular exclusion
- t. vascular isolation (TVI)
- t. wrist arthroplasty
- t. wrist fusion

totally
- t. extraperitoneal (TEP)
- t. extraperitoneal inguinal herniorrhaphy
- t. intrathoracic stomach
- t. stapled restorative proctocolectomy

Toti
- T. operation
- T. procedure

Toti-Mosher operation

touch
- 3-point t.

touch-up procedure

Toupe
- T. method
- T. procedure
- T. technique

Toupet
- T. fundoplasty
- T. hemifundoplication
- T. hemifundoplication fundoplication
- T. procedure

Tourette syndrome

tourniquet
  chemical t.
  t. control
  t. ischemia
  t. ischemic pain
  t. occlusion
  t. pain
  t. paralysis
  t. pressure
  t. test
  t. time
tourniquet-induced pain
tourniquet-related nerve damage
Tourtual
  T. canal
  T. membrane
Towako method
Towne projection
Townley-Paton operation
toxemia
toxic
  t. epidermal necrolysis
  t. granulation
  t. multinodular goiter
toxicity
  acute t.
  aminoglycoside t.
  endocrine t.
  extramedullary t.
  glutamate t.
  neostigmine t.
  oxygen t.
  radiation-induced pulmonary t.
  transient t.
toxic-traumatized patient
toxin
  botulinum A t.
  t. exposure
  extracellular t.
Toynbee muscle
TPC
  target plasma concentration
TPN
  total parenteral nutrition
TPR
  temperature, pulse, respiration
trabecula, pl. **trabeculae**
trabecular
  t. arachnoid component
  t. bone fracture
  t. membrane
  t. network

trabeculated
  t. bladder
  t. bone lesion
trabeculation
trabeculectomy
  Cairns t.
  t. operation
  Smith t.
trabeculopexy
  argon laser t.
trabeculoplasty
  argon laser t.
  laser t.
trabeculotomy
trace anesthetic
tracer dilution
trachea, pl. **tracheae**
  saber-sheath t.
tracheal
  t. adenoma
  t. agenesis
  t. aspiration
  t. bifurcation angle
  t. block
  t. blood flow (TBF)
  t. branch
  t. cartilage
  t. compression
  t. extubation anesthetic technique
  t. fenestration
  t. fracture
  t. gland
  t. intubation
  t. intubation anesthetic technique
  t. ligation
  t. node
  t. reconstruction
  t. repair
  t. resection
  t. ring
  t. safety stitch
  t. secretion
  t. stenosis
  t. suction anesthetic technique
  t. topical analgesia
  t. triangle
  t. tug
  t. tumor
  t. ulceration
  t. web
trachealis muscle
trachelectomy

T

NOTES

trachelematoma
trachelian
tracheloclavicularis
tracheloclavicular muscle
trachelomastoid
trachelomastoideus
trachelopexy
tracheloplasty
trachelorrhaphy
trachelos
tracheloschisis
trachelotomy
tracheoaerocele
tracheobiliary fistula
tracheobronchial
    t. anomaly
    t. foreign body
    t. node
tracheobronchoesophageal fistula
tracheobronchoscopy
tracheocele
tracheocutaneous fistula
tracheoesophageal (TE)
    t. fistula (TEF)
    t. puncture
tracheolaryngeal
tracheopharyngeal
tracheoplasty
tracheostomy
    definitive t.
    elective dilatational t.
    emergency t.
    flap t.
    Great Ormond Street t.
    Montgomery t.
    percutaneous dilational t.
    t. stoma
    tube-free t.
tracheotomy
trachoma gland
track
    pin t.
    radial suture t.
tracking
    electromagnetic t.
    optical t.
Tracrium
tract
    abnormal fetal urogenital t.
    aerodigestive t.
    alimentary t.
    Arnold t.
    association t.
    atriodextrofascicular t.
    atriofascicular t.
    atrionodal bypass t.
    auditory t.
    bile t.
    biliary t.

bronchial t.
Burdach t.
bypass t.
central tegmental t.
cerebellorubral t.
cerebellothalamic t.
cholinergic t.
Collier t.
concealed bypass t.
corticobulbar t.
corticopontine t.
corticospinal t.
crossed pyramidal t.
cuneocerebellar t.
dead t.
deep liver t.
deiterospinal t.
dental sinus t.
dentatothalamic t.
dermal sinus t.
digestive t.
t. dilation
direct pyramidal t.
dopaminergic t.
dorsolateral t.
extrapyramidal t.
fastigiobulbar t.
fetal urogenital t.
fistulous t.
Flechsig t.
frontopontine t.
frontotemporal t.
gastrointestinal t.
geniculocalcarine t.
geniculotemporal t.
genital t.
genitourinary t.
GI t.
Gowers t.
habenulointerpeduncular t.
hepatic outflow t.
high blind t.
Hoche t.
hypothalamohypophysial t.
ileal inflow t.
ileal outflow t.
iliopubic t.
iliotibial t.
infected t.
inflammatory sinus t.
inflow t.
intestinal t.
intramural fistulous t.
lateral corticospinal t.
left ventricular outflow t. (LVOT)
Lissauer t.
liver t.
Loewenthal t.
mamillothalamic t.

Marchi t.
mesolimbic-mesocortical t.
Monakow t.
t. of Münzer and Wiener
nasal t.
needle t.
nerve t.
nigrostriatal t.
nodoventricular t.
occipitocollicular t.
occipitopontine t.
occipitotectal t.
olfactory t.
olivocerebellar t.
olivospinal t.
optic t.
ororespiratory t.
outflow t.
pancreaticobiliary t.
parietopontine t.
perineal sinus t.
portal t.
posterior spinocerebellar t.
prepyramidal t.
pulmonary outflow t.
pyramidal t.
reproductive t.
respiratory t.
reticulospinal t.
retrochiasmal optic t.
right ventricular outflow t. (RVOT)
rubrobulbar t.
rubroreticular t.
rubrospinal t.
t. of Schütz
seminal t.
sensory t.
septomarginal t.
serotonergic t.
sinus t.
solitary t.
sphincteroid t.
spinal dermal sinus t.
spinocerebellar t.
spinoolivary t.
spinotectal t.
spiral foraminous t.
Spitzka marginal t.
sulcomarginal t.
supraopticohypophysial t.
t. tamponade
tamponade needle t.

tangential t.
tectobulbar t.
tectopontine t.
tectospinal t.
temporofrontal t.
temporopontine t.
tree-barking urinary t.
T-tube t.
tuberoinfundibular t.
Türck t.
UGI t.
upper aerodigestive t.
upper gastrointestinal t. (UGI)
upper respiratory t.
urinary t.
urogenital t.
uveal t.
ventral spinocerebellar t.
ventral spinothalamic t.
ventricular outflow t.
vestibulospinal t.
vocal t.
Waldeyer t.
Wolff-Parkinson-White bypass t.
wound t.

traction
t. alopecia
t. aneurysm
t. application
t. atrophy
t. detachment
t. diverticulum
t. epiphysis
t. fracture
gentle t.
t. headache
t. suture technique
t. test

tractotomy
anterolateral t.
bulbar cephalic pain t.
dorsal column t.
intramedullary t.
medullary spinothalamic t.
mesencephalic t.
pontine spinothalamic t.
pyramidal t.
Schwartz t.
Sjöqvist intramedullary t.
spinal t.
spinothalamic t.
stereotactic trigeminal t.

NOTES

tractotomy *(continued)*
    subcaudate t.
    trigeminal t.
    Walker t.
traditional method
trafficking
    membrane t.
tragicus muscle
tragus, pl. **tragi**
training
    joint protection t.
    stabilization t.
train-of-four (TOF)
    t.-o.-f. stimulation
    t.-o.-f. stimulus
    t.-o.-f. transmission
Trainor operation
trajector
trajectory
    bullet t.
    missile t.
TRALD
    transfusion-related acute lung injury
TRAM
    transverse rectus abdominis muscle
    TRAM flap
    TRAM flap procedure
tram line
trampoline fracture
trance coma
tranquilization
tranquilizer
transabdominal
    t. approach
    t. laparoscopic herniorrhaphy
    t. mucosectomy
    t. preperitoneal
    t. preperitoneal hernioplasty
    t. preperitoneal repair
    t. proctopexy
    t. properitoneal (TAPP)
transacromial approach
transactivation
transaminase
    alanine amino t. (ALT)
    glutamic oxaloacetic t.
    glutamic pyruvic t.
    serum alanine amino t.
transampullary septectomy
transanal
    t. approach
    t. endoscopic microsurgery (TEM)
    t. endoscopic microsurgical
      resection
    t. excision
    t. mucosectomy
    t. mucosectomy with handsewn
      anastomosis
    t. pouch advancement

    t. stapling technique
    t. ultrasonography
transanimation
transantral
    t. approach
    t. ethmoidal approach
    t. ethmoidectomy
transaortic valve gradient
transarterial
    t. anesthetic technique
    t. chemoembolization
transarticular wire fixation
transaxial scan plane
transaxillary
    t. apical bullectomy
    t. approach
transbrachioradialis approach
transbronchial
    t. lung biopsy
    t. needle aspiration
transcallosal transventricular approach
transcanine approach
transcaphoid fracture
transcapillary hydrostatic pressure
   gradient
transcapitate
    t. fracture
    t. fracture-dislocation
transcapitellar wire fixation
transcardiac membranotomy
transcarpal amputation
transcatheter
    t. ablation
    t. arterial embolization therapy
    t. closure
transcavernous transpetrous apex
   approach
transcerebellar hemispheric approach
transcervical
    t. approach
    t. balloon tuboplasty
    t. femoral fracture
    t. intrafallopian tube transfer
    t. resection
    t. thymectomy
    t. tubal access
transchondral fracture
transclavicular approach
transcoccygeal approach
transcochlear
    t. approach
    t. cochleovestibular neurectomy
    t. vestibular neurectomy
transcondylar fracture
transcortical transventricular approach
transcranial
    t. Doppler (TCD)
    t. electrical stimulation

t. electrical stimulation anesthetic technique
t. frontal-temporal-orbital approach
t. stimulation (TCS)
transcranial-supraorbital approach
transcriptional control
transcubital approach
transcutaneous
t. access
t. acupoint electrical stimulation (TAES)
t. biopsy
t. cranial electrical stimulation (TCES)
t. electrical nerve stimulation
t. electric stimulation (TES)
t. electrode nerve stimulation
t. oxygen monitoring
t. oxygen pressure measurement
t. partial pressure of oxygen
t. tetanic stimulus
transcylindrical cholecystectomy
transcystic
t. approach
t. choledochoscopy
t. drain
t. drainage
transdermal
t. administration
t. analgesic
t. anesthesia
t. anesthetic technique
t. sympathectomy
transdiaphragmatic approach
transducer
differential variable reluctance t.
transduction
complex signal t.
transduodenal
t. approach
t. endoscopic decompression
t. pancreatectomy
t. sphincteroplasty
t. sphincterotomy
transect
transected
t. ductule
t. vertical gastric bypass
transection
aortic t.
atlantooccipital t.
esophageal t.

hepatic parenchymal t.
t. incision
parenchymal t.
t. plane
step-cut t.
Sugiura esophageal variceal t.
traumatic aortic t.
transendoscopic
t. electrocoagulation
t. laser photocoagulation
t. procedure
t. sphincterotomy
transepiphysial fracture
transesophageal
t. atrial pacing (TEAP)
t. atrial stimulation
t. color Doppler echocardiography
t. echocardiograph-guided left ventricular oximetry
t. echocardiograph-guided right ventricular oximetry
t. echocardiography (TEE)
t. echocardiography scan
t. echocardiography with pacing
t. endoscopy
t. ligation of varix
t. varix ligation
t. ventricular pacing (TEVP)
transethmoidal
transfemoral
t. liver biopsy
t. venous catheterization
transfer
adenoviral t.
barber pole stripe t.
composite free tissue t.
dermal fat free tissue t.
free flap t.
free tissue t.
gamete intrafallopian tube t. (GIFT)
in vitro fertilization-embryo t.
island nail t.
maternal-placental-fetal drug t.
microvascular free flap t.
Ober-Barr procedure for brachioradialis t.
placental t.
pronuclear stage t. (PROST)
saturation t.
single-stage tissue t.
split anterior tibial tendon t.

T

NOTES

transfer *(continued)*
    tissue t.
    transcervical intrafallopian tube t.
    wraparound neurovascular composite
      free tissue t.
    zygote intrafallopian t. (ZIFT)
transferrin
    melanoma t.
transfibular approach
transfixation
transfixing suture technique
transfixion
transforaminal passage
transform
    driven equilibrium Fourier t.
      (DEFT)
transformary mass
transformation
    hemorrhagic t.
    malignant t.
    neoplastic t.
    t. zone
transforming growth factor (TGF)
transfrontal approach
transfuse
transfusion
    acute blood t.
    allogenic blood t.
    arterial t.
    blood product t.
    coagulation factor t.
    direct t.
    double-volume exchange t.
    drip t.
    exchange t.
    exsanguination t.
    homologous blood t.
    immediate t.
    indirect t.
    intraperitoneal blood t.
    intraperitoneal fetal t.
    intrauterine intraperitoneal fetal t.
    mediate t.
    perioperative t.
    peritoneal t.
    simple t.
    subcutaneous t.
    substitution t.
    t. therapy
    total t.
transfusion-related
    t.-r. acute lung injury (TRALD)
    t.-r. air embolism
    t.-r. lung injury (TRLI)
transgastric
    t. fine-needle aspiration biopsy
    t. ligation
    t. plication
transgastrostomic enteroscopy

transgenic therapy
transglomerular hydrostatic filtration
  pressure
transgluteal approach
transhamate
    t. fracture
    t. fracture-dislocation
transhepatic
    t. antegrade biliary drainage
      procedure
    t. approach
    t. catheterization
    t. stenting
transhiatal
    t. blunt esophagectomy
    t. esophagectomy (THE)
    t. esophagectomy approach
    t. esophagojejunostomy
    t. pyloroplasty
transhyoid pharyngotomy
transient
    t. auditory evoked response
      (TAER)
    t. azotemia
    t. bone marrow edema syndrome
    t. cavitation
    t. compartment syndrome
    t. edema
    t. hiatal hernia
    t. hyperemic response
    t. hypocalcemia
    t. ischemic attack (TIA)
    t. lesion
    t. neurologic deficit
    t. neurologic symptom (TNS)
    t. osteoporosis of hip
    t. profound neurologic deficit
    t. toxicity
    t. visual obscuration
transiliac
    t. amputation
    t. bar technique
    t. fracture
    t. rod fixation
transilluminated power phlebectomy
transillumination test
transischiac
transit
    2D t. time
transition
    cervicothoracic t.
transitional
    t. cell carcinoma
    t. epithelium
    t. respiration
    t. zone biopsy
transjugular
    t. hepatic biopsy
    t. insertion

t. intrahepatic portosystemic shunt (TIPS)
t. liver access
t. liver biopsy
translabyrinthine
t. and suboccipital approach
translaryngeal
t. guided intubation anesthetic technique
t. tracheal intubation
translation
anterior t.
anteroposterior t.
caudal t.
cephalad t.
coronal plane deformity sagittal t.
dorsal t.
force t. (FTR)
t. injury
t. mobility
t. motion
posterior t.
pure t.
t. of torque
ulnar t.
vertical t.
translational
t. fracture
t. position
translocation
bacterial t.
t. Down syndrome
transluminal
t. coronary angioplasty
t. extraction atherectomy
transmandibular-glossopharyngeal approach
transmandibular projection
transmastoid approach
transmeatal
t. approach
t. tympanoplasty incision
transmembrane hydraulic pressure
transmesenteric
t. hernia
t. plication
transmetatarsal amputation
transmigration
ovular t.
transmission
double-burst t.
t. electron microscopy

iatrogenic t.
t. image
neuromuscular t.
pressure t.
train-of-four t.
transmucosal
t. delivery
t. drug administration anesthetic technique
transmural
t. approach
t. closure
t. hydrostatic pressure gradient
t. inflammation
t. pressure
transmutation
transmyocardial
t. carbon dioxide laser revascularization
t. laser revascularization (TMLR, TMR)
t. perfusion pressure
transnasal
t. administration
t. bile duct catheterization
t. biopsy
t. endoscopy
transocular
transodontoid screw fixation
transolecranon approach
transoral
t. approach
t. endoscopy
t. odontoid excision
t. odontoid resection
t. radiofrequency treatment
t. technique
transorbital
t. leukotomy
t. lobotomy
t. projection
transosseous suture
transpalatal
t. approach
t. exposure
transpapillary
t. approach
t. biopsy
t. cannulation
t. catheterization
t. endoscopic cholecystotomy
transparietal

NOTES

transpedicular
  t. approach
  t. screw-rod fixation
transpelvic
  t. amputation
  t. gunshot wound
transperineal palladium 103
transperineurial passage
transperitoneal
  t. approach
  t. cesarean section
  t. exposure
  t. hand-assisted laparoscopic surgery
  t. laparoscopic adrenalectomy
  t. laparoscopic nephrectomy
  t. laparoscopic nephroureterectomy
transplacental hemorrhage
transplant
  acute rejection of liver t.
  adult-to-adult living related donor
    living t.
  autologous bone marrow t.
    (ABMT)
  auxiliary t.
  bilateral sequential lung t.
  cadaveric hand t.
  cadaveric whole organ t.
  corneal t.
  domino t.
  double-lung t.
  fetal tissue t.
  Gallie t.
  heart t.
  heart and lung t.
  hepatic t.
  lamellar corneal t.
  liver t.
  living-related small bowel t.
  lung t.
  t. lung syndrome
  t. nephrectomy
  orthotopic liver t. (OLT)
  pancreas t. (PTX)
  pancreas after kidney t. (PAK)
  penetrating corneal t.
  placental tissue t.
  primarily vascularized organ t.
  reduced liver t. (RLT)
  reduced-size t.
  t. rejection
  rejection cardiomyopathy t.
  single-lung t.
  SPK t.
  split-liver t.
  tissue t.
transplantation
  adrenal medulla t.
  allogenic t.
  allograft t.

anhepatic stage of liver t.
autogenous tooth t.
autologous blood stem cell t.
autologous bone marrow t.
  (ABMT)
autologous osteochondral allograft t.
autologous ovarian t.
auxiliary partial orthotopic liver t.
  (APOLT)
bone marrow t.
Bosworth femoroischial t.
brain t.
bridge organ t.
cardiac t.
clinical intestinal t.
composite tissue t.
corneal t.
Cowen-Loftus toe-phalanx t.
cryopreserved extrapelvic ovarian t.
femoroischial t.
fetal cell t.
fetal liver t.
fetal thymus t.
fresh extrapelvic ovarian t.
heart t.
heart-lung t.
hepatic t.
hepatocyte t.
heterotopic t.
homogenous tooth t.
homotopic t.
intestinal t.
kidney t.
liver t.
living donor renal t.
living-related donor t.
living-related liver t. (LRLT)
lung t.
muscle-tendon t.
neonatal pulmonary t.
organ t.
orthoptic t.
orthotopic heart t.
orthotopic liver t. (OLT)
osteoarticular allograft t.
pancreas t.
pancreas after kidney t. (PAK)
pancreas-kidney t.
pancreatic t.
pancreaticoduodenal t.
piggyback liver t.
pigment cell t.
pituitary gland t.
pulmonary t.
renal t.
simultaneous kidney-pancreas t.
simultaneous pancreas-kidney t.
SPK t.
split-liver t.

syngeneic t.
syngenesioplastic t.
T-cell depleted bone marrow t.
tendon t.
tissue t.
toe-phalanx t.
tooth t.
vein valve t.
whole organ pancreas t. (WOP)
xenograft t.
transplantectomy
transplanted stamp graft
transpleural
t. approach
transpleurodiaphragmatic
transport
air critical care t.
alveolar fluid t.
transportation
transposition
carotid t.
t. flap
omentum-to-brain t.
penoscrotal t.
Strombeck nipple t.
vein segment t.
Z-plasty t.
transpubic incision
transpupillary cyclophotocoagulation
transpyloric plane
transradial approach
transrectal
t. approach
t. surgical treatment
t. ultrasound-guided sextant biopsy
transrectus incision
transsacral
t. fracture
t. proctectomy
transscaphoid
t. dislocation fracture
t. perilunate dislocation
transscrotal
transseptal
t. approach
t. left heart catheterization
t. orchiopexy
t. puncture
transsexualism
transsexual surgery
transsinus approach

transsphenoidal
t. approach
t. evacuation
t. hypophysectomy
t. microsurgical resection
t. operation
t. pituitary resection
t. removal
t. surgery
transsphincteric
t. anal fistula
t. approach
t. surgery
**transstenotic pressure gradient
measurement**
transsternal approach
transsylvian approach
transtentorial
t. approach
t. herniation
transthermia
transthoracic
t. approach
t. discectomy
t. dissection
t. echocardiography
t. esophagectomy
t. mediastinoscopy
t. needle aspiration
t. needle aspiration biopsy
t. Nissen fundoplication
t. percutaneous fine-needle
aspiration biopsy
t. route
t. vertebral body resection
transthoracotomy
transtorcular approach
transtracheal
t. aspirate
t. aspiration
t. jet
t. jet ventilation (TTJV)
t. jet ventilation anesthetic
technique
transtriquetral
t. fracture
t. fracture-dislocation
transtrochanteric
t. approach
t. rotational osteotomy
transtubercular plane
transtympanic neurectomy

T

NOTES

transubstantiation
transudation
transudative
    t. ascites
    t. inflammation
transumbilical breast augmentation
  (TUBA)
transureteroureteral anastomosis
transureteroureterostomy (TUU)
transurethral
    t. ablative prostatectomy
    t. balloon dilatation
    t. balloon dilation
    t. collagen injection therapy
    t. electrical bladder stimulation
    t. laser incision
    t. marsupialization
    t. microwave thermotherapy
      (TUMT)
    t. needle ablation (TUNA)
    t. resection
    t. resection of bladder tumor
      (TURBT)
    t. resection of prostate (TURP)
    t. resection syndrome
    t. sphincterotomy
    t. ultrasound-guided laser-induced
      prostatectomy (TULIP)
    t. ureterorenoscopy
    t. vaporization of prostate (TUVP)
transvaginal
    t. approach
    t. Burch procedure
    t. fallopian tube catheterization
    t. oocyte retrieval (TVOR)
    t. tubal catheterization
    t. ultrasonically guided oocyte
      retrieval
    t. ultrasonographic examination
    t. urethrolysis
transvalvular gradient
transvector
transvenous
    t. approach
    t. liver biopsy
    t. therapy
transventricular
    t. approach
    t. mitral valve commissurotomy
transversalis fascia
transverse
    t. abdominal muscle
    t. anthelicine groove
    apical t. (AP-T)
    t. aponeurotic arch
    t. approach
    t. arytenoid muscle
    t. cervical artery
    4-chamber t. (4C-T)

5-chamber t. (5C-T)
    t. colectomy
    t. colon
    t. colostomy
    t. comminuted fracture
    t. costal facet
    t. duodenotomy
    t. facial
    t. facial artery
    t. facial fracture
    t. fascia
    t. fixation
    t. fixator application
    t. foramen
    t. fundal incision
    t. fundal incision of Strassman
    t. head
    t. ligament rupture
    lower uterine segment t. (LUST)
    t. magnetization phase
    t. mastectomy
    t. mastectomy incision
    t. maxillary fracture
    t. mesocolon
    mitral valve-t. (MV-T)
    t. oval pelvis
    t. palatine fold
    t. pancreatic artery
    t. pericardial sinus
    t. plane
    t. plane motion insufficiency
    t. process
    t. process fracture
    t. projection
    t. rectal fold
    t. rectus abdominis muscle
      (TRAM)
    t. rectus abdominis muscle flap
    t. rectus abdominis muscle flap
      procedure
    t. relaxation
    t. relaxation rate
    t. resection
    t. scan
    t. scanning
    t. scapular artery
    t. section
    t. section of heart
    t. section imaging
    t. skin incision
    t. suture of Krause
    t. tarsotomy
    t. tenotomy
    t. venous sinus
    t. vesical fold
transversectomy
transverse-loop rod colostomy
transversely oriented endplate
  compression fracture

transversocostal
transversospinal muscle
transversostomy
transversovertical index
transversus
    t. abdominis aponeurosis
    t. abdominis muscle
transxiphoid approach
Trantas operation
trapdoor
    t.-d. approach
    t.-d. fragment
    t.-d. thoracotomy
trapezia (*pl. of* trapezium)
trapezial
trapeziform
trapeziometacarpal
    t. fusion
    t. silicone arthroplasty
trapezium, pl. **trapezia**
    t. fracture
trapezius
    t. flap
    t. stimulation anesthetic technique
trapezoid
    t. body
    t. line
    t. method
    t. ridge
trapezoidal
    t. incision
    t. keratotomy
    t. osteotomy
trapezoideum
trap incision
trapped lung
trapping
    gas t.
Traube-Hering curve
Traube semilunar space
trauma, pl. **traumas, traumata**
    American Association for the
      Surgery of T. (AAST)
    avulsion t.
    blunt hepatic t.
    t. care
    t. center
    corneal t.
    external t.
    foreign body t.
    genital tract t.
    head t.

    hepatic t.
    inadvertent t.
    intraoral t.
    pancreatic t.
    t. patient
    penetrating t.
    perineal impact t.
    t. room
    T. Score and Injury Severity Score
      (TRISS)
    t. service
    spinal t.
    t. surgeon
    t. surgery
    surgical t.
    t. system
    t. team
    thoracoabdominal t.
    tissue t.
    truncal t.
    t. victim
trauma-related death
traumasthenia
traumata (*pl. of* trauma)
traumatic
    t. amputation
    t. anesthesia
    t. aortic rupture
    t. aortic transection
    t. atlantooccipital dislocation
    t. brain injury (TBI)
    t. cardiac arrest
    t. cervical disc herniation
    t. choroidal rupture
    T. Coma Data Bank
    t. corneal abrasion
    t. diaphragmatic hernia
    t. false aneurysm
    t. fistula
    t. fracture
    t. gangrene
    t. inflammation
    t. internal carotid artery dissection
    t. intracranial hematoma
    t. lesion
    t. optic neuropathy
    t. perforation
    t. progressive encephalopathy
    t. pseudomeningocele
    t. renal mass
    t. tetanus
traumatism

T

NOTES

traumatize
traumatologist
    orthopaedic t.
traumatology
traumatonesis
traumatopathy
traumatopnea
traumatosepsis
traumatotherapy
Trautmann triangular space
Traverso-Longmire technique
Treacher Collins syndrome
treadmill
    t. exercise
    t. exercise capacity
treatment
    acidification t.
    acorn t.
    allocation of t.
    alternative t.
    anoplasty t.
    antifungal t.
    bioelectric t.
    Boyd-Ingram-Bourkhard t.
    brain arteriovenous malformation t.
      (BAVM)
    Carrel t.
    chemotherapeutic t.
    cholecystectomy t.
    chronic anoplasty t.
    cognitive behavior t. (CBT)
    complementary t.
    compression rod t.
    computer-assisted t.
    conservative surgical t.
    continuous medical t.
    Dakin-Carrel t.
    definitive t.
    diabetic retinal t.
    dialysis t.
    distraction/compression scoliosis t.
    dual compression scoliosis t.
    early active t.
    endoscopic t.
    endovascular graft t.
    esophageal dilation t.
    extracorporeal shock wave t.
      (ESWT)
    ex utero intrapartum t. (EXIT)
    ex vivo marrow t.
    ferromagnetic microembolization t.
    Gelfoam particles transarterial
      embolization t.
    graft t.
    hemodialysis t.
    hepatic intraarterial yttrium-90
      microspheres t.
    insulin coma t.
    intracavernosal injection t.

    intravesical chemotherapeutic t.
    iodine t.
    laparoscopic t.
    lipiodol transarterial embolization t.
    local t.
    locoregional t.
    medical t.
    mitomycin transarterial
      embolization t.
    t. modality
    multidisciplinary pain t. (MPT)
    nonsurgical t.
    open surgical t.
    operative t.
    t. option
    percutaneous endovascular t.
    photocoagulation t.
    prophylactic antifungal t.
    radiation t.
    radioiodine t.
    rectovaginal surgical t.
    t. regimen
    retinal t.
    root canal t.
    t. strategy
    surgical t.
    transoral radiofrequency t.
    transrectal surgical t.
    ureteral surgical t.
tree
    biliary t.
    bronchial t.
    cannulation of biliary t.
    endobronchial t.
    extrahepatic biliary t.
    iliac arterial t.
    intrahepatic biliary t.
tree-barking urinary tract
trefoil
    t. deformity
    t. tendon
Treitz
    T. arch
    T. fascia
    T. fossa
    T. hernia
    T. ligament
    T. muscle
trellis formation
trema
trematode infection
tremor
    essential t.
    parkinsonian t.
    pill-rolling t.
Trendelenburg
    T. operation
    T. position
    T. tilt

trepanation
    corneal t.
    dental t.
trephination
    dental t.
    open-sky t.
trephine needle biopsy
Treponema
    microhemagglutination *T. pallidum*
      (MHA-TP)
    T. pallidum immobilization
Trethowan metatarsal osteotomy
Trethowan-Stamm-Simmonds-Menelaus-
  Haddad technique
Treves
    T. fold
    T. operation
triad
    acute compression t.
    Beck t.
    Charcot t.
    hepatic t.
    t. knee repair
    portal t.
    Virchow t.
    wall-echo shadow t.
triadic therapy
triage
triaging
trial
    t. cementation
    t. of conservative therapy
    European Carotid Surgery T.
      (ECST)
    neuraxial medication t.
    neurostimulation t.
    North American Symptomatic
      Carotid Endarterectomy T.
      (NASCET)
    t. point
    t. reduction
triangle
    anal t.
    Assézat t.
    auricular t.
    axillary t.
    Béclard t.
    Burow t.
    Calot t.
    carotid t.
    cephalic t.
    cervical t.

Charcot t.
digastric t.
Elaut t.
facial t.
Farabeuf t.
femoral t.
frontal t.
Grynfeltt t.
Henke t.
Hesselbach t.
inferior carotid t.
inferior occipital t.
infraclavicular t.
inguinal t.
interscalene t.
Labbé t.
Langenbeck t.
Lesser t.
Lesshaft t.
Lieutaud t.
lumbar t.
lumbocostoabdominal t.
Macewen t.
Malgaigne t.
Marcille t.
muscular t.
occipital t.
omoclavicular t.
omotracheal t.
Petit lumbar t.
Pirogoff t.
pubourethral t.
retromolar t.
sacral t.
Scarpa t.
sternocostal t.
subclavian t.
subinguinal t.
submandibular t.
submaxillary t.
submental t.
suboccipital t.
superior carotid t.
supraclavicular t.
suprahyoid t.
suprameatal t.
tracheal t.
umbilicomammillary t.
urogenital t.
vesical t.
Weber t.

T

NOTES

triangular
    t. advancement flap
    t. aponeurosis
    t. bone
    t. capsulotomy
    t. cartilage
    t. fascia
    t. fibrocartilage complex (TFCC)
    t. fold
    t. fossa
    t. ligament
    t. ligament of liver
    t. muscle
    t. space
triangular-shaped skin
triangulation
    indirect t.
    t. stapling method
    t. technique
triarticular complex
triaxial total elbow arthroplasty
tributary
    venous t.
triceps
    t. bursa
    t. flap
    t. tendon
trichangion
trichiasis repair
trichilemmoma
    desmoplastic t.
trichion
trichodiscoma
tricholemmoma
trichoma
Trichomonas **infection**
trichoscopy
tricipital
trick
    cough t.
triclofos
tricorn
tricornute
tricorrectional bunionectomy
tricuspid
    t. position
    t. valve anuloplasty
    t. valve anulus
    t. valve area
    t. valve disease
    t. valve flow
    t. valve repair
    t. valvuloplasty
tridermoma
Trieger test
triethiodide
    gallamine t.
trifacial nerve
trifid stomach

trifurcation
    t. injury
    t. involvement
    popliteal artery t.
trigastric
trigeminal
    t. cave
    t. cavity
    t. decompression
    t. dermatome
    t. ganglion
    t. impression
    t. nerve
    t. nerve root
    t. neuralgia
    t. rhizotomy
    t. tractotomy
trigeminus
trigger
    t. point
    t. point deactivation
    t. point injection
triggered ventilation
trigger-point inactivation
trigona (*pl. of* trigonum)
trigonal ring
trigone
    habenular t.
    inguinal t.
    Lieutaud t.
    right fibrous t.
    vertebrocostal t.
trigonectomy
trigonitis
trigonocephaly
trigonum, pl. trigona
Trillat procedure
trilobate
trimalleolar ankle fracture
trimming
    tissue t.
trimodality therapy
triophthalmos
triotus
triphalangeal thumb deformity
triphenyltetrazolium staining method
triphosphate
    adenosine t. (ATP)
Tripier
    T. operation
    T. operation throw square knot
triplane
    t. osteotomy
    t. tibial fracture
triple
    t. anastomosis
    t. arthrodesis
    t. hemisection
    t. innominate osteotomy

t. intrathecal therapy
t. ligamentous repair
t. lobe hepatectomy
t. loop pouch
t. point
triple-balloon valvuloplasty
triple-lumen infusion
triple-throw square knot stitch
triple-wire
t.-w. procedure
t.-w. technique
triplication
tripod
t. fracture
Haller t.
tripodia
tri-point
triquetral
t. bone
t. fracture
triquetrolunate dislocation
triquetropisiform articulation
triquetrous cartilage
triquetrum
triradial
triradiate
t. acetabular extensile approach
t. line
t. transtrochanteric approach
triradius
triscaphe fusion
trisection
pulse t.
trisectorectomy
trisegmentectomy
trisomy
t. 8 syndrome
t. C, D syndrome
trisplanchnic
TRISS
Trauma Score and Injury Severity Score
TRISS probability of survival
tristichia
triticeal cartilage
triticeum
trituration
trivalve
TRLI
transfusion-related lung injury
trocar
t. cystostomy
t. drainage method

t. gas leak
t. injury
2-t. laparoscopic cholecystectomy
t. site hernia
t. technique
3-t. technique cholecystectomy
t. wound
t. wound bleed
t. wound site complication
trocar-cannula technique
trocar-related injury
trochanter
greater t.
lesser t.
t. major
t. minor
small t.
third t.
trochanterian
trochanteric
t. bursa
t. crest
t. migration
t. osteotomy
trochanterica
trochanterplasty
trochantin
trochantinian
trochlea, pl. **trochleae**
trochlear
t. fossa
t. fovea
t. nerve
t. process
t. synovial bursa
trochleariform
trochleariformis
trochlearis
trochleiform
trochoid
t. articulation
t. joint
Trolard vein
Tronzo intertrochanteric fracture classification
trophectoderm biopsy
trophic
t. fracture
t. lesion
trophoblastic tissue
tropic hormone

NOTES

tropism
>facet t.

Trotter syndrome
trough line
Trousseau point
Troutman operation
Truc
>T. flap
>T. operation

Tru-Cut needle biopsy (TCNB)
true
>t. aneurysm
>t. diverticulum
>t. exfoliation
>t. hernia
>t. knot
>t. muscle
>t. mutation
>t. negative
>t. pelvis
>t. positive
>t. rib
>t. size
>t. vertebra
>t. vocal cord

true-negative result
true-positive result
Trumble talectomy
trumpet
>nasal t.

truncal
>t. lesion
>t. melanoma
>t. trauma
>t. vagotomy
>t. vagotomy and gastroenterostomy
>t. vagotomy and pyloroplasty

truncated
>t. exponential voltage
>t. tarsometatarsal wedge arthrodesis

truncated-wedge arthrodesis
truncation
>t. phenomenon
>protein t.
>uterine positioning via ligament
> investment fixation and t.
> (UPLIFT)

truncus, pl. **trunci**
trunk
>accessory nerve t.
>anterior vaginal t.
>brachiocephalic t.
>bronchomediastinal t.
>celiac t.
>costocervical t.
>t. duplication
>hepatic venous t.
>t. incurvation test
>intestinal t.

>jugular lymphatic t.
>linguofacial t.
>lumbar t.
>lumbosacral t.
>nerve t.
>posterior vaginal t.
>pulmonary t.
>subclavian lymphatic t.
>sympathetic t.
>thoracoacromial t.
>thyrocervical t.
>upper t.
>vagal t.
>venous t.

Trusler
>T. aortic valve technique
>T. technique of aortic valvuloplasty

trypsin
>crystallized t.

trypsinization
Tsai-Stillwell procedure
Tscherne classification
Tscherne-Gotzen tibial fracture
> **classification**

T-shaped
>T-s. capsulotomy
>T-s. constriction ring
>T-s. incision

TSRH
>Texas Scottish Rite Hospital
>TSRH crosslink stabilization
>TSRH double-rod construct
>TSRH rod fixation

Tsui Test
Tsuji laminaplasty
T-tack gastropexy
TTI
>total time to intubation

TTJV
>transtracheal jet ventilation

TTS
>tight-to-shaft
>TTS balloon dilation

TTTS
>twin-twin transfusion syndrome

T-tube
>T-t. drainage
>T-t. placement
>T-t. study
>T-t. tract
>T-t. tract choledochofiberoscopy
>T-t. tract choledochoscopy

TUBA
>transumbilical breast augmentation

tuba, pl. **tubae**
tubage
tubal
>t. branch
>t. cannulation

t. insufflation
t. ligation
t. ligation band technique
t. reconstruction surgery
t. rupture
t. sterilization
tubaria
tubariae
tubatorsion
tube
auditory t.
t. cecostomy
cholecystostomy t.
t. decompression
diagnostic t.
digestive t.
t. dilution test
double-lumen endotracheal t.
embryonic neural t.
end t.
endothelial t.
eustachian t.
t. exchange technique
t. extrusion
fallopian t.
t. feeding
t. flap graft
t. gastrostomy
germ t.
knuckle of t.
t. leakage
medullary t.
t. migration
molar t.
nasotracheal tube fixation using
  infant feeding t.
neural t.
t. placement
t. precipitin test
t. removal
t. replacement
t. thoracostomy
tube-carina distance
tubectomy
tubed
t. free skin graft
t. groin flap
t. pedicle flap
t. urethroplasty
tube-fed patient
tube-free tracheostomy

tube-patient distance
tuber, pl. **tubera**
calcaneal t.
cortical t.
frontal t.
omental t.
parietal t.
tubercle
accessory t.
anatomical t.
anterior t.
auricular t.
calcaneal t.
carotid t.
Chassaignac t.
conoid t.
corniculate t.
cuneiform t.
dental t.
dissection t.
dorsal radius t.
genial t.
genital t.
Gerdy t.
hard t.
iliac t.
inferior thyroid t.
infraglenoid t.
jugular t.
labial t.
Lisfranc t.
Lister t.
mamillary t.
marginal t.
maxillary t.
mental t.
Morgagni t.
obturator t.
t. osteotomy
pharyngeal t.
Princeteau t.
prosector t.
pterygoid t.
pubic t.
quadrate femoral t.
scalene t.
soft t.
superior thyroid t.
supraglenoid t.
supratragic t.
wedge-shaped t.
Whitnall orbital t.

NOTES

T

tubercle *(continued)*
    Wrisberg t.
    Zuckerkandl t.
tubercula *(pl. of* tuberculum)
tuberculation
tuberculization
tuberculocele
tuberculoma
tuberculosis
    central nervous system t.
    endobronchial t.
    endometrial t.
    extraarticular t.
    extrapulmonary t.
    extrathoracic t.
    exudative t.
    t. granulation tissue
    inhalation t.
    peritoneal t.
    reactivation t.
    reinfection t.
    surgical t.
tuberculous
    t. abscess
    t. arthritis
    t. caseation
    t. empyema
    t. infiltration
    t. lesion
tuberculum, pl. **tubercula**
    first-degree t.
    Zuckerkandl t.
tuberoinfundibular tract
tuberositas
tuberosity
    costal t.
    t. fragment
    masseteric t.
    pterygoid t.
    reduction t.
    t. reduction
tuberous
    t. sclerosis
    t. sclerosis-associated renal cell
      carcinoma
    t. sclerosis-associated tumor
    t. sclerosis complex
tube-shift technique
tube-to-film distance
tube-within-tube technique
tubi *(pl. of* tubus)
tuboabdominal
tuboligamentous
tuboovarian abscess
tuboperitoneal
tuboplasty
    balloon t.
    transcervical balloon t.
    ultrasound transcervical t.

tubotorsion
tubouterine implantation
tubovaginal
tubular
    t. aneurysm
    t. basement membrane
    t. carcinoma
    t. colonic duplication
    t. excretory mass
    t. reconstruction
    t. regeneration
    t. respiration
    t. vertical gastroplasty
tubularized
    t. bladder neck reconstruction
    t. cecal flap
tubulation
tubule
    Albarran y Dominguez t.
    convoluted seminiferous t.
    Henle t.
    mesonephric t.
    paragenital t.
    straight seminiferous t.
    uriniferous t.
tubuli *(pl. of* tubulus)
tubulization
tubulovillar lesion
tubulovillous adenoma
tubulus, pl. **tubuli**
tubus, pl. **tubi**
tuck
    t. position
    t. procedure
Tudor-Thomas
    T.-T. graft
    T.-T. operation
Tuffier morcellement technique
tuft fracture
tug
    tracheal t.
Tukey post-hoc correction
TULIP
    transurethral ultrasound-guided laser-
      induced prostatectomy
Tullos technique
tumbler
    t. flap
    t. graft
tumbling
    t. procedure
    t. technique
    t. technique operation
tumescent
    t. liposuction technique
    t. technique breast reduction
tummy tuck flap
tumor
    abdominal t.

t. ablation
Abrikosov t.
adenoid t.
alveolar t.
ampullary t.
t. angiogenesis
t. antigen
antral t.
aortic body t.
t. ascites
t. bed
benign bone t.
benign germ cell t.
biliary tract t.
bleeding t.
blood t.
t. blood supply
blood vessel t.
t. blush
body t.
bone t.
brain t.
brown fat t.
t. bulk
t. burden
Buschke-Löwenstein t.
t. capsule
carcinoid t.
cardiac t.
carotid body t.
celiac t.
t. cell
t. cell-host bone relationship
t. cell purging
cervical t.
colon t.
colorectal primary t.
debulking of t.
deep t.
t. defect
diffuse t.
discrete t.
distal t.
t. dormancy mode
t. doubling time
dumbbell t.
duodenal t.
t. embolism
embryonal t.
t. encapsulation
endocrine t.
t. erosion

esophageal t.
extrahepatic t.
eye t.
eyelid t.
t. feature
focal t.
focus of t.
fungating t.
gastric stromal t.
gastrointestinal stromal t. (GIST)
genital tract t.
glial t.
t. grade
t. grading
gritty t.
t. growth
gynecologic t.
hepatic t.
hyperplastic t.
t. hypoxia
t. imaging
t. infiltration
infratentorial t.
t. initiation
intracranial t.
intraductal papillary mucinous t.
  (IPMT)
intraluminal t.
intramedullary t.
intramyocardial t.
t. invasion
invasive t.
islet cell t.
isolated metastatic t.
t. kinetic model
lacrimal gland t.
liver t.
t. location
lumbar t.
lung t.
t. lysis syndrome
malignant t.
t. marker
t. mass
mediastinal t.
metastatic t.
midbody t.
mixed t.
mucoepidermoid t.
multifocal t.
musculoskeletal t.
t. necrosis

NOTES

T

tumor (*continued*)
t. necrosis factor (TNF)
t. necrosis factor-alpha (TNF-alpha)
t. necrosis factor-binding protein
(TNF-bp)
t. neovasculature
neuroendocrine t.
t., node, metastasis (TNM)
t., node, metastasis carcinoma
classification
nonfamilial malignant endocrine t.
nonfunctional malignant t.
nonfunctioning islet cell t.
nonseminomatous testicular t.
ocular t.
optic nerve t.
oral cavity t.
orbital t.
t. origin
ovarian t.
t. oxygenation
Pancoast t.
pancreatic endocrine t.
parathyroid t.
phyllodes t.
pituitary t.
t. ploidy
t. plop
t. polysaccharide substance
potato t.
primary parathyroid hyperplastic t.
t. progression
t. promoter
proximal t.
pulmonary t.
t. receptor protein negative
t. recurrence
recurrent t.
t. registry
t. regression
t. removal
renal t.
t. resectability
resectable t.
t. resection
sacral bone t.
sacrococcygeal t.
salivary gland t.
t. seeding
sellar t.
t. shrinkage
sinonasal t.
t. site
t. in situ
t. size
t. skin test
skull base t.
solid t.
t. specific

t. spillage
spinal cord t.
sporadic islet cell t.
t. stage
t. stage grouping
stage II$_E$ t.
t. staging
t. stenting
t. subtype
t. suppressor
t. suppressor gene
t. suppressor oncogene
supratentorial t.
t. surgery
synchronous t.
tail t.
t. targeting
temporal bone t.
testicular t.
t. therapy
t. thrombus
thyroid t.
tracheal t.
transurethral resection of bladder t.
(TURBT)
tuberous sclerosis-associated t.
t. ulceration
unresectable t.
t. vascularity
vasoactive intestinal polypeptide t.
t. vessel
t. volume
von Hippel-Lindau t.
Wilms renal t.
tumor-bearing kidney
tumor-cell product
tumor:cerebellum ratio
tumorectomy
tumor-free margin
tumorigenesis
foreign body t.
tumorlike bone condition
tumor-related death
tumor-targeting ability
TUMT
transurethral microwave thermotherapy
TUNA
transurethral needle ablation
tunable dye laser lithotripsy
tunic
mucosal t.
muscular t.
tunica, pl. **tunicae**
tunicary hernia
tunnel
catheter t.
t. creation
t. graft
t. infection

t. and sling fixation
t. of Wertheim
tunneled ventriculostomy
tunneling
Tupper arthroplasty
turbid peritoneal fluid
turbinal
turbinate
turbinated bone
turbinectomy
turbinoplasty
turbo spin-echo sequence
TURBT
transurethral resection of bladder tumor
Türck
T. bundle
T. tract
Turco
T. clubfoot release technique
T. procedure
Turco-Spinella tendo calcaneus repair
Turcot syndrome
Turkish saddle
Turk line
turn-and-suction biopsy technique
Turnbull
T. colostomy
T. end-loop ileostomy
T. multiple ostomy operation
T. technique
turned-down tendon flap
turned-up pulp deformity
Turner
T. operation
T. syndrome
turnover flap
TURP
transurethral resection of prostate
turunda
tutamen, pl. **tutamina**
TUU
transureteroureterostomy
TUVP
transurethral vaporization of prostate
TVI
total vascular isolation
TVOR
transvaginal oocyte retrieval
Tweed method
twelfth cranial nerve
twilight sleep

twin
t. bracket tooth rotation
t. formation
t. method
t. operating theater
thoracopagus t.
Twining line
twin-twin transfusion syndrome (TTTS)
twirling method
twisted
t. fundoplication
t. suture technique
twist-off technique
twitch
t. depression
evoked t.
t. height
t. height test
t. response
t. suppression
t. tension
Tycos pressure infusion line
tylectomy
tylion
tyloma
tympani
chorda t.
t. sinus
tympanic
t. bone
t. canal
t. canaliculus
t. cavity
t. membrane
t. membrane measurement
t. neurectomy
t. notch
t. plexus
t. ring
t. thermometry
tympanitic abdomen
tympanohyal bone
tympanomastoid
t. fissure
t. suture
tympanomastoidectomy
tympanomeatal flap
tympanoplasty
t. mastoidectomy
t. ossiculoplasty
staged t.
type I–V t.

T

NOTES

tympanosquamosal suture
tympanosquamous fissure
tympanotemporal
tyndallization
type
    t. B-1, -2 lesion
    t. C pelvic ring fracture
    depressed t.
    histologic t.
    t. I, II, III, IIIA, IIIB, IIIC open
      fracture
    t. I–IV canal
    t. I–V tympanoplasty
    macroscopic t.
    superficial t.
    ulcerated t.
typhlectasis

typhlectomy
typhlodicliditis
typhloempyema
typhlolithiasis
typhlon
typhlopexy
typhlorrhaphy
typhlostomy
typhlotomy
typhloureterostomy
typhoidal cholecystitis
typical skin lesion
typing
      tissue t.
tyroma
Tyrrell fascia
Tyson gland

UA
umbilical arterial
UA blood
UAL
ultrasonic-assisted liposuction
UC
ulcerative colitis
Uchida technique
UGCR
ultrasound-guided compression repair
UGI
upper gastrointestinal tract
UGI endoscopy
UGI tract
Uhl
U. anomaly
U. malformation
UICC
Union Internationale Contre le Cancer
UICC tumor classification
UID
unilateral interfacetal dislocation
ulcer
aphthous u.
bleeding duodenal u.
cervical u.
collar-button-like u.
Cruveilhier u.
duodenal u.
gastric u.
genital u.
ischemic u.
neuropathic u.
oral aphthous u.
penetrating u.
peptic u.
perforated peptic u.
postsclerotherapy u.
ring u.
scrotal skin u.
skin u.
solitary rectal u.
ulcerated
u. mucosa
u. type
ulceration
acute hemorrhagic u.
anal u.
anastomotic u.
aphthous u.
ASA-induced gastric u.
catarrhal marginal u.
CMV-associated u.
CMV-induced esophageal u.
collar-button u.

corneal u.
diffuse u.
duodenal u.
esophageal u.
gastric u.
gastrointestinal u.
genital u.
herpes epithelial tropic u.
intertrigo with u.
intestinal u.
ischemic infected u.
labial u.
linear u.
marginal u.
mucosal u.
mucous membrane u.
nasal mucosal u.
necrotic u.
oral u.
patchy colonic u.
postbulbar u.
radiation-induced u.
rectal u.
rheumatoid-related u.
serpiginous u.
stasis u.
stercoral u.
stomal u.
stress u.
stress-induced gastric u.
sublesional u.
tracheal u.
tumor u.
ulcerative
u. colitis (UC)
u. inflammation
ulcerogenic fistula
ulcerogranuloma
ulectomy
ulegyria
uletomy
Ullmann line
Ulloa operation
ulna, pl. **ulnae**
ulnar
u. artery
u. branch
u. bursa
u. collateral ligament rupture
u. deviation deformity
u. drift deformity
u. fracture
u. head
u. head excision

ulnar *(continued)*
    u. hemiresection interposition
      arthroplasty
    u. motor neurectomy
    u. translation
ulnari
ulnaris
    extensor carpi u. (ECU)
ulnocarpal abutment syndrome
ulocarcinoma
uloid
ulotomy
Ultane
ultrabrachycephalic
ultrafast
    u. CT electron beam tomography
    u. magnetic resonance imaging
      (UMRI)
    u. spiral computed tomography
ultrafiltration
    continuous arteriovenous u.
    dialytic u.
    extracorporeal u.
    glomerular u.
    modified u.
    spontaneous dialytic u.
ultra-high-frequency ventilation
ultra-high-magnification endoscopy
ultraligation
ultralow
    u. anterior resection
    u. anterior resection parastomal
      infection
ultramicroscopy
ultrarapid subthreshold stimulation
ultrasonic
    u. aspiration
    u. attenuation
    u. cutting
    u. dissection
    u. endovaginal finding
    u. fragmentation
    u. lithotresis
    u. lithotripsy
    u. nebulizer
    u. therapy
ultrasonic-assisted liposuction (UAL)
ultrasonication
ultrasonographic
    u. data
    u. examination
    u. technique
ultrasonographically-guided injection
ultrasonographic examination
ultrasonography
    carotid duplex u.
    color duplex u.
    contrast-enhanced u.
    Doppler duplex u.

    duplex u.
    endoanal u.
    endoscopic u. (EUS)
    high-resolution u.
    intraoperative u. (IOUS)
    laparoscopic u. (LUS)
    laparoscopic intracorporeal u.
      (LICU)
    laparoscopic intraoperative u.
      (LIOUS)
    open intraoperative u.
    transanal u.
ultrasonography-guided fine-needle
  aspiration biopsy
ultrasonosurgery
ultrasound
    u. anesthetic technique
    cervical u.
    Doppler u.
    endoscopic esophageal u. (EUS)
    u. examination
    u. guidance
    u. image
    in vivo duplex u.
    intraoperative u. (IOUS)
    laparoscopic u.
    preoperative u.
    u. therapy
    u. transcervical tuboplasty
ultrasound-assisted percutaneous
  endoscopic gastrostomy
ultrasound-guided
    u.-g. anterior subcostal liver biopsy
    u.-g. automated large-core breast
      biopsy
    u.-g. bronchoscopy
    u.-g. caudal epidural needle
      placement
    u.-g. compression
    u.-g. compression repair (UGCR)
    u.-g. core breast biopsy
    u.-g. core needle biopsy (US-CNB)
    u.-g. echo biopsy
    u.-g. fine-needle aspiration
    u.-g. fine-needle aspiration biopsy
      (US-FNAB)
    u.-g. lumbar facet nerve block
    u.-g. needle biopsy
    u.-g. nephrostomy puncture
    u.-g. shockwave therapy
    u.-g. stereotactic biopsy
ultraterminal excementosis
ultraviolet (UV)
    u. blood irradiation
    psoralens, u. A (PUVA)
ultropaque method
umbilectomy
umbilical
    u. arterial (UA)

u. artery
u. artery blood
u. artery catheterization
u. circulation
u. cord
u. cord anomaly
u. cord hematoma
u. fissure
u. fistula
u. flap
u. fossa
u. hernia
u. hernia rupture
u. herniorrhaphy
u. mass
u. notch
u. plane
u. plate
u. port
u. prevesical fascia
u. region
u. ring
u. skin-knife incision
u. vein (UV)
u. vein blood
u. vein catheterization
u. vein to maternal vein (UV/MV)
u. vein recanalization
u. venous
umbilicate
umbilication
umbilici (*pl. of* umbilicus)
umbilicomammillary triangle
umbilicovesical fascia
umbilicus, pl. **umbilici**
umbo
umbrascopy
umbrella closure
UMRI
ultrafast magnetic resonance imaging
unanticipated hepatic disease
unattended laboratory operation
unavoidable hemorrhage
unbanded gastroplasty
uncal herniation
unci (*pl. of* uncus)
unciform bone
uncinate
u. bundle of Russell
u. groove
u. pancreas
u. procedure

u. process fracture
u. process mass
uncinectomy
uncipressure
uncomminuted fracture
uncommitted metaphysial lesion
uncomplicated
u. acute cholecystitis
u. angiomyolipoma
unconstrained shoulder arthroplasty
uncontrollable glaucoma
uncovertebral joint
uncus, pl. **unci**
uncut
u. Collis-Nissen fundoplication
u. Collis-Nissen fundoplication
method
u. Collis-Nissen fundoplication
procedure
u. Collis-Nissen fundoplication
technique
underangulation
undercorrection
undercut
soft tissue u.
underlay fascia technique
underlying
u. cardiomyopathy
u. cause
u. structure
underresuscitated
underresuscitation
undersensing
pacemaker u.
underventilation
undescended testis
undifferentiated
u. adenocarcinoma
u. connective tissue disease
u. embryonal sarcoma
u. lesion
u. squamous cell carcinoma
undifferentiation
undisplaced fracture
undiversion
Undritz anomaly
undulating membrane
unfiltered
u. preparation
u. radioisotope
unfractionated
u. heparin antibody

U

NOTES

unfractionated *(continued)*
  u. heparin-induced thrombocytopenia
  u. heparin reversal
  u. heparin therapy
ungual
  u. fibroma
  u. labia
unguis, pl. **ungues**
uniaxial joint
unicaliceal kidney
unicanalicular sphincter
unicompartmental knee arthroplasty
unicondylar fracture
unification
unifocal optic nerve lesion
unilateral
  u. amputee
  u. anesthesia
  u. cyst
  u. diaphragmatic elevation
  u. hemidysplasia cornification
    disorder
  u. hemilaminectomy
  u. hernia
  u. hypophysectomy
  u. inguinal hernia repair
  u. inguinal hernia repair method
  u. inguinal hernia repair procedure
  u. inguinal hernia repair technique
  u. interfacetal dislocation (UID)
  u. laryngeal paralysis
  u. lavage
  u. lobectomy
  u. neck exploration
  u. nephrectomy
  u. pallidotomy
  u. parathyroidectomy
  u. pedicle cannulation
  u. pneumoretroperitoneum
  u. resection
  u. sacroiliac approach
  u. salpingo-oophorectomy
  u. subcostal incision
  u. supraglottic edema
  u. testicular torsion
unilobar disease
unilocular
  u. cyst
  u. cystic lesion
  u. joint
unimalleolar fracture
uninhibited neurogenic bladder
uninterrupted suture technique
union
  delayed fracture u.
  fibrous u.
  U. Internationale Contre le Cancer
    (UICC)
  osteonal bone u.

  primary u.
  secondary u.
  vicious u.
unipedicled flap
unipennate muscle
unipolar cauterization
uniportal arthroscopic microdiscectomy
unique
  u. NCRLM
  u. noncolorectal liver metastasis
unit
  autologous blood u.
  autologous RBC u.
  day care surgical u. (DCSU)
  electrosurgery u. (ESU)
  Hounsfield u. (HU)
  inpatient dialysis u.
  intensive care u. (ICU)
  low-grade suction u.
  u. of mass
  u. membrane
  neurosurgical intensive care u.
    (NICU)
  postanesthesia care u. (PACU)
  surgical admitting u.
united
  U. Kingdom Heart Valve Registry
  U. Network for Organ Sharing
    (UNOS)
  U. States Renal Data System
uniting
  u. canal
  u. cartilage
  u. duct
unitunnel technique
Universal Spine System (USS)
**University of Pennsylvania Smell
  Identification Test**
unlocking spiral technique
unmonitored local anesthesia
UNOS
  United Network for Organ Sharing
unplanned valgus osteotomy
unreamed nailing
unreduced dislocation
unremitting symptom
unrepositioned flap
unresectability
unresectable
  u. extrahepatic disease
  u. hepatoblastoma
  u. lesion
  u. metastasis
  u. periampullary cancer
  u. tumor
unresuscitated
unroofing
unsaturated chemical vapor sterilization
unsex

unshuntable portal hypertension
unstable
    u. angina
    u. bladder
    u. fracture
    u. fracture-dislocation
unstrained jaw relation
unstriated muscle
untethering procedure
untreated
    u. HPT
    u. hyperparathyroidism
ununited fracture
unusual opportunistic infection
Unverricht-Lundborg syndrome
unwanted screw torque
up-and-down staircases procedure
upgated technique
UPJ
    ureteropelvic junction
UPLIFT
    uterine positioning via ligament
    investment fixation and truncation
    UPLIFT procedure
U pouch
U-pouch construction
upper
    u. abdominal evisceration
    u. adenoma
    u. aerodigestive tract
    u. airway obstruction
    u. alimentary endoscopy
    u. arm straight graft
    u. cervical spine anterior exposure
    u. cervical spine fusion
    u. cervical spine procedure
    u. dorsal sympathectomy
    u. end
    u. endoscopy and colonoscopy
    u. esophageal sphincter relaxation
    u. extremity
    u. extremity nerve block
    u. eyelid
    u. gastrointestinal bleeding
    u. gastrointestinal endoscopy
    u. gastrointestinal hemorrhage
    u. gastrointestinal panendoscopy
    u. gastrointestinal series
    u. gastrointestinal tract (UGI)
    u. gastrointestinal tract foreign
      body
    u. gastrointestinal tract surgery

    u. genital tract infection
    u. incisor angulation
    u. intestinal endoscopy
    u. jaw
    u. jaw bone
    u. jejunal motility
    u. jejunal motor pattern
    u. jejunum
    u. lateral quadrant
    u. lid
    u. lip
    u. lip bite test
    u. medial quadrant
    u. mediastinum
    u. midline incision
    u. respiratory tract
    u. respiratory tract infection
    u. respiratory tract mucosa
    u. small bowel motor disturbance
    u. sternal split
    u. subscapular nerve
    u. thoracic wall
    u. thorax aperture
    u. tract disease
    u. trapezius flap
    u. trunk
up-regulation of receptor
upright
    u. position
    u. reflux
upright-Y incision
upside-down stomach
upsiloid
uptake
    local lymphatic u.
    lymphatic u.
    placental u.
    radioactive iodine u.
    radioisotope u.
urachal
    u. carcinoma
    u. fistula
    u. fold
    u. ligament
uraniscoplasty
uraniscorrhaphy
uranoplasty
    Wardill-Kilner 4-flap u.
uranorrhaphy
uranostaphyloplasty
uranostaphylorrhaphy
uraroma

NOTES

urate
urate-associated inflammation
uratoma
urban
    U. operation
    u. trauma center
Urbaniak
    U. neurovascular free flap
    U. scapular flap
urea hydrolysis
urea-impermeable membrane
urecchysis
uredema
urelcosis
uremia
uremia-related coagulopathy
uremic
    u. coma
    u. gastrointestinal lesion
    u. inflammation
ureter
    curlicue u.
    ectopic u.
    extravesical infrasphincteric
      ectopic u.
    u. implantation
    postcaval u.
    retrocaval u.
    retroiliac u.
ureteral
    u. bladder augmentation
    u. branch
    u. carcinoma
    u. catheterization
    u. colic
    u. duplication
    u. ectopia
    u. fistula
    u. injury
    u. meatotomy
    u. meatus
    u. patch procedure
    u. perforation
    u. pressure
    u. reimplantation
    u. spatulation
    u. stent placement
    u. stoma
    u. stoma removal
    u. surgical treatment
ureteralgia
ureterectasia
ureterectomy
    distal u.
ureteric
    u. branch
    u. fold
    u. pelvis

    u. plexus
    u. stoma
ureteris
ureteritis
ureterocalicostomy
ureterocele
    ectopic u.
    orthotopic u.
    pyoureter ectopic u.
ureterocelorraphy
ureterocolic fistula
ureterocolonic anastomosis
ureterocolostomy
ureterocutaneous fistula
ureterocystoplasty
ureterocystostomy
ureteroendoscopy
ureteroenteric
ureteroenterostomy
ureterohydronephrosis
ureteroileal anastomosis
ureteroileocecoproctostomy
ureteroileoneocystostomy
ureteroileostomy
    Bricker u.
ureterolithiasis
ureterolithotomy
    laparoscopic u.
ureterolysis
    combined u.
    extravesical u.
    intravesical u.
    Lich-Gregoir u.
    Pacquin u.
    Politano-Leadbetter u.
ureteroneocystostomy
    Glen Anderson u.
    u. herniation
    Politano-Leadbetter u.
    reoperative u.
ureteroneopyelostomy
ureteronephrectomy
ureteropelvic
    u. junction (UPJ)
    u. obstruction
ureteroperitoneal fistula
ureteroplasty
    ileal patch u.
ureteroproctostomy
ureteropyelitis
ureteropyeloneostomy
ureteropyelonephrostomy
ureteropyeloplasty
ureteropyeloscopy
    flexible u.
ureteropyelostomy
ureteropyosis
ureterorectostomy

ureterorenoscopy
    transurethral u.
ureterorrhagia
ureterorrhaphy
ureteroscopy
    rigid u.
ureterosigmoid anastomosis
ureterosigmoidostomy
    ileocecal u.
    Maydl u.
ureterostenoma
ureterostenosis
ureterostoma
ureterostomy
    cutaneous loop u.
    Davis intubated u.
    high-loop cutaneous u.
    low-loop cutaneous u.
    retroperitoneal cutaneous u.
ureterotomy
    Davis intubated u.
    intubated u.
ureterotrigonoenterostomy
ureterotubal anastomosis
ureteroureteral anastomosis
ureteroureterostomy
ureterouterine fistula
ureterovaginal fistula
ureterovesical obstruction
ureterovesicoplasty
    Leadbetter-Politano u.
ureterovesicostomy
urethra
    anterior u.
    female u.
    fixed drain pipe u.
    male u.
    membranous u.
    penile u.
    posterior u.
    prostatic u.
    spongy u.
urethral
    u. artery
    u. atresia
    u. calculus
    u. carcinoma
    u. caruncle
    u. closure mechanism
    u. closure pressure profile
    u. coaptation
    u. crest

    u. dilation
    u. diverticulectomy
    u. gland
    u. groove
    u. lacuna
    u. opening
    u. papilla
    u. pressure
    u. pressure measurement
    u. sphincter
    u. sphincterotomy
    u. suspension
    u. syndrome
    u. vesicle suspension procedure
urethralgia
urethralis
urethrectomy
urethremorrhagia
urethrism
urethritis
urethrobalanoplasty
urethrobulbar
urethrocavernous fistula
urethrocele
urethrocystometry
urethrocystopexy
urethrocystoscopy
urethrodynia
urethrohymenal fusion
urethrolysis
    retropubic u.
    transvaginal u.
urethropenile
urethroperineal fistula
urethroperineoscrotal
urethropexy
    Gittes u.
    Lapides-Ball u.
    Marshall-Marchetti-Krantz u.
    retropubic u.
    Stamey u.
urethroplasty
    Badenoch u.
    Cantwell-Ransley u.
    Cecil u.
    modified Young u.
    onlay island flap u.
    pedicle flap u.
    prostatic u.
    retrograde transurethral prostatic u.
    Tanagho bladder flap u.

U

NOTES

urethroplasty *(continued)*
    Thiersch-Duplay u.
    tubed u.
urethroprostatic
urethrorectal fistula
urethrorrhagia
urethrorrhaphy
urethrorrhea
urethroscopic
urethroscopy
    retropubic u.
urethrospasm
urethrostaxis
urethrostenosis
urethrostomy
    perineal u.
    Poncet perineal u.
urethrotomy
    direct-vision internal u.
    endoscopic optical u.
    external u.
    internal u.
    perineal u.
    Syme external u.
urethrovaginal fistula
urethrovesical
urethrovesicopexy
urge incontinence
uricosuria
urinariae
urinarius
urinary
    u. apparatus
    u. bladder
    u. bladder rupture
    u. calcium excretion
    u. calculus
    u. catheterization
    u. conduit
    u. EGF
    u. exertional incontinence
    u. extraversion
    u. fistula
    u. organ
    u. retention
    u. sand
    u. stuttering
    u. tract
    u. tract abnormality
    u. tract anomaly
    u. tract disease
    u. tract disorder
    u. tract infection
    u. tract injury
    u. tract obstruction
    u. tract reconstruction
urinary-umbilical fistula
urinary-vaginal fistula

urination
    delayed u.
urine specimen collection
uriniferous tubule
urinogenital
urinogenous
urinoma
urinoscopy
urinosexual
urocele
urocheras
urochesia
urocyst
urocystic
urocystis
urodynamics
urodynia
urogenital
    u. anomaly
    u. apparatus
    u. canal
    u. cleft
    u. diaphragm
    u. fistula
    u. membrane
    u. region
    u. ridge
    u. septum
    u. sinus
    u. tract
    u. triangle
urogenous
urokinase thrombolysis
urolith
urolithiasis
urolithic
urolithology
urologic
    u. anesthesia
    u. complication
    u. laparoscopic surgical procedure
    u. oncology
    u. operation
    u. surgery
    u. system cancer
urological evaluation
urologist
    pediatric u.
urology
    pediatric u.
Uromat dilation
uroncus
uronephrosis
uronoscopy
uropathy
    obstructive u.
uropoiesis
uropoietic
uropsammus

urorectal
    u. membrane
    u. septum
uroscheocele
uroschesis
uroscopy
urosepsin
urosepsis
urostomy
urothelial
    u. basement membrane
    u. carcinoma
urothelium
urothorax
urticaria
urtication
US-CNB
    ultrasound-guided core needle biopsy
use
    off-label u.
use-dependent sodium channel blocker
US-FNAB
    ultrasound-guided fine-needle aspiration
    biopsy
U-shaped
    U-s. incision
    U-s. jejunal pouch
    U-s. scalp flap
Usher syndrome
USS
    Universal Spine System
Ussing chamber technique
uterectomy
uteri (*pl. of* uterus)
uterine
    u. adenocarcinoma
    u. anomaly
    u. artery
    u. aspiration
    u. cavity
    u. compression
    u. evaluation
    u. fibromyoma
    u. gland
    u. hernia
    u. hernia syndrome
    u. incision
    u. infection
    u. lysosome level
    u. mass
    u. papillary serous carcinoma
    u. perforation

    u. positioning via ligament
    investment fixation and truncation
    (UPLIFT)
    u. relaxation
    u. rupture
    u. sarcoma metastasis
    u. suspension
    u. vein
    u. venous plexus
    u. window
uteroabdominal
uterocervical
uterocystostomy
uterofixation
uterolysis
    laparoscopic u.
uteroovarian
uteroparietal
uteropelvic
uteroperitoneal fistula
uteropexy
uteroplacental circulation
uteroplasty
uterosacral
    u. block
    u. fold
    u. ligament
uteroscopy
uterotomy
uterotubal
uterovaginal
    u. canal
    u. plexus
uteroventral
uterovesical
    u. fold
    u. ligament
    u. pouch
uterus, pl. **uteri**
    masculine u.
utilization
    impaired oxygen u.
    oxygen u.
utricle
    prostatic u.
utricular spot
utriculitis
utriculosaccular duct
U-turn maneuver
UV
    ultraviolet
    umbilical vein

U

NOTES

UV *(continued)*
    UV blood
    UV irradiation
uveal
    u. metastasis
    u. tract
uveitis
    anterior u.
    endogenous u.
    posterior u.
uveoencephalitic syndrome
uveoplasty
uviofast
uvioresistant
uviosensitive

UV/MV
    umbilical vein to maternal vein
    UV/MV ratio
uvula, pl. **uvuli**
    Lieutaud u.
uvular muscle
uvulectomy
uvuli (*pl. of* uvula)
uvulopalatal flap
uvulopalatopharyngoplasty
uvulopalatoplasty
    laser u.
    laser-assisted u. (LAUP)
uvulotomy
Uyemura operation

V_A
V_A
VAC
    vacuum-assisted closure
vaccinia
    v. infection
    v. melanoma oncolysate (VMO)
vaccinization
VACTERL
    vertebral, anal, cardiac, tracheal,
    esophageal, renal, limb
        VACTERL anomaly
vacuolation
vacuole
vacuolization
    basket-weave v.
    isometric tubular v.
vacuum
    v. aspiration
    constant v.
    v. extraction
    v. extractor delivery
vacuum-assisted closure (VAC)
VAE
    venous air embolism
vagal
    afferent v.
    v. arrest
    v. body
    v. nerve stimulation
    v. trunk
vagectomy
vagi (*pl. of* vagus)
vagina, pl. **vaginae**
    azygos artery of v.
    v. fibrosa tendinis
    v. masculina
    posterior fornix of v.
    v. processus styloidei
vaginal
    v. adenocarcinoma
    v. anomaly
    v. artery
    v. birth after cesarean delivery
    v. birth after cesarean section
    (VBAC)
    v. carcinoma
    v. celiotomy
    v. column
    v. condyloma
    v. cone biopsy
    v. construction
    v. cornification test
    v. cuff
    v. cystourethropexy

    v. ectopic anus
    v. electrical stimulation
    v. examination
    v. fistula
    v. fixation
    v. foreign body
    v. fornix
    v. gland
    v. hernia
    v. hysterectomy
    v. hysterotomy
    v. infection
    v. inflammation
    v. laceration
    v. lithotomy
    v. mass
    v. mucification test
    v. myomectomy
    v. needle suspension procedure
    v. nerve
    v. opening
    v. orifice
    v. perineorrhaphy
    v. process
    v. rhabdomyosarcoma
    v. surgery
    v. venous plexus
    v. vesicostomy
    v. wall approach
    v. wall repair
    v. wall sling procedure
vaginal-psoas suspension repair
vaginapexy
vaginate
vaginectomy
vaginitis
vaginoabdominal
vaginocele
vaginofixation
    Dührssen v.
vaginogram
vaginohysterectomy
vaginolabial hernia
vaginoperineal
vaginoperineoplasty
vaginoperineorrhaphy
vaginoperineotomy
vaginoperitoneal
vaginopexy
    Norman Miller v.
vaginoplasty
    cutback-type v.
    Fenton v.
    posterior flap v.

V

vaginoscopy
  pediatric v.
vaginotomy
vaginourethroplasty
vaginovesical
vaginovulvar
vagoaccessorius
vagoglossopharyngeal
vagolysis
vagotomy
  v. and antrectomy with
    gastroduodenostomy
  bilateral v.
  gastric v.
  highly selective v. (HSV)
  laparoscopic v.
  laser laparoscopic v.
  medical v.
  parietal cell v.
  posterior truncal v.
  proximal gastric v.
  v. and pyloroplasty
  Roux-en-Y procedure with v.
  selective proximal v.
  superselective v.
  surgical v.
  total bilateral v.
  truncal v.
vagovagal reflex
vagus, pl. **vagi**
  v. nerve
  v. nerve root
Vaino MP arthroplasty
Valentine position
valgus
  v. angulation
  v. deformity
  v. extension overload syndrome
  v. wedge-prop osteotomy
  v. Y-shaped prop osteotomy
valgus-external rotation injury
validation
  histopathologic v.
vallate papilla
vallecula, pl. **valleculae**
Valleix point
**Valls-Ottolenghim-Schajowicz needle
  biopsy**
**Valpar whole body range of motion
  test**
Valsalva
  V. maneuver
  V. muscle
value
  acid-base v.
  diagnostic v.
  high predictive v.
  intracranial pressure v.
  negative predictive v. (NPV)

postprandial v.
predictive v.
pressure v.
prognostic v.
standardized uptake v. (SUV)
supranormal v.
valva, pl. **valvae**
valve
  v. ablation
  v. of Bauhin
  v. bladder
  Cabot trumpet v.
  Carpentier-Edwards stented bovine
    pericardial v.
  Carpentier-Edwards stented porcine
    xenograft v.
  v. cinefluoroscopy
  v. cusp
  v. debris
  expiratory v.
  v. of Guérin
  v. of Hasner
  v. of Heister
  v. of Houston
  ileocecal v.
  v. leaflet
  left coronary v.
  mitral v.
  v. orifice area
  v. patency
  positive predictive v. (PPV)
  pressure relief v.
  v. replacement
  right coronary v.
  right septal v.
  v. of Rosenmüller
  v. rupture
  slit v.
  v. of Sylvius
  v. of Vieussens
  v. wrapping
valvectomy
valved conduit anastomosis
valve-sparing aortic root replacement
valvoplasty
valvotomy
  aortic v.
  balloon aortic v.
  balloon mitral v.
  balloon pulmonary v.
  balloon tricuspid v.
  double-balloon v.
  Inoue balloon mitral v.
  Longmire v.
  mitral balloon v.
  mitral valve v.
  percutaneous mitral balloon v.
  rectal v.
  repeat balloon mitral v.

single-balloon v.
thimble v.
valvula, pl. **valvulae**
Amussat v.
Gerlach v.
valvular
v. aortic disease
v. competency
v. heart disease
v. heart surgery
v. septum
valvule
lymphatic v.
valvulectomy
valvuloplasty
aortic v.
bailout v.
balloon aortic v.
balloon dilation v.
balloon mitral v.
balloon pulmonary v.
Carpentier tricuspid v.
catheter balloon v.
double-balloon v.
intracoronary thrombolysis
  balloon v.
mitral v.
multiple-balloon v.
percutaneous balloon aortic v.
percutaneous balloon mitral v.
percutaneous balloon pulmonic v.
percutaneous transluminal balloon v.
pulmonary v.
single-balloon v.
tricuspid v.
triple-balloon v.
Trusler technique of aortic v.
valvulotomy
balloon v.
v. procedure
VAMP
venous/arterial management protection
Baxter VAMP
van
v. Buren disease
v. Buren operation
v. de Kramer fecal fat procedure
v. Herick modification
v. Hoorne canal
v. Hoorn maneuver
v. Lint anesthesia
v. Lint flap

v. Lint injection
v. Lint lid block
V. Lint lid block
v. Lint modified technique
v. Ness procedure
v. Ness rotationplasty
Vancouver fracture
vanished testis syndrome
vanishing lung syndrome
Vannas capsulotomy
vapor
anesthetic v.
v. density
partial pressure of water v.
v. pressure
vaporization
contact laser v.
laser v.
vaporize
vaporizer
draw-over v.
flow-over v.
temperature-compensated v.
VAPS
visual analog pain score
variability
heart rate v. (HRV)
index of v.
interpretation v.
variable
v. positive airway pressure
v. screw placement
variable-dose patient-controlled
  anesthesia (VDPCA)
variable-release compression
variation
anatomic v.
anatomical v.
biliary anatomic v.
varication
variceal
v. band ligation
v. bleeding
v. column
v. decompression
v. hemorrhage
v. pressure
v. sclerotherapy
v. wall
varicella infection
varicella-zoster virus infection
varicelliform lesion

V

NOTES

varices (*pl. of* varix)
varicocele
varicocelectomy
    laparoscopic v.
    microsurgical inguinal v.
    subinguinal microsurgical v.
varicose
    v. aneurysm
    v. vein stripping and ligation
varicotomy
variety
    diffuse v.
    multifocal v.
variocele
variolation
variolization
varix, pl. **varices**
    actively bleeding varix
    aneurysmal v.
    coil-shaped v.
    ectopic v.
    esophageal v.
    v. ligation
    Okuda transhepatic obliteration
      of v.
    percutaneous transhepatic
      obliteration of esophageal v.
    peristomal v.
    transesophageal ligation of v.
Varolius sphincter
varus
    v. hindfoot deformity
    v. rotation shortening osteotomy
varus-valgus plane
VAS
    visual analog scale
vas, pl. **vasa**
vascular
    v. abdominal surgery
    v. abnormality
    v. access
    v. access patient
    v. access thrombosis
    v. accident
    v. anastomosis
    v. anatomy
    v. anomaly
    v. bed
    v. bundle
    v. cannulation
    v. circle
    v. complication
    v. compression
    v. control
    v. decompensation
    v. disease
    v. disease death
    v. ectasia

    v. endothelial growth factor
      (VEGF)
    v. endothelium
    v. exclusion
    v. fold
    v. injury
    v. invasion
    v. isolation technique
    v. laceration
    v. laceration repair
    v. loop
    v. malformation
    v. manifestation
    v. medicine
    v. metastasis
    v. neoplasm
    v. nerve
    v. net
    v. occlusion
    v. pedicle
    v. perforation
    v. plexus
    v. pressure
    v. procedure
    v. radiologist
    v. reconstruction
    v. rejection
    v. renal mass
    v. ring
    v. ring division
    v. ring syndrome
    v. sheath
    v. space
    v. structure
    v. surgeon
    v. system
    v. tissue
    v. watershed
    v. zone
vascularity
    tumor v.
vascularization
vascularize
vascularized
    v. bone graft
    v. free flap
    v. pericranial flap
vasculature
    extracranial cerebral v.
vasculitic lesion
vasculitis
    diffuse v.
    leukocytoclastic v.
    widespread v.
vasculo-Behçet disease
vasculobiliary pedicle
vasculocardiac
vasculogenesis
vasculomyelinopathy

vasculopathy
 graft v.
vas deferens
vasectomy
 no-scalpel v.
 v. reversal
vasoactive
 v. intestinal polypeptide tumor
 v. medication
 v. substance
vasoconstriction
 hypoxic pulmonary v. (HPV)
 isoflurane-induced v.
 thermoregulatory v.
vasocutaneous fistula
vasodilation, vasodilatation
 afferent v.
 efferent v.
vasodilator
 v. administration
 v. agent
 arterial-selective intravenous v.
 v. infusion
 mesenteric v.
vasodilator-stimulated rCBF single photon emission computed tomographic measurement
vasodilatory property
vasoepididymostomy
vasoganglion
vasoligation
vasomotor nerve
vasoneuropathy
vasoneurosis
vasopressin
 intravenous v.
vasopressor
vasoproliferation
vasopuncture
vasoreflex
vasorelaxation
vasorum
vasosection
vasostimulant
vasostomy
vasotomy
vasovagal
vasovasostomy
vasovesiculectomy
Vastamäki technique
vastus medialis tendon

VATER
 vertebral, anus, tracheoesophageal, radial, and renal
  VATER association
  VATER association syndrome
Vater
 V. ampulla
 V. fold
 V. papilla
VATS
 video-assisted thoracoscopic surgery
 video-assisted thorascopic surgery
  VATS procedure
  VATS wedge resection
Vaughan Williams antiarrhythmic drug classification
vault
 cranial v.
VBAC
 vaginal birth after cesarean section
V-banded gastroplasty
VBG
 vertical banded gastroplasty
  VBG pouch
VCP
 vocal cord paralysis
VDPCA
 variable-dose patient-controlled anesthesia
Veau classification
Vecchietti
 V. method
 V. operation
VECO$_2$
 carbon dioxide elimination
vection
vector
 v. phase
 v. product
 v. profile
 v. quantity
vecuronium neuromuscular blocking
vegetative lesion
VEGF
 vascular endothelial growth factor
veil
 aqueduct v.
vein
 aberrant obturator v.
 accessory cephalic v.
 adrenal v.
 anastomotic v.

V

NOTES

vein *(continued)*

angular v.
appendicular v.
aqueous v.
arcuate v.
arterial v.
ascending lumbar v.
auricular v.
autogenous v.
autologous internal jugular v.
axillary v.
azygos v.
basal v.
basilic v.
basivertebral v.
brachiocephalic v.
bronchial v.
Browning v.
buccal v.
Burow v.
canaliculus v.
capillary v.
cardiac v.
central v.
cephalic v.
cerebellar v.
cerebral v.
cervical v.
choroid v.
ciliary v.
circumflex v.
colic v.
collateral v.
comitans v.
common basal v.
common facial v.
condylar emissary v.
v. confluence
coronary v.
costoaxillary v.
cremasteric v.
v. cuff
v. decompression
deep cervical v.
descending genicular v.
digital v.
diploic v.
dorsispinal v.
emissary v.
epigastric v.
esophageal v.
ethmoidal v.
facial v.
femoral v.
fetal intrahepatic v.
frontal v.
v. of Galen malformation
gastric v.
gastroepiploic v.

gonadal v.
v. graft
great saphenous v.
hemiazygos v.
hemorrhoidal v.
hepatic portal v.
human umbilical v. (HUV)
hypogastric v.
hypophyseoportal v.
ileal v.
ileocolic v.
iliac v.
inferior alveolar v.
inferior interosseous v.
inferior lateral genicular v.
inferior medial genicular v.
infraorbital v.
innominate cardiac v.
intercapitular v.
intercostal v.
internal auditory v.
internal jugular v.
internal maxillary v.
internal pudendal v.
internal thoracic v.
intervertebral v.
intestinal v.
intraportal v.
jugular v.
juxtahepatic v.
Labbé v.
labial v.
labyrinthine v.
lacrimal v.
laryngeal v.
left brachiocephalic v.
left subclavian v. (LSV)
lingual v.
long thoracic v.
lumbar v.
Marshall oblique v.
mediastinal v.
meningeal v.
mesenteric v.
musculophrenic v.
nasofrontal v.
native portal v.
v. obstruction
occipital cerebral v.
occipital emissary v.
v. occlusion
ophthalmic v.
orbital v.
v. orifice
ovarian v.
palatal v.
pancreatic v.
pancreaticoduodenal v.
paratonsillar v.

paraumbilical v.
parietal emissary v.
parotid v.
v. patch
v. patch angioplasty
patent portal v.
pericardiacophrenic v.
pericardial v.
peripheral v.
peritoneal v.
peroneal v.
petrosal v.
pharyngeal v.
phrenic v.
popliteal v.
portal v.
portal-systemic collateral v.
posterior anterior jugular v.
posterior auricular v.
posterior facial v.
posterior intercostal v.
posterior interosseous v.
posterior labial v.
posterior parotid v.
posterior scrotal v.
prepyloric v.
proximal v.
pudendal v.
pulmonary v.
pyloric v.
rectosigmoid v.
renal v.
reticular v.
retrohepatic v.
retromandibular v.
rolandic v.
Rolando v.
Rosenthal v.
Santorini v.
saphenous v.
scrotal v.
v. segment transposition
short gastric v.
short hepatic v.
short saphenous v.
spermatic v.
sphenoid emissary v.
spigelian v.
spinal v.
splenic v.
sternocleidomastoid v.
v. stone

stylomastoid v.
subclavian v.
subcostal v.
sublingual v.
submental v.
subscapular v.
supraorbital v.
suprarenal v.
suprascapular v.
supratrochlear v.
supreme intercostal v.
sylvian v.
v. system
temporal v.
temporomaxillary v.
testicular v.
thalamostriate v.
thebesian v.
thoracic v.
thoracoacromial v.
thoracoepigastric v.
thymic v.
thyroid v.
Trolard v.
v. tumor thrombus
umbilical v. (UV)
umbilical vein to maternal v.
  (UV/MV)
uterine v.
v. valve transplantation
v. valve wrapping
vertebral v.
vertical v.
Vesalius v.
vesical v.
vestibular v.
vidian v.
Vieussens v.
vitelline v.
vorticose v.
v. wall
Veirs canaliculus repair
vela (*pl. of* velum)
velamen, pl. **velamina**
velamentous insertion
velamentum, pl. **velamenta**
velamina (*pl. of* velamen)
velar
Veleanu-Rosianu-Ionescu
  V.-R.-I. adductor tenotomy
  V.-R.-I. technique
veliform

NOTES

Vella fistula
vellication
vellus
velocardiofacial syndrome
velocity
    v. catheter technique
    migration v.
velopharyngeal
    v. closure
    v. port
    v. sphincter
veloplasty
    functional v.
    intravelar v.
Velpeau
    V. canal
    V. deformity
    V. fossa
    V. hernia
velum, pl. vela
    corneal v.
vena, pl. venae
venacavaplasty
    face-to-face v.
venectomy
venereal
    v. condyloma
    v. disease
    v. sore
venereology
venesection
venipuncture
Venn-Watson classification
venoablation
    percutaneous v.
venobiliary fistula
venoconstriction
    mesenteric v.
    reflex v.
venodilation
    nitrate-induced v.
    systemic v.
venogram
venographic study
venography
    contrast v.
    wedge hepatic v.
venolysis
    circumferential v.
venom extract
venoperitoneostomy
venostasis
venostomy
venosus
    sinus v.
venotomy
venous
    v. access
    v. access technique

    v. admixture
    v. air embolism (VAE)
    v. anastomosis
    v. angioma
    v. angle
    v. blood gas
    v. cannulation
    v. channel
    v. circulation
    v. collateral
    v. compression
    v. confluence
    v. cutdown
    v. dialysis pressure (VPd)
    v. drainage
    v. effort thrombosis
    v. embolization
    v. foramen
    v. gangrene
    v. groove
    v. hemorrhage
    v. hypercarbia
    v. injury
    v. insufficiency
    v. interposition graft
    v. intravasation
    v. invasion
    v. leak syndrome
    v. ligament
    v. line
    v. loop
    v. malformation
    maternal v. (MV)
    v. occlusion
    v. outflow
    v. outflow recording
    v. pathology
    v. plexus
    v. pressure
    v. puncture
    v. return
    v. sampling
    v. saturation
    v. segment
    v. sheath patch
    v. sinus
    v. stasis
    v. stasis disease
    v. study
    v. system
    v. thromboembolism
    v. tributary
    v. trunk
    umbilical v.
    v. web
    v. web disease
venous/arterial management protection (VAMP)

**venous-occlusion volume
  plethysmography**
venous-related complication
venous-to-venous anastomosis
venovenostomy
venovenous
  v. bypass (VVB)
  v. extracorporeal bypass
venter
ventilation
  v. agent
  airway pressure release v. (APRV)
  alveolar v.
  artificial v.
  assist-control mode v.
  assisted v.
  bag-and-mask v.
  bagged mask v.
  bag-valve-mask-assisted v.
  v. circuit
  v. collateralization
  continuous flow v.
  continuous mandatory v.
  continuous positive pressure v.
    (CPPV)
  control of v.
  controlled v.
  controlled mechanical v. (CMV)
  control-mode v.
  cuirass v.
  v. defect
  difficult v.
  emergency v.
  v. equivalent
  extended mandatory minute v.
    (EMMV)
  forced mandatory intermittent v.
  hand v.
  heart synchronized v.
  HFJ v.
  high-frequency v. (HFV)
  high-frequency jet v.
  high-frequency oscillation v.
  high-frequency oscillatory v.
    (HFOV)
  high-frequency percussive v.
  high-frequency positive-pressure v.
    (HFPPV)
  hyperoxic v.
  v. index (VI)
  inspired v. (VI)
  intermittent demand v.

  intermittent mandatory v. (IMV)
  intermittent mechanical v.
  intermittent positive pressure v.
    (IPPV)
  inverse-ratio v.
  jet v.
  local exhaust v.
  low-frequency jet v.
  1-lung v. (OLV)
  2-lung v.
  v. lung scan
  manual v.
  maximal voluntary v.
  maximum voluntary v. (MVV)
  mechanical v.
  mouth-to-mouth v.
  negative pressure v. (NPV)
  neonate v.
  noninvasive positive-pressure v.
    (NPPV)
  oscillatory v.
  partial liquid v.
  v. peak pressure
  percutaneous transtracheal v.
  percutaneous transtracheal jet v.
    (PTJV, PTV)
  positive-pressure v. (PPV)
  postoperative v.
  pressure control v. (PCV)
  pressure control inverse ratio v.
    (PCIRV)
  pressure-controlled inverse ratio v.
    (PCIRV)
  pressure-regulated volume control v.
  pressure support v. (PSV)
  pressure-supported v. (PSV)
  prolonged postoperative v.
  proportional assist v.
  pulmonary v.
  regional v.
  single lung v.
  split-lung v.
  spontaneous v.
  spontaneous intermittent
    mandatory v. (SIMV)
  synchronized intermittent
    mandatory v. (SIMV)
  synchronized intermittent
    mechanical v. (SIMV)
  synchronous intermittent
    mandatory v.
  v. threshold

V

NOTES

ventilation *(continued)*
  time-cycled v.
  transtracheal jet v. (TTJV)
  triggered v.
  ultra-high-frequency v.
  volume-cycled decelerating-flow v.
ventilation/perfusion (V/Q)
  v./p. abnormality
  v./p. defect
  v./p. distribution
  v./p. imaging
  v./p. inequality
  v./p. lung scan
  v./p. mismatch
  v./p. quotient
  v./p. ratio
  v./p. relation
  v./p. relationship
ventilator
  v. breathing
  v. dependency
  high-frequency jet v.
  high-frequency positive-pressure v.
  v. management
  proportional assist v. (PAV)
  v. support
  v. time
  v. weaning
ventilator-assisted respiration
ventilator-associated pneumonia
ventilator-induced
  v.-i. lung injury (VILI)
  v.-i. pneumopericardium
  v.-i. pneumothorax
ventilatory
  v. depression
  v. response
  v. support
venting percutaneous gastrostomy
ventral
  v. bending technique
  v. hernia
  v. herniorrhaphy
  v. incisional hernia
  v. root
  v. sacrococcygeal ligament
  v. sacrococcygeus muscle
  v. spinocerebellar tract
  v. spinothalamic tract
  v. tegmental decussation
ventricle
  laryngeal v.
  lateral v.
  left v.
  Morgagni v.
  right v.
ventricular
  v. aberration
  v. access

v. activation time
v. canal
v. depolarization abnormality
v. diastolic pressure
v. dilation
v. dysrhythmia
v. endoaneurysmorrhaphy
v. endomyocardial biopsy
v. end-systolic pressure-volume
  relation
v. filling pressure
v. fold
v. inflow anomaly
v. inflow tract obstruction
v. ligament
v. outflow tract
v. outflow tract obstruction
v. perforation
v. peritoneal (VP)
v. peritoneal shunting
v. phonation
v. preexcitation
v. puncture
v. relaxation
v. septal defect closure
v. septal rupture
v. septal wound defect
v. septum
v. tachycardia/ventricular fibrillation
ventricularization
ventricular-programmed stimulation
ventriculectomy
  partial left v.
ventriculi (*pl. of* ventriculus)
ventriculoarterial concordance
ventriculocisternostomy
  Torkildsen v.
ventriculocordectomy
ventriculography
  bubble v.
ventriculomastoidostomy
ventriculomegaly
ventriculoperitoneal
  v. shunting
  v. shunting procedure
  v. shunt placement
ventriculoplasty
  reduction v.
ventriculopuncture
ventriculoscopy
ventriculostomy
  straight-in v.
  terminal v.
  third v.
  tunneled v.
ventriculotomy
  encircling endocardial v.
  partial encircling endocardial v.
ventriculus, pl. **ventriculi**

ventrocystorrhaphy
ventroinguinal
ventrolateral hernia
ventroposterolateral (VPL)
ventroptosis
ventroscopy
ventrotomy
ventrum penis flap
Venturi principle
venula, pl. venulae
venular lesion
venule
    high endothelial v.
verapamil
veratridine
verbal descriptor scale
verbal-rank scale
verbotonal method
Verdan
    V. osteoplastic thumb reconstruction
    V. technique
Verga
    accessory venous sinus of V.
verge
    anal v.
Verhoeff
    V. operation
    V. suture technique
Verhoeff-Chandler
    V.-C. capsulotomy
    V.-C. operation
verification
    intraoperative v.
Vermale operation
vermian fossa
vermicular colic
vermiculation
vermiform
    v. appendage
    v. appendix
    v. body
    v. process
vermiformis
vermilion border
vermilionectomy
Vermont spinal fixator articulation
Vernet syndrome
Verneuil
    V. canal
    V. operation
vernix membrane

verrucous lesion
vertebra, pl. vertebrae
    basilar v.
    caudal v.
    cervical v.
    coccygeal v.
    dorsal v.
    false v.
    lumbar v.
    picture frame v.
    v. plana fracture
    sacral v.
    tail v.
    thoracic v.
    true v.
    wedge-shaped v.
vertebral
    v., anal, cardiac, tracheal, esophageal, renal, limb (VACTERL)
    v., anus, tracheoesophageal, radial, and renal (VATER)
    v. arch
    v. artery
    v. artery disease
    v. artery reconstruction
    v. aspiration
    v. body
    v. body anterior cortex
    v. body corpectomy
    v. body decompression
    v. body fracture
    v. bone mass
    v. canal
    v. column
    v. compression
    v. dissection
    v. epidural space
    v. exposure
    v. foramen
    v. fusion
    v. ganglion
    v. groove
    v. interbody fusion
    v. notch
    v. osteosynthesis
    v. osteosynthesis fusion rate
    v. region
    v. resection
    v. rib
    v. ring apophysis
    v. rotation

V

NOTES

vertebral *(continued)*
  v. stable burst fracture
  v. subluxation complex
  v. subluxation syndrome
  v. vein
  v. venous plexus
  v. wedge compression fracture
vertebrated
vertebrectomy
  Bohlman anterior cervical v.
  cervical spondylotic myelopathy v.
vertebroarterial foramen
vertebrochondral rib
vertebrocostal trigone
vertebrofemoral
vertebroiliac
vertebropelvic ligament
vertebrosacral
vertebrosternal rib
vertex, pl. **vertices**
  v. position
vertical
  v. adjustable banded gastroplasty
  v. angulation
  v. banded gastroplasty (VBG)
  v. banded gastroplasty pouch
  v. canal
  v. compression
  v. compression test
  v. condensation root canal filling
    method
  v. divergence position
  v. flap
  v. gastric bypass
  v. illumination
  v. index
  v. lip biopsy
  v. mastopexy
  v. mattress suture technique
  v. maxillary excess
  v. midline incision
  v. osteotomy
  v. partial laryngectomy
  v. pedicle technique breast
    reduction
  v. plane
  v. relation
  v. ring gastroplasty (VRG)
  v. section
  v. shear fracture
  v. Silastic ring gastroplasty
  v. suspension reflex
  v. tooth fracture
  v. translation
  v. uterine incision
  v. vein
  v. vein system
  v. versus horizontal preparation

vertical-cut
  v.-c. method
  v.-c. technique
vertically acquired infection
vertices (*pl. of* vertex)
verticomental
vertiginous migraine
vertigo
  benign paroxysmal positional v.
    (BPPV)
  cyclic v.
  positional v.
verumontanum
Verwey eyelid operation
very
  v. large scale integration
  v. late activation
Vesalius
  V. bone
  canal of V.
  V. foramen
  V. vein
vesica, pl. **vesicae**
vesical
  v. calculus
  v. diverticulectomy
  v. fistula
  v. flap
  v. gland
  v. lithotomy
  v. nerve
  v. plexus
  v. triangle
  v. vein
vesication
vesicle
  air v.
  brush-border membrane v.
  v. hernia
  optic v.
  otic v.
  seminal v.
vesicoabdominal
vesicoacetabular fistula
vesicobullous lesion
vesicocele
vesicocervical space
vesicoclysis
vesicocolic fistula
vesicocutaneous fistula
vesicoenteric fistula
vesicofixation
vesicointestinal fistula
vesicolithiasis
vesicomyectomy
vesicomyotomy
vesicoovarian fistula
vesicoprostatic
vesicopubic

vesicorectal fistula
vesicorectostomy
vesicosalpingovaginal fistula
vesicosigmoid
vesicosigmoidostomy
vesicospinal
vesicostomy
    cutaneous v.
    preputial continent v.
    vaginal v.
vesicotomy
vesicoumbilical ligament
vesicoureteral reflux
vesicourethral
    v. anastomosis
    v. canal
vesicouterine
    v. fistula
    v. ligament
    v. pouch
vesicouterovaginal
vesicovaginal
    v. fistula
    v. repair
vesicovaginorectal fistula
vesicovaginostomy
vesicovisceral
vesicula, pl. **vesiculae**
vesicular
    v. acute inflammation
    v. appendage
    v. granulomatous inflammation
    v. venous plexus
    v. viral infection
vesiculation
vesiculectomy
    prostatoseminal v.
    total prostatoseminal v.
vesiculitis
vesiculocavernous respiration
vesiculoprostatectomy
    retropubic v.
vesiculoprostatitis
vesiculotomy
Vesling line
vessel
    aberrant v.
    abnormally feeding blood v.
    absorbent v.
    afferent lymphatic v.
    anterior great v.
    bleeding v.

    blood v.
    celiac v.
    chyle v.
    collateral v.
    deep lymphatic v.
    v. distention
    ectatic v.
    endosteal v.
    v. exposure
    gastric v.
    gastroepiploic v.
    inflow v.
    infrapopliteal v.
    innominate v.
    intercostal v.
    lacteal v.
    v. ligation
    lumbar v.
    lymph v.
    lymphatic v.
    nutrient v.
    pancreaticoduodenal arcade v.
    parent v.
    periesophageal blood v.
    portal v.
    posterior great v.
    renal v.
    right subclavian v.
    segmental v.
    short gastric v.
    splanchnic v.
    v. stenosis
    superficial lymphatic v.
    thoracic great v.
    tumor v.
    v. wall
vessel-containing plate
vestibula (*pl. of* vestibulum)
vestibular
    v. blind sac
    v. canal
    v. canaliculus
    v. crest
    v. fissure
    v. fold
    v. ganglion
    v. gland
    v. labyrinth
    v. ligament
    v. membrane
    v. nerve
    v. nerve section

V

NOTES

vestibular *(continued)*
v. neurectomy
v. vein
v. window
vestibule
esophagogastric v.
gastroesophageal v.
labial v.
nasal v.
vestibulitis
vestibulocochlear nerve
vestibuloplasty
vestibulospinal tract
vestibulourethral
vestibulum, pl. **vestibula**
vestige
vestigial muscle
vest-over-pants
v.-o.-p. hernia repair
v.-o.-p. herniorrhaphy
Veterans Administration Cooperative study
V-flap meatoplasty
VI
inspired ventilation
ventilation index
viability
flap v.
viable tissue
vial
multidose v.
scintillation v.
vibrating line
vibration
v. condensation
v. disease
v. neuritis
v. syndrome
v. threshold test
vibrational angioplasty
vibrator hand syndrome
Vibrio fetus **infection**
vibrissa, pl. **vibrissae**
vibroacoustic stimulation
vicarious respiration
vicious union
Vicq d'Azyr bundle
victim
trauma v.
Victor Gomel method
Vidal-Ardrey fracture technique
video
v. image
v. mediastinoscopy
v. small bowel enteroscopy
v. thoracoscopic drainage
v. thoracoscopy
v. transurethral resection technique

video-assisted
v.-a. excisional biopsy
v.-a. gastrectomy
v.-a. technique
v.-a. thoracic surgical procedure
v.-a. thoracoscopic surgery (VATS)
v.-a. thoracoscopic thymectomy
v.-a. thorascopic surgery (VATS)
v.-a. transsternal radical esophagectomy
videoendoscopic-assisted microsurgery
videoendoscopic thyroidectomy
videoendoscopy
videoesophagogoscopy
videoesophagram
videofluoroscopic technique
videofluoroscopy
videolaparoscopic cardiomyotomy
videolaparoscopic guidance
videolaparoscopy
videolaseroscopy
videomicroscopy
videoscopic
v. evaluation
v. fundoplication
v. hernia surgery
v. repair
videoscopy
3-dimensional v.
videostroboscopy
videothoracoscopy
videourodynamic evaluation
vidian
v. canal
v. nerve
v. neuralgia
v. vein
Viers operation
Vieussens
V. ansa
V. ganglion
V. limbus
V. ring
valve of V.
V. vein
view
abdominal v.
anterior v.
apical lordotic v.
Boehler calcaneal v.
Boehler lumbosacral v.
Breuerton v.
cine v.
coned-down v.
decubitus v.
frontal x-ray v.
laparoscopic transhiatal v.
lateral x-ray v.
1-plane v.

vigil
    coma v.
vigilance monitoring
vigorous hydration
VILI
    ventilator-induced lung injury
Villaret syndrome
villous
    v. atrophy
    v. epithelium
villus, pl. **villi**
    arachnoid v.
    intestinal v.
    peritoneal v.
    pleural v.
    synovial v.
villusectomy
Vim-Silverman
    V.-S. technique
    V.-S. technique for liver biopsy
Vim thalamotomy
Vincent infection
vinculum, pl. **vincula**
Vindelov method flow cytometry analysis
Vineberg procedure
vinyl chloride exposure
violaceous lesion
violation
    peritoneal v.
    pleural v.
VIPoma
Virag operation
viral
    v. marker
    v. respiratory infection
Virchow
    V. metastasis
    V. triad
Virchow-Robin
    V.-R. space
    V.-R. space dilatation
virginal membrane
virginity
virgin neck
virilia
virilization
virtual
    v. colonoscopy
    v. cystoscopy
    v. endoscopy
    v. implantation

    v. point
    v. reality
virus
    adenoidal-pharyngeal-conjunctival v.
    coxsackievirus A, B v.
    Epstein-Barr v. (EBV)
    hepatitis C v. (HCV)
    human immunodeficiency v. (HIV)
viscerad
visceral
    v. anesthesia
    v. angiomyolipoma
    v. edema
    v. hamartoma
    v. herniation
    v. hyperalgesia
    v. injury
    v. layer
    v. lesion
    v. muscle
    v. nerve
    v. node
    v. pain
    v. pelvic fascia
    v. perfusion
    v. pericardiectomy
    v. pericardium
    v. peritoneum
    v. pleura
    v. postsurgical disturbance
    v. pouch
    v. rotation
    v. space
    v. sympathectomy
    v. traction reflex
visceralgia
viscera retention
viscerobronchial cardiovascular anomaly
viscerocranium
visceroinhibitory
visceroparietal
visceroperitoneal
visceropleural
visceroptosis
viscerosensory
visceroskeletal
visceroskeleton
viscerosomatic
viscerotomy
viscoelastic tissue
viscosity
viscosupplementation

NOTES

V

viscus
  abdominal v.
  abdominopelvic v.
  herniated v.
  hollow v.
  v. injury
  intraperitoneal v.
  retroperitoneal v.
Visick dysphagia classification
vision
  central v.
  direct laparoscopic v.
  laparoscopic v.
  presbyopic v.
visiting nurse
visor flap
visual
  v. analog pain score (VAPS)
  v. analog scale (VAS)
  v. analysis
  v. association area
  v. closure
  v. compromise
  v. deprivation syndrome
  v. direction
  v. extinction
  v. fixation
  v. function evaluation
  v. laser ablation
  v. laser ablation of prostate
  v. laser-assisted prostatectomy
  v. line
  v. method
  v. orientation
  v. pathway
  v. plane
  v. point
  v. preservation
  v. projection
  v. stimulation
visualization
  contrast v.
  direct fluoroscopic v.
  double-contrast v.
  endoscopic v.
  fluoroscopic v.
  4-gland v.
  inadequate v.
visually triggered headache
Visual-Motor Integration Test
vital
  v. capacity
  v. knot
  v. tissue
vitamin D supplementation
vitelline
  v. duct anomaly
  v. fistula
  v. membrane

  v. sac
  v. vein
vitellointestinal cyst
vitiation
vitreal
  v. hemorrhage
  v. membrane
vitrectomy
  anterior v.
  closed system pars plana v.
  core v.
  open-sky v.
  port v.
  posterior v.
  Weck-cel v.
vitreolysis
vitreoretinal
  v. surgery
  v. traction syndrome
vitreoretinopathy
  exudative v.
  familial exudative v.
vitreous
  v. aspiration
  v. breakthrough hemorrhage
  v. cavity
  v. foreign body
  v. hernia
  v. herniation
  v. humor
  v. membrane
  v. neovascularization
  v. surgery
  v. table
vitreum
vitrification
vividialysis
vividiffusion
vivification
vivo
  ex v.
  in v.
VLDL
V line
VMO
  vaccinia melanoma oncolysate
  polyvalent VMO
vocal
  v. cord
  v. cord atrophy
  v. cord damage
  v. cord injection
  v. cord movement
  v. cord palsy
  v. cord paralysis (VCP)
  v. dysfunction
  v. fold
  v. fold approximation
  v. fold fixation therapy

v. ligament
v. muscle
v. process
v. shelf
v. tract
vocalis muscle
Vogel method
Vogt-Koyanagi-Harada syndrome
Vogt operation
voice
v. disorder
v. disorder of phonation
v. restoration
v. termination time
v. therapy
voiding
v. flow rate
v. urethral pressure measurement
Voigt line
vola
volar
v. angulation
v. angulation deformity
v. aspect
v. epineurolysis
v. finger approach
v. interosseous artery
v. midline approach
v. midline oblique incision
v. plate
v. plate arthroplasty
v. plate arthroplasty technique
  fracture-dislocation
v. plate repair
v. radial approach
v. semilunar wrist dislocation
v. synovectomy
v. ulnar approach
v. V-Y flap
v. zig-zag finger incision
volaris
volarward approach
volatile
v. anesthesia
v. anesthetic
v. anesthetic agent
volatilization
volitional saccade
Volkmann
V. canal
V. clawhand deformity

V. fracture
V. ischemic contracture
Volpicelli functional ambulation scale
volsella
voltage
truncated exponential v.
volume
abdominal v.
biopsy v.
blood transfusion v.
circulation v.
compartmental v.
drain v.
end-expiratory lung v. (EELV)
end-inspiratory v.
v. expansion
expiratory reserve v.
expiratory residual v.
extracellular fluid v. (ECFV)
fiber bundle v.
forced expiratory v.
gland v.
gross tumor v. (GTV)
injection v.
intraperitoneal v.
intravascular v.
liver v.
maximal expiratory flow v.
median biopsy v.
minute v.
peritoneal exchange v.
v. plethysmography
presystolic pressure and v.
v. reduction surgery (VRS)
remnant liver v.
respiratory minute v.
resuscitated by v.
rib-cage v.
v. segmentation
specimen v.
stroke v. (SV)
v. therapy
tidal v.
timed forced expiratory v.
total erythrocyte v.
tumor v.
weight-based peritoneal exchange v.
volume-assured pressure support
volume-cycled decelerating-flow
  ventilation
volumetric
v. analysis

V

NOTES

volumetric *(continued)*
- v. capnometry
- v. method
- v. solution
- v. stereotaxis
- v. study
- v. technique

volumetry
- CT v.

voluntary
- v. area
- v. guarding
- v. sterilization

volutrauma

volvulus
- cecal v.
- gastric v.
- midgut v.
- organoaxial v.
- v. reduction
- sigmoid v. (SV)

Volz arthroplasty

Volz-Turner reattachment technique

vomer

vomerine canal

vomerobasilar canal

vomeronasal
- v. cartilage
- v. nerve

vomerorostral canal

vomerovaginal
- v. canal
- v. groove

vomit
- bilious v.

vomiting
- postoperative nausea and v. (PONV)

vomitus
- coffee-ground v.

von
- V. Ammon operation
- V. Bergman hernia
- v. Blaskovics-Doyen operation
- v. Claus chronometric method
- V. Ebner gland
- V. Ebner line
- v. Economo disease
- V. Frey test
- v. Graefe operation
- V. Haberer-Finney anastomosis
- V. Haberer-Finney gastrectomy technique
- V. Haberer gastroenterostomy
- v. Hippel-Lindau disease
- v. Hippel-Lindau tumor
- v. Hippel operation
- v. Kossa method
- V. Langenbeck bipedicle mucoperiosteal flap
- V. Langenbeck palatal closure
- V. Langenbeck pedicle flap
- v. Noorden incision
- v. Willebrand factor

vortex, pl. **vortices**

vorticose vein

Vostal radial fracture classification

V-osteotomy
- Japas V-o.
- off-set V-o.

VP
- ventricular peritoneal

VPd
- venous dialysis pressure

VPL
- ventroposterolateral
- VPL pallidotomy

V/Q
- ventilation/perfusion

VRG
- vertical ring gastroplasty

VRS
- volume reduction surgery

V-shaped
- V-s. incision
- V-s. osteotomy

V-sign of Naclerio

V-slope method

V-to-Y closure

Vulpius-Compere tendon technique

Vulpius procedure

Vulpius-Stoffel procedure

vulsella

vulva, pl. **vulvae**

vulvar
- v. adenoid cystic adenocarcinoma
- v. biopsy
- v. carcinoma
- v. infection
- v. pigmented lesion
- v. slit
- v. vestibulitis syndrome

vulvectomy
- Basset radical v.
- Parry-Jones v.
- radical v.
- simple v.
- skinning v.

vulvitis

vulvocrural

vulvoplasty

vulvouterine

vulvovaginal
- v. carcinoma
- v. cystectomy
- v. gland

v. lesion
v. premenarchal infection
vulvovaginoplasty
Williams v.
VVB
venovenous bypass
V-Y
V-Y advancement

V-Y advancement flap
V-Y advancement technique
V-Y gastroplasty
V-Y Kutler flap
V-Y plasty
V-Y procedure
V-Y quadricepsplasty

NOTES

V

W

W hernia
W pouch
W procedure

Wachendorf membrane
Wackenheim clivus canal line
Wadsworth

W. elbow approach
W. posterolateral approach
W. technique

Wagener-Clay-Gipner classification
Wagner

W. classification
W. closed pinning
W. modification of Syme
amputation
W. open reduction technique
W. skin incision
W. 2-stage Syme amputation

Wagoner

W. cervical technique
W. posterior approach

wagon-wheel fracture
Wagstaffe fracture
wake-up

w.-u. evaluation
w.-u. testing

Walcher position
Waldeyer

W. fossa
W. gland
W. ring
W. ring lesion
W. sheath
W. space
W. tract

Waldhauer operation
Waldhausen

W. procedure
W. subclavian flap technique

Walker tractotomy
walking

w. epidural
w. epidural anesthetic
w. program
w. ventilation test

wall

anterior abdominal w.
anterior aortic w.
anterior rectus sheath w.
anterior thoracic w.
aortic w.
bile duct w.
w. of body
bowel w.

cavity w.
chest w.
cyst w.
deep anterior w.
duct w.
edematous bowel w.
fibrotic w.
gastric w.
gingival cavity w.
intermediate anterior w.
w. invasion
lateral w.
nail w.
nasal w.
nontumoral gastric w.
orbital w.
oropharyngeal w.
parietal w.
peripheral cavity w.
posterior oropharyngeal w.
posterior rectus sheath w.
pulpal w.
w. push maneuver
rectus sheath w.
soft w.
splanchnic w.
superficial anterior w.
thoracic w.
upper thoracic w.
variceal w.
vein w.
vessel w.

wallaby pouch
Wallace technique
wall-echo shadow triad
wallet stomach
Walsh radical retropubic prostatectomy
Walter

W. Reed classification
W. Reed classification for HIV
infection
W. Reed operation

Walther

W. canal
W. duct
W. fracture
W. ganglion
W. plexus

waltzed flap
wandering

w. abscess
w. kidney
w. liver
w. organ
w. spleen

W

Wangensteen drainage
Wanger reduction technique
Wang pleural stoma
ward
    observation w.
Wardill
    W. 4-flap method
    W. pharyngoplasty
Wardill-Kilner
    W.-K. advancement flap method
    W.-K. 4-flap uranoplasty
    W.-K. procedure
Ward-Mayo vaginal hysterectomy
Wardrop method
warm
    w. condensation
    w. ischemia
    w. ischemic time
warmer
    fluid w.
    high-capacity fluid w.
    inspiratory w.
warming
    forced air w.
    preanesthetic skin-surface w.
    preoperative skin-surface w.
Warner-Farber ankle fixation technique
Warren
    W. flap
    W. incision
Warren-Marshall classification
Wartenberg syndrome
Warthin-Starry staining method
wartlike excrescence
Warwick and Ashken technique
washed
    w. clot
    w. field technique
    w. intrauterine insemination
washing
    cytologic w.
    endometrial jet w.
    peritoneal w.
washout
    peritoneal w.
    seminal tract w.
    w. test
wash technique
Wasmann gland
Wassel
    W. thumb duplication
    W. thumb duplication classification
wasting
    muscle w.
    w. syndrome
Watanabe
    W. classification of discoid
      meniscus
    W. discoid meniscus classification

watchband incision
water
    degasified distilled w.
    w. density line
    w. displacement
    w. dissection
    distilled w.
    extravascular lung w.
    hydration layer w.
    lung w.
    total body w.
    w. vapor monitoring
Waterhouse transpubic procedure
Waterman osteotomy
watermelon stomach
Waters
    W. operation
    W. projection
watershed
    vascular w.
water-soluble
    w.-s. contrast enema
    w.-s. contrast esophagogram
Waterston
    W. extrapericardial anastomosis
    W. method
    W. operation
Waterston-Cooley procedure
water-suppression technique
Waters-Waldron position
watertight closure
water-trap stomach
Watkins fusion technique
Watson
    W. capsule
    W. capsule biopsy
    W. method
    W. operation
    W. scaphotrapeziotrapezoidal fusion
    W. technique
Watson capsule
Watson-Cheyne-Burghard procedure
Watson-Cheyne technique
Watson-Crick method
Watson-Jones
    W.-J. anterior approach
    W.-J. fracture repair
    W.-J. incision
    W.-J. lateral approach
    W.-J. procedure
    W.-J. reconstruction
    W.-J. tenodesis
    W.-J. tibial tubercle avulsion
      fracture classification
Watzke operation
Waugh-Clagett pancreaticoduodenostomy
Waugh operation
wave
    abdominal fluid w.

contraction w.
phasic pressure w.
pressure w.
waveform
    aortic root velocity w.
    electrical stimulator w.
    epidural pressure w. (EPWF)
    photoplethysmographic w.
    pressure w.
wavelength frequency
wavy respiration
wax
    w. expansion
    w. pattern thermal expansion
    technique
wax-matrix technique
waxy
    w. exudate
    w. kidney
    w. liver
Wayne County reduction
Way operation
weakened bowel
weakness
    contralateral w.
    muscle w.
weaning
    ventilator w.
weapon
    stand-off w.
wear
    3-body w.
Weaver-Dunn
    W.-D. acromioclavicular technique
    W.-D. procedure
    W.-D. resection
weaving
    head w.
web
    antral w.
    cell w.
    w. corn
    duodenal w.
    esophageal w.
    w. eye
    finger w.
    w. formation
    hepatic w.
    intestinal w.
    laryngeal w.
    mucosal w.
    postcricoid w.

pulmonary arterial w.
w. space
w. space flap
w. space incision
w. space infection
terminal w.
thumb w.
tracheal w.
venous w.
webbed penis
Weber
    W. humeral osteotomy
    W. organ
    W. physical injury classification
    W. point
    W. procedure
    W. subcapital osteotomy
    W. triangle
Weber-Brunner-Freuler-Boitzy technique
Weber-Brunner-Freuler open reduction
Weber-Danis ankle injury classification
Weber-Fergusson
    W.-F. incision
    W.-F. procedure
Weber-Vasey traction-absorption wiring technique
Webril immobilization
Webster operation
Weck-cel vitrectomy
Weckesser technique
weddellite calculus
Wedensky facilitation
wedge
    arterial w.
    ball w.
    bone w.
    w. bone
    closing base w.
    compensatory w.
    w. compression fracture
    dental w.
    disconnect w.
    w. excision
    w. graft
    w. hepatectomy
    w. hepatic biopsy
    w. hepatic venography
    w. incision
    light-reflecting w.
    w. liver biopsy
    Livingston peribulbar w.
    mediastinal w.

NOTES

wedge *(continued)*
    open w.
    w. osteotomy
    w. pressure
    pulmonary artery w.
    w. resection
    temporal w.
wedge-and-groove joint
wedged
    w. hepatic vein pressure (WHVP)
    w. hepatic venous pressure
wedge-shaped
    w.-s. erosion
    w.-s. fasciculus
    w.-s. osteotomy
    w.-s. tubercle
    w.-s. uncomminuted tibial plateau fracture
    w.-s. vertebra
Weeker operation
Weeks operation
weeping lesion
Wegner line
weight
    body w.
    w. estimation and assessment
    graft w.
    gut mucosal w.
    ideal body w.
    lean body w.
    mucosal w.
    w. reduction
    w. reduction surgery
    total body w. (TBW)
weight-based peritoneal exchange volume
Weiland
    W. classification
    W. iliac crest bone graft
Weinberg
    W. modification
    W. modification of pyloroplasty
Weinstein-Ponseti technique
Weinstock desyndactylization
Weir
    W. incision
    W. operation
Weisinger operation
Weiss logarithmic method
Weissman classification
Weitbrecht
    W. cartilage
    W. cord
Welch technique
Welcker method
weld
    laser tissue w.
welding
    fusion w.

    laser tissue w.
    pressure w.
    tissue w.
well-circumscribed lesion
well-defined mass
well-localized adenoma
Wells posterior rectopexy
Wendell Hughes operation
Wepfer gland
Werb operation
Wernekinck decussation
Wernicke radiation
Wertheim
    W. operation
    tunnel of W.
Wertheim-Bohlman technique
Wertheim-Schauta operation
Wesenberg-Hamazaki body
Westberg space
Westcott Pyramid Program
Westergren sedimentation rate method
Western blot infection
Westin-Hall incision
West operation
West-Soto-Hall
    W.-S.-H. patellar technique
    W.-S.-H. patellectomy
wet
    w. colostomy
    w. field cautery
    w. gangrene
    w. lung
    w. technique with liposuction breast reduction
wetting solution
Weve operation
Weyers-Thier syndrome
Wharton duct
Wharton-Jones operation
Wheeler
    W. halving repair
    W. method
    W. operation
    W. procedure
Wheeler-Reese operation
Wheelhouse operation
wheel rotation
wheezing
    expiratory w.
whewellite calculus
whip
    catheter w.
whiplash
    w. injury
    w. technique
whipping condensation
Whipple
    W. incision
    W. operation

W. pancreatectomy
W. pancreaticoduodenectomy
W. pancreaticoduodenostomy
W. pancreatoduodenectomy
W. procedure
W. resection
whipstitch suture technique
whipworm infection
whispered pectoriloquy
whistle-tip
whistling deformity
Whitaker pressure-perfusion test
white
    w. cell
    w. classification
    w. clot syndrome
    w. dot syndrome
    w. epidermoidoma
    w. fixation
    w. gangrene
    w. graft
    w. lesion
    w. line
    w. line response
    w. matter
    w. muscle
    w. patch
    w. point
    w. posterior ankle fusion
    w. pulp
    w. ring
    w. slide procedure
    w. without pressure
white-centered hemorrhage
Whitecloud-LaRocca fibular strut graft
whitegraft reaction
Whitehead
    W. classification
    W. deformity
    W. operation
Whitesides-Kelly cervical technique
Whitesides technique
white-spot lesion
whitlow
    melanotic w.
Whitman
    W. femoral neck reconstruction
    W. osteotomy
    W. talectomy procedure
Whitman-Thompson procedure
Whitmore-Jewett (W-J)
    W.-J. classification

W.-J. classification for staging of
    prostate cancer
Whitnall
    W. ligament
    W. orbital tubercle
    W. sling operation
WHO
    World Health Organization
    WHO gastric carcinoma
    classification
whole
    w. abdominal radiation
    w. abdominopelvic irradiation
    w. blood lysis technique
    w. lobar graft
    w. organ pancreas transplantation
    (WOP)
whole-abdomen irradiation
whole-arm fusion
whole-body
    w.-b. cooling
    w.-b. extract
    w.-b. hyperthermia
    w.-b. irradiation
    w.-b. scanning
    w.-b. titration curve
wholebody radiation
whole-brain radiation therapy
whole-cell patch clamp recording
whole-gut
    w.-g. irrigation
    w.-g. lavage activating solution
whole-pelvis irradiation
whorl
    coccygeal w.
whorled appearance
WHVP
    wedged hepatic vein pressure
Wiberg patellar classification
Wicherkiewicz eyelid operation
Wick catheter technique
Wickham technique
wide
    w. elliptical anastomosis
    w. internal inguinal ring
    w. local excision
    w. mucosa-to-mucosa Roux-en-Y
    hepaticojejunostomy
    w. plane
wide-field
    w.-f. radiation therapy
    w.-f. total laryngectomy

W

NOTES

wide-mouth sac
widened retrogastric space
wide-open anastomosis
wide-range radiation therapy
widespread
    w. portal system thrombosis
    w. vasculitis
Widman flap
width
    line w.
    pulse w.
Wiener
    W. operation
    tract of Münzer and W.
Wies
    W. operation
    W. procedure
Wigand maneuver
Wigby-Taylor incision
Wilcoxon signed-rank test
Wilde incision
Wiley-Galey classification
Wilkie artery
Wilkinson synovectomy
Wilkins radial fracture classification
will
    living w.
Willett-Stampfer method
William
    W. Dixon Cratex point
    W. microlumbar disc excision
Williams
    W. copulating pouch operation
    W. discectomy
    W. procedure
    W. vulvovaginoplasty
Williams-Haddad technique
Willi glass crown technique
Willis
    W. antrum
    artery of W.
    W. cord
    W. pancreas
    W. pouch
willow fracture
Willy Meyer mastectomy incision
Wilmer operation
Wilms
    W. amputation
    W. renal tumor
    W. thoracoplasty
Wilson
    W. ankle fusion
    W. bone graft
    W. bunionectomy
    W. fracture
    W. muscle
    W. oblique displacement osteotomy

    W. procedure
    W. technique
Wilson-Jacobs
    W.-J. patellar graft
    W.-J. tibial fracture fixation
      technique
Wilson-McKeever
    W.-M. arthroplasty
    W.-M. shoulder technique
Wilson-White method
Wiltberger
    W. anterior cervical approach
    W. fusion
Wiltse
    W. ankle osteotomy
    W. bilateral lateral fusion
    W. system double-rod construct
    W. system H construct
    W. system single-rod construct
    W. varus supramalleolar osteotomy
Wiltse-Spencer paraspinal approach
Winberger line
Winchester syndrome
windblown deformity
window
    aortic-pulmonic w.
    aortopulmonary w.
    dilating w.
    oval w.
    pericardial w.
    peritoneal w.
    soft tissue w.
    w. technique
    uterine w.
    vestibular w.
windpipe
windsock deformity
Windson-Insall-Vince
    W.-I.-V. bone graft
    W.-I.-V. grafting technique
windswept deformity
wind-up
    second pain w.-u.
winged V double flap
Winiwarter-Buerger disease
Winiwarter operation
Winkelmann rotationplasty
Winkler body
Winkler-Waldeyer
    closing ring of W.-W.
Winnie landmark
Winograd
    W. nail plate removal
    W. partial matrixectomy
    W. procedure
    W. technique
Winquist femoral shaft fracture
classification

Winquist-Hansen femoral fracture classification
Winslow pancreas
Winston-Lutz method
Winter
    W. classification
    W. convex fusion
    W. procedure
    W. spondylolisthesis technique
Wintrobe
    W. and Landsberg method
    W. sedimentation rate method
wire
    w. arch
    w. contour preparation
    w. extrusion
    w. insertion
    w. knot
    w. localization
    w. osteosynthesis
    w. passage
    w. removal technique
    w. stabilization
    4-w. trochanter reattachment
wire-guided
    w.-g. balloon-assisted endoscopic biliary stent exchange
    w.-g. biopsy sample
    w.-g. breast biopsy
    w.-g. dilation
    w.-g. endobronchial blocker
    w.-g. placement
wire-loop
    w.-l. fixation
    w.-l. lesion
    w.-l. test
wiring
    compression w.
    continuous loop w.
    craniofacial suspension w.
    facet fracture stabilization w.
    facet subluxation stabilization w.
    interspinous w.
    Ivy loop w.
    sublaminar w.
Wirsung
    W. canal
    W. dilation
    W. duct
Wirth-Jager tendon technique
Wise
    W. mastopexy

    W. operation
    W. pattern mammaplasty
within-list recognition (WLR)
Witzel
    W. duodenostomy
    W. gastrostomy
    W. jejunostomy
    W. operation
W-J
    Whitmore-Jewett
    W-J classification for staging of prostate cancer
WLR
    within-list recognition
WOB
    work of breathing
Wolfe
    W. breast carcinoma classification
    W. method
    W. ptosis operation
Wolfe-Kawamoto bone graft
Wolfe-Krause graft
wolffian
    w. body
    w. cyst
    w. duct
    w. duct carcinoma
Wolff-Parkinson-White bypass tract
Wolf full-thickness free graft
Wölfler
    W. gastroenterostomy
    W. gland
    W. suture technique
Womack procedure
womb
wood
    w. light examination
    w. point
    w. wool
Woods screw maneuver
Woodward
    W. esophagogastroscopy
    W. esophagogastrostomy
    W. operation wound
    W. procedure
    W. technique
Woofry-Chandler
    W.-C. classification
    W.-C. classification of Osgood-Schlatter lesion
Woofry-Chandler classification
Wookey reconstruction

NOTES

W

wool
  wood w.
Wooler-type anuloplasty
Woolf method
WOP
  whole organ pancreas transplantation
work
  w. of breathing (WOB)
  w. hardening program
  preload recruitable stroke w.
    (PRSW)
working bite relation
workup
  diagnostic w.
  hematologic w.
World
  W. Health Organization (WHO)
  W. Health Organization
    classification
wormian bone
Worst operation
Worth ptosis operation
wound
  abdominal gunshot w.
  abraded w.
  w. abscess
  acute w.
  anterior w.
  w. approximation
  avulsed w.
  back gunshot w.
  w. biopsy
  bullet w.
  w. cavity
  central hepatic gunshot w.
  w. closure
  w. complication
  crease w.
  w. dehiscence
  w. disruption
  w. drainage
  w. dressing
  exit w.
  w. failure
  flank gunshot w.
  w. fluid
  fresh w.
  glancing w.
  gunshot w. (GSW)
  gutter w.
  w. healing
  w. hematoma
  hepatic gunshot w.
  w. hernia
  incised w.
  w. infection
  w. irrigation
  laparoscopic trocar w.
  lateral w.

  nonpenetrating w.
  open w.
  penetrating w.
  perforating w.
  precordial w.
  w. problem
  puncture w.
  w. recurrence
  remodeling of w.
  w. retraction
  seton w.
  shotgun w.
  w. site
  skin deficit w.
  stab w.
  sucking chest w.
  superficial w.
  surgical w.
  tangential w.
  thoracoabdominal gunshot w.
  w. tract
  transpelvic gunshot w.
  trocar w.
  Woodward operation w.
wound-breaking strength
W-plasty
W-pouch
  ileal W-p.
wrap
  cardiac muscle w.
  gastric w. (GW)
  gastric fundus w.
  w. hematoma
  Nissen fundoplication w.
  rectus fascial w.
  smooth w.
  total gastric w.
wraparound
  w. neurovascular composite free
    tissue transfer
  w. neurovascular free flap
  w. periapical lesion
wrapping
  fascial w.
  omental pedicle w.
  pedicle w.
  valve w.
  vein valve w.
Wright
  W. maneuver
  W. operation
Wright-Giemsa evaluation
wrinkler muscle
wrinkling membrane
Wrisberg
  W. cartilage
  W. lesion
  W. nerve
  W. tubercle

wrist
- w. block
- w. deformity
- w. disarticulation
- w. dislocation
- w. extensor
- w. extensor tendon

Wroblewski method
wryneck
W-shaped
- W-s. ileal pouch-anal anastomosis
- W-s. incision

W-sitting position

NOTES

xanthoastrocytoma
xanthogranuloma
xanthogranulomatous
 x. cholecystitis
 x. pyelonephritis (XCP)
xanthomatosis
 cerebrotendinous x.
xanthosarcoma
Xase complex
X body
XCP
 xanthogranulomatous pyelonephritis
¹³³Xe intravenous injection technique
xenogeneic
 x. graft
 x. tissue
xenogenic
 x. cell therapy
 x. infection
xenograft
 x. graft
 stented bovine pericardial x.
 stented porcine x.
 x. transplantation
xenografting
xenon
 x. arc photocoagulation
 x. gas
 x. lung ventilation imaging
 x. method
xenon-enhanced cerebral blood flow
xenon-washout technique
xenotransplantation
 cellular x.
 x. thymus
xenozoonosis

xerography
 soft tissue x.
xeroma
xeroradiogram
xerosis
xerostomia
xiphisternal
 x. joint
 x. junction
 x. junction chondritis
xiphisternum
xiphocostal
xiphodynia
xiphoid
 x. cartilage
 x. process
xiphoidalgia
xiphoid-to-pubis midline abdominal incision
xiphoid-to-umbilicus incision
xiphosternalis
 synchondrosis x.
x-line method
X-pattern exotropia
x-radiation
x-ray
 abdominal x-r. (AXR)
 anteroposterior chest x-r.
 barium contrast x-r.
 chest x-r.
 x-r. control
 frontal x-r.
 lateral chest x-r.
 x-r. therapy
X, Y dimension

X

Y

Y body
Y cartilage
Y configuration
Y fracture
Y graft
Y incision
Yacoub and Radley-Smith classification
YAG
yttrium-aluminum-garnet
Yale Optimal Observation Score
Yancey osteotomy
Y angle
y-angle
Yasargil craniotomy
Yates correction
yeast infection
Yee posterior shoulder approach
yellow
y. atrophy
y. body
y. hepatization
y. lesion
y. ligament
y. nail
y. nail syndrome
y. point
yellow-ochre hemorrhage
Yentl syndrome
yield
nodal y.
Y mesh hernia repair
yoke
alveolar y.
y. block
y. bone
cricoid y.
y. hanger
y. transposition procedure
yolk
y. membrane
y. sac
y. sac carcinoma
y. space
York-Mason
Y.-M. incision

Y.-M. procedure
Y.-M. repair
Y-osteotomy
Pauwels Y-o.
young
y. cyst
y. onset cancer
y. operation
y. pelvic fracture classification
y. procedure
y. technique
y. type epispadias repair
Young-Dees
Y.-D. bladder neck reconstruction
Y.-D. operation
Y.-D. procedure
Y.-D. technique
Young-Dees-Leadbetter
Y.-D.-L. bladder neck
reconstruction
Y.-D.-L. operation
Youngwhich modification
Yount
Y. fasciotomy
Y. procedure
yo-yo weight fluctuation phenomenon
Y piece
Y-plasty
ypsiliform
Y-shaped
Y-s. fracture
Y-s. incision
Y-shaped fracture
Y-suture technique
Y-T fracture
yttrium-90
yttrium-aluminum-garnet (YAG)
Yu
Yu osteotomy
Yu pyloroplasty
Y-V
Y-V anoplasty
Y-V plasty
Y-V-plasty incision

Y

ζ (*var. of* zeta)
Z
    Z direction
    Z fashion
    Z incision
    Z line
    Z marginal tenotomy
    Z myotomy
    Z point
    Z procedure
    Z technique
Zadik total matrixectomy
Zaglas ligament
Zahn
    anomaly of Z.
    Z. line
    striae of Z.
Zaias nail biopsy
Zancolli
    Z. capsuloplasty
    Z. clawhand deformity repair
    Z. procedure for clawhand
      deformity
    Z. reconstruction
    Z. rerouting technique
    Z. static lock procedure
Zancolli-Lasso procedure
Zanelli position
Zang space
Zarins-Rowe
    Z.-R. ligament technique
    Z.-R. procedure
Zavala technique
Zavanelli maneuver
Zazepen-Gamidov technique
Z-dimension
ZEEP
    zero end-expiratory pressure
Zeier transfer technique
Zeis gland
Zemuron
Zenker
    Z. diverticulum
    Z. pouch
zero
    z. end-expiratory pressure (ZEEP)
    z. end-inspiratory pressure
    z. line
zeta, ζ
    z, sedimentation ratio method
zeugmatography
    rotating-frame z.
Z-flap incision

Zickel
    Z. classification
    Z. subtrochanteric fracture operation
Ziegler
    Z. operation
    Z. puncture
Zielke technique
ZIFT
    zygote intrafallopian transfer
zig-zag
    z.-z. approach
    z.-z. compensatory deformity
    z.-z. finger incision
Zimany bilobed flap
Zimmerman-Brittin exchange model
Zimmerman operation
zinc sulfate flotation method
Zinn
    Z. ligament
    Z. membrane
    tendon of Z.
    Z. zonule
zipped canal
zipper
    fascial z.
    z. sphincterotomy
Zlotsky-Ballard acromioclavicular injury classification
Zoellner-Clancy procedure
Zollinger classification
Zöllner line
zona, pl. **zonae**
zonal anatomy
zone
    abdominal z.
    adherent z.
    anal transition z. (ATZ)
    arcuate z.
    barrier z.
    basement membrane z.
    calcification z.
    cervical transformation z.
    chemoreceptor trigger z.
    ciliary z.
    dorsal root entry z. (DREZ)
    echo z.
    entry z.
    exudative z.
    gingival z.
    Head z.
    hemorrhoidal z.
    high pressure z. (HPZ)
    normal transformation z.
    orbicular z.
    pectinate z.

Z

zone *(continued)*
    proliferation z.
    pupillary z.
    transformation z.
    vascular z.
zonoskeleton
zonula, pl. **zonulae**
zonular
    z. band
    z. fiber
    z. space
zonulares
zonule
    ciliary z.
    Zinn z.
zonulolysis
    Barraquer z.
    enzymatic z.
zonulotomy
zoodermic
zoograft
zoografting
zoonotic infection
zooplastic graft
zooplasty
zoospermia
Z-osteotomy
    scarf Z-o.
Z-osteotomy-bunionectomy
    scarf Z-o.-b.
Z-plasty
    Z-p. approach
    Broadbent-Woolf 4-limb Z-p.
    Cozen-Brockway Z-p.
    4-flap Z-p.
    Gudas scarf Z-p.
    Z-p. incision
    4-limb Z-p.
    Z-p. local flap graft
    Peet Z-p.
    Z-p. procedure
    scarf Z-p.
    Spencer-Watson Z-p.
    Z-p. tenotomy
    Z-p. transposition
z-point pressure
Z-shaped
    Z-s. anastomosis
    Z-s. incision
    Z-s. suture line
Z-suture technique
Z-track intramuscular injection method

Z-type deformity
Zuckerkandl
    Z. diverticulum
    Z. fascia
    Z. perforating canal
    Z. tubercle
    Z. tuberculum
Zuker and Manktelow technique
Zung Depression Scale
zygapophysial, zygapophyseal
    z. joint
zygapophysis
zygion
zygoma
zygomatic
    z. arch
    z. arch fracture
    z. bone
    z. branch
    z. fossa
    z. maxillary complex fracture
    z. nerve
    z. region
zygomaticoauricular index
zygomaticofacial
    z. artery
    z. branch
    z. canal
    z. foramen
zygomaticofrontal suture
zygomaticomaxillary
    z. fracture
    z. suture
zygomaticoorbital
    z. artery
    z. foramen
zygomatico-orbitalis
zygomaticosphenoid
zygomaticotemporal
    z. branch
    z. canal
    z. foramen
    z. space
    z. suture
zygomaticus
    z. major muscle
    z. minor muscle
zygomaxillary point
zygopodium
zygote intrafallopian transfer (ZIFT)
Zylik operation

Contents: The Appendices

Appendix 1
Anatomical Illustrations

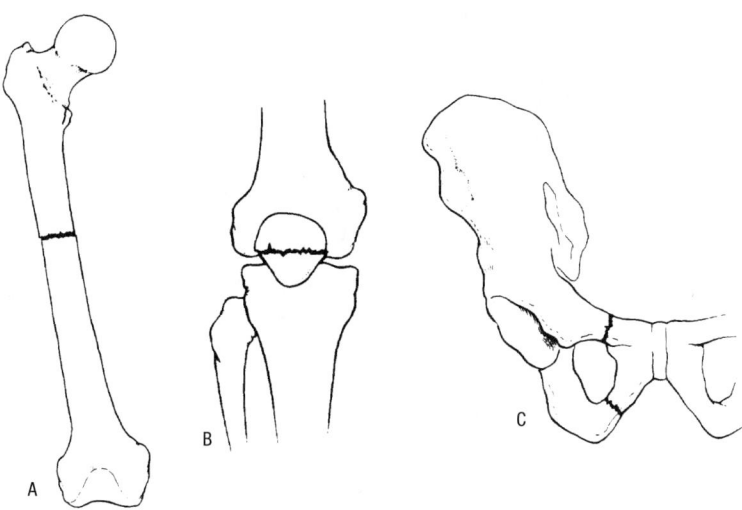

transverse fractures: (A) transverse fracture of the middle third of the femur; (B) transverse fracture of the midpatella; (C) transverse fracture of the superior and inferior pubic rami

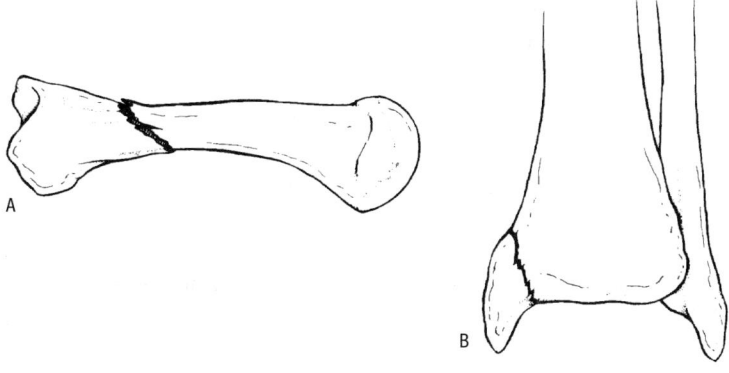

oblique fractures: (A) oblique fracture of the proximal third of metacarpal; (B) oblique fracture of the medial malleolus

spinal fractures

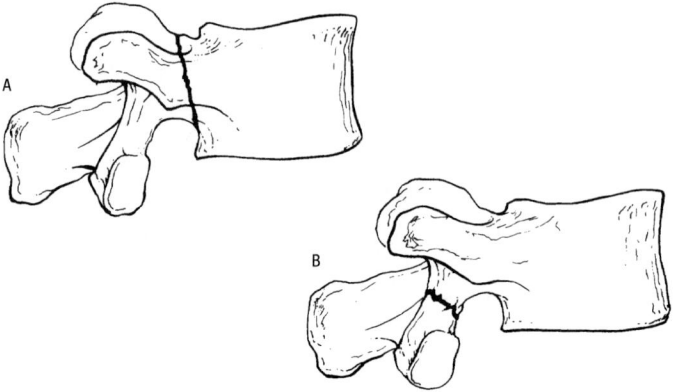

(A) fracture through the pedicle; (B) fracture through the pars interartricularis

shoulder fractures

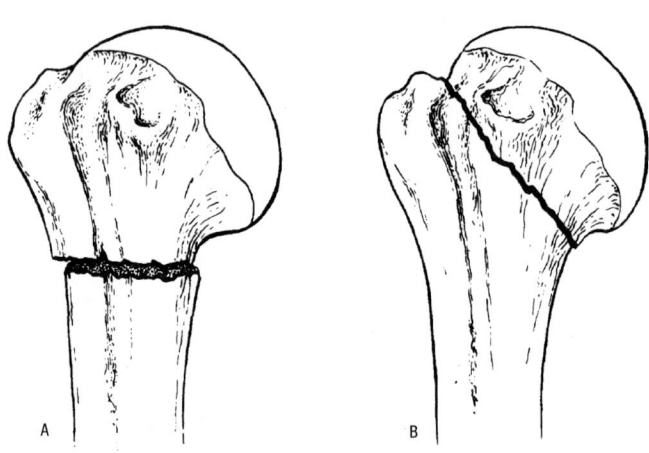

(A) transverse fracture of the surgical neck of the humerus; (B) fracture of the anatomic neck of the humerus

elbow fractures

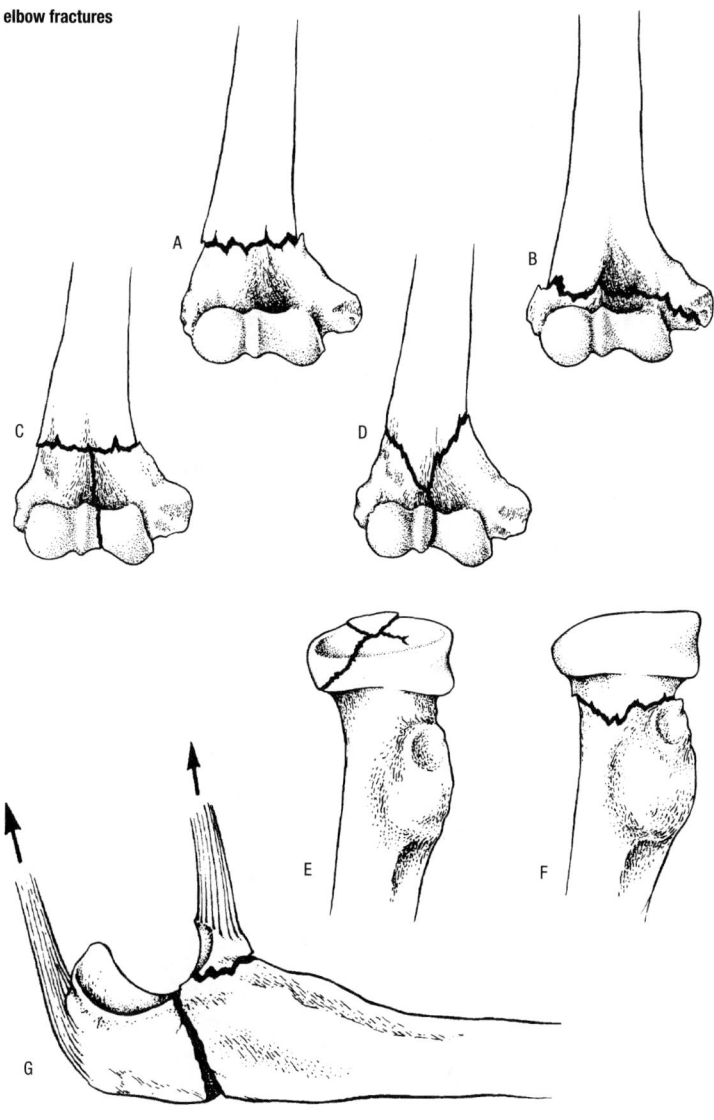

(A) supracondylar fractures are fractures that occur above the level of the condyles; (B) transcondylar fracture. note that the fracture extends through both condyles. comminuted intraarticular fractures of the distal humerus; (C) T-shaped fracture; (D) Y-shaped fracture; (E) comminuted fracture of the head of the radius; (F) transverse nondisplaced fracture of the neck of the radius; (G) fracture of the olecranon and coronoid process. muscle contraction can cause distraction of fracture fragments.

pelvic fractures

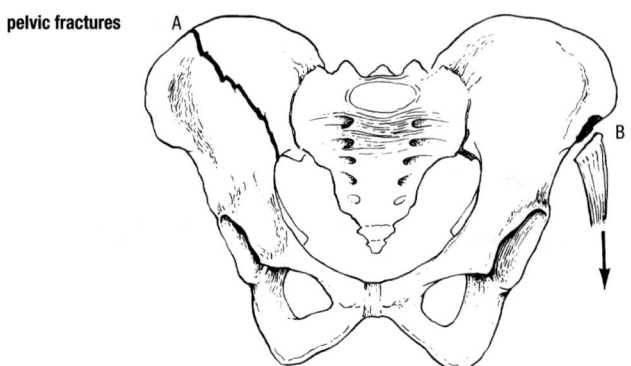

fractures of the ilium: (A) oblique fracture through the wind of the ilium; (B) avulsion fracture of the anteroinferior iliac spine

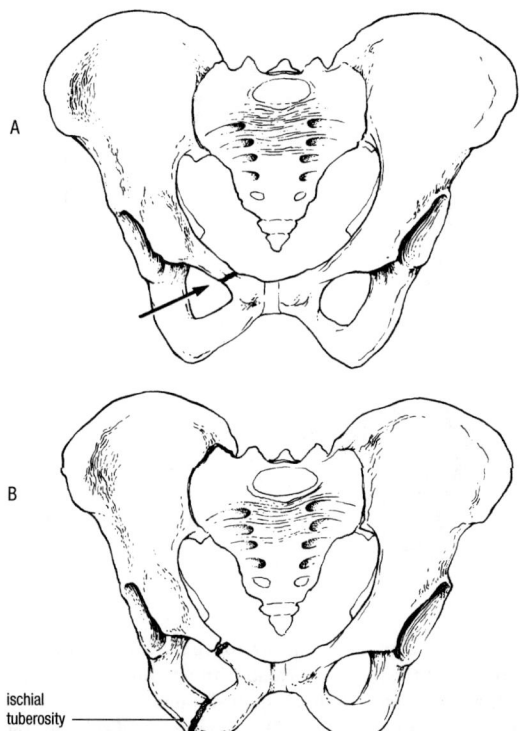

(A) oblique fracture of the superior pubic ramus; (B) transverse fractures of the inferior ischial ramus and superior pubic ramus

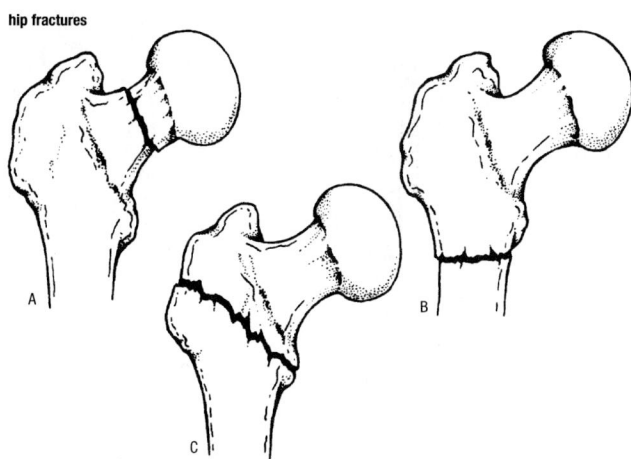

fractures of the hip described by the location in which they occur: (A) transverse intracapsular fracture; (B) oblique intertrochanteric fracture; (C) transverse subtrochanteric fracture

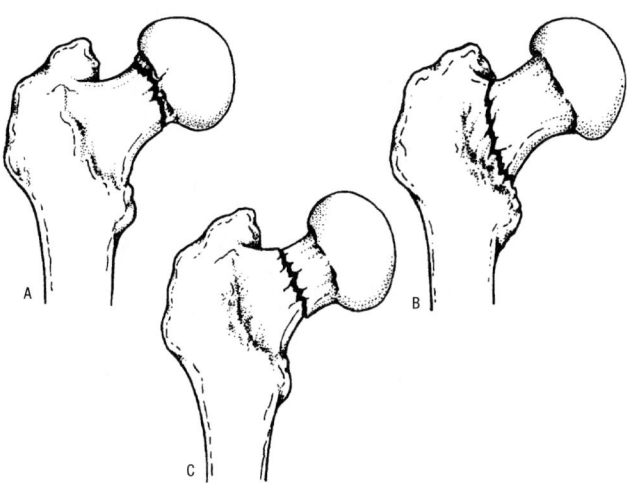

subclassification of intracapsular fractures: (A) subcapital fracture; (B) transcervical fracture; (C) base of neck fracture

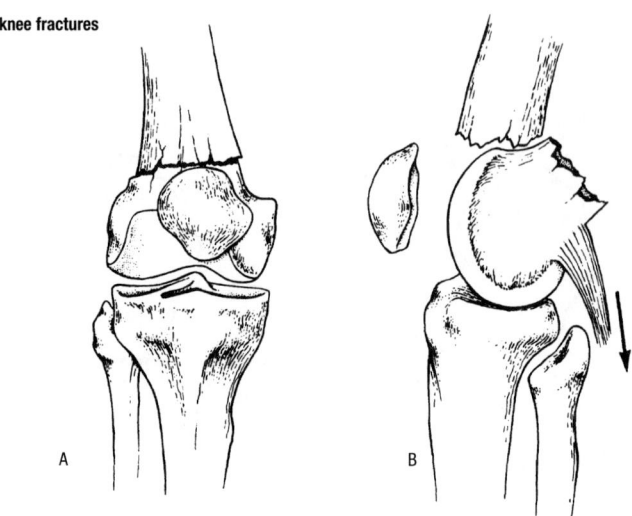

knee fractures

supracondylar fracture: transverse supracondylar fracture of the femur. note the pull of the gastrocnemius muscle, causing the distal fragment to be rotated posteriorly.

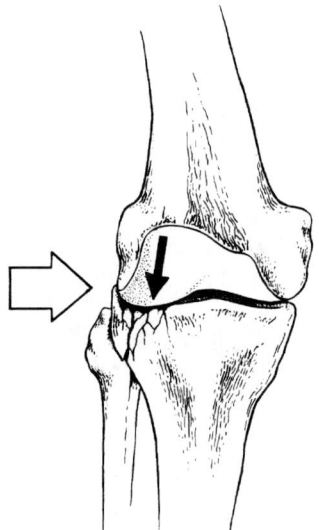

a valgus force applied to the knee causes the hard femoral condyle to be driven into the softer tibial plateau, resulting in depression of the tibial plateau

ankle fractures

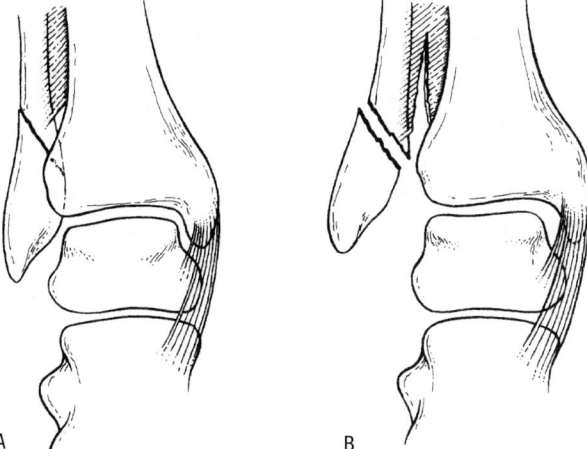

(A) fracture of the lateral malleolus occurring above its articular surface; thus, the ankle mortise is not involved; (B) similar fracture as in (A), above the articular surface with disturbance of the mortise is due to separation of the syndesmosis

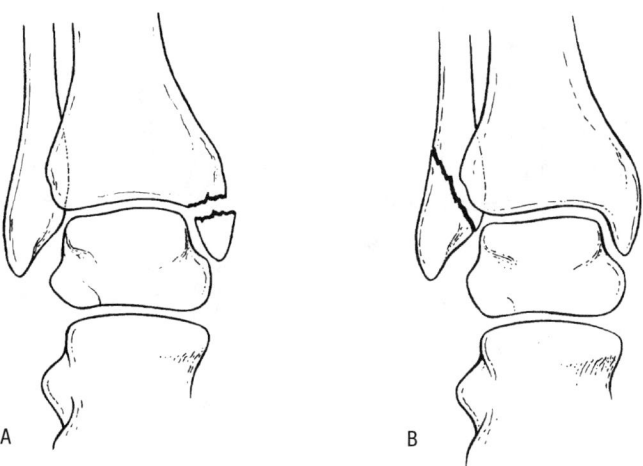

fractures of the malleoli: (A) transverse fracture of the medial malleolus; (B) oblique fracture of the lateral malleolus

ankle fractures

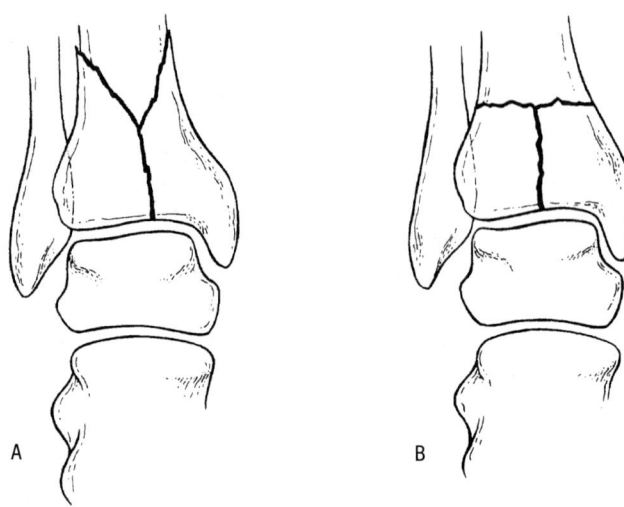

(A) Y-shaped comminuted intraarticular fracture of the distal tibia; (B) T-shaped comminuted in-traarticular fracture of the distal tibia

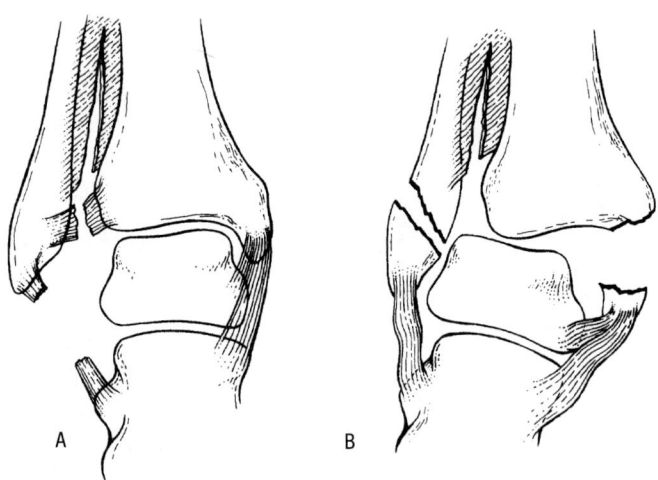

separation of the distal tibiofibular syndesmosis: (A) separation of the tibiofibular syndesmosis without an accompanying fracture; (B) separation of the syndesmosis associated with fracture of the medial and lateral malleoli

leg fractures

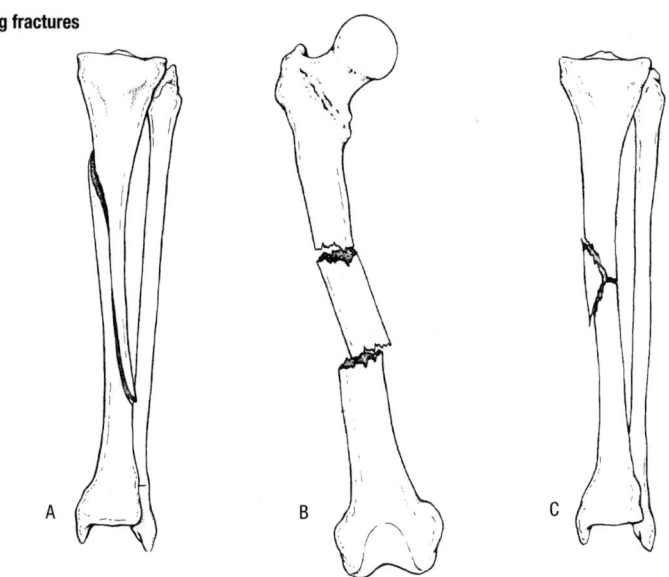

(A) spiral fractures of the middle third of the tibia; (B) segmental fracture of the femur; (C) butterfly fragment

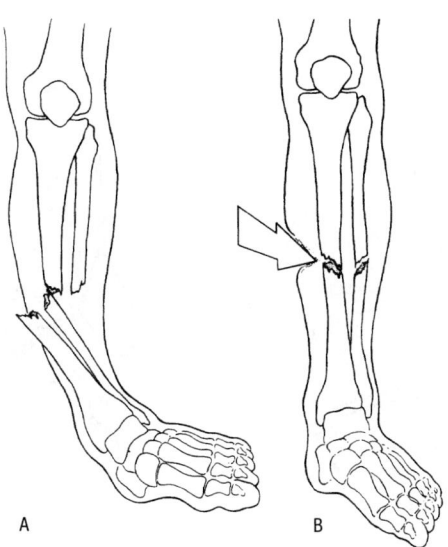

(A) compound fracture caused by an inside-out injury. the skin defect is caused, following the fracture, by the bone perforating the skin from within; (B) outside-in compound fracture. in this injury, the skin defect is produced by the fracturing agent entering from without.

ankle fractures

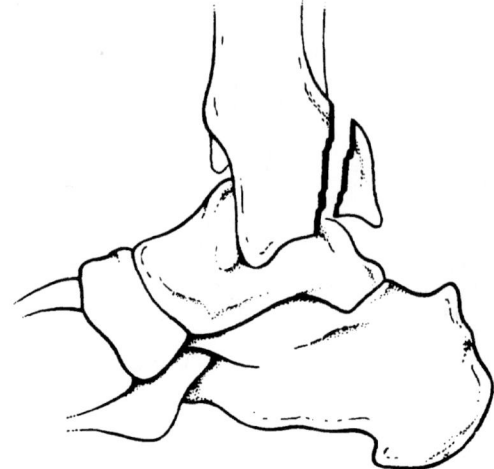

fracture of the posterior malleolus

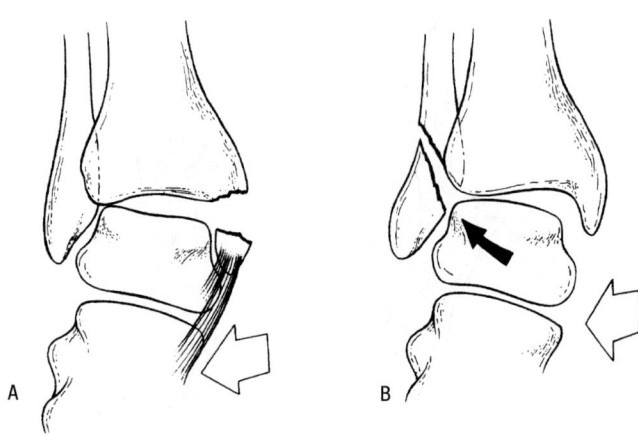

(A) avulsion fracture of the medial malleolus; (B) oblique fracture of the lateral malleolus

foot fractures

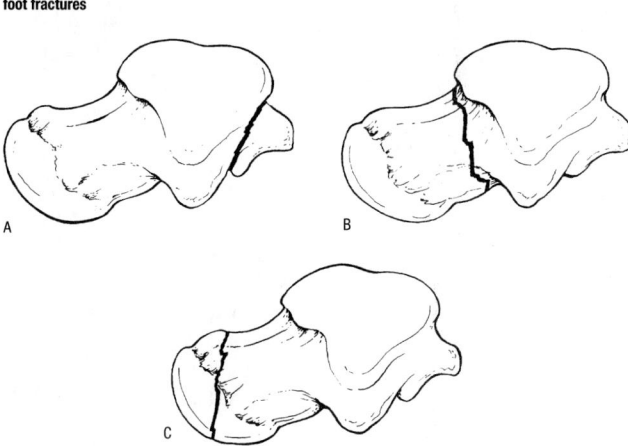

fractures of the talus can be described by the anatomic area involved; (A) fracture of the posterior process; (B) fracture of the body; (C) fracture of the head

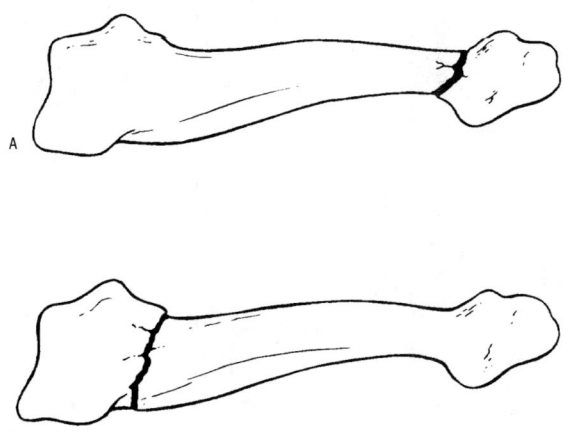

(A) fracture of the head of a metatarsal; (B) fracture of the base of a metatarsal bone.

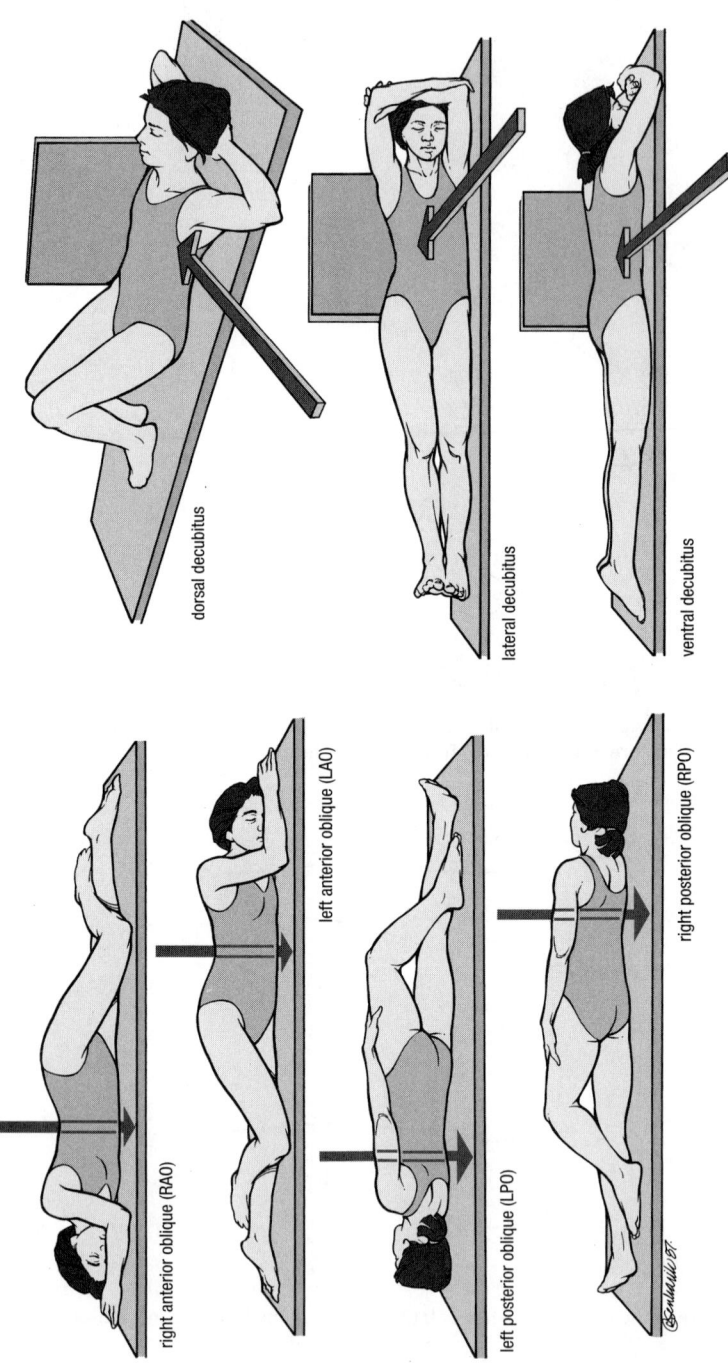

dorsal decubitus

lateral decubitus

ventral decubitus

right anterior oblique (RAO)

left anterior oblique (LAO)

left posterior oblique (LPO)

right posterior oblique (RPO)

patient positions

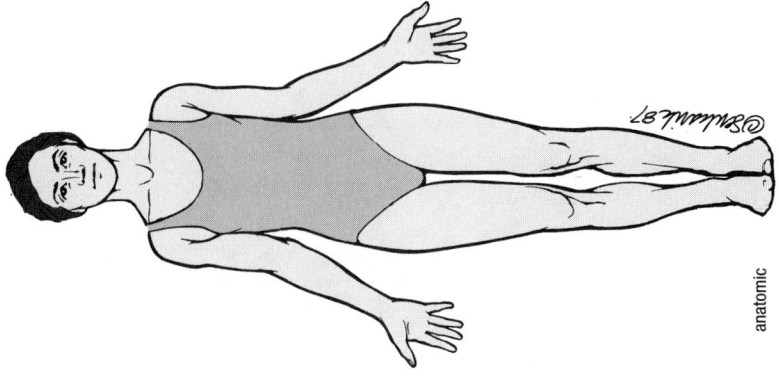

anatomic

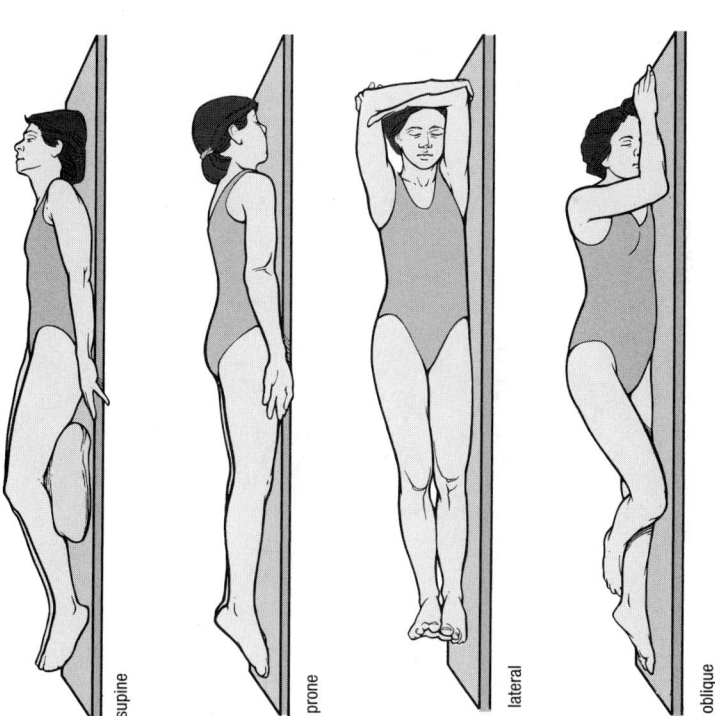

supine

prone

lateral

oblique

patient positions

A13

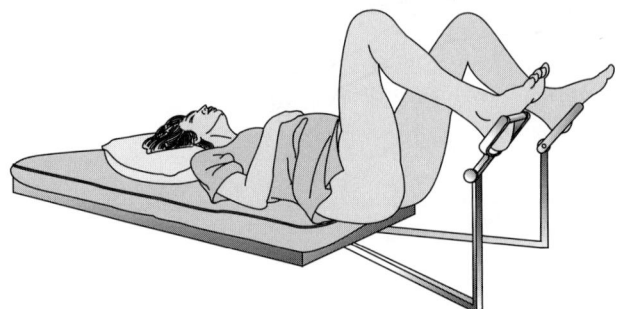

lithomy position, inferolateral view

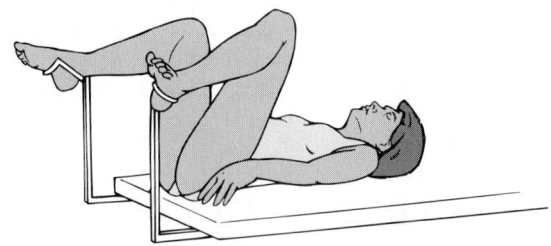

dorsal lithomy position

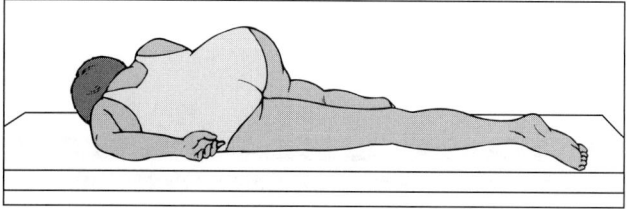

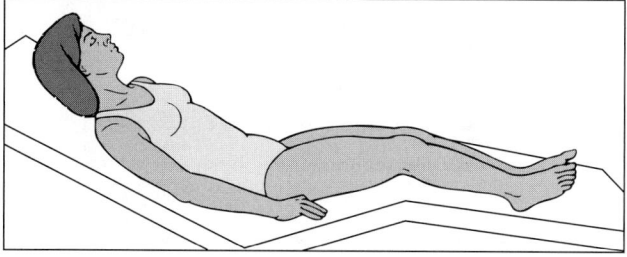

Fowler position

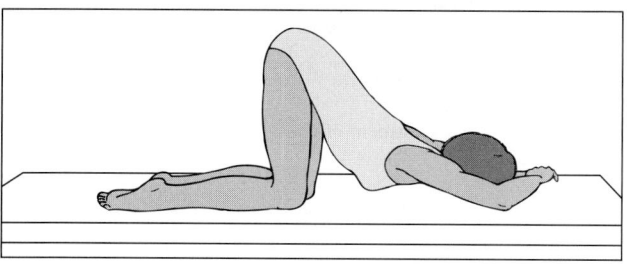

knee-chest position

Assessment of chest pain				
Ailment	**Character, location, and radiation**	**Duration**	**Precipitating conditions**	**Relieving measures**
angina pectoris	Substernal or retrosternal pain spreading across chest May radiate to inside of arm, neck, or jaws	5–15 min	Usually related to exertion, emotion, eating, cold	Rest, nitroglycerin, oxygen
myocardial infarction	Substernal pain or pain over precordium May spread widely throughout chest Painful disability of shoulders and hands may be present	>15 min	Occurs spontaneously but may be sequela to unstable angina	Morphine sulfate, successful reperfusion of blocked coronary artery
pericarditis	Sharp, severe substernal pain or pain to the left of stenum May be felt in epigastrium and may be referred to neck, arms, and back	Intermittent	Sudden onset Pain increases with inspiration, swallowing, coughing, and rotation of trunk	Sitting upright, analgesia, antiinflammatory medications
pulmonary pain	Pain arises from inferior portion of pleura May be referred to costal margins or upper abdomen Patient may be able to localize the pain	30+ min	Often occurs spontaneously Pain occurs or increases with inspiration	Rest, time Treatment of underlying cause, bronchodilation
esophageal pain (Hiatus hernia, reflux esophagitis, or spasm)	Substernal pain May be projected around chest to shoulders	5–60 min	Recumbency, cold liquids, exercise May occur spontaneously	Food, antacid Nitroglycerin relieves spasm
anxiety	Pain over left chest May be variable Does not radiate Patient may complain of numbness and tingling of hands and mouth	2–3 min	Stress, emotional tachypnea	Removal of stimulus, relaxation

assessment of chest pain

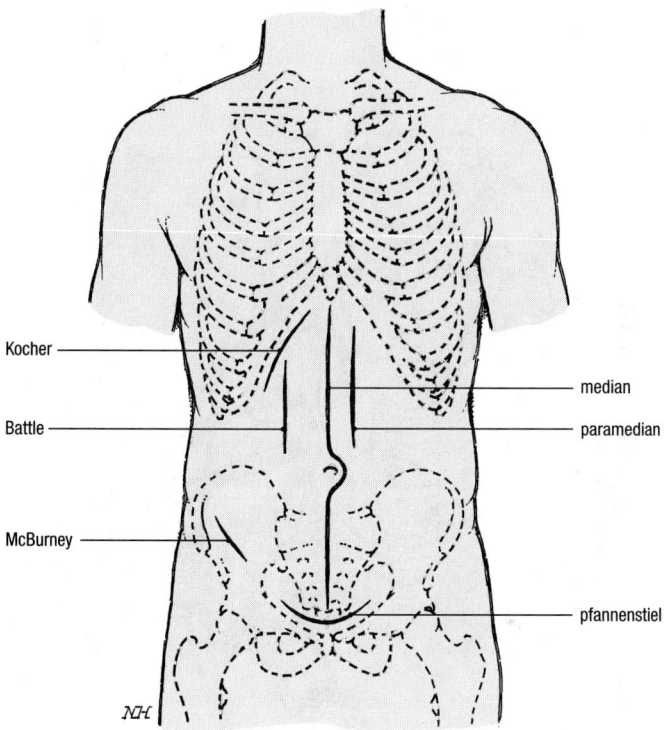

Kocher

Battle

McBurney

median

paramedian

pfannenstiel

surgical incisions

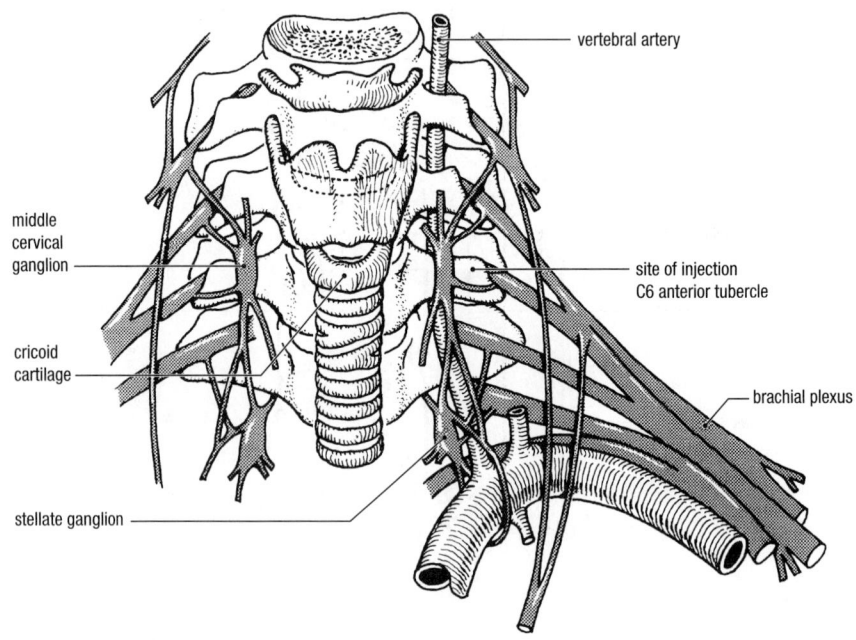

vertebral artery

middle
cervical
ganglion

site of injection
C6 anterior tubercle

cricoid
cartilage

brachial plexus

stellate ganglion

site of injection for the C6 paratracheal approach to the stellate ganglion block

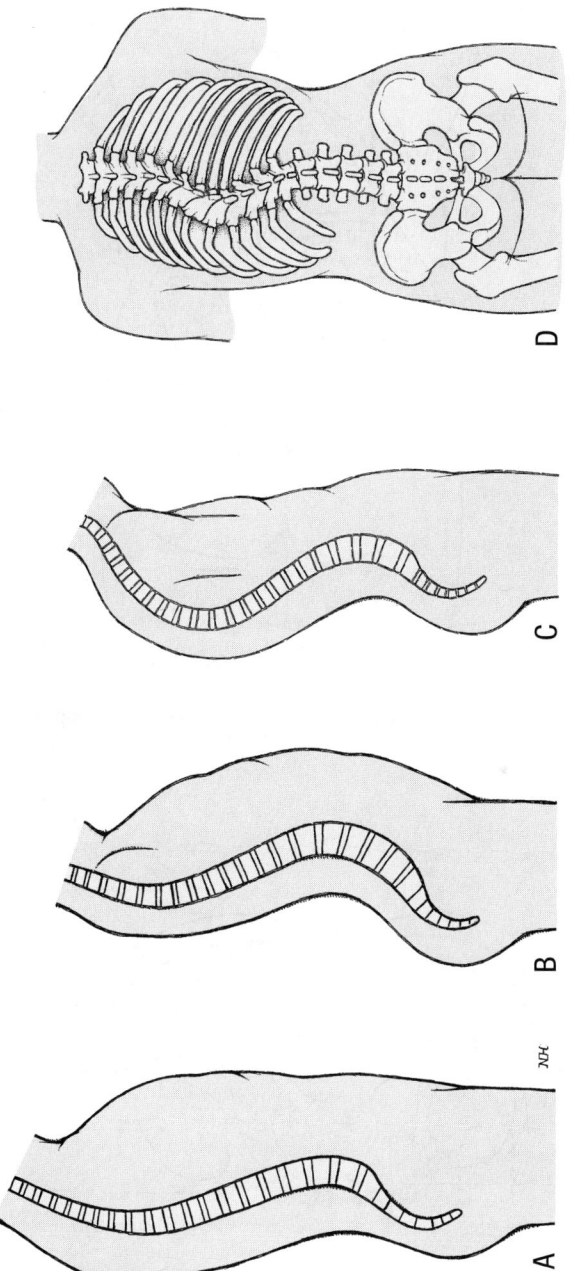

spinal curvatures: (A) normal; (B) lordosis; (C) kyphosis; (D) scoliosis

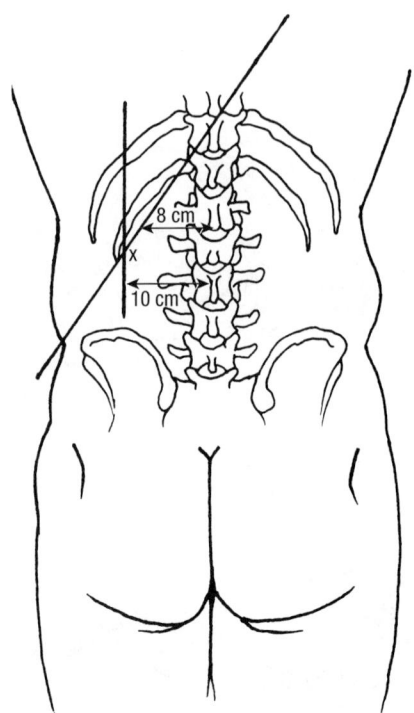

8 cm

x

10 cm

landmarks for the lumbar sympathetic block (L2 paravertebral approach)

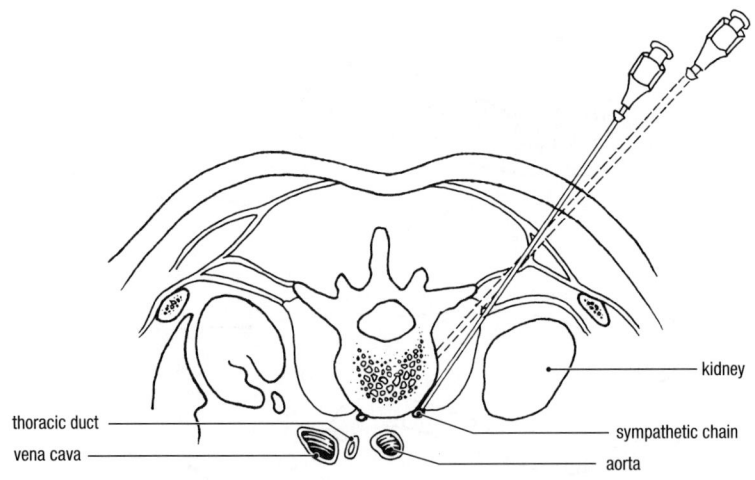

kidney

thoracic duct

sympathetic chain

vena cava

aorta

initial and final needle position for the lumbar sympathetic block

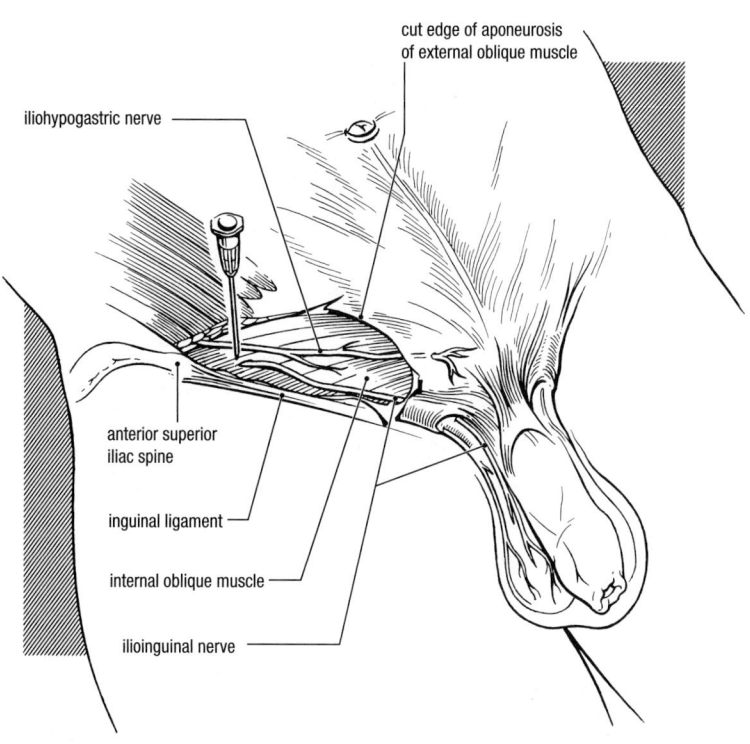

ilioinguinal and iliohypogastric nerve block

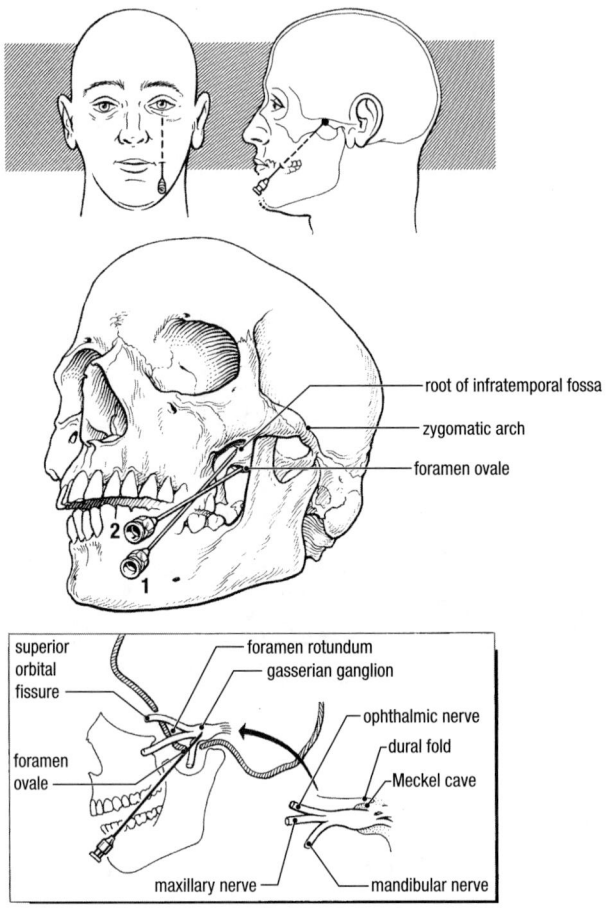

root of infratemporal fossa

zygomatic arch

foramen ovale

superior orbital fissure

foramen rotundum

gasserian ganglion

ophthalmic nerve

dural fold

Meckel cave

foramen ovale

maxillary nerve

mandibular nerve

gasserian ganglion block: top panel: needle is inserted in the cheek about 1 cm posterior to the angle of the mouth as shown and directed toward the pupil in the anterior view and the midpoint of the zygoma in the lateral view. in patients with teeth, needle insertion in the cheek is superficial to the teeth of the upper jaw. in edentulous patients, this may lie a variable distance between the angle of the mouth and the line midway between upper lip and nose. a palpating finger in the mouth helps to prevent needle penetration into the mouth. middle panel: (1) as the needle is advanced into the infratemporal fossa, it will usually strike the roof of the infratemporal fossa initially; this is the correct depth to seek the foramen ovale; (2) the needle is then directed slightly posteriorly to obtain a mandibular nerve (V3) paresthesia. lower panel: the needle can then be advanced through the foramen ovale into the middle cranial fossa, where it will be adjacent to the gasserian ganglion, as shown. note the relationships of the dural fold and Meckel cave, containing cerebrospinal fluid. a needle advanced too far through the foramen ovale can enter the Meckel cave, and subsequent injections could enter the cranial CSF and produce total spine anesthesia.

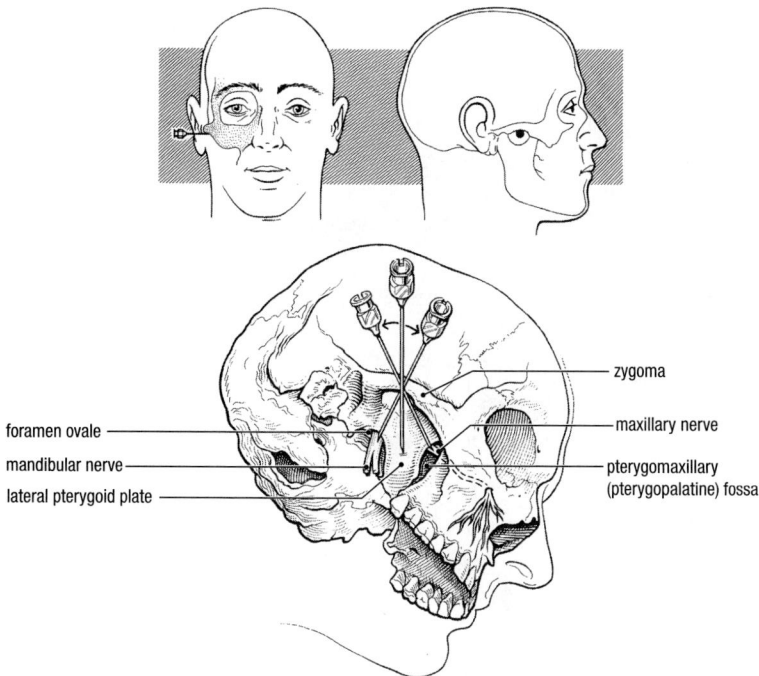

gasserian ganglion block

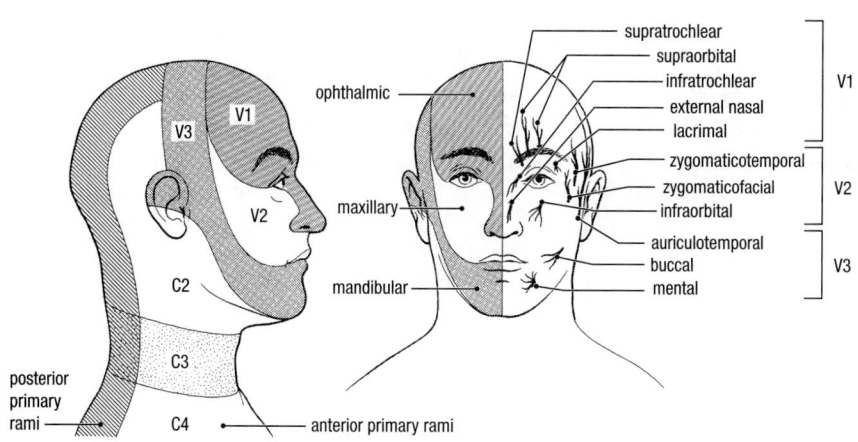

dermatomes and cutaneous nerves of head, neck, and face

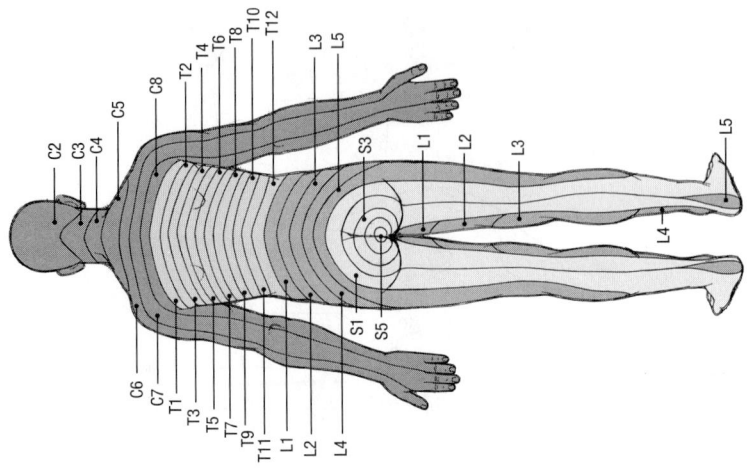

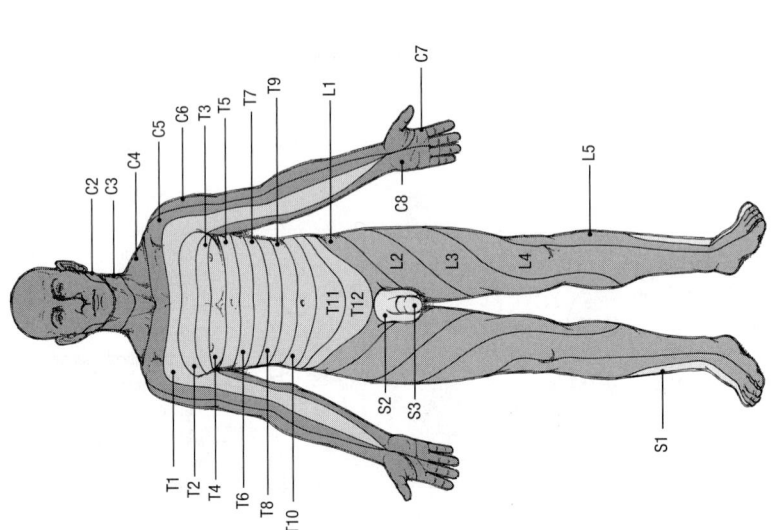

dermatomes

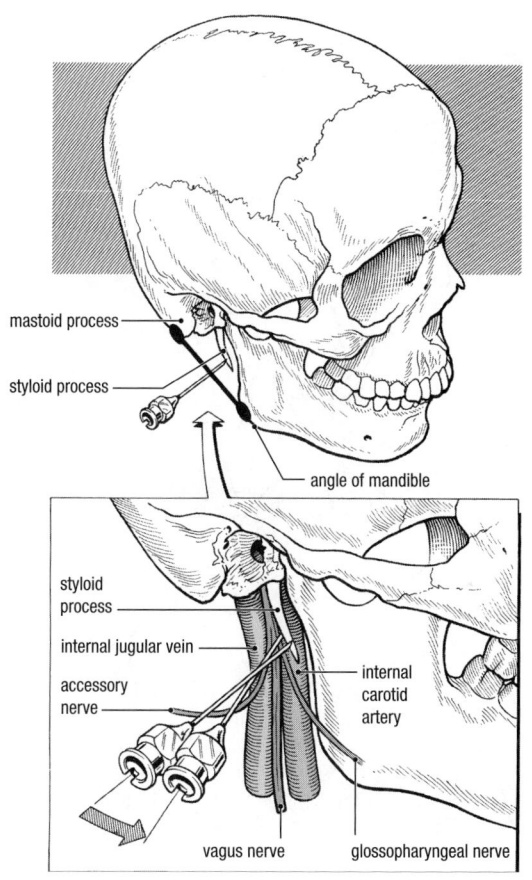

mastoid process

styloid process

angle of mandible

styloid process

internal jugular vein

accessory nerve

internal carotid artery

vagus nerve

glossopharyngeal nerve

glossopharyngeal nerve block

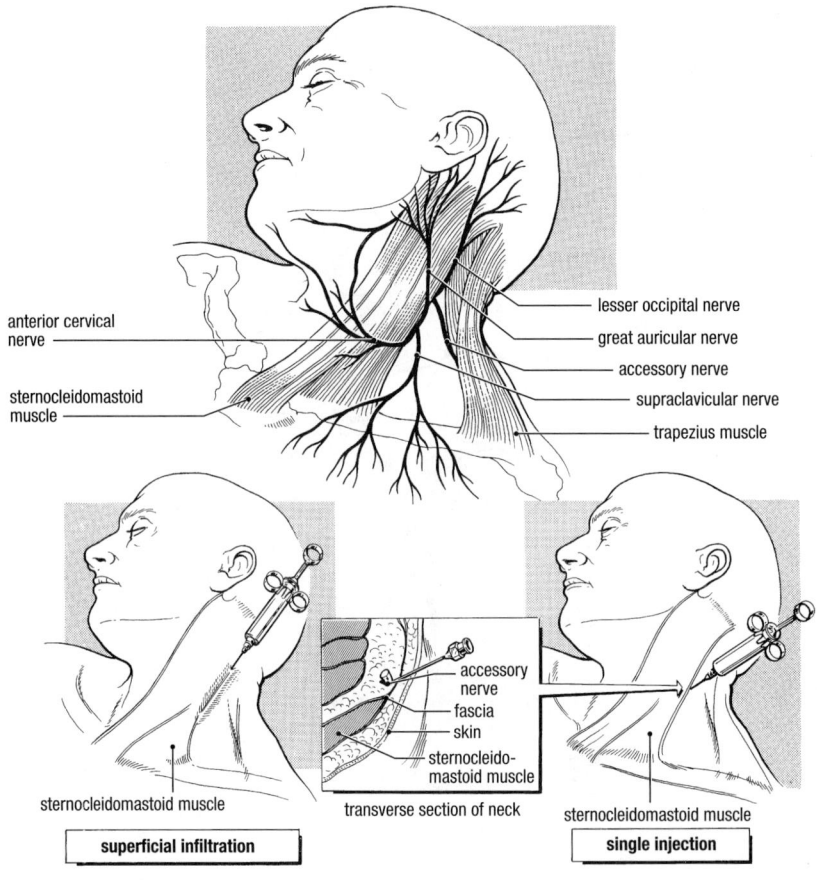

anterior cervical nerve

sternocleidomastoid muscle

lesser occipital nerve

great auricular nerve

accessory nerve

supraclavicular nerve

trapezius muscle

sternocleidomastoid muscle

superficial infiltration

accessory nerve

fascia

skin

sternocleido-mastoid muscle

transverse section of neck

sternocleidomastoid muscle

single injection

the superficial cervical plexus, which is blocked in the posterior triangle of the neck as it emerges adjacent to the midpoint of the posterior border of the sternocleidomastoid muscle

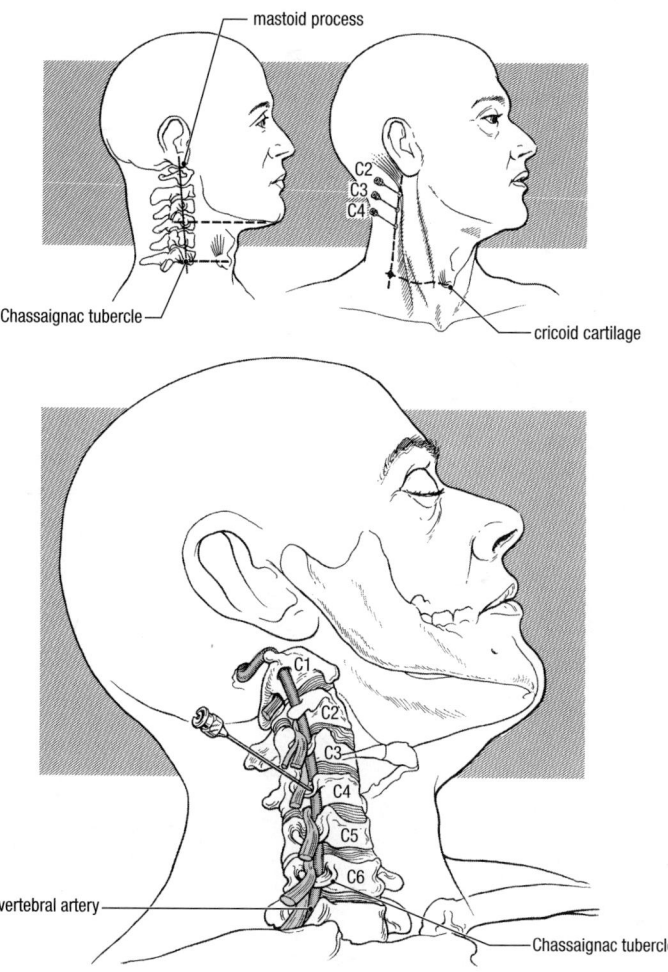

deep cervical plexus block

3-part illustration showing the regions affected by 3 types of anesthesia: (left) general, (middle) regional, and (right) peripheral

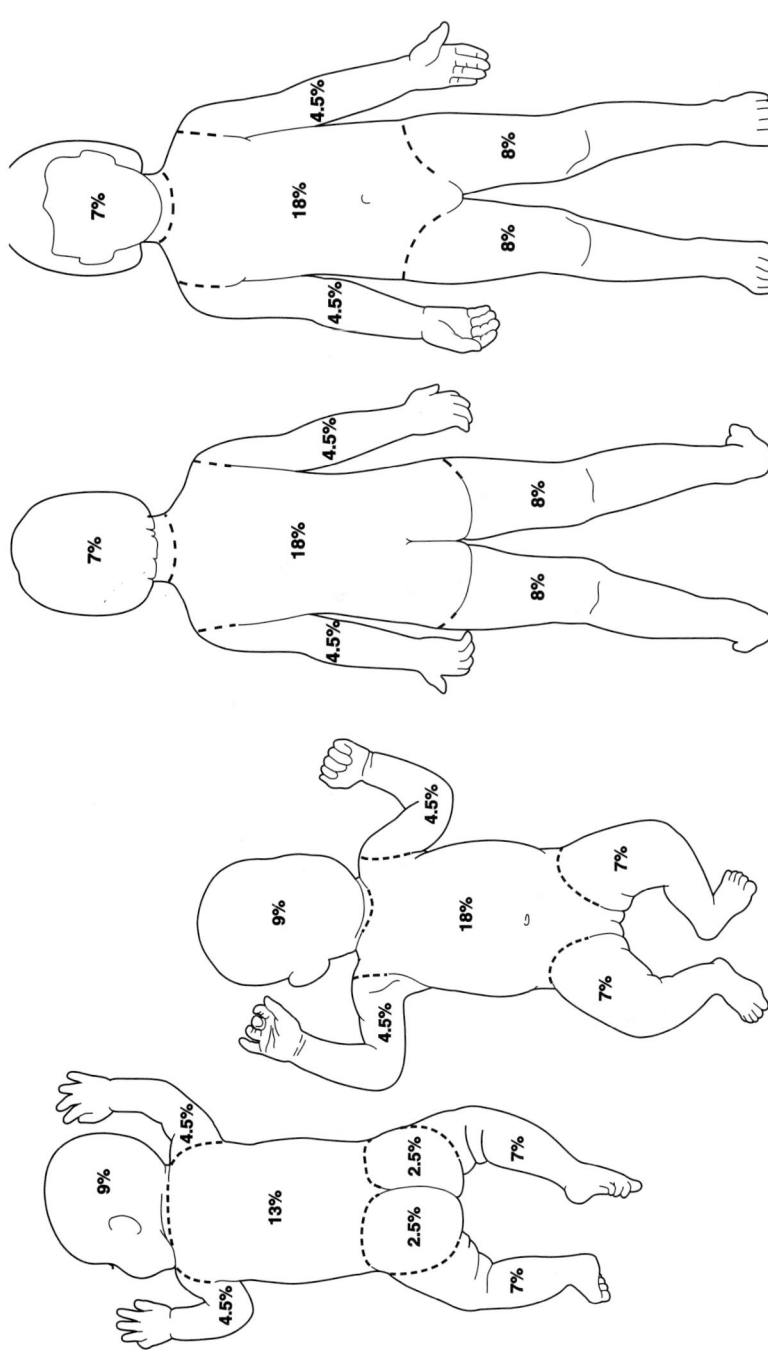

rule of nines (child, 5–9 years): outline of child's body with areas and percentages indicated to calculate total burn surface area

rule of nines (infant): outline of infant's body with areas and percentages indicated to calculate total burn surface area

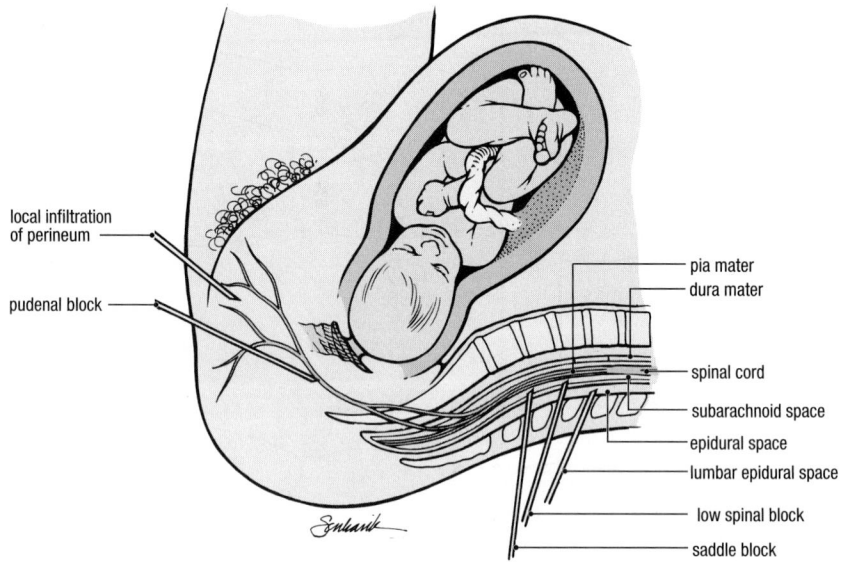

local infiltration
of perineum

pudenal block

pia mater
dura mater

spinal cord

subarachnoid space

epidural space

lumbar epidural space

low spinal block

saddle block

regional anesthesia for chid birth, sites of injection

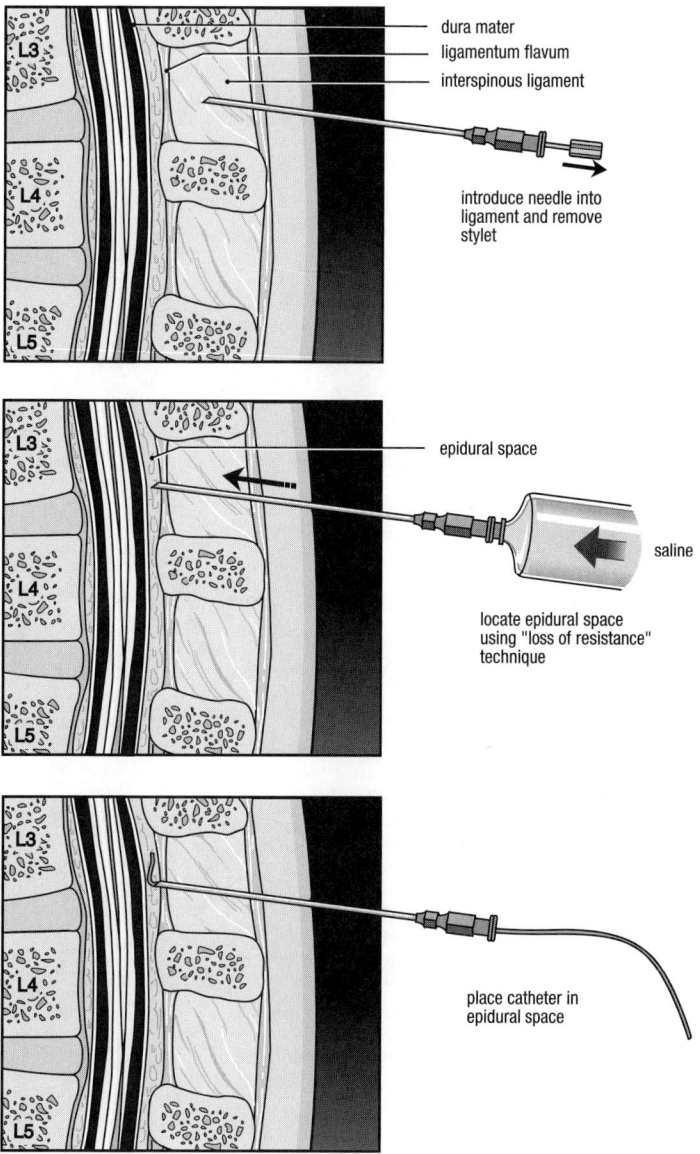

3-step illustration showing the procedure used in giving an epidural

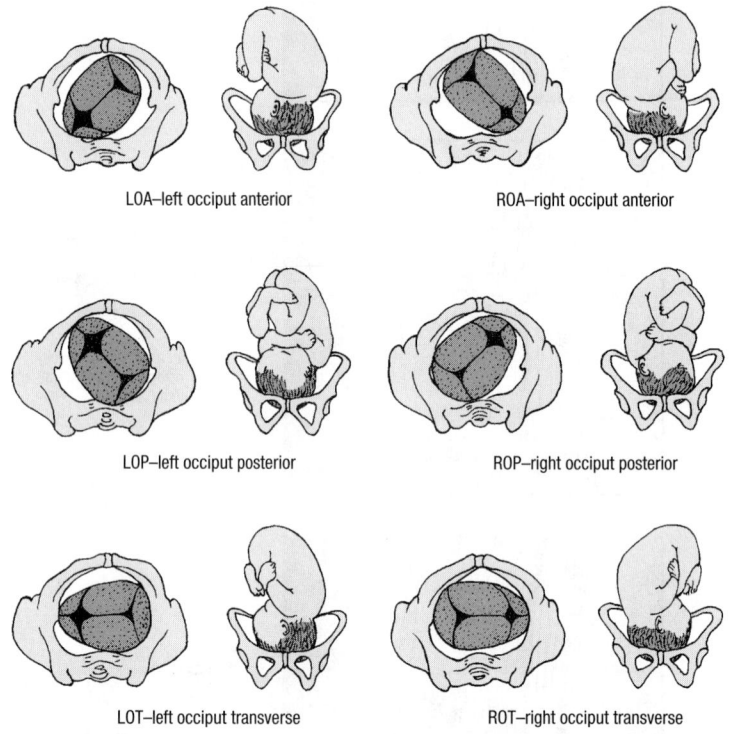

LOA–left occiput anterior

ROA–right occiput anterior

LOP–left occiput posterior

ROP–right occiput posterior

LOT–left occiput transverse

ROT–right occiput transverse

vertex presentation: fetal head positions within the pelvic girdle in a vertex presentation

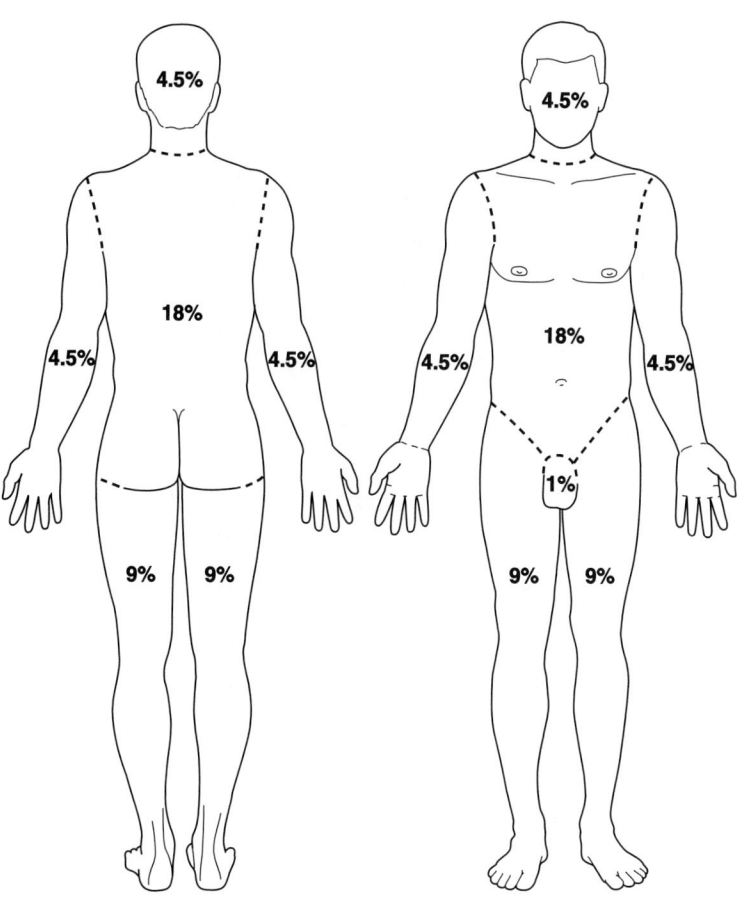

rule of nines (adult): outline of adult's body with areas and percentages indicated to calculate total burn surface area

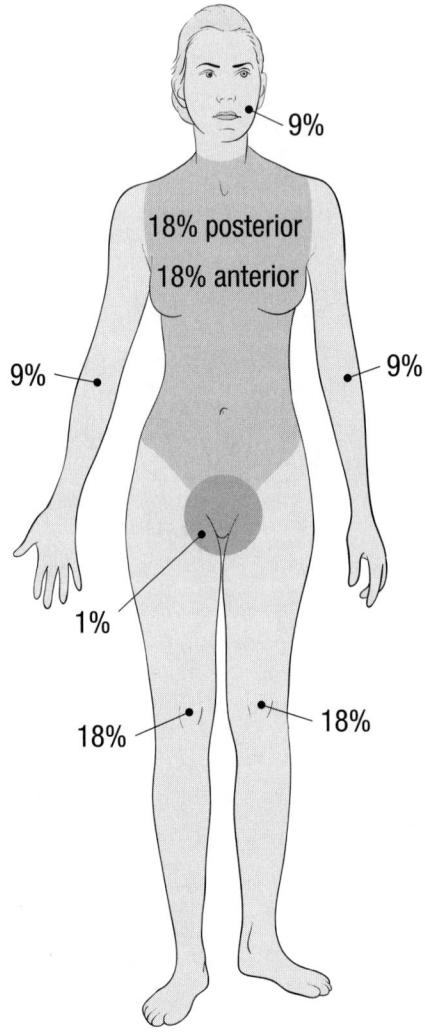

adult female illustrating the rule of nines used when assessing burn damage to various body parts

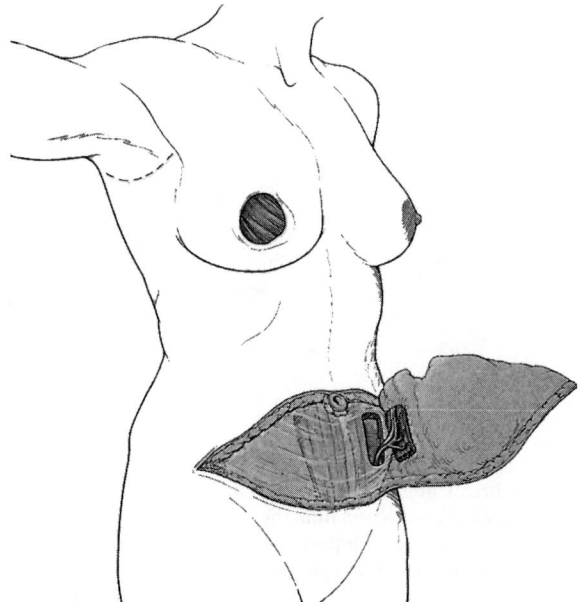

concept of the skin-sparing mastectomy by using the periareolar approach: in this case, the depicted free TRAM flap is based on the deep inferior epigastric artery and vein

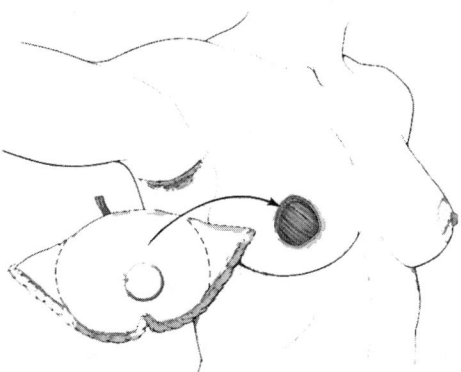

the flap is then passed through the periareolar incision, with the microvascular anastomoses performed through small separate axillary incision

A35

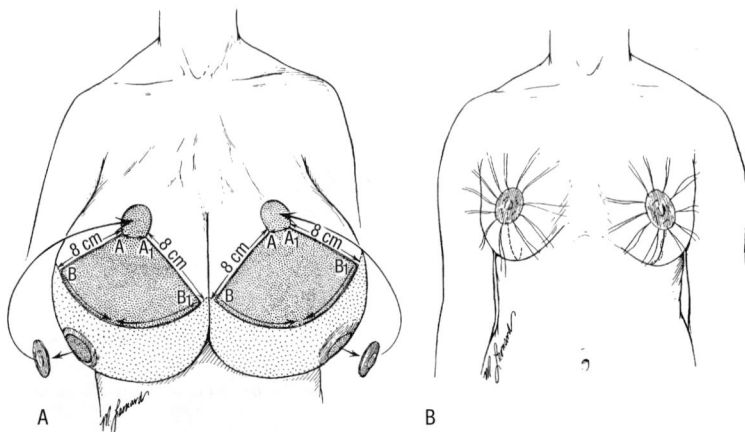

(A) the width of the breast amputation and dermal pedicle may vary depending on the size of each breast. The nipple-areolas are excised from the breast tissue specimen; (B) the position of the new nipple-areola site is determined with the patient in a semi-upright position and the nipple-areola specimen placed on the dermal base as a free graft

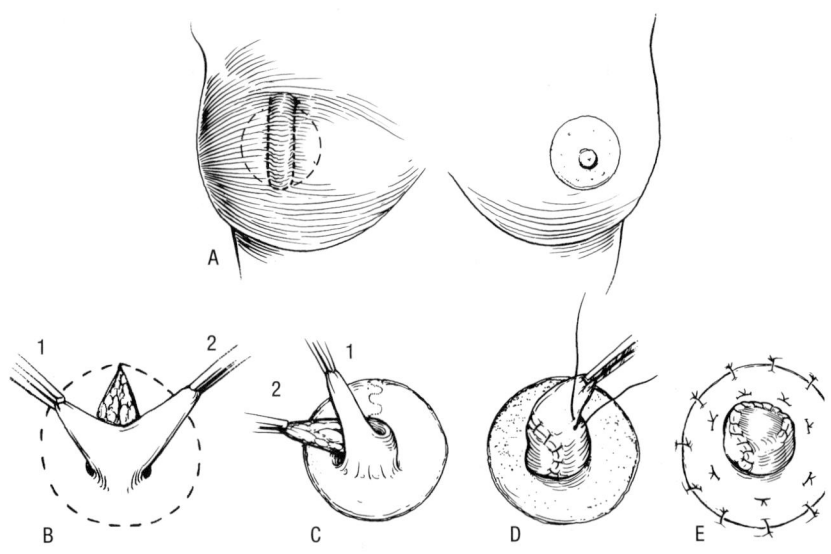

(A) the redundant area of a TRAM flap is marked for the position of a new areola; (B) flaps 1 and 2 are elevated utilizing the redundant TRAM flap tissue; (C) flaps 1 and 2 are now interpolated; (D) the position of new flaps 1 and 2. the surrounding area is deepithelialized; (E) the newly reconstructed nipple and full-thickness skin graft

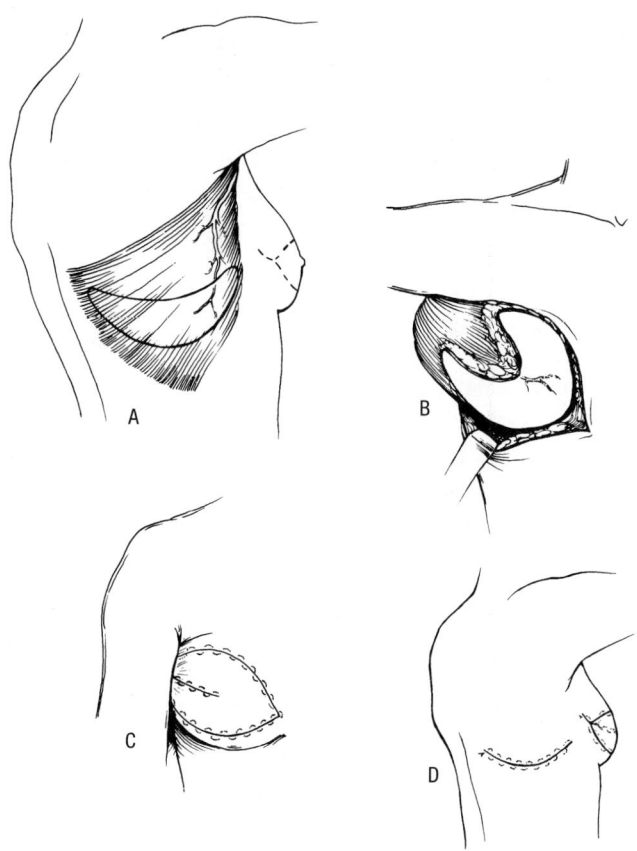

(A) the latissimus myocutaneous flap outline; (B) myocutaneous flap being transferred beneath a lateral axillary skin bridge; (C) transferred flap in its new position; (D) location of the final incisions

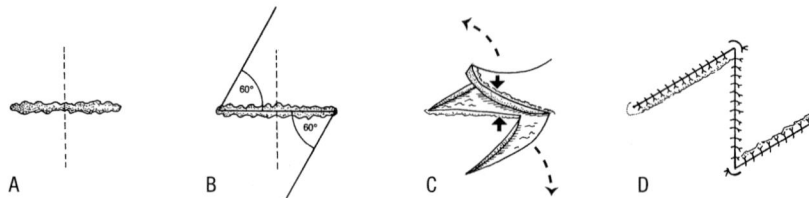

the classic Z-plasty: (A) a thick, contracted scar crosses a skin fold. design is begun by drawing a perpendicular line at the midpoint of the scar; this line helps establish flap incisions, but it is not itself incised; (B) completing the design, the limbs of flaps are equal to each other and to the length of the scar. angles of the flaps are 60°; (C) flaps are elevated, preserving the subdermal plexus. undermining is accomplished around flap bases. the scar is excised unless it is too wide; here a portion of the scar is left for clarity in showing flap transposition; (D) flaps are transposed and sutured. a 3-corner suture (half-buried horizontal mattress) is used to anchor narrow tips, avoiding necrosis that could result from simple sutures near tips.

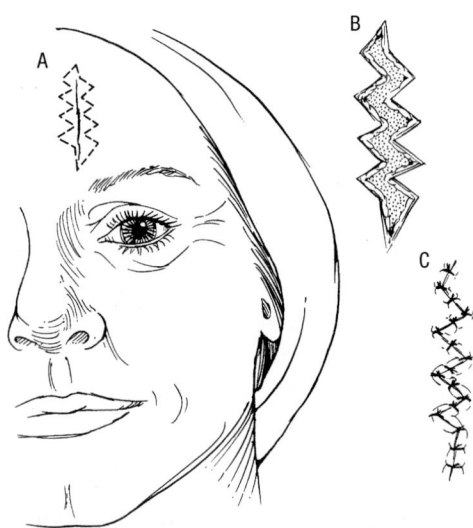

the W-plasty: (A) dotted lines show the design for the excision of the scar; (B) flaps have now been developed and are ready for interdigitation; (C) the W-flaps are in position

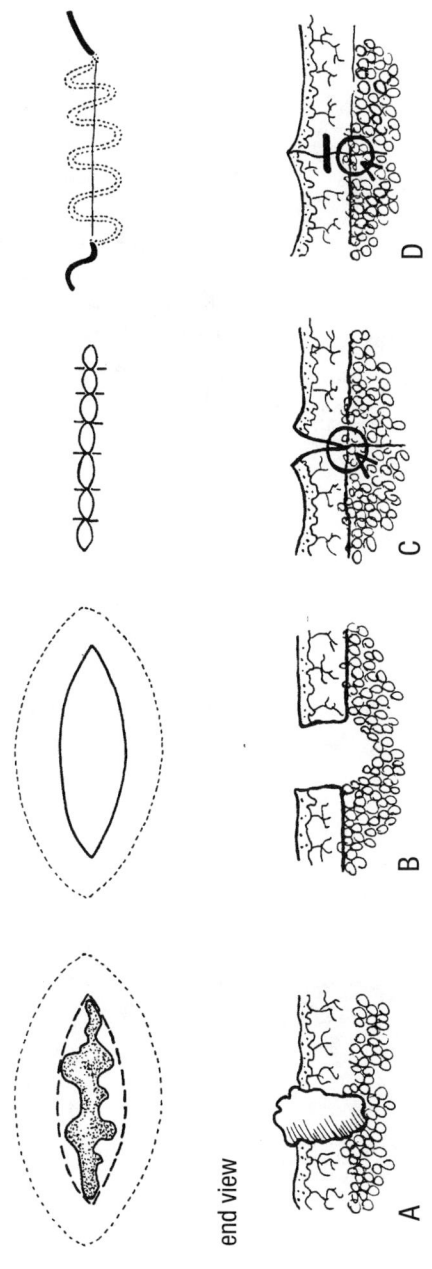

end view

linear scar revision: (A) outline for planned repair; (B) excision and undermining; (C) deep layer closure. the end view shows that the wound should be almost fully closed. (D) final closure, buried running subcuticular Prolene. the top view shows suture weaving back and forth across wound in dermis, piercing the epidermis only at each end. the thickness of the suture is exaggerated for clarity.

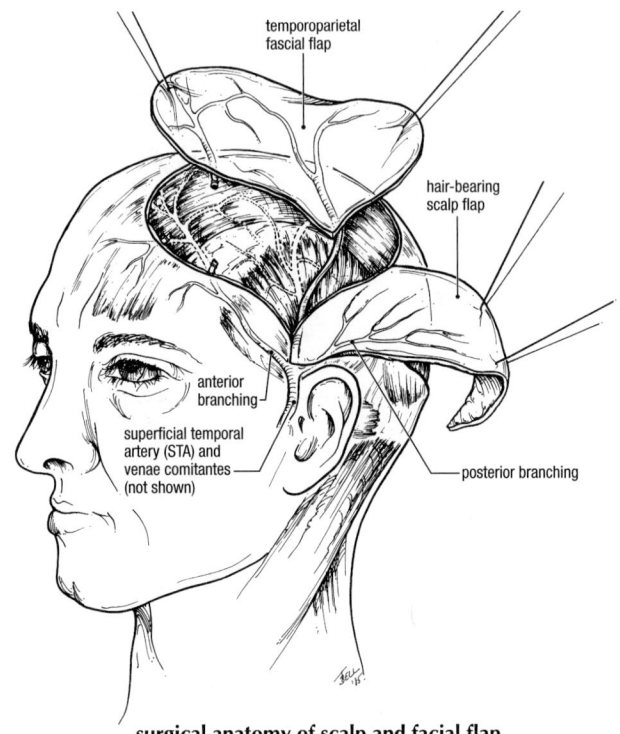

surgical anatomy of scalp and facial flap

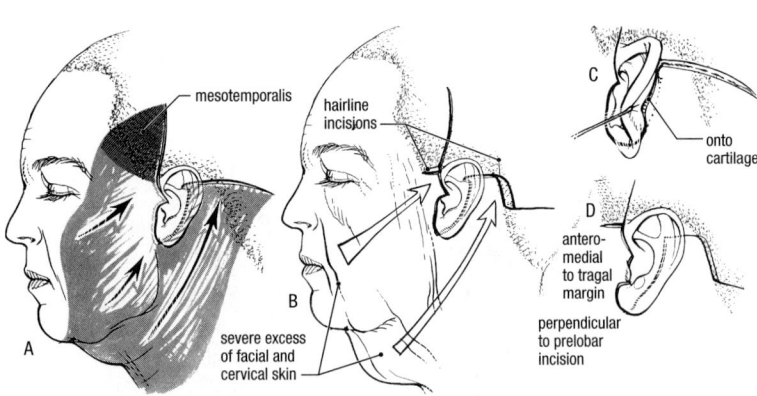

classic facelift incisions: (A) areas of incision; (B) hairline incisions; (C) postauricular incision for re-drape; (D) retrotragal approach for redrape

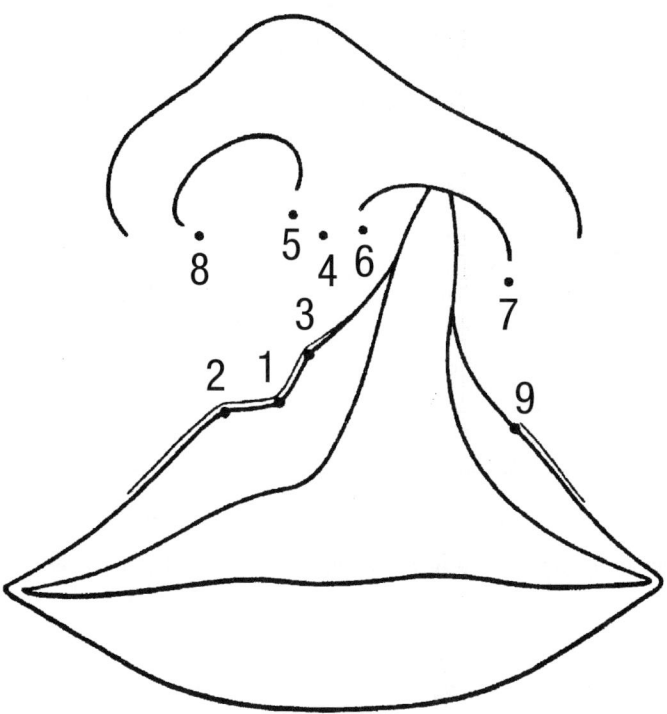

anatomy of the normal and unrepaired unilateral cleft lip indicating key points used for planning repair: (1) lowest point in arch of Cupid's bow, midline of the lip; (2) peak of Cupid's bow on the noncleft side; (3) proposed peak of Cupid's bow; (4) midpoint of the columella; (5, 6) base of columella laterally; (7, 8) inset of alar base into nostril sill; (9) a point on the well-developed vermilion cutaneous roll of the lateral lip and the same horizontal plane as the peak of Cupid's bow on the noncleft side

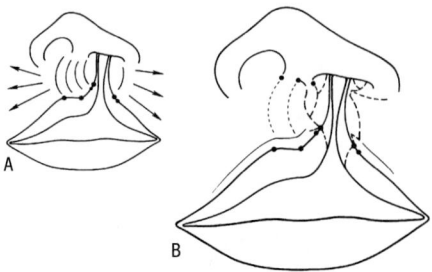

cleft lip repair: (A) unrepaired cleft lip stresses; (B) incorporating stresses into repair

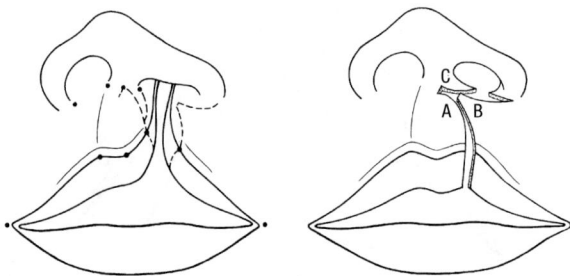

rotation advancement flap technique: (A) medial lip element; (B) lateral lip element; (C) small medial flap

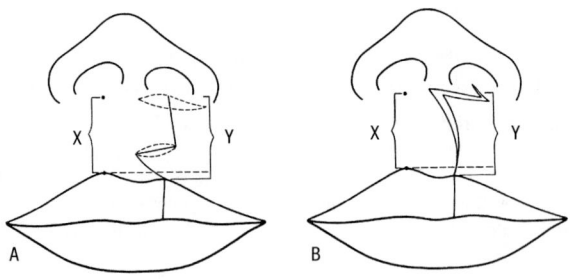

cleft lip redo surgery: (A) previous triangular or quadrangular repair flap; (B) rotation advancement flap redo technique

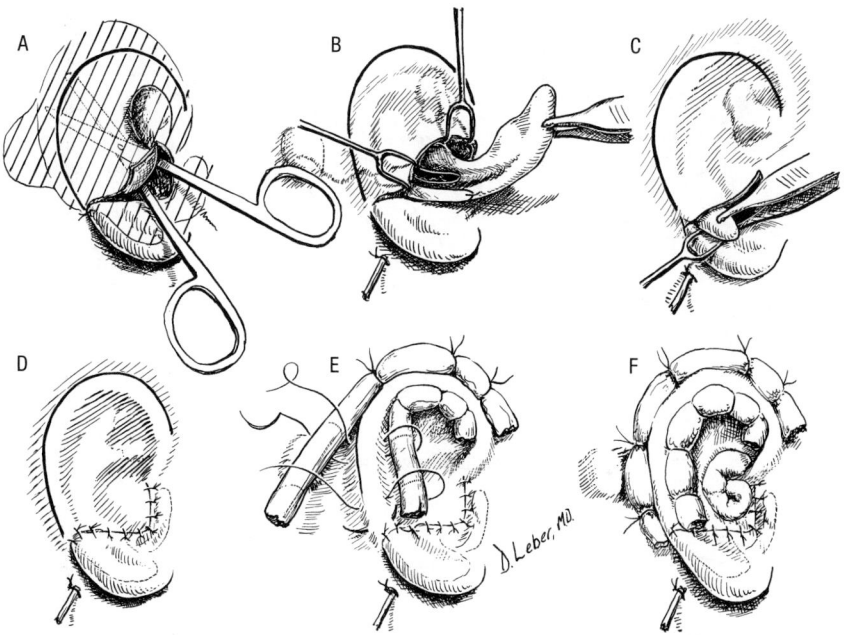

otoplasty techniques: (A) preparing subcutaneous pocket; (B) placing cartilage graft material; (C) incorporating helix; (D) separate placement of tragal material; external sutures; (E) stent placement for external shaping; (F) conchal floor pressure dressing

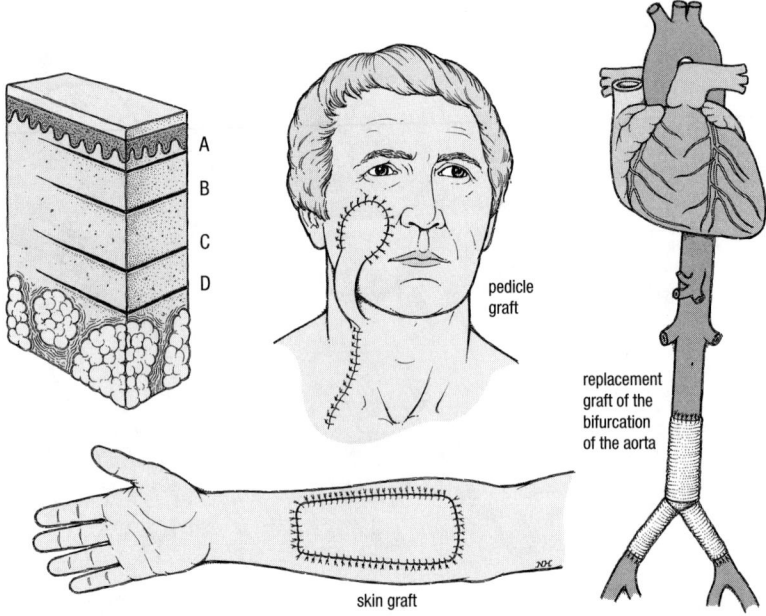

A
B
C
D

pedicle
graft

replacement
graft of the
bifurcation
of the aorta

skin graft

graft types: (A,B,C) split-thickness grafts; (D) full-thickness graft

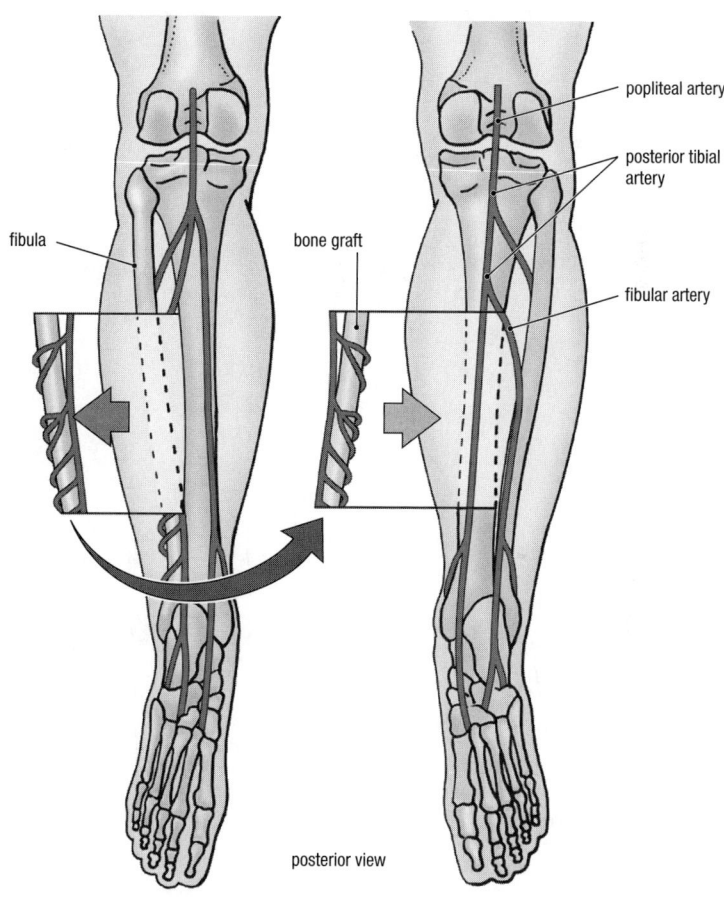

bone grafts: the fibula is a common source of bone for grafting

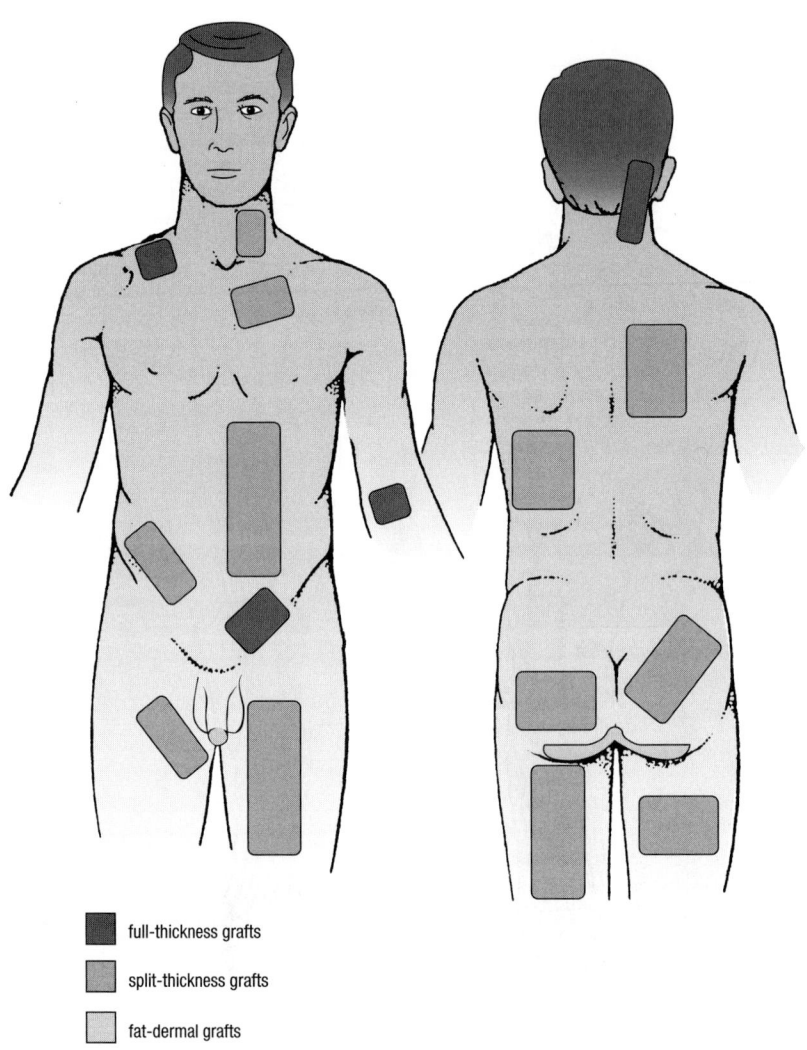

common donor skin graft sites: dark gray skin areas are appropriate for full-thickness grafts; medium gray areas are used for split-thickness grafts, and light gray sites are used for fat-dermal grafts

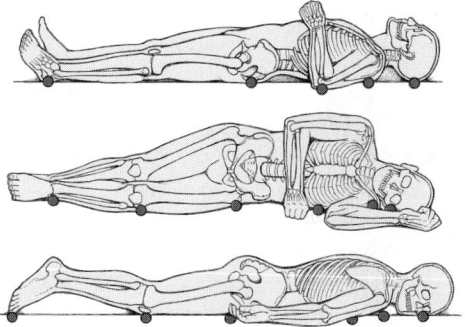

decubitus ulcer: dots indicate most common sites due to proximity of bone to skin

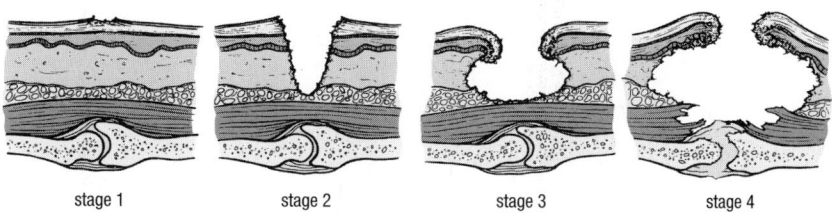

cross-section of skin showing 4 stages of pressure sore and ulcer classification: stage 1: inflammation, redness of epidermis; stage 2: loss of epidermis, damage to dermis; stage 3: involvement of subcutaneous tissue; stage 4: damage to tendon, muscle and bone

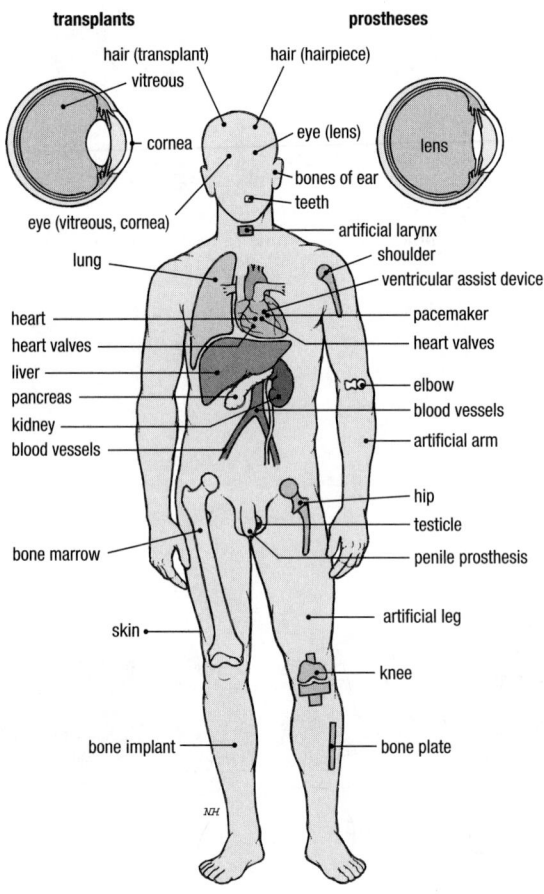

transplants and prostheses

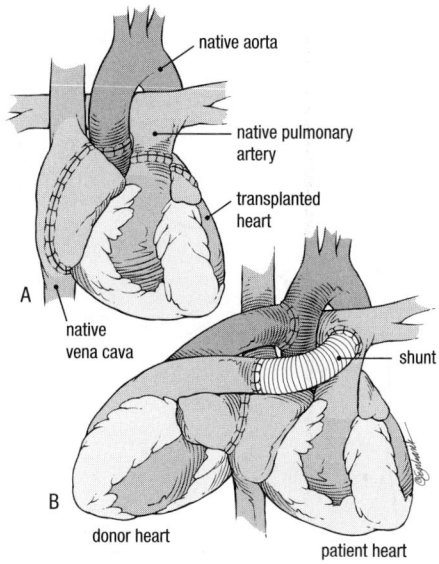

native aorta

native pulmonary artery

transplanted heart

native vena cava

shunt

donor heart

patient heart

heart transplantation: (A) orthotopic method; (B) heterotopic method

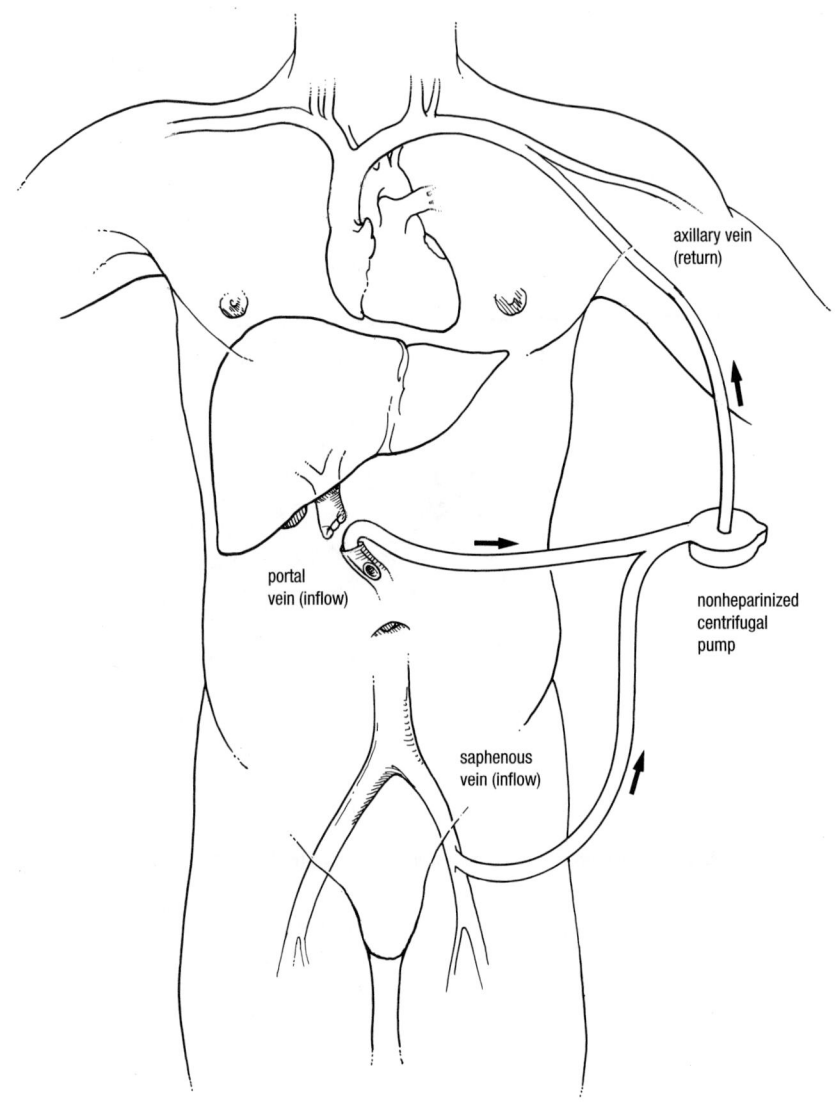

venous bypass: the portal vein is divided and cannulated, and a second cannula is placed into the inferior vena cava. the blood is pumped in a nonheparinized system and returned to the patient via cannula in the axillary vein.

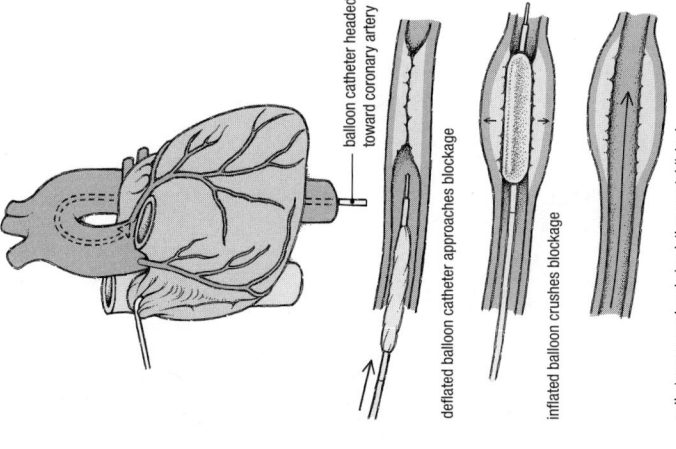

balloon catheter headed
toward coronary artery

deflated balloon catheter approaches blockage

inflated balloon crushes blockage

catheter removed and circulation reestablished

percutaneous transluminal angioplasty

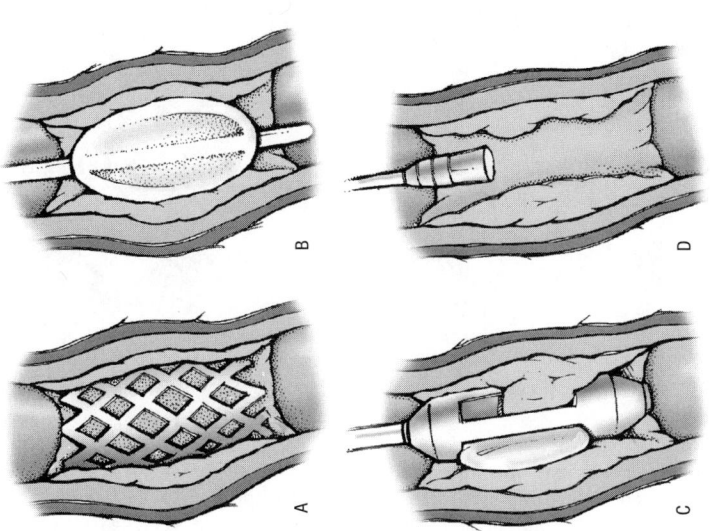

close-up views of coronary arteries showing a variety of procedures to improve blood supply to the heart: (A) stent; (B) balloon angioplasty; (C) atherectomy; (D) laser ablation

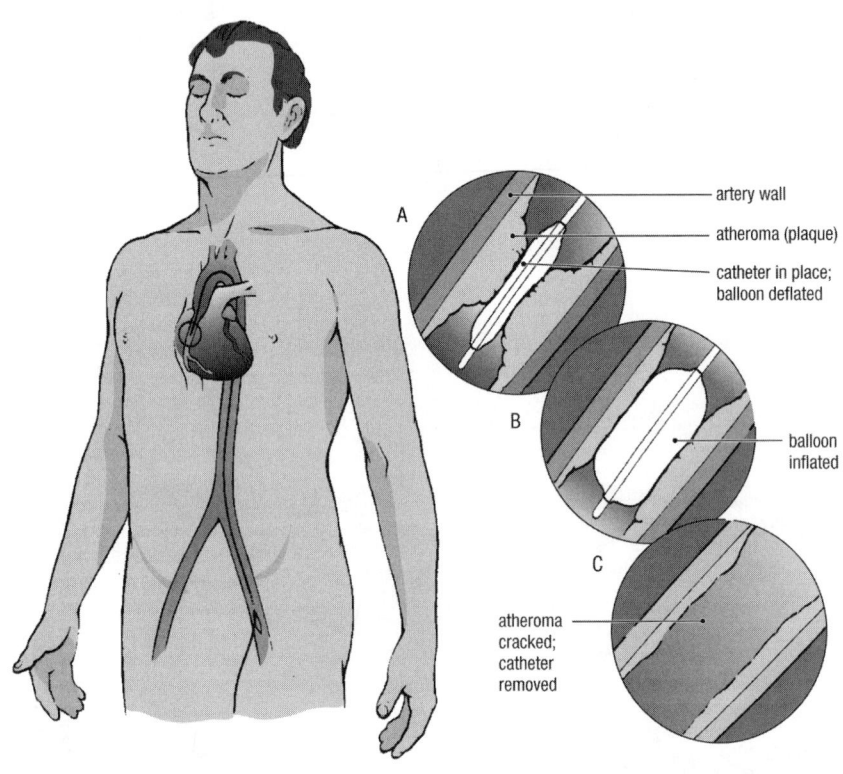

artery wall

atheroma (plaque)

catheter in place; balloon deflated

A

B

balloon inflated

C

atheroma cracked; catheter removed

percutaneous transluminal coronary angioplasty: (A) a balloon-tipped catheter is passed into the affected coronary artery and placed within the area of the atheroma (plaque); (B) the balloon is then rapidly inflated and deflated with controlled pressure; (C) after the atheroma is cracked, the catheter is removed, and blood flow improves

algesthesia	hypersensitivity to pain
allodynia	condition in which ordinarily nonpainful stimuli evoke pain
analgesia	neurologic or pharmacologic state in which painful stimuli are so moderated that, though still perceived, they are no longer painful
anesthesia dolorosa	severe spontaneous pain occurring in an anesthetic area
causalgia	persistent severe burning pain, usually following injury of a peripheral nerve (especially median and tibial) or the brachial plexus, accompanied by trophic changes
central pain syndrome	neurological condition caused by damage to or dysfunction of the central nervous system, which includes the brain, brainstem, and spinal cord
dysesthesia	impairment of sensation short of anesthesia; a condition in which a disagreeable sensation is produced by ordinary stimuli, caused by lesions of the sensory pathways, peripheral or central; abnormal sensations experienced in the absence of stimulation
hypalgesia	decreased sensibility to pain
hyperalgesia	extreme sensitivity to painful stimuli
hyperesthesia	abnormal acuteness of sensitivity to touch, pain, or other sensory stimuli
hyperpathia	exaggerated subjective response to painful stimuli, with a continuing sensation of pain after the stimulation has ceased
hypesthesia	diminished sensitivity to stimulation

intractable pain	pain resistant or refractory to ordinary analgesic agents
neuralgia	pain of a severe, throbbing, or stabbing character in the course or distribution of a nerve
neuritis	inflammation of a nerve
neuropathy	a disease involving the cranial nerves or the peripheral or autonomic nervous system
nociceptor	a peripheral nerve organ or mechanism for the reception and transmission of painful or injurious stimuli
noxious stimulus	stimulus that is potentially or actually damaging to body tissue
pain	unpleasant sensation associated with actual or potential tissue damage and mediated by specific nerve fibers to the brain where its conscious appreciation may be modified by various factors
pain threshold	the smallest intensity of a painful stimulus at which the individual perceives pain
pain tolerance	the greatest intensity of painful stimulation that an individual is able to tolerate
paralgesia	painful paresthesia; any disorder or abnormality of the sense of pain
paralgia	abnormal or unusual pain
paresthesia	an abnormal sensation, such as of burning, pricking, tickling, or tingling
rest pain	pain occurring, usually in the extremities, during rest in the sitting or lying position
telalgia	referred pain

Appendix 3
Pain Management Techniques

I. Pharmacologic Therapy
    A. Nonsteroidal antiinflammatory drugs (NSAIDs)
    B. Opioids
    C. Adjuvant analgesics
        1. Anticonvulsants
        2. Local anesthetics
        3. Corticosteroids
        4. Antispasmodics
        5. Clonidine
        6. Topical agents
    D. Psychopharmacology
    E. Antidepressants
    F. Antipsychotics
    G. Mood stabilizers
    H. Anxiolytics
    I. Psychostimulants

II. Nonpharmacologic Therapy
    A. Blocks
        1. Epidural steroid injections
        2. Central nerve blocks
        3. Sympathetic nerve blocks
        4. Visceral nerve blocks
        5. Peripheral nerve blocks
        6. Facet joint blocks
        7. Sacroiliac joint blocks
        8. Trigger point injections
    B. Intravenous lidocaine injections
    C. Intravenous phentolamine infusions
    D. Intravenous regional sympathetic blocks (Bier blocks)

III. Interventional Therapy
    A. Spinal cord stimulation
    B. Intrathecal therapy
    C. Discography
    D. Intradiscal electrothermal therapy
    E. Vertebroplasty
    F. Cryosurgery

G. Angiogenesis inhibitor therapy
H. Bone marrow transplantation
I. Gene therapy
J. Hyperthermia
K. Laser therapy
L. Photodynamic therapy
M. Targeted cancer therapy

IV. Neurosurgical Therapy
A. Ablative procedures
B. Augmentation procedures

V. Physical Therapy
A. Stretching exercises
B. Strengthening exercises
C. Endurance exercises
D. Electrical stimulation
E. Ultrasound
F. Local heat
G. Local cooling
H. Joint mobilization
I. Soft tissue mobilization

VI. Acupuncture

VII. Radiotherapy and Radiopharmaceuticals for Cancer Pain
A. Palliative treatment
B. Radiation therapy for bone metastases
C. Chemotherapy for reduction of tumor size
D. Hemibody irradiation
E. Systemic radioisotopes

Sample Reports and Dictation

ABDOMINAL WOUND DÉBRIDEMENT AND HEMATOMA EVACUATION

PREOPERATIVE DIAGNOSIS: Incisional hematoma, abdomen.

POSTOPERATIVE DIAGNOSIS: Incisional hematoma, abdomen.

PROCEDURES PERFORMED: Débridement of abdominal wound and evacuation of hematoma.

ANESTHESIA: General.

INDICATIONS FOR PROCEDURE: This woman is about 2 weeks following a lower abdominal scar revision for a small amount of skin redundancy following abdomino-plasty and subsequent weight loss. When reviewed several days following surgery, there was mild bruising, but no evidence of any fluid collection. At that point, the patient returned to her winter home down south. She called me late last week complaining of swelling and pain. She was instructed to seek medical attention to rule out the presence of either a hematoma or infection. After exploring her options, the patient decided to return home, as this was the best option for her financially. She was seen in the emergency room and a diagnosis of an incisional hematoma was made clinically and confirmed with ultrasound. She was brought to the operating room today for evacuation of the hematoma. There was no clinical evidence of infection.

DESCRIPTION OF PROCEDURE: The procedure was done under a general anesthetic. Perioperative antibiotics were used. We reopened the central part of the abdominal incision for a distance of about 8 cm. There was a very superficial hematoma, which flowed freely from the wound with a mixture of liquefied and solid clots. There was no fresh blood. There was no evidence of pus. There was no odor. The cavity was evacuated manually and thoroughly irrigated with saline and cleaned with gauze.

Once we were satisfied with the thoroughness of the evacuation and having not caused any further bleeding, the wound was closed over a Jackson-Pratt drain using deep dermal and intracuticular Monocryl sutures. Steri-Strips were applied, as was a light dressing. The patient was returned to recovery in good condition.

ANTERIOR COLON RESECTION

PREOPERATIVE DIAGNOSIS: Diverticular disease.

POSTOPERATIVE DIAGNOSIS: Diverticular disease.

PROCEDURE PERFORMED: Anterior colon resection for diverticular disease.

ANESTHESIA: General.

INDICATIONS FOR PROCEDURE: This woman was admitted to the hospital late last year with documented diverticulitis on CT scan clinically. She has since had 3 admissions for left lower quadrant abdominal pain without sepsis. She was brought to the operating room for anterior colon resection.

DESCRIPTION OF PROCEDURE: The patient was brought to the operating room, general anesthesia was induced, Foley catheter was placed, and she was prepped and draped in standard fashion. A midline incision was made. The abdomen was entered without any difficulty. The colon was mobilized proximally and distally down to just beyond the peritoneal reflection. We isolated and divided the rectal mesentery to completely isolate the rectum. We divided the mesentery of the sigmoid in an appropriate location to allow good approximation of our 2 ends without tension. We divided the mesentery and tied it with 2-0 Vicryl suture.

We placed the TA stapler across the distal rectum, right-angle clamp proximally, fired the stapler, divided the bowel, and delivered this end of the bowel out with the bowel clamp and Kocher clamp on the proximal tip and divided between. We used our sizer, and chose a #25 sizer, so we took a 25 EEA stapler. We took the anvil and sewed it in with continuous 2-0 Prolene suture.

We then went down below, introduced the EEA stapler and brought the point out just inferior to the staple line, replaced it with the anvil, closed the device, and fired it through the EEA. The rectum was inspected with sigmoidoscope. The anastomosis was at about 12 cm. The bowel was insufflated and with the pelvis full of water, there was no air bubble leakage. There were two good doughnuts.

A Jackson-Pratt drain was placed. The peritoneum was closed with 2-0 Vicryl and the incision was closed with continuous #1 Prolene and with interrupted #1 PDS sutures. The skin was closed with staples.

APPENDECTOMY

PREOPERATIVE DIAGNOSIS: Appendicitis.

POSTOPERATIVE DIAGNOSIS: Appendicitis with perforation.

PROCEDURE PERFORMED: Appendectomy.

ANESTHESIA: General.

DETAILS OF PROCEDURE: Under general anesthesia, the abdomen was prepared and draped. The CT scan showed a large pelvic appendix, so a Pfannenstiel incision was made and the abdomen was entered. There was a foul smell in the abdomen and a modest amount of pus was suctioned away. The appendix was lying across the midline in the pelvis, across the top of the uterus. It was delivered into the wound. It was attached to the posterior aspect of the cecum, immediately adjacent to the ileocecal valve on the posterior aspect. We mobilized the cecum by dividing its lateral attachments to bring the entire area up into the wound. We took down the mesoappendix and stripped it right back to the cecum in order to try and prepare a site to repair the cecum following appendectomy.

Because of the proximity of the appendiceal opening to the ileocecal valve, it was not feasible to staple off the cecum. Accordingly, the base of the appendix was tied off and the appendix amputated and passed off as a specimen. The stitch actually cut through the base of the appendix easily, as it was somewhat gangrenous.

We then closed the cecal defect with 2 layers of sutures into healthy tissue, imbricating the diseased tissue back into the cecal lumen. The 1st layer was with interrupted 3-0 Vicryl simple sutures and the 2nd layer with 3-0 silk Lembert sutures to imbricate the entire original suture line. We used a bit of mesentery and serosa of the small bowel to patch it as well.

The pelvis was suctioned dry, and a Jackson-Pratt drain was left to lie beside the cecum. Closure was done with heavy Vicryl for the rectus sheath transversely and clips for the skin.

The patient tolerated the procedure well and went to recovery in good condition.

BILATERAL BREAST AUGMENTATION AND ABDOMINOPLASTY

PREOPERATIVE DIAGNOSES
1. Mammary involution.
2. Dermatochalasis, abdomen.

POSTOPERATIVE DIAGNOSES
1. Mammary involution.
2. Dermatochalasis, abdomen.

PROCEDURES PERFORMED
1. Bilateral breast saline implant augmentation.
2. Abdominoplasty.

ANESTHESIA: General.

DESCRIPTION OF PROCEDURE: This woman elected to have both procedures under 1 anesthetic. Markings were done preoperatively. The breast markings were made in the usual fashion, marking the midline of the chest, the meridian of each breast, and the inframammary fold. We then laid out the footprint of the implant for an 11-cm diameter to match the previously chosen implant. The plan was to do a retropectoral augmentation using an inframammary incision. Markings were also made for the abdominoplasty again with the midline, the xiphoid prominence, and a planned incision along the lower abdominal and inguinal skin creases. The incision was brought out just below the anterior superior iliac spine on both sides. The procedure was done under a general anesthetic. Perioperative antibiotics were given.

The augmentation was done first. The short inframammary incisions were made, and the retropectoral plane identified. The lower costal and sternal attachments of the pectoralis major muscle were divided, and the pocket was dissected to the limits of the markings and not further. Each pocket was irrigated with bacitracin solution and temporarily packed with gauze to ensure hemostasis.

Mentor number 350-3290 implants were used, serial number XXXXXXX-124 for the right and serial number XXXXXXX-052 for the left. The implants were rinsed with bacitracin and partially filled with saline using a closed filling system and a bag of sterile IV saline. All air was then evacuated and the implants were inserted. They were filled in situ to a final volume of 300 mL each, and excellent balanced result was achieved with the desired size and shape.

The incisions were then closed with 3-0 Monocryl for the deep fascia and deep dermis, followed by a fine intracuticular 4-0 Monocryl.

Attention was then turned to the abdomen. We made the lower abdominal incision and carried it down to the suprafascial areolar plane. Superficial inferior epigastric vessels and other larger vessels were clipped. Cautery was used for small vessels. We dissected in a cephalad direction using clips for fascial perforators. Once the level of the umbilicus was reached, we made a periumbilical incision in a circular fashion keeping a small cuff of skin. The lower flap was then split to allow dissection up to the costal margin and the xiphoid.

Meticulous hemostasis was secured both on the abdominal wall and the undersurface of the flap. We marked and made a rectus fascia plication with a maximum width of about 5 cm. The plication was done with inverted figure-of-8 sutures of #1 Ethibond; an excellent plication was achieved.

We then flexed the bed to allow easier transposition of the upper flap. The position of the new umbilical incision was marked, checked, and re-marked until we were satisfied with the position. We then made a concave upward semicircle. The upper flap was defatted and a core of fatty tissue was removed. The flap was then inverted to allow hemostasis again.

We then secured the umbilicus to the skin and fascia using 3 o'clock, 6 o'clock, and 9 o'clock positions dermal fascial sutures of 2-0 Vicryl suture. An excellent result was achieved. At the end of the procedure, we finished the skin closure of the umbilicus with intracuticular 3-0 Monocryl suture.

The flap was then secured in the midline to the suprapubic incision. With tension being taken up at level of Scarpa fascia, 2-0 Vicryl sutures were used along Scarpa fascia after tailoring the flap to fit. The excised tissue was normal skin with a thinned fatty subcutaneous layer and weighed approximately 330 g. The tissue was discarded. Scarpa layer was closed with Vicryl sutures moving from lateral to medial to take up tension laterally and to prevent dog ears. Deep dermal 3-0 Monocryl sutures were placed. A single Hemovac drain was brought out through the suprapubic skin. Final skin closure was with 3-0 intracuticular Monocryl. Steri-Strips were applied. All flaps were viable, and an excellent appearance was achieved.

Sterile dressing was applied along with an abdominal binder. The patient was returned to recovery room in good condition.

BILATERAL VASOVASOSTOMY

PREOPERATIVE DIAGNOSIS: Requested reconstruction of previous vasectomy performed 11 years ago.

POSTOPERATIVE DIAGNOSIS: Requested reconstruction of previous vasectomy performed 11 years ago.

PROCEDURE PERFORMED: Bilateral vasovasostomy.

ANESTHESIA: General.

INDICATIONS FOR PROCEDURE: The patient is a 41-year-old gentleman who is admitted to the hospital for elective vasovasostomy. He clearly understands the pros and cons of the operation. He had undergone a vasectomy 11 years ago and had fathered 2 children. His present spouse had 1 child before. They understand the fact that results could not be guaranteed at all, and the success rate after 10 years is in the neighborhood of 20% to 25%.

DESCRIPTION OF PROCEDURE: Under satisfactory general anesthesia, the patient was prepped and draped. A transverse incision was performed through the scrotum and carried right down to the tunica vaginalis and both testicles were exposed.

On the right side, the vasectomy was done very close to the convoluted portion of the vas. A segment was removed and sent for histopathology. The distal end of the vas was confirmed to be patent by passing a #1 Prolene suture through it, and then the anastomosis was accomplished with interrupted 7-0 Maxon sutures using the microscope. There was a very nice anastomosis on the right side, even though it was in a convoluted portion of the vas. We had a nice apposition of the ends of the vas together. We could actually see some fluid coming out of the proximal end of the vas.

On the left side, the vasectomy had been done very high on the spermatic cord. This was in the straight portion above the vas. We got a very nice alignment and again the proximal and distal ends of the vas were divided and then reanastomosed without any tension, and we were able to prevent tension on the suture line. The vas ends were approximated with a single 4-0 chromic suture, and using 7-0 Maxon suture we were able to do the anastomosis with a microscope. The lumen of the vas was confirmed to be patent distally with a Prolene suture.

After this, the spermatic cords were infiltrated with Marcaine 0.5% with adrenaline. The testicles were placed back into the scrotum, and the scrotum was closed in 2 layers, the 1st layer with continuous running suture of 3-0 chromic suture in the dartos muscle, and the 2nd layer mattress sutures of 4-0 plain. The area was covered with

Tegaderm, a scrotal support was placed, and the patient was transferred to the recovery room in satisfactory condition. In the operating room he received 1 g of Ancef.

The patient will be going home with a prescription for Keflex 500 mg 4 times a day and will take Tylenol No. 3 for postoperative discomfort. We will see him in the office for followup exam in 6 weeks, and we will obtain a semen sample at that point. He is to refrain from being sexually active for 3 weeks and from doing any lifting or straining for at least 2 weeks.

COLONOSCOPY

PREOPERATIVE DIAGNOSIS: Colocutaneous fistula.

POSTOPERATIVE DIAGNOSIS: Minimal colonic opening only.

PROCEDURE PERFORMED: Colonoscopy.

ANESTHESIA: IV sedation.

INDICATIONS FOR PROCEDURE: This pleasant woman had a gastric revision and gastric bypass a few months ago and developed numerous complications including splenectomy, MI, renal failure, and a leak from her anastomosis. Although she was home for 1 to 2 months, she had a persistent draining sinus in the left midabdomen. The nurses found a dressing sponge during wound changes here on her 2nd admission. It is unclear when or how that ended up in the wound during her 1st admission. This may have kept the abscess going for awhile.

Then radiology performed a percutaneous drainage of the upper part of the cavity. There was a colocutaneous fistula demonstrated on the 1st sinogram, and the etiology of this fistula is not quite clear. The patient has been on TPN now for a couple of weeks with slow improvement in how she is feeling and slow decrease in the amount of drainage. Unfortunately, the last sinogram still showed a connection between the bowel and the abscess cavity.

FINDINGS: The patient's rectum was completely normal. The sigmoid colon showed no diverticular disease, strictures or neoplasms. In the lower descending colon, there was a single area which did not go over 1 cm or 2 cm in length, This area showed some spasm but no real erythema, no blood, and no obvious opening to suggest fistulous site. This was the only abnormal area; however, the remainder of the descending colon and the transverse colon were completely normal. We did not persist with the scope past the hepatic flexure.

DESCRIPTION OF PROCEDURE: With the patient under intravenous sedation with 10 mg of midazolam and 50 mg of meperidine, the flexible colonoscope was inserted into the anus and was advanced up to the proximal transverse colon. The scope was then withdrawn, retroflexed and removed.

PLAN: The patient will be continued on conservative therapy for now since this colonic hole must be very small and should close on its own, given there is no distal obstruction or foreign body to keep it open.

DISTAL GASTRECTOMY

PREOPERATIVE DIAGNOSIS: Gastric cancer.

POSTOPERATIVE DIAGNOSIS: Gastric cancer.

PROCEDURE PERFORMED: Distal gastrectomy.

ANESTHESIA: General endotracheal.

INDICATIONS FOR PROCEDURE: The patient is a 56-year-old male with a history of weight loss and decreased p.o. tolerance. On endoscopic evaluation he was found to have a distal pancreatic lesion. He presents now for elective partial gastrectomy.

DESCRIPTION OF PROCEDURE: The patient was taken to the operating room and placed in the supine position. General anesthesia was administered. Endotracheal intubation was achieved. The patient was prepped and draped in standard sterile fashion. Using a 10-blade knife, a chevron incision was created and subcutaneous tissues were divided through to the peritoneum. The peritoneum was then opened using a blade and further divided using electrocautery with care not to injure the underlying abdominal content. The falciform ligament was divided. We began with exploration. There was no evidence of lesions in the large bowel. The liver was palpated and was found to be without lesions.

At this point we directed attention toward the large, palpable lesion in the distal stomach. The lesser sac was then opened using both electrocautery and Kelly clamps, with silk ties for vessels. After completion of opening the lesser sac, a small opening was made in the gastric mesentery on the opposing lesser curvature side. After creating a tunnel posteriorly on the stomach, a GIA stapler was used to proximally transect the stomach. The proximal duodenum was then cleared of surrounding tissues and transected in a similar fashion. The specimen was then sent for pathological evaluation. Peritoneal washings were also sent for pathology and cytology. Celiac nodes were also identified and sent for further evaluation. Frozen section performed on the margins of the specimen sent was negative for carcinoma.

We then proceeded with reanastomosis. The ligament of Treitz was identified and, approximately 30 cm distal from the ligament, the jejunum was brought up to the remaining gastric sac. The jejunum was opened sharply to the level of the serosa and further opened using electrocautery into the lumen. The jejunum was then anastomosed in the anterior stomach in an antecolic fashion. The anastomosis was then achieved using interrupted 3-0 silk popoff sutures. After completion of anastomosis, the wound bed was evaluated. Hemostasis was seen to be adequate.

The abdomen was then closed using running #2 PDS in 2 layers. The wound was then irrigated and skin was reapproximated using surgical staples. The wound was then cleaned and dressed using sterile dressing. The patient was extubated without difficulty. There were no noted intraoperative complications. All counts were correct at the end of the case. The patient tolerated the procedure well.

EXPLORATORY LAPAROTOMY FOR GUNSHOT WOUND

PREOPERATIVE DIAGNOSIS: Right flank gunshot wound.

POSTOPERATIVE DIAGNOSIS: Perforation of the 2nd portion of the duodenum, descending colon injury.

PROCEDURES PERFORMED
1. Exploratory laparotomy.
2. Primary duodenal perforation repair.
3. Right colon resection with primary anastomosis.
4. Appendectomy.
5. Umbilical hernia repair.

ANESTHESIA: General.

URINE OUTPUT: 100 mL.

DRAINS: None.

ESTIMATED BLOOD LOSS: 100 mL.

SPECIMENS: Right colon and appendix.

INDICATIONS FOR PROCEDURE: The patient is a 15-year-old male, status post gun-shot wound to right flank, who presented to the emergency department after the accident. At this point a chest x-ray was obtained which showed no hemothorax and bullets in the left upper quadrant under the diaphragm. At this point the patient was taken emergently to the operating room.

DESCRIPTION OF PROCEDURE: The patient was brought to the operating room, placed in a supine position, and put under general anesthesia. Foley catheter was placed. Using a #15 blade, a midline incision was made from the xiphoid process down to the pubic symphysis. All 4 quadrants were packed with laparotomy pads.

Next, the small bowel was examined from the ligament of Treitz to the terminal ileum. No obvious injuries were identified. The right retroperitoneal area was examined. There was a retroperitoneal hematoma identified as well as contusion involving the right colon. Next, the entire right colon was mobilized. The 2nd portion of duodenum was examined, and Kocher maneuver was performed. The 2nd portion of duodenum was found to have 2 perforations. They were thought to be entry and exit wounds. They were both repaired in 2 layers using simple 3-0 chromic stitches on mucosa, followed by simple Lembert 3-0 silk stitches on serosa. Inferior vena cava and aorta were exposed and examined. There were no injuries identified. Liver and spleen were examined. There were no injuries identified there either. A bullet was palpated in the left upper quadrant in the retroperitoneum; however, it was very immobile and we were unable to retrieve it. The left diaphragm was palpated, and it was found to be intact. The lesser sac was opened. The pancreas was examined. There were no obvi-ous injuries to this area.

At this point, attention was turned back to the contusion of the large bowel. Upon further examination, we felt there was a defect in the large bowel. At this point, a decision was made to excise a segment of the small bowel, which was done with GIA-55 stapler, followed by primary anastomosis with the 55-mm GIA and TA staplers. A couple of simple 3-0 silk stitches were placed at the crotch of the anastomosis. The defect in the mesentery was closed with a running 3-0 chromic stitch.

Next, attention was turned to the appendix. Taking into account the fact that the patient had an extensive operation and a right colon resection, we decided to proceed with appendectomy. At this point, mesoappendix was divided and tied with 3-0 chromic ties. Next, the appendix itself was tied off with 0 chromic ties and amputated. This mucosa was electrocauterized, a pursestring stitch of 3-0 chromic was placed around it, and the appendiceal stump was buried.

The resected portion of the right colon was opened on the side and it was found to have a defect in the mucosa in one area the approximate size of a penny with only serosa preventing the bowel contents from spilling outside. At this point the peritoneal cavity was profusely irrigated. Next we closed it with a running double-stranded PDS stitch.

In the process of closure, an umbilical hernia was incorporated in the closure. It was obliterated and repaired. At the end of the procedure, the skin was closed with staples.

The patient tolerated the procedure well, was extubated in the operating room, and transferred to pediatric ICU in stable condition.

EXPLORATORY LAPAROTOMY RULE OUT ISCHEMIC BOWEL

PREOPERATIVE DIAGNOSIS: Ischemic bowel.

POSTOPERATIVE DIAGNOSIS: Ischemic bowel.

PROCEDURE PERFORMED: Exploratory laparotomy.

ANESTHESIA: General endotracheal.

DRAINS: None.

ESTIMATED BLOOD LOSS: Minimal.

SPECIMEN: None.

INDICATIONS FOR PROCEDURE: This patient is a 78-year-old female status post aortobifemoral bypass with an IMA right implantation postoperative day #1 who, since her 1st operation, remained hemodynamically unstable with significant lactic acidosis requiring vasopressors. A decision was made to take the patient back to the operating room for a second-look operation to rule out ischemic bowel.

DESCRIPTION OF PROCEDURE: The patient was brought to the operating room and placed in the supine position. Abdominal and bilateral groin dressings were removed. The patient was prepped with Betadine and draped in the usual sterile fashion. Staples were removed from the abdominal incision. The abdominal incision was reopened. The patient's large and small bowels were examined. They were found to be friable and pink with no obvious ischemic changes. On entry into the anterior peritoneal cavity, a large amount of ascites, approximately 1 liter, was suctioned out. At the time the small bowel was examined, it was noted that patient had a mass in her ileum approximately 1.5 cm in diameter, intraluminal, with some puckering of small bowel serosa. The patient's small bowel lumen was found to be open.

At this point small bowel resection of the segment of small bowel involving the tumor was entertained. General surgery intraoperative consultation was obtained. At this point, considering the recent graft placement and possible enteral content contamination of the peritoneal cavity as a result of the small bowel resection, it was decided to not to proceed with small bowel resection.

The peritoneal cavity was then closed with a double-stranded running PDS suture followed by stapling of the skin. A dressing was placed and patient was transferred to surgical ICU intubated but in stable condition.

HERNIA REPAIR WITH KUGEL PATCH

PREOPERATIVE DIAGNOSIS: Left inguinal hernia.

POSTOPERATIVE DIAGNOSIS: Left inguinal hernia.

PROCEDURE PERFORMED: Left inguinal hernia repair with Kugel patch.

ANESTHESIA: Local intravenous sedation.

DESCRIPTION OF PROCEDURE: The patient was brought to the operating room and placed on the table in supine position. After administration of intravenous sedation, the left groin was prepped and draped in the usual sterile fashion. The skin and subcutaneous tissue in the left groin were infiltrated with local anesthetic, and a 4-cm transverse skin incision was made midway between the pubic tubercle and the anterior superior iliac spine. The incision was carried down through the subcutaneous fat with electrocautery, and the external oblique aponeurosis was longitudinally incised. The internal oblique and transversus abdominis muscles were bluntly split, and the transversalis fascia was incised. A preperitoneal pocket was then developed using blunt finger dissection, beginning immediately under the belly of the rectus muscle. Dissection was taken superiorly to the level of the anterior superior iliac spine and inferiorly down to the symphysis pubis. Dissection was then turned laterally along the deep aspect of the superior ramus of the pubic bone. During this portion of dissection no evidence of direct defect was identified. The spermatic cord was then isolated and encircled with a Penrose drain.

Examination of the anteromedial aspect of the cord revealed the presence of a moderate-sized indirect sac. The sac was dissected away from the cord structures and dissection was then continued further up where the peritoneal envelope was dissected away from the more proximal cord structures. The hernia sac was then suture ligated at its neck with a stitch of 0 Vicryl, and the distal portion of the sac was amputated and passed off the field.

Following this, a small oval Kugel patch was introduced into the preperitoneal pocket. Once the patch was properly positioned, it was fixed in place with a single stitch of 0 Vicryl between the anterior layer of the patch and Cooper ligament. Following this, the spermatic cord was returned to its anatomical position and then the internal oblique and transversus abdominis muscles were closed over the patch with interrupted figure-of-8 sutures of 0 Vicryl.

The external oblique aponeurosis was closed with a running suture of 0 Vicryl and Scarpa fascia was approximated with interrupted 3-0 Vicryl stitches. The skin incision was then closed with a running subcuticular tissue of 4-0 Monocryl, and skin closure was reinforced with 1/2-inch Steri-Strips. Sterile dressing was then applied to the wound, and the patient was transported to the recovery room in stable condition, having tolerated the procedure well. All postoperative counts were correct.

LEFT THYROID LOBECTOMY

PREOPERATIVE DIAGNOSIS: Left thyroid mass.

POSTOPERATIVE DIAGNOSIS: Left thyroid mass, benign disease on frozen section.

PROCEDURE PERFORMED: Left thyroid lobectomy.

ANESTHESIA: General.

INDICATIONS FOR PROCEDURE: This patient has had an ultrasound of her neck done. Ultrasound demonstrated a 2-cm lesion in the left lobe of her thyroid. Aspiration biopsy demonstrated cells suspicious for papillary carcinoma. We decided to proceed with thyroid lobectomy.

DESCRIPTION OF PROCEDURE: The patient was brought to the operative room and a general anesthetic was administered. Airway was maintained with the use of an endotracheal tube. A nerve monitor was used. The neck was prepped and draped in an extended position.

A skin crease incision was made above the sternal notch. Dissection was carried through the subcutaneous and platysmal layers. Flaps were elevated superiorly and inferiorly. The strap muscles were then split in the midline, and the face of the thyroid gland was isolated on each side. Dissection was carried around the left lobe of the gland. The upper pole vessels were skeletonized and doubly tied. Posteriorly, the gland was cleared. The recurrent laryngeal nerve was identified. This was confirmed with a nerve stimulator. The gland was gradually dissected inferior to the nerve. We felt that 2 definite parathyroid glands were identified and preserved in the neck. These had good blood supply. There was a relatively large vein entering the midportion of the gland. This was tied with chromic and cut. The gland was then rotated forward off the upper trachea and larynx. It was cut across at the isthmus and sent for frozen section.

Frozen section suggested benign disease. Therefore, it seemed apparent that nothing further should be done.

A Jackson-Pratt drain was brought out through a separate stab wound on the right side. The strap muscles and platysmal layer were closed with interrupted sutures of 3-0 chromic. The skin was closed with a running suture of 4-0 nylon and the procedure terminated.

The patient tolerated the procedure well and left the operative room in good condition.

LIGATION AND STRIPPING OF VARICOSE VEINS

PREOPERATIVE DIAGNOSIS: Varicose veins, left leg.

POSTOPERATIVE DIAGNOSIS: Varicose veins, left leg.

PROCEDURE PERFORMED: Ligation and stripping of varicose veins, left leg.

ANESTHESIA: General.

INDICATIONS FOR PROCEDURE: This man has had trouble with varicosities. He had a chronic ulcer on the right leg that needed to be skin grafted after removing his veins. He was brought to the operating room today for repair of the varicose veins on his left lower extremity.

DESCRIPTION OF PROCEDURE: The patient was brought to the operating room, general anesthesia was induced, and endotracheal tube was placed. He was prepped and draped in the standard fashion.

We identified the saphenous vein in the groin through a groin crease incision, dividing multiple little branches between ties. We then identified the saphenous vein at the ankle, tied it off distally and circled it open. We passed the stripper from the ankle to the groin, tied the stripper into the vein, tied the saphenofemoral junction, divided the vein proximally and distally so the stripper was lying in the leg and disconnected in the vein.

We then made incisions over the previously marked varicosities, stripping out segments. Once we had completed that, we pulled the stripper from the leg, closing incisions with staples and placed our dressings as we pulled the stripper through the leg. We wrapped the leg with sterile gauze, Kerlix and applied elastic dressings. He tolerated the procedure well and was transferred to recovery in good condition.

LIPOSUCTION FOR BILATERAL GYNECOMASTIA

PREOPERATIVE DIAGNOSIS: Bilateral gynecomastia.

POSTOPERATIVE DIAGNOSIS: Bilateral gynecomastia.

PROCEDURE PERFORMED: Liposuction, bilateral gynecomastia.

ANESTHESIA: General.

INDICATIONS FOR PROCEDURE: This man had mostly fatty gynecomastia with no significant element of true gynecomastia. Markings were made with the patient seated preoperatively. There was periareolar fullness in an area measuring about 6 x 10 cm, about 3 cm thick. This tapered upward over the pectoral muscle and laterally just above the inframammary fold. There was about 1.5 cm of fatty thickness above the pectoralis major muscle and about 1 cm or less below the inframammary fold. Contour markings were made. Surgical plan was to go ahead with ultrasonic liposuction initially and then to make a periareolar incision to remove the remaining fibrous tissue centrally. The procedure was done under a general anesthetic. Perioperative clindamycin was given, as the patient is allergic to penicillin.

DESCRIPTION OF PROCEDURE: We made small lateral inframammary fold incisions and infiltrated each side with a mixture containing 1000 mL of Ringer lactate, 1 mg of adrenaline, and 20 mL of 0.75% bupivacaine; a total of 150 to 200 mL was used on each side. Time was allowed for vasoconstriction. We then proceeded with the ultrasonic liposuction on 40% power using a 3-mm cannula. Limited ultrasound was used in the peripheral areas and over the pectoralis major muscle. Additional ultrasound was used in the more fibrofatty tissue in the central areolar region. Care was taken to keep the tip moving so as not to generate hot spots in the tissue, especially near the skin. We were very pleased with the suctioning. The aspiration produced a pure yellowish fat, which had some globules but was mostly homogenized tissue. The area was suctioned thoroughly, especially in the central thicker area. The procedure was done bilaterally. A total of 3 minutes of ultrasound was used on each side, and approximately 100 mL of tissue was removed from each side. We had a very uniform thickness as a result.

The patient was seated upright to almost 90 degrees and examined. We did not feel that there was enough residual tissue or significant retroareolar fibrous tissue to warrant making a periareolar incision. We elected to halt the procedure at that stage without going ahead with the formal resection.

We think that the patient will have a good result from this, and we should expect some skin tightening and further reduction over the next couple of weeks. A single 5-0 plain catgut suture was placed in each of the small incisions covered by a small Coverlet dressing and an abdominal pad. A binder was used, and the patient was returned to recovery in good condition.

RAMSTEDT PYLOROMYOTOMY

PREOPERATIVE DIAGNOSIS: Congenital hypertrophic pyloric stenosis.

POSTOPERATIVE DIAGNOSIS: Congenital hypertrophic pyloric stenosis.

PROCEDURE PERFORMED: Ramstedt pyloromyotomy.

ANESTHESIA: General endotracheal and 0.25% Marcaine local.

COMPLICATIONS: None.

ESTIMATED BLOOD LOSS: Minimal.

SPECIMEN: None.

DESCRIPTION OF PROCEDURE: The patient was brought to the operating room and placed on the table in supine position. General endotracheal anesthesia was induced. The abdomen was prepped and draped. A subcutaneous injection of Marcaine was given.

A transverse right upper quadrant incision was made, carried through the subcutaneous tissues using cautery for hemostasis. The anterior rectus sheath was opened transversely. The muscle was split and the posterior sheath opened longitudinally. The pylorus was delivered into the wound. The anterior surface of the pylorus was scored with a scalpel and then split with the Benson spreader. The mucosa pouched out nicely. Completion of the myotomy was done by inspection and palpation. Antegrade milking of the stomach and retrograde milking of the duodenum failed to demonstrate any leaks. A minimal amount of venous oozing was noted to stop spontaneously on replacement of the pylorus back into the abdomen.

The abdomen was then closed in layers, closing the posterior rectus sheath and peritoneum with a running 4-0 Vicryl. The anterior rectus sheath was closed separately with interrupted 4-0 Vicryl, and Scarpa fascia was closed with 5-0 Monocryl. The skin was closed with a running subcuticular pullout suture of 5-0 Monocryl. Mastisol and Steri-Strips were applied. The patient was awoken from anesthesia and extubated, brought to the recovery room having tolerated the procedure well. All counts are correct.

RIGHT INGUINAL HERNIA REPAIR

PREOPERATIVE DIAGNOSIS: Large right inguinal hernia.

POSTOPERATIVE DIAGNOSIS: Large right inguinal hernia.

PROCEDURE PERFORMED: Right inguinal hernia repair.

ANESTHESIA: Intravenous sedation and local anesthesia.

INDICATIONS: This pleasant young man had a large indirect right inguinal hernia.

FINDINGS: The patient had multiple omenta stuck in a typical, somewhat chronically inflamed sac which went right down into the scrotum.

DESCRIPTION OF PROCEDURE: With the patient under intravenous sedation and local anesthesia with 2% Xylocaine with adrenaline and 0.5% Marcaine, a transverse incision was made in the right groin, excising a mole and sending it to the lab en bloc.

The fascia was opened at the external ring, and the ilioinguinal and genitofemoral nerves were identified and preserved. The cremaster was opened anteriorly, and the sac was dissected out. It was opened, and any residual omentum in it was invaginated back into the abdomen. The sac was then suture ligated with 2-0 Prolene suture, and then the excess was divided and removed. The stump was allowed to return to the abdomen.

The internal ring was then tightened with a running layer of 0 Prolene suture along the posterior canal in a modified Bassini repair. The external oblique was closed with running 2-0 Vicryl suture and the skin was closed with running 4-0 Vicryl subcuticular sutures and Steri-Strips.

The patient tolerated the procedure well, and there were no complications. Sponge and instrument counts were correct.

RIGHT PYELOPLASTY

PREOPERATIVE DIAGNOSES: Right ureteropelvic junction obstruction with significant hydronephrosis and intermittent episodes of pain.

POSTOPERATIVE DIAGNOSES:
1. Right ureteropelvic junction obstruction with significant hydronephrosis and intermittent episodes of pain.
2. Malrotation of the right kidney.

PROCEDURE PERFORMED: Right pyeloplasty.

ANESTHESIA: General.

INDICATIONS FOR PROCEDURE: The patient is a 44-year-old gentleman who was admitted to the hospital with a grossly distended kidney causing him a tremendous amount of pain. In fact, this kidney was palpable in the right upper quadrant. A retrograde pyelogram confirmed that he had a true ureteropelvic junction obstruction, but his renal pelvis was rotated and it was facing outwardly. A stent was placed into the right collecting system and that improved the pressure in his kidney dramatically. The kidney function was very good. As he obviously needed repair, he was taken to the operating room today for reconstruction of the ureteropelvic junction.

DESCRIPTION OF PROCEDURE: Under satisfactory general anesthesia, the patient was prepped and draped with his right side up. The table was flexed to approximately 35 degrees and the patient was placed at 90 degrees on the table.

A submucosal incision was performed and external oblique, internal oblique, and transversus muscles were divided, and the retroperitoneal area was entered. The peritoneum was reflected medially. The Gerota fascia was well developed. We were able to open that up and identified that, indeed, there was a very large renal pelvis, which was facing laterally. We were able to identify the ureter coming in laterally, and there was a leash of blood vessels coming from the renal pelvis down the ureter which were divided and tied off with 3-0 Vicryl. We were then able to detach the renal pelvis, and the ureteropelvic junction was completely removed after we demarcated the renal pelvis medially and laterally with 4-0 Biosyn sutures. We were able to spatulate the ureter and close the redundant portion of the renal pelvis above. The ureter was then attached to the renal pelvis after a part of the renal pelvis had been closed. We replaced the stent that he had in his right collecting system with a new 26-cm double-J stent. Fluoroscopy revealed it was in very good location.

The closure appeared to be very satisfactory. We closed the renal pelvis and then anastomosed the ureter to the renal pelvis with continuous running sutures of 4-0 Biosyn medially and laterally and this actually should provide him with excellent apposition and good drainage. This patient's perinephric space was drained with a 1/2-inch Penrose drain, and this was brought out through the end of the incision. The closure was accomplished by approximating the Gerota fascia with a few interrupted 0 Vicryl sutures. The transversus muscle was then approximated with continuous running suture of 0 Vicryl, then the internal oblique, and finally the external oblique. Subcostal nerve blocks were performed on the 9th, 10th, 11th, and 12th ribs using 0.5% Marcaine with adrenaline. The skin was approximated with staples, and the Penrose drain was secured to the skin with 0 Vicryl suture.

It is anticipated that this gentleman will have an uneventful recovery. He was sent to recovery room in satisfactory condition.

SCROTAL EXPLORATION WITH BILATERAL TESTICULAR FIXATION

PREOPERATIVE DIAGNOSIS: Left testicular torsion.

POSTOPERATIVE DIAGNOSIS: Torsion, left testis, with spontaneous detorsion.

PROPOSED PROCEDURES: Exploration of left scrotum, bilateral testicular fixation, possible left orchidectomy.

PROCEDURES PERFORMED: Exploration left scrotum with bilateral testicular fixation.

ANESTHESIA: General.

DESCRIPTION OF PROCEDURE: Following general anesthesia, the patient was prepped and draped in the routine fashion. A transverse incision was made in the left hemiscrotum carried down through the dartos fascia onto the tunica. Testis and associated hydrocele were brought out through the incision. There was a lot of congestion in the scrotal tissues, and on opening the hydrocele sac the testis was quite congested but obviously spontaneous detorsion had occurred.

Apical sutures of 3-0 silk were placed into the testis and tied to the corresponding position within the left hemiscrotum. A running 3-0 Dexon suture was then used to close the dartos, followed by interrupted 3-0 Monocryl suture to the skin.

A short incision was then made on the right side. The window of tunica was removed and apical silk sutures were placed through the tunica albuginea of the testis and through the corresponding position inside the scrotum.

A 3-0 Dexon suture was used to close the dartos incision, followed by several interrupted Monocryl sutures to skin. Then 7.5 mL of 0.5% Marcaine were instilled as a superficial inguinal ring block on either side. OpSite spray was applied to the incision.

The nurses reported the counts as correct, and the patient was returned to the recovery room in a satisfactory condition.

SIGMOID COLON RESECTION FOR OBSTRUCTION

PREOPERATIVE DIAGNOSIS: Sigmoid volvulus, redundant sigmoid colon.

POSTOPERATIVE DIAGNOSIS: Sigmoid volvulus, redundant sigmoid colon.

PROCEDURE PERFORMED: Sigmoid colon resection for obstruction.

ANESTHESIA: General endotracheal.

INDICATIONS FOR PROCEDURE: This 74-year-old gentleman came in with an acute large bowel obstruction secondary to sigmoid volvulus. He underwent endoscopic decompression and subsequently tolerated full bowel prep for his surgery today.

DESCRIPTION OF PROCEDURE: With the patient appropriately monitored, general anesthetic with endotracheal intubation was administered. The abdomen was prepped and draped in the usual fashion. A lower midline incision was used to gain entry into the abdominal cavity. A laparotomy revealed a normal liver and no other palpable abnormalities in the colon or small bowel.

The sigmoid colon was brought up and out into the wound and found to be quite redundant. There was an area of scarring, presumably at the area of torsion. A site 1 cm distal to this was chosen as the distal resection margin. Proximal resection margin was at the beginning of the sigmoid colon. Windows were created in the mesentery and 1/4-inch Penrose drain placed. The mesentery was divided sequentially between snaps and secured with 0 chromic ties by staying close to the bowel.

Once divided, Kocher clamps were placed, and the bowel was divided after Glassman bowel clamps were placed proximal and distal to the resection margins. The proximal and distal colon was suctioned out and hemostasis was obtained at the anastomosis site. An end-to-end anastomosis was fashioned with interrupted Gambee suture technique of 4-0 PDS suture. The blood supply was excellent. There was no tension on the anastomosis, and there was no contamination of the field. The mesenteric defect was closed with a running 4-0 PDS suture. One small vessel was inadvertently punctured with a needle, but pressure and suture ligation were used to control this. The abdomen was then thoroughly irrigated with 1-1/2 liters of saline.

The midline incision was closed with running #2 Vicryl suture, and the skin was closed with staples after the wound was irrigated.

The estimated blood loss during the procedure was less than 100 mL. There were no complications and all sponge, needle, and instrument counts were correct on both occasions.

The patient was extubated and safely transferred to the recovery room in stable condition.

Note a central line was inserted at the end of the case. Initially, right subclavian line was attempted. Inadvertently, the subclavian artery was punctured twice, pressure was placed, and a left subclavian line was placed with the first-pass effort. A 7.5-French triple-lumen catheter was used.

Chest x-ray at the end of the case revealed no evidence of hemothorax or pneumothorax bilaterally. Note that the dissection, anastomosis and surgery were well away from the area of the ureter.

SMALL BOWEL RESECTION AND PRIMARY REANASTOMOSIS

PREOPERATIVE DIAGNOSIS: Perforated viscus.

POSTOPERATIVE DIAGNOSIS: Perforated jejunum.

PROCEDURE PROPOSED: Laparotomy for perforated viscus.

PROCEDURE PERFORMED: Small bowel resection and primary reanastomosis.

ANESTHESIA: General endotracheal.

FINDINGS
1. Small, 0.5-cm perforation of jejunum, 20 cm from ligament of Treitz.
2. Copious enteric contents within abdomen.

INDICATIONS FOR PROCEDURE: This 63-year-old diabetic gentleman presented with sudden onset of pain of 12 hours' duration. He had an acute abdomen with generalized peritonitis and underwent a CT scan, which revealed a thickened loop of jejunum with air in the bowel wall and moderate free fluid in the abdomen. He was prepared for urgent laparotomy.

DESCRIPTION OF PROCEDURE: With the patient appropriately monitored, general anesthetic with endotracheal intubation was administered. The abdomen was prepped and draped in the usual fashion. A midline incision was used to gain entry into the abdominal cavity, which revealed copious enteric contents. This was suctioned out and the small bowel run and a perforation found at 20 cm from the ligament of Treitz. The remainder of the abdomen was examined, and no other abnormalities were found.

Two windows in the mesentery were created on either side of the perforation, to effectively remove 5 cm of small bowel. The mesentery was divided in continuity and secured with 0 chromic sutures. The GIA-55 stapler was used to divide the bowel and fashion a side-to-side stapled anastomosis. The TA-30 stapler was used to close the resultant defect. The mesenteric defect was minimal and not closed.

The abdomen was thoroughly irrigated with several liters of normal saline until effluent was clear. No drain was placed and the abdominal wall was closed with running #1 Vicryl suture.

The wound was irrigated and packed open with the umbilicus reapproximated with staples.

The estimated blood loss was minimal and there were no complications during the procedure. All sponge, needle and instrument counts were correct on both occasions, and the patient was extubated and safely transferred to the recovery room in stable condition. However, in the recovery room, the patient experienced respiratory deterioration requiring reintubation and ICU admission.

SPLENECTOMY

PREOPERATIVE DIAGNOSES: Hemoglobinopathy and splenomegaly.

POSTOPERATIVE DIAGNOSES: Hemoglobinopathy and splenomegaly.

PROCEDURE PERFORMED: Splenectomy.

ANESTHESIA: General.

ESTIMATED BLOOD LOSS: 15 mL.

SPECIMEN: Spleen.

DESCRIPTION OF PROCEDURE: This 8-year-old with an inherited hemoglobinopathy has been evaluated by the hematology service and was recommended for splenectomy at this time. The patient was brought to the operating room, given general anesthetic, then prepped and draped with Betadine solution. Ancef antibiotic was given. Foley and NG tube were placed.

Transverse incision was made from the costal margin to the midline and the peritoneal cavity opened. The spleen was broad, long, and free of any particular adhesions. The inferior pole was freed up by ligating a couple of attachments to the omentum with silk ties. The splenic ligament was opened, mobilizing the spleen up to the level of the short gastrics. The incision was enlarged because visibility could not be adequately accomplished.

The room became very warm after the anesthesiologist changed the setting on the thermostat. The OR team had to stop for a short time. Gowns and gloves were changed, and the room became cool enough to start again.

The spleen was brought out through the incision. The vessels were exposed, doubly ligated proximally, singly ligated distally including the splenic artery, the short gastrics, the inferior pole, and the splenic vein, in that order. The spleen was then freed and removed. No bleeding occurred. Subsequent to this, the area was irrigated. No accessory spleen was seen in the lesser sac near the pancreatic tail or near the hilum of the liver. There was no bleeding.

The abdominal wall was closed with a running 2-0 Vicryl in the peritoneum, extended into the posterior rectus fascia, also another layer in the internal oblique onto the anterior rectus fascia, and another 2-0 Vicryl placed in the external oblique, 4-0 Vicryl subcutaneously, 5-0 Monocryl subcuticularly, and Steri-Strips were applied. The patient was taken to recovery.

Common Terms by Procedure

Abdominal Wound Débridement and Hematoma Evacuation
abdominal scar revision
abdominoplasty
fluid collection
general anesthetic
incisional hematoma
intracuticular Monocryl suture
Jackson-Pratt drain
light dressing
perioperative antibiotic
skin redundancy
Steri-Strips
superficial hematoma

Anterior Colon Resection
air bubble leakage
anastomosis
anterior colon resection
anvil
bowel clamp
diverticular disease
EEA stapler
Foley catheter
general anesthesia
insufflated
Jackson-Pratt drain
Kocher clamp
left lower quadrant abdominal pain
midline incision
#1 PDS suture
peritoneal reflection
peritoneum
prepped and draped in standard fashion
2-0 Prolene suture
rectal mesentery
right-angle clamp
sigmoidoscope

staple line
2-0 Vicryl suture

Appendectomy
appendectomy
appendiceal opening
appendix
cecal defect
cecal lumen
cecum
computed tomography (CT)
CT scan
good condition
ileocecal valve
imbricating
interrupted 3-0 Vicryl simple sutures
Jackson-Pratt drain
mesentery
mesoappendix
Pfannenstiel incision
prepared and draped
rectus sheath
serosa
3-0 silk Lembert suture
small bowel
suctioned dry
suture line
uterus

Bilateral Breast Augmentation and Abdominoplasty
abdominal binder
abdominal wall
abdominoplasty
bacitracin solution
bilateral breast saline implant
    augmentation
breast markings
cautery

cephalad direction
circular fashion
clip
closed filling system
concave upward semicircle
core of fatty tissue
costal margin
cuff of skin
deep dermis
deep fascia
defatted
dermal fascial suture
dermatochalasis
#1 Ethibond suture
fascial perforator
fine intracuticular 4-0 Monocryl suture
footprint of the implant
general anesthetic
hemostasis
Hemovac drain
inframammary fold
inframammary incision
inguinal skin crease
in situ
intracuticular 3-0 Monocryl
intravenous (IV)
inverted figure-of-8 sutures
lower abdominal crease
lower abdominal incision
lower costal attachment
lower flap
mammary involution
Mentor implant
meridian
meticulous hemostasis
midline of the chest
3-0 Monocryl suture
3 o'clock, 6 o'clock, and 9 o'clock
    positions
pectoralis major muscle
perioperative antibiotic
periumbilical incision
plication

pocket
retropectoral augmentation
retropectoral plane
rectus fascia plication
Scarpa fascia
Scarpa layer
short inframammary incision
skin closure
sterile dressing
sterile IV saline
sternal attachment
subcutaneous layer
superficial inferior epigastric vessel
suprafascial areolar plane
suprapubic incision
thinned fatty subcutaneous layer
umbilical incision
umbilicus
upper flap
usual fashion
2-0 Vicryl suture
xiphoid prominence

Bilateral Vasovasostomy

anastomosis
apposition
approximated
bilateral vasovasostomy
3-0 chromic suture
convoluted portion of the vas
dartos muscle
distal end
elective vasovasostomy
followup exam
general anesthesia
histopathology
interrupted 7-0 Maxon sutures
Keflex 500 mg
Marcaine 0.5% with adrenaline
microscope
operating room
4-0 plain mattress suture
postoperative discomfort

prepped and draped
#1 Prolene suture
reanastomosed
recovery room
satisfactory condition
scrotal support
scrotum
semen sample
sexually active
single 4-0 chromic suture
spermatic cord
suture line
Tegaderm
testicle
4 times a day
transverse incision
tunica vaginalis
Tylenol No. 3
vasectomy

Colonoscopy
abscess cavity
anastomosis
anus
colocutaneous fistula
colonic hole
colonoscopy
conservative therapy
descending colon
distal obstruction
diverticular disease
draining sinus
dressing sponge
fistulous site
flexible colonoscope
foreign body
gastric bypass
gastric revision
hepatic flexure
intravenous (IV)
IV sedation
lower descending colon
myocardial infarction (MI)

neoplasm
percutaneous drainage
proximal transverse colon
renal failure
sigmoid colon
sinogram
splenectomy
stricture
total parenteral nutrition (TPN)
transverse colon
withdrawn, retroflexed and removed
wound change

Distal Gastrectomy
10-blade knife
celiac node
chevron incision
counts were correct
distal gastrectomy
divided using electrocautery
endoscopic evaluation
endotracheal intubation
falciform ligament
frozen section
gastric cancer
gastric mesentery
gastric sac
general endotracheal
GIA stapler
hemostasis
interrupted 3-0 silk popoff suture
intraoperative complication
jejunum
Kelly clamp
lesser curvature
lesser sac
ligament of Treitz
lumen
pancreatic lesion
partial gastrectomy
pathological evaluation
pathology and cytology
running #2 PDS sutures

peritoneal washing
peritoneum
prepped and draped
proximal duodenum
reanastomosis
silk tie
standard sterile fashion
subcutaneous tissue
supine position
surgical staple
tolerated the procedure well
wound bed

Exploratory Laparotomy for GunshotWound

appendectomy
appendiceal stump
#15 blade
bowel content
0 chromic tie
descending colon
electrocauterized
exit wound
exploratory laparotomy
Foley catheter
general anesthesia
GIA-55 stapler
gunshot wound
hematoma
hemothorax
intensive care unit (ICU)
inferior vena cava
Kocher maneuver
laparotomy pad
large bowel
left diaphragm
left upper quadrant
Lembert 3-0 silk stitch
lesser sac
ligament of Treitz
mesentery
mesoappendix
midline incision

pediatric intensive care unit
peritoneal cavity
2nd portion of the duodenum
primary anastomosis
pubic symphysis
pursestring stitch
retroperitoneal area
retroperitoneum
running double-stranded PDS stitch
simple 3-0 chromic stitch
small bowel
supine position
TA stapler
terminal ileum
umbilical hernia repair
xiphoid process

Exploratory Laparotomy Rule Out Ischemic Bowel

abdominal dressing
abdominal incision
aortobifemoral bypass
ascites
double-stranded running PDS suture
draped in the usual sterile fashion
estimated blood loss
exploratory laparotomy
friable
general endotracheal
groin dressing
hemodynamically unstable
ileum
internal mammary artery (IMA)
intraluminal
ischemic bowel
ischemic change
lactic acidosis
large bowel
peritoneal cavity
prepped with Betadine
second-look operation
small bowel lumen
small bowel resection

Common Terms

small bowel serosa
supine position
surgical intensive care unit
vasopressor

Hernia Repair with Kugel Patch

administration of intravenous sedation
anatomical position
anterior superior iliac spine
belly of the rectus muscle
blunt finger dissection
Cooper ligament
cord structure
electrocautery
external oblique aponeurosis
figure-of-8 suture
hernia sac
indirect sac
infiltrated with local anesthetic
internal oblique muscle
interrupted figure-of-8 suture
Kugel patch
left inguinal hernia
local intravenous sedation
4-0 Monocryl suture
operating room
Penrose drain
peritoneal envelope
postoperative counts were correct
preperitoneal pocket
prepped and draped
pubic bone
pubic tubercle
recovery room
running subcuticular tissue
Scarpa fascia
skin and subcutaneous tissue
skin closure
skin incision
spermatic cord
stable condition

sterile dressing
Steri-Strips
subcutaneous fat
superior ramus
supine position
suture ligated
symphysis pubis
tolerated the procedure well
transversalis fascia
transverse skin incision
transversus abdominis muscle
usual sterile fashion
0 Vicryl suture

Left Thyroid Lobectomy

aspiration biopsy
benign disease
3-0 chromic suture
endotracheal tube
face of the thyroid gland
frozen section
general anesthetic
good condition
interrupted sutures
isthmus
Jackson-Pratt drain
nerve monitor
nerve stimulator
4-0 nylon suture
operative room
papillary carcinoma
parathyroid gland
platysmal layer
prepped and draped
recurrent laryngeal nerve
running suture
skeletonized
skin crease incision
stab wound
sternal notch
strap muscle
thyroid gland

thyroid lobectomy
thyroid mass
tolerated the procedure well
ultrasound
upper pole vessel

Ligation and Stripping of Varicose Veins

chronic ulcer
elastic dressing
endotracheal tube
general anesthesia
groin crease incision
Kerlix
left lower extremity
ligation and stripping
operating room
prepped and draped
saphenofemoral junction
saphenous vein
skin grafted
standard fashion
sterile gauze
stripper
tolerated the procedure well
varicose vein
varicosity

Liposuction for Bilateral Gynecomastia

abdominal pad
adrenaline
aspiration
bilateral gynecomastia
binder
bupivacaine
cannula
contour marking
Coverlet dressing
fatty gynecomastia
fibrofatty tissue
fibrous tissue
general anesthetic

good condition
homogenized tissue
inframammary fold incision
limited ultrasound
liposuction
pectoralis major muscle
pectoral muscle
periareolar fullness
periareolar incision
5-0 plain catgut suture
residual tissue
retroareolar fibrous tissue
Ringer lactate
skin tightening
true gynecomastia
ultrasonic liposuction
vasoconstriction

Ramstedt Pyloromyotomy

anterior rectus sheath
Benson spreader
cautery
congenital hypertrophic pyloric stenosis
counts are correct
extubated
general endotracheal anesthesia
hemostasis
0.25% Marcaine
Mastisol
milking of the duodenum
milking of the stomach
5-0 Monocryl suture
myotomy
operating room
palpation
peritoneum
posterior rectus sheath
prepped and draped
pyloric stenosis
pylorus
Ramstedt pyloromyotomy
recovery room
running subcuticular pullout suture

running 4-0 Vicryl suture
Scarpa fascia
Steri-Strips
subcutaneous injection
subcutaneous tissue
supine position
tolerated the procedure well
transverse right upper quadrant incision
venous oozing

Right Inguinal Hernia Repair

Bassini repair
cremaster
en bloc
external oblique
external ring
fascia
genitofemoral nerve
groin
ilioinguinal nerve
inguinal hernia repair
internal ring
intravenous sedation
invaginated
large indirect right inguinal hernia
local anesthesia
0.5% Marcaine
modified Bassini repair
multiple omenta
patient tolerated the procedure well
posterior canal
2-0 Prolene suture
residual omentum
right inguinal hernia
running layer of 0 Prolene suture
running 4-0 Vicryl subcuticular suture
running 2-0 Vicryl suture
scrotum
sponge and instrument counts
Steri-Strips
suture ligated
transverse incision
2% Xylocaine with adrenaline

Right Pyeloplasty

anastomosed
approximated with staples
4-0 Biosyn suture
continuous running sutures
demarcated
distended kidney
double-J stent
external oblique muscle
fluoroscopy
Gerota fascia
hydronephrosis
internal oblique muscle
interrupted 0 Vicryl sutures
kidney function
malrotation
0.5% Marcaine with adrenaline
nerve block
operating room
Penrose drain
perinephric space
peritoneum
prepped and draped
recovery room
redundant portion
renal pelvis
retrograde pyelogram
retroperitoneal area
right collecting system
right pyeloplasty
right upper quadrant
satisfactory condition
satisfactory general anesthesia
spatulate the ureter
stent
subcostal nerve block
submucosal incision
transversus muscle
uneventful recovery
ureter
ureteropelvic junction obstruction
3-0 Vicryl suture

Scrotal Exploration with Bilateral Testicular Fixation

apical silk suture
bilateral testicular fixation
congestion
corresponding position
counts as correct
dartos fascia
3-0 Dexon suture
exploration of left scrotum
general anesthesia
hemiscrotum
hydrocele sac
inguinal ring block
interrupted 3-0 Monocryl suture
left hemiscrotum
left orchidectomy
0.5% Marcaine
OpSite spray
prepped and draped in the routine
    fashion
returned to the recovery room
routine fashion
running 3-0 Dexon suture
satisfactory condition
scrotal tissue
3-0 silk suture
spontaneous detorsion
superficial inguinal ring block
testicular torsion
testis
transverse incision
tunica albuginea
window of tunica

Sigmoid Colon Resection for Obstruction

abdominal cavity
acute large bowel obstruction
anastomosis site
appropriately monitored
blood supply

bowel prep
central line
chest x-ray
0 chromic tie
colon resection
distal resection margin
divided sequentially between snaps
endoscopic decompression
endotracheal intubation
end-to-end anastomosis
estimated blood loss
extubated
7.5-French triple-lumen catheter
full bowel prep
gain entry
general anesthetic with endotracheal
    intubation
Glassman bowel clamp
hemostasis
hemothorax
interrupted Gambee suture technique
Kocher clamp
laparotomy
large bowel obstruction
lower midline incision
mesenteric defect
mesentery
midline incision
no complications
normal liver
palpable abnormality
4-0 PDS suture
Penrose drain
pneumothorax
proximal resection margin
recovery room
redundant sigmoid colon
resection margin
right subclavian line
running 4-0 PDS suture
running #2 Vicryl suture
sigmoid colon
sigmoid colon resection

sigmoid volvulus
skin was closed with staples
small bowel
sponge, needle, and instrument counts
    were correct
stable condition
subclavian artery
suture ligation
thoroughly irrigated
triple-lumen catheter
wound was irrigated

Small Bowel Resection and Primary Reanastomosis

abdominal cavity
abdominal wall
acute abdomen
appropriately monitored
bowel wall
0 chromic suture
copious enteric contents
computed tomography (CT)
CT scan
diabetic gentleman
drain
effluent
endotracheal intubation
enteric content
estimated blood loss
extubated
free fluid
general anesthetic
generalized peritonitis
GIA-55 stapler
ICU admission
intensive care unit (ICU)
laparotomy
ligament of Treitz
mesenteric defect
mesentery
midline incision
no complications
normal saline

perforated viscus
perforation of jejunum
prepped and draped
primary reanastomosis
reapproximated with staples
recovery room
reintubation
respiratory deterioration
resultant defect
running #1 Vicryl suture
safely transferred
side-to-side stapled anastomosis
small bowel resection
sponge, needle and instrument counts
    were correct
stable condition
suctioned out
sudden onset of pain
TA-30 stapler
thickened loop of jejunum
thoroughly irrigated
umbilicus
urgent laparotomy
usual fashion

Splenectomy

abdominal wall
accessory spleen
Ancef antibiotic
anterior rectus fascia
Betadine solution
costal margin
doubly ligated
estimated blood loss
external oblique muscle
Foley catheter
general anesthetic
hematology service
hilum of the liver
inferior pole
inherited hemoglobinopathy
internal oblique muscle
lesser sac

5-0 Monocryl suture
nasogastric (NG) tube
omentum
operating room
pancreatic tail
peritoneal cavity
peritoneum
posterior rectus fascia
prepped and draped
running 2-0 Vicryl suture
short gastric vein

silk tie
singly ligated
splenectomy
splenic artery
splenic ligament
splenic vein
splenomegaly
Steri-Strips
subcuticular
transverse incision
2-0 Vicryl suture

Common Terms

Dermatomal Explanation

Dermatome	Area Innervated and Reflex Elicited	Nerve Affected
C2	occiput, top part of neck	greater occipital and anterior cutaneous of neck
C3	lower part of neck to clavicle	supraclavicular
C4	area just below the clavicle, deltoids	supraclavicular
C5	lateral arm, at and above the elbow, brachioradialis, infraspinatus, supraspinatus, deltoid, biceps	axillary
C6	forearm, radial side of hand wrist extensors	radial and median
C7	pronator teres, flexor carpi ulnaris, latissimus dorsi, triceps, long finger, elbow extensors	median
C8	lateral aspect of hand, wrist extensors and flexors, finger flexors	ulnar
T1	medial forearm, little	medial brachial cutaneous finger adductors
T2	sternal notch	intercostal and medial cutaneous
T3-T12	chest and back to hip girdle	
T4	nipples	intercostal

Dermatome	Area Innervated and Reflex Elicited	Nerve Affected
T6	xiphoid process	intercostal
T10	umbilicus	intercostal
L1	inguinal ligament	ilioinguinal, iliohypogastric
L2	iliopsoas, hip flexors	anterior femoral, lateral femoral
L3	adductor longus, hip adductors, quadriceps, patellar reflex, knee extensors	obturator
L4	vastus lateralis, knee extensors, vastus medialis, ankle dorsiflexors, anterior tibialis, patellar reflex	saphenous
L5	hip abductors, ankle dorsiflexion, eversion and inversion, long toe extensors, hallucis longus	lateral cutaneous
S1	hip extensors, ankle plantar flexors, gastrocnemius, heel, middle of back of leg, Achilles reflex	sural
S2	back of thigh	posterior cutaneous
S3	medial side of buttocks	posterior cutaneous
S4/5	perineal region, anal sphincter	pudendal
S5	skin at and adjacent to anus	pudendal

Appendix 7
American Academy of Pain Management (AAPM) Accredited Pain Programs

This list includes facilities that have passed the American Academy of Pain Management's rigorous pain program accreditation testing and on-site inspection and participate in additional AAPM services and status For additional information, please visit www.aapainmanage.org.

COLORADO
Craniofacial Diagnostic Center
1660 S. Albion, Ste. 1008
Denver, CO 80222

FLORIDA
Wuesthoff Pain Management Center
2400 N. Courtenay Pkwy.
Merritt Island, FL 32953

GEORGIA
Pain Control and Rehabilitation
    Institute of Georgia
2784 N. Decatur Rd., Ste. 120
Decatur, GA 30033

ILLINOIS
Advanced Pain Management Institute
7309 N. Knoxville Ave.
Peoria, IL 61614

Central Illinois Pain Center
OSF Center for Health
8600 N. State Route 91, Ste. 250
Peoria, IL 61615

Kishwaukee Community Hospital Pain
    Management Program
c/o Kishwaukee Community Hospital
626 Bethany Rd.
DeKalb, IL 60115

INDIANA
Oliver Headache and Pain Clinic
2828 Mt Vernon Ave.
Evansville, IN 47712

KENTUCKY
Ephraim McDowell Regional Medical
    Center
Pain Management Center
217 S. Third St.
Danville, KY 40422

Murphy Pain Center
3020 Eastpoint Pkwy.
Louisville, KY 40223

Spine & Brain Neurosurgical Center
1721 Nicholasville Rd.
Lexington, KY 40503

MASSACHUSETTS
Catholic Memorial Home Pain
    Management Program
2446 Highland Ave.
Fall River, MA 02720

Madonna Manor Pain Program
85 N. Washington St.
North Attleboro, MA 02760

Marian Manor Pain Management Program
33 Summer St.
Taunton, MA 02780-3491

Our Lady's Haven Pain Management
  Program
71 Center St.
Fairhaven, MA 02719

Sacred Heart Home Pain Management
  Program
359 Summer St.
New Bedford, MA 02740

MINNESOTA
United Pain Center
280 N. Smith Ave., Ste. 600
St. Paul, MN 55102

MISSISSIPPI
Pain Treatment Center
Rush Foundation Hospital
1314 19th Ave.
Meridian, MS 39301

MISSOURI
Headache Care Center
3805 S. Kansas Expressway
Springfield, MO 65807

St. Francis Medical Center Pain
  Management Center
211 St. Francis Dr.
Cape Girardeau, MO 63703

MONTANA
Frances Mahon Deaconess Hospital
621 Third St. S.
Glasgow, MT 59230

NEW HAMPSHIRE
Cottage Hospital Pain Clinic
PO Box 2001
90 Swiftwater Rd.
Woodsville, NH 03785

NEW YORK
Healthworks of Staten Island
1428 Victory Blvd.
Staten Island, NY 10301

OHIO
Blatman Pain Clinic
10653 Techwoods Circle, Ste. 101
Cincinnati, OH 45242

Grandview Hospital & Medical Center
405 Grand Ave.
Dayton, OH 45405-4796

The St. Joseph Pain Management
  Center
662 Eastland Ave.
Eastland Medical II Building, #201
Warren, OH 44484

PENNSYLVANIA
Gettysburg Rehabilitation Services
124 Carlisle St.
Gettysburg, PA 17325

Jefferson Pain & Rehabilitation Center
4735 Clairton Blvd.
Pittsburgh, PA 15236

Dr. Joseph L. Kaczor, INC. P.C.
2606 Broad Ave.
Altoona, PA 16601

Latrobe Area Hospital-Pain Control
  Center
121 W. Second Ave.
Latrobe, PA 15650

Michael S. Melnick, D.M.D., M.A.G.D.
The Park Plaza, Ste. 207
128 N. Craig St.
Pittsburgh, PA 15213

Pain Management Programs

Montgomery Surgical Center
One Abington Plaza, Ste. 100
Jenkintown, PA 19046

Sarah and Benjamin Lincow Pain
  Foundation
7622 Ogontz Ave.
Philadelphia, PA 19150

TEXAS

Acute & Chronic Pain Management
  Center
24 Care Circle
Amarillo, TX 79124

American College of Acupuncture &
  Oriental Medicine
9100 Park West Dr.
Houston, TX 77063

Center for Rehabilitative Medicine
1307 8th Ave., Ste. 610
Ft. Worth, TX 76104

Central Imaging of Arlington
1015 W. Randol Mill Rd.
Arlington, TX 76012

North Texas Pain Recovery Center
6702 W. Poly Webb Rd.
Arlington, TX 76016

Tri-County Pain Management Centre
PO Box 758
200 N. Arch St.
Royse City, TX 75189

Drugs by Indication

ABORTION

Antiprogestin
  Mifeprex® [US]
  mifepristone
Oxytocic Agent
  oxytocin
  Pitocin® [US/Can]
Prostaglandin
  carboprost tromethamine
  Cervidil® [US/Can]
  dinoprostone
  Hemabate® [US/Can]
  Prepidil® [US/Can]
  Prostin E2® [US/Can]

ANESTHESIA (GENERAL)

Barbiturate
  Brevital® Sodium [US/Can]
  methohexital
General Anesthetic
  Amidate® [US/Can]
  desflurane
  Diprivan® [US/Can]
  enflurane
  Ethrane® [US/Can]
  etomidate
  Forane® [US]
  halothane
  isoflurane
  Ketalar® [US/Can]
  ketamine
  propofol
  sevoflurane
  Sevorane AF™ [Can]
  Suprane® [US/Can]
  Ultane® [US]

ANESTHESIA (LOCAL)

Local Anesthetic
  AK-T-Caine™ [US]
  Alcaine® [US/Can]
  Americaine® Anesthetic Lubricant [US]
  Americaine®[US-OTC]
  Ametop™ [Can]
  Anbesol® Baby [US-OTC/Can]
  Anbesol® Maximum Strength [US-OTC]
  Anbesol® [US-OTC]
  Anestacon® [US]
  Anusol® Ointment [US-OTC]
  Babee® Teething(R) [US-OTC]
  Band-Aid® Hurt-Free(TM) Antiseptic Wash [US-OTC]
  benzocaine
  benzocaine, butyl aminobenzoate, tetracaine, and benzalkonium chloride
  benzocaine, gelatin, pectin, and sodium carboxymethylcellulose
  Benzodent® [US-OTC]
  Betacaine® [Can]
  bupivacaine
  Burnamycin [US-OTC]
  Burn Jel [US-OTC]
  Burn-O-Jel [US-OTC]
  Carbocaine® [Can]
  Cepacol® [Can]
  Cepacol® Gold [US-OTC]
  Cepacol® Maximum Strength [US-OTC]
  Cepacol Viractin® [US-OTC]
  Cetacaine® [US]
  cetylpyridinium
  cetylpyridinium and benzocaine
  Chiggerex® [US-OTC]

Chiggertox® [US-OTC]
chloroprocaine
Citanest® Plain [US/Can]
cocaine
Cylex® [US-OTC]
Detane® [US-OTC]
dibucaine
Diocaine®[Can]
dyclonine
ethyl chloride
ethyl chloride and
    dichlorotetrafluoroethane
Flucaine®[US]
Fluoracaine® [US]
Fluro-Ethyl® [US]
Foille® Medicated First Aid [US-
    OTC]
Foille® Plus [US-OTC]
Foille® [US-OTC]
Gebauer's Ethyl Chloride® [US]
HDA® Toothache [US-OTC]
hexylresorcinol
Hurricaine® [US]
Itch-X®[US-OTC]
Kank-A® [Can]
Lanacane® [US-OTC]
LidaMantle® [US]
lidocaine
lidocaine and epinephrine
Lidodan™ [Can]
Lidoderm® [US/Can]
LidoSite™ [US]
L-M-X™ 4 [US-OTC]
L-M-X™ 5 [US-OTC]
Marcaine®Spinal [US]
Marcaine®[US/Can]
mepivacaine
Mycinettes® [US-OTC]
Naropin® [US/Can]
Nesacaine®-CE [Can]
Nesacaine®-MPF [US]
Nesacaine® [US]

Novocain® [US/Can]
Nupercainal® [US-OTC]
Ophthetic® [US]
Opticaine® [US]
Orabase®-B [US-OTC]
Orajel® Baby Nighttime [US-OTC]
Orajel® Baby [US-OTC]
Orajel®Maximum Strength [US-
    OTC]
Orajel® [US-OTC]
Orasol® [US-OTC]
Polocaine® MPF [US]
Polocaine® [US/Can]
Pontocaine® [US/Can]
Pontocaine® With Dextrose [US]
pramoxine
Prax® [US-OTC]
Premjact® [US-OTC]
prilocaine
procaine
ProctoFoam® NS [US-OTC]
proparacaine
proparacaine and fluorescein
ropivacaine
Sensorcaine®-MPF [US]
Sensorcaine® [US/Can]
Solarcaine® Aloe Extra Burn Relief
    [US-OTC]
Solarcaine® [US-OTC]
Sucrets® Original [US-OTC]
Sucrets® [US-OTC]
tetracaine
tetracaine and dextrose
Topicaine® [US-OTC]
Trocaine® [US-OTC]
Tronolane®[US-OTC]
Xylocaine® MPF [US]
Xylocaine® MPF With Epinephrine
    [US]
Xylocaine® [US/Can]
Xylocaine® Viscous [US]
Xylocaine®With Epinephrine [Can]

Xylocard® [Can]
Zilactin® Baby [US-OTC/Can]
Zilactin®-B [US-OTC/Can]
Zilactin® [Can]
Zilactin-L® [US-OTC]
Local Anesthetic, Amide Derivative
Chirocaine® [Can]
levobupivacaine
Local Anesthetic, Injectable
Chirocaine® [Can]
levobupivacaine

ANESTHESIA (OPHTHALMIC)
Local Anesthetic
Flucaine® [US]
Fluoracaine® [US]
proparacaine and fluorescein

ANGIOGRAPHY (OPHTHALMIC)
Diagnostic Agent
AK-Fluor [US]
Angiscein® [US]
Diofluor™ [Can]
fluorescein sodium
Fluorescite® [US/Can]
Fluorets® [US/Can]
Fluor-I-Strip-AT® [US]
Fluor-I-Strip® [US]
Ful-Glo® [US]

ANXIETY
Antianxiety Agent
Apo-Buspirone® [Can]
BuSpar® [US/Can]
Buspirex [Can]
buspirone
Gen-Buspirone [Can]
Lin-Buspirone [Can]
Novo-Buspirone [Can]
Nu-Buspirone [Can]
PMS-Buspirone [Can]

Antianxiety Agent, Miscellaneous
meprobamate
Miltown®[US]
Novo-Mepro [Can]
Antidepressant/Phenothiazine
amitriptyline and perphenazine
Etrafon® [Can]
Triavil® [US/Can]
Antidepressant, Tetracyclic
maprotiline
Novo-Maprotiline [Can]
Antidepressant, Tricyclic (Secondary Amine)
amoxapine
Antidepressant, Tricyclic (Tertiary Amine)
amitriptyline and chlordiazepoxide
Apo-Doxepin® [Can]
doxepin
Limbitrol® DS [US]
Limbitrol® [US/Can]
Novo-Doxepin [Can]
Prudoxin™ [US]
Sinequan® [US/Can]
Zonalon® [US/Can]
Antihistamine
Aler-Dryl [US-OTC]
Allerdryl® [Can]
AllerMax® [US-OTC]
Allernix [Can]
Apo-Hydroxyzine® [Can]
Atarax® [US/Can]
Banophen® [US-OTC]
Benadryl® Allergy [US-OTC/Can]
Benadryl® Dye-Free Allergy [US-OTC]
Benadryl® Gel Extra Strength [US-OTC]
Benadryl® Gel [US-OTC]
Benadryl® Injection [US]
Compoz® Nighttime Sleep Aid [US-OTC]
Diphen® AF [US-OTC]

Diphen® Cough [US-OTC]
Diphenhist [US-OTC]
diphenhydramine
Diphen® [US-OTC]
Genahist® [US-OTC]
Hydramine® Cough [US-OTC]
Hydramine® [US-OTC]
hydroxyzine
Hyrexin-50® [US]
Novo-Hydroxyzin [Can]
Nytol® Extra Strength [Can]
Nytol® Maximum Strength [US-OTC]
Nytol®[US-OTC/Can]
PMS-Diphenhydramine [Can]
PMS-Hydroxyzine [Can]
Siladryl® Allergy [US-OTC]
Silphen® [US-OTC]
Simply Sleep® [Can]
Sleepinal® [US-OTC]
Sominex® Maximum Strength [US-OTC]
Sominex® [US-OTC]
Tusstat® [US]
Twilite® [US-OTC]
Unisom® Maximum Strength SleepGels® [US-OTC]
Vistaril(v [US/Can]
Barbiturate
  butabarbital sodium
  butalbital, aspirin, caffeine, and codeine
  Butisol Sodium® [US]
  Fiorinal®-C 1/2 [Can]
  Fiorinal®-C 1/4 [Can]
  Fiorinal® With Codeine [US]
  Phrenilin® With Caffeine and Codeine [US]
  Tecnal C 1/2 [Can]
  Tecnal C 1/4 [Can]
Benzodiazepine
  alprazolam
  Alprazolam Intensol® [US]
  Alti-Alprazolam [Can]

Apo-Alpraz® [Can]
Apo-Bromazepam® [Can]
Apo-Chlordiazepoxide® [Can]
Apo-Clorazepate® [Can]
Apo-Diazepam® [Can]
Apo-Lorazepam® [Can]
Apo-Oxazepam® [Can]
Apo-Temazepam® [Can]
Ativan® [US/Can]
bromazepam (Canada only)
chlordiazepoxide
clorazepate
CO Temazepam [Can]
Diastat® [US/Can]
Diazemuls® [Can]
diazepam
Diazepam Intensol® [US]
Gen-Alprazolam [Can]
Gen-Bromazepam [Can]
Gen-Temazepam [Can]
Lectopam® [Can]
Librium® [US]
lorazepam
Lorazepam Intensol® [US]
Novo-Alprazol [Can]
Novo-Bromazepam [Can]
Novo-Clopate [Can]
Novo-Lorazem® [Can]
Novo-Temazepam [Can]
Novoxapram® [Can]
Nu-Alprax [Can]
Nu-Bromazepam [Can]
Nu-Loraz [Can]
Nu-Temazepam [Can]
oxazepam
PMS-Lorazepam [Can]
PMS-Oxazepam [Can]
PMS-Temazepam [Can]
ratio-Temazepam [Can]
Restoril® [US/Can]
Riva-Lorazepam [Can]
Serax® [US]
temazepam

Tranxene® SD™-Half Strength [US]
Tranxene® SD™[US]
Tranxene® [US]
T-Tab® [US]
Valium® [US/Can]
Xanax TS™ [Can]
Xanax® [US/Can]
Xanax XR® [US]
General Anesthetic
Actiq® [US/Can]
Duragesic® [US/Can]
fentanyl
Sublimaze® [US]
Neuroleptic Agent
Apo-Methoprazine® [Can]
methotrimeprazine (Canada only)
Novo-Meprazine [Can]
Nozinan® [Can]
Phenothiazine Derivative
Apo-Trifluoperazine® [Can]
Novo-Trifluzine [Can]
PMS-Trifluoperazine [Can]
trifluoperazine
Sedative
Apo-Bromazepam® [Can]
bromazepam (Canada only)
Gen-Bromazepam [Can]
Lectopam® [Can]
Novo-Bromazepam [Can]
Nu-Bromazepam [Can]

BACK PAIN (LOW)

Analgesic, Narcotic
codeine
Codeine Contin® [Can]
Analgesic, Nonnarcotic
Asaphen [Can]
Asaphen E.C. [Can]
Ascriptin® Extra Strength [US-OTC]
Ascriptin® [US-OTC]
Aspercin Extra [US-OTC]
Aspercin [US-OTC]
Aspergum® [US-OTC]

aspirin
Bayer® Aspirin Extra Strength [US-OTC]
Bayer® Aspirin Regimen Adult Low Strength [US-OTC]
Bayer® Aspirin Regimen Children's [US-OTC]
Bayer® Aspirin Regimen Regular Strength [US-OTC]
Bayer® Aspirin [US-OTC]
Bayer® Extra Strength Arthritis Pain Regimen [US-OTC]
Bayer® Plus Extra Strength [US-OTC]
Bayer® Women's Aspirin Plus Calcium [US-OTC]
Bufferin® Extra Strength [US-OTC]
Bufferin® [US-OTC]
Buffinol Extra [US-OTC]
Buffinol [US-OTC]
Easprin® [US]
Ecotrin® Low Strength [US-OTC]
Ecotrin® Maximum Strength [US-OTC]
Ecotrin® [US-OTC]
Entrophen® [Can]
Halfprin® [US-OTC]
Novasen [Can]
St Joseph® Adult Aspirin [US-OTC]
Sureprin 81™ [US-OTC]
ZORprin® [US]
Benzodiazepine
Apo-Diazepam® [Can]
Diastat® [US/Can]
Diazemuls® [Can]
diazepam
Diazepam Intensol® [US]
Valium® [US/Can]
Nonsteroidal Antiinflammatory Drug (NSAID)
Doan's® Extra Strength [US-OTC]
Doan's® [US-OTC]
magnesium salicylate
Momentum® [US-OTC]

Skeletal Muscle Relaxant
  methocarbamol
  methocarbamol and aspirin
  Robaxin® [US/Can]

BLADDER IRRIGATION
Antibacterial, Topical
  acetic acid

BOWEL CLEANSING
Laxative
  castor oil
  Citro-Mag® [Can]
  Colyte®[US/Can]
  Fleet® Enema [US-OTC/Can]
  Fleet® Phospho®-Soda Accu-Prep™
    [US-OTC]
  Fleet® Phospho®-Soda Oral
    Laxative [Can]
  Fleet® Phospho®-Soda [US-OTC]
  GlycoLax™ [US]
  GoLYTELY® [US]
  Klean-Prep® [Can]
  Lyteprep™ [Can]
  magnesium citrate
  MiraLax™ [US]
  NuLYTELY® [US]
  PegLyte® [Can]
  polyethylene glycol-electrolyte
    solution
  Purge® [US-OTC]
  sodium phosphates
  TriLyte™ [US]
  Visicol™ [US]
Laxative, Bowel Evacuant
  HalfLytely® and Bisacodyl [US]
  polyethylene glycol-electrolyte
    solution and bisacodyl

BOWEL STERILIZATION
Aminoglycoside (Antibiotic)
  Myciguent [US-OTC]
  Neo-Fradin™ [US]

  neomycin
  Neo-Rx [US]

CARDIAC DECOMPENSATION
Adrenergic Agonist Agent
  dobutamine
  Dobutrex® [Can]

CARDIOGENIC SHOCK
Adrenergic Agonist Agent
  dobutamine
  Dobutrex® [Can]
  dopamine
  Intropin® [Can]
Cardiac Glycoside
  Digitek® [US]
  digoxin
  Digoxin CSD [Can]
  Lanoxicaps® [US/Can]
  Lanoxin® [US/Can]
  Novo-Digoxin [Can]

CATARACT
Adrenergic Agonist Agent
  Neo-Synephrine® Ophthalmic [US]
  phenylephrine

COLONIC EVACUATION
Laxative
  Alophen® [US-OTC]
  Apo-Bisacodyl® [Can]
  Bisac-Evac™ [US-OTC]
  bisacodyl
  Bisacodyl Unisert® [US-OTC]
  Carter's Little Pills® [Can]
  Correctol® Tablets [US-OTC]
  Doxidan® (reformulation) [US-OTC]
  Dulcolax® [US-OTC/Can]
  Femilax™ [US-OTC]
  Fleet® Bisacodyl Enema [US-OTC]
  Fleet® Stimulant Laxative [US-OTC]
  Gentlax® [US-OTC]

Modane Tablets® [US-OTC]
Veracolate [US-OTC]

CONGESTION (NASAL)
Adrenergic Agonist Agent
Afrin® Extra Moisturizing [US-OTC]
Afrin® Original [US-OTC]
Afrin® Severe Congestion [US-OTC]
Afrin® Sinus [US-OTC]
Afrin® [US-OTC]
Allersol® [US]
Balminil® [Can]
Balminil® Decongestant [Can]
Benzedrex® [US-OTC]
Biofed [US-OTC]
Claritin® Allergic Decongestant [Can]
Contac® Cold 12 Hour Relief Non Drowsy [Can]
Decofed® [US-OTC]
Decongest [Can]
Dimetapp® 12-Hour Non-Drowsy Extentabs® [US-OTC]
Dimetapp® Decongestant [US-OTC]
Dionephrine® [Can]
Dristan® Long Lasting Nasal [Can]
Drixoral® Nasal [Can]
Drixoral® ND [Can]
Duramist® Plus [US-OTC]
Duration® [US-OTC]
Eltor® [Can]
ephedrine
Formulation R™ [US-OTC]
Genaphed® [US-OTC]
Genasal [US-OTC]
Kidkare Decongestant [US-OTC]
Kodet SE [US-OTC]
Medicone® [US-OTC]
naphazoline
Nostril® [US-OTC]
oxymetazoline
phenylephrine
propylhexedrine

pseudoephedrine
Pseudofrin [Can]
Silfedrine Children's [US-OTC]
Sudafed® 12 Hour [US-OTC]
Sudafed® 24 Hour [US-OTC]
Sudafed® Children's [US-OTC]
Sudafed® Decongestant [Can]
Sudafed® [US-OTC]
Sudodrin [US-OTC]
tetrahydrozoline
Triaminic® Allergy Congestion [US-OTC/Can]
Twice-A-Day® [US-OTC]
Tyzine® Pediatric [US]
Tyzine® [US]
Vicks® Sinex(R) 12 Hour Ultrafine Mist [US-OTC]
Vicks® Sinex(R) Nasal [US-OTC]
Vicks® Sinex(R) UltraFine Mist [US-OTC]
4-Way® Long Acting [US-OTC]
xylometazoline

CYCLOPLEGIA
Anticholinergic Agent
AtroPen® [US]
atropine
Atropine-Care® [US]
Buscopan® [Can]
Cyclogyl® [US/Can]
cyclopentolate
Cylate® [US]
Diopentolate® [Can]
Dioptic's Atropine Solution [Can]
Diotrope® [Can]
homatropine
Isopto® Atropine [US/Can]
Isopto® Homatropine [US]
Isopto® Hyoscine [US]
Minim's Atropine Solution [Can]
Mydriacyl® [US/Can]
Opticyl® [US]
Sal-Tropine™ [US]

scopolamine
Tropicacyl® [US]
tropicamide

DE-BRIDEMENT OF CALLOUS TISSUE

Keratolytic Agent
trichloroacetic acid
Tri-Chlor® [US]

DE-BRIDEMENT OF ESCHAR

Protectant, Topical
Granulex® [US]
trypsin, balsam peru, and castor oil

DECUBITUS ULCER

Enzyme
collagenase
Santyl® [US/Can]
Enzyme, Topical De-bridement
papain and urea
Protectant, Topical
Granulex® [US]
trypsin, balsam peru, and castor oil
Topical Skin Product
papain and urea

DEPRESSION (RESPIRATORY)

Respiratory Stimulant
Dopram® [US]
doxapram

EROSIVE ESOPHAGITIS

Proton Pump Inhibitor
esomeprazole
Nexium® [US/Can]

ESOPHAGEAL VARICES

Hormone, Posterior Pituitary
Pitressin® [US]
Pressyn® AR [Can]
Pressyn® [Can]
vasopressin
Sclerosing Agent
Ethamolin® [US]
ethanolamine oleate
Variceal Bleeding (Acute) Agent
somatostatin (Canada only)
Stilamin® [Can]

ESOPHAGITIS

Gastric Acid Secretion Inhibitor
lansoprazole
Losec® [Can]
omeprazole
Prevacid® SoluTab™ [US]
Prevacid® [US/Can]
Prilosec OTC™ [US-OTC]
Prilosec® [US]
Zegerid™ [US]

GAG REFLEX SUPPRESSION

Analgesic, Topical
lidocaine
Xylocaine® Viscous [US]
Local Anesthetic
Americaine® Anesthetic Lubricant [US]
Americaine® [US-OTC]
benzocaine
benzocaine, butyl aminobenzoate, tetracaine, and benzalkonium chloride
Benzodent® [US-OTC]
dyclonine
Hurricaine® [US]
Pontocaine® [US/Can]
tetracaine

GALL BLADDER DISEASE (DIAGNOSTIC)

Diagnostic Agent
  Kinevac® [US]
  sincalide

GASTRITIS

Antacid
  Alamag [US-OTC]
  aluminum hydroxide and
    magnesium hydroxide
  Diovol® [Can]
  Diovol® Ex [Can]
  Gelusil® [Can]
  Gelusil® Extra Strength [Can]
  Mylanta® [Can]
  Rulox No. 1 [US]
  Rulox [US]
  Univol® [Can]
Histamine H2 Antagonist
  Alti-Ranitidine [Can]
  Apo-Cimetidine® [Can]
  Apo-Ranitidine® [Can]
  cimetidine
  Gen-Cimetidine [Can]
  Gen-Ranitidine [Can]
  Novo-Cimetidine [Can]
  Novo-Ranidine [Can]
  Nu-Cimet [Can]
  Nu-Ranit [Can]
  PMS-Cimetidine [Can]
  PMS-Ranitidine [Can]
  ranitidine hydrochloride
  Rhoxal-ranitidine [Can]
  Tagamet® HB 200 [US-OTC/Can]
  Tagamet® [US]
  Zantac® 75 [US-OTC/Can]
  Zantac® [US/Can]

GASTROESOPHAGEAL REFLUX DISEASE (GERD)

Cholinergic Agent
  bethanechol
  Duvoid® [Can]
  Myotonachol® [Can]
  PMS-Bethanechol [Can]
  Urecholine® [US]
Gastric Acid Secretion Inhibitor
  Aciphex® [US/Can]
  lansoprazole
  Losec® [Can]
  omeprazole
  Pariet® [Can]
  Prevacid® SoluTab™ [US]
  Prevacid® [US/Can]
  Prilosec OTC(TM) [US-OTC]
  Prilosec® [US]
  rabeprazole
  Zegerid(TM) [US]
Gastrointestinal Agent, Prokinetic
  Apo-Metoclop® [Can]
  cisapride
  metoclopramide
  Nu-Metoclopramide [Can]
  Propulsid® [US]
  Reglan® [US]
Histamine H2 Antagonist
  Alti-Ranitidine [Can]
  Apo-Cimetidine® [Can]
  Apo-Famotidine® [Can]
  Apo-Nizatidine® [Can]
  Apo-Ranitidine® [Can]
  Axid® AR [US-OTC]
  Axid® [US/Can]
  cimetidine
  famotidine
  Gen-Cimetidine [Can]
  Gen-Famotidine [Can]
  Gen-Nizatidine [Can]
  Gen-Ranitidine [Can]
  nizatidine

A103

Novo-Cimetidine [Can]
Novo-Famotidine [Can]
Novo-Nizatidine [Can]
Novo-Ranidine [Can]
Nu-Cimet [Can]
Nu-Famotidine [Can]
Nu-Nizatidine [Can]
Nu-Ranit [Can]
Pepcid® AC [US-OTC/Can]
Pepcid® I.V. [Can]
Pepcid® [US/Can]
PMS-Cimetidine [Can]
PMS-Nizatidine [Can]
PMS-Ranitidine [Can]
ranitidine hydrochloride
ratio-Famotidine [Can]
Rhoxal-famotidine [Can]
Rhoxal-ranitidine [Can]
Riva-Famotidine [Can]
Tagamet® HB 200 [US-OTC/Can]
Tagamet® [US]
Zantac® 75 [US-OTC/Can]
Zantac® [US/Can]
Proton Pump Inhibitor
Panto™ IV [Can]
Pantoloc™ [Can]
pantoprazole
Protonix® [US/Can]

HEMORRHAGE

Adrenergic Agonist Agent
Adrenalin® [US/Can]
epinephrine
Antihemophilic Agent
Bebulin® VH [US]
factor IX complex (human)
Profilnine® SD [US]
Proplex® T [US]
Ergot Alkaloid and Derivative
ergonovine
Hemostatic Agent
Amicar® [US/Can]
aminocaproic acid

aprotinin
Avitene® Flour [US]
Avitene® Ultrafoam [US]
Avitene® UltraWrap™ [US]
Avitene® [US]
cellulose, oxidized regenerated
collagen hemostat
EndoAvitene® [US]
gelatin (absorbable)
Gelfilm® [US]
Gelfoam® [US]
Helistat® [US]
Instat™ MCH [US]
Surgical® Fibrillar [US]
Surgicel® NuKnit [US]
Surgicel® [US]
SyringeAvitene™ [US]
Thrombin-JMI® [US]
thrombin (topical)
Thrombogen® [US]
Thrombostat™ [Can]
Trasylol® [US/Can]
Progestin
Alti-MPA [Can]
Apo-Medroxy® [Can]
Aygestin® [US]
CamilaTM [US]
Crinone® [US/Can]
Depo-Provera® Contraceptive [US]
Depo-Provera® [US/Can]
Errin™ [US]
Gen-Medroxy [Can]
hydroxyprogesterone caproate
Jolivette™ [US]
medroxyprogesterone acetate
Micronor® [US/Can]
Nora-BE™ [US]
norethindrone
Norlutate® [Can]
Nor-QD® [US]
Novo-Medrone [Can]
Prochieve™ [US]
Progestasert® [US]

progesterone
Prometrium® [US/Can]
Provera® [US/Can]
Vitamin, Fat Soluble
AquaMEPHYTON® [Can]
Konakion [Can]
Mephyton® [US/Can]
phytonadione

HEMORRHAGE (POSTPARTUM)

Ergot Alkaloid and Derivative
ergonovine
Methergine® [US/Can]
methylergonovine
Oxytocic Agent
oxytocin
Pitocin® [US/Can]
Syntocinon® [Can]
Prostaglandin
carboprost tromethamine
Hemabate® [US/Can]

HEMORRHAGE (PREVENTION)

Antihemophilic Agent
Cyklokapron® [US/Can]
tranexamic acid

HEMORRHAGE (SUBARACHNOID)

Calcium Channel Blocker
nimodipine
Nimotop® [US/Can]

HEMOSTASIS

Hemostatic Agent
Crosseal™ [US]
fibrin sealant kit
Tisseel® VH [US/Can]

HYPERTENSION

Adrenergic Agonist Agent
inamrinone
Alpha-Adrenergic Agonist
Apo-Clonidine® [Can]
Carapres® [Can]
Catapres-TTS® [US]
Catapres® [US]
clonidine
Dixarit® [Can]
Duraclon™ [US]
guanabenz
guanfacine
Novo-Clonidine [Can]
Nu-Clonidine® [Can]
Tenex® [US/Can]
Wytensin® [Can]
Alpha-Adrenergic Blocking Agent
Alti-Doxazosin [Can]
Alti-Terazosin [Can]
Apo-Doxazosin® [Can]
Apo-Methyldopa® [Can]
Apo-Prazo® [Can]
Apo-Terazosin® [Can]
Cardura-1™ [Can]
Cardura-2™ [Can]
Cardura-4™ [Can]
Cardura® [US]
Dibenzyline® [US/Can]
doxazosin
Gen-Doxazosin [Can]
Hytrin® [US/Can]
methyldopa
Minipress® [US/Can]
Novo-Doxazosin [Can]
Novo-Prazin [Can]
Novo-Terazosin [Can]
Nu-Medopa [Can]
Nu-Prazo [Can]
Nu-Terazosin [Can]
phenoxybenzamine
phentolamine

PMS-Terazosin [Can]
prazosin
Regitine® [Can]
Rogitine(® [Can]
terazosin
Alpha-/Beta- Adrenergic Blocker
  Apo-Labetalol® [Can]
  labetalol
  Normodyne® [US/Can]
  Trandate® [US/Can]
Angiotensin-Converting Enzyme (ACE)
    Inhibitor
  Accupril® [US/Can]
  Altace® [US/Can]
  Alti-Captopril [Can]
  Apo-Capto® [Can]
  Apo-Lisinopril® [Can]
  benazepril
  Capoten® [US/Can]
  captopril
  cilazapril (Canada only)
  enalapril
  fosinopril
  fosinopril and hydrochlorothiazide
  Gen-Captopril [Can]
  Inhibace® [Can]
  lisinopril
  Lotensin® [US/Can]
  Mavik® [US/Can]
  moexipril
  moexipril and hydrochlorothiazide
  Monopril-HCT® [US/Can]
  Monopril® [US/Can]
  Novo-Captopril [Can]
  Nu-Capto [Can]
  PMS-Captopril [Can]
  Prinivil® [US/Can]
  quinapril
  ramipril
  spirapril
  trandolapril
  Uniretic® [US/Can]
  Univasc® [US]

Vasotec® [US/Can]
Zestril® [US/Can]
Angiotensin II Antagonist Combination
  eprosartan and hydrochlorothiazide
  Teveten® HCT [US/Can]
Angiotensin II Receptor Antagonist
  Atacand® [US/Can]
  Avapro® [US/Can]
  Benicar HCT™ [US]
  Benicar™ [US]
  candesartan
  Cozaar® [US/Can]
  Diovan® [US/Can]
  eprosartan
  irbesartan
  losartan
  Micardis® [US/Can]
  olmesartan
  olmesartan and hydrochlorothiazide
  telmisartan
  Teveten® [US/Can]
  valsartan
Antihypertensive Agent
  diazoxide
  eplerenone
  Hyperstat® I.V. [Can]
  Hyperstat® [US]
  Inspra™ [US]
  Proglycem® [US/Can]
Antihypertensive Agent, Combination
  Accuretic™ [US/Can]
  Aldactazide 25® [Can]
  Aldactazide 50® [Can]
  Aldactazide® [US]
  Aldoril® D [US]
  Aldoril® [US]
  amlodipine and benazepril
  Apo-Methazide® [Can]
  Apo-Triazide® [Can]
  Atacand HCT™ [US]
  Atacand® Plus [Can]
  atenolol and chlorthalidone
  Avalide® [US/Can]

benazepril and hydrochlorothiazide
bisoprolol and hydrochlorothiazide
candesartan and
   hydrochlorothiazide
Capozide® [US/Can]
captopril and hydrochlorothiazide
clonidine and chlorthalidone
Clorpres® [US]
Diovan HCT® [US/Can]
Dyazide® [US]
enalapril and felodipine
enalapril and hydrochlorothiazide
Enduronyl® Forte [US/Can]
Enduronyl® [US/Can]
eprosartan and hydrochlorothiazide
hydralazine and hydrochlorothiazide
hydralazine, hydrochlorothiazide,
   and reserpine
hydrochlorothiazide and
   spironolactone
hydrochlorothiazide and triamterene
Hyzaar® DS [Can]
Hyzaar® [US/Can]
Inderide® [US]
irbesartan and hydrochlorothiazide
Lexxel® [US/Can]
lisinopril and hydrochlorothiazide
losartan and hydrochlorothiazide
Lotensin® HCT [US]
Lotrel® [US]
Maxzide®-25 [US]
Maxzide® [US]
methyclothiazide and deserpidine
methyldopa and
   hydrochlorothiazide
Micardis® HCT [US]
Micardis® Plus [Can]
Minizide® [US]
Novo-Spirozine [Can]
Novo-Triamzide [Can]
Nu-Triazide [Can]
Penta-Triamterene HCTZ [Can]

prazosin and polythiazide
Prinzide® [US/Can]
propranolol and hydrochlorothiazide
quinapril and hydrochlorothiazide
Riva-Zide [Can]
Tarka® [US/Can]
telmisartan and hydrochlorothiazide
Tenoretic® [US/Can]
Teveten® HCT [US/Can]
trandolapril and verapamil
valsartan and hydrochlorothiazide
Vaseretic® [US/Can]
Zestoretic® [US/Can]
Ziac® [US/Can]
Beta-Adrenergic Blocker
  acebutolol
  Alti-Nadolol [Can]
  Alti-Timolol [Can]
  Apo-Acebutolol® [Can]
  Apo-Atenol® [Can]
  Apo-Metoprolol® [Can]
  Apo-Nadol® [Can]
  Apo-Pindol® [Can]
  Apo-Propranolol® [Can]
  Apo-Timol® [Can]
  Apo-Timop® [Can]
  atenolol
  Betaloc® [Can]
  Betaloc® Durules®
  betaxolol
  Betimol® [US]
  Betoptic® S [US/Can]
  bisoprolol
  Blocadren® [US]
  Brevibloc® [US/Can]
  carteolol
  Cartrol® Oral [Can]
  carvedilol
  Coreg® [US/Can]
  Corgard® [US/Can]
  esmolol
  Gen-Acebutolol [Can]

Gen-Atenolol [Can]
Gen-Pindolol [Can]
Gen-Timolol [Can]
Inderal® LA [US/Can]
Inderal® [US/Can]
InnoPran XL™ [US]
Istalol™ [US]
Kerlone® [US]
Lopressor® [US/Can]
metoprolol
Monitan® [Can]
Monocor® [Can]
nadolol
Novo-Acebutolol [Can]
Novo-Atenol [Can]
Novo-Metoprolol [Can]
Novo-Nadolol [Can]
Novo-Pindol [Can]
Nu-Acebutolol [Can]
Nu-Atenol [Can]
Nu-Metop [Can]
Nu-Pindol [Can]
Nu-Propranolol [Can]
Nu-Timolol [Can]
Ocupress® Ophthalmic [Can]
oxprenolol (Canada only)
Phoxal-timolol [Can]
pindolol
PMS-Atenolol [Can]
PMS-Metoprolol [Can]
PMS-Pindolol [Can]
PMS-Timolol [Can]
propranolol
Propranolol Intensol™ [US]
Rhotral [Can]
Rhoxal-atenolol [Can]
Sectral® [US/Can]
Slow-Trasicor® [Can]
Tenolin [Can]
Tenormin® [US/Can]
Tim-AK [Can]
timolol
Timoptic® OcuDose® [US]

Timoptic® [US/Can]
Timoptic-XE® [US/Can]
Toprol-XL® [US/Can]
Trasicor® [Can]
Visken® [Can]
Zebeta® [US/Can]
Calcium Channel Blocker
Adalat® CC [US]
Adalat® XL® [Can]
Alti-Verapamil [Can]
amlodipine
amlodipine and atorvastatin
Apo-Nifed® [Can]
Apo-Nifed PA® [Can]
Apo-Verap® [Can]
bepridil
Caduet® [US]
Calan® SR [US]
Calan® [US/Can]
Cardene® I.V. [US]
Cardene® SR [US]
Cardene® [US]
Chronovera® [Can]
Covera® [Can]
Covera-HS® [US]
DynaCirc® CR [US]
DynaCirc® [US/Can]
felodipine
Gen-Verapamil [Can]
Gen-Verapamil SR [Can]
Isoptin® [Can]
Isoptin® I.V. [Can]
Isoptin® SR [US/Can]
isradipine
nicardipine
Nifedical™ XL [US]
nifedipine
nisoldipine
Norvasc® [US/Can]
Novo-Nifedin [Can]
Novo-Veramil [Can]
Novo-Veramil SR [Can]
Nu-Nifed [Can]

Plendil® [US/Can]
Procardia® [US/Can]
Procardia XL® [US]
Renedil® [Can]
Sular® [US]
Vascor® [Can]
verapamil
Verelan® PM [US]
Verelan® [US]
Diuretic, Combination
    amiloride and hydrochlorothiazide
    Apo-Amilzide® [Can]
    Moduret® [Can]
    Moduretic® [Can]
    Novamilor [Can]
    Nu-Amilzide [Can]
Diuretic, Loop
    Apo-Furosemide® [Can]
    bumetanide
    Bumex® [US/Can]
    Burinex®[Can]
    Demadex® [US]
    Edecrin® [US/Can]
    ethacrynic acid
    furosemide
    Lasix® Special [Can]
    Lasix® [US/Can]
    torsemide
Diuretic, Miscellaneous
    Apo-Chlorthalidone® [Can]
    Apo-Indapamide® [Can]
    chlorthalidone
    Gen-Indapamide [Can]
    indapamide
    Lozide® [Can]
    Lozol® [US/Can]
    metolazone
    Mykrox® [Can]
    Novo-Indapamide [Can]
    Nu-Indapamide [Can]
    PMS-Indapamide [Can]
    Thalitone® [US]
    Zaroxolyn® [US/Can]

Diuretic, Potassium Sparing
    Aldactone® [US/Can]
    Dyrenium® [US]
    Novo-Spiroton [Can]
    spironolactone
    triamterene
Diuretic, Thiazide
    Apo-Hydro® [Can]
    Aquatensen® [US/Can]
    Aquazide® H [US]
    bendroflumethiazide
    Benicar HCT™ [US]
    chlorothiazide
    Diuril® [US/Can]
    Enduron® [US/Can]
    eprosartan and hydrochlorothiazide
    hydrochlorothiazide
    Metahydrin® [Can]
    Metatensin® [Can]
    methyclothiazide
    Microzide™ [US]
    moexipril and hydrochlorothiazide
    Naqua® [US/Can]
    Novo-Hydrazide [Can]
    olmesartan and hydrochlorothiazide
    Oretic® [US]
    polythiazide
    Renese® [US]
    Teveten® HCT [US/Can]
    Trichlorex® [Can]
    trichlormethiazide
    Uniretic® [US/Can]
Ganglionic Blocking Agent
    Inversine® [US/Can]
    mecamylamine
Miscellaneous Product
    Aceon® [US]
    Coversyl® [Can]
    perindopril and indapamide (Canada only)
    perindopril erbumine
Rauwolfia Alkaloid
    reserpine

Selective Aldosterone Blocker
  eplerenone
  Inspra™ [US]
Vasodilator
  Apo-Gain® [Can]
  Apo-Hydralazine® [Can]
  Apresoline® [Can]
  hydralazine
  Loniten® [US]
  minoxidil
  Nipride® [Can]
  Nitropress® [US]
  nitroprusside
  Novo-Hylazin [Can]
  Nu-Hydral [Can]

HYPERTENSION (ARTERIAL)

Beta-Adrenergic Blocker
  Levatol® [US/Can]
  penbutolol

HYPERTENSION (CEREBRAL)

Barbiturate
  Pentothal® [US/Can]
  thiopental
Diuretic, Osmotic
  mannitol
  urea

HYPERTENSION (CORONARY)

Vasodilator
  nitroglycerin

HYPERTENSION (EMERGENCY)

Antihypertensive Agent
  Corlopam® [US/Can]
  fenoldopam

HYPERTENSION (OCULAR)

Alpha-2-Adrenergic Agonist Agent, Ophthalmic
  Alphagan® P [US/Can]
  brimonidine
  PMS-Brimonidine Tartrate [Can]
  ratio-Brimonidine [Can]
Beta-Adrenergic Blocker
  Apo-Levobunolol® [Can]
  Betagan® [US/Can]
  levobunolol
  Novo-Levobunolol [Can]
  Optho-Bunolol® [Can]
  PMS-Levobunolol [Can]

HYPOTENSION

Adrenergic Agonist Agent
  Adrenalin® [US/Can]
  Aramine® [Can]
  dopamine
  ephedrine
  epinephrine
  Intropin® [Can]
  isoproterenol
  Isuprel® [US]
  Levophed® [US/Can]
  metaraminol
  norepinephrine

INTRACRANIAL PRESSURE

Barbiturate
  Pentothal® [US/Can]
  thiopental
Diuretic, Osmotic
  mannitol

INTRAOCULAR PRESSURE

Ophthalmic Agent, Miscellaneous
  glycerin
  Osmoglyn® [US]

LABOR INDUCTION
Oxytocic Agent
  oxytocin
  Pitocin® [US/Can]
  Syntocinon® [Can]
Prostaglandin
  carboprost tromethamine
  Cervidil® [US/Can]
  dinoprostone
  Hemabate® [US/Can]
  Prepidil® [US/Can]
  Prostin E2® [US/Can]

LABOR (PREMATURE)
Adrenergic Agonist Agent
  Brethine® [US]
  terbutaline

MUSCLE SPASM
Skeletal Muscle Relaxant
  Apo-Cyclobenzaprine® [Can]
  carisoprodol
  carisoprodol and aspirin
  carisoprodol, aspirin, and codeine
  chlorzoxazone
  cyclobenzaprine
  Flexeril® [US/Can]
  Flexitec [Can]
  Gen-Cyclobenzaprine [Can]
  metaxalone
  methocarbamol
  methocarbamol and aspirin
  Mivacron® [US/Can]
  mivacurium
  Norflex™ [US/Can]
  Norgesic™ Forte [US/Can]
  Norgesic™ [US/Can]
  Novo-Cycloprine [Can]
  Nu-Cyclobenzaprine [Can]
  orphenadrine
  orphenadrine, aspirin, and caffeine
  Orphengesic Forte [US]
  Orphengesic [US]
  Parafon Forte® [Can]
  Parafon Forte® DSC [US]
  Rhoxal-orphenadrine [Can]
  Robaxin® [US/Can]
  Skelaxin® [US/Can]
  Soma® Compound [US]
  Soma® Compound w/Codeine [US]
  Soma® [US/Can]
  Strifon Forte® [Can]

MYDRIASIS
Adrenergic Agonist Agent
  AK-Dilate® [US]
  Mydfrin® [US/Can]
  Neo-Synephrine® Ophthalmic [US]
  Phenoptic® [US]
  phenylephrine
Anticholinergic/Adrenergic Agonist
  Cyclomydril® [US]
  cyclopentolate and phenylephrine
  Murocoll-2® [US]
  phenylephrine and scopolamine
Anticholinergic Agent
  atropine
  Atropine-Care® [US]
  Cyclogyl® [US/Can]
  cyclopentolate
  Cylate® [US]
  Diopentolate® [Can]
  Dioptic's Atropine Solution [Can]
  Diotrope® [Can]
  homatropine
  Isopto® Atropine [US/Can]
  Isopto® Homatropine [US]
  Minim's Atropine Solution [Can]
  Mydriacyl® [US/Can]
  Opticyl® [US]
  Tropicacyl® [US]
  tropicamide

NAUSEA
Anticholinergic Agent
  Buscopan® [Can]
  scopolamine
  Transderm Scop® [US]
  Transderm-V® [Can]
Antiemetic
  Aloxi™ [US]
  aprepitant
  dronabinol
  droperidol
  Emend® [US]
  Emetrol® [US-OTC]
  Especol® [US-OTC]
  Formula EM [US-OTC]
  fructose, dextrose, and phosphoric
    acid
  Inapsine® [US]
  Kalmz [US-OTC]
  Marinol® [US/Can]
  Nausea Relief [US-OTC]
  Nausetrol® [US-OTC]
  palonosetron
  Tigan® [US/Can]
  trimethobenzamide
Antihistamine
  Apo-Dimenhydrinate® [Can]
  dimenhydrinate
  Dramamine® [US-OTC]
  Gravol® [Can]
  Novo-Dimenate [Can]
  TripTone® [US-OTC]
Gastrointestinal Agent, Prokinetic
  Apo-Metoclop® [Can]
  metoclopramide
  Nu-Metoclopramide [Can]
  Reglan® [US]
Phenothiazine Derivative
  Apo-Chlorpromazine® [Can]
  Apo-Perphenazine® [Can]
  Apo-Prochlorperazine® [Can]
  chlorpromazine

Compazine® [Can]
Compro™ [US]
Largactil® [Can]
Novo-Chlorpromazine [Can]
Nu-Prochlor [Can]
perphenazine
Phenadoz™ [US]
Phenergan® [US/Can]
prochlorperazine
promethazine
Stemetil® [Can]
Trilafon® [Can]
Selective 5-HT3 Receptor Antagonist
  Aloxi™[US]
  granisetron
  Kytril® [US/Can]
  ondansetron
  palonosetron
  Zofran® ODT [US/Can]
  Zofran® [US/Can]

NERVE BLOCK
Local Anesthetic
  AK-T-Caine™ [US]
  Ametop™ [Can]
  Anestacon® [US]
  Band-Aid(® Hurt-Free™ Antiseptic
    Wash [US-OTC]
  Betacaine® [Can]
  bupivacaine
  Burnamycin [US-OTC]
  Burn Jel [US-OTC]
  Burn-O-Jel [US-OTC]
  Carbocaine® [Can]
  Cepacol Viractin® [US-OTC]
  chloroprocaine
  Citanest® Plain [US/Can]
  LidaMantle® [US]
  lidocaine
  lidocaine and epinephrine
  Lidodan™ [Can]
  Lidoderm® [US/Can]
  LidoSite™ [US]

L-M-X™ 4 [US-OTC]
L-M-X™ 5 [US-OTC]
Marcaine® Spinal [US]
Marcaine® [US/Can]
mepivacaine
Nesacaine®-CE [Can]
Nesacaine®-MPF [US]
Nesacaine® [US]
Novocain® [US/Can]
Opticaine® [US]
Polocaine® MPF [US]
Polocaine® [US/Can]
Pontocaine® [US/Can]
Pontocaine® With Dextrose [US]
Premjact® [US-OTC]
prilocaine
procaine
Sensorcaine®-MPF [US]
Sensorcaine® [US/Can]
Solarcaine® Aloe Extra Burn Relief
   [US-OTC]
tetracaine
tetracaine and dextrose
Topicaine® [US-OTC]
Xylocaine® MPF [US]
Xylocaine® MPF With Epinephrine
   [US]
Xylocaine® [US/Can]
Xylocaine® Viscous [US]
Xylocaine® With Epinephrine [Can]
Xylocard® [Can]
Zilactin® [Can]
Zilactin-L® [US-OTC]

NEURALGIA

Analgesic, Topical
   Antiphlogistine Rub A-535
      Capsaicin [Can]
   Antiphlogistine Rub A-535 No
      Odour [Can]
   ArthriCare® for Women Extra
      Moisturizing [US-OTC]
   ArthriCare® for Women Multi-
      Action [US-OTC]
   ArthriCare® for Women Silky Dry
      [US-OTC]
   ArthriCare® for Women Ultra
      Strength [US-OTC]
   Capsagel® [US-OTC]
   capsaicin
   Capzasin-HP® [US-OTC]
   Mobisyl® [US-OTC]
   Myoflex® [US-OTC/Can]
   Sportscreme® [US-OTC]
   triethanolamine salicylate
   Zostrix®-HP [US-OTC/Can]
   Zostrix® [US-OTC/Can]
Nonsteroidal Antiinflammatory Drug
   (NSAID)
   Asaphen [Can]
   Asaphen E.C. [Can]
   Ascriptin® Extra Strength [US-OTC]
   Ascriptin® [US-OTC]
   Aspercin Extra [US-OTC]
   Aspercin [US-OTC]
   aspirin
   Bayer® Aspirin Extra Strength [US-
      OTC]
   Bayer® Aspirin Regimen Adult Low
      Strength [US-OTC]
   Bayer® Aspirin Regimen Children's
      [US-OTC]
   Bayer® Aspirin Regimen Regular
      Strength [US-OTC]
   Bayer® Aspirin [US-OTC]
   Bayer® Extra Strength Arthritis Pain
      Regimen [US-OTC]
   Bayer® Plus Extra Strength [US-OTC]
   Bayer® Women's Aspirin Plus
      Calcium [US-OTC]
   Bufferin® Extra Strength [US-OTC]
   Bufferin® [US-OTC]
   Buffinol Extra [US-OTC]
   Buffinol [US-OTC]

Easprin® [US]
Ecotrin® Low Strength [US-OTC]
Ecotrin® Maximum Strength [US-OTC]
Ecotrin® [US-OTC]
Entrophen® [Can]
Halfprin® [US-OTC]
Novasen [Can]
St Joseph® Adult Aspirin [US-OTC]
Sureprin 81™ [US-OTC]
ZORprin® [US]

OPHTHALMIC SURGERY
Nonsteroidal Antiinflammatory Drug
    (NSAID)
    Cataflam® [US/Can]
    Voltaren Ophthalmic® [US]
    Voltare Ophtha® [Can]

OPHTHALMIC SURGICAL AID
Ophthalmic Agent, Miscellaneous
    Cellugel® [US]
    GenTeal® Mild [US-OTC]
    GenTeal® [US-OTC/Can]
    Gonak™ [US-OTC]
    Goniosoft™ [US]
    hydroxypropyl methylcellulose
    Tears Again® MC [US-OTC]

OVULATION INDUCTION
Gonadotropin
    chorionic gonadotropin (human)
    chorionic gonadotropin
        (recombinant)
    menotropins
    Ovidrel® [US]
    Pergonal® [US/Can]
    Repronex® [US/Can]
Ovulation Stimulator
    chorionic gonadotropin
        (recombinant)
    Clomid® [US/Can]

clomiphene
Milophene® [Can]
Ovidrel® [US]
Serophene® [US/Can]
urofollitropin

PAIN
Analgesic, Miscellaneous
    acetaminophen and tramadol
    Ultracet™ [US]
Analgesic, Narcotic
    acetaminophen and codeine
    Actiq® [US/Can]
    alfentanil
    Alfenta® [US/Can]
    Anexsia® [US]
    Apo-Butorphanol® [Can]
    aspirin and codeine
    Astramorph/PF™ [US]
    Avinza™ [US]
    Bancap HC® [US]
    belladonna and opium
    B&O Supprettes® [US]
    Buprenex® [US/Can]
    buprenorphine
    butalbital, aspirin, caffeine, and
        codeine
    butorphanol
    Capital® and Codeine [US]
    Ceta-Plus® [US]
    codeine
    Codeine Contin® [Can]
    Co-Gesic® [US]
    Coryphen® Codeine [Can]
    Damason-P® [US]
    Darvocet A500™ [US]
    Darvocet-N® 50 [US/Can]
    Darvocet-N® 100 [US/Can]
    Darvon-N® [US/Can]
    Darvon® [US]
    Demerol® [US/Can]
    DepoDur™ [US]
    dihydrocodeine, aspirin, and caffeine

Dilaudid-HP-Plus® [Can]
Dilaudid-HP® [US/Can]
Dilaudid® Sterile Powder [Can]
Dilaudid® [US/Can]
Dilaudid-XP® [Can]
Dolophine® [US/Can]
Duragesic® [US/Can]
Duramorph® [US]
Endocet® [US/Can]
Endodan® [US/Can]
fentanyl
Fiorinal®-C 1/2 [Can]
Fiorinal®-C 1/4 [Can]
Fiorinal® With Codeine [US]
hycet™ [US]
hydrocodone and acetaminophen
hydrocodone and aspirin
hydrocodone and ibuprofen
Hydromorph Contin® [Can]
hydromorphone
Hydromorphone HP [Can]
Infumorph® [US]
Kadian® [US/Can]
Levo-Dromoran® [US]
levorphanol
Lorcet® 10/650 [US]
Lorcet®-HD [US]
Lorcet® Plus [US]
Lortab® [US]
Margesic® H [US]
Maxidone™ [US]
meperidine
meperidine and promethazine
Meperitab® [US]
M-Eslon® [Can]
Metadol™ [Can]
methadone
Methadone Intensol™ [US]
Methadose® [US/Can]
Morphine HP® [Can]
Morphine LP® Epidural [Can]
morphine sulfate

M.O.S.-Sulfate® [Can]
MS Contin® [US/Can]
MSIR® [US/Can]
nalbuphine
Norco® [US]
Nubain® [US/Can]
Numorphan® [US/Can]
opium tincture
Oramorph SR® [US]
Oxycocet® [Can]
Oxycodan® [Can]
oxycodone
oxycodone and acetaminophen
oxycodone and aspirin
OxyContin® [US/Can]
Oxydose™ [US]
OxyFast® [US]
OxyIR® [US/Can]
oxymorphone
paregoric
pentazocine
pentazocine and acetaminophen
Percocet®-Demi [Can]
Percocet® [US/Can]
Percodan® [US/Can]
Phrenilin® With Caffeine and
    Codeine [US]
PMS-Butorphanol [Can]
PMS-Hydromorphone [Can]
PMS-Morphine Sulfate SR [Can]
PMS-Oxycodone-Acetaminophen
    [Can]
Pronap-100® [US]
propoxyphene
propoxyphene and acetaminophen
propoxyphene and aspirin
ratio-Emtec [Can]
ratio-Lenoltec [Can]
ratio-Morphine SR [Can]
remifentanil
RMS® [US]
Roxanol 100® [US]

Roxanol®-T [US]
Roxanol® [US]
Roxicet® 5/500 [US]
Roxicet™ [US]
Roxicodone™ Intensol™ [US]
Roxicodone™ [US]
Stadol NS™ [Can]
Stadol® [US]
Stagesic® [US]
Statex® [Can]
Sublimaze® [US]
Subutex® [US]
sufentanil
Sufenta® [US/Can]
Supeudol® [Can]
Synalgos®-DC [US]
642® Tablet [Can]
Talwin® NX [US]
Talwin® [US/Can]
Tecnal C 1/2 [Can]
Tecnal C 1/4 [Can]
Triatec-8 [Can]
Triatec-8-Strong [Can]
Triatec-30 [Can]
Tylenol® Elixir with Codeine [Can]
Tylenol® No. 1 [Can]
Tylenol® No. 1 Forte [Can]
Tylenol® No. 2 with Codeine [Can]
Tylenol® No. 3 with Codeine [Can]
Tylenol® No. 4 with Codeine [Can]
Tylenol® with Codeine [US/Can]
Tylox® [US]
Ultiva™ [US/Can]
Vicodin® ES [US]
Vicodin® HP [US]
Vicodin® [US]
Vicoprofen® [US/Can]
Zydone® [US]
Analgesic, Nonnarcotic
Abenol® [Can]
Acephen® [US-OTC]
acetaminophen

acetaminophen and
    diphenhydramine
acetaminophen and
    phenyltoloxamine
acetaminophen and tramadol
acetaminophen, aspirin, and caffeine
Acular LS™ [US]
Acular® P.F. [US]
Acular® [US/Can]
Advil® Children's [US-OTC]
Advil® Infants' [US-OTC]
Advil® Junior [US-OTC]
Advil® Migraine [US-OTC]
Advil® [US-OTC/Can]
Aleve® [US-OTC]
Alti-Flurbiprofen [Can]
Amigesic® [US/Can]
Anaprox® DS [US/Can]
Anaprox® [US/Can]
Ansaid® [US/Can]
Apo-Acetaminophen® [Can]
Apo-Diclo® [Can]
Apo-Diclo Rapide® [Can]
Apo-Diclo SR® [Can]
Apo-Diflunisal® [Can]
Apo-Etodolac® [Can]
Apo-Flurbiprofen® [Can]
Apo-Ibuprofen® [Can]
Apo-Indomethacin® [Can]
Apo-Keto® [Can]
Apo-Keto-E® [Can]
Apo-Ketorolac® [Can]
Apo-Ketorolac Injectable® [Can]
Apo-Keto SR® [Can]
Apo-Mefenamic® [Can]
Apo-Nabumetone® [Can]
Apo-Napro-Na® [Can]
Apo-Napro-Na DS® [Can]
Apo-Naproxen® [Can]
Apo-Naproxen SR® [Can]
Apo-Oxaprozin® [Can]
Apo-Piroxicam® [Can]

Apo-Sulin® [Can]
Asaphen [Can]
Asaphen E.C. [Can]
Ascriptin® Extra Strength [US-OTC]
Ascriptin® [US-OTC]
Aspercin Extra [US-OTC]
Aspercin [US-OTC]
Aspergum® [US-OTC]
aspirin
Aspirin Free Anacin® Maximum
  Strength [US-OTC]
Atasol® [Can]
Bayer® Aspirin Extra Strength [US-
  OTC]
Bayer® Aspirin Regimen Adult Low
  Strength [US-OTC]
Bayer® Aspirin Regimen Children's
  [US-OTC]
Bayer® Aspirin Regimen Regular
  Strength [US-OTC]
Bayer® Aspirin [US-OTC]
Bayer® Extra Strength Arthritis Pain
  Regimen [US-OTC]
Bayer® Plus Extra Strength [US-
  OTC]
Bayer® Women's Aspirin Plus
  Calcium [US-OTC]
Bufferin® Extra Strength [US-OTC]
Bufferin® [US-OTC]
Buffinol Extra [US-OTC]
Buffinol [US-OTC]
Cataflam® [US/Can]
Cetafen Extra® [US-OTC]
Cetafen® [US-OTC]
choline magnesium trisalicylate
Clinoril® [US]
Comtrex® Sore Throat Maximum
  Strength [US-OTC]
Daypro® [US/Can]
diclofenac
Diclotec [Can]
diflunisal

Dolobid® [US]
Easprin® [US]
EC-Naprosyn® [US]
Ecotrin® Low Strength [US-OTC]
Ecotrin® Maximum Strength [US-
  OTC]
Ecotrin® [US-OTC]
ElixSure™ Fever/Pain [US-OTC]
Entrophen® [Can]
etodolac
Excedrin® Extra Strength [US-OTC]
Excedrin® Migraine [US-OTC]
Excedrin® P.M. [US-OTC]
Feldene® [US/Can]
Fem-Prin® [US-OTC]
fenoprofen
FeverAll® [US-OTC]
flurbiprofen
Froben® [Can]
Froben-SR® [Can]
Genaced™ [US-OTC]
Genapap® Children [US-OTC]
Genapap® Extra Strength [US-OTC]
Genapap® Infant [US-OTC]
Genapap® [US-OTC]
Genebs® Extra Strength [US-OTC]
Genebs® [US-OTC]
Genesec® [US-OTC]
Gen-Nabumetone [Can]
Gen-Naproxen EC [Can]
Gen-Piroxicam [Can]
Genpril® [US-OTC]
Goody's® Extra Strength Headache
  Powder [US-OTC]
Goody's® Extra Strength Pain Relief
  [US-OTC]
Goody's PM® Powder [US]
Halfprin® [US-OTC]
Ibu-200 [US-OTC]
ibuprofen
Indocid® [Can]
Indocid® P.D.A. [Can]

Indocin® I.V. [US]
Indocin® SR [US]
Indocin® [US/Can]
Indo-Lemmon [Can]
indomethacin
Indotec [Can]
I-Prin [US-OTC]
ketoprofen
ketorolac
Legatrin PM® [US-OTC]
Lodine® [US/Can]
Lodine® XL [US]
Mapap® Arthritis [US-OTC]
Mapap® Children's [US-OTC]
Mapap® Extra Strength [US-OTC]
Mapap® Infants [US-OTC]
Mapap® [US-OTC]
meclofenamate
Meclomen® [Can]
mefenamic acid
Menadol® [US-OTC]
Midol® Maximum Strength Cramp
   Formula [US-OTC]
Mono-Gesic® [US]
Motrin® Children's [US-OTC/Can]
Motrin® IB [US-OTC/Can]
Motrin® Infants' [US-OTC]
Motrin® Junior Strength [US-OTC]
Motrin® Migraine Pain [US-OTC]
Motrin® [US/Can]
nabumetone
Nalfon® [US/Can]
Naprelan® [US]
Naprosyn® [US/Can]
naproxen
Naxen® [Can]
Norgesic™ Forte [US/Can]
Norgesic™ [US/Can]
Novasen [Can]
Novo-Difenac® [Can]
Novo-Difenac-K [Can]
Novo-Difenac® SR [Can]
Novo-Diflunisal [Can]

Novo-Flurprofen [Can]
Novo-Keto [Can]
Novo-Keto-EC [Can]
Novo-Ketorolac [Can]
Novo-Methacin [Can]
Novo-Naproc EC [Can]
Novo-Naprox [Can]
Novo-Naprox Sodium [Can]
Novo-Naprox Sodium DS [Can]
Novo-Naprox SR [Can]
Novo-Pirocam® [Can]
Novo-Profen® [Can]
Novo-Sundac [Can]
Nu-Diclo [Can]
Nu-Diclo-SR [Can]
Nu-Diflunisal [Can]
Nu-Flurprofen [Can]
Nu-Ibuprofen [Can]
Nu-Indo [Can]
Nu-Ketoprofen [Can]
Nu-Ketoprofen-E [Can]
Nu-Mefenamic [Can]
Nu-Naprox [Can]
Nu-Pirox [Can]
Nu-Sundac [Can]
Ocufen® [US/Can]
orphenadrine, aspirin, and caffeine
Orphengesic Forte [US]
Orphengesic [US]
Orudis® KT [US-OTC]
Orudis® SR [Can]
Oruvail® [US/Can]
oxaprozin
Pain-Off [US-OTC]
Pamprin® Maximum Strength All
   Day Relief [US-OTC]
Pediatrix [Can]
Pennsaid® [Can]
Percogesic® Extra Strength [US-
   OTC]
Percogesic® [US-OTC]
Pexicam® [Can]
Phenylgesic® [US-OTC]

piroxicam
piroxicam and cyclodextrin (Canada only)
PMS-Diclofenac [Can]
PMS-Diclofenac SR [Can]
PMS-Mefenamic Acid [Can]
Ponstan® [Can]
Ponstel® [US/Can]
ratio-Ketorolac [Can]
Redutemp® [US-OTC]
Relafen® [US/Can]
Rhodacine® [Can]
Rhodis™ [Can]
Rhodis-EC™ [Can]
Rhodis SR™ [Can]
Rhoxal-nabumetone [Can]
Rhoxal-oxaprozin [Can]
Riva-Diclofenac [Can]
Riva-Diclofenac-K [Can]
Riva-Naproxen [Can]
Salflex® [US/Can]
salsalate
Silapap® Children's [US-OTC]
Silapap® Infants [US-OTC]
sodium salicylate
Solaraze™ [US]
St Joseph® Adult Aspirin [US-OTC]
sulindac
Sureprin 81™ [US-OTC]
Tempra® [Can]
Tolectin® DS [US]
Tolectin® [US/Can]
tolmetin
Toradol® IM [Can]
Toradol®[US/Can]
tramadol
Tylenol® 8 Hour [US-OTC]
Tylenol® Arthritis Pain [US-OTC]
Tylenol® Children's [US-OTC]
Tylenol® Extra Strength [US-OTC]
Tylenol® Infants [US-OTC]
Tylenol® Junior Strength [US-OTC]

Tylenol® PM Extra Strength [US-OTC]
Tylenol® Severe Allergy [US-OTC]
Tylenol® Sore Throat [US-OTC]
Tylenol® [US-OTC/Can]
Ultracet™ [US]
Ultram® [US/Can]
Ultraprin [US-OTC]
Utradol™ [Can]
Valorin Extra [US-OTC]
Valorin [US-OTC]
Vanquish® Extra Strength Pain Reliever [US-OTC]
Voltaren Ophthalmic® [US]
Voltaren Rapide® [Can]
Voltaren® [US/Can]
Voltaren®-XR [US]
Voltare Ophtha® [Can]
ZORprin® [US]

Decongestant/Analgesic
  Advil® Cold, Children's [US-OTC]
  Advil® Cold & Sinus [US-OTC/Can]
  Dristan® Sinus Tablet [US-OTC/Can]
  Motrin® Cold and Sinus [US-OTC]
  Motrin® Cold, Children's [US-OTC]
  pseudoephedrine and ibuprofen
  Sudafed® Sinus Advance [Can]

Local Anesthetic
  Alcaine® [US/Can]
  Diocaine® [Can]
  ethyl chloride
  ethyl chloride and dichlorotetrafluoroethane
  Fluro-Ethyl® [US]
  Gebauer's Ethyl Chloride® [US]
  Ophthetic® [US]
  proparacaine

Neuroleptic Agent
  Apo-Methoprazine® [Can]
  methotrimeprazine (Canada only)
  Novo-Meprazine [Can]
  Nozinan® [Can]

Nonsteroidal Antiinflammatory Drug
(NSAID)
    Doan's® Extra Strength [US-OTC]
    Doan's® [US-OTC]
    magnesium salicylate
    Momentum® [US-OTC]
Nonsteroidal Antiinflammatory Drug
(NSAID), Oral
    floctafenine (Canada only)

PAIN (ANOGENITAL)

Anesthetic/Corticosteroid
    Analpram-HC® [US]
    Enzone® [US]
    Epifoam® [US]
    Pramosone® [US]
    Pramox® HC [Can]
    pramoxine and hydrocortisone
    ProctoFoam®-HC [US/Can]
    Zone-A Forte® [US]
    Zone-A® [US]
Local Anesthetic
    AK-T-Caine™ [US]
    Americaine® Anesthetic Lubricant
      [US]
    Americaine(R) [US-OTC]
    Ametop™ [Can]
    Anbesol® Baby [US-OTC/Can]
    Anbesol® Maximum Strength [US-
      OTC]
    Anbesol® [US-OTC]
    Anusol® Ointment [US-OTC]
    Babee® Teething® [US-OTC]
    benzocaine
    Benzodent® [US-OTC]
    Cepacol® Maximum Strength [US-
      OTC]
    Cepacol Viractin® [US-OTC]
    Chiggerex® [US-OTC]
    Chiggertox® [US-OTC]
    Cylex® [US-OTC]
    Detane® [US-OTC]
    dibucaine

    dyclonine
    Foille® Medicated First Aid [US-OTC]
    Foille® Plus [US-OTC]
    Foille® [US-OTC]
    HDA® Toothache [US-OTC]
    Hurricaine® [US]
    Itch-X® [US-OTC]
    Lanacane® [US-OTC]
    Mycinettes® [US-OTC]
    Nupercainal® [US-OTC]
    Opticaine®) [US]
    Orabase®-B [US-OTC]
    Orajel® Baby Nighttime [US-OTC]
    Orajel® Baby [US-OTC]
    Orajel® Maximum Strength [US-
      OTC]
    Orajel® [US-OTC]
    Orasol® [US-OTC]
    Pontocaine® [US/Can]
    pramoxine
    Prax® [US-OTC]
    ProctoFoam® NS [US-OTC]
    Solarcaine® [US-OTC]
    Sucrets® [US-OTC]
    tetracaine
    Trocaine® [US-OTC]
    Tronolane® [US-OTC]
    Zilactin® Baby [US-OTC/Can]
    Zilactin®-B [US-OTC/Can]

PAIN (BONE)

Radiopharmaceutical
    Metastron® [US/Can]
    strontium-89

PAIN (DIABETIC NEUROPATHY NEURALGIA)

Analgesic, Topical
    Antiphlogistine Rub A-535
      Capsaicin [Can]
    ArthriCare® for Women Extra
      Moisturizing [US-OTC]

ArthriCare® for Women Multi-
Action [US-OTC]
ArthriCare® for Women Silky Dry
[US-OTC]
ArthriCare® for Women Ultra
Strength [US-OTC]
Capsagel® [US-OTC]
capsaicin
Capzasin-HP® [US-OTC]
Zostrix®-HP [US-OTC/Can]
Zostrix® [US-OTC/Can]

PAIN (LUMBAR PUNCTURE)
Analgesic, Topical
EMLA® [US/Can]
lidocaine and prilocaine

PAIN (MUSCLE)
Analgesic, Topical
dichlorodifluoromethane and
trichloromonofluoromethane
Fluori-Methane® [US]

PAIN (SKIN GRAFT HARVESTING)
Analgesic, Topical
EMLA® [US/Can]
lidocaine and prilocaine

PAIN (VENIPUNCTURE)
Analgesic, Topical
EMLA® [US/Can]
lidocaine and prilocaine

PEPTIC ULCER
Antibiotic, Miscellaneous
Apo-Metronidazole® [Can]
Flagyl ER® [US]
Flagyl® [US/Can]
Florazole ER® [Can]
metronidazole
Nidagel™ [Can]
Noritate® [US/Can]

Novo-Nidazol [Can]
Rozex™ [US]
Trikacide® [Can]
Anticholinergic Agent
Anaspaz® [US]
Apo-Chlorax® [Can]
atropine
belladonna
Cantil® [US/Can]
clidinium and chlordiazepoxide
Cystospaz-M® [US]
Cystospaz®[US/Can]
Dioptic's Atropine Solution [Can]
Donnatal Extentabs® [US]
Donnatal® [US/Can]
glycopyrrolate
hyoscyamine
hyoscyamine, atropine,
scopolamine, and phenobarbital
Hyosine [US]
Isopto® Atropine [US/Can]
Levbid® [US]
Levsinex® [US]
Levsin/SL® [US]
Levsin® [US/Can]
Librax® [US/Can]
mepenzolate
methscopolamine
Minim's Atropine Solution [Can]
NuLev™ [US]
Pamine® Forte [US]
Pamine® [US/Can]
Propanthel™ [Can]
propantheline
Robinul® Forte [US]
Robinul® [US]
Spacol T/S [US]
Spacol [US]
Symax SL [US]
Symax SR [US]
Antidiarrheal
bismuth

bismuth subsalicylate,
metronidazole, and tetracycline
Children's Kaopectate®
(reformulation) [US-OTC]
Diotame® [US-OTC]
Helidac® [US]
Kaopectate(R) Extra Strength [US-OTC]
Kaopectate® [US-OTC]
Pepto-Bismol® Maximum Strength
[US-OTC]
Pepto-Bismol® [US-OTC]
Gastric Acid Secretion Inhibitor
lansoprazole
lansoprazole and naproxen
Losec® [Can]
omeprazole
Prevacid® NapraPAC™ [US]
Prevacid® SoluTab™ [US]
Prevacid® [US/Can]
Prilosec OTC™ [US-OTC]
Prilosec® [US]
Zegerid™ [US]
Gastrointestinal Agent, Gastric or
Duodenal Ulcer Treatment
Apo-Sucralfate® [Can]
Carafate® [US]
Novo-Sucralfate [Can]
Nu-Sucralfate [Can]
PMS-Sucralfate [Can]
sucralfate
Sulcrate® [Can]
Sulcrate® Suspension Plus [Can]
Histamine H2 Antagonist
Alti-Ranitidine [Can]
Apo-Cimetidine® [Can]
Apo-Famotidine® [Can]
Apo-Nizatidine® [Can]
Apo-Ranitidine® [Can]
Axid® AR [US-OTC]
Axid® [US/Can]
cimetidine

famotidine
Gen-Cimetidine [Can]
Gen-Famotidine [Can]
Gen-Nizatidine [Can]
Gen-Ranitidine [Can]
nizatidine
Novo-Cimetidine [Can]
Novo-Famotidine [Can]
Novo-Nizatidine [Can]
Novo-Ranidine [Can]
Nu-Cimet [Can]
Nu-Famotidine [Can]
Nu-Nizatidine [Can]
Nu-Ranit [Can]
Pepcid® AC [US-OTC/Can]
Pepcid® I.V. [Can]
Pepcid® [US/Can]
PMS-Cimetidine [Can]
PMS-Nizatidine [Can]
PMS-Ranitidine [Can]
ranitidine hydrochloride
ratio-Famotidine [Can]
Rhoxal-famotidine [Can]
Rhoxal-ranitidine [Can]
Riva-Famotidine [Can]
Tagamet® HB 200 [US-OTC/Can]
Tagamet® [US]
Zantac® 75 [US-OTC/Can]
Zantac® [US/Can]
Macrolide (Antibiotic)
Biaxin® [US/Can]
Biaxin® XL [US/Can]
clarithromycin
ratio-Clarithromycin [Can]
Penicillin
amoxicillin
Amoxil® [US/Can]
Apo-Amoxi® [Can]
DisperMox™ [US]
Gen-Amoxicillin [Can]
Lin-Amox [Can]
Moxilin® [US]

Novamoxin® [Can]
Nu-Amoxi [Can]
PMS-Amoxicillin [Can]
Trimox® [US]

PERCUTANEOUS TRANSLUMINAL CORONARY ANGIOPLASTY (PTCA)

Anticoagulant (Other)
Angiomax® [US/Can]
bivalirudin

POSTPARTUM HEMORRHAGE

Uteronic Agent
carbetocin (Canada only)

PREECLAMPSIA

Electrolyte Supplement, Oral
magnesium sulfate

PREOPERATIVE SEDATION

Analgesic, Narcotic
Demerol® [US/Can]
Levo-Dromoran® [US]
levorphanol
meperidine
Meperitab® [US]
Antihistamine
Apo-Hydroxyzine® [Can]
Atarax® [US/Can]
hydroxyzine
Novo-Hydroxyzin [Can]
PMS-Hydroxyzine [Can]
Vistaril® [US/Can]
Barbiturate
Luminal® Sodium [US]
Nembutal® Sodium [Can]
Nembutal® [US]
pentobarbital
phenobarbital
PMS-Phenobarbital [Can]

Benzodiazepine
Apo-Midazolam® [Can]
midazolam
General Anesthetic
Actiq® [US/Can]
Duragesic® [US/Can]
fentanyl
Sublimaze® [US]

SHOCK

Adrenal Corticosteroid
A-HydroCort® [US]
A-methapred® [US]
Apo-Prednisone® [Can]
Aristocort® Forte Injection [US]
Aristocort® Intralesional Injection [US]
Aristocort® Tablet [US/Can]
Aristospan® Intraarticular Injection [US/Can]
Aristospan® Intralesional Injection [US/Can]
betamethasone (systemic)
Celestone® Soluspan® [US/Can]
Celestone® [US]
Cortef® Tablet [US/Can]
corticotropin
cortisone acetate
Cortone® [Can]
Decadron® [US/Can]
Deltasone® [US]
Depo-Medrol® [US/Can]
Dexamethasone Intensol® [US]
dexamethasone (systemic)
DexPak® TaperPak® [US]
Diodex® [Can]
H.P. Acthar® Gel [US]
hydrocortisone (systemic)
Hydrocortone® Phosphate [US]
Kenalog® Injection [US/Can]
Medrol® [US/Can]
methylprednisolone
Orapred™ [US]

Pediapred® [US/Can]
PMS-Dexamethasone [Can]
Prednicot® [US]
prednisolone (systemic)
Prednisol® TBA [US]
prednisone
Prednisone Intensol™ [US]
Prelone® [US]
Solu-Cortef® [US/Can]
Solu-Medrol® [US/Can]
Sterapred® DS [US]
Sterapred® [US]
triamcinolone (systemic)
Winpred™ [Can]
Adrenergic Agonist Agent
Aramine® [Can]
dopamine
Intropin® [Can]
isoproterenol
Isuprel® [US]
Levophed® [US/Can]
metaraminol
norepinephrine
Blood Product Derivative
Albumarc® [US]
albumin
Albuminar® [US]
Albutein® [US]
Buminate® [US]
Plasbumin®-5 [Can]
Plasbumin®-25 [Can]
Plasbumin® [US]
Plasmanate® [US]
plasma protein fraction
Plasma Volume Expander
dextran
Gentran® [US/Can]
Hespan® [US]
hetastarch
Hextend® [US/Can]
LMD® [US]

SKELETAL MUSCLE RELAXANT (SURGICAL)

Skeletal Muscle Relaxant
atracurium
cisatracurium
doxacurium
Nimbex® [US/Can]
Norcuron® [Can]
Nuromax® [US/Can]
pancuronium
Quelicin® [US/Can]
rocuronium
succinylcholine
Tracrium® [US]
vecuronium
Zemuron® [US/Can]

SURGICAL AID (OPHTHALMIC)

Ophthalmic Agent, Viscoelastic
chondroitin sulfate and sodium hyaluronate
sodium hyaluronate
Viscoat® [US]

TOPICAL ANESTHESIA

Local Anesthetic
AK-T-Caine™ [US]
Americaine® Anesthetic Lubricant [US]
Americaine® [US-OTC]
Ametop™ [Can]
Anbesol® Baby [US-OTC/Can]
Anbesol® Maximum Strength [US-OTC]
Anbesol® [US-OTC]
Anestacon® [US]
Anusol® Ointment [US-OTC]
Babee® Teething® [US-OTC]
Band-Aid®Hurt-Free™Antiseptic Wash [US-OTC]
benzocaine
Benzodent® [US-OTC]

Betacaine® [Can]
Burnamycin [US-OTC]
Burn Jel [US-OTC]
Burn-O-Jel [US-OTC]
Cepacol Viractin® [US-OTC]
Chiggerex® [US-OTC]
Chiggertox® [US-OTC]
Citanest® Plain [US/Can]
cocaine
Cylex® [US-OTC]
Detane® [US-OTC]
ethyl chloride
ethyl chloride and
    dichlorotetrafluoroethane
Fluro-Ethyl® [US]
Foille® Medicated First Aid [US-OTC]
Foille® Plus [US-OTC]
Foille® [US-OTC]
Gebauer's Ethyl Chloride(R) [US]
HDA® Toothache [US-OTC]
Hurricaine® [US]
Itch-X® [US-OTC]
Lanacane® [US-OTC]
LidaMantle® [US]
lidocaine
Lidodan™ [Can]
Lidoderm® [US/Can]
L-M-X™ 4 [US-OTC]
L-M-X™ 5 [US-OTC]
Mycinettes® [US-OTC]
Opticaine® [US]
Orabase®-B [US-OTC]
Orajel® Baby Nighttime [US-OTC]
Orajel® Baby [US-OTC]
Orajel® Maximum Strength [US-OTC]
Orajel® [US-OTC]
Orasol® [US-OTC]
Pontocaine® [US/Can]
pramoxine

Prax® [US-OTC]
Premjact® [US-OTC]
prilocaine
ProctoFoam® NS [US-OTC]
Solarcaine®Aloe Extra Burn Relief
    [US-OTC]
Solarcaine® [US-OTC]
tetracaine
Topicaine® [US-OTC]
Trocaine® [US-OTC]
Tronolane® [US-OTC]
Xylocaine® MPF [US]
Xylocaine® [US/Can]
Xylocaine® Viscous [US]
Xylocard® [Can]
Zilactin® Baby [US-OTC/Can]
Zilactin®-B [US-OTC/Can]
Zilactin® [Can]
Zilactin-L® [US-OTC]

TRANSURETHRAL SURGERY
Genitourinary Irrigant
    sorbitol

ULCER (DUODENAL)
Proton Pump Inhibitor
    Panto™ IV [Can]
    Pantoloc™ [Can]
    pantoprazole
    Protonix® [US/Can]

ULCER (GASTRIC)
Proton Pump Inhibitor
    Panto™ IV [Can]
    Pantoloc™ [Can]
    pantoprazole
    Protonix® [US/Can]